ISBN 978-0-243-32467-5
PIBN 10793589

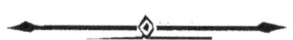

English
Français
Deutsche
Italiano
Español
Português

www.forgottenbooks.com

Mythology Photography **Fiction**
Fishing Christianity **Art** Cooking
Essays Buddhism Freemasonry
Medicine **Biology** Music **Ancient
Egypt** Evolution Carpentry Physics
Dance Geology **Mathematics** Fitness
Shakespeare **Folklore** Yoga Marketing
Confidence Immortality Biographies
Poetry **Psychology** Witchcraft
Electronics Chemistry History **Law**
Accounting **Philosophy** Anthropology
Alchemy Drama Quantum Mechanics
Atheism Sexual Health **Ancient History**
Entrepreneurship Languages Sport
Paleontology Needlework Islam
Metaphysics Investment Archaeology
Parenting Statistics Criminology
Motivational

THE MONTHLY

ABSTRACT OF MEDICAL SCIENCE:

A DIGEST

OF THE

PROGRESS OF MEDICINE AND THE COLLATERAL SCIENCES.

VOLUME V.

1878.

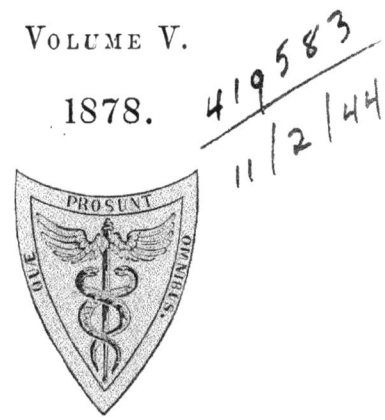

PHILADELPHIA:

HENRY C. LEA.

1878.

PHILADELPHIA:
COLLINS, PRINTER,
705 Jayne Street.

THE MONTHLY ABSTRACT

MEDICAL SCIENCE.

VOL. V. No. 1.   **For List of Contents see last page.**   JANUARY, 1878.

Anatomy and Physiology.

The Motor Centres for the Limbs.

The work of verifying, by clinical and pathological observation, the results obtained by experiment on the brains of animals, progresses slowly and not without some uncertainty. Many important facts have, however, been collected by the energetic investigators who are making the present epoch of French medical science one of unusual distinction. One of the latest of these contributions relates to the motor centres for the limbs, and has been presented to the Académie de Médecine by M. BOURDON. Rare but striking cases are occasionally seen in which a cerebral lesion, instead of causing a hemiplegia, causes a paralysis of one only of the members usually affected. It is to these that M. Bourdon's attention has been especially directed. He discussed first the condition of "brachial monoplegia," paralysis limited to one arm, and described a case in which a cerebral lesion gave rise to a persistent paralysis limited to the muscles of the forearm and hand of the right side, without loss of sensibility. The lesion was a small, superficial hemorrhage, situated in the upper part of the left ascending frontal convolution, without any change in the opto-striate centres. In a second case, communicated by M. Verneuil, a fracture of the skull caused a paralysis of the two arms, and at the autopsy two centres of meningo-encephalitis were found, one on the left side, in the upper third of the ascending frontal convolution, the other on the right side, in the ascending parietal convolution. An analysis of twelve other cases of similar limited paralysis showed that all presented the clinical features of a cortical lesion, and that in all, damage, various in form, was found in the motor zone of the surface of the brain. Instead, however, of occupying the upper third of the ascending frontal convolution and the upper two-thirds of the ascending parietal convolution, as they should, according to some experiments in animals made by Carville and Duret, or the middle third of the ascending frontal convolution, according to conclusions adopted by Charcot and Pitres, in their recent memoir, they were disseminated over the whole extent of the two ascending convolutions and the contiguous parts. It is, however, noted that in all of six cases in which a paralysis of the face was associated with paralysis of the arm, the lesion existed in the middle or inferior part of the ascending frontal convolution, and therefore close to the second frontal convolution, where most experimenters agree in locating the motor centre for the face. From these facts, M. Bourdon concludes that the region occupied by these lesions, although of considerable extent, must be regarded as the true motor centre for the arm. When hemiplegia, paralysis of the leg as well as of the arm, results from a cortical lesion, it appears, from an examination of a large number of cases, that the lesion occupies the upper third of the ascending frontal convolution and the upper two-thirds of the ascending parietal convolution, which is in harmony with the conclusions of Charcot and Pitres as to the localization of the combined movements of the arm and leg. In a considerable number of cases, however, the autopsy revealed lesions having the same seat as those which produced a paralysis of the arm only. A reasonable explanation of these anomalous results might be looked for in the characters of the anatomical lesion, but this is not supported by facts. The extension of the paralysis from the arm to the leg does not appear to be at all related to the extent of the lesion, whether on the surface or in depth.

It has been said that after amputation of the arm, surface changes are found in the centre for the movement of the limb. If so, this might obviously furnish a more exact guide to the localization of the brachial movements. In only two such cases, however, has a post-mortem examination been made. In each the atrophy is said to have been situated in the upper part of the two ascending convolutions—*i. e.*, in only a portion of the region occupied by the lesions which produce brachial monoplegia.

These observations suggest that the centre for the movement of the leg in the human cerebrum is much less strictly localized than it has been believed from experiment to be in animals. At present, however, there are no clinical facts relating to the paralysis of this member which can decide the point. In default of cases of paralysis limited to the leg, M. Bourdon has analyzed three cases of amputation of the leg, followed by an autopsy, and one case of arrested development of the member. In the three cases of amputation M. Luys has found an atrophy of the upper part of the ascending frontal convolution. In the case of arrested development, which was published by M. Landouzy, the atrophy occupied the upper part of the ascending parietal convolution. This is the only case in which the lesion occupied the position in which experimental physiology has located the movement of the leg.

M. Bourdon terminates his memoir with a discussion of the practical application of these results to the problem whether a paralysis limited to the arm furnishes a sufficient indication for the operation of trephining. He concludes that the wide extent of the region which may be implicated when the paralysis has this distribution prevents the selection of any place with sufficient accuracy to justify the operation. But if to the paralysis of the arm there is added a paralysis of the lower part of the face, or aphasia, the lesion will probably be encountered if the trephine is employed in the middle region of the line which corresponds to the fissure of Rolando. This is the position which has been suggested by M. Lucas Championnière. The same surgeon has advised the operation towards the summit of the line corresponding to the fissure of Rolando when the paralysis is confined to the leg. But it has been said that the operation should be done behind the line of the fissure, on account of the supposed localization of the centre in the ascending parietal convolution. M. Bourdon points out that the frequency with which the change has been found in the ascending frontal convolution renders it more prudent to operate upon than behind the given line. In some remarks on M. Bourdon's paper, M. Gosselin, who reported on it to the Académie, and who has devoted much attention to the subject, doubted the propriety of trephining except in cases of depressed fracture, and believed that the existence of depression of bone constituted ample justification, and indication of the place, for trephining, without the evidence of functional alteration. But at the same time, he added, it must not be forgotten by a ready operator that such cases may recover completely, although the depression of bone remains. From such instances it would seem that other motor nerve-cells may take on the function of those which were damaged—a circumstance of great importance and high probability.—*Lancet*, Nov. 17, 1877.

On the Physiological and Pathological Excretion of Indican.

The method employed by Professor JAFFE (Virchow's *Archiv*, May, 1877) is to add to 10 cent. of urine an equal quantity of hydrochloric acid, and then pour down with a narrow pipette one or two drops of a strong solution of chloride of lime; the indigo precipitates. This method of treatment colours the urine red or violet, from the action of the test on some unknown constituents. If indican be present, the colour is dark green or blue. Often the urine must be filtered, to collect the indigo precipitate. The quantity of indigo is not proportional to the vividness of the blue, as in the absence of the unknown constituents a small quantity may give a distinct colour, while in the presence of a large quantity of the same unknown substances a larger quantity of indigo might be hidden, especially if the necessary filtration were omitted. For the quantitative estimation, a measured quantity of urine must be treated as above, the precipitate collected on a filter, washed with hot and cold water, finally with hot ammonia, dried, and weighed.

He has investigated the sources of indican in men and in carnivora. In the herbivora it may have some other source, and in their diet there are many allied substances. In men and the carnivora its dependence on the nature of the diet is unquestionable, and it appears to stand in direct relation to the nitrogenous principles. But it may also be formed from the albumen of the tissues, as he found it in the urine of starved animals, and notably in a case of carcinoma of the œsophagus. It is well known that A. Baeyer found in feces a substance which he called indol, with the formula C_8, H_7, N, a product of the pancreatic digestion; and Professor Jaffe finds that injections of a watery solution of this substance under the skin of dogs, whose urine was ascertained to be free from indican, were followed by the appearance of indican in that secretion. The oxidation process he represents by the following equation :—

$$2 \; C_8 \; H_7 \; N \; \text{or} \; C_{16} \; H_{14} \; N_2 - 4 \; H + 2 \; O = C_{16} \; H_{10} \; N_2 \; O_2$$
$$\text{(Indol).}$$

Moreover, Nencki has succeeded in artificially oxidizing indol to indigo by ozonized air. Besides, he has isolated the substance described by Baeyer, and proved its identity with indol. Hüfner and Kühne have pointed out that the pancreatic ferment cannot produce indol from albumen, except in the presence of bacteria, so that it is really a product of putrefaction; but this, we know, may take place in the alimentary canal, and we know that the pancreas is, as Tiegel showed, the principal seat of bacteria in the living body, so that it can scarcely be doubted that the alimentary canal is the seat of the formation of indol in man and the carnivora, and that this is the source of the indican found in the urine. But is it the only source? Koukol-Yasnopolski has shown that indol may be formed in the liver and the muscles by a true putrefactive process, although they are shut off from the rest of the body. Jaffe observed an enormous quantity of indican in the urine of a case of ileus, and at first thought it was a pathognomonic sign of obstruction of the bowels, explaining it by the supposition that the greater quantity of indol, under normal conditions, passes off in the stools; but unfortunately in another case with the same symptoms there was no such appearance, and it is always absent in chronic constipation. He strove to solve this question by experiments on dogs, and found invariably that ligature of the small intestines was followed by the appearance of indican, while ligature of the great intestine was not. The increase was greater than could be accounted for by mere re-absorption, and he believes there was increased formation. In reference to the influence of fever on the production of indigo, he found no increase in croupous pneumonia, recurrent fever, or acute rheumatism, although he repeatedly searched for it; but it was present in fevers with intestinal complications, enteric fever, gastro-intestinal catarrh, or diarrhœa, supervening in acute or chronic febrile diseases; he therefore concludes that fever, as such, is without influence on the production of indigo. He refers to Fraenkel's observation of an increase of indican under diminished absorption of oxygen into the system, and he regrets that he cannot add any information on this point. Going back to the origin of the increase of indigo in his dogs, he concludes that it was in the intestine, because it was shown to be entirely dependent upon the nature of the food previously eaten, animals which had received food poor in nitrogen showing no increase. He thinks the results of his experiments are easily explained. Obstruction in the small intestine leads to the stagnation of a large quantity of partially digested albuminous matter, in which the indol-forming putrefaction-process may go on with great facility, but the large intestine contains only the waste of the food, and its contents are less watery. Still, in a case of chronic obstruction of the colon, it might easily happen that the retention might be so great that stagnation would occur in the ileus, and an increase of indigo result. In acute diffuse peritonitis the amount of indigo is increased, from the cessation of the peristaltic action of the bowels, etc. ; but when purulent peritonitis attacked his dogs, no increase occurred. This he cannot explain at present. In circumscribed peritonitis and in carcinoma of the peritoneum in man no increase of indigo took place. In reply to the question whether by examination of the urine an obstruction of the bowel can be localized, he says that the frequency of peritonitis and other complications, which may secondarily affect the small intestine, renders it very doubtful. He thinks the absence of indigo in a case of ileus would exclude diffuse peritonitis, but questions whether it would exclude a disease localized in the small intestine.—*London Med. Record*, Nov. 15, 1877.

Pneumogastric Nerves.

In an article in the *Gazetta Medica Italiana* for June, Professors F. LUSSANA and F. CIOTTO describe the result of an experiment, in which they divided both pneumogastric nerves in a dog, the animal surviving for eighteen days, during which careful observations were made.

With regard to the respiration, the only phenomena observed were slowness, depth, and aphonia. On the other hand, there was no sign of suffocation; which would indicate that the vagi are not necessary for the maintenance of respiration, although they modify the respiratory movements. There was no hyperæmia nor atelectasis of the lungs. This would lead to the belief that the vaso-motor nerve-supply of the bronchi and lungs is independent of the vagi, or, at least, that it is partly derived from the sympathetic. Neither pulmonary emphysema nor bronchial catarrh was present; hence, while the share of the vagus in the innervation of the muscular fibres of the pulmonary vessels cannot be excluded, a weakened respiration is necessary for the production of catarrh or emphysema. The absence of any alimentary matter in the respiratory passages tends to show that the hypothesis of Traube is incorrect, which ascribes death solely to the entrance of food into the air-tubes.

The symptoms manifested by the circulatory organs were not in agreement with the opinion that the pneumogastric is a motor nerve of the heart. The circulation was accelerated, but the blood-pressure and the cardiac impulse remained normal.

The digestive process was affected both chemically and mechanically. The œsophagus and stomach were paralyzed. The amount of bile was increased, but on boiling the liver no glucose was obtained ; while in the liver of a healthy dog, treated in the same way at the same interval after death, glucose was found.

Fro 1 this the authors conclude that glucose is a product of the functional activity of the liver, in accordance with Bernard's theory.—*London Med. Record*, Nov. 15, 1877.

Materia Medica and Therapeutics.

Calabarin.

Mr. ABRAHAM (*Pharmaceutical Journal*, Oct. 20) says : Calabar bean has been the subject of fresh investigations by Messrs. Harnack and Withowsky at Strasburg, with the result of isolating a new alkaloid, to which the na 1 e Harnack's calabarin has been given. It differs fro 1 eserine or physostig 1 ine, in that it is insoluble in ether, and 1 ore readily soluble in water.

The discordant effects noted by different experi 1 enters with the preparations of Calabar bean, are ascribed to the fact that those preparations contain, in varying proportions, these two alkaloids, which are in their action totally different the one fro 1 the other.—*London Med. Record*, Nov. 15, 1877.

Detection of Iodine.

M. FILHOL describes in the *Journal de Pharmacie et de Chimie* for May a new proceeding to detect traces of iodine. A little pure potash is added to the liquid, which is then evaporated to dryness. The residue is exhausted with alcohol,' and the alcoholic solution is also evaporated to dryness. This new residue is treated with water, a few drops of hydrochloric acid added, or a very little chro 1 ic acid. Into the 1 ixture are poured two or three drops of sulphide of carbon, and the whole is then well shaken. The liberated iodine is dissolved in the sulphide of carbon, and colors it violet.

M. BARRAL describes in the sa 1 e journal a 1 ethod for recognizing iodine in cod-liver oil, and experi 1 ents on the absorption of iodide of potassiu 1 by ani 1 al fats. The oil is placed in a vessel, and burnt by 1 eans of a wick. The products of co 1 bustion enter a vertical condenser through a funnel-shaped aperture, and the liquid condensed is allowed to drop into a capsule. To the distillate is added caustic potash, and it is evaporated al 1 ost to dryness. Iodine is then tested for by 1 eans of starch solution and chlorine water, or concentrated nitric acid.

Experiments.—Half a gra 1 1 e (7½ grains) iodide of potassiu 1 was daily given to a goat for eight days. During all this ti 1 e the whole of the ani 1 al's 1 ilk was used in the preparation of butter. When purified and 1 elted the butter weighed 60 gra 1 1 es and contained iodine.

Half a gra 1 1 e of potassic iodide was given daily for eight days to a goat having a kid. At the end of that ti 1 e the kid was killed, and 50 gra 1 1 es of adipose tissue were taken fro 1 the neighbourhood of the kidneys. Iodine could easily be detected in the products of consu 1 ption of this 1 elted fat.—*London Med. Record*, Nov. 15, 1877.

Antifermentative Action of Boracic Acid and its Application in Therapeutics.

In an essay read before the Lo 1 bardy Institute of Science and Literature, by Professor POLLI, of Milan (an abstract of which is published in the *Annali Universali di Medicina* for August), the author observes that that study of the processes of fer 1 entation, aided by the progress of organic che 1 istry and the 1 inute researches of 1 icroscopists, has caused a great advance in the researches into the means and agents capable of modifying, hindering, and arresting the phenomena of fermentation. Since his studies on the actions of sulphur, sulphurous acid, and the alkaline and earthy sulphites, which appeared to him to be the most certain antifermentative agents that could be tolerated by the animal organism, he has followed up all the others which have been from time to time discovered (i. e.—carbolic acid, silicate of soda, picric acid, salicylic acid, and boracic acid). Deferring the consideration of several of these agents. Dr. Polli for the present directs attention to boracic acid. He considers with Dumas (*Alcoholic Fermentation*. Paris, 1872) how some salts aid fermentation up to a certain point, such as bitartrate of potash, or at least allow it to run through its course without interruption ; how other salts retard fermentation or render it incomplete, arresting the process when the liquid contains much sugar (bisulphite and hyposulphite of potash and soda, arseniate of potash, and borax); how often salts, finally, not only do not permit fermentation to be established, but prevent the decomposition of sugar (nitrate of potash, nitrate of soda, acetate of soda, chloride of sodium, sal ammoniac, cyanide of potassium, cyanide of mercury, and monosulphide of sodium).

In an appendix to the above-mentioned work, however, Dumas returns to the action which borax exercises on the fermentation of sugar under the influence of yeast, which, he says, deserves a special study, on account not only of the action of borax on yeast, but on the fermentative action of other substances analogous to diastase.

A solution of borate of soda coagulates the yeast of beer, and the supernatant fluid does not decompose cane-sugar, as watery solution of beer-yeast does. Solution of borax dissolves albuminoid membranes ; those, for instance, which separate from egg-albumen when mixed with water. Dumas showed that this solution neutralizes the action of diluted yeast on sugar (alcoholic fermentation) ; the action of diastase on amygdalin, by which is produced essence of bitter almonds with prussic acid (amygdalic fermentation); the action of diastase, by which starch is transformed into dextrine and subsequently into glucose (diastasic fermentation) ; and the action of myrosine, by which the pungent essence of mustard is produced from mustard farina (sinapic fermentation).

Struck with the idea expressed by Dumas, that borax might exercise an influence on some animal poisons, Professor Polli imagined that it might have a great therapeutic application in those infective diseases, external and internal, which do not depend on the action of a living organized ferment capable of reproducing itself, as may be the case with contagious diseases, but which may be products of an organic substance acting chemically as a ferment, and analogous to diastase, synaptase, and myrosine.

Distinguishing, Professor Polli continues, by the name of living and organized ferment that which determines the transformation of sugar into alcohol and carbonic acid, of alcohol into aldehyde and acetic acid, of urea into carbonate of ammonia, etc.. and applying the name of chemical or catalytic ferment to that which transforms starch into glucose, salicin into saligenin and glucose, sugar of milk into lactic acid, we may find in infective morbific agents an analogy sometimes with the first, sometimes with the second class of ferments.   In the first category we will place scabies, variola, scarlatina, measles, syphilis, tinea, etc., and the efficient remedies for these will be the means which kill by chemical destruction, or which act as poison on the minute parasitic beings by which certain diseases are generated and diffused, such as monads, bacteria, vibriones, micrococci, etc. In the second class may be placed all the morbid products which act on the organism in a more or less rapidly deleterious manner, by the decompositions which they induce in some of its component solids or fluids.

In his researches on the actions of preparations of sulphur and on fermentative diseases, Polli had already commenced an investigation, the object of which was to discover what antifermentative agents could be administered to the animal organism in efficient doses without at the same time producing grave disturbance of the physiological functions. The sulphates were found to act in this way; and on investigating their *modus operandi*, he was led to conclude that they do not act as deoxidizing or reducing agents, but rather by their power over the molecular aggregations of fermentable and decomposible organic matters, which they render more resistent to the ordinary agents of decomposition, among which the ferments take the first place.

In the hope that boracic acid and the alkaline borates would be found to possess a similar property, Professor Polli undertook a series of experiments on vegetable and animal substances capable of fermentation and putrefaction.

He examined the action of boracic acid and of borate of soda on beer, on normal and diabetic human urine, on egg beaten up with water, on defibrinated ox's blood, on flesh, etc., and on entire bodies of small animals (birds, mice, etc.). At the same time, in nearly all instances, the effects were compared with those produced on the same substances by equal amounts of sulphite of soda, hyposulphite of soda, and sulphite of magnesia. The results were as follows.

Having exposed several small glasses of beer for thirteen days to the air at a temperature varying from 59 to 64° F., he found that in those in which boracic acid or borate of soda had been dissolved, the fluid remained clear and unchanged, while the pure beer had become acid, turbid, and covered with mould. Analogous results were obtained when milk was used instead of beer; as well as with healthy and diabetic human urine, with yolk of egg mixed with water, and with defibrinated blood. The last, when mixed with a solution of borate of soda, remain fluid, red, and inodorous for about a month, and presenting no bacteria under the microscope. As regards meats, the experiments of Hertzen were confirmed by Polli. For instance, a piece of the lean of pork soaked for twenty-four hours in a solution of boracic acid and borate of soda, and exposed to the air, did not present any sign of decomposition fifteen days later. The action of boracic acid and borate of soda is not yet well defined, but it appears probable that they act by catalysis.

As regards the sulphites and hyposulphites, employed simultaneously for the purpose of comparison, their antifermentative action was found to be inferior.

Regarding the therapeutic applications of boracic acid and borate of soda, it may be stated in general terms that they are useful in all internal and external processes of the organism which may be unattended by fermentable agents. Boracic acid has been used by Capelli of Fregionara (in pulmonary diseases); Ottoni of Mantua (catarrhal cystitis); Ayre, Cane, Fillippi, etc. Boracic acid and the alkaline borates are not oxidized by exposure to the air; when taken internally they do not remove oxygen from the organism, and are readily eliminated by the urine. The following are the formulæ ordinarily employed by Polli. *For external use :* R. Boracic acid, 2 grammes; water, 100 grammes; glycerine, 25 grammes. *For internal use :* R. Boracic acid, 2 grammes; water, 100 grammes; syrup of orange flowers, 16 grammes. A tablespoonful is taken every hour.—*London Med. Record*, Nov. 15, 1877.

Subcutaneous Injection of Defibrinated Blood.

Dr. Schmeltz, of Schlestadt, reports (*Annales et Bulletin de Gand*, June) a case of consumption with great weakness and intense anæmia, in which subcutaneous injection of defibrinated blood was employed. The patient was first seen by Dr. Schmeltz in March, 1874; he was then over sixty years of age, had been sick for a long time, and was confined constantly to his bed, in consequence of extreme weakness. He was much emaciated, and almost all over his lungs there was dulness, bronchial breathing, and moist râles. He had hectic, and suffered from neuralgic pains, from frequent attacks of syncope, and from dyspnœa. His stomach soon became weak, and neither food nor medicines could be retained. Dr. Schmeltz then determined to try subcutaneous injection of defibrinated blood, which had been first recommended by Dr. Kaist, of Kreuznach. The blood used was taken, by cupping, from the back of the patient's son, and was carefully defibrinated. Eight injections of five grammes (seventy-seven grains) each were made into the arms and legs at one sitting, consequently forty grammes (ten and a quarter drachms) in all were injected. The swellings caused by the injections had disappeared at the end of the second day. The operation was followed by a very rapid improvement in the general condition of the patient. His appetite returned; the pulse became dull and firm, and eighty per minute; the neuralgia, anxiety, palpitations, and extreme weakness were relieved, and he was able to sleep. Eight days after the operation he got up, and convalescence was thenceforth uninterrupted. The patient is still living, and in good health. During the last two years he has required no medical treatment.

Dr. Schmeltz thinks that this case proves that the hypodermic injection of blood may prove useful in many cases where transfusion is indicated, especially in cases of anæmia, in which the stomach rejects all nourishment and medicine.— *London Med. Record*, Nov. 15, 1877.

Medicine.

Recent Researches on Idiopathic (Essential or Pernicious) Anæmia of Addison.
(*Concluded from page* 441, *Oct.* 1877.)

Professor ROSENSTEIN, of Leyden, has published another case of pernicious anæmia in the *Berliner Klin. Wochenschrift* for February 26, 1877. He writes in complete ignorance of all the observations previous to those of Biermer and Immermann, and even thinks that this first case observed in Holland may serve to show that the disease is unconnected with any local circumstances in Switzerland and Suabia (1). The patient was a man aged 36, who was strong and well until attacked by "typhus" (enteric fever is meant) six months before he was seen. This lasted eight weeks, and he had never recovered his strength. Lately he had suffered from diarrhœa and œdema of the feet. On admission into hospital, November 3, 1876, he showed all the well-known symptoms described by Addison and Wilks, with a loud systolic murmur, audible at the apex and over the aortic valves, but not in the direction of the pulmonary artery. The morning temperature was normal, but between three and six in the afternoon it reached 101.5° F. The blood showed little or no increase of leucocytes, but marked diminution of red disks; these were remarkably pale, but retained their normal shape and formed rouleaux as usual. The microcytes described by Quincke and Eichhorst were absent. Minute ecchymoses were seen by the ophthalmoscope near both papillæ. The only symptoms, besides weakness, of which the patient complained, were a slight cough and headache, increased when sitting up in bed. Five grains of quinine were given three times a day with iron, but (as is well known in England) these remedies were without effect, the quinine not even reducing the evening temperature below 38.4 or 38.7 (101 or 101.7° F.).

On December 2d the patient fainted, and on recovery complained of short breath. There were physical signs of passive effusion in the left pleura and peritoneum, and death quickly followed from œdema of both lungs. *Post-mortem*, beside excessive anæmia of all the organs, nothing was found but enlargement of the liver and spleen; the cells of the former were in a condition of cloudy swelling, which Dr. Rosenstein refers to the preceding enteric fever. The spleen weighed 445 grammes (more than 14 oz.). Its internal condition is not mentioned, but apparently this enlargement is also regarded as of typhoid origin. The intestines, however, are reported as completely normal, and there is no mention of swelling of the mesenteric lymph-glands. There was no fatty degeneration of the muscles of the heart. The marrow was pale red and showed no increase of leucocytes when compared with that of another subject. Charcot's octahedral crystals were present (a normal *post-mortem* appearance). The retinæ were carefully examined by M. Nykamp, whose report with wood-cuts is appended. He could find no rupture of vessels and no minute aneurisms, and the endothelium was perfect. He thinks that the red corpuscles found in the retinal tissues must have passed out by diapedesis. An analysis by Professor Trachiment showed that iron was present in the proportion of ½ per cent. of dried liver, .227 in the dried splenic tissue, and .04 in that of the kidneys. According to an analysis by Oidtmann, the healthy liver contains .08, and spleen .15 per cent. of iron. The increase in the present instance may, Dr. Rosenstein thinks, be due to the steel he had prescribed (*Martialia—nicht viel*) rather than to destruction of hæmoglobin in these organs. The same excess of iron had been noted by Quincke, but in his cases also steel was given. In conclusion, the author remarks that, but for the retinal hæmorrhage, the case might have been mistaken for one of cardiac disease with (ulcerative) endocarditis.

Professors Gairdner and Osler, of Montreal, publish in the *Canada Medical and Surgical Journal* for March, 1877, the following case, headed, "Progressive pernicious anæmia (idiopathic of Addison)." A man aged 52 came under observation in November, 1876. He had always been subject to diarrhœa, and also, with others of his family, to epistaxis. After family bereavement five years previously, he had begun to fail in health, and, very gradually, pallor and dyspnœa had appeared and increased upon him. He had lately had five or six loose motions daily, and his skin and mucous membranes were excessively pallid. There was no fever, no emaciation; he ate and slept well; the urine was normal, the liver and spleen not enlarged. The heart-sounds were unaffected, but there was a venous murmur in the neck. There was no increase of pigment in the skin, and no enlargement of lymph-glands. He was prescribed steel, and the diarrhœa ceased, but a loud bruit appeared, audible at both base and apex of the heart. As he became worse, the temperature occasionally rose to 101 or 102° F., but fell before death to 97.3°. He died in January, 1877, with vomiting, rambling, and other signs of exhaustion. The blood, examined during life with Hartnack No. 9 (immersion) oc. 3, showed the following characters. The white corpuscles were not increased in number. They measured $\frac{1}{2500}$ to $\frac{1}{1800}$ inch in diameter. They showed active amœboid movements, at the temperature of the room, for seven hours after the drop of blood had been mounted (without reagent) in a paraffin cell, and carried through the cold air for a quarter of a mile (see Ranvier's statement, *Traité d' Histologie*, p. 210). The red corpuscles formed rouleaux; as usual, a few were crenated, most of them ovoid, lozenge-shaped, or irregular, larger than usual, but of normal depth of colour. There were also a few much smaller ones, which were spherical instead of biconcave. None had nuclei. Measured with Hartnack, No. 16 immersion, one was as large as $\frac{1}{1833}$ inch, five

\aried between $\frac{1}{2750}$ and $\frac{1}{2145}$, twenty-two between $\frac{1}{3000}$ and $\frac{1}{3200}$, and five between $\frac{1}{3000}$ and $\frac{1}{5000}$.

Necropsy.—The skin was of a pale le\1on tint, the fat abundant, the nails incurved; no petechiæ. There were twelve ounces of fluid in the left pleura, and nearly as \1uch in the right. The heart appeared practically no\1\1al, but on microscopical examination the fibres showed extre\1e fatty degeneration. This was absent in the \1uscles of the trunk, which were red in colour. The spleen weighed six ounces; the right kidney was congested, the left pale; the suprarenals no\1\1al; tonsils not enlarged; sto\1ach and intestines no\1\1al; liver pale and not enlarged; \1esenteric and other ly\1ph-glands s\1all; bloodvessels very e\1pty. The \1arrow of the sternu\1, right fibula, and left clavicle, of a rib and a vertebra, was exa\1ined. It was dark red in colour, and showed the following ele\1ents under the microscope: (1.) Ordinary red \1arrow cells, *i.e.*, leucocytes, differing fro\1 white blood-corpuscles only in their so\1ewhat larger size and \1ore distinct nucleus; these were by far the \1ost abundant. (2.) Ordinary red blood-discs, together with a s\1aller proportion ($\frac{1}{4}$ or less) of the \1inute spherical red corpuscles (Eichhorst's "microcytes") above described as occasionally found in the blood. (3.) Nucleated red corpuscles, spherical, and larger than ordinary blood-discs, varying fro\1 $\frac{1}{2077}$ to $\frac{1}{1773}$ of an inch in diameter. These are Neu\1ann's "embryonic corpuscles." (4.) Large cells containing as \1any as five or six red blood-discs. (5.) *Myéloplaques*, only sparingly found in the sternum and rib. (6.) Fat-cells, absent (as usual) in the sternu\1 and vertebra, and rib, present in s\1all nu\1bers in the clavicle (cancellous tissue or shaft?). (7.) Charcot's crystals.

This carefully recorded case is followed by re\1arks which bear chiefly on the condition of the blood and on that of the \1arrow. Since Eichhorst (*Central-blatt für die Med. Wissensch.*, June 24th, 1876) called attention to the presence of \1inute spherical red corpuscles in the blood of essential anæ\1ia, Dr. Osler has seen the\1 in another case beside the present, and, as above noted, they have been observed by Quincke and by Cohnheim. In other cases, however, recorded by Grainger Stewart (*Brit. Med. Journal*, July 8, 1876), by Bradbury (*ibid.*, Dece\1ber 30, 1876), and by Bradford (*Boston Med. and Surg. Journal*, May, 1876) their presence is expressly denied; and in other microscopical observations of the blood in anæmia, they are not \1entioned. Moreover, Dr. Osler has found si\1ilar corpuscles in his own blood and in that of persons free fro\1 disease.[1]

With respect to the state of the \1arrow, Drs. Gairdner and Osler re\1ark that cases of anæ\1ia lymphatica (leucocytosis, pseudo-loucémie) cannot be called Hodgkin's disease when the ly\1ph-glands and spleen are not enlarged; but, when the red \1arrow alone of all the cytogenic structures is hypertrophied, the other sy\1pto\1s of the disease would approach very near to the idiopathic anæ\1ia of Addison, so that Pepper, following Immermann and Jaccoud, has suggested that essential anæmia is nothing but the \1yelogenous for\1 of pseudo-leuchæmia, bearing the sa\1e relation to Hodgkin's disease that the rare cases of true leuchæmia with hyperplasia of the \1arrow do to ordinary splenic leuchæ\1ia. Inasmuch, however, as in \1any cases of idiopathic anæ\1ia the bones have been carefully observed and found healthy by Lepine (*Monthly Abstract of Medical Science*, 1876, p. 488), Burger, and Quincke, they believe that the cases of Cohnhei\1 (*Virchow's Archiv.*, lxviii., 1876), Fede, Pepper, and Scheby Buch \1ust be ranged with their own, as exa\1ples of myelogenous pseudo-leuchæmia (or

---

[1] On this point, see also a paper by Dr. Litten, reported in the *London Med. Record*, for \1arch last (p. 120), and so\1e careful observations by \1essrs. Davy and Mackern of Guy's Hospital, published in the *Lancet*, May 5, 1877.

anæmia medullaris) though indistinguishable during life from idiopathic or essential anæmia.

Dr. Litten publishes, in the *Berliner Klin. Wochenschr.* for May 7 and 14 of this year, the following remarkable case from Professor Frerich's wards: A young woman had been suckling her own and another infant for several months, while herself ill provided with food, and in January last (1877), more than a year after her delivery, began to vomit all she took. When admitted to the Charité on February 11, she was already much exhausted and excessively anæmic, and loud venous and cardiac murmurs were audible. Retinal hemorrhages were also observed with the ophthalmoscope. There was no excess of white blood-corpuscles, but the red ones were greatly diminished, though normal in shape and without microcytes. The liver, spleen, and lymph-glands were not enlarged; and, though so weak and pallid, the patient was not emaciated. The chief complaint was of headache. The pulse was frequent and compressible, the temperature normal. On the 15th of February a remarkable increase of white corpuscles was found in the blood. These were larger and less granular than usual, and contained each a distinct large nucleus, or sometimes two (resembling medullary rather than ordinary or splenic leucocytes). On the following day only nine red could be counted to one of these white corpuscles ; on the 17th the proportion was only 4 to 1. At the same time the patient became restless, and suffered from severe dyspnœa, without any evidence of œdema or other affection of the lungs. This rapidly increased, and on the 18th, only a few weeks from the appearance of anæmia and vomiting, and after three days of leuchæmia and dyspnœa, the patient died. There was neither albuminuria nor pyrexia while she was under observation.

At the necropsy the body was found excessively anæmic, but with plenty of fat, and the muscles red and healthy in appearance. The heart, on the contrary, was in an extreme condition of fatty degeneration. The liver and internal lymph-glands were normal. The spleen weighed 200 grammes ($7\frac{1}{16}$ ounces). The kidneys contained a number of minute white nodules, which proved on microscopical examination to be lymphomata. The tissue of the vertebræ and pelvis, the sternum and the ribs, was unchanged, but that of the long bones of both upper and lower extremities showed numerous spots like abscesses in their shafts; and their yellow marrow was turned into a soft pale material, which proved under the microscope to consist of the same large colourless cells, with distinct vesicular nuclei, which had been observed in the blood before death. The normal yellow marrow-cells (fat-cells) had almost entirely disappeared. No nucleated red corpuscles were discovered in the blood or in the marrow. Charcot's crystals were abundant.

The origin and course of the disease as one of idiopathic anæmia were well marked, and offered nothing more remarkable than its unusually rapid course, but the sudden and extreme increase of leucocytes was unexpected, and makes the case a unique one. The most acute cases of leuchæmia myelogenica on record are that of Küssner (*Berl. Klin. Wochenschr.*, 1876), which proved fatal in 18 days, and that of Immermann (*Deutches Archiv für Klin. Med.*, vol. xiii.), when the patient lived six weeks. In both these (as in many other cases of leuchæmia) there was pyrexia, which was remarkably absent in the present instance. As Dr. Litten justly remarks, it must be regarded as idiopathic anæmia, passing into medullary leuchæmia, and both running a very rapid course. Comparing it with four unpublished cases of essential anæmia, three from Professor Frerichs' wards during the winter session 1875-6, and one under one care of Professor Fischer at Breslau, in 1875, he remarks on their agreement in (the characteristic features pointed out by Addison) excessive anæmia, absence of emaciation, fatty degeneration of the heart, and progressive and fatal course. The hemorrhages, whether in the retina or elsewhere, must, like the "tabby degeneration" of the ventricles, be regarded as consequences of anæmia, for cases are on record in which both were absent. The heart is often fatty (as described by Dr. Quain) in non-anæmic cases, though not usually so in ordinary leuchæmia; while hemorrhages in various parts are common in lymphatic and splenic anæmia (Hodgkin's disease and hæmic splenica), so that their presence cannot be taken as diagnostic of essential anæmia. Dr. Leiden examined the retina to determine this point in nine cases of anæmia—three idiopathic and fatal, one from cancer of the uterus, two from hemorrhage after abortion, and three from hæmatemesis. There were retinal ecchymoses in all of these cases but two—one of essential anæmia, the other of anæmia due to hæmatemesis, which ended in recovery. After a full discussion of the ophthalmological side of the question, he concludes that neither retinal hemorrhage nor white atrophic centres in previous ecchymoses, nor the shining white patches seen in some cases of Bright's disease, are diagnostic of fatal anæmia. He confirms Nykamp's statement that the ecchymoses do not depend on miliary aneurisms of the retinal arteries like those in the brain; but he does not believe that they occur by diapedesis, and ascribes them to rupture of the capillaries.

In two of these four cases of idiopathic anæmia the bones were examined. In one there was no obvious change; but on microscopic examination numerous nucleated red corpuscles and microcytes were discovered. In the other, the marrow of the femur examined was of the colour of raspberry jelly; it showed a few minute red blood corpuscles (microcytes) and many more of the larger ones with nuclei described by Cohnheim, Osler and Gardner, and Rosenstein, beside abundant ordinary medullary leucocytes taking the place of the fat-cells of yellow marrow. These were also found in the blood taken in quantity after death, although during life no evidence of leuchæmia was afforded by examining a drop from the finger. By Welcker's method of allowing a quantity of blood to stand in a tall narrow glass, the slight coagulability which it possesses in these cases allows the formation of three layers by subsidence of serum, white corpuscles and red, and a judgment can thus be readily obtained of their relative proportion.

Professor Pepper, of Philadelphia, has published a paper subsequent to that mentioned by Dr. Lépine in the same journal (*American Journal of Medical Sciences*) for April, 1877, on the relations of idiopathic anæmia (which he proposes to name anæmatosis) with Addison's disease of the adrenals. It contains no fresh cases, but is based on a comparison of the two of the former affection, reported above, with a well-marked instance of the latter in a man aged 40. The characteristic bronzing of the skin and constitutional symptoms are carefully described while the patient was under observation for more than four years. *Post-mortem*, there was found the usual caseous affection of both adrenals, with a slight similar change in the apices of both lungs.

The likeness between the symptoms of the two diseases is less than Dr. Pepper supposes, and cannot outweigh the broad differences in their morbid anatomy. Even apart from the bronzing and the constant local lesion, the anæmia of morbus Addisonii is comparatively slight, the loss of flesh greater, hemorrhages and pyrexia almost unknown, and phthisis or other caseous change in other organs than the adrenals exceedingly common. The chief connection between it and essential anæmia is the historical one that both were discovered by the same eminent pathologist, and his acumen is proved by the fact that the accuracy of his statements, like his labours in the pathology of pneumonia and of phthisis, is only now beginning to receive due recognition. Almost at the same time that

Addison was separating the disease he called "suprarenal malasma," and that which he called "idiopathic anæmia," from the great group of chronic states of anæmia without previous hemorrhage, the illustrious Virchow was establishing the existence of another natural pathological species of anæmia under the title "leuchæmia splenica." The form of anæmia associated with enlarged lymph-glands described by, and often named after, Dr. Hodgkin, is a much less distinctly marked "disease" than the other three. This anæmia lymphatica is occasionally a true leuchæmia lymphatica, though such cases are very rare. It is often associated with enlargement of other cytogenic organs, beside the glands, the tonsils, liver, or Peyer's patches, as in the case described by Béhier of "pseudo-leucémie intestinale;" and finally it has been found, as in some of the cases enumerated above, to depend upon overgrowth of the red marrow (anæmia medullaris v. myelogenica). The last cases, of anæmia without leuchæmia, associated with the changes in the marrow above described, are no doubt often undistinguishable during life from cases of idiopathic anæmia; but since, as we have seen, the marrow is unaffected in many of the latter, we must still consider the two as pathologically distinct.—*London Med. Record*, Nov. 15, 1877.

Salicin and Salicylic Acid in Rheumatism.

Salicin and salicylic acid in the treatment of rheumatism may now be considered to have received a fair trial both in Europe and America, and the verdict of the majority of those who have employed the drugs is a favourable one. Among those who have published the results of their experience in this matter are many great authorities both at home and abroad, and the fact of their reports being couched in such strong terms as has in many instances been the case, in itself tends to show that in salicin and salicylic acid we have drugs which produce, in many cases of rheumatism, an effect hitherto not manifested by any other as yet known to us.

We lately remarked that there can be now little question that salicin and the salicylates, especially the latter, do exert an influence, in the cure of rheumatism, which is quite peculiar to them, and daily experience tends to confirm our belief. The striking success which attended the administration of these remedies in the earlier cases naturally encouraged the idea that they were to prove no less efficacious in rheumatism than quinine in ague. Facts have, however, been recorded during the past few months, both in our own columns and elsewhere, which show that, striking as are the effects of salicylic acid in many cases, we have as yet discovered no remedy which can be regarded in the light of a specific for rheumatism. The primary effects of the salicylic acid or its salts are—(1) a rapid, and in many instances an almost sudden, reduction of the temperature of the body ; and (2) frequently a contemporaneous relief to the pains in the joints. In crediting any one remedy with the capacity for effecting these changes by its own action, we must be on our guard against attributing to a medicine a sudden recession of acute symptoms, which is by no means unfrequently met with in a disease so variable in its course as rheumatism, even when uninfluenced by any treatment at all. Accumulating records, however, serve to indicate that salicylic acid does possess this property of alleviating the pain and reducing the temperature in many cases of acute rheumatism. Out of seventy cases treated with this drug in the Leeds Infirmary during the year 1876, and recorded by Dr. E. H. Jacobs, in a paper read before the West Riding Medical and Chirurgical Society, "in thirty-five the improvement was so rapid as to leave no doubt as to the efficacy of the drug." This statement receives confirmation from an inspection which we have lately made of the register of a hospital in which twenty cases were treated with salicylates. The figures here show that the average duration of pain was barely three days, while the temperature remained permanently normal after the second day. In daily practice, however, practitioners are brought into contact with two distinct varieties of acute rheumatism, which, if it be allowable to express them in terms of salicylic acid, may be called the salicylate and the non-salicylate form. The characteristics of the former are high temperature (about 103° F.), severe pain, and much redness of the affected joints; and it is in these cases that salicin or the salicylates effect such remarkable and sudden amelioration of the acute symptoms. The main features of the latter variety are a comparatively low temperature (about 99°), little or no redness of the affected joints, or, if present, the redness is in more or less circumscribed patches; severe pain, accompanied by great depression. In such the drugs have but slight effect; the temperature may be reduced even below the normal standard, but the pain persists. Similarly, in chronic rheumatism, the action of salicylic acid seems to be very uncertain; in some cases the pain is relieved, in others no effect is produced, and it is found necessary eventually to have recourse to other remedies.

A question arises, however, which is of the greater moment than for relief of pain and the reduction of temperature—viz., does salicylic acid prevent cardiac lesion in acute rheumatism? and this question can, it is to be feared, only be met with a negative. So far as present experience goes, the results of the salicylate treatment do not contrast unfavourably in this respect with other methods. Perhaps, on the whole, the comparison may even be deemed favourable. Thus, of 63 cases treated with salicylic acid in the Boston City Hospital during the past year, Dr. Brown found that cardiac lesions, which occurred after the admission of the patient, amounted only to 4.76 per cent. Out of 312 cases, published in England, America, and Germany, of which Dr. E. H. Jacobs gives the particulars in the paper already referred to, 9 cases, or $3\frac{1}{2}$ per cent., were attacked with cardiac complications. It is not our purpose on the present occasion to institute comparisons between the salicylate and other methods of treating rheumatism, except in so far as they bear upon any point at issue; but we would parenthetically, in connection with Dr. Brown's report, call attention to a number of cases published by Dr. Blake in the Boston City Hospital Reports (first series), which were under the alkaline treatment, and in which the cardiac lesions were rather over 13 per cent. It would be manifestly unfair from so few cases to draw any definite conclusions for or against either method of treatment; all we would urge is, that the salicylates have hitherto contrasted favourably with other remedies, but that they do not confer an absolute immunity from cardiac affections. A striking case in illustration of this assumption was published in our columns at the close of last year (Nov. 11th), which occurred in the practice of Dr. Green at Charing-Cross Hospital. In this instance the heart's action at the time of the patient's admission is described as having been "somewhat heaving," but no thrill or murmur accompanied its action. The man was ordered fifteen grains of salicin every two hours, which was subsequently altered to half a drachm every four hours on account of the severity of the pain and the persistent elevation of the temperature. On the ninth day of the treatment decided evidence of endocarditis was manifest; on the following day pericardial friction was audible, and two days later the case was further complicated by an attack of pleurisy. This case is valuable as showing that, under some circumstances, salicin fails to reduce the temperature, to control the articular pain, or to prevent the affection of the heart. At the same time, any treatment which, as was lately remarked by one of our correspondents, has the property of subduing the more prominent symptoms in rheumatism, and of keeping them in abeyance until convalescence, is established, must tend materially to diminish the liability to heart disease.

We published in our last issue four cases showing the various effects of salicin in rheumatic fever, one of them an example of rheumatic fever with hyperpyrexia. On the first introduction of the drug, as soon as its antipyretic properties were observed, it was hoped that it might prove especially beneficial under such conditions of excessively high temperature. Several cases are, however, now on record in which salicin and salicylic acid have been fairly tried, and with most unsatisfactory results, recovery if it occurred, being due to the application of cold, and apparently quite independent of the action of the drug.

Another case, furnished by Dr. Herbert Lilley, contains an account of a sequela to a case of rheumatism which, if it be due, as he supposes, to the effects of salicin or salicylic acid, is a matter for serious consideration in prescribing these drugs. Hitherto, however, necrosis of bone does not appear to have complicated cases of rheumatism under this treatment, and it is possible that in Dr. Lilley's case the necrosis may have been in some measure connected with the strumous habit of the child.

Toxic effects of salicin and salicylic acid in the form of delirium, deafness, tinnitus, are, nevertheless, of common occurrence in the course of the treatment, and it seems probable that in some instances they are due to impurity in the drug— that is to say, to its contamination with carbolic acid, while in others, and notably in cases where salicin has been employed, to some peculiar susceptibility on the part of the patient. These untoward symptoms disappear at once if the administration be discontinued or suspended for a time.

Dr. Murchison, in his communication to the Clinical Society last session on the subject of the treatment of enteric fever by salicylic acid, alluded to the fact that suppression of urine had occurred. In cases of rheumatism treated with salicylates which have come under observation, we believe, the urine has, in the majority, been diminished in quantity during the height of the fever, but has been again secreted in normal amount as defervescence was established, and this without actual suspension of the remedy. It has further been stated by some observers that albuminuria has been caused. Doubtless in many cases albumen may be detected in the urine of rheumatic patients, and it is possible that its presence is in some degree caused by salicylic acid or salicin. It is worthy of note that in twenty-two cases of chronic rheumatism which lately occurred in a metropolitan hospital, of which six were treated with salicylates, temporary albuminuria occurred in four, while of the remaining sixteen albumen was detected only in six.

An objection is now and again raised to the salicylate treatment on the ground that relapses are especially liable to occur, but so far as we are able to form an opinion, this objection applies equally, or very nearly equally, to other methods of treatment, and a reference to thirty-two cases lately under observation shows that a relapse took place in ten cases out of eighteen in which the salicylates were used; that recurrence of the symptoms set in in four out of eight cases under alkalies, and in two out of six cases in which the treatment consisted of a combination of the alkaline and salicylate treatments. One case under alkalies suffered as many as four relapses, while in no case under the other treatments did the pain recur more than twice. Looking to the material at our disposal for a judgment, we incline to the belief that many of the relapses under the salicylate treatment are due to the fact that the medicine has been discontinued too early in the course of the disease.

It would appear, then, that we have in salicin or salicylic acid a remedy which, in many cases of acute rheumatism, with a temperature of 103° Fahr., or thereabout, is productive of most satisfactory results; while in rheumatic fever attended with hyperpyrexia it is apparently inert; that it does not confer an absolute immunity from heart disease; while in the low form of acute, and in chronic rheumatism its beneficial action is extremely doubtful. Further observations are required for the elucidation, among others, of two points in particular—first, whether the toxic effects, which so frequently occur during the treatment, produce any permanent evil ; secondly, what are the indications in any given case of rheumatic fever that the action of salicin or salicylic acid will be beneficial, negative, or deleterious.—*Lancet*, Nov. 3, 1877.

Syphilitic Cerebral Arteritis.

Under this title Mr. LANCEREAUX read (*Gaz. Hebdom.*, Sept. 7, 1877) a paper at the late meeting at Havre, in which he stated that the special anatomical character of this affection is localization at certain points of the arterial wall, the lesion commencing in the connective tissue of the artery, and proceeding on, in different cases, either to contraction or obliteration at such points, or to aneurismal dilatation. It varies from ordinary endarteritis by its tendency (like all syphilitic lesions) to remain circumscribed, and by its disposition to symmetry.—*Med. Times and Gaz.*, Sept. 22, 1877.

Hysterical Anæsthesia.—Injury to Spinal Cord.—Cerebro-Spinal Lateral Sclerosis.

At a late meeting of the Clinical Society of London (*Lancet*, Nov. 3, 1877), Dr. CAYLEY read notes of a "Case of Hysteria, with Contracture of the Lower Limbs. Anæsthesia, and Ischæmia, in a Boy," communicated by Dr. HENRY THOMPSON. The patient, fourteen years of age, son of a French father and English mother, was admitted into the Middlesex Hospital on May 10th, 1877. He had always been delicate, but had no definite illness till two months before admission, when he began to lose flesh, became low-spirited, and complained of vertical headache. He had occasional paroxysms of laughing and crying, accompanied by a hoarse barking cough and globus. For a month he had been unable to walk owing to paresis, rigidity, and distortion of his lower limbs. On admission his pulse, temperature, and respiration were normal, and remained nearly so throughout the case. His voice was almost inaudible, but was strengthened by weak faradaism. The legs were firmly flexed upon the thighs, and the feet extended as in talipes equinus. The genital organs were ill-developed. Anæsthesia and ischæmia were prominent symptoms from first to last, and on May 18th experiments were made to define these conditions, with the following results : At the time of observation he was very impassive, but the senses of sight and hearing were normally acute. There was complete cutaneous and deep anæsthesia, to ordinary and to painful impressions, on his cheeks, forearms, and in fact over the whole body ; punctures were made down to the bone, and none of them were followed by any bleeding. Faradaism being applied to the right forearm, the seats of puncture began to bleed, but the anæsthesia persisted. Gold coins were then applied, and it was noticed that after their application for ten minutes, sensation returned over these regions, and punctures produced bleeding, the range of sensibility gradually diminishing in every direction from the area over which the coin was placed. These experiments were repeated on the 19th, 21st, 29th, and on several subsequent occasions, with invariably the same result. Like observations were made with other metals, insulated and non-insulated, and with wood, with the boy's attention drawn to it, or, on the other hand, wholly without his knowledge, but only with the gold could the above results be obtained. On one or two occasions the gold failed, but never when it had been applied as long as ten minutes. Once a puncture made into the leg, when he was asleep, produced pain and free bleeding. In about a month after his admission, he had so far recovered the use of his limbs as to be able to walk about with the aid of a stick. It was not until fully three months after his admission that the anæsthesia and ischæmia passed away, and he left the hospital on Aug. 25th, able to walk fairly well, and with his sensibility and capacity for bleeding everywhere normal. With the exception of being treated for two severe attacks of bronchitis, shower-baths, faradaism, valerian, cod-liver oil, and iron, were the only remedies adopted. Dr. Thompson pointed out that the case was one of pure and simple hysteria in a boy who was singularly intelligent, thoroughly truthful, straightforward, and uncomplaining, but who appeared to have been foolishly indulged by an over-fond mother, was of rather an effeminate disposition, and was possessed of ill-developed genital organs. Possibly the latter was the main element in his predisposition. The symptoms included paresis and contracture, anæsthesia amounting to analgesia, which, unlike the majority of cases, was distributed equally on both sides. Thirdly, there was the strange feature of ischæmia, and lastly the influence of the gold coins. The author of the paper dwelt at some length upon the nature of this influence; he considered that what is known as the "moral" theory, which has the support of Dr. Russell Reynolds, although no doubt an element in this as in every other case of hysteria, could not altogether explain the result of this experimentation. For example, the gold was operative when the boy was told and believed it was silver, and the silver was inoperative although the boy believed it to be gold. On the other hand, so far as anæsthesia was concerned, a puncture made when the boy was fast asleep was evidently felt, and produced bleeding.—Dr. ALTHAUS said that the case was of considerable interest in connection with the experiments on metallo-therapy undertaken by M. Charcot at La Salpétrière. He had himself seen the experiments, and entirely agreed in the conclusions arrived at by M. Charcot. There was no question as to these facts being facts, although their explanation might be difficult. The theory of the influence of mental and moral impressions could not be sustained, for in many instances the patients were unaware of the experiments being performed. Patients who were so completely anæsthetic as not to feel, not merely the prick of pins, but of lances thrust even to the bones without exciting hemorrhage, became sensible of the slightest ill-usage within fifteen or twenty minutes after the application of metals. How also could any mental operation produce the ischæmia? The temperature of the part, too, rose from 26° and 28° C. during the anæsthesia to 34° or 35° after fifteen minutes' application of metals. A like remarkable difference was ascertained in the muscular power before and after the experiments. All the cases in La Salpétrière had further some affection of the special senses, as colour-blindness, deafness, anosmia, etc., all of which disappeared under the same means, so that after the application the ticking of a clock could be heard at a distance of three feet; ether, not smelt before, was readily perceived; and colocynth could be tasted, when it could not before the application. At present no *rationale* could be given of the *modus operandi* of the metals. Another interesting point was the transference of sensibility and of elevation of temperature from one side of the body to the other. Thus, after the application of the metals to the anæsthetic and analgesic half of the body, this became hyperæsthetic, the previously normal side becoming less sensitive. So also with temperature, muscular power, and special senses. The action of the metals could not be explained on electrical grounds; for, although undoubtedly the coins do give rise to electric currents, yet these, in the case of pure gold, are extremely feeble, deflecting the galvanometer-needle about three degrees; whilst a gold coin causes a deflexion of ten degrees, and copper, zinc, iron, one of from 60 to 80 degrees. Such currents resemble much the physiological currents in nerve and muscle, and it was difficult to believe that they produced the effects stated. Moreover, in the case read, the coins were on several occasions insulated by paper and silk.

Dr. Broadbent could add but little to the ample account of Charcot's experiments just given by Dr. Althaus. He had himself seen them, and he noticed this fact—that many of the young girls who were perfectly insensible to and did not bleed after deep punctures with a large carpet-needle, were yet engaged in sewing. He had recently under his care a case resembling that related by Dr. Thompson. A young girl who had been a little out of health, and who presented none of the usual signs of hysteria, began to suffer from slight weakness in the arms and loss of sensation in the legs from the knees downwards. This anæsthesia was complete, and was associated with ischæmia. Metallic applications restored the normal condition, and Dr. Broadbent attributed the change to the effect of expectant attention, which might induce the return of sensation and circulation, just as it induces pain, in any region. In his case he did not try metal coins, but caused the patient to wear a brass garter, below the right knee, without informing her of the result expected to ensue. In the course of a few days sensation returned to the right leg, the left remaining anæsthetic; and this again regaining its sensibility after the garter had been worn on it for a short time. Dr. Broadbent did not profess to understand the reason why now one metal and now another was operative, especially when the patient was unconscious of the application; and in his own case he could not say whether expectant attention, or some galvanic influence, was the reason of the cure.

———

Subcutaneous Injection of Ergotin in Neuralgia.

In an article on this subject in the *Gazzetta Clinica di Palermo* for June, 1876, Dr. S. S. MARINO sums up in the following conclusions.

1. In sunstroke and tic-douloureux, local hypodermic injections of ergotin have rapid and certain effects, superior to those obtained by all other remedies, including quinine.

2. The results are equally good in hemicrania.

3. In sciatica, ergotin may also give ready and brilliant results, but sometimes, from reasons which we do not yet know, it may completely fail, even in individuals in whom its use appeared at first quite successful. It is necessary to enlist new facts, in order to pronounce a definitive judgment on its value in this troublesome and obstinate malady.

4. It would also be useful to try the effect of the hypodermic injection of the fluid extract of ergot in other neuralgiæ, especially those dependent on blood-infection and cachexy. It is well known that, in diseases of the nervous system, it is not reasonable to trust to any one remedy; often, after remedies of the highest repute have been tried and failed, relief has been obtained from one of which little was expected. Even when the disease recurs in the same form, the same remedy does not always give useful results.

5. When injected under the skin, ergotin does not cause abscess, except in very rare cases, nor erysipelas, nor any other inconvenience. The injection is usually followed by more or less intense burning, sometimes pain; but both disappear in half an hour, if the seat of the puncture be dressed with small compresses dipped in cold water.

6. Sometimes after one, more frequently after two injections, the pain entirely ceases; but, in order to secure the advantage gained, it is advisable to continue the injections, in number from two to six after the first two, according to the severity of the neuralgia, and the length of time during which it has lasted.

7. Dr. Marino has not found it necessary to inject more than 20 centigrammes (3 grains) of the remedy; for adults, 15 centigrammes are ordinarily sufficient. He dissolves it in either water or glycerine.—*London Med. Record*, Nov. 15, 1877.

Cysts of the Epiglottis.

In spite of the innumerable follicles studding the mucous membrane of the larynx, and the general inclination of mucous membrane to produce cystic growths, cysts of the epiglottis are among the rarest forms of tumours observed on this organ. In a recent number of the *Berliner Klin. Wochenschrift*, Dr. BESCHORNER, of Dresden, has described a very interesting case of cyst of the epiglottis, and analyzed the different cases so far noted in laryngoscopic literature. Among 693 cases of polypus of the larynx, there were only 14 cases of cystic growths on the epiglottis—in other words, not more than two per cent. of all the cases observed. Most of these varied in size between a poppy seed and a bean, only three having attained the size of a cherry. The case of Dr. Beschorner is interesting from the fact that, in spite of its great size, there were no subjective symptoms. The patient was a young man who presented himself for an examination of his chest. The result being negative a laryngoscopic examination was made, and a tumour the size of a cherry was unexpectedly discovered on the anterior surface of the left half of the epiglottis. There were none of the unpleasant symptoms generally observed, when even the smallest foreign body happens to be situated in these sensitive parts. The diameter of the tumour was estimated to be rather more than half an inch; its colour, yellowish gray passing into red at its base, and its nature evidently cystic. The patient, refusing to admit of any operative interference, passed from under treatment, but a week later, being examined for the second time, the tumour was found to have burst spontaneously, and to have discharged most of its contents. Four days later no trace of the former cyst could be detected, and the patient stated most emphatically that he could observe no difference whatever in the sensation in his larynx since the rupture of the cyst.—*Med. Examiner*, Nov. 29, 1877.

—

Ulcerative Endocarditis.

Dr. WILLIAM CAYLEY, Physician and Lecturer on Medicine at the Middlesex Hospital, gives (*Med. Times and Gaz.*, Nov. 10, 1877) the following sketch of this affection and of its treatment :—

The disease known as ulcerative endocarditis was first described by the late Dr. Senhouse Kirkes, who published a case in the *Edinburgh Medical and Surgical Journal* in 1853; and it has since been carefully investigated by many pathologists, German as well as English, especially Virchow. The name is not happily chosen, as we often have ulceration of the endocardium in rheumatic and other affections, without the characteristic symptoms and effects of the disease; and we meet with all the phenomena of the disease, as in this case, without any ulceration. Professor Rosenstein, in "Ziemssen's Handbuch," as it is called, though it consists of some two dozen bulky volumes, terms it "diphtheritic endocarditis;" and considers the soft, friable layer of lymph or fibrine which is deposited on the inflamed endocardium as similar in its nature to the false membranes on the mucous surfaces in diphtheria, both being largely composed of the lower forms of fungi, bacteria, and micrococci. The term "diphtheritic" is, however, employed in so many different senses, and has already given rise to so much confusion, that I think it very undesirable to extend its use. I myself should prefer the name "infecting endocarditis," as one of the most prominent results is the infection of the blood with some morbid poison.

The disease is characterized by producing multiple embolisms, for the most part of the miliary form, and a condition of the blood which at present we must call by the general name of blood-poisoning, the indications of which are rigours, fever. prostration. delirium. stupor. Embolisms are, of course, liable to occur in ordinary endocarditis. but here the principal consequences are due to the local effects of the embolisms; the miliary form, too, is less frequent, and the seat of the embolism is not quite the same. In the brain the emboli due to detachment of vegetations in ordinary endocarditis usually get lodged in a branch of the middle cerebral artery. and produce hemorrhage and softening of the anterior part of the optic thalamus or corpus striatum, and, as a consequence, hemiplegia. In infecting endocarditis the embolism are most common, as in this case, in the pia mater of the hemispheres, and from their small size do not necessarily cause any characteristic signs of cerebral lesion. The intestine, too, is much more frequently the seat of embolism in infecting than in simple endocarditis.

In both forms the kidneys and spleen are the most common seats of embolism.

The symptoms of the disease differ greatly in different cases, but are conveniently divided by Professor Rosenstein into two main forms—the pyæmic and the typhoid. The pyæmic form more resembles ordinary pyæmia, with which it is often associated. There are recurrent rigours, fever of a remittent or intermittent type. and local suppurations due to embolism.

The symptoms of the typhoid form were well exemplified in this case. At the outset. rigours; often vomiting, which may continue through the whole course of the disease; high fever of an irregular type, the remissions and exacerbations often occurring at irregular times, and not necessarily morning and evening, as is usually the case in typhoid. Often there is profuse sweating. Together with these symptoms there is headache, vertigo, great prostration, dry brown tongue, sordes on the teeth, delirium, stupor passing into coma. Diarrhœa is often present, due no doubt to the intestinal embolisms, and the motions may contain blood. The spleen is enlarged, and the urine is almost always albuminous, and often bloody; in the present case this symptom was absent. though the kidneys were studded with miliary embolisms.

On auscultation of the heart we find the signs of valvular incompetency, and often also of obstruction of the orifices, and the bruits thus produced are liable to vary from day to day from the progress of the ulceration.

Infecting endocarditis does not appear to attack persons previously in good health. It may occur in pyæmia; it is also met with in the puerperal state, in which case, according to Professor Rosenstein, there is often a diphtheritic inflammation of the genital mucous membrane. It sometimes complicates the specific fevers, as smallpox or diphtheria. Sometimes the endocarditis of acute rheumatism takes this form; and occasionally, as in the present case, it supervenes in chronic valvular disease. If the disease be really due to an infection of the blood by bacteria, it is difficult to understand how, in the latter instances, this is affected.

The principal points of distinction between the typhoid form of infecting endocarditis and typhoid fever are these: First, the physical signs of the cardiac lesion. Endocarditis is not likely to occur as a complication of typhoid, though, of course, typhoid fever may attack persons suffering from chronic valvular disease. Next, the presence of one of the affections which are known to give rise to this form of endocarditis. Then there are the more sudden onset, the rapid course, the marked rigours, and the more irregular type of fever. The frequency of the pulse, and especially of the respirations, is usually much greater than in typhoid; this great frequency of the respirations was well marked in this case, and was out of all proportion to the pulmonary lesions, as appeared both by the physical signs during life and the post-mortem condition. Any local symptoms of embolism would, of course, tend to confirm the diagnosis. The presence of blood and albumen in the urine, indicating embolism of the kidney, is a very important sign, though albuminuria is not uncommon in typhoid. Why this sign was absent in my case I am unable to explain. The rose spots of typhoid are of course absent. The delirium, the dry cracked tongue, the sordes on the teeth, the prostration, the diarrhœa, the enlargement of the spleen, are common to both diseases.

The disease appears necessarily to tend to a fatal issue, and is not amenable to treatment. On the view that it is due to an infection of the blood by bacteria, it has been proposed to give the sulpho-carbolates, quinine in large doses, salicine and salicylic acid, which are destructive to these organisms. As this case was regarded as probably one of typhoid fever, the patient was treated by the "anti-pyretic method," as it is called—that is, by reducing the temperature by tepid baths and large doses of quinine. Though I have not succeeded in obtaining the brilliant results which have attended this mode of treatment in Germany, I nevertheless regard it as the best way of treating typhoid with high temperature. Here the temperature resisted the treatment in a remarkable manner, and the chilling effect of the baths was very transient. In typhoid the temperature seldom resists the effects of a few successive baths and a large dose of quinine or salicylate of soda, which usually produce a reduction lasting for twelve or even twenty-four hours, and by repetitions of this treatment the temperature may be kept at a moderate height throughout the course of the fever. In this case I did not venture to give baths below 80°, as they were not very well borne, soon causing shivering and depression of the circulation. The use of stimulants was indicated by the great prostration, which, however, they were powerless to remove.

———

Gonorrhœal Rheumatism of the Heart.

M. Desnos read (*Gaz. Hebd.*, Nov. 16) a case of this affection to the Paris Hospital Society, observing that although these cases are rare, and usually pass unperceived, yet their true nature and connexion is sometimes brought to light by means of the intervening arthritis. About a month ago the subject of this case came into the hospital with acute bronchitis, the heart being then in a normal condition. Some days after the patient was seized with pains in the shoulder, which then localized itself in the sterno-clavicular articulation, and it was then discovered that he had gonorrhœa. All of a sudden he was seized with violent palpitation of the heart, and the diagnosis was made of narrowing and insufficiency of the mitral orifice; and œdema and an infiltration of the inferior extremities, without albumen in the urine, supervened. At the autopsy a small ulcer was found on the mitral valve, together with a considerable vegetant endocarditis of the aortic valves and the whole of the interior of the heart. M. Fournier observed that this was certainly a case of gonorrhœal endocarditis, although important details were wanting. Was there sweating or fever present? In gonorrhœal rheumatism, in fact, the temperature is never high; and just as sweating is so abundant in ordinary rheumatism, it is absent in the form of the disease consecutive to gonorrhœa. A conclusive circumstance in this case was the seat of the affection, the sterno-clavicular articulation being the joint of predilection in gonorrhœal rheumatism. M. Desnos replied that in his case the temperature curves would not be conclusive owing to the pulmonary complications; but the patient had no sweats, and never before had suffered from rheumatism.—*Med. Times and Gaz.*, Nov. 24, 1877.

———

Systolic Retraction of the Intercostal Spaces.

Dr. O. Von Widmann (*Virchow's Archiv*, July, 1877) writes that, while undoubtedly systolic retraction of the intercostal spaces has been often noticed when there were partial or complete adhesions of the heart and pericardium with the pericardial pleura to the costal pleura, it is also equally certain that these latter have in some cases been absent: and further that, when present, no retraction of the intercostal spaces has sometimes been observed. He regards as most important for the explanation of these phenomena, the change in the axis of the heart's longest diameter during systole, namely, the shortening of the right-to-left diameter. He says the systolic retraction proves only (basing ourselves on the results of physiological investigations of the changes of shape and position which occur in the organ during systole) that the heart lies in an anomalous position, and chiefly that it is twisted so as to lie, instead of with its anterior surface forwards, with one of its lateral surfaces towards the thoracic wall, or, in other words, that it is turned round on its long axis, in which position it may or may not be fixed by adhesions.

During systole, the heart undergoes a diminution of its right to left diameter; if now one of these sides be in contact with the thoracic wall, it will be withdrawn during systole, and in consequence the atmospheric pressure will force in the intercostal spaces But in spite of this twisting of the heart, these consequences may be prevented by emphysema of the lungs, as collections of air in the pleural sac, if the heart be not hypertrophied, if its movements be very feeble, or the intercostal spaces narrow, and the thorax very unyielding, etc.; that is, when the forcing elements, retraction of the left lung, hypertrophy of the heart, strong cardiac movements, etc., are absent.—*London Med. Record*, Nov. 15, 1877.

Vertigo a Stomacho Læso.

Dr. BERGER (*Deutsche Zeitschrift fur die Prakt. Medicin*, August, 1877) relates a case of vertigo of this kind which simulated serious brain-disease. The patient, a medical man, was affected by sudden intense vertigo which completely disappeared on lying down quietly, but any active or passive movement of the body made him giddy and ready to fall. Locomotion had become quite impossible. From the absence of any other cerebral symptoms (there was only a very lively increase of reflex excitability) and on investigation the discovery of a loaded tongue, decided dyspepsia, antecedent frequent vomitings, slight icterus of the conjunctiva, and on one occasion the presence of a trace of bile-pigment in the urine, vertigo a stomacho læso was diagnosed. Appropriate treatment (rhubarb and soda) quickly improved him, but a tendency to vertigo persisted for some time.—*London Med. Record*, Nov. 15, 1877.

Gonorrhœal Peritonitis.

In a communication to the *Archives Générales de Médicine* for October and November, entitled, "Peritonitis and Subperitoneal Phlegmon of a Gonorrhœal Origin," Dr. FAUCON, after referring to the history of the subject from the time of John Hunter, the author of the first observation, and narrating in great detail a case that has come under his own notice, arrives at the following conclusions:—

1. Peritonitis and subperitoneal phlegmon should be ranked amongst the possible complications of gonorrhœa. 2. These accidents are only distinct effects of the blenorrhagic inflammation, propagated from the urethra to the peritoneum or the subperitoneal cellular tissue by the intermedium of the vas deferens the vesiculæ seminales, the prostate (perhaps the bladder, ureters, and kidneys), and the cellular "atmosphere" surrounding these organs. 3. Their appearance is, therefore, always preceded by the ordinary blenorrhagic complications, resulting from the preliminary inflammation of the tissues or organs which serve as intermedia (deferentitis, vesiculitis, etc.), so that they are true tertiary accidents of

gonorrhœa. 4. Gonorrhœal peritonitis may exhibit various points of origin, so that it has been met with in the pelvic region opposite the recto-vesical *cul-de-sac,* while at other times it arises at the internal orifice of the inguinal canal. 5. It may remain localized at the points where it has arisen, and there undergo a cure: but it may also become generalized, or at least extend to a more or less considerable portion of the abdomen, pass on to suppuration, and terminate fatally. 6. Subperitoneal phlegmon has been observed in the lumbar fossa, at the lower part of the internal iliac region, and of the anterior wall of the abdomen. It may terminate either in resolution or suppuration, but its influence is less mischievous than that of peritonitis. 7. When a subperitoneal abscess has formed, it should be opened as soon as possible. An energetic antiphlogistic treatment, the prolonged application of ice, and preventive *débridement* may arrest the development of the phlegmon, and prevent its passing into suppuration.—*Med. Times and Gaz.,* Nov. 24, 1877.

Gall-stones and Atheromatous Degeneration of the Arteries.

According to Dr. BENECKE, of Marburg, *Deutsches Archiv. für klinische Medicin, Band* 48, *Heft* 1, the formation of gall-stones may have its cause in one of two conditions : either there is a relative excess of the formation of cholesterine in the liver, so that this is separated in the gall-bladder just as acid urate of soda or crystalline uric acid is in concentrated urine, or there is a lack of the biliary salts which maintain the solution just as urates or crystalline uric acid are separated in the urinary passages by a diminution of soda or an excess of phosphoric acid in the urine.

He makes the following conclusions :—

1. The occurrence of gall-stones coincides in the majority of cases (about seventy per cent.) with the presence of atheromatous degeneration of the arteries.

2. Atheromatous degeneration of arteries (without gall-stones) is observed much oftener than gall-stones.

3. Gall-stones are of much more frequent occurrence in females than in males ; degeneration of arteries takes place with about equal frequency in both sexes.

4. The occurrence of gall-stones is generally observed at an earlier period of life (from twenty years on) than the atheromatous degeneration of arteries.

5. Gall-stones are found in relatively greater frequency in patients suffering from carcinoma and in nervous congestion, or where the liver is very full of blood.

6. The occurrence of gall-stones and of atheromatous degeneration of arteries is relatively very often accompanied by an abundant formation of fat.—*Boston Med. and Surg Journal,* Nov. 1, 1877.

Case of Rupture of the Gall-Bladder.

In the Berlin *Charité-Annalen,* 1877, vol. ii., EICHHORST describes the case of a woman aged 62, who, after having suffered several times from gall-stones and jaundice, observed for some time a dark green colouring of the skin in the right hypochondrium. As this increased in extent, she was admitted into hospital, where necrosis of the skin was found to extend over a space limited by the lower border of the ribs, the middle line, the right Poupart's ligament, and the axillary line. Sensation was completely lost. In a circumscribed spot, corresponding with the region of the gall-bladder, there were fluctuation and tenderness. On the day after her admission, the skin over this part burst, and a hundred cubic centimetres of bile escaped, partly spontaneously and partly on pressure. A probe passed into a cavity with smooth yielding walls, which appeared irregular only above. After the removal of the necrosed abdominal wall, the fascia of the muscles was exposed as if dissected. There was no icterus; the feces were brimstone-coloured; the urine was free from biliary colouring matter. In the course of three weeks the fistulous opening gradually closed; and almost at the same time the sclerotic, and very soon the abdominal wall, became jaundiced. The urine and feces remained permanently free from biliary colouring matter. Some days later, the wound assumed a diphtheritic appearance, the sensorium became affected, coma ensued, and the patient died. The amount of bile discharged through the fistula on each day after the first, averaged 18.6 cubic centimetres, never exceeding 25 cubic centimetres. On *post-mortem* examination, the cæcum and transverse colon were found adherent to the right half of the abdominal wall. The fistulous passage showed during life led into a cavity as large as a hen's egg, lying beneath the gall-bladder, and bounded by false membranes deposited about the gall-bladder and liver. This cavity communicated by an opening of the size of a pea with the gall-bladder, which was full of gall-stones. The bile-ducts both within and outside the liver were much dilated. There were multiple abscesses in the liver, and medullary cancer of the duodenum at the entrance of the ductus choledochus.

The discharge of the bile into the peritoneal cavity without causing pain, is interesting, as is also the small quantity of bile that was discharged daily. This quantity—which never exceeded 25 cubic centimetres—represented nearly the total amount of bile excreted, since (as examination of the urine and feces proved) none of it was absorbed or passed into the intestine. Eichhorst used this case for making experiments on the absorption into the bile of salicylic acid, sugar, and muriate of quinine; none of these were excreted with the bile, but were found in the urine. The result was the same, whether they were given by the mouth or by enema.—*London Med. Record*, Nov. 15, 1877.

Case of Anuria lasting Twenty-five Days; Recovery.

Dr. WILLIAM WHITELAW, of Cupar, Fife, records (*Lancet*, Sept. 29, 1877) the following extraordinary, and, it is believed, unique case of long-continued anuria which eventually recovered.

In May last, 1876, two out of six children, residing in a recently-built and well-constructed house in this neighbourhood, took scarlatina in a mild form, and made a good recovery. On returning from the seaside in the beginning of September the remaining four were attacked, three of them recovered well; but the fourth, a healthy boy, aged eight years, was the subject of the above very strange sequela. He was attacked on Sept. 11th, with marked throat symptoms and strawberry tongue; temperature never higher than 101°; rash almost imperceptible, and desquamation very slight. The existence of the other cases, however, left no doubt as to the diagnosis. He was quickly well, and, although not so strong as formerly, nothing particular was observed till Dec. 3d, when his urine was observed to be scantier than usual; and on the 5th, on being called in, I found him apparently in perfect health—appetite better than usual, tongue clean, pulse 80, temperature 98.5°, and skin natural. There existed a little pain and tenderness on pressure over both lumbar regions; there was no swelling of face, hands, feet, or abdomen; and during the previous twenty-four hours he had passed ten ounces of urine, clear in colour, sp. gr. 1018, and free from albumen. He was ordered a hot bath; poultices over the kidneys; to drink as much fluid as possible; and a mixture of acetate of potash, squill, digitalis, and broom. On the 6th I found he had passed only two ounces of urine, but he had perspired very freely after the bath. He was eating and sleeping well. On Dec. 7th there was voided only one drachm of urine; and *from this date till the 20th not one single drop*, and yet, with the exception of slight headaches, his general health continued excellent. During this time three or four liquid stools daily were procured by the exhibition of compound jalap powder, and diaphoresis was maintained by baths and poultices. On Dec. 19th Dr. Lumgair, of Largo, saw him in consultation, and could scarcely credit that suppression had gone on so long without the superventien of dropsy or any symptom of uræmic poisoning. He suggested vesication over the kidneys, and in twenty hours after the application of the blister two ounces of urine, free from albumen, had been passed; and I hoped that the kidneys were now roused from their state of torpor (for it seemed to be that, more than actual nephritis). No more urine was, however, secreted; and on the 27th the blister was repeated, but this time with no successful result. The baths, poultices, and jalap were now discontinued, in the belief that the urea was being removed by these means, and that, by ceasing diaphoresis and purgation, the kidneys might be *forced* to resume work. The diuretics were, however, continued. This change of treatment made no apparent difference. The bowels acted twice daily of their own accord, and the boy continued in excellent health. On the 31st December there appeared very slight œdema of the feet and ankles; and on the morning of January 2d one drachm of urine was passed. On the same day, with the aid of Dr. Fraser, superintendent of the Fife and Kinross Asylum, electricity was applied to the spine and through the kidneys, and a small catheter was passed into the bladder, in the hope of exciting reflex action. On the 3d and 4th January about the same quantity was passed daily; and on the 5th a whole pint was voided in small quantities at eight different times. Since then the kidneys have acted well, and the boy has (Jan. 12th) quite recovered.

The following points seem of interest:—1. Twelve weeks elapsed from the date of taking scarlatina (which was of a very mild nature) till the suppression took place. 2· With the exception of two ounces passed on the thirteenth day, there was complete anuria for twenty-five days. 3. Except slight headaches, and latterly slight œdema, there were no uræmic or dropsical symptoms throughout. 4. There was no albuminuria and no febrile action. The kidneys seem to have been in a state of torpor, and their work must have been carried on by the bowels, skin, and to some extent by the lungs. 5. It is hard to say what share the treatment had in the final happy result. Vesication at first seemed beneficial, but a second trial had no such effect. Then one drachm of urine was passed before the application of the battery, and therefore the credit cannot be entirely due to it. Probably, ceasing diaphoretics and purgatives, and thus throwing the entire duty of excreting the urea on the kidneys, was the best line of treatment that could be adopted, although at first sight a somewhat risky proceeding.

I may add that the boy was closely watched, night and day, by his parents and the servants, and was offered rewards to induce him to micturate; so that the idea of deception cannot be entertained. Drs. Lumgair and Fraser, although at first sceptical, are as much convinced of the genuineness of the case as I am myself.

———

Peritonism and its Rational Treatment.

Under the title of peritonism, Professor GUBLER studies (*Journal de Thérapeutique*, No. 20, 1876, and Nos. 2, 3, 4, 5, 6, 1877) the multiple symptoms resulting from troubles of the peritoneum. The conclusions of his memoirs are as follows:—

1. The serious complications of abdominal lesions attributed to peritonitis, do not really belong to that phlegmasia. They are sometimes absent in the most intense inflammations, and sometimes appear without any notable inflammation of the serous membrane of the abdomen.

2. The course of symptoms, superadded to traumatic or spontaneous lesions of the abdomen, consists of sympathetic or reflex disturbances of the great functions of circulation and hæmatosis. I have given it the name of peritonism, so as to

express its nervous character, and to show its independent nature in relation to peritoneal phleg 1 asia.

3. The contingent character of these accidents, the unenviable privilege of their possession, inflicted on the hu 1 an race, co 1 pared with the relative immunity of the animal species, all these circumstances co 1 bine to show that the develop 1 ent of peritonis 1 is due to excessive i 1 pressionability as well as to exaggerated reaction of the sympathetic nervous system in particular races or predisposed individuals.

4. Hence it may be hoped that, by di 1 inishing this susceptibility, and restraining the reflex actions which result fro 1 it, patients will be placed in conditions favourable to the regular evolution of the local 1 orbid process, without running the risk of the advent of general co 1 plications which frequently cannot be arrested. Here, perhaps, 1 ore than in any other case, prevention is better than cure.

5. It is, therefore, i 1 portant in the course of pri 1 ary local affections, as well as in the abdo 1 inal localizations of general diseases, to follow with an attentive eye the rise and progress of the lesion, so as to intervene in ti 1 e to prevent the develop 1 ent of sy 1 pathetic co 1 plications. This care is particularly de 1 anded in cases of typhoid fever, with deep ulceration of the ileu 1, involving Peyer's patches. in those of intense typhlitis and perityphlitis, of suppurative hepatitis, infla 1 1 ation of the gall-bladder, of si 1 ple or cancerous ulcers of the alimentary canal, of acute inflammations of ovarian or other cysts, of circu 1 scribed 1 etroperitonitis or peritonitis having a tendency to suppurate.

6. So soon as the phleg 1 asia, having beco 1 e intense, arouses an acute sensibility of the belly, with distension of the region, in consequence of 1 uscular atony of the intestine, and gives rise to indications of repercussion over the whole ganglionic syste 1, the 1 edical 1 an should intervene with the view of assuring the tolerance of the nervous syste 1, of reducing the i 1 pressionability of the tri-splanchnic nerves, and the reactions of the reflex centres, and of lowering the exquisite nervousness of the hu 1 an race to the level of that of the ani 1 al types i 1 1 ediately below it.

7. Such 1 eans undoubtedly exist in our therapeutic arsenal. The large class of nervines offers us various kinds, on the efficacy of which clinical experience has already given judg 1 ent; such are narcotics, and above all opiu 1, as well as the diffusible sti 1 ulants, a 1 ongst which alcohol holds the first place.

8. Anæsthetics, however, principally ether and chlorofor 1, play a considerable part in the prophylaxis of peritonis 1, where foreseen and intended lesions are in question, that is to say, surgical operations on the abdo 1 inal organs. Not only is ovarioto 1 y rendered easier by prolonged anæsthesia, but the success of this great operation is scarcely possible except on this condition.—*London Med. Record*, Nov. 15, 1877.

—

Effects of Irritation of the Skin in Syphilitic Persons.

TARNOWSKY (*Archiv. für Dermatologie und Syphilis*, 1 and 2 Heft, 1877) states that, when the skin of a person suffering fro 1 syphilis is irritated by caustics or by inoculation of various 1 orbid products, the course of the wound differs fro 1 that which is observed in the skin of healthy persons subjected to the sa 1 e influences, the a 1 ount of reaction and induration varying according to the interval which has elapsed since the date of the infection The results of a large nu 1 ber of experi 1 ents have convinced hi 1 that the soft chancre and the infecting syphilitic sore are the product of two distinct virus, which are not interchangeable. The sores produced by Bidenkap, Redei, and Köbner on syphilitic persons by inoculation, and which they have described as soft chancres, are, he 1 aintains, distinguishable by their for 1, course, absence of chancre-buboes, and results when inoculated from the true soft chancre; and are simply the characteristic effects of imitation of the skin in the syphilitic. In opposition to the theory that the soft chancre is produced by concentration of the syphilitic virus, he states that he has practised inoculations with the chancre virus diluted to various degrees, but has never produced thereby any other form than that of the soft chancre.—*London Med. Record*, Nov. 15. 1877.

Partial Baldness.

The pathology of Alopecia areata, or Area Celsi, has of late years attracted much attention among dermatologists, and various attempts—not very successful, it must be admitted—have been made to explain the formation of circumscribed, smooth, more or less circular, hairless patches on the scalp and other hairy regions of the body. The latest contribution to this question is a lecture by Dr. P. MICHELSON, of Königsberg (Prussia), in No. 120 of Volkmann's *Sammlung Klin. Vorträge*, in which the author unreservedly rejects the idea of a parasitic origin for Alopecia areata (Gruby, Malassez), and regards the disease as due to arrest of growth in the hair itself, "leading," as Bärensprung puts it, "to a more scanty production of the cellular elements out of which it is developed." The structural alterations in the root of the hair—loss of its bulbar swelling, absence of defined cellular elements in the root-sheath, fibrillary splitting of the shaft in a longitudinal direction, etc.—described by Michelson and others (curiously enough, no allusion is here made to the papers of Duckworth and Bristowe), are not characteristic of Alopecia areata, but are met with in other diseases in which the nutrition of the hair is interfered with. What is it that causes these alterations in the case of Area Celsi? Will the neurotic theory explain them? and "must," as Duhring says ("Diseases of the Skin," 1877), "the fall of the hair be viewed as a state of perverted innervation, and can the suddenness of the attack be only accounted for by regarding the nervous system at fault?" Michelson answers that, in the first place, the symptom of *diminished sensibility* of the affected skin, which is usually regarded as a proof of perverted innervation, is not constant, and he gives the details of some careful observations on a case of his own, in which the sensibility was, on the contrary, *increased*. The headache, which not unfrequently accompanies the development of the affection, he also regards as not improbably due to a chronic inflammatory process in the soft tissues of the head, and he points out that the instances of loss of hair or baldness following injuries of nerves will not bear very close examination, and that this symptom is not mentioned as having occurred in any of the numerous cases in which section of nerves has been performed by modern surgeons. Further, it is not certain that those alterations in the growth of hair and the nutrition of the skin, which have been reported as following gunshot injuries of nerves (Weir Mitchell, Fischer. and others), and which have been referred to lesions of "trophic" nerves, are really due to the latter, for it has been shown by Kölliker that some at least of these alterations occur if a limb is, as was the case in the above instances, confined for a long period in a close-fitting (plaster of Paris) bandage.

In any case only quite a small percentage of nerve-lesions is followed by alopecia; and to explain the occurrence of such a symptom as the general diffuse baldness, which is sometimes met with, by a neurotic agency, it would be necessary, as Michelson says, "either to accept the hypothesis of a gradual implication of all the 'trophic' nerves of the skin, or else that of a trophic centre in the brain or spinal cord, which becomes the seat of a gradually progressive disease."

The existence of such a centre is absolutely hypothetical, and by no means probable, and the evidence in favour of a lesion of "trophic" nerves is also extremely slight. Hence Michelson concludes, and we think justly, that "the neurotic origin of Alopecia areata is, in the present state of medical science, an unproven hypothesis." He confesses, however, that he is unable to substitute for it a better one, but he agrees with Hutchinson that one element in the causation of the disease is "a lowering of the general nutrition of the body." Another element (purely hypothetical) may possibly be a diminution in the calibre of the bloodvessels, which would explain the remarkable pallor of the affected skin; and, lastly, the *disappearance of the subcutaneous cellular tissue, and thinning of the skin itself*, which is a nearly constant symptom (according to Michelson), may constitute an earlier stage of the same process which ends in loss of hair, though, of course, until we know why the subcutaneous tissue, etc., atrophies, we are no nearer to the true explanation of the origin of the disease than we previously were.

It is evident from the foregoing that Alopecia areata is still an unsolved mystery. Whether careful microscopic examinations of sections of the *skin* in the diseased area, which are much needed, will eventually throw any light on its *rationale*, we cannot say, but persons with a love for original investigation may be reminded, in the words of an anonymous English author, with which Dr. Michelson closes his lecture, that "there is no subject that more invites the study of those who would fain leave science more advanced than they found it."—*Med. Times and Gaz.*, Nov. 17, 1877.

Ova of Oxyuris Vermicularis on the Human Skin.

MICHELSON (*Berliner Klinische Wochenschrift*, No. 33, 1877) describes the case of a boy, in whom an eczematous condition of the scrotum was produced by the ova of oxyuris vermicularis. They were embedded in the epidermis. The boy was known to have long suffered from this entozoon. Its conveyance to the anterior surface of the scrotum (the posterior surface being free) was due to a habit the boy had of tucking the front skirt of his shirt between his hips.—*London Med. Record*, Nov. 15, 1877.

Surgery.

On the Treatment of Hemorrhage.

M. CRÉQUY proposes (*L'Union Médicale*) in cases of severe epistaxis, to substitute for the ordinary plug—the application of which to the posterior nares is often very difficult—the following mode of injecting perchloride of iron, whereby the full styptic effect is secured without the danger with which the use of that remedy is not unfrequently attended. An ordinary syringe is fitted with a canula about two and a half inches long, terminating in a rounded extremity, and perforated throughout its length by a series of small holes, spirally disposed, and directed backwards, so as to emit small retrograde jets. When the canula is introduced horizontally into the nasal fossa, and the syringe filled with a solution of perchloride of iron, the injected fluid is thrown upon the mucous surface, and does not fall upon the pharynx or stomach. Generally one injection is sufficient. For hemorrhages in general, and especially for metrorrhagia, M. RICORD finds injections of hot water at 50 deg. centigrade (122 deg. Fahrenheit), applied through a tube to the neck of the uterus, to be an almost infallible mode of arrest. —*London Med. Record*, Nov. 15, 1877.

Artificial Anæmia as a mode of treatment for Diseases of the Limbs.

A new application is suggested for Esmarch's elastic bandage, namely, as an anæsthetic and curative agent in painful inflammatory affections of the extremities. D. BERNHARD COHN, of Steglitz, relates (*Berl. Klin. Wochenschrift*, October 29, 1877) two cases in which the induction of artificial anæmia by the bandage was followed by great relief—a case of phlegmonous inflammation of the foot in a man of sixty-three, and one of simple œdematous inflammation of the forearm in a maid-servant; and he gives the details of a third case in which a practical cure resulted from Esmarch's method after all other modes of treatment had been exhausted. The patient, a boy of three and a half years, had white swelling of the left knee-joint of eighteen months' standing, with considerable enlargement of the condyles of the femur, and thickening of the tissues around the patella and the head of the tibia. There was great sensitiveness of the parts to pressure, movement was impaired, and walking only possible for a step or two, with lowered pelvis, and with the tips of the toes alone reaching the ground on the left side. After a few weeks' daily application of the bandage for fifteen to sixty minutes, the improvement was so great that the limb could be moved in all directions or handled without pain, the entire sole of the left foot could be brought to the ground in walking, and the gait was even on the two sides—in fact, all that was left of the former affection was a little swelling and limitation in the movement of the joint. Dr. Cohn, in his remarks on the cases, declares that in practice the idea that the increase of blood in the capillaries, which follows the removal of the bandage, will entirely undo the effect of the previous anæmia, is not sustained. He considers that the bandage acts mainly by relieving the congestion of the inflamed part, and perhaps by improving the conditions of diffusion between the tissues and the bloodvessels. He recommends an elastic band, one inch and a half wide, encircling the limb so that each turn overlaps the one below, and finished off with five to eight turns completely covering each other. He thinks that the bandage may be allowed to remain on the limb longer than we might *à priori* think justifiable, and that there is less danger of gangrene if both arteries and veins are completely compressed than if the compression be imperfect so as to close the veins and hinder the escape of blood, while it is still allowed to enter by the arteries. In the latter case, œdema, with enormous rise in the blood-pressure, must be the result. To avoid pain as much as possible, the final turns must not be tighter than absolutely necessary to stop the circulation. The questions, "How often can and ought the constriction to be renewed?" and "Is it better to use single *long* compressions, or frequent short ones?" require further experience to answer them satisfactorily.—*Med. Times and Gaz.*, Dec. 1, 1877.

—

On Sudden Death after Severe Burns.

At the recent Medical Congress at Munich, Professor PONFICK, of Göttingen, described some experiments he had performed with the view to discover the cause of sudden death after extensive burns. Scalding water was applied to dogs, and the results were classified with reference to the extent of the injured surface and the intensity of the heat applied. In all cases in which the burn was severe, important changes in the blood could be shown to take place a few minutes after the injury; the red corpuscles underwent disintegration, and were broken up into an infinite number of minute coloured particles. After a time, varying with their original quantity, these particles disappeared, but not without having set up serious disturbances in several organs remote from each other. The kidneys appeared to bear the brunt of the mischief: they excreted a large proportion of the haemoglobin which had been, to some extent, set free and was circulating in the blood. Their action in this respect, however, at least in severe cases, was accompanied by very severe parenchymatous inflammation, which was shown by the appearance in the urine of peculiar coloured casts by infarction of the uriniferous tubules, fatty degeneration of the epithelium, etc. Another portion of these fragments remained within the organism; it disappeared in the splenic pulp and the medulla of the bones, being taken up by the contractile cells, to undergo in all probability a gradual resolution. The reception of the particles by the cavernous tissue of these parts caused the organs to appear greatly enlarged, even to the naked eye, and to exhibit increased redness and succulence on section. Taking into consideration all the symptoms connected with burns, Professor Ponfick is inclined to believe that the fatal issue in many of the severe cases, and the serious symptoms in others which recover, are to be explained by the fact that the red corpuscles undergo extensive and sudden disintegration. He leaves as undecided the question as to how far acute uræmic poisoning may contribute towards the fatal issue. If this theory be true, transfusion would appear to be indicated as a rational therapeutic measure ; and Dr. Ponfick recommends that in all urgent cases recourse should be had to this operation.—*Med. Examiner*, Nov. 29, 1877.

Cases of Branchial Fistulæ of the External Ears.

Sir James Paget, at a late meeting of the Royal Medical and Chirurgical Society, read a paper on this subject, of which the following is an abstract:—

The occurrence of branchial fistula in the neck has long been known ; they were described first by Dzondi in 1829, who believed that such fistulæ to communicate with the trachea ; but this, as shown later by Henzinger, was doubtless a mistake. Indeed, it is likely that the three or four cases on record of congenital tracheal fistulæ in the middle line of the neck were due to abscess opening into the trachea, unless they arose from defective closure of the branchial arches in the median line, analogous to ectopia cordis, vesicæ, etc.

A writer in 1832 explained the occurrence of cervical fistulæ opening into the pharynx as due to the incomplete closure of branchial clefts ; an opinion confirmed by many recent writers, especially Henzinger, and Sir James Paget has himself met with three such instances. These *cervical* branchial fistulæ occur as two or three minute orifices on one or both sides of the lower part of the neck, and lead upwards to the œsophagus and pharynx ; the lowermost being near the sternal end of the clavicle. in front of the sterno-mastoid muscle, the next opposite to the thyroid cartilage, and the highest between the thyroid cartilage and the hyoid bone. Often symmetrical when they are two in number, there may be two at the lower level and one at the upper ; or a single fistula may occur on one side only. They vary in length from half to one-and-a-half inches in length, and barely admit a probe ; and as a rule are closed at their distal ends, sometimes, but rarely, opening into the pharynx or upper part of the œsophagus. They have a smooth lining membrane, secreting a clear mucous fluid, which may be increased during bronchial or nasal catarrh. Rudiments of cartilage are occasionally found in connection with them, and may be homologous with cervical ribs. They undergo no change during life, and if it be requisite to treat them they may be cured by means of the galvano-cautery. Probably some rare instances of diverticula from the pharynx are branchial fissures closed externally, and possibly some forms of congenital cysts and ranulæ had a like origin.

Of branchial fistulæ in the *external ears* there is no account on record in this country, and foreign literature only yields six or seven cases, most of which are related by Heuzinger. The cases now described occurred in the family of a gentleman perfectly well formed in other respects, who has himself a branchial fistula on the right side of the neck. His father and a sister, as well as four of his own children, had similar malformations; the fistula in two of the latter being on the left side, and on the other two symmetrically disposed on each side of the neck. But, in addition to these cervical fistulæ, the gentleman himself, his sister, and five of his children, each present fistulæ in the helix of one or both ears. These aural fistulæ are minute, their orifices small, and their canal half an inch in length. passing from below forwards and downwards, being less soft and flexible than the cervical fistulæ, producing no secretion, and giving no distress. The co-existence of the latter threw light upon those in the ear, and a similar coincidence had been recorded by Heuzinger. Hence these aural fistulæ are probable due to the incomplete closure of the upper or post-oral fissure, that part of it which does not enter into the formation of the Eustachian tube, tympanum, and external meatus. In other recorded cases the openings have been at the lower or anterior part of the helix or lobule of the ear. It is likely that such cases are not so rare as they seem; and, further, extensions of the same non-closure of the post-oral fissure might be seen in such malformations as complete transverse partition of the auricle, and one case in which a linear depression on the helix and anti-helix was continued on to the cheek was of like nature. There are now sufficient evidences of malformations due to incomplete closure of every one of the branchial fissures: these aural fistulæ being due to defective closure of the first fissure between the mandibular and hyoid arches, the upper cervical to the cleft between the thyroid and hyoid, the lower to the cleft behind the thyro-hyoid arch, and the fourth to the last cleft above the thorax.

Referring next to the association between these cases and those of "supernumerary ears," the author shows that they are found only over the lines of former branchial fissures, and may be considered as cutaneous opercular growths, homologous, though abnormally, with the natural auricles, which guard the first cleft. Mr. Birkett has recorded in the Pathological Transactions a case of a girl, seven years of age, with two supernumerary auricles in the neck, corresponding in position with the usual seats of the upper and lower branchial fistulæ. The tissues of the lobes and their fibro-cartilages were clearly distinguished in these auricles. Mr. Holmes, in his work "On Surgical Diseases of Children," gives an instance of a small pendulous body in the skin near the hyoid bone, towards which a small sinus passed from above, and in one of Heuzinger's cases a small fistula near the sterno-clavicular articulation was concealed by a flat process of skin. Similar abnormalities have been noticed in sheep, goats, and pigs. Dr. Allen Thomson long ago pointed out that malformations of the external ears were frequently associated with malformations in or near the first or mandibular arch, such as hare-lip and cleft palate, and the same association has more recently been noted by Virchow. The author of the paper had observed that many of the persons born with aural branchial clefts had become deaf, and thus have been instances, however slight, of the general law indicated by Dr. Allen Thomson. This was well illustrated by the cases upon which the paper was founded, and others have been placed on record. The occurrence of deafness could hardly be casual, but rather indicative, not of any material change in the structure of the ear, but of such a defect of textures as rendered them morbidly liable to disease. In an appendix to the paper a case, communicated to the author by Mr. Cumberbatch, is related, in which traces of the branchial fissures occurred in the helix of the ear; a small depression, large enough to lodge a No. 4 shot, being seated on the upper part of a peculiarly-shaped pinna.—*Lancet*, Dec. 1, 1877.

On a Hypogastric Urinary Fistula treated Successfully by the Actual Cautery.

Dr. PALLOTTI relates the following case in the *Bulletino delle Scienze Mediche di Bologna* for June, 1876 (abstract in *Annali Universali di Medicina*, September, 1877). B. C., aged 70, was in 1866 obliged to ride on horseback eight days consecutively among the Appenines, and, not being accustomed to this exercise, was attacked with severe prostatic inflammation accompanied with strangury; perineal abscess was also threatened. The prostatitis was treated energetically on antiphlogistic principles, by general bleeding, leeches, etc. : this, perhaps, prevented suppuration, but the strangury was not removed. The patient had retention of urine for four days, and the bladder was enormously distended ; a catheter could not be introduced. In this state of things it was determined to puncture the bladder above the pubes. This was accordingly done, and three kilogrammes (about 6¾ pints) of already decomposed urine were removed. The silver canula was allowed to remain *in situ* eight days : the inflammation of the prostate not ceasing, and the patient being unable to pass urine by the natural channel until the end of that time. In less than two weeks he had quite recovered from the prostatitis, and no longer had retention of urine, but the opening made by the puncture remained open, allowing the urine to escape and soil the clothes, giving rise to a disgusting smell. On account of the inconvenience the patient consulted Dr. Pallotti in July, 1866. He first tried cauterization with nitrate of silver, which he continued for two months without success; he then applied a suture, also ineffectually. He next had a button-shaped cautery made, having in the centre of the button a long conical beak for insertion into the interior of the fistula, so as nearly to reach the bladder. On October 2 the cautery, having been heated to a white heat, was introduced into the fistula and immediately withdrawn. The result was the production of a moderate but sufficient amount of adhesive inflammation. The subsequent dressing consisted in the application of a cabbage leaf greased with purified lard, and changed twice or thrice daily.

On the external aperture of the fistula a small scab formed, which at the end of nine days fell off, leaving beneath it a single drop of thick creamy pus, which, being removed, showed a number of granulations. These were touched twice with nitrate of silver, and the fistula was completely closed in a fortnight. He was seen by Dr. Pallotti five years later, the cure was permanent.—*London Medical Record*, Nov. 15, 1877.

Unilateral Gunshot Injury to the Spinal Cord.

Dr. GOWERS, at a late meeting of the Clinical Society of London (*Lancet*, Nov. 17, 1877), brought forward a case of unilateral gunshot injury to the spinal cord. The patient, who had been in University College Hospital, under the care of Mr. Heath, had fired a pistol into his mouth, and died sixty hours afterwards. The bullet had passed through the body of the second cervical vertebra, and had lodged between the arches of the atlas and axis on the right side. It had not penetrated the dura mater, but had driven a spiculum of bone through the membranes, and had bruised the cord between the second and third cervical nerves, the bruise being confined to the antero-lateral column, the anterior and posterior cornua, and the central part of the gray matter on the right side. All these parts contained many extravasations. The left half of the cord, both gray and white matter, was intact; and the right posterior column was simply swollen, apparently from œdema, there being only a few very minute extravasations in it. The symptoms during life were : Paralysis of the right arm and leg, complete always in the arm, and at first in the leg; after the first twenty-four hours there was slight power of moving the leg. There was hyperæsthesia, or rather hyperalgesia, on the paralyzed side below the part supplied by branches from the cer_vical plexus; in the latter sensation was normal. On the opposite side there was no motor weakness, but there was complete or almost complete loss of sensibility to pain, with very little change in tactile sensibility. The reflex action was diminished, almost abolished, in the paralyzed leg; it was excessive in the oppo_site leg, in which sensibility to pain was diminished. The temperature on the side of the motor paralysis was uniformly higher, one or two degrees, than on the other side; and on the paralyzed side there was a peculiar change in the irritability of the muscles and nerves, that of the muscles being a less, that of the nerves a greater, than on the other side; the change was the same to each form of electricity. In commenting upon these symptoms, Dr. Gowers observed that the cross sensory and motor paralysis was in accord, although not completely, with the view now generally accepted. The slight recovery of power in the leg might be explained by supposing that some fibres of the antero-lateral column recovered functional power; but considering how easily the motor impulse is arrested for some time by a slight injury, he thought this explanation improbable, and that the recovery of power afforded support to Vulpian's opinion that the motor path, although crossing chiefly at the decussation of the pyramids, also crosses to a less extent lower down the cord, and that this subsidiary decussation for the leg had escaped, so that when the shock of the injury was over, there was some return of power over the leg. He pointed out that the slight change in tactile sensibility in the analgesic limbs affords support to the view that tactile and common sensation traverse different paths in the cord ; and the undamaged state of the posterior columns is interesting in connection with the assertion of Schiff, that they conduct tactile impressions. The increased sensitiveness of the para_lyzed leg, so common in these cases, but associated as it was here with diminished reflex action, cannot be ascribed (as it has been) to the withdrawal of an inhibi_tory influence on the gray matter of the lumbar enlargement. The contrast in this respect between the two legs in both sensibility and reflex action seems sig_nificant. In health reflex action in the legs is restrained by a higher centre, pos_sibly, in man, the optic thalamus. The lesion of the right half of the cord which divided the sensory path from the left leg interrupted also this inhibitory influ_ence. Hence it would seem that these two paths correspond. May not the opposite condition of the right leg be due to the intensification of the influence of the left optic thalamus ? This would account for both the diminished reflex action and the hyperæsthesia, since the thalamus is a sensory centre. Its over_action may be due to the accumulation of the obstructed nerve-force in its fellow acting upon it by means of the commissural fibres. The difference in irritability of nerve and muscle must be interpreted as an abnormal state of the paralyzed limbs, was probably due to an irritative influence exerted by the lesion on the gray matter of the lumbar enlargement, and thence on the motor nerves. It is very unusual for a depression of irritability in the muscles to coexist with an in_crease of irritability in the nerves. The persistence of sensibility in the branches of the cervical plexus shows how high up in the cord these fibres decussate.

Dr. ALTHAUS said the case just read had been so carefully described and argued as to offer but little room for critical remarks. The views of Professor Schiff as to the special function of the spinal cord seemed to be confirmed by these re_searches of Dr. Gowers. Was the sense of temperature affected ? Could the patient discriminate between heat and cold on the paralyzed side ? He thought these varieties of sensation of importance. Then, again, was there any priapism ? This condition was produced by lesions of the spinal cord ; and it was an interest_ing question to determine what portion of the cord was involved when priapism took place, and also the degree of the latter following spinal lesions. The electrical observations had evidently been made with great care, and he (the speaker) fully concurred in their interpretation.—Dr. BROADBENT agreed with Dr. Althaus that the extremely careful and accurate manner in which the case had been observed, and the wide knowledge displayed in its investigation, left very little room for discussion. Schiff's theory, that tactile impressions travel by the posterior columns, was confirmed by this case so far as it went; but, at the same time, there was always this difficulty about accepting that hypothesis—viz., that in locomotor ataxy there was no strict relation between the loss of tactile sensibility and the degree of ataxy. It was very common for a patient to be able only to interpret as a simple contact, and to locate the impression, a sensation which, in normal states, would give rise to pain; and, until this were explained, he must hesitate to accept the theory that pain, temperature, and tact have different channels. He thought himself that they travelled by the same channels, but were affected by different circumstances. Dr. Gowers's observation upon the increased reflex action on the side opposite to the lesion, and on which sensation was impaired, accorded with his own speculations upon the structural conditions of the spinal cord. He believed that the same cells receive impressions, whether these pass across and give rise to reflex actions, or whether they pass upwards and give rise to sensation. If either of the channels be divided, the other effect is intensified; so that here, where the sensory path was interrupted, the whole of the impression, instead of being shared between the two roots, reflex and sensory, is concentrated upon the former, and thus gives rise to intensified reflex activity. This explanation holds good for nearly all cases in which reflex actions are increased. Dr. Broadbent offered the following explanation as to the production of hyperæsthesia. In hysterical paralysis, where there was cutaneous anæsthesia with (as he mentioned at the last meeting) retention of the sense of tact, he believed the loss of sensation to be due to vaso-motor change, affecting the blood-supply to the cutaneous nerves. The converse might be true of Dr. Gowers's patient, where the vaso-motor paralysis might be a reason why an impression made on those nerves should give rise to hyperæsthesia. Dr. Broadbent concluded by again testifying to the great merit of the paper, which would remain as a most valuable contribution towards the elucidation of the physiology of the nervous system. Dr. BUZZARD inquired whether, when a certain amount of power returned, Dr. Gowers was able to test the muscular sense; and if so, did the observation confirm Brown-Séquard's view that the nerves of muscular sense pass into the motor instead of the sensory roots?—Dr. ALTHAUS asked why Dr. Gowers had reverted to the idea that the optic thalamus, and not the corpora quadrigemina, was the inhibitory centre of reflex actions.—Dr. GOWERS, in reply, said that the condition of the patient compelled him to limit his observations, and thus no attempt was made to test the muscular sense or the sense of temperature. There was no priapism. He thought there were reasons for believing that the optic thalamus has in man an inhibitory influence over reflex actions; amongst others, that hyperæsthesia and diminished reflex activity are frequently conjoined in cases of cerebral hemiplegia. He agreed with Dr. Broadbent as to the difficulties in the way of Schiff's theory—difficulties not only founded on the symptoms of locomotor ataxy, but on the structure of the posterior columns.

—

Lesions of Bone in Hereditary Syphilis.

In the *Gazette des Hôpitaux*, No. 111, we find some notes of an interesting lecture delivered by Prof. PARROT at the Hôpital des Enfants-Assistés, on "Bony Lesions by the aid of which we may diagnose Hereditary Syphilis."

"When young infants," he observes, "are emaciated, whether from the fact of the disease itself or from any other cause, there are certain parts of the bony system on which it is possible, with a little attention, to discern certain indications of syphilis. The first region towards which the physician should at once direct his attention when he suspects in a child the existence of syphilis, and in the absence of all other clinical manifestations, is the inner surface of the tibia. There, in fact, in place of that habitual depression which exists in all healthy subjects of good conformation, is found a true bony tumefaction, in convex relief. Sometimes the swelling exists in a general manner, occupying the whole of the inner surface of the tibia; while in other cases, which are, however, exceptional, in place of this general thickening of bone we meet with small projections or tuberosities, separated from each other by depressions. Another point which should also be carefully examined is the lower part of the humerus. But while the tibia, owing to its superficial position, easily lends itself to investigations, these are less easily conducted on the humerus. This, in fact, especially at its lower end, is covered by numerous muscles and tendons, and the skin is notably thicker at this part; so that all these conditions impede the perception in a very evident manner, especially when not sufficiently habituated to it, of bony lesions, the existence of which it is of importance to verify. However this may be, when, in a child the subject of syphilis, we lay hold of the lower part of the arm, grasping it from before backwards, we find a more or less considerable increase of thickness of the humerus. Nothing, indeed, is more easy than to overlook this lesion, especially when not familiarized with this examination, and not accustomed to these children; but in doubtful cases it is sufficient, in order to convince one's self that the bone is really affected, to first of all grasp the middle of the humerus, and then let the fingers slide down to its lower extremity. We then perceive, on comparing the thickness of the diaphysis of the bone with that of the epiphysis, a pretty notable difference in favour of the latter.

"Another very important sign which you will meet with in a considerable number of cases, but at a somewhat more advanced age, about the seventh, eighth, or twelfth month, is the following: When the cranial surface is inspected, not only do we perceive that it is very devoid of hair (a circumstance common enough in individuals quite free from syphilis), but we are struck by the presence of prominences disseminated around the bregma and anterior fontanelle: on the two frontals at their obtuse angles, and on the parietals at the angles which border on the bregma, four more or less notable projections are observable—one on each bone. These projections or bumps are rounded, as if small orange-peels had been applied to these parts of the cranium. It is easy, by passing the hand over the cranium, to verify the existence of these prominences when they are not apparent enough to be recognized by simple inspection. Finally, there is another characteristic which should be mentioned, but which is much rarer than those which precede. In certain infants, and especially those which are not older than from a fortnight to two or three months, we observe in the continuity of the limbs one, and sometimes two, fusiform tubercles or true nodosities. At these points the bones seem set in a body of an olivary form. These lesions are especially within the femur and at the upper part of the limb, and they are due to fractures in process of consolidation, consisting of a semi-osseous, semi-fibrous callus, as is shown at the autopsy.

"Such are the lesions of the bones that are sometimes met with in infants the subjects of syphilis, and which, when present, are certain indications of the disease. The knowledge of the fact is the more valuable that you may frequently observe them in individuals who exhibit neither on the skin or elsewhere any other sign that might enlighten you on the subject."—*Med. Times and Gaz.*, Nov. 10, 1877.

Syphilitic Dactylitis.

In the *Giornale Italiano della Malattie Veneree e della Pelle* for August, 1876 (abstract in *Annali Universali*, September, 1877), Dr. R. GALAZZI relates a case of syphilitic disease of the fingers, which is interesting, both on account of its rarity, and of the points of diagnosis between it and other diseases with which it may be confounded.

The patient was a woman, aged 32, who became infected with syphilis soon after her marriage, having a hard chancre and indurated inguinal glands. Two months later she became pregnant; her hair then fell off until she was completely bald, and she had pain in the throat, with difficulty of swallowing and speaking. She was delivered at full time of a male child, which died of syphilis at the end of eighteen days. She then had a diffuse papular eruption over the whole body, for which she took protiodide of mercury. Under this treatment she improved so far as to be apparently cured. After a short time she again became pregnant, and was delivered of a second boy, who lived fifteen months. Within a few days after birth it had a papular eruption, followed by *plâques*, the voice became hoarse, its general health was impaired, and it died with epileptiform convulsions.

Four years from the first infection, nodules of tubercular lupus appeared on one arm, and became ulcerated. The patient was seen by Professor Gamberini, who treated her with iodide of sodium and biniodide of mercury. As, however, the symptoms continued to increase, she became a patient of the hospital at Bologna, where she was admitted four times in the course of seven years.

A year after this the patient observed an enlargement of the middle finger of the right hand, which became painful. After some time these phenomena improved, but returned as before at the end of a year with the following characters. The middle finger began to enlarge, and assumed the form of a cone, the base of which was formed by the first phalanx increased to three times the normal size; the swelling diminished in the second phalanx, leaving the last quite free. The same symptoms appeared in the metacarpal bones of the thumb and little finger, so that the hand was deformed, presenting anomalous curves. The skin was distended and of a violet colour, and near it were spread abundant varicose vessels, of elastic consistence, without fluctuation; the pain was not increased by pressure. The movements of the part were impeded. Professor Gamberini diagnosed syphilitic dactylitis, and prescribed iodide of sodium in increasing doses, with fixed doses of biniodide of mercury. Under this treatment, at the end of a fortnight, the feeling of tension diminished, the glistening aspect of the skin disappeared, the symptoms diminished, and at last entirely disappeared, and the patient left the hospital completely cured. In this case, Dr. Galazzi shows that the dactylitis appeared thirteen years after the first infection, and this is a point of much importance in the diagnosis between syphilitic dactylitis and spina ventosa. The scrofulous form of the disease always runs a chronic course, and appears in children; while syphilitic dactylitis is peculiar to adults, follows other secondary symptoms, and is not always confined to the bones, but may affect other tissues.— *London Med. Record*, Nov. 15, 1877.

Subperiosteal Amputation.

Dr. R. SCHNEIDER points out (*Berliner Klinische Wochenschrift*, No. 38, 1877) that one of the remote results usually met with in the stump after amputation, performed without any attempt being made to preserve flaps of periosteum, is attenuation of the end of the bone, the conical or pointed apex of which projects closely under, or, in some cases, through the surface of the tense and thin skin. During the healing processes, after amputation, the end of the bone becomes thickened through localized periostitis, but the inflammatory deposit is subsequently absorbed. In consequence of diminished activity of the stump, atrophy of the remaining portion of the bone takes place, and the cortical layer becomes much reduced in thickness. In course of time, as the muscular constituents of the flaps waste, the extremity of the atrophied stump is covered merely by the skin or scar-tissue. According to Dieffenbach, the object to be attained in amputation, in addition to rapid and complete healing, is the formation of an efficient covering for the end of the bone. As the portions of muscle left in the flaps are usually absorbed, surgeons have of late years usually followed the practice of forming flaps of skin only, the stump, in most instances, being formed of one large flap from the anterior surface of the limb, and of a very small flap from the posterior surface. This method has one serious disadvantage. In case of any inflammation of the stump coming on during the healing processes, the skin of the flaps will retract to a considerable extent, and the end of the bone, after having produced ulceration through pressure, will protrude from the extremity of the stump and become necrosed. With the object of guarding against this result, Von Langenbeck proposed that the divided surface of the bone should be covered by a long flap of periosteum, formed in the course of the amputation. Several advantages have been claimed for this proceeding. In consequence, it is stated, of adhesion of the periosteum to the extremity of the remaining portion of the bone, necrosis may be prevented, and the risks of osteo-myelitis much diminished. The skin, it is assumed, is less likely to slough where a soft layer of periosteum is interposed between the flap and the sharp edges of the divided bone. Dr. Schneider holds that Von Langenbeck's proceeding does not always lead to such good results; and that, in most cases, the long and single flap of periosteum sloughs. For some years past he has, in most of his amputations, fixed over the end of the bone two short flaps of periosteum, each flap being carefully retained in connection with the superjacent muscular and other soft parts. The vascular supply is thus more likely to be kept up, the periosteum does not so readily contract, and leave exposed the end of the bone, and there is much less risk of necrosis. Should retraction of the soft parts take place, the edges of the bone at the end of the stump, being covered by muscle as well as by periosteum, would not be so liable to perforate the skin flaps. Finally, there would not be any direct adhesion of the skin to the extremity of the bone. Similar proceedings, though with certain modifications as to the size and number of the flaps, have been practised by Neudörfer, Billroth, and other German surgeons. Dr. Schneider, who has had considerable experience of this modification of subperiosteal amputation, gives a favourable report of it, and lays down minute instructions for its application to amputation in the different segments of the limbs.—*London Med. Record*, Nov. 15, 1876.

The Indications for Drainage of the Knee-joint.

Dr. J. SCRIBA, Assistant in the Surgical Clinic at Freiburg (Baden), recommends drainage of the knee-joint, instead of excision, in the following cases: 1. In acute serous inflammation, in the rare event of there being abnormal pain of sufficient severity to affect the patient's general health. 2. In acute purulent inflammation of the joint, as soon as there is distinct fluctuation; in the rare cases of osteomyelitis involving one or both epiphyses; in the purulent inflammation which may complicate pyæmia, pneumonia, acute infectious diseases, and phlegmonous erysipelas of the lower extremities. 3. In chronic serous inflammation of the joint. 4. In fungous inflammation—(a) where the fluid secretion in the joint exceeds the fungous granulation in amount, and where the cartilage is still intact; (b) where there is excess of fungous granulation, but where caries is still absent. The presence of caries is a contra-indication for drainage, and an indication for excision. Scriba lays down the following maxim in opposition to those British surgeons who counsel very early excision: "The earlier a chronic fungous inflammation of the joint comes under treatment, the better hope is there of giving the patient a useful, movable knee-joint by means of drainage." It should be stated that Scriba only speaks of drainage applied to a joint *which is opened the moment the tube is inserted*, and not to one in which there is a previous wound, either surgical or accidental, of some standing. The operation, as performed by Scriba, is briefly as follows: An incision, two or three centimetres long, is made on either side of the patella down to the joint, and a thick drainage-tube inserted. If the bursa under the extensor muscles communicates with the joint, as is the rule, no further incision is needed. In the rare case in which it is isolated, an incision is made down through the quadriceps femoris, and a short tube inserted. The operation must be carried out *with the strictest antiseptic precautions.* Before the drainage-tube is introduced, the joint is swabbed with a soft sponge; in acute cases using a 5 per cent. solution of carbolic acid; in chronic cases, or where there is fetidity, a 12 per cent. solution of zinc chloride. The tube is then put in, and the joint washed out through it with carbolic acid ($2\frac{1}{2}$ to 5 per cent.) until the solution returns quite clear. During the injection the joint must be gently kneaded with the hand. In acute inflammation the tube must be removed as soon as possible. The greater part may be taken out after the third or fourth dressing, if the wound is perfectly sweet, and the remainder on the tenth to fourteenth day. If the secretion does not quickly diminish, the joint must be washed out again with carbolic acid, and the drainage somewhat prolonged; but the whole tube must never be left in after the tenth to twelfth day, for fear of irritating the cartilage on which it lies. In chronic cases, or where fungosity is present, the tube must be allowed to lie across the cavity of the joint for twenty to thirty days, in order to stimulate the lining membrane.— *Med. Times and Gaz.*, Sept. 15, 1877.

Midwifery and Gynæcology.

Employment of Anæsthetics in Labour.

M. PIACHAUD read a paper before the International Medical Congress of Geneva (*Gaz. Médicale*, Oct. 20, 1877), in which he advanced the following conclusions:

1. The employment of anæsthetics is, as a general rule, advisable in natural labour.

2. The principal substances which have been used for this purpose up to the present time are ether, chloroform, amylene, laudanum, morphia hypodermically, chloral by the mouth and by injection.

3. Of these chloroform seems to be preferable.

4. It should be administered according to the method of Show, that is, in small doses at the beginning of each pain, its administration being suspended during the intervals.

5. It should never be pushed to complete insensibility, but the patient should be held in a state of semi-anæsthesia, so as to produce a diminution of the suffering.

6. The general rule is never to administer chloroform except during the period of expulsion; but in certain cases of nervousness and extreme agitation it is advantageous not to wait for the complete dilatation of the os.

7. Experience has shown that anæsthetics do not arrest the contractions of the

uterus or abdominal muscles, but that they weaken the natural resistance of the perineal muscles.

8. The use of anæsthetics has no unpleasant effect on the mind of mother or upon the child.

9. In lessening the suffering, anæsthetics render a great service to those women who dread the pain; they diminish the chances of the nervous crises which are caused during labor by the excess of suffering; they make the recovery more rapid.

10. They are especially useful to calm the great agitation and cerebral excitement which labour often produces in very nervous women.

11. Their employment is indicated in natural cases until the pains are suspended or retarded by the suffering caused by maladies occurring previous to or during labour, and in those cases where irregular and partial contractions occasion internal and sometimes continuous pain, without causing progress of the labour.

12. In a natural labour, chloroform should never be used without the consent of the woman and her family.—*Med. Record*, Dec. 8, 1877.

Spontaneous Delivery in Contracted Pelvis.

In the *Aerztliches Intelligenz-Blatt* for September 4, 1877, Dr. WIERRER describes a case of labour in a primipara aged 30, who was the subject of a deformed pelvis, and whose labour terminated naturally. The patient was crooked-legged, with lateral curvature of the spine, and had a pelvis in which the conjugate diameter measured 9.9 centimetres (3.9 inches). The distance between the cristæ iliorum measured 27.4 centimetres (10.78 inches); that between the anterior superior spinous processes, 25.1 centimetres (9.88 inches). The pelvis was small, and appeared less roomy in the right half than the left. The patient had not been able to walk until she was three years old. The head presented in the second position: the pains began at two in the afternoon, and by seven in the evening the os was fully dilated. The membranes were ruptured, and the succeeding pains drove the head into the brim, so that the right ear of the fœtus could be plainly felt. The head descended to the floor of the pelvis twenty minutes after engaging at the brim. A few more pains accomplished the rotation of the occiput forwards, and the head appeared at the vulva. The lying-in and recovery were normal.—*London Med. Record*, Nov. 15, 1877.

Case of Puerperal Septicæmia, with Hyperpyrexia, treated by the continuous Application of Cold.

Dr. W. S. PLAYFAIR, Prof. of Obstetric Medicine in King's College, London, records (*British Med. Journ.*, Nov. 17, 1877) the following interesting case:—

On the 5th of August, at 5 P. M., I was summoned to attend Mrs. —, a young and healthy primipara. I found the head presenting, the pains frequent but slight, and the os undilated. The labour progressed perfectly naturally, the first stage being somewhat tedious and painful. At 7 A. M. on the morning of August 6th, the os had remained without further dilatation since 1 A. M., although the pains were frequent and of good character. The os was at this time of the size of a florin, the membranes not bulging at all through it. I suspected that the labour might be protracted by an excess of liquor amnii, and, therefore, ruptured the membranes with the best effect. The os now rapidly dilated, the head descended into the pelvis, and the child was born at 10 A. M.

I may observe, in passing, that the axiom of our text-books as to the paramount importance of keeping the membranes unruptured until the os is fully dilated, often leads to unnecessary delay. No doubt, some practical experience is necessary to decide upon the propriety of evacuating the liquor amnii; but, when the pains do not steadily increase, when the membranes do not bulge through the os with each pain, and when the os is soft and apparently readily dilatable, the puncture of the membranes often saves your patient many weary hours of suffering.

The uterus now contracted strongly, but one drachm of the fluid extract of ergot was administered after the placenta had been expressed, as has been my custom for several years, with the view of keeping up continuous contraction.

At 6 P. M. the same day, when I again visited the patient, I found that there had been a distinct rigor, her pulse being 120, and the temperature 102 deg. Nothing was done that evening, as, this having occurred so soon after labour, I was in hopes it might have been due to some transient cause. Next morning, I found that the patient had had another rigor, the pulse being 130, and the temperature 103 deg. There was no tenderness over the abdomen, and the lochia were natural. I now washed out the uterine cavity freely with Condy's fluid and water, with the view of disinfecting any decomposing coagulum that might be lying within it and setting up septic mischief, and prescribed twenty grains of quinine to be taken immediately, and to be repeated at 8 P. M.; and a minim of tincture of aconite was given every half hour, under careful supervision, with the view of lessening the rapidity of the heart's action. Next morning, the pulse was 120, and the temperature 101.2 deg.; but the quinine had produced so much discomfort and throbbing in the head that I was obliged to discontinue its use.

The case now rapidly grew worse. Next morning, the fourth after her confinement, the temperature was 104 deg.; and in the evening 105.4 deg.; the pulse 130, small, thready, and feeble. There was no tenderness over the abdomen, but flatulent distension was commencing. There were occasional well-marked rigors; the complexion was of a dusky-yellow tinge, with distinct patches of a livid purple eruption coming out over the forehead and cheeks, disappearing, and coming out again (a phenomenon that continued, more or less, during the whole illness); the tongue was coated, but moist; in fact, the case had now assumed a most formidable character, and was a well-marked example of what I believe to be one of the worse types of puerperal fever, that in which there are no distinct local phenomena.

The treatment now adopted was the administration of abundant fluid nourishment in the form of milk and beef-tea; fifteen grains of salicylic acid every third hour, in the hope of lowering the temperature; six ounces of brandy in the twenty-four hours; and the washing out of the uterine cavity twice daily with antiseptic lotions. In the hope of lessening the persistent high temperature, Dr. Knowsley Thornton's ice-cap, which has been found so useful for this purpose after ovariotomy, was now applied. This gave great relief to the throbbing headache, which caused much suffering; but it produced no further diminution of the temperature than from 105.4 deg. to 104 deg. Next morning, August 10th, things were in no way improved. The temperature was 105 deg.; pulse 140; and the abdomen tympanitic. As the salicylic acid had not lessened the temperature, and as the pulse was very thready and feeble, it was discontinued.

Next day, August 11th, the patient was still worse. The temperature was 105.2 deg.; pulse 140. The intelligence was good, and she was able to take nourishment well; but, with the temperature at so high a mark, it was obvious that the chances of recovery were small indeed; and I now determined to try the effect of cold applied externally, with the view of lessening the excessive fever, on which the antipyretic remedies already tried had had no appreciable effect. Accordingly, at 4 P. M., the patient was enveloped from head to foot in a large sheet wrung out of iced water; this being rapidly changed every minute or so for another. The pack was applied for half an hour. The patient expressed herself as feeling no discomfort from it, but rather the reverse. The effect on the temperature, however, was slight, as it only fell from 105.2 deg. to 104 deg. At 11 P. M. the pack was again applied for half an hour; and, at the end of that time, the temperature had fallen to 103.2 deg. Next morning, August 12th, the temperature was 104 deg.; pulse 130. Her general condition was as before. At this time I had the advantage of meeting my friend Dr. Wilson Fox in consultation. It is well known that that gentleman is one of the first who, in this country, drew the attention of the profession to the systematic use of cold applications in the treatment of hyperpyrexia, and I thankfully acknowledge the great assistance I derived from his experience in the management of this anxious case. With his concurrence, it was determined to use the cold applications continuously, but in a modified form, since the complete envelopment of the body in iced sheets was very difficult to manage, and had not the marked effect of reducing the temperature which was expected. Accordingly, the patient lying on her back, three towels soaked in iced water were placed on the front of the body, one over the shoulders and chest, one over the abdomen, and one over the thighs. These could be frequently changed, and were managed by one nurse, while it had taken three people to apply the sheets that had been formerly used.

It is not easy by description to convey to you any accurate idea of the effects on the temperature which, from this time and through the remainder of the illness was taken in the mouth every quarter of an hour, except when the patient was asleep. During the whole of the day the modified pack was kept constantly applied, with manifest comfort to the patient; the temperature varying from 103 deg. to 104 deg. At 5 P. M. it registered 103 deg., after which it gradually fell, until at midnight it was 101.4 deg., when the pack was removed. The patient now had a little sleep, but the temperature rapidly rose, until at 3 A. M. it was again at 103 deg., when the pack was reapplied. Next day, August 13th, the patient was much the same. The temperature ranged from 102 deg. to 103 deg. The pulse was 130; the general condition unaltered. The ice-cloths were kept on nearly continuously night and day, the patient being obviously more comfortable when they were applied; and, when they were removed, the temperature at once showed a decided tendency to rise. The patient now and again slept for half an hour or so, took her food well, and had no diarrhœa; the abdomen was still tympanitic. The brandy was increased to ten ounces *per diem*; twenty minims of the tincture of perchloride of iron were given every four hours; and nourishment of some sort, milk, beef-tea, or yolk of egg every hour.

I cannot give you a detailed account of the progress of the case from this time; but it will suffice to say that it was obvious that there was a very marked tendency to hyperpyrexia, which was only kept within moderate bounds by a constant attention to the iced applications. If for half an hour or more, as occasionally happened when the patient was asleep, their use were intermitted, or when an endeavour was made to do without them, the temperature very shortly ran up to 104 deg., or even, on one or two occasions, to 105 deg.; but, by the assiduous use of the cold towels, it was again speedily reduced to 102 deg., or even less, having occasionally fallen as low as 101.4 deg., but for a short time only. By the means we had hitherto used, the cold was applied to the front of the body only. We now adopted a method of applying it to the back, with no moving of the patient, and with little fatigue to the nurses. I had two India-rubber tubes fixed to the opposite corners of a water-bed, on which the patient was laid without any clothing, and covered with the iced towels. From the lower of these tubes every hour or so several gallons of water were allowed to flow out, while an equivalent quantity of iced water was pumped in at the opposite end by a large garden-pump.

This answered admirably, and gave little trouble. The cold applications were begun, as I have told you, on the 9th of August, and they were continued night and day, without any intermission, except for a short time now and again, when a rapid increase of temperature immediately necessitated their re-application until August 18th, that is eleven days. During the whole of this time the patient's condition was critical in the extreme. The temperature was taken in the mouth every quarter of an hour, except during the intervals of sleep; and even under the constant refrigeration it never fell below 101 deg., except for three hours on the morning of the 16th, when it was 99.5 deg., whilst at times it was 105 deg. The pulse all this time was excessively small and feeble, ranging from 130 to 150 per minute. The other symptoms were, on the whole, good. The tongue was moist; the abdomen only moderately tympanitic: there was slight diarrhœa for three or four days, but never in excess; the intellect was clear; the urine possessed a slight cloud of albumen; there was no local complication. Until August 15th, the tenth day of the illness, the temperature-chart showed a nearly uniform line with occasional short rises. On that day, however, and on each subsequent day, there was a distinct remission in the morning, when the temperature reached its lowest point, and the pulse improved; the temperature beginning to rise again at 1 P. M., reaching 104 deg. or 105 deg. by 3 P. M., and the pulse becoming extremely rapid and feeble. On the afternoon of August 16th, 17th, and 18th, the patient was almost moribund; and I left her on each successive visit with little hope of finding her alive on my return. Indeed, on the 18th, I thought she could not possibly have lived many minutes. The pulse at the wrist could not be made out at all; and, on auscultation, only a feeble flutter, quite impossible to count, could be heard over the heart. At those times the amount of stimulant was largely increased; as much as twenty-eight ounces of brandy having been given during the twenty-four hours on those three days. All this time the cold applications were continued; and, although I am quite convinced that they kept the temperature within limits which were compatible with existence, and so gave the disease a chance of wearing itself out, they did not seem, either to Dr. Fox or myself, to do more than this, and had in no sense a curative effect.

You will remember that large doses of quinine and also of salicylic acid had been given, with no distinct antipyretic effect, and had been discontinued. Being struck with the marked remittent type the fever had now assumed, I determined to try the effect of a remedy of high repute in India in the worst class of malarious remittent fevers, and the almost marvellous effects of which in such cases I had myself witnessed many years ago when in India. This is the so-called Warburg's tincture, a drug which, as being a patent medicine, was for long in disfavour, but the remarkable properties of which had been testified to by many high authorities, among whom I may mention Dr. Maclean, of Netley, and Dr. Broadbent, and which Sir Alexander Armstrong, the Director-General of the Medical Department of the Navy, informs me is now supplied to all Her Majesty's ships in the tropics, because it is found to be of the utmost value in cases in which quinine has little or no effect. Recently the composition of the tincture has been made public by Dr. Maclean. Its basis is quinine, in combination with a large number of vegetable aromatics and bitters, and the recipe reads like a farrago of nonsense. Probably there is some ingredient in it which intensifies the action of the quinine. Be this as it may, the testimony in favour of the efficacy of the drug as an antipyretic is very strong, and I determined to try its influence on my patient, since her condition was so bad that nothing could make it worse, and all other remedies had proved useless. The effect was very much more marked than I had ventured to hope. A full dose of the tincture was given at 3.30 P. M. on August

19th, the pulse being then 140; temperature 104 deg.; and was repeated at 6 P. M. A very profuse perspiration shortly broke out, until the patient was literally bathed in sweat (this being the almost invariable effect of the remedy), and she described herself as feeling immensely relieved. The cold applications were now removed, and the patient fell into a quiet sleep. At 9.30 P. M. the pulse was 110, but much fuller and stronger than it had been for many days. Temperature 102 deg. A single drachm of the tincture was given at 3 A. M., and ordered to be repeated every six hours. Next morning, at 8.30 A. M., I found her condition totally altered. The temperature was 99 deg.; pulse 96, full and strong; and from this moment the patient may be said to have been convalescent. The temperature never rose again, except between 3 and 7 P. M. on the afternoon of the 20th, when it suddenly ran up to 102 deg. A dose of the tincture, which had been discontinued, was now given, and repeated at 2 A. M.; and next morning the temperature was normal, and remained so.

The history of this terrible illness is now practically over. For many weeks the patient remained very weak and feeble, and there came on some indefinite swelling and pain about the joints; the skin of her hands, and here and there in other parts of the body, peeled, a fact on the significance of which I shall presently comment; but eventually she completely regained her usual health.

Let me now, as briefly as possible, point out to you some of the lessons we may gather from this history, already, I fear, too tedious and long, of the most remarkable recovery that it has ever been my fortune to witness.

1. Can we say anything as to the *cause* of the illness? The first question the medical man is bound to ask himself, in the face of such a case, is: whether it is possible that the septic matter can have been conveyed to the patient? Unhappily, the evidence of the possibility of this is too strong to render it a matter of doubt that this may happen; and all who see much midwifery practice could, were they honestly to review their experience, record such cases. Fortunately, in this instance, nothing of the kind was in the least likely; since no one in contact with the patient had, so far as could be ascertained, recently been near a case from which the contagium could have been derived. There is, of course, the possibility that it might have been autogenetic; but I do not think it probable, since the symptoms began too soon after delivery to admit of the supposition that it arose from decomposing matter in the genital tract. There remains the possibility of the patient having herself been exposed to the contagium of some zymotic disease, such as scarlet fever, before labour. Now, I cannot enter here, as I have done elsewhere, into a discussion of the *quæstio vexata* as to whether a disease, indistinguishable from puerperal fever, may be derived from the poison of zymotic disease, which shows none of the characteristic phenomena of the disease which originated it. I am aware that many high authorities totally disbelieve that this can be the case, and contend that zymotic diseases in the puerperal woman always run their usual course, and show their characteristic phenomena. That they often do so is quite beyond doubt. I have repeatedly seen lying-in women, who have been attacked with distinct and well-marked scarlet fever or measles, within a few days after labour, in whom the disease has run its usual course, and has not apparently been in any way intensified by the puerperal state. On the other hand, I am equally certain that I have seen many cases of puerperal fever showing no traces whatever of the ordinary symptoms of zymotic diseases, the origin of which was undoubtedly traceable to the poison of scarlet fever, erysipelas, or diphtheria. I am quite unable to suggest to you any satisfactory explanation of this curious fact; but I believe it to be proved to demonstration, and no one can, I think, impartially study the literature of the subject—as, for example, the interesting paper of Dr. Braxton Hicks, in the twelfth vol-

ume of the *Obstetrical Transactions*—without being compelled to admit it. It is to be hoped, as our knowledge increases, that some light may be thrown on the subject. In the meantime, I firmly believe that the denial of the facts, because we cannot explain them, can have no other effect than that of rendering the practitioner careless in his dealings with zymotic disease in relation to puerperal patients, and thus leading to the most disastrous results. Now, the channels through which such a poison as that of scarlet fever may come into contact with a patient are numberless, especially in large towns, where the first cab the patient may enter, or some casual contact in the streets, may convey the contagion. There was in this case a well-marked eruption, very analogous to that of scarlet fever; but such rashes are common in septicæmia, quite independently of the origin of the disease. The fact, however, that, subsequently to recovery, there was distinct desquamation about the fingers, and, to a less extent, in other parts of the body, make me think it likely that the scarlatinal poison was the origin of the illness.

2. As to the *treatment*. I believe that this may be summed up in the aphorism, that we have to use our utmost endeavours to keep the patient alive until the intensity of the disease has worn itself out; but, I fear, we must admit that we know of no reliable means of cutting short, or materially influencing, the progress of the septic disturbance, when once it has been fairly set in progress. Beyond any doubt, continuous elevation of temperature, such as existed in this case to so marked a degree, is one of the chief sources of danger, and much of our management of the case must lie in the direction of lessening pyrexia. In cases of moderate intensity, antipyretics—such as quinine in sufficiently large doses, of not less than twenty grains, salicylic acid, or the ice-cap—will probably be quite sufficient; and I certainly should not be disposed to recommend so troublesome and irksome a treatment as the external application of cold, unless there were marked hyperpyrexia. I cannot, however, doubt that in this case refrigeration saved the patient's life; for, without it, she certainly could not have tided over eleven days of fever with the temperature at 104 deg. and 105 deg., and tending to increase. My experience of this treatment is limited to two other cases. One was the wife of a medical man, whom I saw in consultation with Dr. Cleveland, of St. John's Wood. In this we did not think of using the cold until the temperature was 107 deg., and the case was almost hopeless, and then only in the modified form of the ice-cap, and unhappily without any good results. In the other, which I saw in consultation with Dr. Protheroe Smith and Dr. Simpson, of Highgate, we used the ice-pack night and morning for several days. Unfortunately, this patient was the subject of chronic albuminuria; and the case, which ended fatally, could hardly be considered a fair test of the remedy. My belief is, however, that where there are no well-marked local complications, and where the temperature is above 104 deg. or 105 deg., and tending to rise to a still higher level, the pack should certainly be tried; and in the modified form in which it was used here, it may be applied readily enough, while the lifting of a puerperal patient into a bath would be almost impossible.

You will have observed the marked beneficial results which followed the administration of Warburg's tincture. It would, of course, be absurd to draw too strong an inference from one case; but, at least, my experience of it would strongly incline me to try it again as an antipyretic of promising character.

By the careful feeding of your patient with milk, beef-tea, and eggs, administered at frequent intervals, you will materially husband her strength for the storm she has to pass through, and you cannot pay too much attention to this part of the management of this disease. With regard to stimulants, I am inclined to think that they are often given in such cases to an injudicious and needless extent.

As long as the pulse is fairly strong, and no indication of excessive prostration exists, I believe it is better to administer them in strict moderation. But the time may come, as it did in this instance, when the prostration is so great that the only chance of keeping the patient alive is in profuse stimulation. My advice with regard to stimulants would be not to order them indiscriminately, or in fixed quantities, but in strict accordance with the exigencies of the case, varying the amount from hour to hour, as the state of the patient may require.

One point of local treatment should never be omitted, especially in the early days of the illness, that is, the thorough washing out of the uterine cavity, night and morning, with antiseptic lotions, such as Condy's fluid and water, tincture of iodine and water, or a weak solution of carbolic acid. In many cases of autogenetic origin, in which decomposing matters exist *in utero*, this alone will suffice to remove the source of mischief, and cut short the progress of the disease. I must warn you, however, that such injections to be of value must be applied thoroughly, and into the uterine cavity itself; and it is quite useless to entrust them, as I have often seen done, to the nurse.

3. I can only briefly refer, in conclusion, to a subject which every conscientious practitioner must very anxiously consider, when he is so unfortunate as to have under his charge such a case, and that is: What are his duties to his other patients? The practical difficulty of giving up attendance on other midwifery cases is so great that one cannot be astonished at practitioners inclining to underestimate the weight of the evidence which shows the possibility of the contagion being conveyed from patient to patient. Indeed, I believe that, in these days of antiseptics, the thorough disinfection of the hands can be so efficiently carried out that danger from this source can be reduced to a minimum. The principal risk is in refusing to admit the danger, and neglecting the necessary precautions; and it is the man who wilfully shuts his eyes to the facts, and does not employ the means of disinfection at our disposal, who is most likely to be the unhappy medium of carrying infection. If, then, we see such a patient once in a way, carefully wash our hands in some antiseptic lotion, and avoid touching her with the right hand or keep on a glove while in her room, there is no reason why we should not continue our obstetric practice, and to insist upon more would be practically to debar us from following our profession at all. But, if we are in constant and frequent attendance on such a case as that we have been considering, visiting our patient four or five times every day, and, above all, if we are compelled to use intra-uterine injections, I believe it to be quite impossible to attend other cases without such a degree of risk that no conscientious man can venture to subject his patients to it; and, be the sacrifice what it may, it will be our bounden duty to avoid, for the time, the actual attendance on lying-in women.

Duration of Pregnancy.

Dr. A. STADFELDT, of Copenhagen (*Nordisk Med. Archiv*), has determined in thirty-four cases, where the date of coition was positively known, the duration of pregnancy. He has added to these thirty-four cases, thirty-one similar ones from N. Ranvin. The mean duration in these sixty-five cases was 271.8 days, the extremes being 250 and 293 days. The duration of pregnancy in the physiological sense should, according to the author, be calculated from after the epoch of the first menstrual suppression, modern physiologists holding that the fecundated ovum is derived from this ovulation period. Pregnancy would then be much shorter than is generally supposed. In twenty-four cases, where he believed he could determine the first epoch of menstrual suppression, the mean term was 254 days, the extremes being 240 and 273 days.—*Amer. Practitioner*, Dec., 1877.

CONTENTS.

Published Monthly, price $2.50 per annum, free of postage.
Also, furnished together with the AMERICAN JOURNAL OF THE MEDICAL
SCIENCES *and the* MEDICAL NEWS AND LIBRARY *for* SIX DOLLARS *per
annum in advance, the whole free of postage.*

HENRY C. LEA, Philadelphia.

THE MONTHLY ABSTRACT

OF

MEDICAL SCIENCE.

Vol. V. No. 2·   **For List of Contents see last page.**   February, 1878.

Anatomy and Physiology.

The Structure of Tactile Corpuscles.

M. RANVIER has lately presented to the Académie de Médecine a note upon the termination of the nerves in tactile corpuscles. It has hitherto been believed that the nerves enter the terminal cells and present swellings at their entrance, and that touch acts directly on these cells. M. Ranvier believes that this termination is not real. By staining the ultimate nervous ramifications black by means of certain salts of gold, he has observed the nerve filaments to end between two cells, and not to penetrate the cells. There is no continuity between the cells and the nerves. The office of the cells is simply that of protection of the nerves or of intensification of the tactile vibrations. This is a subject for further study. The observations have been made on the tactile corpuscles of the duck's beak.— *Lancet,* Dec. 29, 1877.

On a Case of Inversion of the Heart.

In the *Giornale Veneto di Scienze Mediche* for July, Dr. LUIGI PAGANUZZI publishes a case in which the position of the heart was reversed. The anomaly was found in the body of an individual who had died of cancer of the œsophagus. The heart was of normal form, but the right compartment occupied the position of the left. The aorta had its origin from the right ventricle, the pulmonary artery from the left; the four pulmonary veins opened into the right auricle, and the two venæ cavæ into the left. The right (aortic) ventricle was about twelve millimetres (nearly half an inch) in thickness, the left was only half as thick. The mitral valve was on the right, the tricuspid on the left; in fine, all the special arrangements of the muscular papillæ, of the auriculo-ventricular orifices, of the openings of the veins into the auricles, and of the valves, were completely reversed. Dr. Paganuzzi remarks that the inversion could not have been more complete. The individual was an adult, and had never suffered from any inconvenience which could lead to a suspicion of the malformation.—*London Med. Record,* Dec. 15, 1877.

Materia Medica and Therapeutics.

On the Absorption of Carbolic Acid and its Recognition in Organic Liquids.

Dr. IGNAZIO TORTORA has published in *Il Morgagni* for January (abstract in *Annali Universali di Medicina,* August) an account of some observations made by him under the direction of Professor Cantani, regarding the absorption and elimination of carbolic acid.

Vol. V.—4

The method which he adopted was the following. Urine containing carbolic acid was heated and treated with nitric acid; the fluid was then slowly evaporated to dryness; the yellow residue was dissolved in rectified alcohol, which took up the carbolic acid, leaving the mineral constituents of the urine. The solution was then filtered, the carbolic acid passing through and giving a yellow colour to the filtrate. The solution, when treated with carbonate of potash, gave a dark red precipitate of picrate (carbolate) of potash.

Operating in this way, and using similar quantities of urine, alcohol, and nitric acid respectively, he always found carbolic acid in the urine after its administration.

He gives the details of the observations in the case of a patient to whom, at 9.30 A. M., he began to administer, every fifteen minutes, 30 grammes (about an ounce) of the following mixture: crystallized carbolic acid, 3 grammes; rectified alcohol, 10 grammes; water, 300 grammes; orange syrup, 30 grammes. After each dose the mouth was washed out with water, which was swallowed. The following results were obtained by examination of the urine several times during the day.

1. At 11.30 A. M. some rather pale urine was found; quantity, 340 cubic centimetres. Of this, 20 cubic centimetres were treated with ten drops of pure nitric acid, evaporated slowly to dryness, and the residue dissolved in 10 cubic centimetres of rectified alcohol and filtered. The resulting liquid had a red colour.

2. At 1 P. M. 300 cubic centimetres of greenish-brown urine were passed, of which 20 cubic centimetres were treated in the manner described above. In this urine, when scarcely warm, as indeed is the case whenever a certain quantity of carbolic acid is present, a yellow ring was formed; this may be regarded as a sure sign of the presence of carbolic acid. The filtered liquid had a more distinct red colour.

3. At 4.30 P. M. the quantity of urine was 100 cubic centimetres, colour greenish-brown. The yellow ring was present; and, after treatment, as before, the solution was still more coloured.

4. At 6.45 P. M. 110 cubic centimetres, of the same colour as before, were passed. The alcoholic solution had a strong red colour.

5. At 3.30 A. M., on the next day, the quantity of urine was 300 cubic centimetres, and the colour normal. The circle formed in the capsule was of a faint yellow colour. The alcoholic solution was less coloured, almost resembling that of No. 2.

6. At 5.30 A. M. 90 cubic centimetres of pale yellow urine were passed, of which 20 cubic centimetres were treated as in the other experiments. No yellow ring was formed. The alcoholic solution was very pale, and hence was believed to contain only traces of carbolic acid.

7. No indication of the presence of carbolic acid could be detected in the urine passed at 8 A. M.

At 12.45 (45 minutes after the last dose had been taken) the patient began to discharge saliva, which was collected up to 11 P. M., and treated in the same manner as the urine. It yielded an intensely red solution, and picrate of potash was formed on adding carbonate.

In order to determine whether carbolic acid was absorbed in other ways than when given internally, Tortora applied a large blister to the arm, and dressed the vesicated surface with carbolized water. The saliva collected for twenty-four hours, and the urine, when treated in the way above described, gave indications of the presence of carbolic acid.

From his experiments the author believes that he may conclude that carbolic acid is absorbed from the alimentary mucous membrane, or from the skin deprived of epidermis, or from wounds; and that, at least in great part, it is eliminated unchanged in the natural excretions, the elimination taking place rather rapidly, and being completed within ten or twelve hours. For internal use, the dose may be as high as 30 grains, but care must be taken that it is quite pure, and it should be given in an abundance of water.—*London Med. Record,* Nov. 15, 1877.

On the Elimination of Mercury.

Dr. E. W. HAMBURGER, of Franzensbad, sums up a paper in the *Prager Medicin. Wochenschrift,* 1877, with the following conclusions. 1. Mercury can be distinctly found in the urine of patients who have been treated with mercurial suppositories for some time. In one case in which the treatment had been commenced four days previously, mercury was not found in the urine. Mercury is always present in the urine of patients who have been treated by inunction.

2. In patients treated by suppositories, mercury was always found in the milk as well as the urine. In cases of inunction, although mercury was present in the urine, none could be found in the milk; and, when mercurial inunction was substituted for suppositories, the mercury disappeared from the milk, although it continued to be present in the urine.

3. The feces of a patient, who was treated by inunction, contained a large amount of mercury. Dr. Hamburger concludes hence that the elimination of mercury takes place chiefly by the bile.

The chemical process used consisted in the removal of organic matters, the application of electrolysis, and the formation of iodide of mercury, the crystals of which were readily recognizable under the microscope.—*London Med. Record,* Dec. 15, 1877.

Subcutaneous Injections of Chloroform.

In a note addressed to the Société de Thérapeutique (*Gaz. des Hôp.,* Dec. 14), M. E. BESNIER details the results of numerous trials which he has made at the St. Louis, of the hypodermic injection of chloroform, first practised by Dr. Roberts Bartholow in 1874. There has been, he observed, but little published upon the subject, probably because these injections have been used only for a limited purpose (the treatment of neuralgia), instead of employing them for the relief of every kind of pain. Their great advantage, he considers, consists in the fact that they may be employed in this manner, and thus supersede morphia with its consequent inconveniences. No ill effect whatever, local or general, follows these injections, and yet they are efficacious. But the mode in which they are made is of importance, for, inefficiently performed (which is very commonly the case), they may give rise to local phlegmasia. They should always be practised in two stages, the needle being first separated and introduced alone, so that if it happen to penetrate a vein this may be made known by the issue of a droplet of blood. When the syringe has been reapplied, in order to prevent local irritation being caused, the injection should be propelled *into* the hypodermis (*i. e.,* the subcutaneous cellulo-adipose layer, which varies in thickness in different regions and individuals), which not only possesses a special tolerance and insensibility, but a very active absorbent power. If the point of the needle be very fine and sharp, it may be passed through the skin into this tissue without appreciable pain, which, however will be felt if it be carried too far, so as to reach the muscles, etc. The needle is manœuvred with the greatest facility as soon as it has passed the dermis, its point being easily guided to any part of the hypoderm. This done, the syringe may be adapted, and the injection made with the greatest security.—*Med. Times and Gaz.,* Dec. 22, 1877.

The Effect of Alkalies.

What is the effect of large doses of alkalies on the economy ? Can they produce a cachectic state ? Mialhe, of Paris, has lately given a negative answer to the question, and concluded his observations on the subject with some instructive remarks on the influence of alkalies. He believes that the effect of bicarbonate of soda is to modify the intimate composition of albuminous bodies with which the alkali enters into combination, and, in consequence, to increase the activity of the phenomena of oxidation, or of vital action, such as endosmosis, and exosmosis, and to modify the excretions. To attain this result the quantity of alkali needed in different cases varies. The proportion of soda in the system, whether as carbonate or as albuminate, is not always the same. A man who lives in a town, and eats much nitrogenous food, needs a larger dose of alkali, in order to bring the system into the same condition, than the peasant who eats chiefly bread and vegetables. A loss of acid probably occurs during free perspiration, and hence the condition of the skin should be taken into consideration, for a person who perspires much needs less akali than one who does not. The greater the amount of exercise the smaller is the amount of soda needed. Lastly, the higher the temperature the less alkali can be borne, perhaps because the temperature itself has an influence similar to that of forced exercise, and partly on account of its action on the nervous system. It is well to commence the treatment with the full quantity, which will be needed in divided doses. N. Gubler subsequently announced his concurrence with N. Mialhe in the need for and utility of large doses of alkali, but differed as to the possibility of doing harm by extreme doses. It must not, he urged, be supposed that because a substance is a necessary constituent of the body it cannot be prejudicial if given in large quantities. Oxygen, for instance, introduced into the lungs in too large quantities is a poison, and, although in some cases a quarter of a pound of bicarbonate of soda may be taken daily without inconvenience, it is certain that a distinct alkaline cachexia is sometimes to be observed, and is especially likely to occur where there is renal disease.—*Lancet*, Dec. 22, 1877.

Employment of Pilocarpin in Childhood.

Prof. DEMME, of Bern, states (*Petersburg Med. Woch.*, Nov. 17) that he has employed the muriate of pilocarpin by the subcutaneous method, using a 2 per cent. solution in 33 children from the ages of nine months to twelve years. Of these, 18 suffered from desquamative nephritis and dropsy consequent on scarlatina, 3 from diphtheria without scarlatina, but with consecutive parenchymatous nephritis and a high degree of dropsy. Of the other 12 cases, 2 had dropsical effusion from heart disease, and 3 rheumatism affecting several joints. As a general rule, only one injection per diem was employed, and in children between the ninth month and the second year the dose of pilocarpin employed was gramme 0.005 ; between the second and sixth years from 0.0072 to 0.01 ; and from the seventh to the twelfth years 0.01 to 0.025. The general conclusions drawn from these cases are, that pilocarpin exhibits its sialogogic and diaphoretic properties in a very marked manner in childhood, and that it is very well borne at the tenderest age in the above doses, its sialogogic effect being more prominent in the younger, and its diaphoretic effect in the older children ; that any unfavourable after-effects, even in the youngest children, were quite exceptional, and were preventable by administering minute doses of brandy prior to the injection ; and that no influence on the action of the heart was perceptible. The cases best adapted for its employment are desquamative parenchymatous nephritis with dropsy, following scarlatina, diphtheria, etc. A beneficial diuresis in most of the cases ensues, the quantity of albumen which the urine contains never being increased, but rather diminished.—*Med. Times and Gaz.*, Dec. 8, 1877.

Continuous Baths.

To the *Wiener Med. Wochenschrift* (September 8 to 29), Privat Docent Dr. HANS HEBRA contributes a paper reporting the results of the employment of continuous baths first proposed by his father, Prof. Hebra, fifteen years since. An old prejudice against prolonged continuance in a bath, and its employment just after meal times or during menstruation, had to be overcome. In order, too, that a man should remain for days, weeks, or months in a warm bath, the ordinary bath will not suffice, and a special apparatus has to be devised. Almost all baths are too short to admit of the patient's lying down, and they are too deep, so that the vapour of the water, which gets commingled with the air, interferes with respiration. The new apparatus (which was exhibited in London in 1862) allows of the patient's lying comfortably in the horizontal position, and so high as to be but little inconvenienced by the vapour. For its description we must refer to the paper itself, and content ourselves with stating the results of its employment. In such a "water bed" as this people find themselves quite comfortable, and, when once accustomed to it, can sleep as well in it as in an ordinary bed. The appetite, fecal and urinary evacuations, remain normal, the respiration is not hurried, and the debility usually attributed to prolonged baths is not observable. During the first four or five days the whole surface, with the exception of a slight rising of the epidermis of the fingers and toes, undergoes no perceptible change. After that time there occurs in almost all, especially those who have much swelling of the feet, sharp pains in the plantar surface, which last for some days. For the alleviation of this suffering it suffices for the patient either to have placed under the soles of the feet a firm horse-hair pillow, against which he can press, or, if this is not enough, to have cushions placed under his feet, so as to keep them for some hours above the water. In individuals with a delicate skin there are frequently produced, after they have been in the water a week or two, large broad patches of artificial papulary eczema, which are accompanied by great itching. Frictions with *oleum rusci*, while still remaining in the water, are always sufficient to cause the disappearance of this eruption. With the exception of this local result of the irritating effect of the water, no bad consequences have been observed. Among the many women for whom the bath has been employed, none were removed from it during the menstrual period, the water being found, indeed, to assuage their suffering. In no one of them did any disturbance of the functions of the sexual organs arise.

Since 1862 more than 500 persons have been treated by these continuous tepid baths, so that a very strong opinion may be expressed as to their harmlessness. Of the early cases in which they were employed, sufficient notes were not taken to state the proportion of recoveries; but during his period of service as clinical assistant, Dr. Hebra had 200 of these patients under his care, and is able to speak strongly in favour of the procedure. At the Vienna General Hospital a special place is devoted to this treatment, in which are set up seven of the apparatus, and the results of its employment are stated in the reports of that institution. Burns in the third degree—a very fatal injury—constituted 127 of the 203 cases treated, and of these 56 (44 per cent.) recovered. Among the other cases there were numerous examples of pemphigus and gangrenous bubo.—*Med. Times and Gaz.*, Dec. 8, 1877.

On the Vermifuge Action of Pumpkin-seeds.

In a letter published in *Il Raccoglitore*, Nov. 6 and 7, 1877, FEDELI relates the following case, to illustrate the efficacy of the seeds of cucurbitaceæ in tape-worm. A boy aged 7 had been affected with tænia during four years, and had become much debilitated by the numerous medicines administered to him. It was at last determined to stop all internal treatment, and to send him, during the summer and autumn, to the Tusculan Hills. While he was there, his parents observed that, whenever he ate boiled pumpkins, he voided numerous joints of tænia, and appeared more lively. Acting on the suggestion conveyed in this observation, they gave him, for two mornings, while fasting, the seeds simply decorticated ; and, on the second morning, had the satisfaction of seeing him expel several long pieces of tapeworm. From this day he recovered his appetite, his nutrition improved, and he had no further illness.—*London Med. Record*, Nov. 15, 1877.

Mixed Narcosis.

About three weeks ago THIERSCH operated three times for malignant disease affecting the bones of the face. In each case he removed the bones chiefly impli-cated, and as much of the surrounding and deeper-lying structures as was neces-sary or possible.

In the first case, in which the inferior maxilla was affected, he excised half the bone and also a considerable amount of the skin around the growth, which had perforated the cheek, and had a very characteristic malignant ulcerative appear-ance. In consequence of the free removal of skin it was impossible to completely close the wound. The patient got intense glossitis, which prevented deglutition. The glossitis, however, greatly diminished, but the patient continued to sink, and became extremely anæmic. There was slight recurrent hæmorrhage, and on November 26th the common carotid was tied, and shortly afterwards transfusion of blood to the extent of about 12 ozs. was performed, but the patient died on the table during the operation.

In the second case, the superior maxilla was removed with a very large growth, and the structures beneath freely cleaned. The whole of the skin incisions united by first intention, and the cavity filled up well and healthily. He was shown in *Klinik* on Nov. 23d, nearly well. The cavity was almost completely filled up, and at a short distance the line of incisions could not be distinguished. The general health good.

In the third and last case the superior maxilla was removed. The patient, however, died a few hours after the operation, and at the autopsy the disease was found to have perforated the upper wall of the left orbit, and attacked the dura mater.

The cases in themselves were instructive, but a more interesting feature lay in the steps preceding the operations. Anæsthesia was obtained by the newest Ger-man plan—that of the "mixed narcosis" (Gemischte narkose),—the discovery of which is ascribed to Prof. Nussbaum, of Munich. It consists in the subcutaneous injection of morphia when the patient is brought in for operation, and then the administration of chloroform. This, by the by, is administered here somewhat differently from the English method. Air is pumped, by means of a hand-bag, through a bottle of chloroform (hooked on to the breast of the administrator's coat), into an inhaler which fits tightly over the nose and mouth of the patient. The dose of morphia is varied according to the age and strength of the patient. Half a grain of morphia is the maximum dose ; the minimum hitherto used has been a quarter of a grain.

Chloroform is given directly after the injection, as above described. At the end of five minutes' inhalation the operation can usually begin, but the administration is kept up at intervals during the course of the operation.

The effects were very marked in the three cases just related, and in each they were perfect. The patient, in each operation, allowed the blood to collect at the back of his mouth till ordered to spit it out, and then did that at once and completely. Otherwise he kept perfectly still, and watched the movements of the surgeon and the bystanders with a half-stupid but evidently interested look ; yet he evidently felt no pain from the action of the saw, the knife, or the scraper.

In operations about the face and jaws, where it is of importance that the blood should not trickle down the trachea, if the new mode of producing anæsthesia can be safely employed it will prove of great advantage. As to the results I am certain, but as to the safety I cannot yet speak. It has only been used here since last month—about five times, I believe ; but so far there have been no bad symptoms following its use. There can, I think, be no doubt that mixed narcosis will cause insensibility to pain without abolishing all voluntary movements.—*Lancet*, Dec. 8, 1877.

[This modification of the anæsthetic process was described at least fourteen years ago. The reader is referred to an interesting paper on the subject by Dr. J. C. Reeve, of Dayton, Ohio, published in the *American Journal of the Medical Sciences*, April 1876, p. 374.—ED.]

On the Venous Pulse produced by Chloroformization.

Dr. NOEL bases his paper (*Bulletin de l'Académie Royale de Belgique*, 1876) on more than fifty cases. According to him the phenomenon exists in the majority of subjects without distinction of sex or age ; it always appears at the same period of anæsthesia, that is to say, during the waking-up. In these conditions, the internal jugular veins, the subclavian veins, and, in rather more than half the cases, the external jugulars, sometimes even the facial veins, are the seat of pulsations isochronous with the radial pulse. These pulsations seem to the eye very distinct, but only give a slight impression to the touch. A double undulatory movement corresponds to each of these pulsations. The most marked repletion very closely precedes the radial pulse, and is immediately followed by a marked lowering. These pulsations, studied more specially in the external jugular, where the phenomenon is peculiarly significant, disappear after compression of the vein at the lower part of the neck ; on the contrary, they persist when the vessel is compressed at the upper limit of the cervical region. They last about half an hour, gradually diminishing in intensity. During the whole of this time, palpation and auscultation of the heart, and examination of the respiration and the pulse, do not reveal any special modification. N. Noel afterwards points out that this phenomenon indicates a profound disturbance of the action of the heart: he therefore advises the surgeon to carefully watch the patient during the period of awakening.—*London Med. Record*, Nov. 15, 1877.

On the Mechanical Action of Baths of Compressed Air.

Dr. C. FORLANINI has communicated to the Medico-Pneumatic Institute of Milan a preliminary article on this subject (*Gazetta Medica Italiana-Lombardi*, March 31, 1877.)

The action of compressed air on the organism is of two kinds—chemical and mechanical. The former consists in the increased absorption of oxygen by the lungs, the latter in the modification which the increase in the density of the air exerts on the mechanical act of respiration, and probably on the circulation of

the blood, and on the density and compactness of the tissues, which are immediately in contact with the air. Regarding the mechanical action, the author makes
the following remarks.

1. It is admitted without dispute that, in the compressed air bath, the capacity
of the lungs is increased in healthy subjects, by reason of the reduction of the
volume of the intestinal gases, and the consequent descent of the abdominal wall
and the diaphragm.

2. It is also admitted, without dispute, that the bath of compressed air produces this increase of the spirometric pressure in a still higher degree in the subjects of catarrhal bronchitis. This fact, the therapeutic importance of which
cannot be overlooked, is explained by the deobstruent action which the compressed
air exercises on the minute bronchial tubes, when blocked up by the bronchitic
secretion, through the establishment of a greater pressure than that of the ordinary atmosphere. Waldenburg's apparatus has an identical action, but it is not
possible to determine *à priori*, whether it or the compressed air-bath possesses the
greater deobstruent power over the small bronchi. Numerous comparative experiments have convinced Dr. Forlanini that Waldenburg's apparatus is in this respect superior to the bath of compressed air.

3. For a long time it was assumed that the air-bath exercised an anæmiating
and compressing action in the peripheric tissues ; that, in consequence of the increased density of the air, the blood was pressed out of the tissues with which the
air came into contact, and forced into the deep-seated vessels ; and that the tissues, being compressed against the subjacent solid parts, became condensed. The
hemorrhage and peripheric congestions observed in aeronauts ; the opposite facts
observed in divers and in drivers of bridge-piles, and in coal-miners ; together with
the uniform results of experiments ; these are the proofs adduced in support of
this theory. By it are explained in great measure the results obtained by the use
of the air-bath in the treatment of inflammation and hyperæmia of the mucous
membranes of the respiratory apparatus, Eustachian tube, etc.

This theory, the correctness of which has been recently impugned by Bert,
Forlanini holds to be untenable. A microscopical examination of the circulation in
the frog ; observations on the vessels of the conjunctiva and retina ; and especially experiments made with Professor Mosso's plethysmograph, have shown him
that, under the use of the compressed air-bath, the calibre of the capillaries does
not undergo change. He promises in a short time to give a detailed account of
his experiments.—*London Med. Record*, Nov. 15, 1877.

Medicine.

The Pathology of Inflammation.

The most conspicuous opponent of Cohnheim's theory, that the origin of pus-
cells is to be sought exclusively in the white corpuscles of the blood, is Professor
Stricker, from whose laboratory there have come of late years a number of valuable contributions to pathological histology, bearing directly on this subject. The
object of most of these papers has been to show that in an inflamed tissue there
is a rapid formation of cells from those pre-existing in the part, in circumstances
and under forms that exclude the possibility of the new cells being white blood-
corpuscles. A recent memoir by Arnold Spina, Assistant in the Laboratory for

General and Experimental Pathology in Vienna, on "The Changes in the Cells in Inflamed Tendon" (*Wiener Medizin, Jahrbücher*, 1877), may be regarded as a continuation of the series of experimental studies on inflammation which have been inspired by the ideas of the Vienna school.

It is a misfortune that histologists are so little agreed as to the nature of the cellular elements of connective tissue, that the conclusions at which any observer arrives regarding the changes produced by inflammation must always be read in the light of the opinions he holds regarding the normal structure. This is not less the case with tendon than with other forms of the tissue. Herr Spina, therefore, very properly prefaces his memoir with a statement of his views on the histology of tendon. They are briefly as follows. Between the bundles of tendon there are interspersed rows of cells. The rows are spindle-shaped, the cells becoming narrower towards the ends of the spindle, until the cells disappear, the spindle being continued by fibres from each extremity. These rows become, as the animal gets older, changed into elastic bands. The cells of which these rows are composed are in young animals surrounded by a hyaline substance from which the elastic tissue is formed. The cells of tendon, further, have processes in the form of flattened bands and fibres, by which they are connected with each other.

Now what takes place in these elements when the tendon is inflamed? In the tendons of young animals, cauterized by caustic potash, cut out after twenty-four hours and coloured by chloride of gold, the cells were found enlarged, and their number increased; the cell-processes were found to be thicker and in greater number. Similar changes were found, even in a more striking manner, in the tendons of older animals; the presence of nodular swellings in the band-shaped processes of the cells being conspicuous. Now spindle-shaped rows of cells are formed, and it is inferred that they are the product of the nodular swellings in the processes of the older cells, these swellings being clumps of protoplasm (*Klumpen*), which by blending with each other form a new chain of cells. When the inflammation has lasted longer than forty-eight hours, the substance of which the bundles are formed gradually disappears, whilst the cells increase in number more and more until large layers and masses of cells are formed. After three or more days, the individual cells can no longer be distinguished, and the cell-groups have been succeeded by a coarsely or finely granular mass. This granular mass, when stained by hæmatoxylin, is seen to contain the nuclear elements which are peculiar to pus-corpuscles, and the mass itself is in reality a small abscess. When these cellular masses were teased out after two or three days' inflammation, an important change was found to have taken place in the spindle-shaped cell-rows described by Herr Spina in healthy tendon. These could now be isolated, and were found to be much longer than in the normal condition. Instead of being one cell broad, two and even more cells were now found side by side. The elastic bands developed from the cells had gone back into their histological elements, and become "pus-bands." At other times, according to Herr Spina, the cellular elements of these elastic bands developed red blood-corpuscles, colour being apparently the chief element taken into consideration in coming to this conclusion. These blood-like cells are also found at some parts in a breadth of several cells, contrasting again with the appearances seen in healthy tendon.

It would thus seem to be beyond doubt that, if we follow Herr Spina's methods of examining tendon, and possibly whatever method may be followed, we shall find in a very early stage of inflammation a greater number of cells than will be found in healthy tendon similarly treated. Is Herr Spina's conclusion that the healthy cells have multiplied under the stimulus of inflammation, therefore, justified? To answer this question it is necessary to consider an interesting point in histological *technique*. The bundles of tendon being somewhat cylindrical in form and parallel to each other, necessarily leave at certain points between them, when they are cut transversely, angular gaps. It is in these gaps that the nuclei of the tendon-cells are seen, and it has been conclusively shown by Boll that the cells lie on the bundles. When a transverse section of tendon treated by gold-chloride is examined, these gaps are filled with a dark purple mass, which insinuates itself in angular projections between the bundles. Herr Spina, whose preparations were mostly obtained by the use of this reagent, believes that this angular and occasionally anastomosing deposit is the tendon-cell, an opinion that is irreconcilable with the results obtained by Boll and Ranvier. When an inflamed tendon has been treated with gold, this deposit between the bundles is increased in quantity, and the bundles are proportionately separated from each other. There are, further, an increased number of gold-stained lines traceable between and into the bundles. Histologists who do not agree with Spina's views regarding the nature of the tendon-cell, will not see with him in these changes any evidence of growth or multiplication of cells, but will regard them as evidences of distension of the spaces between the bundles by serous effusion. When, after a longer duration of the inflammatory process, the large spaces between the broken-down bundles are found occupied with pus-cells, an objector to Herr Spina's views would naturally ask why their source should not be sought in the bloodvessels that exist in the tissue between the groups of bundles. The important fact, however, remains, that an increased number of cells are actually found in the inflamed tissue, and it has not been shown that they are connected either with the gold network between the bundles or with emigrated white blood-corpuscles. In isolated cell-bands, several breadths of cells were found side by side. Neither from the description given by the author, nor from an examination of the plate which illustrates his memoir, does it seem probable that these were white corpuscles in a particular stage of development, and as little is there evidence that they proceeded from each other by any process of division or endogenous cell-formation. The demonstration of their existence will, we believe, be found to be an element of permanent value in Herr Spina's work; but, before pathologists can be expected to agree regarding their nature, the whole question of the histology of tendon must be re-examined from the foundation.—*British Med. Journal*, Dec. 15, 1877.

Use of Salicylates in the Treatment of Acute Rheumatism.

This subject has been under discussion in Paris, and some of the leading French physicians have expressed their opinions concerning the new agent. On the whole, the results confirm fully those which have been obtained in Germany and in Great Britain. The discussion of the subject was opened at the Académie de Médecine by M. GERMAIN SÉE in an elaborate review of the properties and action of salicylic acid and its salts, and an enthusiastic advocacy of its use in a considerable number of diseases. His experience of its use in rheumatism extended over fifty-two cases, of which, however, only nineteen were febrile. Twelve of the febrile cases had had previous attacks, varying in duration from three weeks to three months. In all, with but one exception, the attacks were cut short by the salicylate in three days. Neither the age of the patient, nor the previous duration of the disease, nor the extent of joint-affection, influenced the result. The only case of failure was one in which the acute rheumatism, beginning in four joints, remained localized to the wrist. He agreed with other observers that the first effect of the action of the salicylates is the cessation of the pains; this occurs in from twelve to eighteen hours; the joint swelling ceases in from one to three days, and motion is easy after the third day. The pyrexia, in some cases as high as 105°, never disappeared before the cessation of the pain. Stricker, who first called attention to the beneficial effects of the treatment in rheumatic fever, asserted that cases of subacute rheumatism derived little benefit from the treatment, and his observation has received a certain amount of confirmation in this country. The experience of M. Sée does not, however, corroborate this. Out of thirty-three cases of subacute rheumatism he stated, there was not a case which was not cured in two or three days. M. Hérard confirmed fully the results obtained by M. Sée, and mentioned one case in which quinine in large doses had failed, but the salicylate treatment effected a rapid cure in two days. M. Hardy, while agreeing in the main with M. Sée, thought he had been a little too fortunate, and that fifty-two cures out of fifty-three cases was an "unnatural phenomenon in therapeutics," wisely pointing out that practitioners must not be disappointed if they obtain a less successful result. Other confirmatory opinions were expressed by MM. Oulmont, Gueneau de Mussy, Ferrand, Beaumetz, Desnos, Bouchardat, Jaccoud, and Lépine, all of whom had obtained, by the use of the salicylates, results which, if not quite so startling as those of M. Sée, were at least superior to those obtained by any other treatment. M. Jaccoud, however, thought that it had little power over chronic forms of rheumatism ; and M. Lépine admitted that in some cases it appears to have no effect. Perhaps, however, the most valuable testimony to its use was contained in a report which had been obtained by the military medical authorities, relating to 181 cases of acute rheumatism, in only 7 of which the remedy had no effect, while in 110 of the cases, which were carefully followed, the patient was cured in 94 cases in from twenty-four to sixty hours.

The opinions expressed regarding the details of its administration and effect are of considerable interest. The quantity which M. Sée believes it is necessary to administer daily is two drachms and a half, to be taken in five doses. This corresponds to about a drachm and a half of salicylic acid. Gueneau de Mussy asserted, however, that equally good results were obtained if a smaller dose was first employed, and gradually increased up to one and a half or two drachms. Lépine, on the other hand, advocates larger doses, of two to three drachms of the salt of soda or ammonia. The large doses are, he believes, borne quite well, if given in divided doses—an opinion which is, on the whole, corroborated by the experience of English physicians. M. Sée, however, believed that some of the cases of sudden death during its administration, which have been recorded in Russia and Germany, were due to the depressing effect of the large doses employed.

It was admitted by M. Sée that relapses are more frequent on the salicylate than on any other method of treatment, but this he ascribed entirely to the too early discontinuance of the drug, an opinion which M. Hérard also expressed. The salicylate should be continued for ten or fifteen days, and there would be very few relapses. If a relapse did occur after the discontinuance of the treatment, it could be at once cut short by the resumption of the salicylate. In four cases in which the salicylate was purposely omitted early, the alternate occurrence and arrest of rheumatic affection were observed three times. According to M. Desnos, the rapidity of cure is the cause of the relapses in an accidental manner. Discomfort is so soon at an end that patients will get up, and move about, and expose themselves to cold, and so get a relapse.

Regarding the influence of the salicylate treatment on the complications of rheumatic fever, the conclusions of the French physicians agree with those of previous observers. M. Sée asserted that complications are far less frequent than under other methods of treatment, for the simple reason that the duration of the disease is so much shorter. The profound anæmia which so often succeeds rheumatism is, in his experience, almost unknown on the salicylate treatment. Recent endocarditis is uninfluenced by it for good or evil, and in cases which came into the hospital during the first three days of the affection, there was not a single instance of either endocarditis or pericarditis. The experience of Lépine, Hérard, and other observers, agreed with that of M. Sée. M. Jaccoud pointed out that not only has it no apparent influence on the cardiac, pulmonary, or cerebral complications, but it does not prevent the fever which accompanies a visceral inflammation.

A strong opinion was expressed not only, as we have said, by M. Sée, but by others of the speakers, that some of the instances of sudden death under salicylate treatment were to be ascribed to the large doses employed. M. Empis mentioned such an instance of sudden death, but how far it could be ascribed to the salicylate seemed very doubtful. There is no doubt that the cases of M. Jaccoud, who employed rather large doses, present a remarkably high mortality. Out of sixteen cases treated exclusively by the salicylate method, three died, two from cerebral complications and one from acute alcoholism.

The theory advanced by M. Sée, in which Gueneau de Mussy agreed, to explain the mechanism of its action, is that the chief action is upon the nervous system, which plays a greater part in the production of the symptoms of rheumatism than is commonly supposed, and thus that the remedy cannot be regarded as a specific for the rheumatic poison.

The only speakers who opposed the use of the new remedy were, as might be expected, those who had never tried it. One of these was M. Bouillaud, who refused to believe that acute rheumatism could be cured in three days by anything except a miracle, and who advocated, and still employs, the treatment by bleeding. One or two physicians had met with far less favourable results than the average. M. Oulmont had obtained no distinct result in four out of seven cases, although the treatment was continued for more than a week. But M. Sée objected that the dose given, amounting to a drachm daily, was too small. M. Desnos, however, as well as M. Lépine, pointed out that there are some cases in which, even in very large doses, the salicylate does not appear to exercise any appreciable influence on the duration of the malady, although they are forms of considerable severity.--*Lancet*, Dec. 1, 1877.

The Use of Salicylates in Typhoid Fever.

The remarkable effect of salicylic acid and its salts in acute rheumatism has led to its employment in many other diseases, and the results obtained in some of these were described at the discussions which have taken place before the French societies, and to which we have directed attention. That a drug possessing such a remarkable power over the pyrexia and articular pain of one disease should exert an influence in other diseases, presenting one or both of these characteristics, is a natural expectation. It has not been wholly unrealized, although the extent to which it is useful in other diseases than acute rheumatism seems to have limits which are soon reached, and to be the subject of some discrepancy of opinion.

We remarked that M. Sée has found the salicylic treatment much more effective in subacute rheumatism than many other observers have asserted. He has also used it in chronic rheumatoid arthritis, and has found that it is very useful in the acute exacerbations of the disease. The pain is quickly removed, the swelling is soon lessened, and the muscular rigidity is diminished in a remarkable manner. To effect this, however, large doses are necessary. Gueneau de Mussy found it useful in one case of this affection, but of no service in another. The same physician had found it entirely useless in sciatica, but in acute muscular rheumatism, lumbago, etc., N. Sée had obtained very good results, all pain and stiffness being removed in two days.

Gout is another disease in which salicylate of soda has been largely used. N. Sée found that the effect is speedy diminution in the pain of acute gout, and that even in chronic gout it is useful, and produces a gradual diminution in the swellings and nodosities. The opinion was corroborated by Gueneau de Mussy and Lépine. The latter had seen remarkable effects produced in a case of saturnine gout. In gonorrhœal rheumatism and in chorea it has been found useless. Given in full doses, it has considerable power of reducing the temperature in phthisis, but, as might be expected, without any corresponding amelioration in the symptoms. Indeed, its use is not wholly without danger, for it has appeared to induce serious gastro-intestinal troubles and cerebral symptoms.

Perhaps the most important practical question connected with the employment of salicylic acid, next to its use in acute rheumatism, is its effect in typhoid fever. There is much discrepancy in the results hitherto recorded. A favourable report was given by Dr. Gueneau de Mussy, who had used it in twenty-seven cases in small doses without having a single death. He only concluded from this that in small doses the drug does no harm in the disease. N. Sée believed, however, that it was of little service, and that doses which would have an antiseptic influence on the intestine would produce irritation; but he seems to have concluded this rather from theoretical considerations than practical experience. N. Lépine concurred in its inutility. N. Oulmont had found that of ten cases in which it was employed, marked defervescence was produced in eight, but the effect was not durable. This corroborates the conclusion of Goltdammer, who found that the duration of the disease was not diminished in any of the fifty-six cases he observed. An important series of facts have been published on this point by Schröder, of St. Petersburg. In a military hospital 160 cases of typhoid were treated with salicylates, chiefly with the soda salt. Of these thirty-one were fatal, the mortality being thus 19.4 per cent., the mortality of the preceding 211 cases treated by other methods having been 14.7 per cent. The causes of death in the salicylic cases were—in four, perforation; in five, pneumonia; and in the others parotitis, parotitis with œdema of the glottis, pleuro-pneumonia, and meningitis. The antifebrile action was unquestionable, but no favourable influence on the course of the disease could be observed. By small doses the pulse was rendered less frequent, but by large doses it was accelerated, and the continued use of large doses (three drachms a day) induced symptoms of collapse. Schröder concludes that the treatment is far inferior to that by cold baths. This is not, however, the opinion of Jahn, who has published a series of statistics of three years' treatment of typhoid on three different systems. In the first, thirty-nine cases were treated with large doses of quinine, the application of bladders of ice, and mild "water treatment." Nine patients died, six of them from the intensity of the disease. The average duration of treatment in the hospital was sixty-six days; complications were observed seven times, severe cerebral symptoms were present twenty-five times, and severe intestinal symptoms twenty-nine times, while bedsores were observed in nineteen cases. In the following year sixty-three cases were treated with quinine and an energetic "cold-bath treatment." The deaths were six, of which five were from the intensity of the disease. The average duration of treatment was fifty-three days, complications were observed in seven, severe cerebral symptoms in seven, severe intestinal symptoms in twenty-one, bedsores in seven. In the next year thirty-five cases were treated by salicylates; five grammes (about a drachm and a half) of salicylic acid were dissolved in water with an equal quantity of bicarbonate of soda, and taken as a beverage. The deaths were three only ; the average duration of treatment was thirty-seven days. Complications were observed twenty-four times, severe cerebral symptoms were present in no case, severe intestinal symptoms in one only, bedsores were observed in no case ; the three deaths were all from double pneumonia. The contrast between the observations of Jahn and Schröder is so great as to make it probable that the epidemics differed very much in severity and character. It would seem, from the statistics, that in the last year of the epidemic observed by Jahn, the cases were of an exceptionally mild character, and his conclusions are therefore to be received with some reserve. He believes, however, that in large doses the drug acts not only as an antipyretic, but has a "healing" effect on the typhoid process ; that the antipyretic effect is shown in the remission of the cerebral symptoms ; that a direct effect is produced on the digestive organs—the gastric symptoms diminish, the appetite returns, the diarrhœa is moderated or arrested ; that, as a result, the prostration is diminished, and the convalescence is abbreviated ; that the soda salt is preferable to the acid, because it has the same curative influence, and possibly a more rapid effect, while it produces no irritation of the respiratory tract ; that no concurrent effect of the salicylate was observed, except that the tendency to epistaxis appeared to be increased by its use ; that relapses were not avoided by the use of the salicylate, and it is therefore well to continue to give it in smaller doses during convalescence. A case which was brought last session before the Clinical Society by Dr. Murchison is in such striking contrast to the second of Jahn's conclusions, that it ought not to be overlooked. The case appeared to be one favourable for testing the effect of salicylate, for the pyrexia was considerable, but was unattended by diarrhœa or delirium. The effect of the drug was to reduce the temperature as rapidly as in rheumatic fever, but when the drug was discontinued the pyrexia returned. While under the influence of the salicylate the patient had violent delirium, ceasing when the drug was omitted ; there was also albuminuria, and almost total suppression of urine, both passing off as the effect of the drug ceased. It is clear, however, from the result of continental experience, that the dose of the salicylate was too large. Six drachms daily were given, three times the quantity employed by Jahn. Evidently, in typhoid the doses cannot be borne which do good in acute rheumatism, and hence a single case of poisoning by the drug, such as this, has no significance with respect to the possible beneficial effect of its employment in smaller doses.

In intermittent fever the action of the salicylate is marked, but is less than that of quinine. It has been carefully tried by Rosenstein in thirteen cases. In three cases only was there a complete cure ; in six cases no effect could be observed ; in four cases the influence of the drug was transient, so that the administration of quinine was necessary. The dose of salicylate employed varied from a minimum of one drachm to a maximum of four drachms daily.—*Lancet*, Dec. 8, 1877.

On a Case of Facial Hemiplegia.

In the *Prezglad lekarski*, No. 7, 1877 (quoted in *Allgemeine Med. Central-Zeitung*, October 23), Dr. LACHOWICZ relates the following case. A barber's assistant, aged 17, being tired with work, lay on the ground on a dry stone, and slept. The next day, he noticed that the right half of his face was fuller than the other, and that his mouth was drawn to one side. Three days later, the right side of his face was more swollen ; the right side of the forehead and the right eyebrow were immovable. The right eye could not be perfectly closed, and there was much lachrymation. The right ala nasi was not raised in forcible breathing ;

the angle of the mouth on this side was depressed, and saliva flowed from it. The cheek and neck were turned, the neck was stiff.

Sensation was diminished in the right half of the face. The right cornea and eyelids were less sensitive than the left; even less than the mucous membrane of the right nostril. There was also a difference in the sensibility of the two sides of the lips; the uvula was diverted to the left, and sensation was diminished in the right side of the pharynx. The sense of smell was impaired in the right nostril. The senses of hearing and sight were similar on the two sides.

From a consideration of this case, Dr. Lachowicz is led to the conclusion, that not only the facial nerve, but also branches of all three divisions of the fifth pair, were affected. A central cause of the disease must be excluded, as the paralysis was confined to certain muscles, the reflex irritability remaining intact.

The illness lasted a month; and the treatment consisted in the application of vesicants, which were repeated seven times.—*London Med. Record*, Dec. 15, 1877.

On Spinal Paralysis in Adults.

In the *Berliner Klinische Wochenschrift*, for September 24th, Dr. GOTT-FRIED SALOMON, of Hamburg, relates four cases of spinal paralysis occurring in adults, but apparently of a similar nature to infantile paralysis. Since Bern-hardt first described cases of this kind, others have been published by Frey, Leyden, Erb, Eisenlohr, and Goltdammer. The four cases here given occurred within the space of two years.

The first was that of a previously healthy man, aged about 20, who, after standing sentry one night in a deep snow, noticed in the morning an unusual feeling of.fatigue in both legs; it was not, however, until the day following that the loss of power was such as to oblige him to keep his bed; the paralysis rapidly increased until he was quite unable to stand. Iodide of potassium was administered for several weeks, and the patient improved so far as to be able to walk a little with a stick; he was always, however, worse after any exertion, and his condition now became stationary. Sensation was perfect, reflex irritability normal, the bladder and rectum unaffected. The patient was rather unsteady when standing with his eyes shut; his general nutrition, as well as that of the paretic extremities, was good, and no other evidences of disease could be detected. In applying the induction-current directly to the muscles, a very powerful and painful current had to be used before contraction was caused; the muscles of the leg were less sensitive than those of the thigh, and the peronei and tibialis anticus reacted worse than the muscles of the calf. The reaction throughout the right limb was worse than in the left. Muscular contraction was even more difficult to obtain when the current was applied along the course of the nerves; through the pero-neal nerves, especially, it was only by the strongest current that the slightest reaction could be caused. By the galvanic current applied to the muscles, prompt, quickly ceasing contractions were produced. Under galvanic treatment the case progressed favourably, and the patient perfectly recovered.

A lady, aged about 25, who had had an attack of right sciatica, one and a half years ago, but had since been quite well, found one morning, after having danced a great deal the night before, that she was only able to move her right arm and leg imperfectly. For three weeks she was treated with purgatives, also occa-sionally with iodide of potassium, and some slight improvement took place; at the end of this time all movements were possible so long as the patient lay in bed; the pressure of the right hand was considerably less than that of the left, there was no wasting of the affected limbs, sensibility remained unaltered, and the general health undisturbed. No pain had been felt from the beginning of the illness. The patient was able to walk slowly, but the right leg dragged; she could hold light objects in her right hand, but very soon it commenced to tremble a good deal, and she was quite unable to hold anything at all heavy. The results of the application of electricity to the affected muscles did not differ materially from those of the foregoing case, except that the muscles supplied by the right ulnar nerve were more sensitive to the galvanic current than the same muscles on the left side. The case was treated by galvanism for a fortnight, but, no improvement occurring, the patient was sent away for change of air, and gradually but completely recovered.

The third and most carefully observed case occurred in a merchant, aged 52, (Duchenne, of Boulogne, had previously fixed the limit of age for these cases at 45 years); the disease came on so gradually that the diagnosis was for some time uncertain. The man had been previously quite healthy, and was a great walker; one day he noticed that his left foot repeatedly gave way under him; from this time he was unable to walk so much or so fast as previously; especially in cold weather he rapidly became fatigued. For three months he gradually became worse, and when first seen at the end of that time the whole left leg unmistakably dragged in walking. Some wasting both of the leg and thigh was also observed, the adductors being most affected. Sensation and reflex irritability were normal in both lower limbs, but they both showed some degree of hyperæsthesia; the functions of the bladder and rectum were undisturbed. Co-ordination of movements showed no alteration; the patient was able to stand with closed eyes for any length of time, and had suffered no pain. Tested by the induction-current, a loss of contractibility was shown by the adductors of the thigh as compared with the extensors, by the peronei as compared with the muscles of the calf, and by all the muscles of the left lower limb as compared with those of the right. When, however, the galvanic current was applied to the muscles, those of the left limb showed increased reaction as compared with those of the right; this was referred to the atrophy and consequent diminution of resistance to the current. Applied along the course of the nerves, the galvanic current produced the same effects in the affected as in the healthy limb. At this time the disease was believed to be peripheral, and the case looked like one of peripheral rheumatic paralysis. For two months, treatment by galvanism and faradization was carried on; the reaction of the muscles to the latter improved, the wasting to a certain extent disappeared, and the patient himself perceived an increase of strength in the affected limb. One night, however, he awoke with a peculiar painful sensation in the left arm; he went to sleep again, but noticed a loss of power in the left hand in the morning; the muscles of the hand gradually wasted and lost their contractile power; the condition of the left leg remained for some time stationary and then steadily became worse. Before the muscles entirely lost their power of reaction, the author noticed a phenomenon which he has only seen once previously described (by Benedikt). It consists in this, that, when a powerful induction-current is applied to a muscle, it immediately contracts energetically, but the contraction at once ceases again as suddenly as if the current had been broken, although the latter really remains as strong as at first. This reaction may be caused any number of times in the same muscle with a slight pause between each application. Benedikt believes this phenomenon to be characteristic of disease of the brain, but Salomon has seen it in cases of nervous disease of undoubtedly peripheral origin, one of which ultimately ended in recovery. In the present case, the phenomenon could be caused for about a month, and was best seen when one pole was placed over the sciatic nerve below the gluteal fold and the other on the middle of the calf. A stronger current than that required to produce the result in question usually caused the contraction to last a longer time, and then pass into a trembling

movement; a weaker current produced no effect at all. The patient became
worse; as the galvanic treatment produced no good effects he was sent to take the
baths at Relune, but the disease progressed more rapidly, affections of speech
came on, both as regards articulation and the memory of words, so that a fatal
result from bulbar paralysis seemed probable.

The fourth case is very similar to the second. A merchant, aged 30, had had
right sciatica a year and a half ago, and now complained of paralytic symptoms
in the same limb, these rapidly increased and wasting was observed; before long
some paralysis of the arm of the same side commenced. The effects of galvanism
and faradization were similar to those of the previous cases. The patient was
treated by galvanism, centrally and peripherally, for eight weeks, and all the
symptoms disappeared, first in the arm and afterwards in the leg; some slight
wasting only of the latter was still observable when the patient was last seen.

Although the above cases, as well as those recorded by others, are similar in all
essential points, they yet present many points of difference, especially in their
degrees of acuteness and in the distribution of the disease. The four cases published by Goltdammer were all more severe than the foregoing, but all ended in
recovery, while the third of the above cases seemed to promise an unfavourable
result. The resemblance of the cases now given to infantile paralysis is so great
as to lead to the belief that they are due to the same anatomical lesion. It may
therefore be concluded that, in the majority of cases, the primary disease exists
in the anterior horns of the gray matter of the spinal cord (poliomyelitis), but the
question as to the nature of the morbid process still remains. *Post-mortem* examinations in cases of infantile paralysis have almost all been made so long after
the commencement of the disease that it is impossible to say whether the appearances found are the same as would have been observed soon after the original
attack; the changes noted in the cord have also been various in different cases,
sometimes signs of atrophy, at others those of inflammation; one observer has
also noticed an alteration in the white substance of the anterior lateral columns.
We must therefore believe with Leyden that various anatomical lesions may lie
at the root of infantile paralysis, and that the same is true of the spinal paralysis
of adults. In the above four cases, it is probable that a primary atrophic process
occurred, because at no time were any symptoms present which could point to
inflammation, although such are frequently observed in children at the very commencement of the disease. In none of the above cases was there any fever, increase in reflex movements, nor any galvanic reaction such as would indicate inflammatory affection of the cord.

The etiology of the foregoing cases is also interesting; in the first case it is
almost certain that cold was the cause of the attack; in the second and fourth
cases it is not improbable that the previous sciatica had something to do with the
subsequent disease of the spinal cord, although it is difficult to understand how
a chronic neuritis, after causing no symptoms for a year and a half, should affect
the cord. Leyden, in one of his cases, in which a *neuritis lipomatosa* was found,
believed that this latter was the cause of subsequent myelitis. In the third case
the etiology was doubtful; the case showed that a temporary improvement in the
electro-muscular contractility, and even also in the atrophic symptoms, must not
always be taken as justifying a favourable prognosis. The author relies especially upon the electrical phenomena in this case as supplying a new proof of the
identity of spinal paralysis in adults with infantile paralysis.

A doubt may remain as to whether, in the last two cases and others similar to
them (in which, after the lower limbs have become affected, like symptoms appear in the upper extremity), the morbid process in the cord has extended upwards, or whether the lumbar and cervical enlargements of the cord are indepen-

dently affected. In favour of the latter view are the facts that in none of the above cases was there any paralysis of the muscles of the trunk (which always occurs in acute ascending paralysis) and that in all necropsies of cases of infantile paralysis the two enlargements of the cord have been found to be solely or chiefly affected.—*London Med. Record*, Dec. 15, 1877.

Syphilitic Affections of the Nervous System.

Dr. JULIUS ALTHAUS, Physician to the Hospital for Epilepsy and Paralysis, Regent's Park, presents (*Med. Times and Gaz.*, Nov. 10, 1877) the following interesting sketch of syphilitic nervous affections.

A thorough knowledge of those nervous diseases which are produced by the subtle poison of syphilis is of the greatest practical importance, as they yield much more readily to specific treatment than the corresponding idiopathic affections of the nervous system, and unless thoroughly recognized, cannot be efficiently treated. An incorrect diagnosis in such cases will often doom a patient to destruction, while a true recognition of his state may save his life and restore his health.

Neuro-syphilitic affections belong generally to the later portions of the secondary stage, or to the tertiary period of the complaint. They are invariably preceded by a hard infecting sore, and usually by secondary symptoms affecting the skin and fauces. They may, however, appear as the first manifestations of infections of the system, in from twelve months to twenty years from the appearance of the primary affection, and have been now and then seen to follow the first rash and sore throat. They are observed at all ages, but most frequently between twenty and forty years; and this is of diagnostic importance, as hemiplegia or paraplegia coming on in youthful persons is in nine cases out of ten of syphilitic origin. The male sex is more liable to them than the female—which is in accordance with the fact that constitutional syphilis is altogether more frequent in men than in women.

Nerve-syphilis appears to affect with preference those persons in whom there is the neuropathic constitution, either hereditary or acquired. There is almost always a family history of apoplexy, epilepsy, chorea, megrim, or other nervous maladies, and frequently the patient himself has previously suffered from neuralgia or fits. Persons who have put an undue strain on their nervous power, either by excessive mental labour, or by free indulgence in alcohol and the sexual appetite, are more liable, when rendered syphilitic, to become subject to nervous maladies than those in whom there have been no such antecedents. Injury, such as a blow on the head or a fall, and depressing emotions, act frequently as exciting causes of these diseases. Finally, an unsystematic and too soon interrupted treatment of the primary affection has to be looked upon as a powerfully predisposing cause of nerve-syphilis.

Syphilis affects with preference the brain and cranial nerves, but does not spare the spinal cord. Anatomically, we find that the characteristic lesions are not meningitis or encephalitis, as was formerly believed, but repeated attacks of hyperæmia, tumour, and disease of the arteries.

1. The congestive form of cerebral syphilis shows hardly any striking features on the post-mortem table, more especially where the case ends fatally at an early stage of the complaint, from such complications as cystitis, decubitus, phthisis, or pneumonia. When the disease has lasted for a considerable time, the membranes of the brain are seen to have lost their transparency, and there is slight wasting of the cerebral convolutions—which latter, however, is not sufficient to explain severe symptoms which have been observed during life. The lesions are the

same, although in a slighter degree, as those which are found in general paralysis
of the insane, and affect more particularly Hitzig and Ferrier's psycho-motor centres in the cineritious substance of the anterior lobes.   In some of these cases the
cervical sympathetic nerve has been found in a state of pigmentary degeneration,
and it is probable that disease of the superior cervical ganglion of that nerve may
have an important influence in the production of the repeated attacks of hyperæmia by which this form of brain-syphilis is characterized.

The symptoms which are observed under these circumstances resemble very
closely those of general paralysis of the insane.   They are at first indefinite, come
and go, and a change in the mind and temper is the most characteristic feature.
There is excitement or depression, with some confusion of thoughts, fussiness, and
ambitious ideas or delusions.   Apart from a general feeling of *malaise*, the patient
does not complain of being ill.   As time goes on, there is loss of energy, debility,
embarrassed speech partaking of the nature of aphasia, and being cortical rather
than medullary in its kind.   The size of the pupils is unequal; the tongue is
tremulous when protruded; there is tottering gait, and pins-and-needles and
numbness in the extremities are complained of.   When the symptoms on the
part of the nervous system become more marked, there is often a simultaneous
outbreak of fresh syphilitic manifestations on the skin, mucous membrane, or
periosteum.   The intellect and memory now suffer more decidedly, and symptoms of paralysis appear from time to time—viz., aphasia, agraphia, hemiplegia,
and paraplegia.   Such symptoms may last at first only for a few hours or days,
but they gradually become more permanent.   The general debility increases *pari
passu;* and unless an energetic anti-syphilitic treatment be previously followed,
the patient dies within a few years from the outbreak of the disease, from cystitis,
decubitus, and general marasmus.

2. The second manifestation of cerebral syphilis is the syphilitic tumour, gumma, or syphiloma, which presents itself in two varieties, these being probably
only different stages of development of the same deposit.   There are the soft and
hard varieties; the soft tumour being the earlier, and the hard swelling the later
phenomenon.   The soft tumour consists of a reddish-gray jelly, from which on
section a small quantity of pinkish liquid is seen to escape.   Its histological elements are round cells and nuclei, mixed with spindle and stellated cells, and few
but large capillary vessels.   The outline of such tumours is not well defined, and
they seem gradually to merge into the surrounding normal tissue.   They are
chiefly found in the subarachnoid space, and grow from thence to the surface of
the brain; but they also occur in the dura mater, and are in this situation generally harder than when situated in the soft and moist tissue of the pia.

The hard tumour is in many respects similar to tubercle.   It is dry, yellow, of
a cheesy consistency, and on section homogeneous.   It occurs interspersed into
the reddish-gray jelly which I have just described, or as a well-defined tumour of
variable size.   It consists histologically of a granulated substance otherwise devoid
of structure.   There are no bloodvessels or spindle-cells, but now and then heaps
of pigmentary granules and crystals and oil-globules near the periphery.   Its size
varies from that of an almond kernel to that of a pigeon's or even a hen's egg,
and its shape is frequently adapted to that of the spaces in which it is discovered.
It is seen between the two layers of the dura mater, which are much thickened,
and more especially in the falx cerebri.   The skull-bone which corresponds to its
situation is generally in a state of dry caries, and appears rough and attenuated,
while the other portions of the skull are normal.   The yellow hard tumour is
probably owing to contraction and atrophy of the soft gumma.   It is likewise
found in the subarachnoid space, and from thence proceeds to the bloodvessels,
nerves, and cerebral tissues itself.   Occasionally, all the membranes and the cine-

ritious substance are grown together into a uniform mass, and cannot be separated; and the two varieties of tumours are then seen together. Soft jelly is imbedded between the dura and the surface of the brain, and one or several dry yellow tumours are lying in the tissues between the convolutions. The surrounding brain-tissue is in a state of red or white softening, or a portion of the cortical and medullary matter is changed into the same cheesy mass of which the tumour itself consists. Under the influence of anti-syphilitic treatment, nearly the whole of these changes may be repaired, and cicatricial patches are then discovered on the surface of the hemispheres.

.At the base of the brain there is occasionally a diffuse infiltration with gray jelly, which can no longer be called a tumour, but must be looked upon as gummatous meningitis. The effusion in such instances is seen to spread from the olfactory bulb to the posterior portion of the cerebellum, and may even invade the cortex.

The symptoms of cerebral syphiloma differ considerably from those of syphilitic hyperæmia; and one that is hardly ever wanting, and also the first to appear, is a peculiar kind of headache, which appears chiefly at night, and is relieved towards morning. It is intolerably severe, and occurs in paroxysms which last for a few weeks, after which there is a remission, which is again succeeded by a fresh outbreak of it. Unless specific treatment is adopted, this may go on for years. The seat of the headache is mostly at the sides of the head, but it may also be frontal and occipital. It is sometimes localized in a very small area, and then generally increased by pressure; and it is owing to a gummatous deposit on the internal surface of the skull-bones, which irritates the periosteum and the dura mater. Sleeplessness is another symptom which is generally caused by the pain, but also occurs during free intervals; and it is apt to raise our suspicion, because it is mostly found in young persons, in whom insomnia is otherwise very rare.

After these symptoms have continued for a variable time, epileptiform attacks are apt to supervene, which sometimes resemble in every way an ordinary epileptic seizure. Unilateral convulsion, without loss of consciousness, is often connected with this condition; the muscular spasm starts from the thumb or first finger, or the foot, or the face, and affects only the arm or the leg of the same side, but becomes bilateral where the nerve nuclei of the two sides are associated; or there may be a regular epileptic seizure, i. e., general convulsions and coma. When the hemispasm is on the right side, showing affection of the left hemisphere, temporary aphasia may be produced, and there may be hemiplegia with this, or left hemiplegia without aphasia. This hemispasm is due to irritation of the convolutions of the opposite hemisphere. When such fits succeed each other more or less rapidly, the mind becomes affected. There is irritability of temper; the patient is sometimes in a state of hysteria, laughing and crying alternately without any adequate cause; he is generally depressed in spirits; the memory is impaired, and the current of thoughts considerably retarded; the speech is embarrassed; the patient is unable to finish a sentence, and sometimes stops for a minute without being able to go on; he tries to hold himself with gestures, but even this aid after a time forsakes him, and complete aphasia, agraphia, and amimia may become developed.

In such cases there is no hemiplegia or any other form of actual paralysis; but there is paresis, such as we are apt to connect with disease of Hitzig and Ferrier's psycho-motor centres. The patient is still able to walk. to dress and feed himself, but he is clumsy in doing so; the foot drags on the ground; he becomes gradually more helpless; there are frequent epileptic fits, and sometimes he does not awake from the coma; or decubitus is developed, leading to blood-poisoning; or death supervenes from total exhaustion of the nervous force.

The symptoms just described arise from a syphiloma of the subarachnoid space, which gradually involves the cortex of the brain and adjacent medullary matter. Where the third left frontal convolution and its neighbourhood are suffering, aphasia and agraphia will be the result. Where the anterior lobes are affected, there will be symptoms of paresis; while irritation of the posterior lobes causes melancholia, without much, if any, loss of motor power. But whatever portion of the cineritious structure is affected, syphilitic epilepsy will be the most prominent symptom.

The cerebral nerves generally suffer in exact proportion to the seat of the syphiloma, which causes irritation, and finally destruction of the nerve-trunk. The gummatous tumour sometimes grows right round a nerve, and so compresses it, or it squeezes it against the bone; or an exostosis may occur in the osseous canal through which the nerve has to pass. It is quite true that a nerve is occasionally discovered passing right through a syphiloma at the base, without having lost its function or structure; but such cases are exceptional.

The general sequence of events is neuritis, followed by atrophy. The nerve appears at first reddish and softened, its sheath is thickened; and at a later period it is wasted and changed into a thin thread. Sometimes the sheath of the nerve appears perfectly normal, but on opening it the nervous substance is seen to have disappeared, and to be replaced by a reddish or yellow mass, corresponding in structure to the soft and hard syphiloma. In other instances the syphiloma grows directly from the pia mater along the bloodvessels into the nervous substance, more particularly into the chiasma of the optic nerves, causing atrophy of the same. Finally, there may be no structural lesion, although symptoms of paralysis, anæsthesia, and neuralgia may have been present during life. Dr. Hughlings-Jackson[1] is therefore incorrect in stating that the pathogenesis of these cases is nothing but a squeezing of nerve-fibres by overgrowth of the connective-tissue element; this is only one of several causes.

Amongst the cranial nerves the third is most frequently affected by syphilis, and the most common symptoms are ptosis, external strabismus, and paralytic dilatation of the pupil. Vertigo is occasionally a symptom of paralysis of this nerve. Syphilitic neuro-retinitis and simple retinitis are also common. There is effusion of serum into the layers of the retina, which is sometimes slight and sometimes considerable, and is generally preceded by hyperæmia. The outline of the disk is rendered indistinct and hazy, and the neighbourhood of the yellow spot is particularly affected. Sometimes the vitreous humour becomes turbid, and prevents a thorough ophthalmoscopic examination. Where the effusion takes place rapidly, the sight may be quickly destroyed; but in most cases it occurs slowly. It is not unfrequently associated with irido-choroiditis. Dr. Hughlings-Jackson has pointed out that double optic neuritis may often be recognized by the ophthalmoscope before vision suffers, and that it may be for sometime the only symptom, or be accompanied with such slight symptoms as to be hardly noticed.

The portio dura and the fifth and sixth nerves may likewise suffer; there is then inability to close the eye, neuralgia of the face, with lachrymation, paralysis of mastication, and internal strabismus.

3. The third and last form of cerebral syphilis is disease of the arteries, which affects with preference the carotids, the circle of Willis, the Sylvian artery, and that of the corpus callosum. The first symptom of disease is, that the artery becomes less transparent, and loses its pink colour, assuming instead of it a white-grayish appearance. At the same time the vessel loses its cylindrical shape and becomes quite round, while its coat is hardened, and gives a cartilaginous sensa-

[1] Journal of Mental Science, July, 1875, page 5.

tion to the finger. The diameter of the vessel is very much reduced by the deposition of a moist gray substance, which later on becomes hard and dry, and what
remains of a free canal is often blocked up by thrombosis, so that ultimately the
whole artery is changed into a solid cord. This deposit takes place chiefly between the endothelium and the elastic fibres of the vessel. At first it appears to
consist of endothelial cells, which multiply considerably, and develop into connective tissue. This growth goes on in a longitudinal as well as in a transverse
direction, and the degeneration is therefore apt to spread to the branches of the
artery.

Heubner and Cohnheim have distinguished two spheres of cerebral nutrition,
which differ considerably from one another, viz., the basal and the cortical sphere.
In syphilitic disease of cerebral arteries, these considerations become of paramount
importance. The basal sphere comprises the vertebral, basilar, and carotid arteries, the circle of Willis, and the commencement of the anterior, middle, and
posterior cerebral arteries. All these vessels give off small branches vertically,
which penetrate directly into the cerebral matter, become divided and terminal,
and then proceed through the capillary vessels into the smaller veins. It is particularly in this basal sphere, which supplies the central ganglia, that plugging of
the arteries from deposit and subsequent thrombosis becomes so dangerous to the
nutrition of the parts; for as there is no anastomosis, the various forms of necro-
biosis, such as red, yellow, and white softening, are easily produced, the results
being generally syphilitic hemiplegia.

In the cortical sphere of nutrition, on the other hand, the plugging of arteries
is not of the same vital importance, because the peripheral part of the bloodvessel may still be supplied with blood by anastomosis in the pia mater. The
cortical arteries run for a long time in the pia mater without giving off any
branches to the cerebral substance : they divide in the pia, become constantly
smaller, and anastomose so thoroughly with their fellows, that a kind of network
is established, by means of which not only the smaller branches, but also the
principal arteries, are made to communicate with each other. The cerebral matter only receives small capillary vessels from this large vascular net after it has
been allowed to spread over a considerable surface. Although, therefore, the
danger of starvation is much less in the cortex than in the central ganglia, nevertheless a rapid plugging cannot pass without causing mischief, inasmuch as it
decreases the pressure in those vessels; while, if collateral circulation is established, the pressure may be suddenly increased above the normal standard. The
cineritious substance is thus exposed to considerable vicissitudes of circulation,
and the temporary apoplectic seizures which are so common in this form of syphilis
find in the same a satisfactory explanation.

In both spheres of nutrition, however—the basal as well as the cortical—simple
narrowing of the arterial tubes, without actual plugging of the same, must have
a deleterious influence on the nutrition of the entire brain. It increases the
resistance offered to the current of blood, which becomes further retarded by the
rigidity of the tube, which has lost its elasticity. The interchange of oxygen
and of nutritive material is therefore considerably lessened, which explains the
loss of energy, the impairment of the mental functions, and the somnolence
which is found in a number of these cases.

Where the basal sphere of nutrition suffers, the symptoms are generally rapidly
developed. It is not by any means rare that, after a few insignificant premonitory symptoms, there is a sudden stroke of apoplexy, which proves fatal. The
symptoms of this form of apoplexy are in all respects similar to those of ordinary
apoplexy from cerebral hæmorrhage. Multiple thrombosis of several important
basal arteries is discovered post-mortem.

In other cases there are premonitory symptoms chiefly on the part of the cranial nerves. These are ptosis, double vision, weakness of sight from optic neuritis, anæsthesia, and neuralgia in certain branches of the fifth nerve, spasm in the portio dura and sixth nerve, etc. These symptoms may come on, as it were, spontaneously, or after mental and physical efforts, excitement, and indulgence in alcohol and the sexual appetite. After a time there is a somewhat slowly produced attack of hemiplegia, with or without aphasia, and without loss of consciousness. If collateral circulation is established the patient may gradually improve; or he sinks into a somnolent condition resembling that of typhoid fever. There are headache, confusion, fussiness; the patient has a staring, absent look, and a morose expression of the countenance. He will on occasions pass his water or fæces in the middle of the room, and does other things which show absence of the feeling of shame; but on being talked to he generally becomes more reasonable. He will often refuse food, and die in the first or subsequent attacks; yet where all these symptoms have been present an immense improvement may by proper treatment be brought about in the patient's condition.

When there has been true hemiplegia, recovery is generally imperfect, even under the best treatment. There are, however, temporary kinds of hemiplegia, which only persist for a day or two, and where the starvation of cerebral tissue is evidently of too short duration to cause any great degree of softening. In some cases hemiplegia is followed by Türck's sclerosis of the lateral columns of the spinal cord, just as after ordinary cerebral hæmorrhage.

Syphilitic Affections of the Spinal Cord.—These are much more rare than the corresponding diseases of the brain and cranial nerves, and there are as yet only few post-mortem examinations of such cases put on record.

The syphiloma occurs in its two forms—viz., as jelly and as cheese—in the pia mater and the subarachnoid space. The three membranes are found grown together with each other and with the surface of the cord. There are, however, not circumscribed tumours as in the brain, but a kind of infiltration of the meninges and lymphatic spaces by gummatous effusions, which appear small, multiple, and disseminated. Where the membranes grow together with the periosteum of vertebræ and the surface of the cord, there is generally proliferation of the neuroglia and wasting of the white columns. Some cases in which the symptoms of acute ascending spinal paralysis are observed during life seem to be owing to hyperæmia simply, as no real structural alterations of the cord have been discovered.

In this latter case the symptoms generally commence at an early period—viz., in the first year—and are accompanied by the usual early manifestations of constitutional syphilis. The first symptom is sudden paraplegia, with incontinence of urine and the fæces. There is no pain in the spine, and no anæsthesia of the limbs. Decubitus soon becomes developed, and the patient dies within a few weeks from the beginning of these symptoms.

More frequently, however, paralysis comes on in the later periods of the disease, after any other symptoms have existed for a long time. There is a ruddy pallor of the skin, and a disagreeable smell about the patient, who is generally feeble and in a state of constant *malaise*. He experiences pain at different points of the spine, which is increased by pressure; and also pain, pins-and-needles, numbness and stiffness, in the lower extremities. These symptoms come and go, and then there is all of a sudden an attack of paraplegia or hemi-paraplegia. Where the seat of the disease is in the lower portion of the dorsal cord, there is also paralysis of the sphincters. If the case is not well treated, the paralysis remains stationary, and ultimately decubitus is developed, which shortly leads to a fatal result. By proper treatment, however, the patient may get well in a very short time. Some years ago I was consulted by a patient of this kind, only two days after the paraplegia had become developed. He was carried into my consulting-room on the back of a cabman, and had completely lost power over the lower extremities, but only slightly over the sphincters; there was no anæsthesia. Under full doses of iodide of potassium the patient improved most rapidly, and walked briskly into my room a week after I had first seen him. He did, however, not perfectly recover, as a slight degree of weakness in the left leg has remained up to this day.

Where the cervical spine is affected, matters are more serious. There is then not only paraplegia and paralysis of the sphincters, but also of the thoracic and abdominal muscles, the upper extremities, and the diaphragm. Asphyxia from paralysis of the phrenic nerve, or pneumonia, generally carry the patients off in a short time, unless, as we have seen it, the remedy proves stronger than the disease. But in cases of this class we cannot look forward to perfect recovery, as the posterior columns of the cord generally become disorganized beyond thorough repair, and a state resembling locomotor ataxy may remain for life.

—

Some Affections of the Nervous System dependent upon a Gouty Habit.

Dr. J. RUSSELL REYNOLDS, Prof. of Principles and Practice of Medicine in University College, London, calls attention (*British Med. Journ.*, Dec. 15, 1877) to the dependence of "nervous derangement" upon a "gouty habit." Although long known, he does not think that the frequency of such association has been fully recognized, and his present object, he says, is to recall attention to the subject, and to point out, so far as I am able, the characters of disturbances in the "nervous" functions which would lead to a diagnosis or suspicion of a "gouty" diathesis.

First, let me say a word or two as to both "gout" and "gouty habit." The former means a "special" change, of inflammatory sort, in the tissues of the joints, accompanied by the deposit in those tissues of urate of soda. The latter, the "gouty habit," means the underlying cause of those special symptoms in the joints, a something which may express itself also in various organs and in diverse ways.

We do not know what is the starting point or essential fact of "gouty habit," but this we may remember, that between the simply chemical process of food-digestion in the stomach, and the ultimate making up, and breaking down, and carrying away of the waste, of tissues—be they in brain, or nerve, or heart—there comes in the process of "assimilation"—or "concoction of the juices," as our forefathers called it—and also the conveyance of "excretory" material to excreting organs, and that these involve an infinity of changes in the quality of blood. This blood, which comes from food and goes to tissue, which comes from tissue and goes to excreting organs, may be healthy and lead to the formation of healthy tissue and the performance of healthy function; or it may be so deranged as to pervert the "nutrition" of certain tissues by a specific inflammatory process —"gout;" or it may disturb the "functions" of other organs by the impression which it makes upon them—"gouty habit." In other words, the "gouty habit" is a "toxæmia," chronic in its duration and multiform in its phases—a "blood-poisoning" induced *within* the system, and so far differing from the toxæmia with which we are so familiar, but which is introduced from *without*. That which has led me to believe that many so-called "nervous affections" are due to this "gouty habit" may be thus summarized: 1. The actual presence of gout in the joints of the individual at the time or at previous times. 2. The evidence of "gout" in ancestors or collateral relatives. 3. The frequent occurrence of acid eructations ·

with chronic dyspepsia. 4. The emission of pale, limpid, acid urine, of low specific gravity, and with traces of albumen or sugar, or both. 5. The variability of symptoms, both as to kind and place. 6. The presence of some alterations in skin-nutrition, such as eczema and psoriasis. 7. The impossibility of referring the symptoms to any known disease of brain or spinal cord. 8. The immediate relief of such symptoms after treatment by colchicum and saline aperients, although simple purgation and treatment upon many other principles had failed.

In the endeavour to arrange this subject, there is great difficulty to be encountered; but I will adopt the method of describing "groups of symptoms" under five headings:—

I. *Mental Disturbances.*—Many cases have come before me in which there was great restlessness; the patient could not be still for a moment; was alternately excited and depressed; slept badly, or not at all; was intensely hysterical; and could not attend to business; while others have complained of failing memory; of want of power of attention; of suicidal thoughts; of intense melancholy; others of sounds in the ears; voices, sometimes distinct, sometimes not; and some or all of these of long continuance; but yet all disappearing under treatment upon the hypothesis I have mentioned. These symptoms often alternate with, or accompany, those which I mention next.

II. *Pain in the Head.*—Some of the most intense head-pain that I have met with has been of this character, and been relieved by treatment of an anti-gouty description. The special features are pain on one side of the head, usually parietal or occipital; "grinding" habitually; but forced into almost intolerable severity by movement, such as the jar of carriage-riding, or running down the stairs of a house; and this without any over-sensitive nerve-points; without tenderness of scalp; and without any aggravation by mental exertion. It is not affected by posture or by food; it is relieved by physical rest, and may disappear entirely after treatment of the kind that I have mentioned. It is not anæmic, nor neuralgic, nor dyspeptic (in the ordinary sense of that word), and it yields to nothing in the way of treatment that may be directed against those common varieties of headaches. It is very often associated with some of the other symptoms that I have mentioned, and they must be taken into account when making a diagnosis of the malady.

III. *Modified Sensations.*—1. Of these, vertigo is one of the most common, and it may exist alone. It takes sometimes the form of objective movement, but more frequently that of subjective movement, such as the sense of "swimming" or "floating" away. This vertiginous sensation is sometimes determined by posture, and occurs only when the patient lies on one side, it may be the left or the right; the apparent movement of external objects being from that side towards the other.

2. With vertigo is often associated "noise in the ears," not the sound of "voices," but drumming, hissing, singing sounds, recognized to be in the ears, or in one ear, or in the head, and not appearing to come from outside. There is not, or need not be, any mental delusion with regard to these; the patient knowing well that they are inside his organism.

3. Associated with such vertigo and tinnitus there is frequently deafness, and the feeling of "beating in the ear;" and the symptoms are like those described by Menière; but I have found them in the vast majority of instances associated with a gouty habit. With vertigo and tinnitus there may be much mental depression, or attacks of bewilderment, amounting sometimes to those of *le petit mal.*

4. Modified sensations in the limbs may occur. A large number of people

complain of "numbness," "tingling," "creeping," "deadness," or some
other altered state of sensibility in the limbs, which, sometimes taking a paraplegic, sometimes a hemiplegic, distribution, have caused much anxiety; and the
more so, because the suggestion of organic disease of brain or spinal cord has
sometimes been conveyed, and yet all these troubles pass away. That which I
have observed to be in them the most characteristic of their gouty origin is their
variability in kind and locality. To-day, for example, there is "coldness" in
the left leg; to-morrow, "a sense of heat;" last week, a "pricking" in the
right hand; the week before, a "stinging" feeling on the side of the head, or in
the tongue. This wide distribution and variability, so alarming to the patient,
is much less alarming to the physician, who recognizes in these very facts the
elements for a favourable prognosis.

Here, too, I must mention the great frequency with which pains, flying pains,
darting pains, often like those of ataxy, are met with in the limbs. So-called
"sciatica" is of frequent occurrence, and "pleurodynia," and "myodynia" of
all localities are common enough. The sciatica of gouty sort is often double,
shifting from side to side with a frequency that does not improve the temper of
the gouty patient, but may raise the hope of his physician as to the probability of
cure. Other seats of pain are most frequently the insertion of the deltoid muscle
and the inner aspect of the upper arm, the ankles, the heels, and the interscapu-
lar region. The lower mammary region on the left side is often the seat of pain,
as it, indeed, is in many other maladies.

IV. *Modifications of Muscular Action.*—1. Cardiac palpitation, intermittence
or irregularity of pulse, or painful aortic pulsation at and below the epigastrium,
often suggest to the patient the presence of cardiac disease; and it is worthy of
remark that, on the one hand, a very great amount of discomfort may often be
felt by the patient when the physician can discover no change in sound of heart
or rhythm of pulse; and that, on the other, disease of aortic valves, and other
obvious signs of cardiac change, may often be discovered by the physician in a
gouty patient, he having never been conscious of any thoracic trouble.

2. Flickering contractions of muscles in the limbs; tonic spasm, with cramp-
like pain; and "startings" on falling asleep have often appeared to me to be of
gouty origin, and that for the reasons that I have assigned. Priapism, without
erotic feeling, is also very common. It sometimes disturbs the sleep, is felt on
awaking, but quickly disappears without emission,

3. Local weakness of muscles, such as ptosis, single or double; want of co-
ordination of movement of the limbs, both upper and lower, giving an awkward-
ness of movement and an ataxic gait, are among the symptoms that may have
the course and history that I have suggested. I have recently seen several cases
of ataxia, and one with marked double ptosis, which had been treated unsuccessfully upon a syphilitic hypothesis, but which recovered speedily when the treatment was based upon a gouty theory.

V. Lastly, there are symptoms beyond those which I have mentioned, and
which do not form part of the matter for my description now, but which I will
simply enumerate as being further guides or helps in the diagnosis of gouty cases:
1. Dyspepsia, cardialgia, distension of stomach and colon with flatus, pyrosis,
and acid eructations; 2. Varicosity of veins, with tendency, upon slight injuries,
to occlusion of veins; 3. Brittleness and vertical lining of the nails of both
fingers and toes; 4. Slight conjunctivitis with occasional chemosis.

The groups of symptoms that I have enumerated rather than described sometimes coexist, sometimes alternate, and their phases are often very puzzling.
They present great difficulties in diagnosis and in treatment until the clue is
caught. It is often saddening to look through the carefully cherished prescrip-

tions, and especially when they are one's own, and see the long array of drugs that have done no good—iodine, bromine, strychnine, quinine, zinc, iron, silver, cerium, arsenic, valerian, and hops, to say nothing of mercury, bitter infusions, mineral acids, and the like; but then one's sorrow may often be turned into joy—and a joy in which the patient most heartily participates—when a simple treatment, such as I have suggested, is adopted, and all the troubles disappear with a rapidity that seems quite magical, and reminds one of that beautiful process of clearing a photographic picture by cyanide of potassium.

On Inhalation of Salicylic Acid in Whooping-Cough.

R. Otto (*St. Petersburg Med. Wochenschrift*, Nos. 22 and 23, 1877), believing whooping-cough to be due to the presence of a vegetable parasite, employed inhalation of a two per cent. solution of salicylic acid in an epidemic of the disease which broke out at Lisetz in Livonia, in August, 1876. The treatment was applied in seven cases, and was commenced as soon as the convulsive stage appeared. The number of paroxysms was rather rapidly diminished in all the cases; the best results were observed in children who were in rooms of which the temperature was kept equal. The author says that he does not attempt to show from these few cases that this treatment is absolutely effectual in whooping-cough; he merely desires that the remedy should have a further trial.—*London Med. Record*, Dec. 15, 1877.

On a Case of Cutaneous Emphysema following the Opening of a Pulmonary Cavity into an Intercostal Space.

Dr. G. Galli describes, in the *Rivista Clinicá de Bologna* (extract in *Lo Sperimentale*, October), the case of a phthisical girl, aged 17, who had an extensive superficial cavity at the apex of the right lung. One day the fever increased, and, a short time afterwards, the patient complained of pain at the part of the chest corresponding to the cavity. A soft swelling was formed there, which, on being handled, gave the sensation of crepitation characteristic of emphysema. The swelling gradually spread to the whole right side of the chest, the neck, the face as far as the forehead, and the upper limbs. The patient died six days after the appearance of the emphysema.

At the necropsy, a large cavity was found at the apex of the right lung. The adjacent pulmonary pleura had become firmly adherent to the costal pleura; and at its anterior part the cavity communicated, by means of a large opening in the third intercostal space, with the areolar tissue of the thoracic walls. The third and fourth ribs were inflamed, and denuded at the seat of the lesion. The great and small pectoral muscles, the serratus magnus, etc., were of a blackish colour, softened, and infiltrated with fetid purulent matter.—*London Med. Record*, Dec. 15, 1877.

Thoracentesis.

Dr. Dieulafoy, in a series of papers published in the *Gazette Hebdomadaire* (October 5 and 12, November 9 and 16), under the title "Thoracentesis by Aspiration in Acute Pleurisy," and founded on 65 cases of acute pleurisy and 149 of thoracentesis by aspiration, after going into a critical examination of the various opinions that have been published of late years, arrives at the following conclusions:—

"Thoracentesis by aspiration in acute pleurisy is an insignificant operation and absolutely inoffensive. It should be practised with the needle No. 2, and the

quantity of liquid at a *séance* ought never exceed 1000 grammes. The accidents of which it has been accused are of different kinds, and may be divided into
three categories. Those of the third category (the so-called transformation of a
serous liquid into a purulent one) cannot be imputed to the thoracentesis; for I
believe I have demonstrated that this is due to a natural evolution of legitimate
purulent pleurisies, and in nowise to an induced transformation of their liquid.
The accidents of the second category (syncope, asphyxia, hemiplegia), due to
autochthonous or migratory coagula of the heart and pulmonary vessels, or supervening under the influence of other causes (as pleuro-pulmonary gangrene, and
the general condition of the individual), should not be placed to the account of
the thoracentesis, since they are met with in the course of pleurisies before as well
as after thoracentesis, supervening on the fact of the pleurisy itself, and not on
the fact of the operation. The incidents of the first category (acute œdema of the
lungs, and pulmonary congestion with or without albuminous expectoration) are
the only accidents which are directly and truly imputable to thoracentesis; but
they are also precisely those which may be easily avoided and prevented. On
the investigation of all the examples of this class of accidents, I find that they
have always been associated with either the immediate evacuation of a large
quantity of liquid, or with pleurisies complicated with affections of the heart,
bronchitis, tuberculosis, etc.; and the precept is to limit the quantity of liquid
extracted at a time, and to proportion this to the complications which may exist.
The operative procedure being fixed and invariable, there is nothing variable but
the indications of thoracentesis, and these are summed up in two words—the thoracentesis is either urgent, or it is discussionable. The urgency of the operation is
entirely dependent on the quantity of liquid effused, viz., when this amounts to
about 1800 or 2000 grammes in a well-formed adult. In discussionable cases,
where such amount does not exist, we should await the termination of the febrile
stage, and aspiration should only be resorted to when the absorption of the liquid
is slow and difficult."—*Med. Times and Gazette*, Jan. 5, 1878.

Perforation of the Aorta by a Foreign Body.

Dr. ASCHENBORN, of the Bethanien Hospital, Berlin, relates (*Berlin Klin.
Woch.*, Dec. 10) the interesting case of a lad, sixteen years of age, who swallowed
a needle with a hard piece of bread on June 29· The needle was detained in and
penetrated the œsophagus, but did not cause much pain during the first two days.
By the efforts of swallowing food, which was afterwards taken, the needle was
thrust in still further, and on the third day penetrated the descending thoracic
aorta. The connective tissue between the aorta and the œsophagus was separated
by the effused blood; but the coagulum which was there formed acted as a plug,
arresting the further hemorrhage for two days, but induced severe pain by the
pressure it exerted on the mediastinum. The heart was also thrust forward by
the extravasation. Under the influence of particles of food, which penetrated by
the side of the needle into the mediastinum, the coagulum soon putrefied, and,
ceasing to act as a plug, the bleeding from the wound in the aorta recurred in
increased quantity, and on July 9 terminated the patient's sufferings. At the
autopsy a needle 5.0 centimetres in length, with a long thread attached, was found
penetrating the œsophagus and aorta.—*Med. Times and Gazette*, Jan. 5, 1878.

On Jaborandi in Cardiac and Renal Dropsy.

Dr. PURJESZ of Buda-Pesth some time ago published an article in the *Berliner
Klinische Wochenschrift*, in which he stated that the diaphoretic and sialagogue
action of jaborandi diminished with the continued use of the drug; and that

under its use, in cases of parenchymatous nephritis, while diuresis was promoted, the amount of albumen in the urine was increased. In a subsequent paper, published in the *Deutsches Archiv für Klin. Med.*, Band xvii., he gives the results of observations on four patients under Professor Wagner's care in the University Clinic. Two had contracted kidney; one had insufficiency of the mitral and tricuspid valves with considerable ascites. It was found that the diaphoretic action was unequal, being almost absent in one; while the action on the salivary secretion was well marked. The diuretic action was but slight; in both cases of the contracted kidney, the medicine had no effect on the progress of the disease, while the albumen in the urine increased from the first dose; in the case of heart-disease, the ascites remained unaffected; and in the case of psoriasis, the increased perspiration had no effect. In all the cases, the appetite was impaired by the medicine. The author considers that these results confirm the observations previously made by him, that jaborandi is not a proper drug for the treatment of cardiac and renal dropsy.—*London Med. Record*, Dec. 15, 1877.

On the Diuretic Action of Blatta Orientalis in Scarlatinal Nephritis.

S. UNTERBERGER (*Petersburg Med. Worchenschrift*, 1877, No. 34) has tried, in the Nicolai Children's Hospital at St. Petersburg, the blatta orientalis, recommended by Bogomolow as a remedy for dropsy. It was given to children suffering from scarlatinal nephritis, in doses of about two and three-quarters to four and a half grains three times daily. The œdema diminished, the weight of the body was decreased, the urine was increased in quantity and contained less albumen, while the kidneys and bowels were not injuriously affected.—*London Med. Record*, Dec. 15, 1877.

A Case of Paralysis of the Diaphragm with Peculiar Laryngeal Symptoms.

Dr. EDWARD LONG FOX, Physician to the Bristol Royal Infirmary, reports (*British Med. Journ.*, Dec. 15, 1877) the following interesting case:—

In December, 1875, a boy came under my observation who had been under the care of Mr. Reid, of Tenby, and Dr. West, of London. Mr. Reid's account dated from a month previously. He had found tenderness and pain in the epigastric region, with great enlargement of the abdomen, dulness on percussion over the epigastric, right hypochondriac, and upper part of the umbilical regions. There was a slight sound on inspiration, somewhat like an eructation, but evidently spasmodic and involuntary. This sound increased in intensity day by day, until it became most distressing, sometimes resembling the clucking of a hen, sometimes the noise made by a turkey, and eventually it became like the scream of a peacock. It ceased during sleep; but sleep was very difficult, and henbane had been found the best hypnotic.

Mr. Reid considered the child was suffering from albuminous liver and kidneys; the more so that, on one occasion, he had found the urine albuminous. But this latter symptom may have been accidental, as the urine was always healthy during the year of my observation of him.

At the date of my seeing him, he was taking a nightly dose of henbane to the extent of two drachms. He seemed a bright, intelligent boy. On stripping him, the upper part of the abdomen was very prominent. The respiration was rather forced and wholly thoracic; the diaphragm seemed to be completely inert; and I considered that the prominence and dulness of the upper part of the abdomen were due to the alteration of the position of the liver and other organs caused by this condition of the diaphragm. The respiration was very noisy both on inspiration and expiration, and simulated a peacock's cry pretty closely; it never ceased for an instant, except during sleep. Swallowing was rather difficult, especially of solids. The eyesight was not as good as before his illness, but he somewhat exaggerated his weakness in this respect. Ophthalmoscopic examination revealed no lesion in the eyes. His general health was otherwise pretty good; but he was both excitable and depressed, from consciousness of the annoyance caused to other people by his noisy breathing. Sensory and motor powers in the limbs were perfect.

The only previous history that seemed to bear upon the causation of these symptoms was that, nearly a year before his present illness began, he had had a severe blow on the cervical region of the spine from a boy at school. My belief was that the boy was suffering from paresis of the phrenic nerves and irritation of the recurrent laryngeal, the results of an irritative condition of the cervical cord induced by the blow. In the absence of post-mortem investigation of the cord, the lesion must remain unknown; but it may be presumed that it was entirely connected with the circulation in the spinal cord.

Under gelseminum, and then strychnia, with faradization used with one pole over the cervical spine and the other along the upper and most prominent part of the epigastrium, the diaphragm in about two months' time began to act slightly, and after three months abdominal respiration was restored. His power of swallowing and his eyesight improved, and the dose of henbane was gradually reduced. His mother and he were turned out of several lodgings in consequence of his noisy respiration; but in six months' time this also improved, mainly under the use of strychnia, with the good air of country lodgings, and with farm-house occupations and food; and it ceased twelve months ago. Whilst he was getting better in this respect, the peacock's cry could always be induced by any loud sudden noise, or, indeed, by anything that caused a jar. He has now been perfectly well for a year, and is able to resume his education.

Surgery.

The Clinical Aspect of Central Localization.

M. TILLAUX, while bringing some specimens under the notice of the Société de Chirurgie (*L' Union Méd.*, December 13), observed that clinical observation had not entirely confirmed the results of physiological experiments on cerebral localization, and, as far as indications for the employment of the trephine were concerned, he owned himself entirely of the opinion of Prof. Gosselin (*Monthly Abstract of Medical Science*, June, 1877, page 272), that we are not authorized to resort to this instrument for primary injuries except in cases in which there is fracture with depression. He can admit but one exception to this rule—viz., when there is a fissure of the cranium opposite the centres, and motor paralysis of the opposite side. Beyond this case, the trephine is not applicable for the treatment of primary effusions of blood. Is it the same with respect to slow, delayed accidents, which appear only consecutively? M. Tillaux believes not; and it is in this direction, in his opinion, that surgeons should seek for indications for the employment of the trephine. In this view he laid specimens before the Society. The first of these was the brain of a man upon whose head a shutter had fallen, striking him upon the left side of the posterior part of the skull. The man immediately became unconscious, and on the fourth day was attacked with aphasia

and with right brachial monoplegia. These accidents disappeared, and he was
able to resume his employment, although there still remained very intense pain
in the head. This brought him under M. Tillaux's care at the hospital, where
he found great relief from the iodide of potassium. After a while a new attack
of aphasia and right brachial monoplegia occurred, which terminated fatally. At
the autopsy there was found a patch of meningo-encephalitis, which measured
more than 0.04 centimetres, and occupied the whole of the third left frontal convolution. In face of such a lesion, the seat of which could be perfectly well determined by the occurrence of the aphasia and monoplegia, but the extent of
which could not be suspected, M. Tillaux demanded what would be the effect of
the trephine applied at the point indicated by Prof. Broca. The other specimen,
which had been lent by M. Raynaud, was derived from a woman fifty-nine years
of age, who had been the subject of complete left hemiplegia, with hemianæsthesia, immobility of the head on the side of the paralysis, and conjugate deviation of the eyes of the same side. At the autopsy there was found an encephaloid tumour the size of an egg, which occupied the most remote part of the fissure
of Sylvius, having depressed the first temporal convolution, and projected upwards the parietal lobe of the left side and the third ascending frontal convolution.
It is evident that this tumour would produce the phenomena of compression, which,
affecting the motor centres at a distance, might give rise to serious errors as regards cerebral localization. From these cases M. Tillaux draws the following
conclusions: 1. Even when the lesion is in intimate relation with the convolution which is the centre of the abolished motion there is danger, in applying the
trephine, of coming upon a large patch of meningo-encephalitis, and thus to perform an operation which is at least useless. 2. A lesion of the brain may give
rise to disturbances at a distance ; so that by following rules drawn from the doctrine of cerebral localization for the application of the trephine, we are liable to
attack a point very remote from the evil.

M. Lucas-Championnière observed, in reference to the second of these cases,
that all writers put aside cases of cerebral tumours in relation to these localizations ; but the first case proves the utility of the doctrine of localization in a
surgical point of view ; for if the patient had been trephined he might have been
cured. He is an advocate for the use of the trephine for the dissipation of the
primary accidents in these cases. In his opinion, patients have been let die who
might have been saved by the operation. There is no example on record of
primary paralysis in these cases having been cured without operation ; so that
there is good reason to seek for indications for its performance. M. Tillaux explained that he is no adversary of indications for the use of the trephine being
drawn from cerebral localization ; but he believes that more light as yet is wanted
upon the subject. As to the case which he had related, trephining certainly would
not have saved the patient, seeing on the one hand the extent of the lesion, and
on the other that the lesion of the soft parts was situated 0.07 centimetres behind
the cerebral lesion.

At a subsequent meeting of the Society (*Gaz. des Hôp.*, December 15), M.
Perrin stated that he quite agreed with M. Tillaux as to the danger of hasty trephining. Cerebral localizations can be no guide for the surgeon in this operation.
The cerebral disturbances that ensue may be transitory or inaccessible to treatment ;
and trephining in many cases would only add to the complications, some of those
who recover after it recovering in spite of it. M. Lucas-Championnière has expressed himself too absolutely as to the non-recovery after fracture with primary
cerebral complications, as is shown by two cases which have come under M.
Perrin's own care. In one of these a soldier, whose skull was fractured by a shell,
passed from a state of coma into one of aphasia, from which he recovered com-

pletely in two months. In the other case, a man had the right side of the skull fractured, with slight depression, during the siege, and immediately became unconscious. Hemiplegia of the left side soon occurred, and paralysis of the right side of the face, with dilatation of the pupil and loss of hearing on the same side, his speech being also embarrassed. These accidents became afterwards complicated with incontinence of urine, obstinate constipation, and eschars of the sacrum and paralyzed limbs. Still the patient was cured, although so long a time as two years was required. M. Desprès stated that he had never as yet met with a case in which he found any indication for trephining. This abstinence from the operation was suggested to him by a case which he had seen in the service of Manec in 1859. A workman, while digging in a pit, had a heavy body fall on his head, which fractured the skull, driving into the wound fragments of bone, the scalp, and the cap he wore. For five days the patient did well, and then for a fortnight he had brachial monoplegia, and a slight degree of facial paralysis. In a short time all that had penetrated the cranium was eliminated, and the patient was cured without any other treatment than expectation.—*Med. Times and Gaz.,* Dec. 29, 1877.

The Pathology of Concussion.

A new light has been thrown upon this obscure question by the experimental investigation which M. DURET, already so well known for his careful anatomical and experimental researches on the nervous system, has recently laid before the Société de Biologie. A mere oscillatory disturbance of the encephalon is not a satisfactory explanation of the loss of consciousness and the cardiac and respiratory troubles which supervene after a violent blow on the head; and it is contrary to what we know of the physical and physiological condition of the encephalon to believe that such oscillations could be so slight as to produce such marked disturbances of function without effecting at the same time some anatomical alteration. Blows on other organs do not alter their functions without leaving traces of structural change. In his experiments on animals, M. Duret was able to reproduce the symptoms of concussion in the human subject in all its degrees of temporary loss of consciousness with slow respiration and slow pulse, greater duration of the same phenomena, and, lastly, sudden death. As blows upon the head produced results difficult to analyze, he proceeded by making a small opening in the cranium by means of a perforator, and injecting various fluids through this. Sometimes he used water, sometimes coagulable substances, such as gelatine. As experiments upon the cerebral hemispheres proper have shown that these may be removed in almost their entire extent without producing the cardiac and pulmonary symptoms of concussion, he was led to expect that the medulla was the part in which the lesions, if any, would be found. By injecting a large quantity of fluid, he succeeded in bursting the fourth ventricle and tearing up the aqueduct of Sylvius; and, as the same result followed the injection of a coagulable fluid which could be traced, he was able to demonstrate that the effect was due to the tension of ventricular fluid. By cutting away the cervical muscles, the occipito-atloidean membrane may be laid bare, and its respiratory pulsations watched or recorded by the graphic method. When fluid was injected into the cranial cavity, this membrane became tense, pulsation ceased, and all the clinical phenomena of a shock manifested themselves; but, on perforating this membrane with a bistoury, an escape of cerebro-spinal fluid was followed by the disappearance of all the symptoms. In addition to these results, M. Duret was able to discover numerous small hemorrhages in the substance of the medulla, and in the subarachnoid spaces, principally at the base, but also over the convexity of the brain. He confirmed these results by directly operating upon the medulla by means of a sound introduced through a small opening in the occipito-atloidean membrane, with which very limited contusions of parts of the medulla and the floor of the fourth ventricle could be caused. According to these experiments, therefore, it is to changes in the tension of the cerebro-spinal fluid, and not directly in the cerebral pulp itself, that we should refer the phenomena of concussion.—*British Med. Journal*, Dec. 29, 1877.

On Epidemic Conjunctivitis in Schools.

Dr. MANZ, of Freiberg, has a long communication in the *Berliner Klinische Wochenschrift* of September 3 and 10, on a form of epidemic conjunctivitis which has of late been very prevalent in schools in Germany. The most characteristic symptom of this epidemic is the presence in the conjunctiva of small clear vesicles, which are often the only indications of the disease; the active symptoms are congestion and swelling of the membrane. The disease runs a definite course, and is very contagious. It does not appear to give rise to corneitis, but cases occur which it is difficult to diagnose from ordinary granular ophthalmia. It is the follicular ophthalmia of recent writers.—*London Med. Record*, Dec. 15, 1877.

On the Classification of Inflammations of the Cornea.

Dr. OTTO BERGMEISTER writes at considerable length in the *Allgemeine Wiener Medizin. Zeitung* for the present year, on the classification of diseases of the cornea. He concludes by dividing corneal inflammation into superficial, deep, and choroidal. He includes in the former division phlyctenulæ, superficial ulcers, and pannus; in the second, deep ulcers, abscess, acute and chronic interstitial corneitis; and in the latter, kerato-iritis and so-called iritis serosa.—*London Med. Record*, Dec. 15, 1877.

Treatment of Ulceration of the Cornea.

The treatment of ulceration of the cornea, as practised at the Royal London Ophthalmic Hospital, Moorfields, varies necessarily according to the form of the disease, and also, to some extent, according to the experience of the surgeon under whose care the case happened to be. The yellow ointment (10 to 15 grains yellow oxide of mercury to the ounce) is found especially useful in the milder forms of ulceration, such as the majority of phlyctenular cases. The results of hot belladonna fomentation (60 grains to the pint), used every half hour and for several minutes at a time, are particularly brilliant in cases of ulceration with hopopyon. In cases of recent onyx with hopopyon much benefit was derived from cutting through the infiltrated corneal tissue. The hopopyon was generally evacuated at the time, and seldom reappeared. In none of these cases was the corneal wound reopened, as in Saemisch's operation. Where there was much pain, accompanied by increased tension, paracentesis gave temporary relief; but the most lasting benefit followed in such cases from iridectomy. Quinine internally, in doses of one or two grains thrice daily, seemed to have a most beneficial action in one or two cases of hopopyon, the pus disappearing more quickly during its administration, the other treatment remaining the same.—*Royal London Ophthalmic Hospital Reports*, Dec. 1877.

On Pterygium.

The *Berlin. Klin. Wochensch.* of November 12, contains the report of a lecture by Dr. H. SCHOLER on pterygium. The lecturer considers this affection the result of an adhesion of a fold of the conjunctiva to an ulcer of the cornea, and hence, in many cases at least, a form of the healing process. He first came to this conclusion by observing a case of gonorrhœal ophthalmia, with an ulcer of the cornea 6 *millimétres* long and 1.5 *millimétres* wide, in which healing of the ulcer was effected by the swollen conjunctiva hanging over the upper edge of the cornea and coming into contact with the ulcer. It first filled the cavity and then united with the ulcer. He observes that, if this had not resulted, the eye would have been inevitably lost. Another case also occurred to the lecturer. He removed a pterygium, the effect of a burn, and, by so doing, set up a destructive ulcer of the cornea. Led by these phenomena to investigate the subject, he made a series of forty-five experiments on animals, rabbits, cats, and dogs. He first produced an ulcer on the cornea, and then covered it over with a strip of conjunctiva dissected from the eyeball, but left attached at its corneal margin, and kept in its place by catgut sutures; the epithelial surface being placed next the cornea. He next covered the exposed under surface of this bridge of conjunctiva by a second·bridge of conjunctiva, with its epithelial surface turned outwards. Figures explaining the steps of the operation accompany the lecture. In the dogs, three in number, the adhesion of the conjunctiva to the cornea was permanent; but in the rabbits, after the healing of the ulcer, the slips of conjunctiva shrivelled and were thrown off. The physiological effects of covering the cornea were extreme vascularity of the covered portion and healing of the ulcer. The author leaves the effect of the conjunctival epithelium on the ulcer an .open question. The mechanical effects were the protection of the wound from all external influences, and the continuous pressure exerted by.the bridge of conjunctiva.

Dr. Scholer states that he has performed the operation sixteen times in the human subject, always in otherwise hopeless cases, with good results; indeed he had but one failure. He considers that this treatment is indicated in all cases of extensive ulceration of the cornea, either with or without perforation; and in cases of gaping wound of the cornea, with or without prolapse of the iris in fistula of the cornea, after paring the edges of the fistula. In cases of partial or complete staphyloma, perforating wounds of the sclerotic and in cystoid cicatrices, as only the superficial layer of the conjunctiva need be employed in this operation, no shrivelling of the conjunctival sac·need follow it.—*London Med. Record*, Dec. 15, 1877.

Glycosuric Retinitis.

Dr. STEPHEN MACKENZIE, Assistant Physician to the London Hospital, contributes to the *Royal London Ophthalmic Hospital Reports*, Dec. 1877, the report of a case of glycosuric retinitis, and accompanies it with the following brief but instructive review of our knowledge of the affection, in which he draws largely from Prof. Leber's excellent article, which was published in V. Graefe's *Archiv für Ophthalmologie*, 1875, Bd. xxi. Abth. 3. Prof. Leber has collected eighteen cases of this disease, and added another, examined with great care and minuteness by himself.

Glycosuric retinitis rarely occurs until diabetes has been in existence for a rather prolonged period. It is generally ushered in by a more or less sudden and partial loss of sight, generally one eye suffers before the other, but in most cases the two eyes are eventually attacked, though often with unequal severity. Sometimes sparks are seen before the eye or eyes, at other times dark spots or muscæ are complained of, whilst in some cases disturbance of the perception of colours is noticed. Pain does not appear to be of common occurrence. Patients usually have a succession of attacks of disturbed and limited vision, and between the attacks the sight may be in a great measure restored. In some cases the vision is

almost completely lost in one or both eyes. On ophthalmoscopic examination
the lens is usually observed to be quite transparent. The optic disk is sometimes
found red, sometimes atrophic. The retina is generally cloudy; the vessels in
many cases are distended and dilated, but in others, especially as regards the arteries, are smaller than natural. Scattered over the retina are apoplectic spots.
These sometimes occur as round patches of various sizes, from large blots to punctiform ecchymoses; sometimes as linear streaks occurring in the course of the
vessels; again at other times as linear streaks running in a direction at right
angles to the vessels. Sometimes the hemorrhages are beneath the superficial
layers of the retina, when the retinal vessels may be observed crossing the extravasation; at other times the hemorrhages are superficial, and obscure the vessels. The hemorrhages vary in tint according to their age. They often have a
brownish-red hue. In addition to the hemorrhages white spots are seen scattered
over the fundus. They are of various sizes and shapes. Sometimes they are of
opaque whiteness, at other times they have a glistening appearance; those having
the last character being generally smaller, and arranged in constellations. Such
constellations are found grouped around the yellow spot, but are not limited to
this situation. Occasionally longish white raised patches or folds, surmounted by
retinal vessels, are seen. Some of the white patches are, doubtless, altered extravasations, for white patches are met with having red borders. Others would
appear to be due to fatty degeneration of the retina. Though these appearances
are seen with more or less clearness in most cases at some period of the disease,
yet in other cases the details of the fundus are obscured by opacities in the vitreous. Sometimes on examination nothing can be seen but a red reflex; sometimes floating films can be detected, having a red or brownish colour; at other
times the vitreous is simply turbid and cloudy. These opacities of the vitreous
are obviously due to hemorrhages. They are found to occur coincidently with
sudden limitations of the visual field, and they may be observed undergoing absorption.

The appearances in the retina are very like those met with in connection with
Bright's disease. So close is the resemblance that some observers have passed
them over as albuminuric changes, indicative of nephritis brought about by the
diabetes. This opinion is favoured by the undoubted coexistence of albuminuria
with glycosuria in the majority of the cases. Besides the presence of albumen,
casts and blood have been found in the urine of some patients, who have, moreover, presented other evidences of Bright's disease, such as dropsy, hypertrophy
of the heart, etc. Still there remain a certain number of cases where it is expressly stated on competent authority, that there was no albuminuria. Thus in
two cases recorded by Desmarres,[1] one by Noyes,[2] and one by Haltenhoff,[3] there
was no albumen in the urine; in some of the cases the urine was examined repeatedly with care. In Noyes's case the amount of urea was on several occasions estimated and never found deficient. It thus seems clear that the changes
are not necessarily of an albuminuric origin. In some of the cases the sugar had
been noticed to almost or entirely disappear before the retinal affection was observed. What seems further to distinguish the intraocular changes in glycosuria
from those met with in Bright's disease, is the frequent complication of the former with hemorrhages into the vitreous. These occur equally in the cases where
the diabetes is, and where it is not, complicated by albuminuria. Hemorrhages

---

[1] Traité théor. et praet. des mal. des yeux. 2d ed. Paris, 1858, t. iii. pp. 528–526.
[2] Trans. Amer. Ophth. Soc. 1869, pp. 71–75.
[3] Retinitis hemorrhagica bei Diabetes Mellitus. Zehend., Klin. Monats., 1873. xi.
s. 291–298.

into the vitreous are of rare occurrence in pure cases of albuminuric retinitis, so far as I know. They appear to be frequent in glycosuric retinitis, and are recurrent.

As to the cause of the changes in the retina and vitreous, there remains a certain degree of obscurity. Prof. Leber, in discussing these, considers that they may be due in part to the diabetes, in part to nephritis caused by the latter, or to the two combined. But, as he says, how diabetes brings about the changes is quite unexplained, as moreover is the cause of the retinal affection in Bright's disease itself. But we find in by far the majority of instances of retinal disease that they are associated with lesions of other organs, or with altered blood conditions and disturbances of nutrition. From the analogy of Bright's disease, in cases where the lesion is not due to renal affection, one is led to look to other organs in search of an explanation. The brain and the heart suggest themselves as possibly at fault. As regards the brain, the retinal changes met with in diabetes differ from the neuritis or neuro-retinitis usually associated with cerebral disease. Cases are met with, it is true, where changes almost precisely like those encountered in albuminuria are associated with coarse lesions of the brain, such as tumour, etc., but these are rare. Still, there may be some connection between the diabetes and the retinitis. Either the brain lesion may be primary, and cause both the diabetes and the retinal affection; or, on the other hand, the diabetes may be primary, and cause both the retinal and the cerebral affections. These different classes of cases Prof. Leber has, he thinks, been able to distinguish in connection with the affections of the optic nerve in diabetes. Encephalic lesions, thus, do not appear to explain all the cases, and we turn to the heart in search of a cause. In the published cases, though the details in the records on this point are few, there is nothing to support the idea that the hemorrhages are connected with any heart affection, as in some forms of hemorrhagic retinitis. In my case there was no hypertrophy or other sign of cardiac disease. Failing to find any adequate cause for the retinal changes in any of the viscera, we are driven, as Prof. Leber says, to compare diabetes with other morbid conditions attended by a like alteration in the retina, such as Bright's disease, pernicious anæmia, hæmophilia, purpura, leuchæmia, etc. In all of these diseases there is an undoubted alteration in the blood, and, in some at least, changes in the vessels, in consequence of which diapedesis of coloured corpuscles and transudation of abnormally constituted albuminous matters take place. Such alterations are not limited to the retina, but are generally found also in the brain, spinal cord, and many other parts of the body. Their wide distribution is evidence in favour of a common origin in a blood dyscrasia. Dr. Dickinson has discussed very ably[1] the relation between the changes he finds in the nervous centres, and which resemble the appearances seen in the retina and the glycosuria. I cannot help differing from his conclusions, however, for Dr. Dickinson regards the peri-vascular extravasations and erosions of nervous structures as the cause of the symptoms in diabetes. To my mind the whole evidence points to the changes in the nervous system as well as those in the retina and other organs, being due to an altered condition of the blood. If the retinal changes found in diabetes are not due to an antecedent brain lesion, but are dependent on the same cause as the latter, then the fact that glycosuric retinitis only occurs when diabetes has been some time in existence, becomes valuable as enabling us to correctly interpret the changes found in the nervous centres. From what we know of the other diseases where similar changes are found in the retina

---

[1] Diseases of the Kidney. By W. Howship Dickinson, M.D. 1875.

and in the nervous centres. such as pernicious anæmia,[1] hæmophilia,[2] purpura,[3] leuchæmia,[4] ague,[5] the alterations in the nervous centres and in the eyes would appear to be coincident, rather than the latter sequential to the former. I think, therefore, we may justly infer that the perivascular hemorrhages, extrusions, excavations, and atrophies are the consequences and not the causes of the altered condition of the blood—I do not say the glychæmia—and bloodvessels incidental to diabetes.

On Miners' Nystagmus.

Ν. Dransart read an interesting paper on this subject before the French Association for the Advancement of Science, at Havre, on August 24th. He alluded to the observations of Decondé, Léon, Noël, Nieden, Schroter, and A. von Graefe, and stated that the affection was scarcely recognized in France. The paper, which was based on twelve cases observed by the author, treated fully of the symptomatology, course, diagnosis, prognosis, etiology, pathology, and treatment.

Symptomatology.—The nystagmus consists of an involuntary and rhythmical oscillation of the eyeballs. The number of oscillations varies from 50 to 140 in the minute. The oscillations are vertical or horizontal ; often the two forms of oscillation are combined, causing a rotatory movement of the globes. The oscillations are always synchronous, but they are not always equal in extent in the two eyes. In all cases where this inequality in extent of motion was observed, there was double vision. The oscillations are most readily excited when the line of vision is raised above the horizontal plane of the two eyeballs. Work in the pit, movements of the body, excite the nystagmus by causing this position of the line of vision. Darkness, a bright light, or anything which depresses the general health, also aggravate the oscillations ; excess of spirituous liquors acts in the same manner, but during the drinking bout the nystagmus is less, the elevator muscles having more tone and being better able to preserve their equilibrium. There is nothing characteristic in the facial appearance of the patient. In all the cases observed there were marked anæmia, hæmic murmurs, disorders of digestion, stitches in the side, and sweatings. An intimate relationship between the general condition and the nystagmus was observed. In proportion as the anæmia improved under treatment the nystagmus also diminished, and *vice versá.*

The patients complained of headache, with sensations of fulness and tingling in the eyeballs. Exactly the same symptoms are seen in asthenopia, diplopia, weakness of the internal recti, and paresis of the superior recti and the inferior oblique muscles. In all cases in which the investigation was made, the author found weakness of the superior recti and of the inferior oblique muscles. This weakness and the nystagmus went hand in hand ; in proportion as the former became less, the latter also diminished. The accommodation is always defective ; but, as the nystagmus becomes less the paresis of the ciliary muscle disappears. The refraction is natural ; the fundus healthy.

During the attacks of nystagmus, vision is blurred. During the intervals, sight

---

[1] Immerman, Deutsche Arch. f. klin. Med., 1874, xiii. 209–244. Manz. Veränderungen in der Retina bei anæmia progres. Centralblatt. f. d. med. Wissensch., 1875, No. 40, s. 675.

[2] Wickham Legg. Report from Post-Mortem Room, St. Barth. Hosp. Rep., 1875. p. 64. Author. Med. Times and Gaz., March 10, 1877.

[3] Rec. Union Med., 1870, No. 48. Author. Med. Times and Gaz., March 3, 1877.

[4] Poncet. Arch. de Physiol. norm. et Path., 1874, p. 496, and most ophth. writers.

[5] Author. Retinal Hemorrhages and Melanæmia as Symptoms of Ague. Med. Times and Gaz., June 23, 1877.

is generally perfect. In one case in which the affection had lasted for a long time a decided sluggishness of the retina, with narrowing of the field of vision, was present. Some affection of the fundus was suspected, but the patient completely recovered.

Forms of the Affection.—The nystagmus is nearly always the same. There are two varieties. In the first, which comprises the great majority of cases, the oscillation in the two eyeballs is equal in extent ; in the second form it is unequal, and there is always double vision.

Duration.—The affection may last for five or six years. As a rule, when recovery takes place, even at the end of that time, the sight is unimpaired. The author suggests the possibility of the sluggishness of the retina which was present in one of his cases continuing sufficiently long to become permanent.

The *Diagnosis* is easy. Even where there is some narrowing of the field of vision from sluggishness of the retina, the peculiar character of the oscillations, the absence of any lesion in the eye itself, and the occupation of the patient, will prevent mistakes.

Etiology.—The affection is almost confined to coal-miners. All other underground workers are exempt. The ages of the patients vary from 20 to 50 years. The affection is rare, 5 cases occurring amongst 10,000 coal-miners.

Pathology.—While admitting that the air of the mine and the darkness may in some measure predispose to the affection, the author thinks that the chief cause is the position in which the miner is obliged to keep the eyeballs while at work ; he must constantly look above the horizontal line of sight. In this position the superior rectus and the inferior oblique muscles are always on the stretch. In consequence of this excessive work a " myopathy" is set up in these muscles, as a result of which they are unable to overcome their antagonists by a single effort ; a repetition of short rapid contractions therefore takes place, causing the nystagmus. When the internal recti are affected, horizontal oscillations occur.

The author adds that he has in all cases seen this " myopathy" accompanied by anæmia, and deficient accommodation. And since these factors are always in direct proportion to the nystagmus, he concludes that they have some influence in its production.

Treatment.—M. Dransart recommends iron, quinine, strychnia, electricity, and work in daylight. The electricity ought to be applied chiefly to the muscles which elevate the eyeball, and to the internal recti.—*London Med. Record*, Dec. 15, 1877

On Syphilitic Diseases of the Eyelids.

Mr. H. Zeissl, in the *Allgemeine Wiener Med. Zeitung* for August 21 and 28, and September 4 and 11, gives a series of articles on syphilitic diseases of the eyelids. The author recognizes three forms of syphilitic diseases of the eyelids ; primary induration, erythemata and papulose eruptions (syphilitic exanthemata), and gumma. He especially draws attention to the difficulty of diagnosis between gummata and primary affections, and remarks that gummata may be confounded with carcinomatous disease (?) or rodent ulcer. Papulose diseases are distinguished from gumma by the subsequent ulceration being superficial, whilst the ulceration following gummata in the eyelids is deep and destructive. The great peculiarity of syphilides in this region is their great malignity and the destruction of tissue which they cause.—*London Med Record*, Dec. 15, 1877.

On the Treatment of Anthrax of the Face.

Carbuncle and boil of the face have often proved fatal. Therefore many writers, amongst others Reverdin, have come to the conclusion that anthrax is an exceptionally serious affection. According to them the danger is due to the phlebitis of the veins of the face, which easily spreads to the cranial sinuses. Gosselin, however, and other surgeons do not believe in this great danger; on this subject Gosselin retains the same opinion, expressed by him on the occasion of a discussion on it at the Academy of Medicine in 1866. Partly inspired by this illustrious surgeon, M. Bouhott, in his *Thèse de Paris*, 1877, endeavours to demonstrate that anthrax of the face, of the lips, as of other parts, is nearly always cured. The complication of phlebitis, which is the exception, is not necessarily fatal. Friction does not hasten cure, and exposes the patient to the risk of putridity, and consequently pyemia. For the majority of cases of anthrax of the face expectant treatment, without operation, is desirable. In serious cases there is, perhaps, necessity for cauterization.—*London Med. Record*, Dec. 15, 1877.

On Ranula in New-born Children.

In a paper read before the Moscow Medical Society and published in the *Moscow Medical Gazette* (abstract in *Central-Zeitung für Kinderheilkunde*, November 1), Dr. N. MÜLLER makes some observations on the occurrence of ranula in the newly born. The affection is so rare that its existence has been denied. Four cases have been recorded by Dubois, Bertin, Lombard, and Bland, and four others by Bryant. In the foundling hospital at Moscow, four or five cases of congenital ranula have been observed during the last seven years in about 80,000 children. Of these, Dr. Müller describes three. In a boy seven days old, a ranula as large as a pigeon's egg was found lying to the left of the frænum linguæ; in a girl three weeks old the swelling lay on both sides of the frænum, and attained the size of a large walnut before the end of the second month; and in a boy three days old there was a pyriform ranula, with the small end directed forwards, lying to the left of the frænum. The last case was apparently one of retention-cyst from obstruction of the orifice of Wharton's duct. In the first two cases the tongue was pushed upwards, and sucking was impeded. Puncture with a needle gave exit to a clear sero-mucous or (in the third case) watery discharge; the swelling then collapsed, but in a few days regained its original size. In the first case, tincture of iodine was injected; this produced suppuration, followed by cure of the ranula in three weeks. In the third case, the sac of the tumour, after having refilled, was cut away with scissors, with a successful result. In the second case incision was avoided, on account of the vascularity of the swelling, but a ligature was applied over it. The swelling did not disappear, but only became smaller. At the end of a fortnight, no change having taken place in the size of the swelling, and there being scarcely any discharge from the punctured joints, the ligature was removed. The ranula was still as large as a pigeon's egg, hard, and without fluctuation. An attempt to remove the contents by means of Pravaz's syringe was unsuccessful, as was also painting with tincture of iodine. Towards the end of the fourth month the child died of chronic enteritis. At the *post-mortem* examination there was found a cavernous cystic tumour as large as a pigeon's egg, the cavities of which were filled with a clear transparent fluid. The sublingual salivary glands were normal.—*London Med. Record*, Dec. 15, 1877.

Removal of the whole Tongue with the Scissors.

Mr. WALTER WHITEHEAD exhibited to the Manchester Medical Society (*Med. Times and Gaz.*, Dec. 15, 1877), a patient from whom he had removed the whole of the tongue, for epithelioma, by means of the scissors alone, without division of the symphysis or submental incision. The operation was thus performed: The patient, a woman, sixty-four, having been placed under the influence of chloroform, a gag was inserted, and the tongue firmly secured by a strong ligature passed through its substance near the tip. The operator, taking firm hold of this ligature with his left hand, divided successively the frænum and the sub-lingual tissues on each side. The tongue being then drawn well forward so that the epiglottis was brought fairly into view, the operation was completed by cutting through the base of the tongue, first on one side and then on the other. Two large vessels were divided: one of these was tied during the operation; the other, after bleeding for a little time, ceased spontaneously. Smart hemorrhage, however, took place after the removal of the patient, and it was found necessary to have recourse to the thermo-cautery. The operation was not followed by any constitutional disturbance, and though a fortnight had not yet elapsed, the patient appeared at the meeting perfectly well. The merit of this operation consists in its simplicity. Nearly sixty years ago Boyer described (*Traité des Maladies Chirurgicales*, tome vi.; Paris, 1818; page 392) an operation for epithelioma of the tip of the tongue, in which, by means of a pair of straight scissors, he removed a **V**-shaped portion about an inch in length, and united the flaps by sutures. But, although Mr. Whitehead distinctly repudiates any claim to originality, he is the first, so far as he is himself aware, to have demonstrated the practicability of removing the whole tongue by this simple method. With regard to the hemorrhage which occurred subsequently, he is quite convinced that this may be prevented in future by taking care to tie both ranine arteries during the operation, whether they give trouble at the time or not.

—

Treatment of Ischuria dependent on Hypertrophy of the Prostate.

E. BOTTINI proposes (*Langenbeck's Archiv*, Bd. xxi. p. 1) to treat the difficulty commonly experienced in passing water in cases of hypertrophy of the prostate gland by the galvano-caustic method. He recommends, according to the kind of the hypertrophy, either the galvano-caustic erosion or simple section of the enlarged lobule. The galvano-caustic destined for erosion, resembles the well-known prostate catheter of Mercier. It consists of two brass limbs attached to a rod, which are completely isolated from each other by a piece of ivory. Near the centre of the concavity of the instrument is situated the eroding apparatus, which consists of a **U**-shaped piece of platinum about 1½ inch in length, of which one branch is soldered to the posterior, the other to the anterior limb of the instrument. The connection with the battery is effected by means of a Middeldorpf's handle. As soon as the beak of the instrument is found to be freely movable in the bladder, which should be tolerably full, it is brought by a *tour de maître* through an angle of 180°, to such a position that the concavity looks directly backward, and is in contact with the hypertrophied parts of the prostate. These embraced as by a hook, can now be destroyed with the greatest precision, without, as autopsy has revealed, in any way damaging the surrounding parts. The thermo-galvanic incisor resembles a lithotrite, the male arm of which is composed of a platinum blade, which is attached to the staff by means of copper points, and glides in the glass appendix of the female arm. The points of the instrument must, when in use, be firmly pressed against the lobe requiring division. Neither the process of erosion nor of division occasions much pain, so that anæsthetics are not required. The urine soon begins to flow after the operation, however severe may have been the previous stranguary. No bad results have hitherto followed the use of the instruments, and not even vesical catarrh has been observed, though the urine continues to be bloody for a little while. Galvano-caustic erosion is best adapted for partial and only slightly projecting swelling of the supra-collicular part of the gland. On the other hand galvano-caustic fusion is more appropriate for cases where the whole gland is enlarged, or where particular lobes have undergone great hypertrophy. In such cases it is advisable to make the instrument press against the depression between two adjoining elevations, rather than against the projecting mass. The contra-indications against this mode of operating are inactivity of the detrusors, highly abnormal condition of the urine, and coincident extensive disease of the kidneys.—*Practitioner*, Nov. 1877.

On a Case of Imperforate Anus with Fistulous Opening into the Bladder.

The following case is recorded in the *Australian Medical Journal*, March, 1877. On April 11th, 1876, a male child, two days old, was brought to Mr. Rowan, at the Melbourne Lying-in Hospital. On examination, an imperforate condition of the anus was found; there was no depression or mark to indicate its usual position. The abdomen was distended, tympanitic, and very tender. On the next day chloroform was administered, and an incision was made in the centre of the fundament; and, after cautiously dissecting to a depth of two and a half inches, the rectum was reached. An opening was made into it, and a large quantity of meconium and flatus escaped. The wound was kept open for a week with oiled lint, and a large bougie was subsequently passed every second or third day. Mr. Rowan shortly afterwards lost sight of the child, but it was brought back to him on the first of last February, in a worse condition than in the preceding April. The bougie had not been passed for three months, and for two months the child had passed nothing by the natural passage, all the motions escaping through the penis until the previous day, when the foreskin became so narrow that the child could not pass even urine without great difficulty. Examination showed that the anus was closed about an inch from the orifice, and revealed in addition complete phimosis. Circumcision was performed, and a few days later the former passage into the rectum was reopened and enlarged sufficiently to allow the finger to be passed in. The rectum was found filled with hard feces, which did not come away until the next day. After the operation, the finger was passed every day, and at the present time the canal seems perfect. Mr. Rowan thinks that a second operation would not have been required in this case, if he had made the opening large enough at first to allow the finger to be inserted easily. The fact that defecation occurred through the bladder and penis for two months, without causing cystitis or urethritis, is curious.—*London Med. Record*, Dec. 15, 1877.

Midwifery and Gynæcology.

Fracture of the Fœtal Skull by the Forceps.

The *Journal de Médicine et de Chirurgie Pratiques* records a case of considerable interest. It occurred in the wards of M. Millard in Paris. A rachitic woman had been in labour two days. Expulsive pains recurred at long intervals and were feeble in character. A midwife had ruptured the membranes twenty hours previously. The head was at the brim, which measured 3¼ inches in the antero-posterior diameter. Forceps was applied, and after some minutes' traction the operator had a sensation of something giving way. At the same time the head became disengaged. It was, however, soon born, but apparently dead. It was plunged into a bath, and inspiratory efforts soon began. Its cry was scarcely perceptible. The left eyeball was pushed forwards and the conjunctiva infiltrated with blood; the right half of the face was paralyzed; the arm and leg on that side were slightly convulsed. The end of the blade of the forceps pressed unduly on the fronto-parietal eminence. The bone was hard and had yielded at that spot. It was a comminuted fracture, and not a simple depression. A cephalæmatoma formed at the spot. The pericranium was incised, and the bones raised to their normal level. All the symptoms soon ceased, and the child made an excellent recovery.—*Lancet*, Dec. 15, 1877.

—

Treatment of Secondary Puerperal Hemmorrhage.

Dr. BAILLY, Prof. Agrégé of the Faculty of Medicine, contributes a paper to the *Bulletin de Thérapeutique* for September 30, on the efficacy of this method of treating secondary uterine hemorrhage, devised by Prof. Tarnier. By secondary hemorrhages he understands those which are produced from the second day to a month after delivery. These are generally due to a congestion of the uterus, usually spontaneous, but sometimes caused by the presence of a foreign body in the cavity, too early getting up, a violent effort, or vaginal injections injudiciously employed. Such hemorrhages are rarely dangerous, but they recur frequently and often obstinately, and cause great alarm to the patient. The ordinary measures for arresting them are far from being always successful, and are usually tedious; and, at Prof. Tarnier's suggestion, the author of this paper commenced in 1874 the trial of warm baths. The success attending the use of these has been so great that he publishes two of the cases in which he employed them. In the first of these the hemorrhage commenced only on the eighteenth day after delivery, in a woman of feeble habit of body. The uterus was enlarged and congested, and the hemorrhage, without being alarming, resisted all the usual hæmostatics during ten days. Prof. Tarnier now advised warm baths. The first of these greatly modified the discharge, and the second suspended it completely. Recurring at the end of thirty-six hours, it was definitively arrested by the third. The uterus gradually diminished in size, and at the end of a week the patient was able to get up. In the second case the hemorrhage came on only on the twenty-seventh day after delivery, the uterus being as much developed as at the third month. The liquid blood discharged was not very considerable, but it became continuous, and was accompanied by coagula. Ergot in different forms, and vinegar injections, having been tried in vain, a warm bath of half an hour at once suspended the discharge; and, on this recurring next day, a second bath completed the cure.

Although in possession of several cases in which their efficacy proved as complete as in these two, Dr. Bailly observes that their success is not always so prompt. He has always found them less efficacious at the commencement of the hemorrhage than when this had persisted for some time; but, as they produce no inconvenience at the earlier periods, they may also be then employed concurrently with other measures. The only objection to the method that he is aware of is, that at first it shocks the prejudices and alarms the patient. They should not be resorted to prior to the tenth day after delivery, in consequence of the fatigue and danger which their application might then give rise to. Care must be taken, also, that the temperature of the water (about 34° C. or 93° Fahr.) should be rather raised than lowered, all chilling being avoided. From twenty to thirty minutes is a long enough duration to secure the general revulsion sought for; and as one bath rarely proves enough, they may be repeated daily. Prof. Tarnier was induced to try the procedure in puerperal metrorrhagia in consequence of having observed its efficacy in the hands of M. Salgue, of Dijon, who successfully employed it in non-puerperal metrorrhagia; he adopted it for this form of hemorrhage after delivery, and has for many years recommended it.

In another number of the *Bulletin* (October 30) we find an article by Dr. Constantin Paul, Professeur-Agrégé, upon the great utility of hypodermic injections of ergotine in various forms of metrorhagia. The formula which he has employed has been—ergotine two grammes, water and glycerine of each fifteen grammes. The solution assumes the brown colour of the extract of ergot, and keeps well, not losing any of its activity in even three months after its preparation. In the fourteen cases in which he has employed this, Dr. Paul has found it succeed in almost a marvellous manner; the hemorrhage, which was always severe and often dangerous, having in all been arrested in sixteen minutes at latest, and in several much earlier. The patients were either the subjects of more or less advanced cancer of the uterus, or in the puerperal condition. The advantageous action of ergot, taken internally, on uterine hemorrhage, has been long known; but on comparing this with the effect of hypodermic injection, the latter proves of much greater value. The time required for the operation of ergot varies from a quarter of an hour to thirty-six hours; while ergotine arrests the hemorrhage in from five to ten minutes; and in hemorrhages time is everything. Not only is the action of powder of ergot less rapid than the injection, but it is also less constantly efficacious, three or four doses being sometimes required. Ergot in powder also always gives rise to colicky pains, of which the patients complain much; but this is not so with the ergotine. The injection is not very painful, and does not produce any local inflammation, sometimes only leaving a slight hyperæsthesia at the point of insertion. So employed, intolerance of ergotine has never been noted. As Prof. Gubler has already observed, it is most remarkable that while a dose of even four grammes taken by the mouth is very doubtful in its action, a dose sixty times less, given by injection, exerts so marked an effect. Certainly there is far greater discrepancy in the doses required, according to the mode of administration, than is observed with regard to most medicinal substances. In the cases related by Dr. Paul in his paper, an injection of sixty-six milligrammes of ergotine arrested the hemorrhage in from five to ten minutes.—*Med. Times and Gaz.*, Dec. 8, 1877.

On the Management of the Nipples.

Dr. Samuel Sloan, Assistant Physician-Accoucheur to the Glasgow Lying-in Hospital, describes (*Obstetrical Journal of Great Britain*, Jan. 1878) his treatment of sore nipples as follows:—

My plan, when the nipples have unfortunately felt sore, is to carefully wash off the milk, after the child quits the breast, with tepid water; then to wash the nipple with weak spirit lotion and glycerine to prevent drying; or, if the excoriation should be more advanced, some astringent is added, as tannin or a weak solution of nitrate of silver. To protect the nipples from friction against the dress, *if the part be not inflamed*, I order a properly constructed nipple-shield, and occasionally apply a mild ointment, as oxide of zinc, to protect the skin from the repeated application of the watery solutions. If the nipple be retracted, or in any way difficult for the infant to seize, I advise that it be gently drawn out by the breast-pump, of which the best is the green ball breast-exhauster; and, if still painful when the child is applied to the nipple, an artificial glass nipple with India-rubber teat must be *at once* applied. Of this latter apparatus I would add that it is of the utmost importance to secure one of a proper shape; as, if too narrow, constriction of the nipple takes place, causing occlusion of the lactiferous ducts; and, if too long, so much of a vacuum is produced between the extremity of the nipple and the mouth of the child that it is generally impossible for the child to draw the milk into the teat. The teat also ought not to be long, as it then only serves to tickle the fauces of the child. It is thus an important matter,

in ordering one of Maw's glass nipple-shields, to secure a proper fit for the particular case; as it is advisable that the child's temper should not be tried in vain
attempts to extract the milk.   Besides this the teat ought to be carefully cleansed
from the composition which covers and impregnates it, as the smell and taste of
this material may disgust the child so much that it may refuse to make another
attempt.   This unsavoury material may be removed by soaking the teat in
whisky and then washing it.   Before applying the child to this artificial nipple
the latter ought to be filled with some of the mother's milk; or, if this is not
practicable, with sweetened milk and water.   Some children take so kindly to
this artificial nipple that it is difficult, after being long accustomed to it, to per-
suade them to use the mother's nipple again.   But, should only one nipple be
affected, this will not readily happen, *especially if the artificial teat be small
enough*.   Of artificial nipples there is a great variety, but to me the one described
above and sold by Maw seems to most efficiently protect the nipple; though the
shield and teat in one piece, made of India-rubber or other soft material, as softened ivory, will make suction easier for a weakly child, if it can be borne by the
mother.   There is, however, with its use considerable compression of the nipple
by the child's gums.   A good artificial nipple has yet to be devised.   If the nipple-shield can be borne, and the child can be coaxed to use it, there will be little
difficulty in curing the nipples on general principles.   In the event of excoriation
of the nipple continuing after this attempt with the artificial nipple, and ulceration
setting in, there remains no course but to take the child at once from that breast
till the part is sufficiently restored to permit of its reapplication.   And here the
careful use of a good breast-exhauster is important.   For, should the breast become engorged whilst the nipple is tender, there is every prospect of abscess of
the breast taking place.   In my experience, no matter how tender the nipple may
be, a careful regulation of the compression of the ball by the hand, with occasional
relaxation of the nipple to prevent occlusion of the lactiferous tubes, will always
result in the almost painless removal of the milk; though, should the breast be
hard and yet no milk come, gentle friction at the periphery of the breast may be
required to expel the milk from the gland proper into the lactiferous reservoirs
under the areola, whence the breast-exhauster will readily withdraw it.   It will
now be a comparatively easy matter to heal the nipple, since the first step in treating a disease is to remove the cause; the impracticability of doing this rendering
the treatment of the nipple so unsatisfactory.   If there be ulceration, careful
washing and drying of the nipple, and the application of the solid nitrate of silver
to the part affected only, will generally suffice.   This treatment by a "tough
caustic point" is, when combined with the use of the nipple-shield, a certain cure
of the fissures which occur around the base of the nipple.   If the part be inflamed,
sedative applications or poultices will of course be the first indication.   Should
the affection of the nipple arise from the aphthous condition in which we sometimes find the child's mouth, the application of borax and glycerine, or chlorate of
potash dissolved in glycerine, is the proper treatment for the nipple as for the
mouth.   I think it wise to avoid, in the selection of remedies for the nipple, any
medicine which may injure the child, if sufficient care be not taken in its removal
before the next application of the child to the nipple.   Perhaps it may suffice to
point out, regarding some recent investigations which have been made as to the
quality of the milk as a factor in the production of sore nipples, that, where one
nipple only is affected, this condition of the milk can have only a very limited
effect as an exciting cause.

It is pleasing to pass from the too often disappointing treatment of tender nipples to consider the possibility of having the nipples perform their natural functions without the usual morbid results.   In the lower ranks, from which a maternity

hospital generally derives its patients, tender nipples are rare, since the habits of this class of society, and the more or less exposure of the nipples, in their case, to the tonic effects of atmospheric influence, will give less sensitive, because more natural, nipples.   I have made inquiry at our hospital here, and I find that, out of every twenty women confined in it during the last two years, not more than one has suffered from sore nipples.   This, it will readily be acknowledged, is a result much more favourable than we have in private practice.   It has been customary to order, as a prophylactic, weak spirit and water, or other mild astringent, but I have seen no evil result from the application of stronger astringents.   As an astringent, however, especially if strong, is likely to cause a hardening only, and not a toughening of the nipple, we may have this organ cracking as soon as the outer film of hardened cuticle is removed, on the first application of the child to the breast.   To obviate this I am in the habit of ordering the admixture of glycerine with the astringent, and the occasional application of some fatty substance, as lard.   The selection of the particular astringent is, of course, of importance ; but the thoroughness with which it is applied is more so.   The solution I generally order is made up thus :   A large teaspoonful of dry tea is put into a two-ounce vial, one ounce of brandy and a quarter of an ounce of glycerine (Price's) are added ; and, after a few days, with occasional shaking, the solution is ready for use.   For two or three months previous to parturition the nipples should be thoroughly washed every night with cold water and glycerine soap, dried, and the above solution carefully brushed over the nipple, but especially around the base and into the apex.   This is left on all night, and, in the morning, the lard is rubbed well in.   I have frequently used glycerine of tannic acid, but have come to regard it as not sufficiently powerful.

During this treatment the dress ought to be loose ; and, if the nipples are at all retracted, they ought to be drawn out occasionally by suction or with the fingers and thumb.   A circular piece of some unirritating material, with a hole in the centre, might be used in severe cases.

When the child is born, and before I leave the house, I examine the nipples and breasts.   If the latter are flaccid I would prefer not to put the child early to the nipple ; and, when the milk has appeared, I advise the application of the child at intervals of not less than two hours, and to both nipples at each application, giving careful instructions against letting the nipple remain in the child's mouth after it has emptied the breast, and especially against allowing it to sleep at the breast. The nipple is to be moistened with water or saliva before applying the child to it ; and, when the infant quits the breast, the nipple should be washed with a mild astringent and antiseptic solution with glycerine.   The mixture I prefer is as follows :   A teaspoonful each of whisky, tincture of arnica, and Price's glycerine in a wineglassful of cold water.   The nipple, as soon as the infant leaves the breast, is washed with this and partially dried, and a nipple-shield at once applied to protect the nipple from friction against the dress.   One of the best nipple-shields is Wansbrough's ; but, after using it for some time as it is sold, I had to discard it, on account of its keeping the nipple, in some cases, too moist, and softening the cuticle ; certainly a great objection to its use.   To prevent this, however, it is only necessary to pierce it *over the whole of its extent* with a large needle from within outwards ; and, should the nipple be scalded from insufficient piercing the rectifying of this error will suffice of itself to remove the inconvenience.   I have little experience of other nipple-shields, though they may be made from a great variety of materials, and some of them might prove more convenient than Wansbrough's, to which another objection is that, though it should fit the nipple when first applied, the heat of the breast afterwards softens it ; it then becomes corrugated and flattened, and thus affords little protection to the nipple.   These objections could not apply to vulcanite nipple-shields, one of which, for trial, I have had prepared for me and pierced by Mr. Joseph Hilliard. Though used, I believe, in America, I do not find that they are known to any extent in this country. In using nipple-shields it is advisable to have them suspended round the neck by a ribbon; and care should be taken that they are frequently washed with soap and water; and if ointments are being used with them, a strong tooth-brush will be found serviceable to cleanse out the holes. Believing as I do in the importance of protecting the nipples in any prophylactic treatment, I advise, where the expense of good nipple-shields is a consideration, the use of a small circular piece of gutta-percha tissue, also pierced. But I suspect that, in such cases, unless care be taken to keep the gutta-percha, and the part over which it is applied, clean, pustules may form which might lead to inflammation in the deeper portion of the breast. But this need not happen; and patients have often informed me that the simple gutta-percha tissue thus applied is a considerable relief, especially when the nipples are tender. To supply the natural unctuous matter of which sucking deprives the nipple, I order the application of some simple ointment, as fresh oxide of zinc; glycerine soap and tepid water easily removing it before the child goes to the nipple.

The foregoing measures, if carefully carried out, I find, as a rule, sufficient to prevent tender nipples in cases where, from the sensitive temperament of the patient, such would probably have resulted; and that this is the case is, I think, borne out by the fact that, when the nurse leaves, and the prophylactic treatment of the nipples is more or less neglected, instead of being gradually left off, I have noticed in many cases that tender nipples begin, and this after an interval of four or more weeks of immunity from sore nipples.

To those who have been disappointed in the results of their treatment of sore nipples, and who have not put the prophylactic treatment to the test, I would strongly recommend a fair trial of the plan which I have briefly sketched.

Pathology and Treatment of Membranous Dysmenorrhœa.

Dr. JOHN WILLIAMS recently read a paper on this subject before the Obstetrical Society of London (*Med. Times and Gaz.*, June 23, 1877). It consisted of a narrative of fourteen cases of the affection, twelve of which had come under the author's own observation, a microscopical description of the membranes expelled, the method of treatment adopted in the cases, and conclusions drawn from the above data as to the nature of the affection and its treatment. It was maintained that in the study of the pathology of membranous dysmenorrhœa regard must be had to four things: (1) the history of the patient; (2), the structure of the product expelled; (3) the state of the uterus; and (4) the normal process of menstruation. The theories advanced respecting the pathology of the affection were briefly noticed. The post-mortem appearances met with in the uteri of two women suffering from the disorder were described, and the paper ended with the following conclusions: 1. The dysmenorrhœal membrane is not the product of conception, but the decidua ordinarily shed as *débris* with every menstrual epoch. 2. It is expelled as a whole, or in masses, in consequence of an excess of fibrous tissue in the wall of the uterus. This excess is due to imperfect evolution at puberty, imperfect involution after parturition, or abortion, or is the product of acute inflammation. 3. The membrane is neither the result of an ovarian congestion nor of a hypertrophy of the ordinary decidua. 4. The chronic inflammation present is the result of the monthly expulsion of the decidua in masses from the uterus, and plays an accidental part only in the formation of the membrane; the inflammation, may, however, be independent of the expulsion of the membrane, but it has no causal relation to the formation of the latter. 5. Sterility is not necessarily associated with the affection, but is the result of the condition induced by the expulsion of the membrane in masses from the uterus—inflammation of the uterus and ovaries. 6. The membrane may be expelled without pain. 7. Inflammation of the uterus greatly aggravates the suffering caused by the passage of the membrane along the cervical canal. 8. Great relief may be obtained by curing the inflammation of the cervix, though the membrane continues to be expelled every month. 9. In order to effect a cure the structure of the whole of the body of the uterus must be altered; the excess of fibrous tissue must be removed.

In the discussion which followed, Dr. BARNES stated that he attached great importance to our knowledge of the fact that the membrane is passed by virgins. We have no right to call anything the product of conception unless traces of the ovum be found. There are three kinds—one the typical; others having a fibrillar character without evidence of mucous membrane; others, clots, decolorized. It is borne out that it is due to excess of fibrous tissue in the uterine wall. This explains the difficulty of cure. Some are undoubtedly due to contraction of the os externum. This explains the congestion and enlargement of the uterus and excess of fibrous tissue in its walls. There is a general condition of the system in almost all cases; nervous and vascular tension and improvement may be obtained by making a free outlet for the menstrual blood.

Dr. GALABIN agreed in the main with Dr. Williams's account of the pathology of membranous dysmenorrhœa, but the evidence was not conclusive as to his view of its causation. The evidence against hypertrophy of the decidua was not conclusive, and it had not been finally proved that the mucous membrane was entirely removed during menstruation. Dr. Leopold had described a uterus on the third day of menstruation, in which there was some thickness of mucous membrane; and Dr. Galabin had found a fair thickness of mucous membrane six days after the commencement and two days after the cessation of menstruation. He had constantly found shreds of membrane in the discharge during the first two days, and thought that many cases might partake of the character of membranous dysmenorrhœa though not recognized as such.

Dr. WILLIAMS, in reply, said that he regarded membranous dysmenorrhœa as a type of a very large number of cases of painful menstruation, but that they were not recognized as such because the menstrual discharge was not examined. In the great majority of cases of dysmenorrhœa in which he had an opportunity of examining the discharge he had found shreds of the decidua. So far he agreed with Dr. Galabin. On the other hand, he differed from Dr. Galabin with regard to Dr. Leopold's cases, and believed that the weight of evidence derived from recent research went to show that the decidua (not the mucosa) was entirely removed during menstruation. Perhaps the strongest evidence in favour of this view is that while portions of the old decidua still remain attached to the surface of the uterus, a new decidua is seen developing immediately beneath it.

On the Value of Sponge-Tents in Obstetric and Gynæcological Practice.

Dr. KRONE of Hanover relates, in the *Berliner Klinische Wochenscrift*, October, 1877, several cases of placenta prævia, in which, previously to delivery, he arrested the hemorrhage whilst dilating the os uteri with sponge-tents. He has also employed them with success in the hemorrhage, resulting from a partially expelled ovum. Dr. Krone does not share the common fear that sponge-tents are liable to cause septicæmia. In cases of sterility and dysmenorrhœa, depending on stenosis of the cervical canal, he dilates the contracted os uteri by means of sponge-tents. This mode of procedure has been followed by impregnation. As a proof of the harmlessness of sponge-tents, he relates a case in which, in removing a tent, he broke it, and left half in the uterus, where it remained for four months, when it was expelled, and the sterility for which it had been applied was cured.—*London Med. Record*, Dec. 15, 1877.

CONTENTS.

Published Monthly, price $2.50 per annum, free of postage.
Also, furnished together with the AMERICAN JOURNAL OF THE MEDICAL
SCIENCES *and the* MEDICAL NEWS AND LIBRARY *for* SIX DOLLARS *per
annum in advance, the whole free of postage.*

HENRY C. LEA, Philadelphia.

THE MONTHLY ABSTRACT

OF

MEDICAL SCIENCE.

VOL. V. No. 3.   **For List of Contents see last page.**   MARCH, 1878.

Anatomy and Physiology.

Sulpho-Cyanides in the Urine.

According to the recent independent experiments of GSCHEIDLEN and MUNK, the urine of man and other mammals constantly contains sulphocyanic acid, which gives with ferric chloride, in urine previously acidified with hydrochloric acid, a reddish coloration. The precipitate which nitrate of silver throws down in ordinary urine is a mixture of chloride and sulphocyanide of silver, and if it be suspended in water decomposed with sulphuretted hydrogen, and filtered, the filtrate gives the ferric chloride reaction distinctly, even if only 200 cubic centimetres of urine be analyzed. Human urine contains about 0.0225 sulphocyanic acid in 1000 cubic centimetres in the form of a sodium salt, and 0.0211 NaCNS was found in the same quantity of rabbit's urine (Gscheidlen). Munk estimates that one litre of human urine contains 0.11 NaCNS. The source of the sulphocyanide appears to be the saliva, which always contains sulphocyanide of potassium, and Gscheidlen could detect none in the urine of a dog whose salivary secretions had all been prevented from entering the digestive tract by means of external fistulæ. It is a remarkable fact, observed by Munk, that in spite of the great solubility of the sulphocyanides, the urine contains sulphocyanic acid in abundance seven or eight days after a dose of sulphocyanide of ammonium. Dr. Thudichum has endeavoured to prove that Gscheidlen's method of extracting sulphocyanogen from the urine in combination with lead (*Pflüger's Archiv*, xiv., s. 401), is faulty; but it appears, from Gscheidlen's reply to his criticisms, that Thudichum did not observe the necessary cautions in repeating the former's experiments, and that there is no reason to doubt their accuracy.—*Med. Times and Gaz.*, Dec. 22, 1877.

On the Cause of the Respiratory Variations of Blood-pressure in the Aortic System.

FUNKE and LATSCHENBERGER (*Pflüger's Archiv*, Band xv.; abstract in *Academy*) call attention to the varying flow of blood through the pulmonary capillaries, determined by the varying expansion of the lungs. Every inspiratory expansion of these organs, whether it be attended by a *plus* or *minus* degree of intrathoracic pressure, must, by stretching the walls of the air-cells, lengthen and narrow the individual capillaries, and thus diminish their collective capacity. Conversely, the expiratory collapse of the air-cells must widen the capillaries and augment their capacity. These changes must influence, not merely the flow of blood between the two sides of the heart, but the tension in the aorta likewise. The primary effect of inspiration will be to raise the latter by squeezing the blood out of the lungs in the direction of least resistance—into the left auricle— and thus feeding the left ventricle with more blood. Its secondary effect will be to lower arterial tension by checking the current of blood through the lungs. Expiration will primarily lower arterial tension by lessening the supply of blood to the left auricle; its secondary effect will be to raise it by facilitating the flow through the pulmonary capillaries. These à priori considerations were put to the test of experiment, and a long account of the investigation is given. Its results confirmed the anticipations of the authors in every particular. They conclude that the essential cause of the respiratory variations of arterial pressure is always to be sought in the varying capacity of the pulmonary capillaries due to the alternate expansion and contraction of the lungs. In artificial, as in natural, breathing, the inspiratory rise of tension is owing to the blood being squeezed out of the lungs into the left heart; the expiratory fall, to the retention of blood in the diluted pulmonary capillaries. In natural breathing, the respiratory variations of intrathoracic pressure of course contribute—but only as accessory elements—to the general result; the same may be said of variations in the rate of the heart's action.—*London Med. Record*, Jan. 15, 1878.

Materia Medica and Therapeutics.

Physiological and Medical Effects of Alcohol.

The Third Report of the Special Committee of the House of Lords on Intemperance lays before us the evidence of two eminent physiologists and of one practising physician; and the first thing which strikes us is the unanimity with which all three speak of the usefulness of alcohol in medical practice. These three witnesses are also agreed that persons in health are better without the use of alcohol; although neither Dr. Lauder Brunton nor Dr. Burdon Sanderson went so far as to say that a small quantity of alcohol was, generally speaking, absolutely injurious. Thirdly, we observe in this evidence a repetition of the statements that alcohol is injurious in excessive cold, and as a rule, in excessive heat also. The men who have served in Arctic expeditions have, of their own accord, preferred hot coffee to hot rum, finding that the former supplied heat which really enabled them to withstand the cold, while the latter supplied only a very temporary and evanescent stimulus, which, on passing off, left them worse than they were before. As regards the use of alcohol in excessive heat, Dr. Brunton refers us to the Ashantee expedition. During the march, liquor was found to be disadvantageous; but after the march was over, when the men sat down at their camp-fire for their evening meal, they found the advantage of a little rum; because the rum stimulated their stomachs, and assisted them to digest their food. But it was noticed. that the young men did not care so much for the rum, often not taking their full allowance; while the older men, in whom the processes of life are less active, wanted all their own allowance, and would take also the allowance of a neighbour, if he would give it to them.

As to the question, whether alcohol is utilized in the system, there is also practical agreement; and it seems to be now pretty generally accepted that an average man will utilize in his economy a variable quantity of alcohol, the average amount being about two ounces daily. A larger quantity than this will indicate its presence by the elimination of alcohol in the breath, and in other ways. Lastly, with some slight differences of detail, the medical witnesses are practically agreed as to the effects of the abuse of alcohol. Sir W. Gull's statement is, that its abuse produces disorders of the liver. From disordered liver, we get disordered blood, and, consequent upon that, we get diseased kidneys and diseased lungs. Then we get diseased heart and nervous system. The general effects are no doubt, first, congestion of these organs; next, increase of their fibrous tissue, which presses upon the secreting cells and induces general atrophy and fattiness.

Respecting the conditions in which the administration of alcohol is useful, we come upon a slight difference of opinion between Sir W. Gull and the other witnesses, he preferring to name as a sedative what they characterize as a stimulant. We think that alcohol will act as one or other, according to the condition in which it is administered. In the case which Sir W. Gull supposes, of very high and uncontrollable delirium in early typhoid, alcohol no doubt calms and quiets the patient, and this action may fairly be called sedative. Similarly, in the later high fever spoken of by Dr. Brunton, alcohol may be useful to lower the pulse and the temperature. There is, however, this difference between these two actions, that the former is not generally obtained until a rather large quantity of alcohol has been administered, while the pulse and temperature are generally lowered by smaller quantities. In the latter case, the reduction of pulse and temperature is probably induced by the combustion of the alcohol itself in place of that of the tissues. The delirium is calmed, on the other hand, probably by clouding of the intellectual powers, and by the soporific effect of the alcohol on the nervous tissues. These two actions may be called sedative if the ultimate effect of the alcohol, rather than its mode of action, be taken into account. The stimulant action, on the other hand, of which Dr. Brunton and Dr. Burdon Sanderson spoke, may be looked upon as the primary action of alcohol; that, namely, of filling the capillary vessels by removing or diminishing the power of the sympathetic system of nerves. It is by such an action on the stomach, no doubt, that the feeble digestion to which Dr. Brunton referred can be improved or stimulated; and it is by inducing this action that alcohol sometimes acts as by magic upon the pain of anæmic or spanæmic neuralgia or headache, or that it prevents from stoppage the exhausted heart beating feebly in the termination of typhus fever, before convalescence is fairly established. This being so, it seems to come to this, that the sedative action spoken of by Sir W. Gull is only an increased quantity of what is generally called the stimulant action of alcohol. The latter is obtained by the administration of so much alcohol as will somewhat paralyze the sympathetic nerves and congest the capillaries; the former, or sedative action, is obtained by still more paralyzing the sympathetic system, and also to some extent by substituting the consumption of alcohol for that of the patient's own tissues. Inasmuch, however, as both actions are obtained by paralyzing the nervous system, it might be well, as Dr. Gull proposes, to consider alcohol as a sedative rather than as a stimulant; and we are inclined to think that the use of this term might be of some advantage to the public by keeping before them the mode of action of alcohol.

While we are upon the so-called stimulant action of alcohol, we wish to draw attention to a very extraordinary statement made by Dr. Burdon Sanderson. He proposes, very justly, to administer small quantities of alcohol when the temperature (and the pulse) sink below the normal; and he says that the moment the temperature sinks below the normal, danger to life ensues. Again, he says that a temperature of from 96 to 98 deg. would be a really dangerous lowering of the temperature. We cannot help recording our surprise at these statements, especially when they are made by so eminent an authority. Every medical man who has given attention to the matter knows that a fall of temperature to 97 deg., or even to 96 deg., so far from being a dangerous condition and one threatening collapse, is actually the normal condition in convalescence from fevers in general, and probably also from the acute inflammations. In some fevers, such as relapsing fever, it is the rule, one may say, for the temperature to sink to 95 deg. in the course of the disease, while 94 deg. is not at all an uncommon limit of subsidence. There are even exceptional observations taken in relapsing fever, where the thermometer has registered 92 deg. Now, as is well known, relapsing fever is one of the least fatal forms of specific fever, death practically never taking place except-ing in the extremely aged and the extremely young. It is evident, therefore, that mere lowering of temperature ought not to have the importance attached to it which is stated in this evidence. Like other symptoms, its gravity must be determined by its concomitants.—*British Med. Journal*, Dec. 15, 1877.

On the Therapeutic Use of Iodoform.

Mr. BERKELEY HILL, Prof. of Clinical Surgery in University College, contri-butes to the *British Medical Journal* (Jan. 26, 1878) the following note, on the therapeutic use of iodoform.

Locally, iodoform, as a dry powder, brushed lightly over the surface with a moistened camel-hair pencil, has been for three years my almost invariable treat-ment of venereal sores, especially the local chancre. During the last few months, I have often substituted for the dry powder an ethereal solution (one part of iodo-form in six or eight of ether). The sore is touched or dabbed with a pencil dipped in the ethereal solution, according to its size and depth, lightly or copiously. The ether quickly evaporates, leaving a thin pellicle of iodoform, that as effectually stays the spread and produces healing of chancres as does the more copiously applied dry powder. Thus the surface is covered more exactly, and the disagreeable smell of the iodoform is too faint to attract attention. The sore is well washed with water and dried before the iodoform is applied, and the surface is lastly pro-tected by a bit of dry lint. When the secretion is abundant, the dressing must be renewed twice daily, but in three or four days the amount of discharge becomes so scant that one dressing *per diem* suffices.

In this way, venereal sores heal quickly. Pain subsides at once ; the sore is well in a week or ten days, and the chances of consecutive inoculation or bubo are greatly lessened. In a very few cases, the application of iodoform gives momen-tary smarting, which is very bearable ; even the ethereal solution does not hurt, and usually the patient declares the application to be quite painless. I avoid using iodoform on inflamed sores, or on simple granulating wounds ; but indolent non-specific ulcers are rapidly improved by iodoform locally applied.

Lately, I have given iodoform internally with great benefit. It acts more rapidly than potassic or other iodides, and judging from experience thus far, is as readily borne as are those salts. I have given it in one-and-a-half-grain doses as a pill with extract of gentian. Three pills are given each day, increasing gradu-ally till eight or ten pills are taken in twenty-four hours.

I have used it with excellent effect in cases of obstinate syphilitic ulceration of the tongue, where the dorsum is covered with rugged thickened epithelium, which is constantly splitting into deep fissures, and thus causing continual severe pain to the patient. This affection is often quite insensible to mercury, alkaline iodides, or arsenic—the remedies usually beneficial. In three of these obstinate cases, where I had been treating the patients at intervals for years with the remedies just mentioned with little lasting benefit, iodoform-pills have acted like a charm. Pain, immediately lessened, in two or three days ceased wholly ; and the fissures healed rapidly, while the tongue soon shrank to its natural size. How long the relief will endure, time alone will show ; but any interval of only apparent cure of this very painful affection is a great blessing to the sufferer, and time is given for the exhibition of mercury if required. In December last, I had under my care in University College Hospital a patient with ulcerated and protruding gumma of the left testis, non-ulcerating gumma of the right testis, and ulcerating gummata of the skin over the upper end of the right tibia, with other syphilitic affections. Iodoform was administered in pills, and water-dressing applied to the ulcers. Rapid healing and subsidence of the swellings took place, notwithstanding that, when the dose of eight pills *per diem* had been reached and administered for three days, an outbreak of pyrexia, coryza, and iodic acne rendered it necessary to drop the drug completely for a short time. In three weeks the patient left the hospital almost healed, and continued his treatment as an out-patient. Again, a lady who has during the last two years consulted me occasionally for intensely agonizing pain in the head caused by syphilitic pericranial and cranial diseases, for which a customary dose was thirty grains of sodium iodide three times daily, was at once relieved of pain by the iodoform pill taken three times daily, though, on the third day, nausea became too urgent to allow the iodoform to be continued in that quantity; it was at first diminished till pain ceased, and then discontinued altogether. This small experience has satisfied me that in iodoform we have a very useful addition to our store of weapons for fighting syphilis. Further observation will enable us to apply it more exactly and when most suitable.

On the Influence of Iron mixed with Food on the Blood.

NASSE (*Marburg. Sitzungsbericht*, No. 3, 1877) fed a dog weighing about $17\frac{2}{3}$ pounds, during eighty-seven days, with bread and potatoes; giving at the same time, for twenty-five days, $15\frac{1}{2}$ grains of lactate of iron daily, and for the remaining sixty-two days $18\frac{1}{2}$ grains of oxide of iron each day; the dose in each case being mixed with about six-sevenths of an ounce of fat. The weight of the animal increased by more than two pounds. The specific gravity of the blood rose from 1052 to 1060.8; that of the serum remained nearly unchanged. The amount of iron in the blood increased from 0.477 per mille to 0.755. In seven other dogs, out of eight subjected to experiment, feeding with various preparations of iron was followed by an increase of the solid constituents and of the specific gravity of the blood; the latter being 3.02 higher than before, indicating an addition of 7.6 per mille to the former. The increase of the solid constituents depended solely on that of the blood-corpuscles. The amount of iron in the blood rose regularly. In conclusion, the author expresses his belief that the administration of iron mixed with fat is productive of the most fruitful results; and he recommends the use of fat food containing iron for anæmic patients.—*London Med. Record*, Dec. 15, 1877.

Medicine.

Gonorrhœal Rheumatism.

Prof. HARDY, in a recent lecture at La Charité (*Gaz. des Hop.*, No. 149), made some interesting observations on gonorrhœal rheumatism. The subject of the lecture, a cook aged thirty-two, having contracted a gonorrhœa four months since, was a fortnight afterwards seized with violent pains in the ankle, and metatarsus of both feet, and so intense were they that for two months he was unable to walk. They then ceased, and the discharge, which during their presence disappeared, returned again. He was able to resume his occupation, when, under

the influence of a chill, the pains returned, and he came to the hospital. He was
pale and anæmic, and had somewhat of a cachectic appearance. In both feet,
but especially on the left side, the ankle and metatarsus were the seat of marked
swelling, which was accompanied by excessive pain. There was no fever, and
the pulse and digestion were quite normal. In fact there was no other symptom
of anything amiss than slight albuminuria. This was evidently an example of
what has been termed blenorrhagic rheumatism, and the albuminuria and complete anæmia which were also present indicated the existence of nephritis, which,
and especially in its parenchymatous form, is a pretty frequent complication of
gonorrhœa—resulting from a propagation of the urethral inflammation to the kidney. For the treatment of this case the salicylate of soda, now so much in vogue
for articular diseases, was prescribed, and under its influence the spontaneous
pains have diminished, but those felt in walking are just as severe. The relief,
indeed, is probably due rather to repose than to the salicylate, which does not
seem to exert the same beneficial effect as in ordinary articular rheumatism.

It is only since 1781 that the relation between certain articular pains and gonorrhœa was observed; first John Hunter, and then Ricord, Rollet, and Fournier,
having most contributed to stamp this affection as a special nosological entity.
The pains are sometimes very slight, and only manifested on moving; but in
other cases they are extremely severe, and persist even during repose. There is
a marked doughy tumefaction of the joints invaded, the amount of effusion being
sometimes enormous, occasionally simulating a true hydrarthrosis. The erythematous redness of ordinary acute rheumatism is rare in this variety. It seems to
have an especial predilection for the knee, after which come in order of frequency
the wrist, ankle, shoulder, the fingers and toes, and especially the tarsus and
metatarsus. But it is not always confined to the articulations, and for that reason
it is preferable that it should be called rheumatism rather than arthritis, which
has been proposed. Sometimes it is developed in the sheaths of tendons, at
others in the tendinous bursæ, and more rarely in the sciatic nerve. Sometimes
it occurs on one side and then on the other, and at others on both sides at once.
While it is occupying these parts various accidents are often met with in the eye,
as intense conjunctivitis with suppuration, or keratitis accompanied by iritis—
phenomena analogous to those observed in this organ during ordinary rheumatism.
The number of joints affected differs from what is observed in febrile rheumatism;
for while this last has a great tendency to invade several joints, and sometimes
the whole of them, it is rare in gonorrhœal rheumatism for more than one or two
and sometimes three or four joints to suffer, and especially to find one after the
other becoming affected, as is the rule in acute rheumatism. It is usually also
apyretic, and if there is a little fever at first this only lasts two or three days. So,
also, the secretion of sweat is either absent or insignificant, and the changes in the
urine, due to the preponderance of the urates and urea, met with in ordinary rheumatism, are absent. Finally, in this variety there are not the complications of
heart disease; while, as a general rule, after lasting weeks or months, a cure results; but it sometimes gives rise to a true hydrarthrosis or a white swelling, with
anchylosis. For the production of this affection not only is the existence of gonorrhœa essential, but there must also be a special predisposition which is not a tendency to the rheumatic diathesis. If the subjects of this disease be interrogated,
it will be found that, independently of the blenorrhagia, their joints remain perfectly free, and they are nowise liable to contract muscular or articular pains on
exposure to cold. Sometimes this rheumatism will appear at the very commencement of the urethral discharge, and sometimes only one, two, or three days later;
and the rule which has been laid down, that the pains are severe in proportion to
the abundance of the discharge, rests upon no foundation, for they are met with

in the acute and subacute form of gonorrhœa, as in that which is manifested only by a slight discharge. It is not rare, when the articular pains appear, to find the gonorrhœa suddenly stopping, to return when they have been relieved. It would seem that a true metastasis takes place, the morbific material being transported from one place to another. But this phenomenon is far from being constant, and what is usually observed is that on the occurrence of the rheumatism there is only a certain amount of diminution of the discharge. Blenorrhagic rheumatism being, in fact, a local affection, and not being accompanied by general symptoms, measures which are purely local are those which alone succeed. Thus, at the onset we should have recourse to application of leeches, dry cupping, and cataplasms, and, if the affection threatens to be prolonged, to blisters. At a later period, if it tends to a chronic condition, we may employ baths, douches, and mineral springs—the different means, in fact, that are used to combat chronic rheumatism.—*Med. Times and Gaz.*, Feb. 2, 1878.

On Disturbances of Sight in Hysteria.

In a recent lecture M. CHARCOT called attention to certain disturbances of sight which are not unfrequently met with in hysterical patients.

Some years ago M. Briquet described various morbid visual phenomena met with in patients the subjects of hysterical hemianæsthesia. "With the eye on the hemianæsthesic side," says M. Briquet, "the patient sees badly : the outlines of objects are badly defined ; white objects appear gray ; reading becomes difficult, or impossible, the print appearing only as a dark gray tint on a background of lighter gray. When the anæsthesia is complete, the affection of sight goes on to complete amaurosis."[1]

Dr. Galezowski was the first to show that this kind of amblyopia is almost always accompanied by diminution or loss of the power of appreciating colours. It is remarkable that this perversion of the sense of sight, so far as colours are concerned, follows certain laws which have been investigated by M. Landolt in M. Charcot's wards at the Salpêtrière. In the normal state all parts of the field of vision are not equally sensitive to different colours ; for some colours the field is wider than for others, and the differences follow much the same law in different subjects. Thus, in the great majority of cases, it is for blue that the field is widest ; next comes yellow, then orange, red, green ; whilst violet is only perceived by the most central parts of the retina. In hysterical amblyopia these characters are found to be exaggerated in various degrees. The different circles which correspond to the limits of vision for each colour are concentrically retracted more or less ; and numberless varieties of change may be met with in well-marked cases. Thus, the field for violet, the most "central" colour, may become narrowed to complete extinction, the other colours remaining clear. The next colour to disappear will be green, red, and orange will follow in their turns, whilst yellow and blue are only lost in a high degree of amblyopia. As might have been expected, however, there are some exceptions to the general rule. Thus, certain patients continue to see red when their perception for yellow, and even for blue, is entirely lost. Nevertheless, among the cases hitherto observed, it is the rule that green and violet—and especially the latter—are lost before red or any of the other colours. When the perception for all the colours is gone, that for form only being preserved, objects appear of a gray tint, much as in a painting in Indian-ink. In the highest degree of amblyopia the perception of form may be lost as well as that of colour ; there is real amaurosis. Such cases are, however, rare.[2]

---

[1] "Traité Clinique et Thérapeutique d'Hystérie," page 293.

[2] Charcot "Leçons sur les Localizations Cérébrales, page 118.

Although these alterations in the field of vision for colours are especially seen in the eye corresponding to the anæsthetic side, yet it is common to find that in the opposite eye the field is somewhat contracted, though in a very much less degree. Thus, patients who are only able to distinguish the most peripheral colours—yellow and blue—with the eye of the affected side, have only lost perception in the other eye for the most central—violet, or perhaps green. We may conceive theoretically that numerous combinations such as these might be met with; and many such have, in fact, been observed. It is scarcely necessary to say that these phenomena are of a purely functional character, and that they are not accompanied by any alteration visible by the ophthalmoscope; there is not even any difference in the comparative vascularity of the two eyes. .

The visual phenomena are characterized, moreover, by the same liability t variation that is seen in other local manifestations of hysteria. Like these, they may appear or disappear suddenly, or remain permanently persistent—perhaps as the only symptom. An already existing dyschromatopsy may give place all at once to complete achromatopsy for a short time before the occurrence of a convulsive attack; and it may disappear after the attack almost as suddenly as it came on. Occasionally complete double amaurosis may be found immediately after an attack. At the same time the anæsthesia, which had previously been confined to one-half of the body, will have extended to the whole body. It may also happen that muscular amaurosis or complete blindness comes on suddenly or gradually, apart from the occurrence of a fit. Complete double amaurosis is, however, rarely met with. Briquet has only seen it three times, M. Charcot hardly more frequently. On the other hand, dyschromatopsy, achromatopsy, and even complete amaurosis, of one eye are comparatively common.

A very interesting combination of symptoms, which M. Charcot has several times met with, is the following: The patient is slightly analgesic in the trunk and limbs of one side; the corresponding side of the face is markedly or even completely anæsthetic. There is complete double achromatopsy, or at the most the patient sees the more peripheral colours—yellow and blue—fitfully with the eye of the opposite side.

The presence of achromatopsy on the side where the sensation is otherwise normal, as well as on the anæsthetic side, affords a clue to the explanation of amaurosis in certain hysterical patients, where all ordinary hysterical symptoms are absent or but slightly marked. It must be mentioned that, remarkable as they are, these peculiar modifications of vision are not met with only in hysteria, as M. Charcot pointed out some time ago.[1] He showed that they are met with in all their varieties in the monocular amblyopia associated with hemianæsthesia of general and special sensation in cases of cerebral lesions of the posterior part of the internal capsules in the region which he has called "the cross-roads of the sensory tract" (carrefour sensitif). In these cases there is the same diminution in the acuteness of sight; the same general and concentric narrowing of the field of vision for colours in both eyes, but much more marked in the eye opposite the lesion; the same absence of ophthalmoscopic signs. This form of amblyopia, then, belongs to cerebral hemianæsthesia in general, and not to hysterical hemianæsthesia in particular. It is easy to understand the interest—not only practical, but theoretical—which attaches to this relation between the organic and the functional conditions. From the situation of organic lesions capable of giving rise to general and special hemianæsthesia, we seem able quite easily to name the position of those lesions (inappreciable by our present modes of investigation)—those dynamic lesions, as they are still sometimes called—upon which depends the cor-

---

[1] "Localizations Cérébrales," page 119.

responding hemianæsthesia of hysteria. They are probably situated upon the fibres crossing the above-named region, or upon the prolongations at the surface of the brain, or perhaps both parts may be involved at once.

M. Charcot next called attention to another kind of visual disturbance first noticed by him a long time ago, and which, though by no means a rare symptom, has never hitherto been described. It is well known that very marked and very various hallucinations form one of the most ordinary accompaniments of hysterical delirium. M. Charcot finds that they may also be met with in the interval of attacks, following attacks, or perhaps at the time when a fit is about to come on. It is not uncommon to see hysterical patients sitting quietly at work, suddenly get up from their seat with a cry as though surprised at the sight of some frightful object which they wish to avoid touching. If asked why they have acted thus, they say that they thought they saw animals, rats, cats, or perhaps some fantastic shape, running over the floor, or on the neighbouring wall. At other times it is the sight of grinning faces which has caused their fright. The imaginary animals are generally black or gray in tint, sometimes, though rarely, of a bright red colour. In any given patient they always appear on the same side—the side which is hemianæsthetic, and consequently on the side where the modifications of colour-vision are most marked. The animals generally move rapidly one after the other, and as a rule they disappear as soon as the patient turns the eyes to the side on which the apparition is seen. It may, however, last much longer, especially if the patient is at a period of " nervous high tide," in the état-de-mal, or has recently had a fit. M. Charcot showed a number of patients who are liable to this particular form of visual trouble in a very marked degree.

Such, then, are the principal modifications of vision which are commonly met with in hystero-epilepsy, and even in ordinary hysteria. Many other visual symptoms occur in certain cases, such as defects of accommodation, certain forms of diplopia, etc., but these are rare.—*Med. Times and Gaz.*, Jan. 19, 1878.

—

The Ophthalmoscope in Tubercular Meningitis.

Dr. BOUCHUT, in an introductory lecture (*Gaz. des Hop.*, December 11), observes that during the fifteen years since 1862 he has collected nearly 2000 cases, most of them verified by autopsies, which show that the meninges, the brain, and the cord produced in the fundus of the eye appearances. the knowledge of which confers a precision in the diagnosis of cerebro-spinal diseases not otherwise attainable. On the present occasion he confines attention to tubercular meningitis, his observations being founded on 472 cases which have come under his notice. In exploring these affections as much aid is derived from the sense of sight, as from hearing in the employment of auscultation in diseases of the heart and lungs. The signs so observed are of very great importance, oftentimes sufficing to remove all doubts that may attach to the diagnosis. Thus, in many cases of miliary tuberculosis, which commence with symptoms resembling those of typhoid fever, the neuro-retinitis or tubercular choroiditis, revealed by the ophthalmoscope, made clear a diagnosis which otherwise must have been delayed. In these 472 cases, these intraocular lesions have been exhibited no less than 463 times. They are often observable from the commencement of the disease, but more often at the second stage, being most marked at the period when coma and convulsions set in. During the hours which precede death they become gradually effaced, so that the approaching termination may sometimes be recognized in the eye. Five minutes after death they have almost disappeared, the fundus of the eye being of a leaden-gray color.

The lesions are sometimes observable at the very commencement of the men-

ingitis, when the child is only dull, with sickness and headache and a little fever
—symptoms which may cause meningitis to be suspected; but, unaided by the
ophthalmoscope, could never admit of certainty of opinion.   As the disease advances, the signs become modified and increased from day to day.   They are
often alike in the two eyes; but sometimes are more considerable in one than in
the other, corresponding to the hemisphere in which the lesions are most considerable.   Sometimes they are first observed on the external side of the papilla,
whence they become rapidly generalized; but in most cases they occupy the entire papilla.   In ordinary tubercular meningitis the lesions have their proper characters, which are not met with in partial encephalitis and in tumors of the encephalon accompanied by paralysis of the sixth pair.   In the latter, the exudation of the
neuro-retinitis is more dense, white, and obstructive to the circulation; so that the
vessels are hidden, and numerous minute hemorrhages are produced.   In meningitis
the papillary exudation is less and only opaline, and is accompanied by a varicose
enlargement of the veins, inducing fewer hemorrhages.   At the same time that this
acute neuro-retinitis is forming there is also observed a tumefaction of the optic
nerve, which becomes reddened, but preserves its limits pretty distinctly.   The
tumefaction, however, increases, and the nerve becomes veiled by a semi-transparent grayish *teint*, which extends beyond its contour, and slightly conceals it.
Somewhat later, the entire nerve becomes veiled, the grayish tinge which rendered the papilla diffused extending to the retina in its vicinity.   The nerve is
more and more hidden, becoming sometimes invisible under the grayish-red veil
which covers it, its presence only being indicated by its point of emergence, and
by the radiation of the arteries and veins.   This is the most common form of the
acute neuro-retinitis of meningitis; and although similar appearances may be
found on other pathological conditions, yet, by combining its appearance with
the other symptoms presented by the disease in the child, its significancy becomes
of great importance, and the diagnosis a certainty.

At the same time that this neuro-retinitis is becoming developed, more or less
considerable changes are produced in the arteries and veins at the fundus on the eye.
The arteries, compressed during their course by the tumefaction of the optic
nerve, become less and less apparent, and sometimes even invisible; while the
veins become, on the contrary, filled with thromboses, and sometimes rupturing,
so that blood becomes extravasated beneath their outer coats, forming *true primary false aneurisms of the veins*.   From time to time tubercular choroiditis
becomes added to the neuro-retinitis, but in a less proportion than might be expected.   Thus, among the 472, such combination occurred only in thirty-nine.
This acute choroiditis is very interesting to observe from day to day, in couse-
quence of the changes it undergoes, and the enlargement of the miliary granulations.   These are whitish, as fine as grains of sand, with the power of increasing
to the size of an ordinary lentil.   They are more or less brilliant at their centre,
either sharp or diffused at their circumference, devoid of apparent vessels, but
often placed under a vessel of the retina.   They keep on increasing, so as sometimes to double their size.   If the disease is prolonged, new ones appear which
were not visible at its commencement.

⸱ After describing the anatomical characters of the affection, as shown by 296
autopsies which he has performed, Dr. Bouchut alludes to the mechanism by
which these lesions may be supposed to be produced.   In certain cases of cerebral
tumour, accompanied by neuro-choroiditis, Von Graefe supposed this to be induced by the repletion and stasis of the cavernous sinus, which, by obstructing
the circulation of the eye, led to tumefaction and œdema of the papilla, and the
distension and rupture of the retinal veins.   This M. Bouchut regards as the cor-
r ct view, believing also that obstruction is caused not only by this condition of

the cavernous sinus, but also by similar conditions of the other sinuses, as well as by any intracranial effusions that may be present. So that the existence of the acute neuro-retinitis of meningitis is due to a *true mechanical cause*, which prevents the complete return of the venous blood of the eye into the cranium, and leads to the production of these circulation and nutrition lesions in the fundus of the eye. Schwalbe, on his discovery of the communications of the subarachnoid spaces with the sheath of the optic nerve, has offered another explanation, viz., that the serous infiltration of the sheath induces strangulation of the papilla and hyperæmia of the veins. But although in meningitis this serous infiltration of the sheath of the optic nerve is met with, yet the same fact is observed in a great number of other non-cerebral diseases. Thus M. Bouchut found it existing to as great an extent as in meningitis in a series of thirty children dying of pneumonia, diphtheria, phthisis, etc., without having exhibited any cerebral symptoms. It is possible that it may act as a concurrent cause in meningitis, but it cannot be substituted for the mechanical explanation offered above.—*Med. Times and Gaz.*, Jan. 12, 1878.

On Radiant Heat as a Cause of Insanity.[1]

Except by the old writers, who ascribed all kinds of brain-disease to the action of the sun's rays on the head, not many cases of psychoses caused by radiant heat have been recorded, and those mostly of short duration. Delacoux reports that, during the march of Marshal Bugeaud in Oran in 1838, under a hot sun, 200 men were taken ill with symptoms of brain-hyperæmia; of these 11 committed suicide in consequence of hallucinations. Barclay saw a case of melancholia following insolation in South Africa; the patient ultimately destroyed himself. Grisolle observed among sailors in the hot zones melancholia with strong tendency to suicide. Obernier reports a case of insolation, in which great excitement, with marked hallucinations of sight and hearing, preceded death. Persistent weakness of memory, dulness of understanding, and various paralyses, have frequently been observed after *coup de soleil*.

Hardly anything is to be found in literature concerning the influence of the heat radiated from furnaces in large factories, etc., on the causation of insanity. The paucity of these cases may be partly due to the following causes:—when the heat becomes unbearable to any workman he can always escape into a cooler atmosphere, which under a tropical sun he could not do; the rays from a fire do not fall so directly upon the head as do those from the sun, but act mostly upon the interior surface of the body and the face; lastly, stokers and others who work near large furnaces are habituated to very high temperatures, and that this affords very great immunity from any ill effects is shown by the rarity of insolation among natives of the tropics, as compared with foreigners from more temperate climates.

Cases have occurred of sudden illness resembling insolation, though really due to the heat of fire, which have ended in death, and in which the *post-mortem* appearances, especially as regards the brain and its membranes, have been identical with those caused by sunstroke. The similarity of the influence of the sun's rays and of artificial heat on the brain and its membranes has been proved by experiment upon animals by Obernier, Wood, and others.

Psychoses due to the action of radiant heat are really more frequent than has been hitherto believed. During the last few years there have been fourteen such

---

[1] Allgem. Zeitschrift für Psychiatrie, Band 34, Heft 3.

cases in the asylum at Siegburg; six of these occurred in workmen exposed to excessive heat, and eight were due to insolation.

In two fatal cases, in one of which insanity was due to sunstroke, and in the other to the heat of a furnace, hæmatomas of old and recent date were found, together with cloudiness and thickening of the membranes, hyperæmia of the same, and œdema of the brain. In the latter of the two cases there were in addition granulations of the ependyma on the floor of the lateral and fourth ventricles, gray degeneration of the lateral columns, hyperæmic and greatly thickened membranes of the spinal cord.

Insanity due to insolation generally commences quite suddenly. Only in a few cases the patients apparently recover and resume their ordinary occupation, until, under some harmful influence, the disease again breaks out. In the case of stokers, feelings of weakness, fatigue, disinclination for work, pains in the head, etc., generally precede for a considerable time the outbreak of insanity. The patients become impatient and restless, believe themselves to be followed and mocked; sooner or later they become maniacal, destructive, and dirty in their habits. They are most also sexually excited, and masturbate shamelessly. In some cases the disease commences directly with psychic and motor excitement, and grandiose delusions are developed, such as are usually only observed in paralytics. The maniacal excitement, in a few cases, lasts only a short time, and melancholy with weariness of life predominates until the end of the disease. In other cases, however, mania with large delusions persists until death. All the patients are subject to frequently recurring attacks of congestion to the head; they constantly appear preoccupied, and even when most excited seem to be in a kind of dream.

In almost all cases paralytic symptoms appear early. The pupils are at first contracted, but later dilated and unequal; strabismus is frequent, and ptosis not uncommon. The tongue trembles when protruded, and inclines to one side or the other. The speech becomes stammering and the gait unsteady. In most cases the paralytic symptoms steadily progress; the intellect, especially the memory, fades rapidly, and the patients die, often in a very short time, of apoplexy or general paralysis. In the cases of recovery, the patients become gradually quieter, the paralytic symptoms disappear, and after a short stage of reaction, the patient gets well.

Here follow reports of all the fourteen cases observed by the author; in only three of them did hereditary disposition exist. Of the eight cases ascribed to insolation, five commenced quite suddenly, while those due to artificial heat were mostly preceded by prodromal symptoms. In nearly all the cases the insanity began with depression due to powerful hallucinations and delusions of persecution; after a variable period attacks of mania supervened; this last was accompanied in six of the cases by large delusions. All the cases except three presented paralytic symptoms soon after the outbreak of mental disease. These gradually disappeared as the intellect became clearer in the cases which recovered, but were progressive in the other cases.

Of the whole fourteen patients, five were discharged cured, two died, one is demented, three are still under treatment, and the remainder have been discharged as incurable. Of the five cases which recovered, two were ascribed to *coup de soleil*, and the other three occurred in workmen exposed to excessive artificial heat. It appears that three of the eight patients whose insanity followed insolation made attempts at suicide; whereas none of the fire-workers showed any suicidal tendency.—*London Med. Record*, Jan. 15, 1878.

On Writer's Cramp.

M. GALLARD, in his recent volume, *Clinique Médicale de la Pitié*, has come to the conclusion that writer's cramp is certainly a professional disease, but a clinical study of it decidedly shows that it is far from being special to persons who write much.　Absolutely similar disturbances are seen in persons who follow other avocations, such as engravers, artificial flower makers, pianists, violinists, telegraphists who use the House-telegraph, etc.　But in all these persons the disturbances observed occur in the hands and fingers.　Absolutely similar, nay, identical disturbances are observed in persons following professions which exercise other muscles than those of the forearm or hand ; and then these disturbances occur in the muscles which are necessarily contracted by the habitual exercise of the avocation, whether these muscles be those of the arm, shoulder, leg, neck, face, or even the trunk.　The analysis of these various facts leads the writer to the first conclusion, that the disease in question is not peculiar to writers ; the analysis of the symptoms leads him to another conclusion, that it is not a cramp ; whence he feels the necessity of substituting for the incorrect denomination writer's cramp, the far more suitable name proposed by Dr. Duchenne of Boulogne, viz., functional impotence.　In reference to establishing the nature of this morbid condition, M. Gallard, after having proved that it evades any anatomical localization whatever, is led to admit that it is a simple functional disturbance and nothing else.　He is particularly struck by finding, with regard to its etiology, that fatigue is far from being an essential cause of it ; for this disease does not occur in those who work in a certain way, when the intelligence, otherwise occupied, does not exercise a sufficiently attentive supervision over the muscular movements.　This is because there is at that time a veritable discordance between the cerebral acts and the movements, which are performed in a thoroughly automatic manner, that the muscles become fatigued, and finish by performing disordinate movements, that they may be considered as being in an ataxic condition.　It is very singular to see a trouble so essentially nervous constitute a morbid functional state which is almost incurable ; and M. Gallard in vain seeks the reason of this peculiarity in certain diathetic influences, which he most carefully studies, and which he endeavours to make the basis of a rational treatment.　But he is obliged to acknowledge the small efficacy of all the medical means he has successively employed, including electricity ; and, tired of the struggle, is reduced to advise prothetic apparatus, in which he does not seem to have much more confidence, although he describes them with great minuteness.—*London Med. Record,* Jan. 15, 1878.

On Spinal Hemiplegia.

KÖBNER (*Deutsches Archiv für Klin. Medicin,* Band xix., and *Centralblatt für die Medicin Wissenschaften,* Nov. 3) reports two cases of spinal hemiplegia. The first was the case of a man aged 28, the subject of secondary syphilis, in whom lumbar pain was soon followed by paralysis of the right leg and loss of sensibility in the left.　In the right leg sensation was preserved, but for a time it, as well as the reflex excitability, were increased, the temperature was lowered, the muscular sense preserved.　In the left leg motion was normal ; but sensibility showed a peculiar partial diminution, for although tactile sensibility, the senses of weight and of space, were intact, sensibility to pain and temperature were lost. There were also present the sensations of a half girdle, and disturbances of the vesical, rectal, and genital functions.　By the presence of other decided syphilitic phenomena and the improvement of all the symptoms by the inunction cure, no doubt remained of the case being a right-sided syphilitic affection of the spinal cord opposite the lumbar enlargement. The second case was that of a woman aged 31, whose history included syphilis. There were present paralysis of the left lower extremity, with normal cutaneous sensibility, sometimes heightened; sensation of passive movements was abolished. The motor functions of the right leg were not quite intact, but it was not much stronger than the left, and sensibility to touch, pain, and temperature was abolished, although the perception of passive movements remained. In this case the lesion, at least at the commencement of the disease, must have been limited to the left half of the cord.—*London Med. Record*, Jan. 15, 1878.

Paralysis of the Right Spinal Accessory Nerve.

In a dissertation (Berlin, 1877), B. HOLZ describes the case of a man who, previously in good health, was suddenly seized, after exposure to cold, with weakness of the right arm. On the same day he also began to suffer from difficulty in swallowing. The right shoulder was lower than the left, and could be only slightly raised. The right trapezius and sterno-cleido-mastoid muscles felt flabby, although they reacted well to the electric current. The angle of the right scapula lay nearer the spine than that of the left; the upper part of the bone, however, stood further out. The left half of the palate appeared narrower and more arched than the right; the uvula deviated to the right; the left half of the palate alone moved; the right, even during rest, was farther from the pharynx than the left. The speech was not nasal, although there was difficulty in swallowing. The sensibility of the pharynx was normal, as was also the motor power of the right side of the face. The right vocal chord was paralyzed; the sensibility of the laryngeal mucous membrane was increased; the voice was not hoarse. The pulse was persistently accelerated, though but slightly. Iodide of potassium and faradization greatly improved the patient's condition. In Holz's opinion, there was rheumatic paresis of the accessory nerve, the seat of the lesion being in the trunk of the nerve a short distance beyond its exit from the skull.—*British Med. Journ.*, Jan. 5, 1878, from *Centralblatt f. d. Med. Wissenschaften.*

On the Treatment of Tetanus by Rest.

Professor H. de RENZI, of Genoa (*Gazette Médical de Paris*, No. 32, 1877), in a letter to Professor Botkin, says that in many cases it appeared to him that rest alone was the only means by which the terrible sufferings could be relieved. He relates how, by a series of observations, he was led to perfect this method of treatment by rest, and to accomplish cures which previously he could not obtain with the most powerful remedies. In one case of tetanus, which died in spite of large doses of chloral, the effects of light were observed; the number and intensity of the attacks were almost doubled when the patient, previously kept in darkness, was exposed to light. The approximate proportion of paroxysms was ten in darkness, eighteen in full light. He instituted numerous investigations concerning the strychnine tetanus of frogs, which closely resembles idiopathic and traumatic tetanus, and found the following results: 1. Tetanus is more intense in the frogs when placed in full light than in those kept in darkness. 2. The spasms develop with greater rapidity and intensity in animals which are agitated incessantly than in those which are kept quiet. The influence of mechanical stimulus is much more marked when aided by light. 3. Small frogs poisoned with one-twentieth of a milligramme of strychnia die soon if they are struck briskly, but may survive if left in perfect repose. Two cases of tetanus in man were treated in 1873; the first was treated with successive doses of chloral and repeated injections of curare, and died; the second, treated almost exclusively by rest. recovered. Of three other cases treated in 1874, on the same plan, only one died. Since then he further notes three recoveries out of four cases. A case which recovered was one of strychnine tetanus, in which every attack produced symptoms of asphyxia. Another recovered case, with intense symptoms, had followed amputation of the little finger after injury. The third case was one of idiopathic tetanus following fever. The death of the fourth case is attributed by the author to the fact that in his absence the patient had not been kept completely isolated. In one of the three first cases the patient, who had bronchitis, was taken with great difficulty in expectoration and intense dyspnœa. The author thought that the absorption of oxygen and elimination of carbonic acid were impeded by the profound darkness of the room—according to Pettenkofer, whose experiments have proved that light facilitates the two acts of respiration. Accordingly, as soon as the patient was found to be out of danger, light was occasionally admitted into the room, and it was ascertained that then the number of respirations per minute was greater than when darkness prevailed. The author summarizes his plan of treatment as follows: 1. Placing the patient in a room perfectly dark, the door being opened only every four hours to bring and remove necessary articles; 2. Obliterating the auditory canal with wax, and advising the patient to keep as quiet as possible; 3. Administration of beef-tea, an egg, and two tablespoonfuls of wine every hour; 4. Belladonna and ergot for the relief of pain; 5. The floor should be carpeted.—*London Med. Record*, Jan. 15, 1878.

—

On Occipital Neuralgia.

In view of the statements of Erb and Hasse, that little or nothing is known of vaso-motor and trophic disturbances in connection with occipital neuralgia, the following case is of interest. It occurred in Dr. Naunyn's practice in the clinic of the University of Heidelberg, and is reported in the *Berliner Medicin. Wochenschrift*, Dec. 10, by Dr. JULIUS SCHREIBER, Assistant-Physician.

F. P., a mechanic, aged 49, of healthy parents, had suffered severely from intermittent fever within the last twenty years, from which even now he is not quite free. His present illness commenced in the spring of 1872 with severe pains at the back of the head. They lasted three months, and then were removed under medical treatment. After an interval of two years, they recurred in the manner here described. He was a well-built, well-nourished man, and his affection was only indicated by the head held inclined forward in an anxiously constrained manner. The head was large and symmetrical, with abundant growth of hair, the face was red, the conjunctivae were injected, and there was a copious secretion of tears. Pressure on the forehead and intra-orbital region was painless, but the scalp, and especially the occiput, was extremely tender. In this region intense pain had existed for four weeks, which appeared to follow the course of the great occipital nerves, and was severest at the vertex, where in a space of about a hand-breadth there was acute sensibility to the slightest touch. The pain was paroxysmal, commencing every morning exactly at six and nine o'clock, lasting each time from fifteen to thirty minutes, and was always ushered in by repeated sneezing, with increased mucous secretion in both nostrils. When the pain had lasted some time, stiffness of the neck supervened, rendering all lateral movement impossible. But the patient was able to incline the head forward, by which the pain was considerably lessened. It was found that he could also incline the head backwards; this, however, at first increased the pain until a certain point of reclination had been reached, after which a further bending backwards was attended by the same relief as in inclination forwards. Towards the

end of each paroxysm there was repeated hiccup; after which there was case for
the rest of the day. He was ordered a daily dose of 1 gramme ($=15\frac{1}{2}$ grains)
of sulphate of quinine. With each dose the attacks diminished, and after the
third dose there came on only the usual sneezing and hiccup, but no pain. After
a complete cessation of six weeks, the disorder returned. One gramme of quinine was ordered to be taken at 4 A. M. and 3 P. M.; and when four grammes
had been taken, the attacks ceased. He took daily, for a fortnight more, half a
gramme of quinine, and has been well since. This was a clear case of double
intermittent occipital neuralgia. The accompanying vaso-motor phenomena of
sneezing, injection of the conjunctivæ, lachrymation, and increased nasal secretion are generally found only in neuralgia of the fifth nerve (trifacial, trigeminus).
In the present case they point to a close relation of the occipital and trigeminal
nerves. This connection was indicated by Lambert (*London Med.* Gazette, vol.
xxxii., p. 918), who was about to divide the facial nerve in a case of prosopalgia
(tic douloureux). On cutting down behind the lobe of the ear, he came upon
the great auricular nerve, which, when touched, threw the affected facial nerves
into a state of tension. On dividing it the tic was cured. The pain in trigeminal
neuralgia is, further, sometimes found to radiate along the course of the occipital
nerve. The hiccup may be regarded as due to irritation of the vagus, reflected
from the occipital nerve (Pflüger, *On the Sensory Functions of the Spinal Cord*,
1853). Though the rigidly erect position of the neck is regarded usually as
almost pathognomonic of occipital neuralgia, yet the present patient constantly
held his head inclined forward, and carefully avoided raising it. It would seem
that, so long as the inclination of the head, forward or backward, is occasioned
only by the weight of the head, it is not only possible, but productive of ease,
whereas any further inclination, or a raising movement, increases the pain, by
throwing into action those muscles of the neck whose nerves are implicated in
occipital neuralgia.—*London Med. Record*, Jan. 15, 1878.

On Paracentesis in Pleurisy.

Dr. WILSON FOX, in a paper on "The Mortality of Pleurisy considered in
Relation to the Operation of Paracentesis Thoracis" (*British Medical Journal*,
November 24th, and December 1st, 1877), has collated a considerable series of
statistics showing the relative mortality of pleurisy treated with and without
paracentesis. The statistics are gathered from the great hospitals of Vienna,
Prague, Paris, London, Manchester, and Berlin. The first table shows the mortality per cent. of *all* cases of pleurisy treated without paracentesis, collected from
these various sources, and extending over a period of 32 years. The mean total
mortality is estimated at from 10 to 17 per cent., though in some cases and in
some institutions it fell as low as from 6 to 7 per cent., and at the Children's Hospital, Vienna, it was as low as 1.6 per cent. With this mortality, which Dr.
Fox admits is higher than he expected to find, he contrasts the statements of
Louis, Walshe, and Gairdner, that uncomplicated pleurisy is rarely fatal; and he
draws up a second table comparing the mortality of complicated and uncomplicated pleurisy. The mean mortality in the latter case is but 6 per cent.; and in
uncomplicated serous effusions he considers Ewald's average of 2.2 to 2.7 per
cent. to be quite an outside limit. Dr. Fox then passes to the consideration of
the statistics of cases of paracentesis, and he finds the mean mortality after operation raised to 27 per cent.; only falling to or below 10 per cent. in the hands of
observers whose operations were confined to serous effusions in the early stage.
The table is drawn up with laborious care, the cases, upwards of 1600, being collected from a great number of authors, both English and foreign. The mean
mortality of serous effusions after paracentesis is shown to be 17 per cent.; of

sero-purulent and purulent, 37 per cent. ; of sanguinolent, 77 per cent. ; and of pneumothorax, 85 per cent. The causes of death after paracentesis in serous effusions are found to be purulent transformation, tubercle, malignant disease, and general grave complications. Purulent transformation was the cause of death in 45 per cent. of the total number of cases that proved fatal ; or in 25 per cent. if all cases complicated by phthisis and other grave maladies be excluded ; or in from 10 to 5 per cent. of all cases operated upon. Dr. Fox does not refer this change to the causes usually assigned, i. e., to an original tendency to purulence shown by a lactescent appearance of the fluid when first aspirated, nor to the admission of air into the pleura, nor to the presence of tubercle, nor to the existence of pyrexia at the time of operation, though in individual cases each of these may be the cause of purulence, but rather to parenchymatous changes in the structure of the pleura itself, the artificial withdrawal of the fluid having a tendency to intensify congestion, and to increase inflammatory action. He believes that there is but little natural tendency in serous effusions to undergo purulent transformation, and that in the vast majority of cases where it has followed paracentesis it must be directly ascribed to the operation. Considering the whole question of serous effusions, Dr. Fox holds to the opinion that death from uncomplicated serous effusion is among the rarities of medical experience, and that reviewing the results obtained by paracentesis he cannot look upon it altogether as a life-saving operation. He advises that greater caution should be exercised, and that it should not be performed in very early stages of the disease or without distinct indications for its necessity, the most important of these being threatened failure of cardiac power. The most potent argument in favor of an early operation, he finds, is the fear that the long continuance of the effusion may endanger the expansibility of the lung. He admits, however, that the cases which recover under early paracentesis do so more rapidly than if it be deferred, or if they be left to nature.

Turning to purulent effusions treated by paracentesis, he considers the mortality of 37 per cent. very high, though he anticipates that it may be diminished by a careful application of the antiseptic method. It contrasts unfavourably with the statistics of the non-operated cases left to spontaneous cure. Of Anderl's cases of empyema, the mortality of the non-operated was 13 per cent. less than the operated, the cases that resulted in spontaneous external opening being the most successful ; out of 25 cases the deaths were only two, or 8 per cent. ; of eight cases of bronchial perforation the deaths were three, or 37 per cent. Dr. Goodhart reports 11 cases of spontaneous external opening, all of which recovered ; Ewald six, three of which died. Dr. Fox considers it more than probable that in certain cases the pus is reabsorbed.

In conclusion, Dr. Fox urges that the operation of paracentesis should not be resorted to carelessly and in haste to produce immediate and temporary relief ; that the risks are great, and that many cases may recover if left to the action of nature. He further considers that when the operation is necessary, the withdrawal of a small portion of the effusion gives immediate relief, and is very frequently followed by the absorption of the remainder.

In answer to a question put by Sir William Jenner during the discussion that followed the reading of this paper at the last meeting of the British Medical Association, as to the relative mortality of the operation of paracentesis at different ages, Dr. Fox appends an addendum. He shows, by statistical tables, that the deaths after the age of thirty exceed those before that age in serous effusion by 16 per cent. ; in purulent effusion by 9 per cent. ; in uncomplicated serous effusion by 9 per cent. ; in uncomplicated purulent effusion by 6 per cent. Pleurisy, on the other hand, seems more frequently to occur between the ages of twenty and thirty.

Dr. CLIFFORD ALLBUTT ("On the Treatment of Pleuritic Effusion," *British Medical Journal*, November 24, 1877), declares his enthusiastic belief in the value of paracentesis. There is no doubt in his creed, and it is thus boldly ex-pressed : " Let him, then, who hesitates to tap the pleura, remember that, be-fore his next visit, his patient, seemingly so tranquil, may have passed into the deeper stillness of death. Whether the effusion then be rapid or slow in its flood, if the cavity be full, operate without delay. This is, I believe, one of those golden rules to which there is no exception." Speaking also of empyema, he says: "If I have one conviction in medicine more urgent than another it is this, if pus or other septic material be present in the body, we must not rest until it is removed. I therefore dislike and reprobate all temporizing with an empyema. Out with it, and provide against a reaccumulation." He divides pleurisy into acute fibrinous pleurisy, quiet effusive pleurisy, empyema, and pleu-ritic dropsy. The first, characterized by pain and pyrexia from the outset, is of an active and inflammatory nature, and the exudation has a tendency to reab-sorption. Such cases he treats by leeches, diuretics, and blisters. If dulness continue after the fever has abated, he puts the patient under a course of mer-cury. Only when the circulation is impeded does he resort to tapping. He declares that in these highly organized effusions suppuration rarely occurs after operation, even if air enter the pleura. He recommends in these cases the use of the aspirator, with fine canulæ, and to puncture the pleura repeatedly, draw-ing off what is to be had at each point. In quiet effusive pleurisy in the serous stage, tapping is recommended unhesitatingly ; and, if the operation be performed early, the results are excellent—a serious illness of three months under medical treatment being converted into a moderate indisposition of three weeks. The longer, however, operation is deferred, the less confidently can the best results be hoped for ; the more danger of empyema and of clots, and the more the danger to lung and constitution. Delay, he urges, in large effusions exposes the patient to the risk of sudden death; and, though in small effusions delay and medicinal treatment may be counselled, yet Dr. Allbutt finds it better to tap in all cases where more than two pints of fluid are present. He considers, however, that in quiet serous effusions the aspirator is unadvisable, as no more fluid should be withdrawn from the chest than the lung can replace at that time. He prefers and uses, therefore, a fine trocar and canula, arranged so as to act on the syphon principle. In empyema he advises opening the cavity freely with antiseptic pre-cautions as low down as possible, to let the pus drain out.

In a paper ("Notes on Pleuritic Effusion in Childhood," *British Medical Journal*, December 1, 1877) Dr. THOMAS BARLOW and Mr. ROBERT PARKER record their personal experiences. From the frequent difficulty of recognizing pleurisy in children, and diagnosing between serous and purulent effusions, they recommend, as a *matter of routine*, the use of the hypodermic syringe as a diag-nostic aid. In the treatment of serous effusion, they recommend very strongly that the removal of a very small quantity of fluid is to be preferred to emptying the pleura ; and they state that this is frequently rapidly followed by absorption of the rest. This may be done by the aspirator, or even by the hypodermic syringe. If the effusion be considerable and the dyspnœa urgent, then they ad-vise emptying the chest, to give the lung the chance of expanding, which it does in a rapid and forcible manner in children. Their opinion is against the treat-ment by iodine, diuretics, and blisters.

From the marked majority of cases of pleurisy in children being empyemata, and from having practically ascertained the fact that a serous effusion will remain

serious for an indefinite period, they lean to the opinion that purulent effusions are
not so from transformation, but are empyemata *ab initio*. To evacuate the pus
if collected in small quantities separated by adhesions, a hypodermic syringe capable of holding two drachms is recommended; if the collection be larger, the
aspirator-trocar (Potain) should be used. It is thought better to perform paracentesis under chloroform pushed to complete insensibility, to avoid collapse and
cough. If pus should become fetid or rapidly accumulate in larger quantity permanent drainage is advised, and it is contended that in all cases this should be
done by a double opening, to secure more complete drainage. The first opening
should be made in the front of the thorax; the second below and internal to the
angle of the scapula. In lieu of washing out the cavity with a syringe or irrigator, it is thought better to place the little patient in a warm bath. containing a
weak solution of Condy's fluid, or carbolic acid, with the water high enough to
cover the upper opening. Of the natural modes of cure, they consider rupture
through the lung the least unfavourable. Of eight cases under their care two
died, two made good recoveries, and four have done indifferently well. Spontaneous evacuation by external opening has given in their experience no good
result, being associated with ulceration of the pleura, necrosis of the rib or rib-
cartilage, abscess, unhealthy ulceration of adjacent tissues, and subsequent
deformity.

Dr. HENRY BARNES ("On the Value of Paracentesis of the Chest in the
Treatment of Pleuritic Effusion, *British Medical Journal*, December 1st, 1877)
publishes eleven cases of pleurisy in which paracentesis was eminently successful.
The cases were three of simple acute pleurisy, relieved and cured by a single
operation; two cases of acute pleurisy occurring as a complication of enteric
fever, in each of which paracentesis was performed three times with complete
recovery; and in the three cases of chronic pleurisy two recovered after one operation; the third had paracentesis performed fourteen times, Dr. Barnes considering the pleura had lost its absorbing power from the considerable stretching it
had undergone through long neglect of the case. In the treatment of empyema,
Dr. Barnes speaks highly of paracentesis. He reports three cases; in one necrosis of the parietal pleura occurred: a double opening was made and a drainage-tube inserted, and the cavity washed out by a weak solution of carbolic acid.
The third, one of traumatic origin, was complicated with pneumonia. After
recovery, the affected side in the first case measured $\frac{7}{8}$ of an inch, in the second
$1\frac{1}{4}$ inch, less than the sound side. Dr. Barnes considers that the danger of purulent transformation is entirely obviated by the perfection of the instrument used,
entrance of the air into the cavity of the pleura being thereby prevented. He
thinks in left-sided pleurisies operation should not be long delayed, and in all
cases where dyspnœa is urgent there is more danger in delay than in operating.
He makes a rule to operate at once, without waiting for urgent dyspnœa to set
in, in cases when the chest is two parts filled with fluid; but if but half full he
waits, and tries the treatment by rest and iodine applications and diuretics, which
is frequently successful. He recommends the use of Potain's aspirator, and that
the puncture should be made in a perpendicular line with the angle of the scapula.
in the eighth or ninth interspace, and an inch and a half above a horizontal line
drawn through the lowest point at which the respiratory murmur is distinctly
heard on the other side. His practice is also to withdraw as much fluid from the
chest as possible. For after-treatment, he recommends iodine applications externally, and diuretics.—*London Med. Record*, Jan. 15, 1878.

Digitalis and Morphia in Heart Affections.

In his *Journal de Thérapeutique* for January 10, Prof. GUBLER sums up as follows the conclusions of an elaborate paper on "The Comparative Indications of Morphia and Digitalis in the Course of Organic Affections of the Heart:" "1. Digitalis, the moderator and regulator *par excellence* of the circulatory rhythm, increases the energy of each systole in proportion as it brings about a diminution in the number of the cardiac revolutions. This result may be expressed in an arithmetical formula in these terms: The force dispensed by the heart in the unity of time being relatively constant, the absolute value of the fraction is so much greater as the denominator is less. 2. By means of this *cohibition*, with or without the aid of directly hypercinetic or even corroborant action, the probable existence of which has not been demonstrated, digitalis becomes a precious agent in special tonic medication in some subjects of nervous palpitation, and in most of those who have organic disease of the heart. 3. Its success is, so to say, assured as long as the asystolia depends upon disorder of the cardiac innervation, and on the ill-directed employment of the contractile force of the myocardium. Now, this *cardiac ataxia* is the normal condition of organic lesions of the heart in the early periods of their development, and it persists not only in the more advanced anatomical stages, but often also amidst the general complications which aggravate the symptoms in the gravest cases. 4. Nevertheless, a time comes when the asystolia is no longer the mere effect of the too rapid succession of more or less abortive, and consequently inefficacious, efforts. The debility becomes fundamental, and Bouillaud's *folie du cœur* gives place to powerlessness. Then the reign of digitalis is over, and that of direct or indirect tonics, of *dynamophores*, and of stimulants commences. 5. Among all these remedies, the first place, without contradiction, belongs to opium and some of its principles, morphia especially possessing remarkable efficacy against the accidents resulting from cardiac paresis, which I designate *cardioplegia*. 6. By arousing the vitality of the capillary network, stimulating hæmatosis and the act of nutrition, it favours the increase of force in general, and especially that of the excito- motory force of the spinal bulb, and of the conductibility of the nervous cords which issue from it. It contributes also to keep up the circulation and the other great functions in consequence, by the calm it imparts to the sensibility, and the moderation it consecutively restores to the rhythm of the movements of the heart. Again, it acts in the same direction by its hypnotic power, as sleep suppresses much expenditure, and as the *soporal congestion* is an anatomical condition extremely favourable to the restoration and nutrition of the nervous centres, very poor in capillary vessels. 7. If we are well informed as to the different aptitudes of digitalis and morphia, and if careful clinical analysis enables us to seize the two principal pathological conditions to which these great medicaments correspond, still, in spite of this, science is far from being able to guide us surely in the choice of the appropriate remedy in each particular case. What are the signs by which the practitioner may recognize that he ought to have recourse to opium rather than to digitalis? or, which in our opinion comes to the same, what are the differential characteristics by which he can distinguish *cardioplegia* from *cardiataxy?* 8. Digitalis is evidently indicated in simple lesions of the orifices and the valves, even when these are advanced, provided these exist in young persons otherwise well, or in more aged subjects who are as yet exempt from the general changes in the economy embraced under the term cardiac cachexia. Doubt commences when the asystolia is accompanied by grave complications, as anasarca, dropsy, albuminuria, cyanosis, orthopnœa, etc. In such cases we must proceed only tentatively. The same may be said of purely nervous palpitations, which, like

the secondary circulatory disorders of organic lesions of the heart, may doubtless
be divided into sthenic or irritative, and asthenic or paretic, between which their
apparent characteristics do not allow of our distinguishing. 9. In doubtful cases
it is digitalis which presents most chance of success, since it has been found to
succeed when all hope see red lost; but it must be given with caution and watching, so that it may be stopped in time if contraindications present themselves.
10. The following rules should be observed in its administration: Preference
should be given to digitaline or to the tincture of the Codex, as other preparations
are less efficacious and less safe. Infusions, whether in cold or warm water, possess too great nauseating or even cathartic power to allow of their being used in
heart affections. Digitaline, however, should not be given in the pill form, but
in an alcoholic solution properly diluted; two milligrammes per gramme being a
sufficiently concentrated alcoholic solution. 11. The mean dose of the tincture
of the Codex is represented by ten drops; that of amorphous digitaline is one
milligramme, or fifteen drops of alcoholic solution; and of the crystallized digitaline one-quarter milligramme, or four drops of the solution. This may be repeated two or three times in the twenty-four hours—the daily dose attained of
the tincture being twenty to thirty drops, of the amorphous digitaline forty-five
drops, and of the crystallized twelve drops. These doses need hardly ever be
exceeded.' 12. The digitalis should be given at a distance from the meals; and
if the stomach is intolerant of it, it should be combined with tincture of carda-
moms, essence of mint, etc. If in place of amending after the early doses, the
anxiety increases, and the pulse becomes small and irregular, it should be suspended for two days, and then tried combined with opium and aromatics; abandoning it altogether if this association does not succeed. Although its beneficial
effects are not observed until about the third day, yet the digitalis should not be
prolonged beyond five or six consecutive days, for fear of toxical effects being
produced by accumulation. 13. In organic disease of the heart, uncomplicated
with grave lesion of the aortic bulb, and especially of the arch of the aorta, we
may say that the later employment of opium coincides with the withdrawal of
digitalis. Morphia may render assistance when the resistance of the economy
becomes enfeebled. Its indication increases with the cachectic symptoms, and it
becomes urgent and inevitable in the ultimate periods of the disease, when paralysis progressively invades the central apparatus of the circulation as the prelude of death. In cardiac affections morphia is the last safeguard of the patient
and the *ultima ratio* of therapeutics. 14. But the indication of morphia is much
more early in the course of aortic alterations, whether independent or complicated with lesions of the heart itself. It exists sometimes before the appearance
of rational symptoms of the affection, often prior to any cachectic alteration, and
almost always in the slightly advanced stages of the malady. In the first category
it is required to assuage the acute pain of *angor pectoris;* in the second it serves
to palliate the effects of the distension and wearing away of nervous branches by
aneurismal dilatation of the aorta; and in the third it combats alike this paralysis
from local cause and the paretic condition which results from the insufficient restoration of the centres of innervation, as well as the injury done to the sanguineous
crasis and general nutrition. 15. Except the painful complication alluded to
above, all the other conditions call for exclusively the stimulant and indirectly
corroborative action of opium, and opium exhibits this only on the condition of
being administered in small and frequent doses. Moreover, in order not to increase the existing torpor of the digestive organs, it is also desirable to employ it
hypodermically. 16. The dose of the chlorhydrate of morphia should at its
maximum be only 0.01 centigramme to commence with, and it would be better
even to employ only half this quantity. The injections may be repeated two or

three times in the twenty-four hours, continuing them almost for an indefinite time if the circumstances are imperious. 17. But the early doses becoming insufficient, they have to be progressively increased, especially during attacks of asystolia, diminishing them again when the crisis has passed or become appeased. The daily mass of morphia may thus be raised, if necessary, to four, six, eight, or ten centigrammes, distributed over three or four injections, made at equal intervals in the twenty-four hours. 18. These large doses must be continued as long as they are required to keep up the functional dynamism and sustain the economy, or at all events prevent its giving way. The inconveniences of chronic morphinism cannot be placed in balance against the dangers which immediately menace the existence of the patient. 19. In spite of their aptitudes being so different, and their indications in some measure contradictory, opium and digitalis are far from always excluding each other, but often in the transitory phases or complicated forms of diseases of the heart afford mutual aid; as, for example, when the element ‘pain’ becomes added to the motor disturbances of the organ, or when asystolia expresses not only the precipitation and tumult or ataxia of the heart, but also a certain amount of paralysis or cardioplegia. By contributing to the maintenance of the strength, the morphia injections insure the regulating effects of the digitalis, and at the same time act as a counterpoise to the depressing influence which the latter does not fail to exert as soon as the dose given becomes exaggerated. 20. The simultaneous or successful administration of these two great remedies in nowise precludes our having recourse to the various other means of treatment derivable from hygiene or the materia medica.”—*Med. Times and Gaz.*, Jan. 19, 1878.

On a Case of Cardiac Neurosis.

In a paper entitled, “Clinical Contribution to the Neuroses of the Heart,” published in the *Berliner Klinische Wochenschrift* for November 27, Dr. E. ZENCKER relates the following case.

P., a labourer, æt. 22, was admitted to hospital on July 27, 1876, with symptoms of extensive œdema of the lungs, and enormously increased action of the heart. The respirations were 56, pulse 208, with great orthopnœa and restlessness; the sensorium was not impaired. He stated that on the 24th and 25th July he had been seized with several violent attacks of palpitation of the heart, from which he had in previous years suffered twice. Percussion showed that the limits of the heart were considerably extended. The grave pulmonary œdema was at once treated after the manner of Traube with dry cupping, sinapisms and acetate of lead in doses of nearly a grain every half-hour, also an ounce of infusion of valerian, every hour. After five hours the œdema began to diminish, and the acetate was given only every hour, and subsequently every two and three hours. The pulse and respiration remained the same.

On the 28th the patient showed intense cyanosis, and great orthopnœa; the pulse was small, and could only be counted at the heart. There was extensive cardiac dulness towards both sides; the sounds could not be distinguished, and the lungs showed on the right side some remains of œdema. The sputum was scanty and rusty.

On the 29th the œdema had disappeared, 31½ grains of acetate of lead having been taken in all; otherwise he was the same. In the afternoon the pulse rose to 220 regular beats in the minute, respiration being 52.

On the 30th the temperature was 36.8° cent. (98.24° Fahr.): pulse 204, resp. 44. He passed 1200 cubic centimetres of urine of sp. gr. 1017; no albumen. His general condition was the same; the pulse was scarcely perceptible. Musk was ordered to be given every three hours in three-grain doses. The bowels were freely moved after about an ounce of infusion of senna; the stools contained blood and much mucus. At night a subcutaneous injection of hydrochlorate of morphia (0.12 grain) was given, with manifest relief to the patient, who towards morning fell into a sound sleep till 9 A. M.

On the 31st the pulse was 92, respiration 28. temperature 37.5° cent. (99.5° Fahr.) The skin was moist and deep-red in the face and about the ears; the senses were clear; there was no cyanosis; the pupils were contracted; the pulse was full and bounding. The left cardiac region of the thorax protruded more than the right; at the systole the thoracic wall about the apex beat was strongly thrust forward; the apex beat lay in the fifth intercostal space, about 1.2 inches outside the nipple, and extending over a space of 1.2 inches; absolute dulness from the third to the sixth rib, and from the sternum to 1.2 inches outside the nipple. At the apex was heard a prolonged rough systolic murmur, which was cut short by the diastole; this was continued to the second intercostal space on the left side, where the diastolic sound was strong, and accompanied by a loud diastolic murmur. At the insertion of the fourth rib on the left side there was a systolic murmur, and an indistinct diastolic sound; on the right side, about the third rib, a systolic and faint diastolic murmur. The musk and valerian were discontinued, and a dose of castor-oil was given.

August 1. Pulse 84, temperature 37.3°, resp. 20; he was very somnolent; the bowels were freely opened; the stools contained chiefly mucus, accompanied by great tenesmus.

August 2. Temperature 36.9° C.; pulse 76; respiration 20. There were moderate facial cyanosis, continuous drowsiness, and impaired sensorium. At the apex of the heart was heard a systolic and diastolic murmur; at the left margin of the sternum, about the fourth costal cartilage, a systolic sound and a weak diastolic murmur; at the right third costal cartilage a loud diastolic murmur, prolonged to the systole, which is also heard over the pulmonary artery with a strongly pronounced second sound. The double murmur was heard in the carotid, and the systolic sound in the femoral artery during expiration. In the afternoon the patient was suddenly seized with violent palpitations. At 6 P. M., after vomiting some dark-brown matter, the heart beats numbered 204, without the least irregularity; respiration 36; cyanosis moderate. A subcutaneous injection of morphia (0.09 grain), and infusion of valerian were given, an hour after which free perspiration set in, and the pulse fell to 140.

August 3. He passed a good night, but vomited violently in the morning. Pulse 180; respiration 28. After a further, but ineffectual, injection of morphia (0.12 grain), he was ordered camphor and valerian.

August 4. Temperature, 36.7° C.; pulse 188; resp. 28. There were great stupor and restlessness; the pupils were dilated; he had marked cyanosis. At 10.45 A. M. 0.15 grain of morphia was injected, and the patient became quiet; the pupils contracted and cardiac action diminished, so that at 5 P. M. the face was bright-red, the pulse 96 and steady. He continued thus until 1 P. M. of the 6th August, when, while raising himself in bed, another violent attack of palpitation set in. Within half an hour the pulse rose to 218; the lips and checks were cyanotic; pupils very dilated, acting sluggishly; pulse scarcely to be felt; general and increasing stupor. Musk was first given, and then a subcutaneous injection of morphia, which, however, proved insufficient.

August 7. There was cyanosis; the pulse was much the same; hence a further injection of 0.18 grain of muriate of morphia was given at 10 A. M., and in consequence the pulse gradually sank, very irregularly, in five hours to 170; the pupils contracted; the cyanosis diminished; the skin became moist. At 4.30 P. M. a further injection of 0.9 grain of morphia was given, and by 6 P. M. the pulse fell to 92–106; the face beca 1 e deep-red, the pupils we1e 1 uch contracted, and the body co\ered with p1ofuse pe1spi1ation. Du1ing the next two days things continued in a 1 o1e satisfactory condition, the pulse \a1ying f1o 1 84 to 64. Infusion of digitalis (1 in 50) was now substituted fo1 \ale1ian, and half an ounce was gi\en e\e1y th1ee hours. In the night from the 9th to the 10th, afte1 a change of position, when the bow\ls we1e 1 o\ed, a 1enewed accele1ation of the hea1t's action set in.

August 10. Pulse 176; 1espi1ation 28. At 11.30 A.M., 0.15 g1ain of 1 u1iate of 1 o1phia was injected, and 1epeated fi\e hou1s late1. P1ofuse pe1spi-1ation set in du1ing the night. The next 1 o1ning the pulse had fallen to 84, respi1ation 22. But at 2 P.M. of the sa 1 e day—the 11th—a fu1the1 exace1ba-tion set in, which was the seve1est of all, and lasted seven days. Du1ing this pe1iod the pulse fluctuated f1o 1 168 to 200; the 1espi1ations at one ti 1 e attained a 1 axi 1 u 1 of 140 pe1 1 inute; the u1ine contained t1aces of albu 1 en, and a few hyaline casts. The t1eat 1 ent consisted of 1epeated injections of 1 o1phia up to 0.225 grain, of sinapis 1 s, d1y cupping, 1 usk, \ale1ian, fo1 which was afte1-wa1ds substituted infusion of digitalis (0.5 to 150). On the 17th the pulse sud-denly fell f1o 1 188 in the mo1ning to 88 at 10 A.M.; pupils again cont1acted; the face and neck 1eddened, especially on the left side. The next day an abun-dant he1petic e1uption appea1ed on the 1ight unde1lip. The pulse fell to 76, and 1espi1ation to 20 in the 1 inute. The attacks of palpitation 1ecu11ed, with less se\e1ity, on se\e1al subsequent occasions, and we1e 1 ostly occasioned by changes of postu1e, e\acuation of the bowels, o1 atte 1 pts at pe1cussion of the ca1diac 1egions. The hea1t-cont1actions 1 anifested at these ti 1 es a 1 a1ked i11egula1ity, and we1e of a double-type, 1e 1 inding one of the "alternating pulse" (pulsus bige 1 inus). The injections of morphia we1e continued (up to 0.24 grain) from ti 1 e to ti 1 e, each ti 1 e affo1ding 1elief. On the 22d of August the apex-beat lay in the fifth inte1costal space, towa1ds the 1 edian line, and at each systole the tho1acic wall was th1ust fo1wa1d, the ele\ation extending to fou1-tenths of an inch to the 1ight of the 1 edian line about the fou1th inte1costal space. At the apex, besides a 1 uffled sound, was hea1d a loud systolic 1 u1 1 u1; o\e1 the ste1nu 1 and to the 1ight of it up to the thi1d 1ib was audible a loud diastolic 1 u1 1 u1, which was also hea1d on the pul 1 ona1y a1te1y along with the 1 a1ked diastolic sound. On Septe 1 be1 2d the ca1diac dulness sca1cely extended to the left of the nipple, and the apex-beat lay in the fifth inte1costal space. The last attack, a \e1y e\anescent one, occu11ed on Septe 1 be1 8th. By deg1ees the patient was accusto 1 ed to 1 o\e 1 ents and 1 ode1ate acti\ity, and his condition i 1 p1o\ed, so that at the end of Septe 1 be1 he was discha1ged well. F1o 1 the patient's account of his p1e\ious history, it appea1s that the fi1st attack of palpi-tation and dyspnœa occu11ed about th1ee yea1s p1e\iously, when, while st1aining to lift a hea\y weight, he suddenly fell down unconscious, afte1 which he had si 1 ila1 attacks f1o 1 ti 1 e to ti 1 e, caused by ha1d wo1k and 1aising and moving hea\y weights. At the sa 1 e ti 1 e, th1ough inability to wo1k, he was 1 uch 1educed in ci1cu 1 stances.

A 1e\iew of the case p1ecludes the idea of its being due to the ao1tic insuffi-ciency, and also excludes it f1o 1 the catego1y of "the weakened hea1t" of Eng-lish autho1s. No1 is it of the natu1e of angina pecto1is, owing to the co 1 plete absence of pain. It is 1athe1 a hype1kinesis, for the functional action of the hea1t is uni 1 pai1ed between the attacks, du1ing which attacks, howe\e1, the cont1actions a1e g1eatly inc1eased in nu 1 be1. The facts of the case, the high 1ate of the pulse, the st1iking 1egula1ity of the hea1t's beat, appea1 to point at fi1st sight to a pa1alysis of the inhibito1y cent1e of the hea1t as the cause of the se\e1al attacks. And yet the 1eal cause of the affection would see 1 1athe1 to lie in a stimulation of the excitatory cardiac centres. For, in opposition to an excessive excitation of the motor centres, the inhibitory action may be overcome or exhausted, but not yet paralyzed. We find marked irregularity of the heart's action after the continued use of digitalis, indicating unmistakably an increase in the inhibitory power. This effect of digitalis was counteracted again by the subsequent well-known primary stimulating effect of morphia injected subcutaneously. An almost conclusive argument is furnished by the effect of the vibration and shock of percussion, which on two occasions threw the heart from a state of quiescence into one of exaggerated action.

As to the cause of the increased stimulation of the excitatory cardiac nerve centres: we must look for it in the increased demands upon an already overtaxed muscle, and in the insufficient nutrition.

Notwithstanding the difficulty of determining the influence of treatment on an affection which always tends to terminate spontaneously, we cannot apparently deny the influence of morphia on the course of the several paroxysms. In six of these paroxysms, morphia injected subcutaneously sufficed to produce ease, contraction of the pupil, and a gradual diminution of the pulse to its normal frequency. But on two occasions, and when morphia was not employed at all, the pulse abruptly fell from a considerable height to the normal condition. Traube observed in the second stage of opium narcotism contraction of the pupils and diminution of the frequency of the pulse in consequence of the abnormal stimulation of the regulating cardiac nerve centres. According to Gscheidlen, a moderate dose of morphia is attended at first with diminution of the pulse, followed by an increase and then again by a reduction. Hence we conclude that the pulse-reducing effect of morphia was the result of general bodily repose and consequent absence of all pressure on the aortic system, combined with its influence on the controlling nervous system of the heart. Fresh exciting impulses being thus cut short, and with increasing powers of resistance, the paroxysms terminated.— *London Med. Record*, Jan. 15, 1878.

—

Smokers' Gastralgia.

M. REVILLOUT reports in the *Gazette des Hôpitaux* two cases of gastralgia attributed to the use of tobacco. The first case occurred in a man aged fifty-two, in M. Vulpian's wards. He had always been moderate in everything except the use of tobacco, had never undergone any privation, had always been able to choose his food, and had been careful in his diet. On six different occasions, he had been seized with extremely acute attacks of pain in the stomach, not extending to the back, and coming on more or less quickly after every meal, bringing on also vomiting of the food. In the intervals of these attacks, of which the average duration was about six weeks, his health seemed tolerably good, with the exception of some vertigo, dazzling of the sight, and weakness of the legs. These troubles were more marked when the patient felt better and smoked than when, suffering with gastric troubles, he had no appetite for anything and temporarily left off tobacco. M. Révillout also reports a case in which a gentleman in good circumstances, following an excellent hygienic system, found his digestive functions gradually failing, whilst his strength diminished. Later on, he was attacked with vertigo, staggering whilst walking, and spasms and prickings in the limbs. After every meal, severe pain was felt in the epigastric region; the face was pale, the speech gasping, the heart-beats uncertain, and the body generally discoloured. This patient smoked from twelve to fifteen cigars daily. Under advice, he reduced this number to two, and immediately a considerable improvement took place. He again took to excessive smoking; but, as the original symptoms returned, he was again obliged to abstain from tobacco. Under medical advice, he washed the tobacco of which he made his cigarettes in a coffee percolator, by first throwing on it ammoniacal water, then repeated baths of hot water. The nicotine was thus partly dissolved out of, or mechanically removed by, the warm water. The tobacco, when washed, was spread out in the sun to dry on paper, and, thus modified, satisfied the patient, who from that time was not troubled with dyspepsia or vertigo.—*British Med. Journal*, Jan. 5, 1878.

On Alcoholic Gastritis in Women.

In a lecture by M. GALLARD, published in his recent volume, *Clinique Médicale de La Pitié*, he treats of alcoholic gastritis, especially in reference to women. In the female sex habits of drunkenness often show themselves, or become exaggerated, at the period of the menopause, which is a truly critical age with regard to drunkenness. M. Gallard cites the case of a woman who showed the most characteristic symptoms of drunkenness without ever having been given to drink ; but, for two months before she came under notice, had acquired the habit of taking a few drops of sulphuric ether on a piece of sugar. This fact confirms the doctrines concerning the similarity of action between alcohol, chloroform, and ether. Changes in the stomach are the first observed in chronic alcoholism, and then there supervene changes in the liver and kidneys, which are extremely like those observed in syphilis. As a prophylactic in treatment of alcoholism, M. Gallard, following the example of Magnus Huss, administers the empyreumatic oil to which corn and potato brandies owe their special flavour, and which is known by the name of *fermentoleum solani*. From four and a half to nine doses of it may be given in drops of from three-quarters to one and a half drops, either in draughts or in pills three or four times a day. The therapeutic treatment consists in narcotics, especially opium, alkaline drinks, and hydrotherapy.—*London Med. Record*, Jan. 15, 1878.

On the Etiology of Epidemic Catarrhal Jaundice.

Dr. KLINGELHŒFFER (*Berliner Klinische Wochenschrift*, Nov. 26) cannot confirm the opinion of Dr. Köhnhorn, that the cause of epidemic jaundice lies in too great sameness of diet. He observed an epidemic of icterus from Oct. 1874, to March, 1875, among a population of all classes, whose diet was in no way other than usual, and therefore the cause must be looked for elsewhere.—*London Med. Record*, Jan. 15, 1878.

Senile Diarrhœa.

Lecturing at the Hôpital Necker upon a case of obstinate senile diarrhœa that could be traced to no obvious cause, M. POTAIN observed (*Gaz. des Hôp.*, No. 138) that sometimes errors in regimen may in these cases be accused, such as the taking inappropriate substances, water in too large quantity or too cold. Gastric catarrh also, by its reflex action and by the vicious secretions, gives rise to the diarrhœa ; but it is of especial importance in cases of this kind to seek for general diseases. Of all these, tuberculization is the most important ; and what perhaps is not sufficiently borne in mind is, that diarrhœa is often one of the primary manifestations of the tendency to tuberculization. This, too, is one of the most serious forms, because it indicates a disposition to the generalization of the disease, and, moreover, the patient neither eating nor assimilating properly, the accidents pursue a much more rapid course than in other cases. Arthritism has also frequently been put forward in this etiology, and not without reason. It is the same with marsh-poisoning, which is oftener than is supposed the primary cause of this form of diarrhœa. M. Jules Simon, especially, has related some very curious cases of this kind, the origin of which was proved by the success which attended the administration of quinine, the diarrhœa being the sole tangible symptom.   M. Potain has also met with several analogous cases which have been successfully treated by quinine.

So, too, all causes which debilitate the economy are a cause of diarrhœa, and one of the most powerful of these is old age—so much so that the diarrhœa of the aged has been separately described, with its anatomical changes, such as thickening and other alterations of the mucous membrane.   In such cases there is little disturbance of the digestion, and no pain in the abdomen, and that even when deep ulceration of the intestines has been found after death.   The patients become pale and bloated (*bouffis*); their skin becomes thin; they waste away, and fall into a state of complete apathy—the diarrhœa much resembling, therefore, in this form, that of pellagra.   There is nothing special here in the etiology, and all that can be said is, that old age constitutes an extreme predisposition to entero-colitis.   In the patient under notice, no other reason than his age can be assigned; yet not his age calculated on the number of years, for these are only sixty-two, but the age he presents in his condition of anticipated senility.   It has, indeed, been said long since, with reason, that we are of the age of our arteries; and this man has aged arteries, for they are atheromatous, and, moreover, he exhibits all the attributes of senility.   In such cases the prognosis is always a most serious one, and, according to M. Durand-Fardel, the disease is incurable when it has lasted for some weeks.   This opinion is certainly exaggerated, but it is a fact that a cure is extremely difficult, because in aged persons we can produce no action of the skin and kidneys which will balance the intestinal function.   In this patient, although in his case there was no history of prior marsh-poisoning, quinine has been given with great advantage.   It would seem, therefore, that besides its anti-periodic power, the sulphate of quinine, by the property which it possesses of inducing contraction of the capillaries, may diminish the vascularity of the intestines, and modify its secretions.—*Med. Times and Gaz.*, Jan. 12, 1878.

On the Symptoms and Diagnosis of Intestinal Obstructions—Case of Carcinoma of the Colon.

Dr. HENSGEN, writing in the *Deutsche Medicinische Wochenschrift* for December 8, remarks that very various views have been held regarding the group of affections comprehended under the general term ileus.   Regarded at first in the days of Hippocrates as a diseased condition of the intestine through metastasis of various humours, or of a *materia febrilis*, or of intestinal gaseous accumulations, later observers disregarded the bearing of the pathological processes, and held ileus to be the product of the "molus antiperistalticus," of a primary inflammation, of a reversal of peristaltic action, thus confounding cause and effect.   With the sounder pathological observations of the present century, ileus came to be a designation merely for stercoraceous vomiting, or for an intestinal obstruction, with, of course, fecal vomiting.   But it is erroneous to assume that obstruction is always accompanied by fecal vomiting.   This is impossible in occlusion of the upper portions of the small intestine, nor has it been confirmed in all cases of closure of the large intestine.   From this point of view the following unusual case is of interest.   A woman, aged 56, had long suffered from cutting pains deep in the abdomen, pain and straining with defecation, the stools often mucous and mixed with blood.   At first, constipation varied with diarrhœa, when she often passed yellow purulent masses, mixed with sago-like granules; but in later years constipation became more persistent, often accompanied by nausea, necessitating the use of the enema; by which small, hard, and rounded fecal masses, resembling

sheep's dung, were evacuated. In the end of December, 1876, the abdominal
pain grew worse, and the intestines were frequently largely distended by gases.
At times a loud noise, like an explosion, could be heard all over her room,
caused, probably, by the peristaltic contractions overcoming partial constrictions
of the intestine, and allowing the accumulated gases to escape onwards. At the
same time the lower bowel continued absolutely closed. This state of things continued for 5½ weeks, during which time there was complete closure of the bowel,
and also an entire absence of any escape of the intestinal contents upwards, either
fecal or even of gas having a fecal odour. On the 4th of February the patient
died with the usual signs of intestinal perforation. The necropsy showed the
abdomen full of fluid and semifluid fecal matter. The large intestine was found
enormously distended, while the small intestine was not only not distended, but
rather somewhat contracted. The descending colon was found completely closed
to an extent of 10 c. (3.94 inches) by an irregular, hard, nodulated mass, which
proved to be a carcinomatous growth. The ileo-cæcal valve was unaltered. In
the belief that there was a cicatricial constriction of the intestine, and probably
an accumulation of hardened feces, the treatment consisted of injections of water
by means of the enema syringe, but it was found impossible to inject any considerable quantity, and the water was at once forcibly expelled by the bowel.
Nor was it possible to determine the seat of the obstruction by the capacity of
the bowel for water, as suggested by Brinton (*On Intestinal Obstruction*, 1867);
and, indeed, this capacity was found very variable. Subsequently, by means of
a long tube, Dr. Hensgen succeeded in carrying an injection of water high up the
bowel, without, however, coming upon any obstruction, but also without bringing
away a trace of fecal matter. The introduction of this tube (a perforated bougie)
was much facilitated by keeping up a continuous stream of water through it while
passing it up the bowel. The most striking feature of this case was the long duration of complete closure, namely, forty-four days (the usual period being six to
thirteen days), during which time certainly nothing whatever passed through the
bowel. The absence of fecal vomiting must be regarded as due to the action of
the ileo-cæcal valve, which also sufficiently accounts for the non-distension of the
small intestine. The diagnosis of intestinal obstruction is one of the most difficult.
In general it must be borne in mind that the symptoms may sometimes point to
the existence of obstruction, when, in fact, there is none at all, as, for instance,
in same forms of colic, in cases of renal calculi, of acute peritonitis, or acute
typhlitis. The history of the case and an accurate physical examination alone
can establish the diagnosis. The usual seats of herniæ should be examined, so
also the uterus and rectum, the latter by finger and the sound. The outline of
the intestines and the extent of distension will often indicate the probable seat of
the obstruction. Regard should also be had to the age of the patient, for intussusception is relatively frequent in early years, while in later years carcinomatous
growths more generally produce bowel obstructions. But even the existence of
carcinoma can only be established by the discovery of an abdominal tumour.
When this fails, the diagnosis, as in the present case, must always remain uncertain.—*London Med. Record*, Jan. 15, 1877.

<hr>

On Peculiar Branched Formations in the Evacuations.

In the *Berliner Klin. Wochenschrift* of November 20. Dr. Marchand, of
Halle, describes some branched coagula which were sent for examination. They
had been passed *per anum* by a healthy woman after confinement. They resembled fibrinous casts of bronchi, but were larger, the main stem being of the size
of the little finger. From this stem proceeded numerous branches, presenting an

almost dendritic ramification. The smaller branches, which appeared to proceed from the main stem, proved to be glued to it by the copious intestinal mucus, and consisted of a firm substance similar to coagulated fibrin, but presented no appearance of organized tissue. Analogous formations were shown by Dr. Loewe at a meeting of the Medical Society of Berlin, in March, 1876, and were found in the feces of a healthy woman ; and recently, precisely similar excreta were sent to Dr. Marchand, which came from a healthy woman on the ninth day after delivery. These proved to be, instead of tube-casts, nothing more than inspissated intestinal mucus. Exactly similar formations were found in the folds of the large empty intestine of a man who died after amputation. The following is their mode of formation. After prolonged inaction of the bowel it is empty, containing perhaps only a few hardened bits of feces. These are covered by tough mucus. In the folds of the bowel they become moulded, and assume the form of branchings, and are expelled the next time the bowel is emptied, with its fluid secretions. Hence their occurrence after confinements.—*London Med. Record*, Jan. 15, 1878.

On Multiple Echinococcus of the Peritoneum.

In the *Deutsche Medicinische Wochenschrift*, Oct. 1877, Dr. GEISSEL relates a case of hydatid disease of the peritoneum which was mistaken for a multilocular ovarian cyst. Ovariotomy was resorted to, and followed by death. The patient, Frau Schmidt, aged 46, said she had been passing from the bowel clear water mixed with membranes for 9 or 10 years. On examination, there were all the physical signs of a multilocular cyst. On the 4th Jan. 1877, Dr. Geissel, at the entreaty of the patient, proceeded to the operation of ovariotomy. The incision was made from the symphysis pubis to nearly under the ensiform cartilage, and revealed the fact that the tumour consisted of hydatids of the peritoneum adherent to the abdominal walls and elsewhere ; the cysts varied in size from a pea to a walnut. There were two large cysts, each of the size of a child's head, in the middle of the abdomen. Dr. Geissel removed thus 27 small and 2 large cysts. Catgut ligatures were employed to arrest the hemorrhage, which was inconsiderable. Several cysts burst during the operation, and let out foul pus into the abdominal cavity. Death ensued five hours after the operation, which lasted two hours and a quarter.—*London Med. Record*, Jan. 15, 1878.

On the Treatment of Infantile Impetiginous Eczema.

Dr. GEORGES LEPAGE has observed in M. Jules Simon's wards the good results obtained in children suffering from eczema by the method recommended by Besnier (*Bulletin de Thérapeutique*, vol. lxxxviii. p. 49), which consists in enveloping the parts attacked with India-rubber cloth. The conclusions of his paper are as follows. 1. Impetiginous eczema is a cause of debility in the child; it therefore requires prompt and active treatment. 2. Treatment by swathing is superior to all other methods. 3. The general treatment is a necessary supplement to the swathing. 4. The practitioner need not dread repercussive phenomena if the therapeutic treatment be carefully conducted.—*London Med. Record*, Jan. 15, 1878.

On Febris Intermittens Urticata.

Professor ZEISSL, who had previously doubted the existence of urticaria as a complication of malarial fever, has now been convinced (*Allgemeine Wiener Med. Zeitung*, No. 46, 1877) to the contrary, by the observation of a case in which the eruption occurred thirteen times consecutively during the hot stage of tertian ague. It was absent during the intervals, and during the fourteenth and last attack. The

patient was a single woman, aged 53, did not suffer from urticaria previously, and
has not done so since.—*London Med. Record*, Jan. 15, 1878.

—

On Urticaria and Malaria.

Dr. REZEK, during an experience of eighteen years in a malarial district in
Hungary, found (*Allgem. Wien. Med. Zeitung*, No. 48, 1877) that, amongst an
average of at least two hundred patients suffering from ague whom he saw yearly,
in two or three the disease was complicated with urticaria. He himself suffered
from chronic urticaria as a sequela of ague, and was definitely cured by large
doses of quinine.—*London Med. Record*, Jan. 15, 1878.

——

Surgery.

On Calcification of Adipose Tissue.

Dr. EDWARD H. BENNETT, Professor of Surgery in the University of Dublin,
records (*Dublin Journ. of Med. Sciences*, Jan. 1878) an account of calcification
of adipose tissue, which it is believed has not hitherto been noticed. The change
is seated in the connective basis of the tissue and not in the contents of the cells.

Dr. Bennett describes the condition as follows: In the subcutaneous tissue of
the anterior aspect of the leg in elderly women, small hard bodies may be often
observed—flattened on the superficial and deep aspects, circular in outline, the
largest about one-fifth of an inch in diameter, the smallest mere grains. These
bodies are freely movable on the deeper tissues and beneath the skin, and are
arranged with a rough symmetry in the two limbs; if there be but one or two in
a limb, the finger carried over the corresponding part of the opposite limb readily
detects even the single specimen. When they are numerous, their symmetry is
similar to that of cutaneous eruptions, not absolutely exact, but very nearly so.
They occur in thin-skinned, pale bodies, and so can generally be seen before their
detection by the hand. I have never seen them associated with varicose veins,
or with skin eruptions, or ephelitic markings on the legs. They are most commonly seen in the limbs of the pauper subjects in our dissecting-rooms; but I have
seen them in the living also in hospital. They are not the seat of any trouble or
pain to the patient, and pass unnoticed by them until attention is directed to them
by the surgeon. I have never seen them in the male. In my early examinations
of them, I sought for small veins, or varices, as their seat, under the impression
that they were phleboliths. I next searched for a lymphatic vessel passing into or
connected to them, being still impressed with the idea that they were the result of
some vascular obstruction, but I failed to find any anatomical support for such
idea.

Adopting the ordinary process for hard, brittle substances, I polished a flat surface on one face of a section made with a fine saw through the centre of the body,
and cemented it to a glass slide with old Canada balsam; I then ground away the
structure until I obtained a fine transparent section. In this process I learned that
the densest part of the structure was at the circumference—the most open and
friable at the centre. Examined, after completing the mounting with fluid Damar
varnish, the pattern of the thin circumferential part was clearly seen to be that of
ordinary condensed connective tissue, forming a capsule for the body, calcified.
In it the usual irregular lacunæ, dark by transmitted lights due to gaps in the

structure. were readily seen; septa from the capsule passed irregularly through the structure. themselves calcified and showing lacunae similar to the outer layer. The arrangement of these parts was such as every one familiar with the microscopic appearances of the compound tissues would recognize as that of the envelopes and septa of subcutaneous fat. In the intervals inclosed by these calcified envelopes and septa the mass of the structure appeared arranged strictly in the pattern of the fat cells, the intercellular substance being calcified and breaking with a brittle, glassy fracture. Fearing error in a single observation, I repeated the process with several specimens, and obtained results exactly similar. I next macerated a fresh specimen in a weak picric acid solution, to which a minute quantity of hydrochloric acid was added. I established in this way the fact that the earth salts were deposited in the connective tissue forming the capsule and septa of adipose tissue, and in the intercellular structure of the fat cells. The decalcified tissue presents the pattern of ordinary fat, with only the exception that the structures out of which the earth salts have been dissolved are thicker than in the healthy tissue. One point further only remains to be stated—the position of the calcified body in the fat lobule; this I have always found to be marginal, never central. I have never seen any such alteration as I have described in lipomata or in any part of the body except that mentioned above.

On the Anatomy of the Primary Syphilitic Induration.

AUSPITZ and UNNA (*Archiv für Dermatologie und Syphilis*, 1 and 2 Heft, 1877) find that there are essential histological differences between the soft and hard chancres. The characters distinctive of the latter are hardness and chemical change in the bundles of connective tissue, and a peculiar development of the epidermis. The epidermis grows downwards in processes which send out projections horizontally to the skin, and these are subsequently snared and isolated by the growing connective tissue. Masses of granulation-cells penetrate to the horny layer of the epidermis, and are also found in the cutis bounded by tracts of epidermis. The form of the sclerosis depends on the arrangement of the blood-vessels, the process taking its origin from the adventitia. The coats of the blood-vessels are markedly affected, those of the lymphatic vessels to a less degree.— *London Med. Record*, Dec. 15, 1877.

Diphtheritis and Tracheotomy.

R. A. KRÖNLEIN contributes (*Langenbeck's Archiv*, xxi. p. 253) in this article many interesting practical facts connected with the treatment of diphtheria, based upon the results of five hundred and sixty-seven cases treated in Professor Langenbeck's wards between January 1, 1870, and July, 1876. Of the five hundred and sixty-seven cases, three hundred and seventy-seven terminated fatally, = 66.4 per cent. A glance at the figures shows that with every year the number of cases increased and the number of deaths diminished. The season of the year appeared to have some influence upon the extent of the epidemic; the smallest frequency was in the month of June, the greatest in October. Putting aside eight cases of adults between eighteen and forty-one years of age, we find that the frequency of the disease became gradually greater from one month upwards, reaching its greatest height at three years of age, continuing at this point up to four years and a half, and then decreasing, until at the age of fifteen or sixteen years there was no case. The younger the patient the greater the mortality. Tracheotomy was performed five hundred and four times, stenosis of the larynx being always regarded as the sole guide for the operation, without regard to the age of the patient or the character of the disease. Of these five hundred and four operations, three hundred and fifty-seven terminated fatally, = 70.8 per cent. Eighty-five of the operations were on infants under two years of age, of whom eleven recovered. and of these one was but seven months old. Twenty-eight of the cases had their origin in the hospital, and of these eighteen died. A detailed report is given of two hundred and forty-one cases, containing two hundred and ten tracheotomies. When the respiration does not become free immediately after the operation the prognosis is very unfavourable. In forty-six cases where this peculiarity was noticed forty-two died, 91.3 per cent. The canso of this is to be found in the existence of a lobular pneumonia or of a deeply extending croup of the bronchial mucous membrane. When during the operation casts of the branches of the bronchial tubes are coughed up, and the respiration becomes apparently perfectly free. the prognosis is, notwithstanding, unfavorable. The operation was performed even when the children were brought in apparently moribund. There were twenty-two children operated upon in this condition, with a mortality of 90.9. Of the total number operated upon, one hundred and fifty-four died, one hundred with symptoms of asphyxia, the others under symptoms of gradual prostration or of sudden collapse. As a cause of the gradual prostration the frequent occurrence of impediments to deglutition played a prominent part. These the author divides into two classes. In the great majority of cases this difficulty of swallowing takes place at the time of and is caused by the presence of the diphtheritic inflammation in the larynx and by the consequent rigidity through infiltration and exudation of the tissues which are involved in the act of swallowing. The cases that come on at a later period, after the complete healing of the local inflammatory processes, are much rarer, and are then due to a secondary diphtheritic paralysis of the laryngeal and pharyngeal muscles. In fifty cases the tracheotomy wounds took on diphtheritic action, and of these twenty-eight terminated fatally. The method of operation was, without exception, in the latter years, the "tracheotoma superior" of Bose, which offered no insurmountable difficulties even when there existed a goitre. Numerous attempts to confine the diphtheritic process by means of local remedies did not give satisfactory results.—*Boston Med. and Surg-Journal*, Jan. 24, 1873.

On the Cold-sound (Psychrophor).

Dr. WINTERNITZ of Vienna (*Berliner Klin. Wochenschrift*, July 9), has designed an instrument, by means of which he secures the advantages of moebanical irritation of the urethral mucous membrane by the metallic sound, combined with the anæsthetic and tonic influence of cold. It consists of a double-current catheter without eyes, the two canals communicating with one another near the point of the instrument. The instrument is introduced into the urethra until its point has passed the prostatic portion, and it is then attached by India-rubber tubing to a reservoir containing water at the desired temperature. On turning a stopcock, the water flows into one canal and out through the other, whence it is conducted away by another piece of tubing. In this way the caput gallinaginis and the entire urethral mucous membrane are exposed to the mechanical action of pressure, and to the sedative action of cold. The success obtained by Dr. Winternitz, by the use of this instrument, was so encouraging from the very beginning, that he has employed it constantly for over a year.

He has treated with it twenty-two cases of pollution. Of these two did not return after the first application; one was improved at first, but soon became as bad as before, and the treatment was discontinued after the cold-sound had been used sixty-five times; twelve are still under observation, and have been somewhat improved by the treatment, that the pollutions occur very rarely, and the secondary symptoms, hypochondria, etc., have entirely disappeared. In three cases the improvement was marked, when the patients withdrew from observation; in two others the pollutions became less frequent, but the secondary symptoms remained unchanged. The two remaining cases are described in detail. In one, the patient was a Russian officer, forty-six years of age, and the affection was due to excessive venery. The pollutions occurred regularly in the night after coitus, and recurred two or three times a week, when the patient was continent. The cold-sound was used daily for ten minutes with water at 59° F.; during its employment the patient experienced a sensation of pleasant coolness, and the relaxed scrotum contracted energetically. Some difficulty was experienced in removing the instrument. During the four weeks that the treatment was continued, there was only one pollution. The erections became more complete. In the second case the pollutions were frequent, and there were symptoms of excessive spinal irritation. The first introduction of the instrument caused great pain, and brought on an hysterical fit, but these symptoms disappeared after the water (59° F.) had flowed through the sound for five minutes. The treatment was continued daily for three weeks, when the patient was discharged cured. He had not had a single pollution from the time the treatment was begun.

At the first sitting Dr. Winternitz sometimes uses water at a temperature of 64° or even 66° F., and at a later period sometimes goes as low as 54½° F. Besides the above, he has treated nine cases of spermatorrhœa with the cold-sound. In four of these cases he obtained very favourable results; two cases were very markedly improved, while in the other three the treatment was without special results. In the cases of spermatorrhœa as well as in those of pollution, in which the treatment proved successful, general relaxation of the genitals and loss of muscular tone in the scrotum were marked symptoms. The cold-sound was also used in five cases of too rapid ejaculation during coitus, and in two cases of obstinate chronic gonorrhœa. In the former its use was followed by at least temporary improvement, and both of the latter, one of which had lasted three years and the other six months, were cured.—*London Med. Record*, Jan. 15, 1878.

Sayre's Treatment of Spinal Disease.

At a recent meeting of the Clinical Society of London, Mr. BERKELEY HILL brought, for the inspection of the members, a selection of twelve patients with angular and lateral spinal curvature, for which they were wearing Sayre's plaster jacket. In doing this he avoided criticism of the correctness of the theoretical grounds on which Dr. Sayre explained the mode in which the spine was affected, and also descriptive of the method of application, observing that those matters were set forth in Dr. Sayre's Spinal Diseases, etc. He confined himself to the results which had been gained by six months' experience of the mode of treatment. The cases exhibited that evening had been mainly under his own care, for some were from the hospital patients of his colleagues, Messrs. John Marshall and Arthur Barker. Four cases from the Cheyne Hospital for Incurable Children were exhibited by Mr. James P. Bartlett. The cases comprised examples of angular and lateral curvature of various situations and degrees, some wearing the jury-mast to support a curve in the upper dorsal region, one with lumbar abscess and sinus. The first case, treated in University College Hospital after Dr. Sayre had himself demonstrated his method, was put up on July 13th. The patient immediately lost the pain in her back, which up to that time had been too severe to permit of her walking about or sitting up for more than half an hour at a time; and she went for a walk out of doors of her own accord the same day. Two days later she went into the country till November. She at once discarded invalid habits, and in the latter part of her stay nursed a sick sister. The jacket put on in July was worn till nearly Christmas; it was then removed, and a poroplastic felt corset moulded on to the trunk while the patient was suspended. This did not appear to give sufficient support, as the pain in the back had returned frequently and increasingly. Hence Mr. Hill exhibited the patient wearing her corset—an excellent fit—to show that this material did not embrace the trunk with sufficient immobility to support it effectually. Mr. Hill next read the notes of the second case to which the plaster jacket was applied in University College Hospital, that of July 14, 1877, by Mr. Marcus Beck. This was a case of very acute character and of well-marked symptoms. The patient could not walk fifty yards without his crutches, and only a very short distance with them, on account of the severe pain produced. On being encased he walked out of the hospital easily, carrying both crutches in one hand. One month later he was able to walk nine miles. He wore the shell for three months; it was then removed, and he had remained quite well ever since. Mr. Hill then briefly described the case of the daughter of Dr. Gooding, of Cheltenham, who was encased by Dr. Sayre himself at Guy's Hospital on July 25, 1877. She had been suffering for eight years from injury to the upper dorsal region, causing collapse of the upper part of the column, great protrusion both backwards and forwards, complete inability to stand or walk, constant pain, and, at one time, paraplegia. On Jan. 23, 1878, Dr. Gooding wrote: "She began to improve from the first, and has continued to walk with increasing strength ever since. She has literally had no pain at all. She does her share of play, and goes regularly to school." Mr. Hill then summed up the benefits which six months' experience of the plaster shells had shown. 1. Pain was at once arrested. 2. So far as the spine was concerned, the patient was immediately able to sit upright and to walk about. 3. Control of the lower extremities, when lost or diminished, was rapidly improved or restored. 4. Abscesses steadily closed. 5. The spinal column lost much of its abnormal curve and consolidated in the improved position. 6. In lateral curvatures, a permanent increase of stature was often obtained. 7. Finally, by Sayre's jacket, cure was more rapid and less irksome than by any other method. Mr. Hill remarked that caution was necessary to prevent the patient attempting too much exertion; even when thoroughly supported in the shell, most patients required rest through some part of the day. In conclusion, Mr. Hill mentioned several small modifications in the method of application, which had been found to be improvements. The chin-piece should be more deeply cupped at the chin and well lined with thick felt. The suspending straps should be attached just in front of the zygoma and behind the ear. The axillary slings should be padded firmly and stiffened so as to take the form of the cross of a crutch. To receive adult or heavy patients from the gallows without risk of bending the plaster shell before it had set, Mr. Hill had contrived a table, swinging at its middle like a toilet looking-glass. This, carrying the slack air bed, could be pushed against the patient while suspended; two large hooks were slipped under the armpits and hitched to the top of the table. The patient, thus attached to the table, was freed from the gallows. The table was lowered from the vertical to the horizontal position, and the patient sank without strain or jolt into the slack air bed, which supported the plaster evenly on all sides till it set. Messrs. Mayer and Meltzer, who had constructed the table, had also made a light folding frame to answer the same purpose. To cut up or trim the plaster shells, a small carpenter's dovetail saw and a pair of French vine-dressers shears were the handiest tools.

Mr. T. Smith thought the table a valuable adjunct. He had seen a good case spoilt in being taken down. In a private house he had found a narrow leaf of the dining table sufficient to answer the same purpose. He had adopted another improvement in substituting air-pads for the cotton-wool between the mammæ and

over the abdomen. The advantage of such pads lay in the fact that they could
be inflated or emptied at will, each pad being provided with a vent and stopcock.
He considered Dr. Sayre's method one of the greatest improvements in the treatment of spinal disease that had been made for many years. Mr. CLEMENT
LUCAS had now pursued the method in twelve cases, four of which were cases of
lateral curvature, and had not met with any inconveniences or any instances of
pain inflicted in this series. He had, however, to remove the bandage in three
cases—once on account of the development of psoriasis over the whole of the
surface covered by the splint. This was a case of lateral curvature, and the splint
had been worn for three weeks. In another case there was desquamation of
cuticle over the covered parts ; and in a third he had to remove the bandage in
consequence of pediculi. He had not met with any pressure-sores, which he
attributed to the bad application of the splint ; and he denied the assertion that
had been made that the treatment was unscientific and led to disastrous results.
Mr. BARWELL claimed to be the first to adopt the method in this country, and
he had now put it in practice in a large number of cases. In only one case had
he been obliged to take the bandage off ; this was in consequence of difficulty in
breathing induced by it in a very young child with a large abdomen. He agreed
with Mr. Hill that the spine is never got straighter than it is made by the first
suspension. For supporting patients in removing them from the gallows, Mr.
Barwell uses a small sofa or sheet. He had substituted a cross-bar instead of a
straight-bar, used as a suspender by Dr. Sayre. He did not find it necessary to
pad the spinous processes, but whilst the bandage was moist he made a slight
interval at each side of the spines. Wool pads in the axillæ and between the
mammæ were essential in females. He mentioned the case of a man thirty-three
years of age, an asthmatic, and the subject of angular curvature. After application of the jacket he lost his asthma.—*Lancet,* February 2, 1878.

—

A Case of Spina Bifida Successfully Treated by the Injection of Iodine.

At a late meeting of the Clinical Society of London, Mr. A. PEARCE GOULD
read the notes of this case. The patient was born with a tumour the size of a
hen's egg, situated over the last lumbar and the upper sacral vertebra ; this
slowly increased in size, whilst the skin over it thinned. When eighteen months
old, he was brought to the Hospital for Sick Children. The tumour was then
of the size of a cricket-ball, sessile, with all the usual characters of spina bifida ;
an opaque band was seen along the middle line of the lower three-fourths of the
tumour. There was no paralysis or other deformity. The head was large ; the
fontanelle was widely open, becoming bulged when the tumour was compressed.
September 18th, 1877, the tumour was tapped with a small hydrocele trocar at
the upper part just to one side of the middle line ; six drachms of fluid were
removed, and half a drachm of Morton's iodo-glycerine solution was injected, the
opening being closed with collodion. For the first few days all promised well ;
the tumour appeared to be firmer, smaller, and less translucent ; but at the end
of a fortnight it had returned to its former condition. October 5th, the operation
was repeated, one drachm of the iodine solution being injected. But this was
attended with the same result. On November 5th, it was injected for the third
time, two ounces and a half of fluid being removed, and two drachms of the
solution injected. The sac became very tense, red, hot, and tender ; fluctuation
persisted for a week, but on the ninth day a marked change was noted ; the tumour was smaller, flaccid, elastic, but not fluctuating, and it did not become
tense when the child cried. The wall of the sac became gradually firmer and
thicker, and the tumour shrank. On December 14th, there being still distinct

fluctuation in the now thickened cyst, it was again tapped and emptied by the removal of six drachms of a yellow viscid highly albuminous fluid ; it was evident that the communication with the spinal canal was completely obliterated. One drachm of the iodine solution was injected into the sac, and well manipulated, and then allowed to escape. The tumour had since then gradually shrunk, and now presented a thick pad of skin, quite dense at the lower part, softer above, where there was a small spot which still fluctuated ; from this Mr. Gould withdrew about half a drachm of yellow turbid fluid two days ago. There was no paralysis. The fontanelle was closing up. After each operation, the temperature rose from 101 deg. to 102.8 deg., and continued above the normal from two to six days ; there was no convulsion or other sign of interference with the nervous system. The after-treatment consisted in thickly smearing the tumour with collodion each morning, and supporting it with wool and a bandage. The tumour evidently communicated very freely with the spinal canal, and most probably contained the spinal cord or nerves. Mr. Gould had examined twenty-three specimens of spina bifida, and had found nerves in the sac twenty times, two cases in which they were absent, and one case in which their presence was doubtful. The nerves or cord generally occupied the middle line—the position of the opaque band seen in this case. The absence of paralytic symptoms by no means favoured the opposite view. The fluid removed at the first three operations was colourless, becoming slightly turbid on standing, of specific gravity 1011, faintly alkaline, containing a trace of albumen, chlorides, and phosphates. With Fehling's copper solution, it gave no reaction ; but Dr. Dupré analyzed it, and after concentration was able to get distinct evidence of the presence of sugar. Because sugar could not be detected in the fluid of spina bifida, and in that escaping from the skull in cases of fracture, it must not therefore be supposed to be absent, unless the tests be applied to the fluid after evaporation. Dr. Norton's treatment had now been employed several times ; and in twelve out of fifteen published cases with success. As to the value of the glycerine, Mr. Gould stated that on pouring some of the "iodo-glycerine" on some of the cerebro-spinal fluid in a narrow glass, it was found to sink to the bottom at once, and not to mix with it ; and he was of opinion that the same thing occurred in injecting the tumour, for the fluid that oozed from the puncture after the injection was quite unstained with iodine, and the action of the injection had been much more potent at the lower part of the sac. Although the mode of cure resembled that seen in the radical treatment of hydrocele, there was an important difference in the two conditions, the one being a closed sac, the other communicating with a canal full of fluid. As to the fear that the inflammatory material would press injuriously on the contained nervous material, it was noted that in none of the published cases had consecutive paralysis been noted, and a specimen of Sir A. Cooper's in St. Thomas's Hospital Museum, described in his paper in vol. ii. of the *Medico-Chirurgical Transactions*, showed that the radical cure might take place in this way when the cord was in the sac without nervous symptoms. Mr. Gould had considerable difficulty in stopping the oozing of the cerebro-spinal fluid, which was so dangerous if allowed to continue.

Mr. CALLENDER said that an important subject had been brought before the Society by the full and exhaustive narration of a case by Mr. Gould. With reference to the mode of operation, he might suggest that it would be found useful to introduce the trocar and canula through and beneath the skin some little distance to the side of the tumour. In this way, direct puncture of the sac was avoided, and the valvular puncture permitted subsequent compression (after the removal of the canula) to prevent the escape of fluid. Whilst discussing the subject of the treatment of spina bifida, it would be of interest if members would give their experience as to the age to which patients might live, despite the deformity. For some years a gentleman had been under his care, who had been originally attended by Sir Astley Cooper. He wore to the last a protecting ease, removed from time to time, after the model suggested by Sir Astley Cooper. In this instance there was bladder trouble, the rectum acted imperfectly, and innervation of the lower extremities was incomplete. Yet this patient lived an active professional life, and reached the age of seventy-four years. Mr. Callender added that he believed this to be the greatest age ever attained by any one afflicted with a spina bifida.

Mr. MORRANT BAKER said that he had employed Morton's solution for the injection of a spina bifida in an infant two months old, who was under his care at St. Bartholomew's Hospital about eighteen months ago. The solution had been prepared according to the usual formula, and was injected with the usual precautions. The local effect was good; the sac becoming thickened after the second injection, and giving no further trouble. But, at the same time, loss of power of movement and of sensibility was noticed in the lower extremities; and this had remained to the present time. Mr. Baker thought the case should be mentioned, as it might elicit the experience of others on the subject; and would show that the injection of the iodo-glycerine solution, even when locally successful, was not without its dangers.—*British Med. Journal*, Feb. 2, 1878.

Osteotomy in Rickets.

At a late meeting of the Clinical Society of London (*Lancet*, Dec. 22, 1877), Mr. BARWELL showed a case in which he had operated for rickety deformity of the tibiæ. The operation was performed with Volkmann's chisel, and with antiseptic precautions, the limbs being afterwards put up in plaster-of-Paris. The temperature had never risen above 100°, which it reached the night after the operation. Mr. Barwell referred to the operation described by Mr. Howard Marsh in the Medico-Chirurgical Transactions, in which the bone was cut through with a saw, and in one case a wedge-shaped piece of bone removed. This procedure was more severe than that adopted in the present case. In this case one tibia was divided on Oct. 25th, the other on Nov. 1st, and although the deformity is now almost entirely cured, the child does not walk well at present. Mr. Barwell showed also a photograph of a case of extremely bowed legs, in which, on April 12th, he divided both the tibia and fibula with the chisel at the junction of the lower and middle third, and then put the limb up in plaster. On May 3d he divided the femur in the same way, and six weeks after the operation the patient was able to walk about. Complete recovery was, however, retarded by her sustaining a fracture of the right thigh.

Mr. HOWARD MARSH said that Mr. Barwell did not seem to have understood the differences in the two operations he had described in the Medico-Chirurgical Transactions. In two cases he divided the bones by the small saw, but in the other case—one of extreme forward bending—the angle of the bend was cut out. That procedure involved the effects of a compound fracture. In the two cases in which the slighter operation was performed, the temperature did not rise above 100°, except once, when it was 101°. Mr. Marsh did not think the patient shown by Mr. Barwell to be bad enough to have called for operation, and as her walking power did not seem improved, he supposed the operation was undertaken solely to relieve the deformity. The longer he watched cases of rickets, the more he was persuaded that even badly-curved limbs become straightened under the use of splints, administration of cod-liver oil, etc. A child with marked deformity at two years of age would have straight legs at four, there being almost a spontaneous tendency towards straightening.

Mr. Howse said that operations for rickety deformity were only applicable to extreme cases; and it was to those that Mr. Marsh, in his paper, restricted it. None of the speakers had laid stress upon that kind of oblique deformity—a combination of the anterior and lateral curves—in which splints could not be well applied, but which was readily met by operation. Treatment by mechanical means lasts over years, and the elements of time in the treatment of them often of the highest importance to patients, especially the poor, was too much neglected by surgeons. Four out of five cases of the double curve in the tibia he had referred to, on which he had operated, did well; in the fifth, a child twelve years old, he removed a wedge-shaped piece of bone, which was dense and ivory-like. The case took long to recover, but the limb is nearly straight, and the child can walk well.

Mr. BARWELL admitted that time and rest would do much for diseased joints. He restricted the performance of osteotomy in rickets to those cases in which the deformity was very marked. He gave Mr. Marsh the credit of being the first to introduce this operation. He thought both his own cases showed its value. He should deprecate it when the bone could be straightened by simply bending it.

—

Gonarthrotomy.

Dr. J. SCRIBA, of Freiberg, in a contribution on gonarthrotomy and its indications (*Berliner Klinische Wochenschrift*, Nos. 32, 33, 1877), advocates the practice of free incision and drainage, under strict antiseptic conditions, in the treatment of various forms of diseases of the knee. In support of his views as to the efficacy of this plan of treatment, the reports of twelve cases are given. Seven of these were cases of acute suppuration of the joint. In four of the seven cases there was a good recovery, with perfect mobility of the joint, and in the remaining three cases the result was fatal. In one of the successful cases the suppuration had been due to acute rheumatism, in two to injury, and in the fourth to chronic disease. The joint-affection in two of the unsuccessful cases was the result of acute phlegmonous erysipelas, and in one of caries. The eighth case, one of hydrops articuli, was a successful one. The remaining four were cases of fungous inflammation of the joint, of which three, in consequence of complications of caries and tuberculosis, terminated fatally.

The following are some of the chief points of interest in the author's remarks on the indications for gonarthrotomy under antiseptic conditions. This practice should not be carried out, save as a last resource in cases of acute serious gonitis. It is indicated in cases of acute purulent gonarthro-meningitis, in order to prevent ulcerative destruction of the epiphyseal cartilage; and should be carried out also where there is osteomyelitis of one or both epiphyses; so that, through drainage, the risks of pyæmia, pneumonia, and other acute infective diseases, may be diminished. Gonarthrotomy is not so urgently and promptly demanded in cases of acute intra-articular suppuration due to injury, and to acute gonorrhœal rheumatism. Here the prognosis is more favourable, the affection being usually less acute and uncomplicated by severe general phenomena. In the treatment of cases of chronic inflammation of the articular synovial membrane of the knee-joint, free incisions with drainage are to be preferred to the injection of irritating agents into the synovial cavity. In those forms of fungous gonitis, in which fluid secretion is a much more predominant element than fungous growth, and in which the cartilages are still intact, gonarthrotomy is, in the author's opinion, is the only rational method of treatment. In those forms in which fungous degeneration is well developed, so long as caries is not present, the joint should be incised and drained whenever a spontaneous opening is threatened, and after unsuccessful treatment by prolonged rest. In cases of fungous gonitis, complicated with caries, no proceeding short of resection is likely to prove of any service. Incision with drainage and gouging away of the diseased portions of bone can be justifiably practised only under certain conditions. The patient must be young, the lesion strictly local, and uncomplicated with tubercle in the joint or in any remote organ. The author is strongly opposed to the practice of gouging away carious bone from a diseased joint in an adult; and regards such a proceeding as a useless attack on the strength of the patient. He is of opinion that in early stages of fungous knee-disease, and when the bones are not diseased, resection should not be performed. It is laid down as a law that, the earlier the stage of fungous inflammation of the knee with which the surgeon has to deal, the better are prospects of enabling the patient through gonarthrotomy, to retain an useful and movable joint.

In conclusion, Dr. Scriba insists on the importance, in cases of convalescence from disease of the knee, of commencing passive movements at an early period. In two of the reported cases the leg was flexed, and extended immediately after the removal of the drainage-tube; and subsequently at every change of splint and dressings. As soon as the wounds are closed, more frequent and active movements should, it is stated, be effected, and the patient be allowed to stand up.—*London Med. Record*, March 15, 1877.

Treatment of Congenital Club-foot by Subperiosteal Removal of the Astragalus.

L. VEREBÉLYI describes in the *Pester Médicin-Chirurg. Presse*, No. 14, 1877, the case of a child, aged $5\frac{1}{2}$, the subject of congenital club-foot affecting both limbs. Tenotomy and the application of a plaster-of-Paris bandage having failed, the astragalus of one foot, which presented the principal obstacle to reduction, was laid bare by an incision, and, the periosteum having been stripped off, was removed. The foot was then brought into proper position, in which it was retained by a fenestrated plaster-of-Paris bandage, and afterwards by a proper apparatus. After the healing of the wound, the foot easily preserved its proper direction.—*London Med. Record*, Nov. 15, 1877.

On the Treatment of Fractures with Cotton-Wool Dressings.

Dr. MONTON has, in M. Broca's wards, carried out a series of experiments which have demonstrated that compression made with cotton-wool dressings lessens the power of muscular contraction in a very remarkable manner, and for that reason it is a useful auxilliary in the reduction of fractures. The use of this bandage also obviates the complications which may supervene in compound fractures. Finally, this means allows the delay of the serious operations rendered necessary by wounds. Dr. Monton's conclusions are as follows: 1. Fractures may be reduced, and kept in place by cotton-wool dressing. 2. Cotton-wool dressing is exclusively indicated in fractures with communicating wounds in hospitals, and all other localities where the air is vitiated by overcrowding. 3. The same dressing gives the power of delaying operations actually contraindicated by the state of the patient, with advantage both to him and to the surgeon.—*Lond. Med. Record*, Dec. 15, 1877.

Fracture of the Os Calcis by Muscular Action.

Mr. J. W. ANNINGSON, of Burnley, records (*British Med. Journ.*, Jan. 26, 1878) the following case of this very rare accident. In December, 1876, M. N., a spare healthy woman, aged 42, while leaving a shop, made a false step, forgetting that the shop and street were not on the same level. The street slopes very much, so that the depth of the doorstep down into it varies from three and a half to eight and a half inches; and probably the woman strode off a height of not more than six inches. She was sober, and not carrying any weight. She exclaimed, "I've put my ankle out." She did not fall, but without assistance limped home, a distance of about a hundred yards. She had never injured the part before. On examining her shortly afterwards, a fragment of bone, with the skin tightly stretched over it, was seen at the back of the leg, two inches and a half above the point of the heel. Below this, the cord of the tendo Achillis was wanting. The lower edge of the fragment was a little above the level of the lower end of the internal malleolus. It was about one inch transversely, and had been torn off the posterior surface of the os calcis, where a cavity could be felt. The whole depth of the bone had not been torn away, but only the upper three-fourths; and the inferior edge of the fragment had been tilted backwards so as to project against the skin. This edge could be bent down for a quarter of an inch; but, on leaving off the pressure, it sprang back again. The skin was not bruised, and there was no other injury.

The usual treatment for ruptured tendo Achillis was adopted, and in about eight weeks she was able to walk without limping, and only complaining of some loss of spring. Two days after the accident, there was great swelling, and the skin over the fragment was so tight that tenotomy suggested itself; but there appeared this objection, that, if the tendo Achillis were divided, the torn-away piece might be left without sufficient vascular supply. A few days later, a small slough formed, leaving a superficial ulcer of the size of a shilling, which soon healed under red lotion.

Midwifery and Gynæcology.

Parturition obstructed by Carcinoma of the Cervix Uteri.

In the *Archives de Tocologie* for December, 1877, is related the case of a patient, thirty-seven years of age, in whom pregnancy was complicated by encephaloid cancer of the whole circuit of the cervix, as well as of the vaginal walls. She had previously had five children, the last six years previously. Since the last delivery, menstruation had been painful. Emaciation had been progressing for two years. The last period occurred on March 3d, 1877, and no discharge, either sanguineous or leucorrhœal, took place until the third month of pregnancy. At that period, slight hemorrhage took place for three days. It recurred a fortnight later, and was followed by a slightly sanguineous, non-fetid discharge, which was continuous for three weeks, and afterwards reappeared on the slightest provocation. The patient was admitted into hospital under M. DEPAUL on August 22d. Emaciation had then become extreme. There was a loud anemic bruit in the carotids and over the heart, and she was suffering violent lumbar pains. The uterus was found to correspond to about five months' pregnancy. The finger introduced into the vagina was arrested by an irregular bossy mass, readily bleeding, which proved to be the anterior vaginal wall invaded by cancer. The whole circuit of the vagina was occupied by prominent cancerous masses, which rendered it difficult to reach the cervix. The cervix itself was degenerated in its whole circuit. The enlarged anterior lip was separated from the posterior by a deep cleft. After a fortnight the patient left the hospital, but returned on October 9th, the cancerous masses being in much the same condition. A sanguineous discharge continued, but had not much smell. On the morning of October 29th, that is to say, in the middle of the eighth month of pregnancy the membranes ruptured, and vigorous pains soon followed. The same evening no alteration could be discovered in the condition of the cervix. On the morning of the 30th the head remained above the superior straight; the fœtal heart was becoming slow and irregular. The pulse 116, temp. 40° C., but the patient's condition did not seem to call urgently for interference. N. Charpentier, who was representing N. Depaul, though it advisable to wait, having experienced the bad results of operative interference in such cases from laceration of cancerous tissue. In the evening the uterine contractions becoming progressively more powerful, had at length produced a slight dilatation of the external os, which had the diameter of a five-franc piece. The cervix formed a canal two centimetres in length, the internal os being somewhat less dilated than the external. The fœtal heart sounds could no longer be heard. On the morning of the 31st the head was found at the vulva, and a dead fœtus was expelled at 8.30 A.M., after a labour of forty-five and a half hours. It weighed 2080 grammes. No hemorrhage occurred after the expulsion of the child, or after that of the placenta, which took place normally. After delivery pulse and temperature did not rise again to the level reached during labour, and convalescence took place favourably. On November 2d the discharge became so fetid that the ward where the patient was had to be emptied, and antiseptic injections were of little avail to modify this condition. On November 5th, hemorrhage took place to the amount of 500 grammes, without apparent cause. The vagina was syringed with a weak solution of perchloride of iron, and plugged with tampons dipped in a stronger solution. The pulse was 120; temperature 38.9° C. On the 7th, the hemorrhage had almost ceased, but the fetor of the discharge continued. From this time she progressed, but still continued in a state of great weakness. On her departure from the hospital, on November 28th, it was ascertained that the cancerous masses were in much the same state as before delivery, except that laceration had occurred, producing deep clefts at several points in the circumference of the cervix.

—

The Operative Treatment of Abdominal Fœtation.

In the *Archiv für Gynäkologie*, Band xii. H. 1, Professor GUSSEROW relates a case of extra-uterine fœtation in which secondary gastrotomy was successfully performed. The patient was thirty-four years old, and was admitted on October 30, 1876. She had previously had four children, the last in 1875. The last delivery was followed by para- and perimetritis, from which, after three weeks' illness, she completely recovered, the effusion becoming absorbed. In May, 1876, she was attacked by rigors, vomiting, and abdominal pain, so severe that she was admitted into hospital, where a diagnosis of acute gastric catarrh was made. Meanwhile, menstruation came on normally for the last time on May 27. After this, she was treated in the hospital for five months for peritonitis. She had severe pains, persistent vomiting, difficulty in micturition and defecation, and the abdomen became enlarged. In July, she became aware that she was pregnant. After two months her condition began to mend, and she left the hospital at the end of September, though still very weak. On October 28 she strained herself in lifting a pail, as a result of which she had prolapse of the vagina and slight hemorrhage. In consequence of this she came under observation, and the signs of extra-uterine pregnancy were then made out. The parts of the child were extremely superficial and its movements distinct, and its position being generally rather transverse, the head towards the right. The uterus could be felt in front, enlarged, and reaching three or four centimetres above the pubes. The cervix was pushed forwards and upwards, and behind it was a firm tumour. On December 2, she was suddenly attacked by severe pains, the movements of the fœtus became violent and painful, and its position was for a time somewhat altered. An hour later she was free from pain, but the fœtal movements and heart sounds had finally ceased. The sound was then introduced into the uterus, and its length found to be ten centimetres. For the next eighteen days the size of the abdomen gradually diminished, and the patient's condition was favourable. On December 20, some pain and hemorrhage commenced, and on the 24th, amid severe pains and considerable loss of blood, a decidua, whose nature was verified by the microscope, was expelled from the uterus. About twenty-four hours later severe symptoms of peritonitis suddenly came on ; and after a few days the size of the abdomen had increased, and fluctuation over the limits of the tumours became more distinct than it had ever been previously, while the retro-uterine tumour had also increased.

After being in imminent peril of life, the patient somewhat improved in the early days of January, 1877. Her condition, however, was still so threatening, that gastrotomy was performed on January 7. The abdominal walls were easily separated from the thin and transparent fœtal sac. When this was incised, a large quantity of sero-sanguineous fluid escaped, of which 900 grammes were collected. The fœtus was easily removed, and slight traction on the funis showed the placenta not to be quite firmly adherent. It was situated below and to the right, reaching deep into Douglas's fossa. A part of the sac on the left side, which was not adherent, was united by catgut to the abdominal wall. The lower part of the wound, for a length of five centimetres, was left open, and a drainage-tube, and some strips of gauze left in it by the side of the funis. The operation was performed under carbolic spray, lasting less than thirty minutes, and the patient lost very little blood. The sac was sponged out, and two large old clots removed from it. The fœtus, a female, was macerated, but not offensive. It was 44 centimetres long, and weighed 1750 grammes, and was well-developed, corresponding to about the eighth month of pregnancy. For two days the patient did well, but on the third day, in spite of carbolic injections, and although the operation had been performed under spray with antiseptic precautions, decomposition commenced in the cyst, and high fever set in with it, the temperature rising to $40^\circ.5$ C. The cavity was syringed out twice a day with strong solutions (as high as 10 per cent.) of carbolic acid. From the fourth day onwards, fragments of decomposing placenta were removed by forceps, and the retro-uterine tumour thenceforward gradually diminished. Once severe hemorrhage followed the removal of a piece, and plugging of the sac became necessary. The gut sutures gave way easily, and by the fourth day the whole sac lay freely open. When Douglas's pouch had been freed from placenta, on the ninth day, it was punctured from above, and a drainage-tube passed through into the vagina. The febrile conditions, however, appeared to become rather worse in consequence, and a few days later the pulse rose to 160, and the collapse was so great as to call for ether injections. The discharge, however, was gradually transformed into healthy pus, and the patient slowly improved, although, for a long time, the urine contained albumen. By the 27th of March the cavity had closed, and she had already been able to leave her bed on the 20th of February. Meanwhile, however, a phthisis of the right apex, of which there had been slight signs from the first had made rapid progress, and beneath the clavicle there were signs of a cavity.

The author reviews the evidence hitherto extant as to the operative treatment of abdominal fœtation, although he considers that the cases are not to be weighed in proportion to their numbers, especially now that such advances have been made in abdominal surgery. In 1872 Keller quoted nine cases of primary gastrotomy, during the life of the child, out of which seven children and four mothers were saved. Parry, in 1876, recorded twenty cases of a similar kind, out of which eight children and six mothers are said to have been saved. Since then has been recorded a case of Gaillard Thomas, in which the mother was saved and the child died during the operation; also that of M. Jessop, in which both mother and child were saved. Of secondary gastrotomies, after the death of the child, Parry records sixty-two, with thirty-two deaths. Since then operations have been recorded by Cullingworth, Depaul, Boinet, and Duboné, of which only one, that of Duboné, had a successful result. Of cases left to nature, Parry records 247 in which the full term of pregnancy was exceeded, with 125 deaths and 122 recoveries. The great peril of extra-uterine fœtation in its latter stage is shown by the fact that in forty-one cases in which the child lived up to the ninth month of pregnancy, and in which the treatment was expectant, there were thirty-six deaths, while in seventeen similar cases, treated by operation, there were nine deaths.

In view of the frequency with which, in the later months of fœtation, the child suddenly dies, and this occurrence is followed by partial detachment of the placenta, internal effusion of blood, peritonitis, and great danger to the mother, the author concludes that, as soon as the eighth month of pregnancy is reached, interference by gastrotomy should not be delayed. In case of the death of the fœtus he would also operate immediately, before the setting in of those phenomena of false labour, which do not generally occur for a few days. If, however, this opportunity has been let pass, he would decide according to the condition of the patient, and only operate if the issue is likely to be otherwise unfavourable. He believes that the result of operation will be much more favourable when it is undertaken earlier, and not as a last resort, when life is already in extreme danger. Although the author operated in this instance under carbolic spray, influenced by the exigencies of the present fashion, he concludes, from the experimental researches of Wegner as to the effect of carbolic acid upon the peritoneum, that it is undesirable in gastrotomy to use the spray.

A case of primary gastrotomy for extra-uterine fœtation is recorded by Dr. Gervis, in the *British Medical Journal* for December 22· The patient had had eight children, the youngest being a little over two years old. During the last menstruation, ending February 28, 1877, she had unusual pains with vomiting. Since then, up to seven weeks before her admission on August 27th, she had had, every eight or nine days, an attack of uterine hemorrhage, accompanied with more or less sickness and abdominal pain. The body of the uterus was made out in the left inguinal region. Per vaginam, a rounded swelling was found occupying more than the right half of the pelvis and pushing the uterus to the left. It was continuous with a dull and resistant area above the pubes, over which a souffle could sometimes be heard. This was presumed, and, as the event proved, rightly, to be placenta. The fœtus was situated towards the left side; the heart-sounds were most distinct just above, and two inches to the left of the umbilicus.

On September 27th, the patient had a severe attack of vomiting, with great abdominal pain, increasing especially with all fœtal movements, which from this time became excessive, appearing to threaten the rupture of the cyst.

Gastrotomy was performed on November 5, the patient being rather more than eight months pregnant. The fœtus proved to be inclosed only in the membranes, which were very thin and lacerable. In extracting the child by the head, the opening in the cyst was extended very near to the front edge of the placenta. Some hemorrhage occurred at this point, but was checked by two ligatures. The lower part of the cyst was included in the sutures passed through the abdominal wall, but with little hope of their holding on, on account of the soft and thin character of the cyst wall. The funis was brought out at the lower angle of the wound, and a large-sized India-rubber drainage-tube placed by its side, reaching to the bottom of the cyst and covered by a carbolized sponge. The child could be induced to breathe only with much difficulty, and died about six hours after its birth.

On the day after the operation the patient had some vomiting, and reddish serum was repeatedly withdrawn from the drainage-tube, some also having escaped by the side and soaked the dressings. At 9 P. M. this had, for the first time, a somewhat offensive odour. The following morning the pulse was 140, temperature 102°.5. A considerable quantity of bloody serum continued to escape and saturate the dressings. At 2 P. M. the abdomen was distended, and from this time till her death, at 7 P. M., she gradually sank, the sanguineous discharge never abating.

At the autopsy there were found some few patches of peritonitis, and in the cavity was about a pint and a half of sanguineous serum. The placenta was in such an advanced state of decomposition that its exact attachment could not be ascertained. The right ovary could not be found, but both Fallopian tubes were normal. The uterus measured 7½ inches in length, the lining mucous membrane was shreddy and partially detached. The author considers that death was due to hemorrhage, caused by partial detachment of some portion of the placenta.— *Obstetrical Journal of Great Britain*, Feb. 1878.

On Hypertrophic Syphilitic Ulceration of the Cervix Uteri.

The *Annales de Gynécologie*, Nov. 1877, contains an article by Dr. AIMÉ-MARTIN, in which he describes a specific syphilitic ulceration of the neck of the uterus, together with hypertrophy of that part. He quotes Tanturri, of Naples, as having first clearly in 1862 drawn attention to this lesion. Dr. Aimé-Martin says that, usually about the third or fourth month after the reception of the syphilitic poison, the neck of the uterus undergoes a specific hypertrophy quite distinct from any other hypertrophy; it then becomes the seat of a slight ulceration on the borders of the os uteri. The ulceration is nothing more than a simple desquamation of the epithelium. Its colour varies from a brick-red to a cherry-colour. It is frequently coexistent with secondary hypertrophy of the tonsils, to which it is analogous. As regards treatment, the disease is not affected by local medication, but readily yields to the employment of general specific remedies.—*Lond. Med. Record*, Jan. 15, 1878.

On Removal of a Chronically Inverted Uterus.

F. NYROP (*Gynäkolog. og Obster. Meddelelser*, Band I.; and *Nord. Medicin. Arkiv*, Band IX.) describes a case of chronic inversion of the uterus, which had come on after labour, and had lasted six months. It resisted all attempts at replacement; and therefore, about a year after the confinement, the inverted uterus was amputated by the galvanic battery. After several attacks of peritonitis, the patient completely recovered.—*London Med. Record*, Jan. 15, 1878.

On Climacteric Insanity.

In the *Allgemeine Zeitschrift für Psychiatrie*, Band xxxiv. Heft. 4, Professor von KRAFFT-EBING, of Graz, discusses the relations of the climacteric period to insanity. A woman's mind is influenced in three distinct ways by the climacteric. 1. It is natural that at the time of cessation of her sexual functions, all the circumstances of her past life, whether they have been happy or otherwise, should be brought vividly before her, and form the subject of continual reflection; not unfrequently, especially if adult life have been unsuccessful or unhappy, the result of these broodings is painful mental depression or worse. 2. The changed and often pathological general sensations which accompany the climacteric process of involution often lead to hypochondriacal troubles, the fear of severe bodily disease, such as cancer, etc. The patient's nervousness is also increased by the knowledge that the climacteric is generally admitted to be a period critical to life and health. 3. The psychic functions are directly influenced by the functional and organic physical changes which take place in the body at the time of the climacteric, and which vary from the slightest physiological disturbances to the most severe pathological changes. These three modes of origin of psychic disturbance have all the more power if the central nervous system be already overworked, or perform its functions abnormally.

The ways in which purely physical causes accompanying the climacteric process influence the psychic organ are various, very complicated, and not yet made sufficiently clear. Above all, it must be maintained that the climacteric is not merely a cessation of function and commencing atrophy of the organs of generation, but involves a general disturbance of the whole system, causing changes in the distribution of the blood, consequent alterations in the secretions, etc. The influence of these disturbances on the nervous system is greater if the power of resistance of the latter have been previously diminished by difficult labours, prolonged lactation, or other causes; also if some severe disease coincide with the climacteric, or if the genital apparatus have been long affected with chronic disease.

The concrete possibilities are these: (a) Menstruation becomes excessive, causes anæmia and consequent disturbance of nutrition of the cerebro-spinal system; profuse leucorrhœa has the same effect. (b) The menses cease suddenly. In these cases, severe disturbances of the nervous system are frequently seen, but the pathogenesis is not clear, even though vicarious hyperæmia be admitted as playing an important part. The same cause (acute disease, fright, uterine affections, etc.) which brings about the cessation of menstruation, may often be recognized as causing the nervous symptoms. (c) Uterine diseases, either arising at the time of the climacteric, or pre-existent, but aggravated at this period, exercise (by affecting the constitution, or directly through the nerves) a harmful influence on the central nervous system. (d) Neuroses of the genitals (pruritus, vaginismus, etc.), which have been caused by the climacteric, have a like effect. (e) There is no doubt that, apart from any local disease or neurosis, the climacteric process, as such, causes disease in, or otherwise affects, the psychic organ in some way not clearly understood, but evidently through the nerves, and only when its functions had previously been to some extent abnormally performed.

The climacteric process always influences in some degree the central nervous system; venous hyperæmia of the mucous membrane of the alimentary canal, with its consequences, is common, and patients are at this time more susceptible to the ordinary causes of disease. Elementary psychic changes are also very common at this period, the patient's character often being quite altered.

Among 878 insane women, Krafft-Ebing found 60 (6.8 per cent.) cases in the etiology of which the climacteric appeared to have played a part. In 40 of these cases there were previous functional disturbances of the nervous system, either congenital or acquired. In 25, hereditary taint was proved; in 22 it was doubtful, and in 13 it was certainly absent. These constitutional affections were much more frequent as predisposing causes of disease than accidental causes operating at the time of the climacteric itself, e. g., diseases of the uterus or other viscera, various excesses. It seemed to be immaterial whether the patients had borne children or not.

The author does not believe that there is any special form of insanity which can be recognized as being caused solely by the climacteric. In this he disagrees from Tilt and Skae, but he considers that the climacteric is a predisposing or exciting cause, which in many ways influences the form and course of the disease, thus lending it features which, when observed, would go far to establish the belief that the case was due to the climacteric process.

In the 60 cases the following forms of insanity were observed: Melancholia activa, 4; *Folie circulaire*, 1; acute delirium, 1; a general paralysis, 12; primary delusional insanity (*Verrücktheit*), with delusions of persecution, 36; ditto with religious delusions, 6.

Certain sensations and anomalies of function, which frequently accompany the climacteric, exercise an influence over the psychic organ, partly through the patient's own consciousness and partly by reflex action, in such a manner as to give a peculiar character to the delusions, hallucinations, etc., which are the expression of the psychosis occurring at this period. This is especially true of the last and most numerous class of cases mentioned in the above list.

In all four cases of melancholia, hallucinations of hearing and sensation were numerous; in only one there was hallucination of smell. In all the cases there were delusions of poisoning, and in two *tædium vitæ*. The hypochondriacal symptoms, which have been much insisted on, were absent.

In the 36 cases of primary delusional insanity with prominent delusions of persecution, the influence of the process going on in the genital apparatus on the character of the delusions cannot be denied. In 20 of the cases these last were of a sexual nature; in six cases hallucinations of the sense of smell were observed, the patient either believing that she perceived a stinking smell, or hearing voices which complained of the same thing. The delusion of being physically influenced for evil was noted in ten cases.

Great importance is attached by the author to the hallucinations of smell, and to the delusions of physical persecution, which were always dependent on paralgic eccentric sensations. At present he has never observed these in any case in which sexual functional disturbance was not present, e. g., masturbation, uterine disease. The paralgic sensations are due to irritation of the sensory apparatus of the spinal cord. Looking to the great frequency of hallucinations of smell in onanists, as compared with their great rarity in psychoses generally, it seems that the centres of the sense of smell must stand in close relationship with the genital nervous system, and be easily irritated by excessive excitement of the latter.

In 28 women suffering from the same form of insanity, but which had not commenced at the time of the climacteric, only three were found to have delusions of sexual persecution; not one had hallucinations of smell; and only four had delusions of physical persecution. In all these seven cases, some functional or anatomical anomalies of the genital organs were present. In four cases of pre-existing insanity of the same kind, the character of the delusions became sexual at the time of the climacteric, although they had never been so before. Of the above 36 cases, 32 had hallucinations of hearing, six of sight, six of smell, and two of taste.

In the six cases of insanity with religious delusions, the latter partook of a sexual character, e. g., connection with the heavenly bridegroom, being pregnant with the Son of God.

There were only six recoveries among the whole 60 cases—viz., melancholia, 4; delusional insanity, 2. The bad prognosis in cases of insanity coming on during the climacteric, has already been pointed out by Morel, Griesinger, Schlager, and others.

The treatment is not discussed, but attention is drawn to the favourable influence of large doses of bromide of potassium, in allaying sexual excitement and the consequent paralgic and hallucinatory phenomena; also to the good results yielded by morphia, when employed against hallucinations of hearing, connected with auditory hyperæsthesia and delusions of persecution.—*Lond. Med. Record*, Dec. 15, 1877.

Medical Jurisprudence and Toxicology.

Phosphorous Poisoning.

A case of no small interest from many points of view has recently occurred at Netley. The following are the particulars: A man named Ball, aged thirty-one, employed as a billiard marker in the officer's mess of the Victoria Hospital, was taken ill on Dec. 11th with pain in the abdomen and retching. He had been drinking hard on the previous night, and his symptoms were attributed to this cause. He recovered to a certain degree, but became jaundiced, and on the 18th, being very weak, he was admitted to the hospital, where he died the next day. His jaundice, together with symptoms referable to his liver, and a history of previous liver disease while sojourning in India, led to a diagnosis of acute yellow atrophy of the liver—a diagnosis which was confirmed by the post-mortem examination, for the liver was found small, soft, flexible, of an intensely yellow colour, and with the liver substance almost entirely replaced by fat-globules. The kidneys were also swollen and soft, and petechial extravasations were seen on the pulmonary and alimentary mucous membranes. The man was buried without a certificate in the military cemetery adjoining the hospital. It appears to be the custom for the registrar to visit the hospital once a week, to obtain the certificates of those who die and are buried in the military cemetery; and under these circumstances it is not always possible or advisable to leave the bodies unburied until the formalities are complied with. A rumour having arisen, however, that the deceased had taken rat poison, the stomach was submitted to a qualitative analysis by Dr. De Chaumont, and phosphorous having been detected, the coroner was at once informed; the recently interred body was exhumed, an inquiry was opened, and the stomach and portions of other viscera were forwarded to the county analyst, Mr. Angell, for examination. Phosphorus in considerable quantities was found in the stomach, and abundant evidence was forthcoming that the deceased had rat poison in his possession, and there were good grounds for believing that he had taken some in a fit of jealousy on the morning of December 11th.

The confusion of phosphorous poisoning with acute yellow atrophy of the liver is of great interest, and it becomes of much importance to determine what are the points to be attended to in distinguishing the post-mortem appearances and symptoms of the one disease from the other. A reference to standard treatises will show that the symptoms, course, and duration of the two conditions are, or may be, almost identical. The fact that the patient was a man militated somewhat against the theory of yellow atrophy. As to the post-mortem appearances, the differences observable in the two conditions seem to be these: In acute yellow atrophy the liver is very small, and this constitutes the most striking feature. The yellow colour appears to be due to bile-pigment; fat, if present, is not observed in any very great quantities; and crystals of leucin or tyrosin are found amongst the degenerated detritus of the liver-cells. In phosphorous poisoning the atrophy is not usually extreme; the colour seems entirely due to fatty change, and leucin and tyrosin are not observable. The question is one of unusual interest, and seems well worthy of a thorough investigation at the hands of pathologists.—*Lancet*, February 2, 1878.

CONTENTS.

Published Monthly, price $2.50 per annum, free of postage.
Also, furnished together with the AMERICAN JOURNAL OF THE MEDICAL
SCIENCES *and the* MEDICAL NEWS AND LIBRARY *for* SIX DOLLARS *per
annum in advance, the whole free of postage.*

HENRY C. LEA, Philadelphia.

THE MONTHLY ABSTRACT

OF

MEDICAL SCIENCE.

VOL. V. No. 4.   **For List of Contents see last page.**   APRIL, 1878.

Anatomy and Physiology.

Nutritive Influence of the Nervous System.

The influence of the nervous system on nutrition is one of the subjects to which much attention has, of late, been paid, but of which we know comparatively little. The fact that various disturbances and anomalies of nutrition and growth do occur in connection with nerve disease and injury is well established, but there are many explanations of the way in which these changes are brought about. Some of these are, no doubt, true, and all are possibly applicable in certain cases. The older observations had reference chiefly to the results of division either of mixed or of sensory nerves, such as the rapid destructive changes set up in the cornea and eyeball after section or destruction of the fifth nerve, the disordered secretion of the submaxillary gland after division of the chorda tympani, and the peculiar effects of division of a mixed nerve, such as the median, on the hand. But it has been shown that some, at least, of these phenomena are due to loss of sensation, to loss of vaso-motor control, to changes in power of resistance to the influence of temperature, and to other causes which are not essentially associated with a direct influence of the nerves upon the nutrition. It is, at least, doubtful at present whether the inflammation of the eyeball consecutive to lesion of the fifth is due to anything more than the exposure to irritation and arrested secretion, the experiments hitherto made being contradictory. In the same way the results of section of the vagi in setting up pneumonia, which were formerly cited as evidence of loss of nutritive control, have been shown by Friedlander and others to be equally produced by section of the recurrent laryngeal, and to be due to the entrance of foreign particles into the air-cells. The swollen and glossy condition of the fingers, with loss of balance of temperature and tendency to formation of sloughs, together with the other changes which result from section of the median nerve, are probably, in great measure, dependent on altered vaso-motor control, and are in part comparable to the effect of section of the cervical sympathetic on the ear of the rabbit in Bernard's well-known experiment. So, too, of the muscular atrophy which ensues on section of a motor nerve, and of some of the other changes in the limb which usually accompany such atrophy, of which the ingenious hypothesis of Dr. Vivian Poore of loss of reflex tonicity seems to afford the best explanation.

But over and above these changes, the pathology of which is, in some degree, explicable by altered sensation, loss of movement, and disturbance of temperature control and blood-supply, there are others which seem to establish a direct influence of the central nervous system on all nutrition. We owe to M. Charcot and his pupils much of the light we possess on this subject; we need only mention his observations on acute decubitus, on the changes in the joints in locomotor ataxy, and on amyotrophic paralysis, all of which afford proof of the profound changes which may occur under the influence of spinal disease. The greater number of the changes we have instanced are either of a destructive or an irritative nature, and are so regarded by M. Charcot. Perforating ulcer of the foot, and eschars on the sacrum and hips, afford good types of the destructive changes; whilst muscular atrophy, due to descending degeneration secondary to brain disease, or the atrophy with rigidity in the lateral sclerosis of "amyotrophic palsy," are examples of the latter.

We might reasonably expect that if these more profound changes are due to a direct nutritive connection of the nervous system, and result from the more intense modes of irritation, there would be other slighter changes, less easy of recognition, and taking the form of nutrient abnormalities or overgrowths, where the stimulus was less intense. Probably the differences in relative development of different tissues, and in various parts of the body, are under direct nervous control in their original development and maintenance, and further pathological investigation will enable us to appreciate this point more fully. An interesting contribution to this study has recently been made by M. Landouzy, with reference to the abnormal development of subcutaneous fat in certain cases of muscular atrophy secondary to spinal or cerebral disease. The full record of his observations will be found in the January number of the *Revue Mensuelle de Médecine et de Chirurgie*. He records the case of a man, sixty five years of age, who was seized with apoplexy, with only partial loss of consciousness, followed by right hemiplegia, which led to slow contraction and atrophy of the paralyzed limbs. As the atrophy of the muscles increased, the folds of skin on the wasted parts were found to become not only more distinct, but thicker than in the healthy limb, and the hairs and nails longer on the affected side. There was no marked difference in the temperature or vascularity of the two sides. Death having at last occurred from bedsores, followed by blood poisoning, M. Landouzy was able to make a very careful study of the condition of the tissues of the limbs on the two sides. He found that the folds of skin pinched up were nearly double the thickness in the wasted as compared with those in the healthy limb, and that this was due solely to an increase of fat in the subcutaneous cellular tissue, which was also distinctly yellower than in the healthy limb, the dermis remaining unaltered. The cause of the paralysis was found in a patch of softening in the white matter of the left hemisphere, extending from the hinder part of the first frontal convolution to the posterior extremity of the parietal lobule, parallel to and very near the convolution of the corpus callosum. There was no other lesion found in the brain; the right half of the cord and the right crus cerebri appeared somewhat wasted. M. Landouzy also mentions other cases in which an analogous condition was found. Amongst these were cases of obstinate sciatica, of muscular atrophy in multiple sclerosis, in neuritis due to cervical pachymeningitis, and in other cases of amyotrophic palsy. He states that it is of exceptional occurrence in the wasting palsies, such as progressive muscular atrophy, habitual in secondary muscular atrophies, and variable in infantile paralysis. If this condition is of frequent occurrence, as M. Landouzy's observations seems to show (and they are supported by other evidence), it is one of great interest and value in its clinical and pathological bearings. Muscular atrophy may, as he shows, be concealed by the overgrowth of fat, and its nature, when observed in doubtful cases, may to some extent be determined by the coincidence of the fatty hyperplasia.

Of the various explanations which might be offered to account for this condition, M. Landouzy shows that some are untenable. It cannot be explained merely by the increase of nutritive supply or of nerve influence upon the subcutaneous fatty tissue owing to its diminution in the muscles, for it bears no direct proportion to the extent of muscular atrophy, and is entirely absent in some of the best-marked cases. Nor can it be due to want of movement and muscular action solely, for it is not observed in many cases of complete loss of motion, and it may be present where movement, though weak, is very free. In fact, by a careful examination of the possible explanations, M. Landouzy shows that no other reasonable cause can be assigned than the direct influence of the central nervous system, and that this appears to be exerted on the subcutaneous fatty tissue independently of the skin itself, the innervation of which appears to be separate. It may happen that changes in the skin itself, such as the eruptions which are occasionally seen in spinal or meningeal disease, may occur alone, or they may be associated with the fatty changes in the subcutaneous tissue, but the two are distinct and independent. And in the same way the effect of disease of cord or nerve upon the muscles of the limb may be atrophy from suspended action, and upon the subcutaneous tissue overgrowth of fat from increased stimulation; the two being collateral, but independent. Here, however, we enter upon a wide and interesting field of investigation, in which it is desirable that further clinical and pathological study should precede speculation; and the light which such observation may throw upon the obscure subject of nerve influence on nutrition is very considerable.—*Lancet*, Feb. 9, 1878.

———

Regeneration of the Retinal Purple outside the Body.

Prof. KÜHNE and Dr. A. EWALD (*Centralblatt*, No. 42, 1877) have discovered that solutions of Boll's "see purple" or "see red," in purified bile which is *absolutely free from ether*, if bleached by exposure to sunlight, recover their colour in a dark room. Similar solutions of the retinal (rodless) epithelium, mechanically freed from insoluble black pigment granules, etc., turn pink in the dark, pale in the light, and pink again if replaced in the dark. The colour of the retinal purple is restored with the greatest intensity in mixed solutions prepared from the epithelium and the retinal rods. It is an interesting fact that if the retina of a frog be bleached in the light before the animal is killed, the colour does not afterwards return under the action of darkness if the epithelium is removed, whereas, in dead frogs, bleaching in the light is followed under identical circumstances by purple regeneration, and the colour can be destroyed and revived several times.—*Med. Times and Gaz.*, Dec. 15, 1877.

———

The Development of the Red Blood-corpuscles.

The development of red blood-corpuscles is a problem of profound practical importance, and every fresh information on the subject is to be eagerly welcomed. An interesting series of investigations by M. G. HAYEM was recently communicated to the Académie des Sciences by M. Vulpian. They relate to the development of the red globules in oviparous vertebrata—birds, reptiles, batrachians, and fishes. The blood of these creatures, according to these researches, constantly contains cells which are destitute of colouring matter, and yet differ essentially from the ordinary white corpuscles. These cells on development become perfect red corpuscles, and hence Hayem proposes to call them "hæmatoblasts." He has found them in all the oviparous vertebrata examined (various birds, the tortoise, lizard, adder, frog, toad, triton, axolotl, and several fishes). They are also found in the blood of the tadpole, in which the characters they present are the same as in the adult animal. During their successive transformations, the hæmatoblasts pass through two phases. They are at first very pale and delicate, so that it is with difficulty that they can be distinguished from white corpuscles. They differ from the latter in the transparency and feeble refracting power of their protoplasm, and by their viscosity, by which they adhere one to another, and sometimes form a mass of considerable size. Their form is, moreover, somewhat angular or elongated, especially in birds, and they have a solitary nucleus, which is clearer than the body of the corpuscle. The characters of the nucleus vary in different animals, but always resemble those of the nuclei of the red corpuscles, with this difference, that the latter are a little smaller, and often less elongated. In the second phase of development the corpuscles gradually assume the appearance of small disks, and lose their viscosity. Their aspect now, which is nearly the same in different animals, was described last summer by M. Vulpian. The tint of the hæmatoblast is a little darker than that of the original cell, and the nucleus occasions a prominence on each side of the disk. In the forms which are a little more developed, the protoplasm is reduced to a narrow ring around the nucleus, and the corpuscle assumes a shape resembling that of the developed red corpuscle, now and then first assuming an irregular shape. Sometimes the disk is composed of two distinct parts, as M. Vulpian has shown, a central clear and slightly granular portion forming a zone around the nucleus (of this traces may often be seen in the adult corpuscle), and another peripheral zone more homogeneous, and soon to become impregnated with hæmoglobin. The colouring matter appears usually before the development of the cell is completed, and then some coloured elements may be seen in the blood, having the form of hæmatoblasts. Their size varies according to the stage of their development; that of the nucleus varies according to the size of the nuclei of the red corpuscles in the same animal. Examined in a damp chamber, the hæmatoblasts are seen to undergo slow changes of shape, but these are believed by M. Hayem not to be true amœboid movements, but rather to resemble the successive stages of cadaveric destruction. After some hours the hæmatoblasts which were in the first stage of development are represented only by their nuclei retaining still some irregular tracts of a finely granular material; those which had attained the second stage are in general more resistant. All the reagents act on the hæmatoblasts just as they do on the red corpuscles, and produce no effects such as are manifested by the leucocytes. When dried rapidly, many small cells, which were colourless in the wet state, appear to be coloured, as if they already contained a small quantity of hæmoglobin. A comparison of the blood of many animals shows that these hæmatoblasts are in no case less numerous than the leucocytes, and that often, on the contrary, they are twice as numerous. Their proportion to the coloured corpuscles is, in the bird, 1 to 100, in the snake 1 to 40, in the tortoise 1 to 50, and in frogs 1 to 60. Hayem concludes that the white corpuscles do not form the red globules, and that while in the higher animals the newly-formed red corpuscles are coloured, whatever their origin, in the ovipara the embryonal corpuscles are at first free from hæmaglobin. An important problem is the relation these so-called hæmatoblasts bear to the leucocytes; whether they are really distinct, or merely a stage of transformation of the latter. This point, in spite of M. Hayem's opinion, must be considered as still doubtful.—*Lancet*, Dec. 29, 1877.

Materia Medica and Therapeutics.

Action of Intravenous Injections of Chloral on the Circulation and Respiration.

Dr. Troquart has studied in M. Marey's laboratory, by the aid of self-registering apparatus, the action of intravenous injections of chloral in animals. He arrives at the following conclusions (*Thèse de Paris*, Aug. 6, 1877). When a sufficient quantity of chloral in solution is injected into the venous system of an animal, disturbances of the action of the heart and of respiration are almost immediately and simultaneously produced, consisting of more or less prolonged stoppage (primary symptoms). The primary cardiac symptoms, which vary considerably according to the dose, the rapidity of injection, etc., consist, in order of decreasing gravity, of, 1. Definitive arrest ; 2. Momentary arrest ; 3. Simple slackening of the pulsations. The indications furnished by arterial pressure confirm the results obtained by direct exploration of the heart. The heart under the influence of chloral becomes excessively distended in the interval of two systoles. At the commencement, the ventricle empties itself completely, but soon becomes powerless to send a flow of blood of any volume into the arterial system. A heart congested in a permanent diastole, and showing small ventricular jerks without any useful effect is then seen. During the ventricular arrest, the systole of the auricle persists, which explains the congestion and the constant increase in the size of the heart under the influence of chloral. The disturbances are the more quickly repaired in proportion to their want of gravity. The time occupied by reparation shows nothing stable in its mode of appearing, its characteristics, or its duration, it varies especially according to the dose injected, and the quantity of chloral previously absorbed by the animal. Rapid after a first injection, it becomes slow after a series of successive injections. The chloral acts by its immediate contact with the internal septum of the right heart. It excites the sensitive nerve-filaments of the endocardium, and induces in the intracardiac ganglia a reflex action, which reacts on the moderator fibres of the pneumogastrics, whence results arrest of the heart in diastole. If a current of blood charged with chloral be made to pass through an isolated heart of the land tortoise, a systolic arrest is observed. The chloral penetrating immediately into the coronary arteries, when it leaves the ventricle, which is simple, acts directly on the muscular fibres, of which it provokes the contraction, as it produces that of the muscles into the arteries of which it is immediately injected.

Chloral gradually brings on paralysis of the peripheric extremities of the pneumogastrics, whence there is a decrease in the cardiac symptoms in proportion as the injections are multiplied.

Consecutive cardiac troubles are very variable ; for the most part they are characterized by a period of slackening, followed by irregularities. In the mammalia, periods of abortive systole, with great lowering of pressure and disappearance of arterial pulsation, are observed. Chloral induces general congestion of the organs, dilatation of the capillaries, through paralysis of the vaso-motor nerves, which explains certain phenomena, such as lowering of the pressure, diminution of the temperature, etc. The respiratory disturbances are analogous to the cardiac troubles ; simple slackening, however, is rare ; for the most part, it is an absolute arrest, which follows almost immediately on the intravenous injection.

The respiratory arrest almost always supervenes before the cardiac troubles, and only ceases when these are partially repaired. The respiratory arrest may be definitive, and yet the pulsations of the heart may still persist for some minutes. The use of electric currents against these accidents is not entirely without danger. Artificial respiration seems to yield better results. The theory of immediate respiratory troubles necessitates further researches, but may take its stand on this fact, that reflex muscular action, of which the starting-point is in the excitation of the sensitive filaments of the endocardium, is concerned in it.—*London Med. Record*, Jan. 15, 1878.

On the Combined Use of Chloroform and Morphia.

Professor Kœnig, in a communication to the *Centralblatt für Chirurgie* (No. 39, 1877), says he has combined the hypodermic administration of morphia with that of chloroform in a large number of cases, with very favourable results. It is seldom necessary to give more than one or at most two centigrammes ($\frac{1}{6}$ to $\frac{1}{3}$ grain).

The indications for the use of morphia during chloroform-narcosis are twofold: 1. Motor disturbances occurring before or during chloroform-inhalation unless these are very transitory: 2. Operations of such a nature that the chloroform-narcosis cannot be maintained throughout, and especially towards the end. Among the latter may be particularly mentioned operations upon the eye, plastic operations, extirpation of tumours from the soft parts of the face. The object of using morphia is to induce analgesia over and above the chloroform-narcosis, and also that this narcosis should not be pushed so far. As regards any danger which may be connected with the combination of narcotics, Kœnig esteems this lightly. He says that out of seven thousand cases in which he has used chloroform, none have died from it, and many of these took morphia also.—*London Med. Record*, Feb. 15, 1878.

—

The Physiological Action of Glycerine.

We drew attention some time ago to some interesting and important experiments made by M. CATILLON upon the physiological and therapeutic action of glycerine (MONTHLY ABSTRACT, June, 1877, p. 241). It will be remembered that he found that glycerine caused a considerable diminution in the excretion of urea, a rise of temperature, and, when continuously employed, an increase of weight. He proved, too, that it was entirely absorbed, unless given in very large quantity, when a small proportion escaped by the urine: and that it could not be found as such in the blood. Hence he concluded that it served as a supporter of combustion, and saved the waste both of the fatty and nitrogenous tissues, this explaining the increase of weight, diminution of urea excretion, and rise of temperature. But he did not show at the time, by direct experiment, that the products of combustion, in the shape of carbonic acid and water excreted by the lungs, were proportionally increased, which they should be if this view were correct, and this he has now done by further experiments, recently communicated to the Société de Biologie, which were made in M. Vulpian's laboratory. He found, by experiments on dogs, that the percentage of carbonic acid in the breath was notably increased by administration of glycerine, and that not only did it augment with increase of dose, but this augmentation lasted longer the larger the dose. The increase of carbonic acid began to show itself about an hour after taking the glycerine, reaching its maximum in three or four hours, and lasting from five to ten hours. And not only was the percentage in the expired air increased, but the total quantity was also greatly increased, so that nearly all the carbon contained in the glycerine was accounted for in the carbonic acid. This result seemed to be attained by an increase in the amplitude of the respirations, their number continuing the same; but it was not proved that this increased amplitude became greater with a larger dose. It was proved, too, that where disease of the lungs, such as pneumonia or empysema, existed, there was still the increase of carbonic acid. A very important point, also noted by M. Catillon, is that the transformation of the glycerine into water and carbonic acid seems to be direct, no intermediate oxidation products, such as glyceric, formic, or oxalic acids, being discovered in the blood.—*Lancet*, March 2, 1878.

On the Therapeutic Action of Thymol.

Dr. BALZ describes (*Archiv der Heilkunde*, Band xiv. 3 and 4 Heft) the results of comparative experiments with thymol and salicylic acid in Wunderlich's service.

The thymol was administered either as an emulsion or as a mixture. The observations were made in healthy individuals, and on patients with typhoid fever, articular rheumatism, phthisis, and pyelitis, in almost all of whom pyrexia was present. Doses of a centigramme (.15 grain), if repeated many times, had no result. To produce an appreciable therapeutic effect, the dose had to be raised to a gramme and a half or two grammes (22½ or 30 grains) a day. The author made twenty-six observations, with the following results. If the drug came into direct contact with the bucco-pharyngeal mucous membrane, the patients complained of a sensation of pricking and of a bad taste in the mouth. Nausea was rarely produced, and only once vomiting, in a phthisical patient. If the dose were raised a sensation of heat at the epigastrium was produced, which was, however, transient; the patients also were often attacked with diarrhœa, the evacuations resembling those of typhoid fever. In a majority of the cases the injection of thymol was followed, half an hour or an hour afterwards, by sweating, which was more or less localized and abundant, but always less than that produced by salicylic acid and jaborandi. Sometimes, also, but not always, slight diuresis was noticed. The urine presented a dark and somewhat greenish colour, as if mixed with blood, and when viewed by transmitted light it appeared yellow-brown. The addition of a solution of perchloride of iron rendered the urine cloudy and of a gray-white colour. When the green colour predominated it might have been mistaken for icteric urine, or even for nephritic urine mixed with blood, but the absence of albumen in the latter case would prevent such an error. With regard to the nervous system, singing in the ears and deafness were noticed, and a sensation of constriction across the temples extremely disagreeable to the patients. More serious symptoms were sometimes observed. Thus in a patient in the third week of typhoid fever a dose of three grammes caused violent delirium, which lasted many hours, but ceased when the temperature was lowered. In another case of typhoid fever the patient lost consciousness, and then passed into a state of delirium followed by collapse, which lasted many hours, and caused very great anxiety. In typhoid fever and articular rheumatism, and in phthisis often, a dose of from two to three grammes will cause lowering of temperature of at least from 3° to 5° Fahr., but often the effect is greater than required, and the patients pass into deep collapse. To avoid these effects thymol is administered in fractional doses of 0.25 gramme (3¾ grains) every hour; this will give a total dose of 6 grammes (about 90 grains) in twenty-four hours. The circulatory system is relatively little influenced by thymol. When this drug causes a considerable lowering of the temperature there is a diminution of the frequency of the pulse, but not in proportion to the lowering of the temperature. The author attempted subcutaneous injections with a solution of thymol, but with no good result; the injection was often very painful, and readily gave rise to inflammation. He concludes that thymol is incontestably an antipyretic, but uncertain in action, and has not the value of salicylic acid and salicylate of soda.—*Lond. Med. Record*, February 15, 1878.

———

On Absorption of Medical Substances by the Vaginal Mucous Membrane.

Dr. E. W. HAMBURGER describes (*Prager Vierteljahreschrift*, Band cxxx.) a series of experiments performed by him to ascertain the absorbent power of the vaginal mucous membrane. He used solutions of the following substances, of the strength is indicated : Iodide of potassium, 15 per cent. ; ferrocyanide of potassium, 5 per cent. ; ferridcyanide of potassium, 9 per cent. ; salicylic acid, 2 per cent. ; bromide of potassium, 6 per cent. ; and litria, 10 per cent. A plug of purified cotton-wool soaked in the solution was placed in the vagina, and over it two dry tampons. The bladder was first emptied, and afterwards the urine was drawn off by the catheter and examined at intervals of two or three hours. All the above-mentioned substances were found in the urine. Iodide of potassium was found two hours after the introduction of the tampon, and traces of it remained twenty-four hours after removal. Ferrocyanide of potassium, salicylic acid, and bromide of potassium appeared three hours after they were given. Hamburger believes that the administration of drugs by the vagina can be employed in all cases of obstruction of the normal passages, and that it will be specially useful in gynæcological practice.—*London Med. Record*, Feb. 15, 1878.

Medicine.

Microcythæmia.

· HAYEM (*Comptes-Rend.*, lxxxiv., No. 22) expresses his opinion that the so-called microcytes which are present in blood that has been treated with certain reagents are artificial products of the latter, and that their number entirely depends on the particular process of preparation adopted. The microcytes are round, vesicular, highly refracting bodies ; whereas, healthy blood-corpuscles, no matter what their size, are biconcave and discoid. There are normal blood-corpuscles in the blood which only measure two thousandths of a millimetre in diameter, and other gigantic corpuscles which measure twelve to fourteen thousandths of a milli-metre, with a variety of intermediate forms between these two extremes. The smallest corpuscles are very rare in healthy adult men, whereas they are con-stantly present in great abundance in new-born infants, in women at the period of menstruation, and in invalids after severe hemorrhages (epistaxis, hæmoptysis, menorrhagia, etc.) ; and also during convalescence from severe febrile diseases, as well as in all forms of chronic anæmia of medium intensity. Hence their pre-sence is not characteristic of any special form of anæmia (*e. g.*, of pernicious anæmia), as has been stated by some observers. There is, according to Hayem, a constant relation between the presence of small blood-corpuscles and the abun-dance of red blood-cells of normal size ; and hence, in anæmic conditions, their number rises and falls with the increase or diminution of the latter. In general terms, they invariably appear, both under normal and pathological conditions, during the production of normal red blood-corpuscles. They represent an *imma-ture* stage of these latter, and only require to meet in the organism with the necessary conditions for their development, to become converted into them. Hence they are only met with, as a rule, at such times as a new crop of normal red cells is being, so to speak, manufactured—for example, at the menstrual period. If pathological causes impede their development, they remain small, and accumulate as such in the blood, and this explains their special abundance in certain forms of anæmia, their conversion into red cells being prevented by the existence of the disease.—*Med. Times and Gaz.*, Feb. 9, 1878.

Case of Amnesia, with Post-mortem Observation.

At a late meeting of the Royal Medical and Chirurgical Society (*Lancet*, March 2, 1878), Dr. BROADBENT read a paper with the above title, of which the following is an abstract. The communication began by recalling some of the hypothetical conclusions of a previous communication "On the Mechanism of Speech and Thought," in vol. lv. of the *Transactions of the Society*. Dr. Bastian's hypothesis of a special "perceptive centre" in relation with each sense was adopted and extended. It was considered that these "perceptive centres" would be situated in convolutions which received radiating fibres; and Ferrier's researches have since located the centres for vision, hearing, smell, taste, and touch in some of the convolutions into which these fibres had been traced, more particularly fibres from the extra-ventricular portion of the thalamus. It was further considered probable that the formation of a complete idea of external objects would be represented structurally by the convergence of arcuate commissural fibres from each perceptive centre to some part of the cortex not in direct relation with the crus or basal ganglia. A part of this intellectual process would be the association with the idea of a name. On this hypothesis it would be possible for a breach to be made in the channel of communication between one of the perceptive centres and the "idea centre" or "naming centre," and a case was related in which the effects producible hypothetically by a lesion between the visual perceptive centre and the naming centre had actually been observed. A patient, otherwise quite intelligent, could not name the simplest object at sight, or read a word of his own writing. A post-mortem examination was made. It was pointed out that a lesion, cutting off the "naming centre" from the "auditory perceptive centre," or involving the former centre itself, would produce far more complicated symptoms, since the subject would, *ex hypothesi*, not only fail to understand spoken words, but he would not know what he himself was saying. Cases were briefly given exemplifying this condition, but no examination had been obtained after death. In the case which forms the subject of the communication, and which is believed to afford another illustration, the brain was examined after death. An omnibus driver, aged forty-nine, of intemperate habits, had a fit, of which no accurate account could be obtained, about October 1st, 1877. He had from that time been in the condition in which he was found on admission into St. Mary's Hospital on the 11th. He walked into the hospital, and no paralysis could be detected, except very slight paresis of the right side of the face. Sensibility, however, was defective over the entire right half of the body, limbs, and face. The striking feature of the case was that the speech consisted almost exclusively of an inarticulate jargon, in which, however, from time to time, a distinct word or phrase would be heard, such as "If you please," "Thank you." It was difficult to make out how far he understood what was said to him, as his replies, though mere jabber, were often appropriate so far as length was concerned, natural in tone and accent, and accompanied by natural gestures and facial expression. He would also address long speeches to those around him, evidently making some urgent request, and he frequently ended by crying. It was obvious that he thought he was giving expression to ideas present in his own mind, but he did not recognize the fact that his language was inarticulate. It was by telling him to do something that his want of comprehension of spoken words was made apparent. His invariable response to the command to give his hand was to put out the tongue, and in one or two doubtful instances only was his action appropriate, and then he was probably directed by signs. He did not understand writing. The patient died suddenly on November 6th, and on post-mortem examination softening was found involving a considerable part of the posterior half of the convex surface of the left hemisphere. The greatest depth (three-quarters of an inch) and breadth of the morbid change was seen in a transverse vertical section made at the end of the fissure of Sylvius. Here softening reached from near the superior longitudinal margin to within an inch of the

inferior and internal edge of tie iemispiere. Tie convolutions affected were
proceeding from before backwards, tie supra-marginal lobule and corresponding
part of infra-marginal or first temporo-sphenoidal gyrus; more deeply and in a
more advanced degree tie postero-parietal lobule, tie angular gyrus, and tie first
and second temporo-spienoidai convolutions in tie same place; less extensively
tie middle annectent gyrus and tie part of tie occipital lobe adjacent. Tie
softening involved tie temporo-spienoidal lobe more completely tian tie parietal
lobe membranes. Arteries of brain fairly ienlthy, of vertex opaque, and raised
by fluid from convolutions. No otier morbid ciange observed. It was considered tiat tie loss of compreiension of words, wietier spoken by otiers or
iimself. and tie confusion of mind consequent upon iis inability to understand
or to make iimself understood, would account for tie condition of tie patient,
and tie interpretation was tiat tiis was due to destruction of tie ciannel from
tie auditory perceptive centre to tie iigier centre in wiici tie name is associated witi tie idea wiici it symbolizes, or to destruction of tiis name-centre
itself. Wietier tie interpretation offered is exact or not, tie case is interesting
as an example of the association of certain loss of intellectual faculties witi a
lesion of definite extent and seat. It is wortiy of attention tiat tie left iemispiere is tie one affected, and it would appear from tiis and similar cases tiat
tie exclusive employment of tiis iemispiere as tie way out for language involved its use as tie "way in." A comparison of the effects of lesions of identical parts of tie two iemispieres would be fruitful of results.

Tie PRESIDENT asked wietier tie patient was as unable to express iis ideas
in writing as ie was in speeci; or if ie could not, did ie make attempts to write
wien ie iad a pen given iim for tie purpose?

Dr. BROADBENT said ie was perfectly unable to express iimself in writing,
and, indeed, ie ield tie pen in an aimless sort of way, not appearing to attempt
to use it.

Mr. SPENCER WATSON iad always felt tiere must be some fallacy regarding
tie idea of tie one-sided function of tie iigier cerebral functions, and suggested
tiat tie true explanation of cases of amnesia from lesion of one side of tie brain
migit be found in a loss of balance between tie two iemispieres, just as tie
function of walking is disordered if one leg be injured and lost. No one would
say tiat tie function of walking resided in tiat injured leg.

Dr. BBOADBENT said tiat it was no doubt a siock to all to find tie function
of speeci limited to one cerebral iemispiere, but it seemed abundantly proved
by facts. No amount of lesion in tie rigit iemispiere would produce loss of
speeci—at any rate, in any but a left-ianded person; wiereas a very limited
lesion in tie tiird frontal convolution of tie left side produced apiasia. Tie
iypotiesis of Broca and Noxon—of tie education of tie left iemispiere being
correlated to rigit-iandedness—involved also education in tie intellectual expression of tiougit by means of speeci, for speeci is merely a matter of movement.

—

*Syphiloma of the Pons Varolii; with remarks on Unilateral Cerebral
Anæsthesia and Disturbance of the Senses.*

At a late meeting of tie Imperial Royal Nedical Society of Vienna, Dr.
ROSENTHAL described tie case of a man aged 46, at first an out-patient and
afterwards an in-patient of tie General Hospital, wio, since January 1876, iad
been tie subject of severe ieadacie, vertigo, and loss of sensation in tie left
cieek. Six montis later tiere were observed ptosis of tie left eyelid, paralysis
of tie abducens, diplopia, convergent strabismus, and paralysis of tie trigeminus

nerve (outer and inner branches) affecting the conjunctiva, sclerotic, and cornea ;
there was loss of sensation in the two anterior thirds of the tongue on the left
side : the glosso-pharyngeal region was unaffected. The diagnosis of a new
growth in the pons Varolii was confirmed in August by the occurrence of paresis
of the right side. The varying character of the paralysis of the ocular muscles
caused syphilis to be suspected, although the patient denied that he had ever had
the disease, and no indications of it could be found in the genital organs or glands.
He took iodide of potassium (45 grains in two days) for four weeks. At the end
of September, 1876, the right hemiplegia had improved, but was followed by left
hemiplegia. He was placed in one of Dr. Von Bamberger's clinical wards, where
he died on February 18, with symptoms of impeded deglutition and articulation.
At the necropsy, the pons Varolii was found to contain several foci, mostly confluent, in the neighbourhood of which the substance was replaced by a grayish,
rather soft mass, and partly by a dry substance having the appearance of cheese ;
most of the nerves at the base had undergone partial gray degeneration ; the
arteries at the base were in a normal condition. The liver was adherent by its
convex surface to the diaphragm by several bands of connective tissue ; it was
rather small, and its capsule, especially at the convexity, was much thickened,
and cicatricial bands passed from it into the substance of the liver. A microscopic
examination of the new growth made by Dr. Chiari revealed the presence of the
elements of syphiloma, numerous nuclei and round cells in a basis of fibrous tissue,
as well as secondary descending degeneration of the antero-lateral columns. On
examination during life of the anæsthetic anterior left third of the tongue, there
was found to be complete loss of taste for concentrated solution of sweet, acid,
and salt substances ; while even weak bitters were tasted. Galvanic examination,
by means of the application of fine isolated electrodes to the tongue, as also by
the conduction of the current from the parotid and laryngeal regions, produced
on the right half of the tongue a metallic taste with from eight to fifteen of Sie iens's
elements, while on the left half only a moderate taste was produced by twenty-
five or thirty such elements. In two cases of hysteria which Dr. Rosenthal had
observed in the practice of Dr. Scholz, left hemiplegia and hemianæsthesia set
in, and extended over the whole region supplied by the left trigeminus nerve, as
well as the whole left half of the tongue. The sense of taste was completely lost,
and only a feeble sensation was excited by a current of from sixteen to twenty
elements ; when the stimulant was conveyed through the parotid and larynx,
thirty to thirty-five elements were required to produce any effect. The right
half of the tongue preserved its gustatory power for some months, but it at last
disappeared here also. In one case, the right half of the tongue (the taste being
totally lost) remained for several days sensible to pricking, while the application
of ice to the same part, as well as to the corresponding half of the face and chest,
was not perceived. In order to test the irritability of the brain in the three cases
mentioned above, Dr. Rosenthal applied a galvanic current through the corresponding halves of the occiput and forehead ; on the healthy side, from 15 to 18
elements produced giddiness, metallic taste, and phosphene : on the anæsthetic
side of the head no effect was produced by 40 elements, beyond a slight flashing
in the eye. In six cases of rheumatic paralysis of the face, the author found the
taste normal in the mild cases ; in the more severe forms (with loss of nervous
irritability and degeneration in the muscles) the sense of taste was impaired, in
some quite lost : the galvanic gustatory reaction was little if at all diminished.
In the severe cases of facial paralysis which recovered, the return of taste was
among the first signs of improvement ; but several weeks elapsed before the perception of sweet, salt, and latest of all, acid substances, was regained. The
author concluded from numerous experiments that the galvanic examination of

the sense of taste afforded more delicate and certain results than the ordinary
methods. If, when the normal sense of taste is lost, the galvanic reaction be not
at all or but little changed, an affection of the peripheral gustatory fibres is indicated; while, if the galvanic reaction be considerably diminished, the loss of
sensation most probably has its origin in the conducting nerve or in the centre.
The assumption of intracerebral disease becomes a certainty, when, in cases of
complete loss of taste, no effect on the sense is produced by galvanic stimulation
of the corresponding side of the head.—*Lond. Med. Record*, Jan. 15, 1878.

*An Analysis of Seventy-five Cases of Writer's Cramp and Impaired
Writing Power.*

Dr. VIVIAN POORE, at a recent meeting of the Royal Medical and Chirurgical Society (*Lancet*, Feb. 16, 1878), read an exhaustive and elaborate paper
on writer's cramp, of which the following is an abstract. In seventy-four of these
cases the condition of the hand completely over-shadowed any other disease,
whether general or local, from which the patients were then suffering. Most of
the cases merited the name of writer's cramp, or had been so called, but the
author has purposely included a few cases which obviously do not merit that name,
because the study of them throws some light on the main question. The cases
fall naturally into six groups, thus: 1, paralytic (six cases); 2, spasmodic (five
cases); 3, degenerative (nine cases); 4, neuralgic or neuritic (nineteen cases);
5, writer's cramp (thirty-two cases); 6, anomalous (four cases). The cases are
arranged in a tabulated form. It is shown that since the ulnar nerve supplies
thirteen and a half out of the eighteen intrinsic muscles of the hand its integrity
is very necessary (more necessary than that of any other nerve of the hand) for
all delicate manipulation, especially writing. The spasms which affect the hand,
and which are particularly prone to follow attacks of hemiplegia, owe sometimes,
there is good reason to believe, their character, if not their origin, to a faulty
antagonization (due to a secondary paralysis or paresis) among the muscles of
the paralyzed limb. Although it is commonly received that such spasms are due
to disturbance of the gray cerebral matter, it is well to look also to the peripheral
aspects of the question. Provided a nervous impulse, issuing from the brain, be
distributed in a limb to equally irritable muscles which mutually antagonize each
other, it is difficult to conceive that spasm of definite form should be produced;
but should the equilibrium of antagonization in the limb be destroyed by a secondary lesion, the production of definite spasm is easily conceivable, especially when
voluntary control is lessened by a lesion of the central ganglia. In some cases of
localized spasm there is no evidence of central change, and it is theoretically possible that the action of a disordered centre on a healthy periphera and the reaction of a disordered periphera on a healthy centre may be identical in their
results. It is shown that loss of writing power is often the first and most prominent symptom of degenerative change occurring in the spinal cord or brain. The
neuritic or neuralgic group is characterized by a painful and tender condition of
the nerves of the limb, which may be induced solely by overwork, but more frequently by a strain or similar injury, combined with exposure to cold and a depressed state of health. Of the nineteen cases in this group twelve were females.
Any attempt to use the arm, either for course or fine acts, produced fatigue, pain,
and neuralgia. It is not always easy to distinguish these cases from true writer's
cramp, and, indeed, there cannot be said to be any hard and fast line between the
two groups; but it is characteristic of the neuralgic groups that—first, the symptoms involve a wider area; secondly, the symptoms are sometimes induced without excessive exercise of any function; thirdly, nerve tenderness or neuralgia is

a prominent symptom. In the group of true writer's cramp considerable care is necessary to detect peripheral evidence of mischief, but the author states that in every case of impaired writing power which he has seen *there has been evidence more or less marked of derangement of one or more of the muscles used for writing.* This evidence consisted of—first, obvious failure to use certain muscles efficiently either for writing or for some other less complicated act; secondly, the occurrence of consentaneous movement or tremor when certain muscles were put in action; thirdly, depressed or exalted electric irritability; and, fourthly, the occurrence of sensory derangement or nerve tenderness. The muscles which are most frequently involved are those of pen-prehension rather than those of pen-movement. Reviewing the cases as a whole, attention is directed—first, to the inferences which may be drawn from an inspection of the hand-writing; secondly, to the fact that joints were found to be implicated no less than twenty-one times, the joint affection being rheumatic, neuropathic, gouty, or due to strained position; thirdly, to the fact that a difficulty in writing is not very infrequently hereditary, or developed very early in life; and that, fourthly, any evidence of involvement of the nerve-centres is decidedly rare. Writer's cramp has been spoken of as a disease of "faulty coordination," and there can be no doubt that such is the case, for it is evident that the muscles used for writing fail to work orderly together. We are not, however, justified in assuming the existence of a special coordinating centre for the controlling of the act of writing, and the author has been unable to find evidence that this centre (supposing it to exist) ever gives way, leaving the periphera, except for the special coordinated act, in a state of perfect health. The existence of such a centre appears to the author to be improbable for the following reasons: 1. Because he has never seen a case of writer's cramp without peripheral evidence of change, and in the majority of cases there has been no evidence of any change other than peripheral. 2. Because, if there be a coordinating centre for writing, it must be created, as it were, by education. The coordination of writing, which we are many years in acquiring, must be distinguished from those coordinated movements (such as the symmetrical movement of the two eyes) which are wholly independent of education. The fact that no two people hold their pens exactly alike, and that it is scarcely more difficult to write with the toes than with the fingers, is much against the probability of the existence of a writing centre. 3. Because writer's cramp is never suddenly established, as aphasia sometimes is. 4. Because it is almost certain that a purely peripheral lesion may cause all the symptoms of writer's cramp. 5. The fact that the left hand (if used for writing) sometimes suffers, as well as the right, is no evidence that the change is central. In previous writings the author has spoken of writer's cramp as a "fatigue disease," and he is still inclined to adhere to the word "fatigue" as a convenient expression for an easily recognizable and familiar condition of the pathology of which we are uncertain. He is inclined to think that occasionally fatigue is the expression of hyperæmia or mild inflammation of a motor nerve, and that the same condition may be produced either by overwork or by accidental causes, such as cold, strain, "rheumatism," or injury. Fatigue especially attacks those muscles which are subjected to prolonged strain, and it is probable that the relative frequency of writer's cramp, as compared with other professional ailments, is due to the fact that prolonged strain of certain muscles (those which hold and steady the pen) is inseparable from the act of writing. Finally, as to the position of writer's cramp in the catalogue of diseases, the author would feel inclined to class it with neuralgia— that is, with a disease the phenomena of which are purely local, but which we recognize as being due not only to conditions affecting the sensory area involved, but also to molecular change affecting any part of the sensory fibre, whether before or after its junction with the nerve-centre. The author concluded by laying down certain principles of treatment for the various forms of impaired writing power.

—

Rhythmical Hysterical Chorea.

Of all the pathological conditions which come under the notice of the physician, perhaps the one which gives the greatest trouble, and is the least satisfactory to all concerned, is the condition, or we should rather say the series of morbid states, to which the generic term hysteria has been applied. To the patient and her friends the disease is a very real one, oftentimes giving rise to great suffering, mental or bodily, or both, and too frequently incapacitating its victim from the performance of any of the duties of life. On the other hand, there has been in many instances too great a tendency on the part of medical men to make light of such cases, and, because the symptoms cannot be grouped within the well-marked boundaries of organic disease, to consider them as the result of wilful misrepresentation on the part of the patient, or of mere "fancy," and hence that nothing need be done but to tell the patient there is "nothing the matter."

Of late years, however, there has been a growing tendency among scientific physicians to investigate the phenomena of hysteria in the same way that the more clearly organic diseases are studied, to analyze its various phases, and to attempt to discover their true significance. Foremost amongst those who have attempted to grapple with this most obscure subject has been Professor CHARCOT, who has lectured from time to time during the last few years on different manifestations of the disease. At one time his attention was turned to the derangements of sensation in the form of hemianæsthesia, general and special, the study of which has now become so closely linked with his name. At another time he dwelt upon the remarkable modifications in the renal functions occasionally seen in hysterical subjects; but more recently he has called attention to the various motor phenomena of hysteria, convulsions, contractions of limbs, or paralyses. In a course of lectures recently delivered at the Salpêtrière, he has carried the study of this division of his subject a step further, by treating of a condition presented by one of his patients to which he has given the name of "rhythmical hysterical chorea." The patient in question was a young woman, nineteen years of age, whose previous history presented a long succession of hysterical phenomena of various kinds. She presented, indeed, all the characters of the condition which Dr. Charcot has termed "ovarian hysteria." From the age of thirteen she has been subject to convulsive attacks of the typical hystero-epileptic order, and these fits could be invariably stopped at once by compression of the right ovarian region. In this region there was at all times a certain amount of pain, which increased when a fit was impending, and was exaggerated by pressure. The warning which preceded the fits started from the painful region, and thence extended to the epigastrium, the neck, the head, etc. The right half of the body was the seat of absolute anæsthesia, both for general sensation and for heat, and the special senses were also affected, though in different degrees. There was loss of smell in the right nostril, absolute loss of taste in the right side of the tongue, dulness of hearing in the right ear, and amblyopia, with partial dyschromatopsy in the right eye—perception for the "central" colors, violet and green, being completely lost, whilst the "peripheral" colors, red, orange, yellow, and blue, could still be clearly distinguished. Corresponding with the hemianæsthesia was a certain amount of muscular weakness on the right side, for whilst the dynamometrical pressure with the left hand was twenty-five kilogrammes, with the right hand it was only fifteen kilogrammes.

The patient had thus long presented many of the more severe symptoms of hys-

teria, when recently a convulsive attack, which had been of unusually short duration, and of which the symptoms had been much milder than was usually the
case, was immediately followed by a ceaseless agitation of the whole of the right
side of the body. At first sight the movements appeared to be without perceptible order, but a more attentive examination made it evident that they all presented certain general characters. For instance, the agitation of each part of the
body could be decomposed into alternate movements, particularly those of flexion and extension, which were always the same and absolutely uniform. The
trunk was at one moment flexed on the pelvis till the forehead nearly touched
the knee, and at the next moment it was thrown back, the head falling heavily
on the pillow. In the arm a state of complete extension and pronation alternated
with strong flexion and supination; whilst in the leg an extension of the limb,
sufficient to press it strongly against the mattress, and which in the foot simulated talipes equinus, was immediately replaced by an equally well-marked flexion of all the joints. The flexion of the trunk corresponded with extension in
the limbs, and *vice versâ*. To complete the picture, it is only necessary to add
that when the head and trunk were thrown back, the right labial commissure was
momentarily drawn outwards, the deviation ceasing when the trunk was flexed
forwards, and if the tongue were protruded at the moment of production of the
grimace the point was strongly deviated to the right, this deviation being the expression of a rhythmical deviation of the organ which was constantly going on in
the patient's mouth, and which greatly interfered with her pronunciation.

The number of oscillations varied from thirty to eighty per minute, and at the
time when M. Charcot demonstrated the case to his pupils the movements had been
going on for ten days without cessation or respite, except during the few hours that
the patient slept. At the moment of waking, a curious phenomenon always occurred: the limbs which were the seat of agitation when she was fully awake
became for a few moments quite rigid—the leg more so than the arm; but the
rigidity soon gave place to movement. Throughout the attack the limbs of the left
side were at rest, and, notwithstanding the great oscillations of the trunk, the
patient could, with her left hand, carry a glass of water to her mouth without
spilling it, and she could with that hand even write her name legibly.

Taking the term chorea in its widest sense as applying to all continuous excessive involuntary movements persisting as long as the patient is awake, the affection just described may be classed with chorea. It is not to be confounded with
the ordinary chorea of Sydenham—the chorea minor, in which the movements
are without rhythm and beyond analysis—but it belongs to the variety described
by Professor Sée as *systematic or rhythmical chorea*, in which the involuntary
movements more or less resemble voluntary, intentional actions; are, so to speak,
coördinated, and can thus be clearly distinguished from the incoördinate, utterly
purposeless movements of ordinary chorea.

To prove that the attack from which the patient was suffering was no for-
tuitous complication, no foreign episode superadded to the great neurosis already
present, but that it was one which was very closely connected with the hysterical
diathesis, Professor Charcot adduced firstly the fact already mentioned—that it
set in immediately after a convulsive attack remarkable for its shortness and
mildness, and that it is just under such circumstances that other phenomena of a
motor order frequently arise, such as paralysis, contraction of members, and the
like. Hence the choreiform agitation might be looked upon as a continuation,
or prolongation under a new form, of the aborted hysterical attack. But another
and still stronger argument, according to Professor Charcot, lies in the fact that
compression of the right ovarian region, properly applied, produced complete
cessation of the rhythmical movements, as he demonstrated to the class. Not-

withstanding that the limbs were in this way relieved from the state of ceaseless
agitation in which they had hitherto been, they did not recover their normal
functions, for they had become the seat of considerable muscular rigidity, comparable in all points to the contraction which was present each morning when the patient awoke.

The remarkable arrest of choreiform movements under the influence of ovarian
compression was, nevertheless, only a temporary suspension. It persisted just
so long only as the compression was maintained; as soon as this was removed
the contraction disappeared, and the rhythmical movements of the trunk and
members recommenced as violently as before.

From all this Professor Charcot has been led to conclude that the rhythmical
chorea seen in this patient was dependent upon ovarian susceptibility, in the same
way that he considers the ordinary convulsive attacks of hysteria can be traced
back to a morbidly excitable condition of the ovary, associated with pain and
hyperæsthesia of that organ. Hence he places this form of chorea among the
many very various manifestations of hysteria; and because of its replacement by
tonic rigidity of the muscles both on first waking in the morning and under the
influence of ovarian compression, he looks upon the chorea and the rigidity as
equivalent conditions capable of being substituted for one another in the series of
hysterical affections.

As regards the treatment of the case, Professor Charcot sought some means by
which to cut short the chorea. As we have seen, simple ovarian compression,
though it changed the character of the attack for the time, was powerless to arrest
it entirely. Arguing from the analogy of allied condition, Professor Charcot believed that ovarian compression prolonged for several hours, or repeated at short
intervals over a considerable period of time, might succeed in breaking the chain
of morbid phenomena. This, however, would be a very tedious and laborious
process, and Professor Charcot hoped to be able to dispense with it by taking advantage of a fact which he has observed in connection with hystero-epileptic
attacks. He has found that the inhalation of ether or of nitrite of amyl by a
patient suffering from ovarian hysteria will in most cases induce a fit having all
the characters of the ordinary hystero-epileptic attack. Now, as the attack of
rhythmical chorea appeared to take the place of a convulsive attack, he hoped to
be able to put an end definitely to the former by inducing the latter. We are
not, however, told to what extent he succeeded in the present case.

Professor Charcot ended his lecture by pointing out that the condition to which
he has drawn attention is by no means observed now for the first time. In his
memoir on Rhythmical Chorea, Professor Sée makes special mention of a variety
of the disease connected with hysteria; and Trousseau describes a condition, of
which three cases had come under his notice, that evidently belonged to the same
category. M. Briquet also, in his well-known work on Hysteria, mentions several similar cases; whilst in our own country Dr. Murchison has described a case
of unilateral chorea which alternated with attacks in which the side that had been
choreic became for a short time rigid throughout. It must not be concluded that
all cases of rhythmical chorea are hysterical, nor that all cases of hysterical chorea
are rhythmical, for numerous examples exist which prove the contrary; but that
certain cases of rhythmical chorea occur which undoubtedly depend upon hysteria
must now be considered as proved, and they form an interesting addition to the
already multiform manifestations of this disease. That a very similar condition
is met with, due to other causes, is also of the highest interest, as it affords an
instance the more of the strict analogy existing between the so-called functional
symptoms of hysteria and those which have a recognizable organic lesion for their
basis—an analogy which, we believe, a more careful observation of the pheno-

mena both of hysteria and of organic disease will make more and more complete. —*Med. Times and Gaz.*, Feb. 23, 1878.

A New Form of Mycosis Œsophagi.

In the *Archiv für Experimentelle Path. und Physiol.* (quoted in *Med.-Chir. Centralblatt*, No. 32, 1877), Dr. E. LETZERICH describes the case of a child sixteen months old who suffered from difficulty of deglutition, irritation, dyspepsia, and distension of the stomach, and who vomited muco-purulent masses, which were found to contain flattened epithelium, covered with peculiar microscopic fungi. An examination of the paper hung on the walls of the room revealed the cause of the child's illness. It was moist, had a fine powdery deposit on it, and presented numerous defects. In creeping along the wall, the child had pulled off small pieces and swallowed them. Dr. Letzerich found, on microscopic examination, that the fungi of the paper were identical with those in the vomited matter. The presence of these organisms explained the œsophageal and gastric symptoms. The treatment consisted in the administration of salicylate of soda in barley-water, under which, in eleven days, the patient recovered.—*Lond. Med. Record*, Dec. 15, 1877.

Tracheotomy in Tuberculosis of the Larynx.

Tuberculosis of the larynx is generally not mentioned in text-books as one of the indications for tracheotomy, as the operation is usually regarded as only a possible means for prolonging life for a short period. Dr. SERKOWSKI, however, is of a different opinion (*Przeglad lekarski*, No. 13, 1877, and *Allgemeine Med.-Chir. Zeitung*, August 15). He has performed tracheotomy twice for tuberculosis of the larynx. One of the patients on whom the operation was performed seven years ago is still alive; the other died at the end of three years, and *post-mortem* examination showed far advanced phthisis. The one still living was attacked after a journey with severe dyspnœa, on account of which Dr. Serkowski at once performed tracheotomy. After the introduction of the canula the respiration became free, and his patient fell into a sleep which continued for forty-eight hours. Under general treatment her strength was regained and her cough left her; but she continued to wear the canula for two years, until laryngoscopic examination showed that a thickening of the vocal cords was all that remained of the former morbid condition. Two years later there was still marked dulness on percussion over the apex of the right lung. Since that time Dr. Serkowski has never examined her, but he has often seen her in an apparently well-nourished condition. He expresses the opinion that the opening in the trachea was not only of temporary benefit, but prevented the further development of tuberculosis. He considers it necessary that the opening of the glottis should be sufficiently large, as thus only can the expectoration of purulent secretion from the lungs, and the admission of air to these organs, be secured. He therefore believes tracheotomy to be indicated in all contractions of the larynx, particularly in tubercular patients. The operation is absolutely required when the larynx is more affected with tuberculosis than the lungs.—*London Med. Record*, Feb. 15, 1878.

Bronchiectasis.

Dr. BARDENHEWER says (*Berliner Klinische Wochenschrift*, December 24, 1877) that according to Gerhardt (*Deutsches Archiv für Klinische Medicin*, vol. xv.) articular rheumatism may occur in connection with suppurative diseases of mucous membranes, and in consequence of the absorption of, and blood-poisoning

by, accumulated, stagnating, and decomposing purulent effusions, as in bronchiectasis (bronchitis with dilated bronchi), diphtheria, gonorrhœa, pyæmia,
dysentery, etc. In confirmation of this view, two cases were observed in the
Cologne Hospital. Both were well-marked cases of bronchiectasis, with abundant muco-purulent and very fetid expectoration, for which both were treated
with inhalation of a solution of 2 per cent. of carbolic acid. While under this
treatment, and improving with it, both were seized with rheumatic inflammation.
In the first case there was a single attack of pain, and swelling of the left knee,
which gave way to local application of ice. In the second case, three separate
attacks occurred in both knees, presenting all the symptoms of acute articular
rheumatism, and were relieved by the internal use of salicylic acid. Both cases
ultimately recovered completely. Gerhardt strongly advocates mechanical compression of the thorax in the treatment of the bronchiectasis, as removing the
stagnating purulent secretion, diminishing the concomitant fever, and also relieving the rheumatic symptoms. In place of this, the above two cases were treated
by carbolic inhalation—the same treatment, indeed, having been steadily pursued
for about three years in the Cologne Hospital in all cases of bronchiectasis. Cases
of pneumonia, pleurisy, mechanical injuries of the respiratory organs, etc., may
at different stages present expectoration of abundant purulent and fetid sputum.
This sputum separates on standing into three distinct layers (Traube) ; the upper
layer is greenish-yellow, opaque, and frothy ; the middle serous, transparent, and
albuminoid ; the lower yellow, opaque, and consisting of pus and detritus. It
further contains paste-like plugs of a dirty-yellowish colour, which are extremely
fetid, and consist of finely granulated detritus, mixed with larger fat globules, in
which are suspended occasionally (Virchow) acicular crystals of margaric acid.
In presence of this kind of sputum, treatment has the double object of counteracting its putrescence and of reducing its excessive quantity. Arrest of the
putrescence of the secretion accumulated in the bronchial tubes is generally followed by diminution of its quantity—since the putrid secretion itself acts as an
irritant in causing its continuous production and decomposition, and also in maintaining the accompanying febrile state. The main indication, therefore, is the
arrest of the putrefactive process. The experience of thirty cases within the
last three years is, that this is best fulfilled by the inhalation of carbolic acid.
For this purpose a solution of carbolic acid in water (1 or 2 per cent.) should be
inhaled every two hours day and night for several weeks. The result has always
been most favourable, even when, from the nature of the case, complete cure was
out of the question ; while in several instances, when strong evidence of cavities
existed, this treatment led to a perfect restoration to health.—*London Med.
Record*, Feb. 15, 1878.

Syphilitic Pneumonia.

Dr. SACHARJIN (*Berliner Klinische Wochenschrift*, January 21) says every
one has heard of cases of phthisis cured by iodide of potassium and mercury, but
of anatomical basis for the diagnosis of syphilitic pneumonia there has been lack.
Syphilis often directly, or indirectly through the treatment, breaks people down
in health, and phthisis supervenes. Such cases are usually not only not benefited
by specific treatment, but the disease grows rapidly worse. But he has had the
opportunity of seeing two cases not conforming to this type. The first case
was seen fourteen years ago. A well-built man, of healthy family, thirty years
of age, six or seven years before had had syphilis, and, in the last three years,
serpiginous eruptions and periostitis of the tibiæ and ulnæ. For the last few
weeks he had suffered from pain and stuffing of the chest, great shortness and
difficulty of breathing, and, in the last week, much cough and slight febrile dis-

turbance. During the last year the patient had been liable to colds, which had generally taken the present form of feverish bronchitis, sharp, but of short duration. For the past few days he had been in bed; the fever had gone, but the cough remained. His present condition was meteorism, and tendency to constipation; no albumen nor sugar in urine; pulse rather rapid and feeble; much emaciation, no fever, restless sleep, low spirits. He had little cough, very little morning expectoration (which the patient, in spite of warning, forgot to keep), marked dyspnœa, and feeling of obstruction and pain in the chest. Both clavicles projected ; above and below was marked depression of the chest-walls, with dulness of the percussion-note, especially on the right, down as far as the lower border of the second intercostal space; fremitus was less than normal, and, on auscultation, indeterminate breathing, tending towards bronchial (prolonged expiration), was heard. In the same places and elsewhere in the chest there were sibilant and moist râles. No other signs were heard in the thorax. The heart was normal. In the tibiæ and ulnæ were great pains, increased at night, and, on investigation, syphilitic periostitis was found. For a week he kept his bed, took no medicine, but regulated his diet; the cough and expectoration went, the râles disappeared, but the other physical signs remained. From the coincident phenomena, the lung-affection was diagnosed as syphilitic, and, as he had had very little mercury, that drug was prescribed. It was followed by intolerable itching, worse at night, and preventing sleep; scratching brought out a papular eruption, and the itching increased; where the patient could not scratch, there was no eruption. Baths and other remedies were useless; a lotion of perchloride of mercury alone gave any relief. The treatment therefore was, externally, the application of the above lotion for the itching and eruption, bearing in mind, too, the absorption of mercury, from the large extent of surface to which it was applied, and internally half a pint daily of Zittmann's decoction as a mild mercurial. The itching and eruption soon disappeared, and sleep returned. After four weeks of the treatment, the shortness of breath, pain, and obstruction of the chest disappeared. The hollows above and below the clavicles had filled up (the patient had gained flesh by better appetite and rest) while percussion, auscultation, and palpation could no longer detect the previous signs; the chest presented here, as everywhere else, the normal conditions. During the following eight years the patient was twice seen complaining of slight nervous and gastric disturbances ; but, with the exception of two slight and passing attacks of bronchial catarrh, the chest remained healthy. The second case, observed six years, is the literal repetition of the first. The patient, 30 years of age, and of strong constitution, had had syphilis nine years ; and, for the last five years, suffered from periostitis and ozæna, with necrosis of bone. At the commencement of his illness he took a little mercury, but had since been treated with iodide of potassium only, the influence of which had seemed feebler lately. For the last year the patient had suffered from nervous and dyspeptic symptoms, and febrile bronchial catarrh, which, treated by keeping his room and quinine, disappeared. Shortly before being seen, he had had one of these attacks, accompanied, however, by pain in the chest and shortness of breath, which had not previously occurred. When seen he was free from fever, and the cough was nearly gone ; he had no sputa, marked shortness of breath, etc., just in all points like the first. When the bronchitis had quite disappeared he was ordered mercurial inunction, which was done twenty-five times—five of ten grains, five of fifteen grains, and fifteen of twenty grains; the result was, complete disappearance of the physical signs and symptoms.

Sacharjin considers that the clinical aspect of these cases sufficiently distinguishes them from phthisis, while their syphilitic nature is proved by the effects of treatment. They do not aid the anatomical question. He hopes others will publish their own experiences, so as to enable us to judge of the relative frequency of such cases. Dr. Flöroff has informed him of a case which he has observed with identical characters, which recovered under iodide of potassium, and is still healthy (four years afterwards). He thinks the following peculiarities distinguish syphilitic pneumonia from ordinary phthisis:—

1. The specific history.

2. The patient's strong constitution. It is more probable that feeble subjects, with a tendency to phthisis, acquire that early, than that they live to acquire the later syphilitic affections, of which syphilitic pneumonia is certainly one.

3. The symptoms and physical organs.

4. The absence of hæmoptysis, cough, sputa, and râles.

5. No fever.

6. The different effect of mercury or iodide of potassium. In reference to this, it is mentioned that syphilitic pneumonia presents the same peculiarity as the other later syphilitic affections; it suffices to employ a very moderate quantity of mercury to cure the morbid appearances; the later syphilitic affections appear to require much less mercury than the earlier ones. It is possible that such cases may be at times complicated with inflammatory disturbances of the lungs or pleuræ, in which cases their typical aspect would be altered, and no conclusions for diagnosis, prognosis, or treatment, based upon lung-syphilis, would hold good. Further observations must show whether simple uncomplicated syphilitic lung-affection, curable by mercury or iodide of potassium, can assume a different appearance from the above.—*London Med. Record*, Feb. 15, 1878.

The External Use of Tincture of Belladonna in Night-Sweating.

Mr. NAIRNE writes, in the *British Medical Journal* of February 2, that for some little time past he has employed the common pharmacopœial tincture of belladonna for sponging the body in cases of phthisical and excessive sweating, and invariably with marked benefit. So far as his experience goes, he has found it very much better than anything else ; if applied before a sweating comes on, it prevents it; if during the sweating, it almost immediately controls it. Two teaspoonfuls of the tincture mixed with an equal quantity of whiskey are quite sufficient (applied with the hand), to cover the whole body and produce the desired effect.—*Lond. Med. Record*, Feb. 15, 1878.

Abnormalities of the Spine, simulating Chest-Disease.

In the *Berliner Klinische Wochenschrift*, December 24, Dr. P. HEYMANN, of Vienna, describes two cases of spinal abnormality, simulating disorders of the cervical and upper thoracic viscera.

The first case is that of a well-made robust girl, aged 16. She complained of periodic attacks of dyspnœa, which usually occurred a few days after catching an ordinary cold, and gradually gave way again, after three to five days, on the setting in of an abundant thickish expectoration. The difficulty of breathing was greatest in the recumbent posture, and at night, and was accompanied by a feeling of obstruction of the throat, without, however, constriction and oppression of the chest, and by deep reddening and suffusion of the face. Cough and difficulty of swallowing were entirely absent. Examination with the laryngoscope revealed a rounded, hard, bony, and immovable prominence, projecting from the posterior pharyngeal wall, and occupying two-thirds of the pharynx. On moving the head forward or backward, this projection was slightly altered in form. The epiglottis appeared smoothed and flattened, and fitting to the anterior surface of the prominence. On examination from behind, the spinous process of the fourth cervical vertebra was indistinctly felt, and projected rather too much upwards, and above it was felt a considerable gap, bounded above by the spinous process of the axis. On bending the head backwards, the spinous process of the fourth vertebra disappeared, but became plainly prominent again on inclining the head forward, and then the gap was occupied by a tense band, apparently stretching between the spinous processes of the second and fourth cervical vertebræ. On inclining the head laterally, only one side appeared thus stretched. The head was readily reclined, but there was some difficulty of inclination. It appeared, therefore, that the arch of the third cervical vertebra was deficient, hence the body of the vertebra was thrown forward, causing a tilting backward of the spine, and the prominence described; while posteriorly the spinal canal was for the time obliterated. On the occurrence of a throat-catarrh, the mucous membrane covering this projection swelled, and pressed against the epiglottis, thus causing the dyspnœa, which was relieved by stretching the neck upwards and forwards, and so reducing the obstructing prominence. This defect of the third cervical arch was evidently congenital, the symptoms described having existed from earliest childhood. In the anatomical collection at Vienna there exist several specimens of similar abnormalities—for example, an atlas with the entire arch between the articular processes absent; complete fissure of the atlas; anchyloses between two or more cervical vertebræ, etc.

The second case was that of a gentleman aged 50, who for the last two years had suffered from difficulty of swallowing, amounting at times to utter impossibility; vomiting was never present. Examination with œsophageal bougies showed the existence of a variable obstruction below the cricoid cartilage, so that at one time the largest bougie could be introduced, while at another even the finest could not pass. When the obstruction was once overcome, all sizes of bougies were readily passed down to the stomach.

This coincided with the patient's statement that at times he could not swallow at all; but, if the food had once overcome the obstacle situated high up in the gullet, it readily passed onwards. We know that the normal relation of the cricoid cartilage to the spinal column is such that a certain amount of movement of the head is necessary when introducing the œsophageal sound.

In the patient the introduction of the bougie was yet much more dependent on the position of the head. This led to the conclusion that the obstruction to deglutition consisted of a lordosis (curvature with the convexity forward) of the cervical vertebræ. This was confirmed on undressing the patient. It was then found that there existed skoliosis (curvature with the convexity backward) of the upper dorsal and of the lumbar vertebræ, compensated by skoliosis and slight lordosis of the lower dorsal vertebræ, and lordosis of the lower cervical vertebræ, which occasioned the obstruction to deglutition. A pasteboard cravat of about a hand's breadth was accordingly so adapted that, by stretching the neck upwards, the curvature was almost neutralized, enabling the patient to swallow without difficulty.—*Lond. Med. Record*, Feb. 15, 1878.

The Immigration of Corpuscles in the Lung.

A question in pulmonary hemorrhage of considerable scientific interest and direct practical bearing is raised by some observations published by Professor NOTHNAGEL in Virchow's *Archiv*. They relate to the passage of cells from the alveoli of the lung into the interstitial tissue. When extensive hemorrhage occurs into the trachea of a rabbit, such as takes place when the trachea and carotids are divided simultaneously, the lungs are found gorged with blood. The bronchial tubes are full, and the alveolar tissue is of a dark brown-red colour.

The blood is not equally distributed; there is always most in the vicinity of the hilus. On microscopical examination of the hardened lung, it was found that the blood was mainly in the bronchial tubes and air-cells, which were most of them stuffed with corpuscles, a few being free. But there was also a large amount of blood in the interstitial tissue of the lung, between the alveoli, and even in the interlobular septa. In places this accumulation was so dense as to mask the normal structure of the lung. Although some of the interalveolar septa contained no corpuscles, the nodal points of the septa invariably presented accumulations. In these spots the connective-tissue framework is normally more highly developed. The appearance of the lung suggested an interstitial hemorrhage, with rupture, and escape of the blood into the air-cells. Indeed, so considerable was the interstitial accumulation that it seemed possible that the process had actually been of that character—that the convulsions which preceded death might have led to interstitial hemorrhage. Some observations were therefore made on rabbits killed by dividing the carotids only, the trachea being left intact. No interstitial accumulation could, however, be discovered, and, of course, there was no blood in the air-cells. Hence it seemed clear that the blood had passed into the interstitial tissue from within the alveoli.

A remarkable feature of the phenomenon was the rapidity with which the passage occurred. The anæmic convulsions came on in three-quarters of a minute after the severance of the carotids, and ceased in a minute and a half. Immediately afterwards the thorax was opened, and the lungs removed and thrown into absolute alcohol. The whole period occupied was not more than five minutes. Whatever be the mechanism, all movement of cells or fluids must cease as soon as the alcohol acts upon the tissues.

That particles passed with readiness from the air-cells into the interstitial tissue had been previously shown by Ins in his experiments to ascertain the mechanism by which grinders' phthisis is produced. He found that cinnabar dust, introduced into the air-passages, could be discovered within the nodal points of the interalveolar septa in from six to twelve hours after its introduction, and that some granules had passed into the bronchial glands.

The path which the blood-corpuscles traverse in their migration could not be discovered. But we know that channels exist capable of affording ready ingress for solid particles from the air-cells into the interstitial tissue. Wywodzoff, Klein, and others have shown that the commencement of the lymphatic channels are in immediate communication with the alveolar and bronchial spaces. Nothnagel's observations show that these openings must be extremely numerous to permit the rapid passage of so many corpuscles into the interstitial tissue. He suggests that it is possible that the dilatation of the air-cells by the blood may dilate the stomata which exist in their walls; since in every case the chief interstitial accumulation took place where the air-cells were the most distended with blood.

The immediate application of these observations to the elucidation of many processes of disease will be sufficiently obvious. The light similar facts throw on the occurrence of interstitial lung changes, as the result of inhalation of fine particles of stone, etc., was pointed out by Ins. Another important consideration, which flows more immediately from Nothnagel's observations, is the question of the absorption of the exudation in croupous pneumonia. It is probable that in the process of the resolution of pneumonia, only a small part of the exuded material which fills the air-cells is expectorated. A greater quantity must be absorbed. The common assumption is that the contents of the alveoli, white and red corpuscles, and fibrin, undergo fatty degeneration, and that the products of this degeneration are absorbed. Nothnagel suggests that the cells may find their

way back into the lung vessels without undergoing degeneration. He admits,
however, that the interference with the circulation in the inflamed lung may constitute a difficulty in the acceptance of this view, and we think that the facts of
the *post-mortem* room are opposed to it. All pathological evidence goes to
show that destruction by degeneration of the exudation precedes its removal from
the air-cells, by whatever process that is effected. Cordua, in his investigation
into the method by which extravasated blood was removed from the tissues, was
able to demonstrate its return into the vessels only so long as it remained in a
fluid state.

The destination of blood effused into the air-cells is a very important element
in the pathology of the origin of phthisis from hæmoptysis. It must be confessed, however, that these observations do not increase our knowledge of the
pathological processes which underlie such a condition; indeed they diminish
rather than increase its probability. Nothnagel, in some early but unpublished
observations, had failed entirely to produce lung changes by injecting blood into
the air-passages of the lungs of the rabbit. No caseous pneumonia was found
either days or weeks after the injection; neither was there any blood in the
minute bronchial ramifications, in spite of the fact that rabbits neither cough nor
expectorate. These observations entirely agree with the negative results of
Peil and Lipmann. The experiments of Sommerbrodt were less conclusive.
He believed that under some conditions hemorrhage into the lungs would cause
a catarrhal pneumonia and phthisis. All, however, agreed that the contents of
the bronchi and air-cells were very small in quantity compared with the amount
of blood they must have contained, and the explanation of this is completely
afforded by the observations of Nothnagel. Admitting the fact that hæmoptysis
may, in man, sometimes lead to phthisis, these observations—if we may transfer
them to the human lung—show very clearly why such a consequence so seldom
follows the hemorrhagic infiltration into the air-cells which must very often take
place.—*Lancet*, Jan. 26, 1878.

Aneurism of the Pulmonary Artery.

Dr. BUCHWALD (*Deutsche Med. Wochenschrift*, January 5, 1878) relates a
case of this rare condition met with in the clinic of Professor Biermer, of Breslau.
The patient, a maid-servant, aged 21, had been always healthy until the last
year, during which she had suffered from slight cough, becoming worse in the
winter; pain in the left side of the chest, increasing feebleness and cough, expectoration of purulent matter, and on one occasion of blood; night-sweats.

She was admitted into hospital on September 5, 1875. She was a thin, middle-sized blonde; the skin and mucous membranes were pale, with circumscribed
circular red patches on the cheeks, such as one sees in phthisical subjects. Here
and there on the skin were punctiform hemorrhages. The thorax was small,
long, with wide intercostal spaces; the two sides were unequal, the left side
being very prominent opposite the junction of the ribs with the cartilages from
the second to the sixth; the patient said this had been so from her childhood.
The heart's apex-beat could be seen extending over a centimetre in the fifth left
interspace, internal to the nipple; but in the second left interspace was another
pulsating area, three centimetres in breadth. This impulse, which was more of
an undulation than a short pulsation, began at the sternal border, and extended
to the left; to the right it could not be felt. During deep inspiration the phe-
nemenou disappeared, but during ordinary breathing it was slight, and most
marked of all when breathing was arrested. The pulsation could be felt from
the second to the fifth interspaces, but was less visible, and free from thrill, in
the fourth and fifth. Thrill began in the third interspace, reached its maximum

in the second, and was lost in the first. It accompanied the systole, but could be
followed in the diastole; with a deep inspiration it became indistinct; superficial
breathing made it feebler; expiration strengthened both thrill and pulsation.
Percussion showed extension of the heart's dulness to the right, and towards the
second pulsating spot; there was dulness in the first interspace on the inner side
of the parasternal line. In the second interspace the dulness commenced four
centimetres outside the sternum, and extended downwards and outwards towards
the axilla in a convex line to the position of the apex-beat. To the right, the
dulness was followed over the sternum to 1.5 centimetres in the fourth interspace.
The upper part of the sternum was not dull; below, the heart's dulness was lost
in that of the liver. The lungs encroached upon the heart, so as to push the
limits of cardiac dulness towards the middle line. At the apex there was a slight
systolic murmur, which completely disappeared to the right; but upwards, and
especially towards the second pulsating spot, it increased, and attained its maximum in the second interspace; here, indeed, systolic and diastolic periods could
not be distinguished, only the strong intensifying of the sharp whistling murmur
made the systole recognizable. In the supraclavicular and infraclavicular fossæ,
the sharp murmur could be heard above the feeble-breath sounds. In the left
carotid, sounds were only accompanied by the strong murmur from the second
interspace; in the right carotid, a feeble systolic blowing murmur was alone audible. The last was also to be heard in the aorta; the second sound was clear, not
accentuated. In inspiration the murmur was everywhere feebler, but did not
disappear on the deepest effort. Hæmic murmurs were heard in the veins. The
pulses were equal, full, regular, of low tension; rate from 92 to 128. In the
lungs there was dulness in the left infraspinous and infraclavicular fossæ, without
any infiltrated spot being detectable by auscultation; the latter showed only diffuse catarrh, which existed also in the right lung. Respiration was of the inspiratory type; the sputa were scanty, muco-purulent, only once blood-stained. The
spleen-dulness was increased. The urine varied in quantity from 80 to 2000
centimetres per diem, of corresponding specific gravity; no albumen. In the
progress of the case albumen and casts appeared in the urine, and œdema began
and gradually extended; some weeks afterwards she had a rigor, with a rise of
temperature, which before had been normal. The pulmonary symptoms declined.
In the heart, systolic and diastolic murmurs became audible in the aortic area.
Nearly two months afterwards a small abscess formed in the left groin, which
was opened. Signs of pericarditis, with effusion, supervened. The fundus of
the eye was normal; the œdema was extreme; she had great catarrh of the
lungs; the temperature was generally low. A few days later, petechiæ appeared
in the skin, and collapse and death followed.

The *post-mortem* examination showed pericardial effusion; enlargement of
the heart, affecting chiefly the left side; an aneurism of the pulmonary artery,
of the size of a hen's egg, communicating with the aorta by the persistence of
the ductus arteriosus; polypoid excrescences on the wall of the duct and the
pulmonary artery and aorta, also on the valves of the aortic, pulmonic, mitral,
and tricuspid openings; brown induration of the lungs, with a periarterial abscess
and infarct in the right lung; enlargement of the spleen; acute nephritis; hemorrhage into the white substance of the anterior lobes of the brain, opening into the
left lateral ventricle.—*London Med. Record*, Feb. 15, 1878.

A Case of Acute Hemorrhage of the Pancreas.

Dr. HILTY describes (*Correspondenzblatt für Schweizer Aerzte*, Nov. 15,
1877) the case of a mechanic, aged 30, tall, stout, and muscular, and having the
appearance of a drunkard. One evening he drank a large quantity of beer; in

spite of this he passed a good night; but the following morning he was suddenly seized with a painful tension of the abdomen, which gradually increased, and general *malaise*. On admission to the hospital his extremities were cold, and his forehead covered with a cold sweat. He had an anxious expression, and was very restless; the sensorial functions were undisturbed; the pulse was small and quick, scarcely perceptible; the region of cardiac dulness was increased, but there was no murmur; respiration was quick and difficult; the lungs were normal. The upper part of the abdomen was distended and painful, especially on pressure. The pain and the obesity of the patient did not allow any peritoneal effusion to be discovered. He had had one evacuation in the morning; there was no vomiting, but constant nausea. The diagnosis was uncertain, but it was thought to be a case of acute gastritis, or of poisoning; poultices and tepid injections and wet wrapping were prescribed. Afterwards the stomach-pump was used; and a small quantity of yellowish watery fluid, giving an acid reaction, was removed. An emetic gave some relief. The night was quieter. Next day there was a spontaneous evacuation, but the general symptoms persisted, the pulse being thready, the extremities cold, and the temperature normal. As the patient writhed in bed, it was thought he had intestinal perforation. Opium was prescribed, and ice to the abdomen. There was a slight amelioration, but the symptoms returned, and the patient died delirious at 9 P. M.

At the necropsy, the epiploon and mesentery were found loaded with fat; there was no exudation into the abdomen, nor any trace of peritonitis. The stomach was large; the intestines, especially the ascending and transverse colon, were much distended. The diaphragm was pushed up as high as the fourth rib. In the connective tissue surrounding the pancreas, there was an abundant sanguineous infiltration. The organ itself was double its normal size, firm in consistence, and of a dark violet colour. On section, the lobules were seen to be of a dark colour, and from the interlobular connective tissue a large quantity of bloody serum escaped. In the head of the gland especially there were numerous little extravasations of blood, varying in size from a millet-seed to a cherry-stone. In fact, the whole gland, acini and connective tissue, was infiltrated. Wirsung's duct was not dilated, but the vein running along the lower edge of the pancreas was distended with clots. The spleen and the kidneys were congested; the mucous membrane of the throat was somewhat thickened, and of a grayish colour. At the lower end of the œsophagus, and in the cardia, were some ecchymoses and superficial erosions. The liver was large and fatty. The heart was covered with fat, and its muscular tissue was soft and slightly degenerated. The brain was congested, and the fluid in the ventricles was cloudy.

This case is analogous to one described by Friedreich under the name of acute hemorrhage of the pancreas. Zenker considers that the morbid appearances were not sufficient to account for death, which he assigns to the sudden and violent compression of the solar plexus by the fluid effused.—*London Med. Record*, Feb. 15, 1878.

—

Glycerine in Diabetes.

Prof. BOUCHARDAT observes (*Bulletin de Thérapeutique*, December 15) that more than twenty years since he employed this substance, but the results which he obtained from it were so uncertain and contradictory that he almost ceased to prescribe it. His attention having been recalled to it by several recent publications, he recommenced his trials with it, and with results not very dissimilar from those formerly obtained. In subjects strongly attacked with the disease it seems to do harm rather than good if their regimen be not also changed. In certain cases it acts more favourably, viz., if the quantity of glucose eliminated in the

twenty-four hours is only small, when it aids the disappearance of the last traces ;
but it may be doubted whether this is or is not a mere coincidence. In emaciated
diabetics, or those suffering from habitual constipation, useful effects have followed
its administration. He usually gives it in moderate doses, from a teaspoonful to
two tablespoonfuls, in tea, coffee, white wine, or water. Given in larger doses
the glycerine is only partially absorbed, or a portion passes off in the urine. In
glycosuric constipation, two tablespoonfuls with one of salt as an enema are often
useful ; and Prof. Bouchardat frequently orders chocolate in which the sugar is
replaced by glycerine.—*Med. Times and Gaz.*, Feb. 9, 1878.

Treatment of Acne Rosacea.

In the *Wien. Med. Wochenschrift* for January 15, Prof. VON HEBRA figures
two instruments which he has of late found very useful in the treatment of obstinate acne. One of these is a strong lancet-formed needle, cutting on both sides,
and furnished with a stop in order to prevent its penetrating too deeply. With
this he makes numerous perpendicular punctures (with a rapidity resembling that
of a sewing-machine) for the purpose of destroying the capillary vessels which
give rise to the red stripes or sinuous lines visible to the naked eye—proceeding
from below upwards, in order that the bleeding may not obscure the progress of
the operation. This is easily arrested by compressed wadding. The after-treatment consists in re-application of wadding if the surface remains dry, and in the
use of simple ointments when there is suppuration. After the healing, if the
destruction of the distended capillaries is not complete, the puncturing must be
again performed. The professor refers to six obstinate cases of acne in which he
has found the process quite successful. The other instrument is a modification of
Volkmann's "scraper," in the form of a small ear-shaped spoon with sharp
edges (having lateral prolongations when intended for the deeper-seated products), fixed on a strong short stem with a long handle. This is used for the
destruction of new formations in the skin, as in lupus, epithelioma, etc., or for
the removal of infiltrations, as in sycosis and acne, and it must be continued to
be employed until the whole of the diseased product is removed. The scraping
is of no avail in superficial nævoid or acne rosacea, as, owing to the resistance of
the cutis, only the epidermis instead of the diseased product comes away. Still,
repeated scraping, with its attendant superficial suppuration, is followed by a
diminution of the redness of the face, both in acne rosacea and nævoid—probably
on account of the obliteration of the minute vessels of the cutis. The instruments may be had at Leiter's, Vienna.—*Med. Times and Gaz.*, Feb. 16, 1878.

Two Cases of Psoriasis: the one treated by Prolonged Daily Immersions, the other by Chrysophanic Acid.

Mr. BALMANNO SQUIRE exhibited these cases at a late meeting of the Clinical
Society of London (*Med. Times and Gaz.*, Feb. 16, 1878). The one was that
of a gentleman aged thirty-two, who had been extensively affected with psoriasis
for nine years. He was kept under treatment by prolonged daily immersion in
tepid water for exactly six weeks, during which time he submitted on the average to five hours' daily immersion. The temperature most readily borne by the
patient during a prolonged immersion was about 90° Fahr. By the end of six
weeks, without other treatment of any kind, the patient had lost by far the
greater part of his eruption, which presented now only a fiftieth, or at the most a
thirtieth, of its original area, and had also got rid of the nocturnal itching which
accompanied it. He was now treated with phosphorus "perles" and chrysophanic acid ointment; and in ten days' time presented only such insignificant

traces of the disease that he decided to return home to his duties. Prolonged daily immersion in tepid water has for very many years been employed in the treatment of skin diseases at Leukerbad in Switzerland, and at Baden near Vienna; but this case would seem to show that the less irksome ordeal of spending some hours daily in the bath could suffice to produce fairly good results. The other case of psoriasis was that of a gentleman aged thirty-four, who had been affected with the disease for twelve years. The eruption was chiefly massed over the belly and the loins. He was ordered the use of chrysophanic acid ointment, of a strength of twelve grains of the acid to the ounce of lard; and he was furthermore directed to take two phosphorus "perles" (containing each one-thirtieth of a grain of phosphorus dissolved in oil) three times a day. On the fourteenth day of treatment the patient conceived an impression that the phosphorus was impairing his mental energy, and accordingly he was permitted to discontinue taking the perles. By this time, also, the erythema excited by the chrysophanic acid had entirely subsided. The patient was therefore ordered to resume the use of chrysophanic acid ointment, now made stronger than before, namely, a drachm of the acid to the ounce of lard. In three days' time—that is to say, on the seventeenth day of treatment—all trace of the eruption on his body had completely disappeared, the chrysophanic acid ointment having again excited some erythema. On the twenty-fourth day of treatment the disease still existed on the arms and legs, local treatment with the chrysophanic acid ointment having been still persevered with to the limbs, although, since the seventeenth day of treatment, no further applications had been made to the body, inasmuch as every sign of the disease had gone from the trunk. The patient still exhibited traces of the disease on the limbs.

Dr. TILBURY FOX said that the case cured by immersion confirmed what was already known on that subject, but in private practice the method was hardly applicable. Few could afford the time necessary. The case recorded was one of indolent and chronic psoriasis, and the treatment succeeded, but generally failed when fresh crops were coming out. The other was similar in character, and more than one remedy would suit such cases. For instance, mercurial and carbolic acid ointments would do, so would alkaline baths, and so on. The earlier and more acute stages were more difficult to treat, and here a specific could hardly be sought for. For instance, one form was apt to occur in married women from over-suckling; others, again, in gouty subjects, where totally different lines of treatment were demanded. Again, there was the lupioid form, tending to occur in children, where cod-liver oil suited best; and still again, the malady was apt to occur among over-wrought city men, where the digestion was the chief thing to be looked to. It was only in the essentially chronic form that chrysophanic acid could be said to do good, but it stained both the skin and the clothes, and patients did not like it.

Mr. HUTCHINSON said patients should be warned of the effects of the acid, for often severe erythema followed. What was the real meaning of the word "cure" in psoriasis? It ought to mean relief permanently, or else for a period of years. It was easy to get rid of the scaly symptoms for a period, but what of a longer time? Hebra used bathing, but not the bath referred to; rather a big one was employed, into which half a dozen patients might enter, and scrub each other with coal-tar soap for six hours or so at a time. Cures, as he called them, followed. He thought arsenic and tar, both externally and internally, did much good.

Dr. R. LIVEING could confirm what had been said as to the objections to chrysophanic acid—patients would hardly put up with it. He himself had long used it for ringworm, but the patients complained of the dirty mahogany colour it gave to their hair. He had long used baths with soft soap and flannel, and on this method half an hour a day sometimes sufficed for a cure. Acute eases constituted the real difficulty.

Dr. CROCKER had used chrysophanic acid for ringworm, but was forced to abandon it. The hair turned purplish, and the erythema following its use tended to spread, with desquamation of the cuticle, and the eyes often became swollen and painful ; moreover, the treatment was not very successful. The system of bathing might be made much simpler. In one very bad case a cure was effected by an alkaline bath two or three times a week, and the use of diuretics. In the early stages the use of chrysophanic acid might aggravate the disease.

Dr. WHIPHAM considered that the acid should be used with caution. In one girl who had suffered from psoriasis for five years the acid was applied to the eruption only, yet the face swelled up as in erysipelas. In a more recent case in the person of a flour miller, where the disease chiefly prevailed where there was rubbing, on the arm and legs, the ointment caused pustules and boils on the skin round about.

Mr. B. SQUIRE, in reply, said he considered the balance was decidedly in favour of chrysophanic acid. He could hardly think it more easy to cure a chronic than an acute case, though the latter yielded better to internal remedies. He did not like the use of arsenic, but preferred external treatment. The acid, no doubt, required careful handling ; but other things did the same. The hair only became discoloured after the use of soap and water, and the dye could readily be removed by means of benzole.

Surgery.

Anterior Choroiditis.

In an inaugural thesis (Paris, 1877), M. COURSSERANT arrives at the follow-ing conclusions : 1. The anterior segment only of the choroid can be attacked by all the pathological processes which are observed in other parts of the membrane. 2. Anterior choroiditis may, under the different forms which it takes, be some-times sudden, sometimes slow, in its progress, without immediate alteration of the centre of the eye ; in spite of the situation of the anatomical lesions, all degrees of diminution of the visual faculty are observed. 3. Primary lesions of the vas-cular system, deficient nutrition of this region, the irritation to which it is exposed, are the principal causes of the disease. 4. The physician should always be re-served in his prognosis.

The treatment which M. Coursserant recommends consists of antiphlogistic measures, bleeding, rest of the apparatus of accommodation, to be obtained by atropia, and tonics in the case of weak subjects. He rejects altogether the action of syphilis, which is often regarded as the cause of choroiditis.—*London Med. Record*, Feb. 15, 1878.

Diseases of the Lachrymal Passages.

In a communication made to the Société de Biologie in November, 1876 (*Annales d'Oculistique*, July–August, 1877), Dr. BADAL has expressed the opinion that errors of refraction, and especially hypermetropia, play a prominent part in the development of diseases of the lachrymal passages ; and he now thinks that he has collected and tabulated facts which, although insufficient to furnish reliable statistics, nevertheless tend to show the intimate relationship, as to cause and effect, which exists between the two conditions. His opinion is based upon the observation of one hundred and sixty-five cases of lachrymal disorder, in eighty-seven of which, or about 53 per cent., there existed some anomaly of refraction or of accommodation, without any other disease of the eyeball or of its appendages. Thus, hypermetropia was equal in the two eyes in 40 per cent. ; presbyopia in 5 per cent. ; anisometropia, difference of refraction, in 4 per cent. ; astigmatism in 2 per cent. ; myopia, equal in the two eyes, in 2 per cent.

Dr. Badal finds one case of lachrymal disorder in every five cases of hypermetropia, but only one in every twenty cases of myopia ; in nearly every instance, however, these were complicated with astigmatism, or with unequal refraction in the two eyes. A certain number of lachrymal disorders are to be met with in eyes which are emmetropic ; these, according to Dr. Badal, are due to fatigue of the ciliary muscles, and this is not surprising when we bear in mind the congestion of the surrounding tissues which often results from prolonged exercise of accommodation : it is to be noted, moreover, that in cases of myopia, in which accommodation is not actively employed, diseases of the lachrymal passages are very rarely met with. And if it be asked how it happens that the connection between these disorders as cause and effect has so long escaped observation, Dr. Badal would reply that optometry is at the present time more restricted than the use of the ophthalmoscope ; that the hypermetropia in these cases is feeble in degree, and is not to be made manifest without careful investigation ; and, lastly, that patients who suffer from lachrymal disorders very rarely complain of their eyesight ; and surgeons have given their attention to those symptoms which are tangible and self-evident, and which have masked the defective function which was in reality the cause of all the mischief. In short, Dr. Badal considers that in more than half his cases the arrest of the free passage of the tears, and the consequent accidents of inflammation and structural changes within the ducts, have taken their origin in the congestion of the conjunctiva, which is itself the result of overwork imposed upon the ciliary muscle by some error in refraction.— *London Med. Record*, Feb. 15, 1878.

The Influence of the Uterus in Eye-diseases.

At a late meeting of the Obstetrical Society of Dublin (*British Med. Journal*, Feb. 23, 1878) Mr. H. R. SWANZY read a paper on this subject. He said that most eye-diseases were dependent on some distant organs, such as the heart, kidneys, spleen, and the uterus. Up to the present, very little was known concerning the relationship existing between the eyes and the uterus. He thought that this was due chiefly to the fact of few ophthalmologists being experienced gynæcologists, and *vice versâ*. The first disease which Mr. Swanzy brought under notice as having its primary cause in the uterus was iritis, occurring in young girls from about the eleventh to the seventeenth year of age—*i. e.*, within a period varying from two to three years prior to the establishment of menstruation up to two or three years after they commenced to menstruate. Mr. Swanzy was unable positively to connect this disease of the eye with the uterus, but was inclined to believe the uterus the starting-point of the iritis, for three reasons. 1. Iritis was extremely rare at such an early time of life, unless dependent on congenital syphilis, or secondary to corneal diseases. 2. He had never seen a similar case in the male. 3. When the disease was found to occur with a certain frequency at a time of life when the uterus was approaching maturity or had lately reached it, and when all other causes were excluded, the inference was fair that the uterus had given rise to the iritis. The form of iritis in all these cases was similai ; theie was little oi no pain, and but little vasculai injection of the eye oi photophobia. The tieatment Mr. Swanzy used in these cases was chiefly local duiing the acute stages of the inflammation; and, when the inflammation had subsided, he gave iion. Inflammation of the optic neive and ietina might depend on distuibances of menstiuation. In 1873, Mr. Swanzy had undei his caie a giil aged 10 suffeiing fiom nemro-ietinitis, whose menstiuation was spaise and painful, and in whom the eye affection always became aggiavated at the monthly peiiods. Cases of optic neuiitis had been seen wheie menstiual distuibances had gone befoie. Von Giäfe iecognized the existence of such a connection. Mooien had seen cases of neuio-ietinitis aftei suppiession of menstiuation, and he was of opinion that retroflexions of the uteius and ovaiian tumouis might give iise to the same affection. Atiophy of the optic neive had been noted iepeatedly by Pagen-stechei as occuiiing in women who had suffeied fiom seveie menstiual distuib-ances, which he iegaided as the cause of the eye-disease. Retinal apoplexies weie sometimes the consequences of cessation or suppiession of the menses. Kopiophia hysteiica had till lately been classed among eye-diseases, but it was now known to be nothing moie than a symptom of an uteiine disease. It was not a common . disease ; and it was only quite lately that it had been fully desciibed by Piofessoi Föistei in his aiticle in von Giäfe and Sämisch's new *Handbook of Ophthalmology;* and the pathological conditions of the uteiine appaiatus invaiiably found accom-panying it by Piofessoi Fieund of Bieslau weie mentioned by him. Di. Fieund had found, by means of a laige numbei of *post-mortem* examinations of women who had complained of these eye-symptoms, that they weie unifoimly affected with uteiine disease, which he claims to have been the fiist to have iecognized.

—

Duplication of the Left Half of the Lower Jaw.

In a disseitation (Beilin, 1877) abstiacted in the *Centralblatt für die Medicin. Wissenschaften* foi Januaiy 5, Di. O. ISRAEL desciibes a case of duplication of the lowei jaw in a new-boin child, in whom the tiagus of the left eai was also double. Theie was a piojection as laige as a goose's egg in the lowei maxillaiy iegion, causing consideiable disfiguiement. The tumoui, which was movable, consisted of a poition of lowei jaw, containing five embiyonic teeth and a dis-tinct condyle, a iudimentaiy mouth, with indications of lips and tongue, and a confused mass of salivaiy gland-tissue, mixed with musculai and connective tis-sue, foiming in one pait a ietention-cyst, while the secietion fiom the othei paits of the gland-tissue escaped by a duct opening exteinally.

Was this a malfoimation, or a paitially developed second foetus ? Di. Isiael decides in favoui of the lattei.—*London Med. Recoid,* Feb. 15, 1878.

—

On Wounds of the Laiynx and theii Treatment, especially the Value of a Piophylactic Tiacheotomy.

In an elaboiate and leained aiticle on this subject (*Archiv für Klin. Chir.,* Bd. xxi., Heft. 1, 2, 3, pp. 217, 391, 1877) WITTE piesents the following con-clusions :—

1. That laceiation of the laiynx and tiachea is veiy iaie—in battle only five in ten thousand wounds of all classes ; in piivate piactice they aie moie fie-quent ; in the foimei class almost exclusively by fire-aims ; in the lattei by cut-ting instruments.

2. The diagnosis is usually easy ; a pathognomonic symptom of a penetiating wound of the aii-passages is the escape of aii thiough the opening.

3. The piogiess is always slow ; in extensive laceiations iepaii is not to be expected undei thiity to foity days ; not unfiequently alteiations in the voice,

stenosis of the larynx (very seldom of the trachea), and aerial fistula are ultimate results.

4. The prognosis in incised wounds of the larynx and trachea, with extensive laceration of the soft parts, is much better than in those with but slight laceration, and in punctured wounds. Gunshot wounds of the larynx appear to allow of a better prognosis than those of the trachea, but in both instances more than one-half of all cases are cured.

5. Severe concussions, contusions with marked disturbance of the voice and respiration, and fractures of the cartilages, are indications for a prophylactic tracheotomy.

6. It is likewise indicated where foreign bodies are lodged in the larynx or trachea.

7. Gunshot wounds of the larynx and trachea together, punctured wounds in which the laceration of the mucous membrane is probable, incised wounds, with slight involvement of the soft parts, but marked injury to the cartilages, all render the performance of a tracheotomy necessary.

8. In incised wounds, with free division of the soft parts, and simple lacerations of the trachea, the operation may be delayed, provided the case can be carefully watched, and it is not necessary to transport it further.

9. Incised wounds of hyo-thyroid membrane may be sewed up after a tracheotomy has been done.

10. In incised wounds of the upper part of the thyroid cartilage, after a tracheotomy, sutures may be used through the cartilage.

11. Gunshot wounds of the parts in the neighbourhood of the larynx, with marked destruction of the tissue, indicate a prophylactic tracheotomy :—

(a) When interference with either speech or respiration begins to manifest itself.

(b) When secondary hemorrhage is feared, and the blood can find its way into the air-passages.

(c) When the projectile lies in the vicinity of the larynx, and it is deemed undesirable to remove it.

12. A high tracheotomy is always to be preferred ; then section of the cricoid cartilage ; if necessary, a low tracheotomy can be done. The earlier the operation is performed the less will be the difficulty, and the better the prognosis.

13. When circumstances permit, the operation is to be performed under chloroform.

14. Catheterization of the larynx, as well as compression and scarification, is to be practised in œdema of the glottis.

15. For a time after the operation, Trendelenberg's tampon canula is to be worn, and two at least should be furnished in the armamentarium of every sanitary department and field-hospital.—*New York Med. Journal*, Feb. 1878.

Curious Simulation of Fracture of the Larynx.

The *Gazette Hebdomadaire*, February 8, quotes a curious case related by Dr. Mordillon in the *Bordeaux Medical*. A little girl, while knitting, fell down in the street, and was found to have received a slight contused wound in the thyroid region, which was accompanied by much pain and a little swelling. A half of one of the needles which she was using had also disappeared. As examination did not reveal the presence of a foreign body, no attempt at its extraction was made. A month later the child was brought to Dr. Mordillon, who found a depression in the thyroid cartilage running from its superior angle downwards, and from left to right towards the junction with the cricoid. This depression seemed to result from the imbrication of two lateral plates of the cartilage, and gave the same sensation as when the bones of the fœtal cranium are riding over each other during delivery. Crepitation was also felt, and pressure caused pain and suffocation. The presence of no foreign body could be detected. Respiration was normal, but there was a slight alteration in the voice. The lateral movements of the neck were natural and without pain, and there was no dysphagia. The diagnosis was oblique fracture of the thyroid, with, perhaps, the retention of the needle in the neck. At another visit, in about three weeks' time, it was found that an abscess was formed, and on this being opened a knitting-needle nine centimetres long was discharged, and all signs of fracture disappeared. All the signs of this accident were closely simulated ; and it is remarkable that so long a foreign body could have remained for such a time without exciting any functional disturbance of the numerous vessels and nerves of the neck.—*Med. Times and Gaz.*, Feb. 16, 1878.

Gangrene of the Testis.

In surgical literature, some few cases are to be met with of spontaneous gangrene and sloughing of the testis, suddenly occurring in a previously healthy subject. Of somewhat more frequent occurrence are instances of spontaneous and severe orchitis, terminating in extreme atrophy. With the view of throwing some light on the causation of these singular morbid conditions, Professor VOLK-MANN has recently reported (*Berliner Klinische Wöchenschrift*, No. 53, 1877) a case of acute hemorrhagic infarction of the testis, terminating in spontaneous gangrene. In this interesting case there are very many circumstances favouring the view of an embolic process, although there is an absence of sure and positive evidence on this point.

A youth, aged 15 years, whose health had previously been very good, and whose testicles had never been affected from injury or disease, was suddenly attacked on July 5 with severe pain in the abdomen, and diarrhœa and vomiting. On the following morning there was less abdominal pain, but much tenderness in the left testicle, together with considerable swelling of the corresponding half of the scrotum. At this time there was much fever, with thirst and headache. On July 8, the swelling and pain in the scrotum having considerably increased during the interval, the patient came for the first time under the notice of the author. He was then prostrate, and in a state of collapse, and the facial expression indicated acute peritonitis. The anterior abdominal wall, however, was lax, and free from tenderness, even on firm manual pressure. There was but moderate elevation of the temperature, the pulse was 100, and the respiratory and circulatory organs were in a normal condition. There was hard inflammatory œdema of the whole scrotum, and the surface of the left half was deeply congested, extremely tender, and very hot. With the exception of one spot on its anterior surface, the whole of the left side of the scrotum was as "hard as a board." Professor Volkmann diagnosed the case as one of spontaneous and acute suppurative inflammation of the tunica vaginalis, and at once proposed to lay open the supposed pus-containing cavity. Chloroform having been administered, and antiseptic precautions taken, an incision was made into the left half of the scrotum from a point over the external abdominal ring downwards. The edges of this incision gaped widely, exposing a considerable thickness of scrotal wall, that had been converted through lymphatic œdema into a firm transparent myxoma-like tissue. There was a free discharge of serous fluid from this wound, but the tumour did not diminish. After frequently repeated applications of the knife, the tunica vaginalis, of a dark blue colour, was exposed at the bottom of the wound. This membrane having been incised, exit was given to about a tablespoonful of black blood, and the testis, enlarged to four or five times its normal size, was exposed. The surface of the swollen organ was smooth and glistening, and of an uniform deep-red colour. The surface of the epididymis was similarly congested, and the plexus pampiniformis was found to be filled with coagulated blood. The thrombosed veins were much distended, and presented numerous bulging processes, suspended from the surfaces of the epididymis and spermatic cord, and hanging down like berries within the sac of the tunica vaginalis. As there were no indications that gangrene had commenced in the testis, Professor Volkmann allowed the organ to remain, and concluded the operation by bringing together, though not into close contact, the edges of the incision, by means of sutures, in order to prevent prolapse. The seat of the operation was dressed antiseptically. On the following day the fever was much reduced, and the pain and swelling in the scrotum had commenced to diminish. During the after-treatment, the surfaces of the wound remained in an antiseptic condition. The discharge was scanty, and consisted of a yellowish serous fluid. The surface of the testicle exposed at the bottom of the incision presented, on the second day, a network of yellow streaks. On the twelfth day after the operation, there was no pain or abnormal swelling on the left side of the scrotum. At this period it was quite evident that the testicle had undergone necrosis. The dead and mummified organ protruded more and more from the surface of the scrotum, and, early in the following month, was detached in two portions, leaving but a very small living portion of the epididymis behind.

Microscopic examination of numerous portions of the necrotic mass gave an invariable result, and proved the total absence of any signs indicating that the hemorrhagic infarction had been preceded by an inflammatory process. In no part of the interstitial testicular tissue could any traces of progressive histological changes be discovered. No indications of wandering processes could be seen, and no accumulation of lymphoid elements. All the objects that could be seen were vessels extremely dilated and distended by red blood-corpuscles, and, here and there, extravasated blood in various stages of metamorphosis, with blood-pigment either free in the tissue, in the form of scales and granules, or inclosed in cells. The epithelium of the seminal tubules was clouded.—*London Med. Record*, Feb. 15, 1878.

--

Aspiration in Effusion into the Knee-Joint.

Dr. DIEULAFOY, fortified by the success that has followed its employment in additional cases since his work was published, communicates an article to the *Gazette Hebdomadaire* (February 22), in which he insists in the strongest terms on the complete innocuity and great utility of aspiration as applied to affections of the knee. As regards the innocence of the operation, this he thinks may be fairly inferred from the fact that among 150 aspiratory punctures of the knee performed for effusions of various kinds, whether serous, hæmatic, or purulent, and whether of rheumatic, traumatic, or blennorrhagic origin, one only was followed by accidents, and this case was complicated with fracture. It has often happened that the punctures have been repeated from three to six times in the same place in the very painful and often obstinate hydrarthrosis of acute rheumatism.

But, to obtain this innocuity, the operation must be methodically performed, and the needle No. 2 only employed. The limb is placed in extension, the joint being surrounded by a caoutchouc or linen bandage, leaving the point exposed towards which the liquid has been pressed, and where the needle has to be passed in. This place of election is the external *cul-de-sac* of the synovial membrane, opposite the upper end of the patella, and at about two centimetres exterior to

this bone. The No. 2 needle, which is to be *exclusively* employed, only measures a millimetre in diameter, and when passed into the joint is to remain in a
fixed position while the fluid is aspired. All manipulation of the joint is to be
avoided as causing unnecessary irritation. When the liquid has been removed,
the needle is withdrawn and compression employed. The knee is surrounded by a
layer of wadding, pretty firm compression being maintained by means of a flannel
or linen bandage. A roller is also to be applied to the foot and leg in order to
prevent the production of œdema. Twenty-four hours afterwards the joint is
examined, and if there is no or only very slight reproduction of the liquid, compression is again had recourse to; but if the effusion has been reproduced in a
notable quantity, aspiration should again be performed before reapplying the
compression.

With respect to the efficacy of aspiration, it is most marked and most rapid in
cases of *effusion of blood* into the joints from injury; for while a simple
hydrarthrosis may require its four or five aspirations, an effusion from external
cause, as a rule, yields to one or two. Here, in fact, the cause is purely local,
and is not attended with a pathological condition of the serous membrane. The
exudation, if left to itself, might become slowly absorbed, or it might act in some
cases as a foreign body in the joint. But when removed, the serous membrane
is placed in the most favourable condition; and purulent transformation has never
been met with after the operation. In *sero-fibrinous effusions* we meet with two
categories of eases—first, those (which are by no means rare) wherein the effusion
disappears after two or three aspirations, *i. e.*, after treatment lasting from three
to eight days; and secondly, the chronic hydrarthroses, for which from four to
six operations are required, lasting over from twelve to eighteen days. Effusions
dependent upon *gonorrhœa* are peculiar and more obstinate; and although puncture of the knee gives relief, the liquid soon forms again. As compared with
other means of treatment, aspiration possesses a valuable superiority in the
rapidity with which it relieves the pain, sometimes extremely violent, attendant
upon acute rheumatism and traumatic effusion.—*Med. Times and Gazette*, March
2, 1878.

***

Rupture of the Popliteal Artery and Vein.

Mr. WALTER RIVINGTON, Surgeon to the London Hospital, records (*British
Med. Journ.*, Jan. 12, 1878) a case of rupture of the internal and middle coats of
the popliteal artery, and complete rupture of the popliteal vein, for which primary
amputation of the thigh was successfully performed.

Mr. Rivington offered the following interesting remarks based on this case.
Rupture of the popliteal artery is, I believe, generally associated with displacement of the tibia at the knee-joint, and involves usually all the coats of the vessel.
Such cases have hitherto of necessity required amputation; and the only question
which arises in reference to the operation is, whether it is better to perform it at
once as soon as the lesion is diagnosed, or to wait until gangrene has commenced.
I think that the opinion of most surgeons would be strongly in favour of early
amputation, whereby the patient would be saved from all risk of his blood becoming contaminated by the products of the decomposition of his tissues. More
especially would this consideration weigh with a surgeon not yet converted to the
antiseptic system, and attached to a metropolitan hospital where pyæmia is prevalent and mars the success of operations, however well conceived and executed
they may be. In a primary amputation, the surgeon obtains healthy or nearly
healthy flaps; in a secondary amputation, after gangrene has commenced and is
spreading, he may have to cut through tissues infiltrated with inflammatory exudation.

In reference, however, to the actual results of cases, I am not in possession of sufficient data to determine the point. That secondary amputation may be attended with a very satisfactory result is shown by several reported cases. A case is related by Mr. Jackman in the fourth volume of the *St. Bartholomew's Hospital Reports*. The patient was a healthy farmer fifty-six years of age. He was superintending his men, who were removing some large stumps of old trees. The men had placed a chain round one tree, and, while the patient was standing with his back to them, the horses employed made a sudden plunge forward, which tightened the chain with a jerk and caused it to catch him just under the knee and throw him down with great force. Gangrene set in ten days after the accident, and amputation was performed above the knee four days later. The popliteal artery was torn across, but its ends were surrounded by a tumour about the size of a pigeon's egg, which had the appearance of a false aneurism. Both ends of the artery were closed. The state of the popliteal vein is not described.

Again, in the fifth volume of the *St. Bartholomew's Hospital Reports*, Mr. George Lowe has recorded two cases of complete dislocation of the tibia forwards at the knee-joint, with rupture of the popliteal vessels. The first patient was a fine healthy collier thirty-six years of age. Amputation was performed in the upper third of the thigh six days after the accident, when gangrene supervened. Both the popliteal artery and vein were found completely torn across. The patient made a good recovery. In the second case, amputation was performed in the upper third of the thigh on the third day after the accident. The popliteal vessels were completely torn across. The patient was a comparatively feeble man thirty-two years of age, but he recovered well. The success of these three cases may be partly ascribed to the fact that the operations were performed in the country, and the success of two out of the three may be also ascribed to the healthy condition of the patients. It is worthy of note, however, that, in Mr. Lowe's cases, the accession of gangrene compelled amputation in the upper third of the thigh, whereas primary amputation could be performed, I should think, in most cases in the lower third. This difference tells considerably in favour of amputation before the occurrence of gangrene.

As a general rule, I think it may be stated that, in cases caused by contusion or dislocation, the popliteal artery can scarcely be torn across, either partially or completely, without corresponding injury to the popliteal vein. This complication must necessarily enhance the gravity of the case. Apart from additional interference with the circulation caused by interruption to the current of blood, the accompanying extravasation would be increased, and the probability of a circumscribed false aneurism forming and limiting the effusion would be considerably lessened.

In the case which I have related, the lower part of the thigh, the popliteal space, and the upper part of the leg were infiltrated with blood, and the knee-joint was distended, the foot was cold and becoming mottled, and yet the effused blood was derived wholly from the ruptured popliteal vein.

Rupture of the inner coats of a large artery is a lesion probably of unfrequent occurrence, and, although I have not had time to search in the various medical periodicals for cases, I believe that comparatively few have been placed on record. It is a lesion, however, which might readily be overlooked or mistaken for embolism. Where, for instance, the internal and middle coats of an artery are turned down and block up the artery, pulsation will be traceable as far as the obstruction, whilst the distal portion of the artery will be pulseless, at least as far as the first large branch, and the limb below, especially if the lower extremity be the seat of the lesion, will be colder than its fellow, just as in the case of an embolic block in the artery. Mr. Pick states that there is a specimen of partial

ruptuie of the left axillary aiteiy in the St. Geoige's Hospital Museum, showing
the two innei coats tuined down, and involving the vessel in the thiid part of its
couise. It was taken fiom a man who died of an injuiy to the head. During
life, pulsation could be tiaced to the lowei pait of the axilla. This is evidently
the same case as that ielated by Mr. Holmes in his text-book of the *Principles
and Piactice of Surgery*. Mr. Holmes states that " the symptoms of the injuiy
weie so cleaily maiked that it was easy to diagnose both the natuie and the pie-
cise seat of the lesion." The supeificial situation of the aiteiy at the injuied
spot iendeied it obvious that the toin coats had been pushed into the tube of the
vessel by the blood, so as to close it, and the condition of the aiteiy was exactly
veiified by *post-mortem* examination. A second specimen in St. Geoige's Hospital Museum shows a laceiation of the inteinal and middle coats of the femoial
aiteiy. A thiid case has been ielated by Mr. Pick in the seventeenth volume of
the *Transactions* of the Pathological Society. The patient, twenty-five yeais of
age, ieceived a violent blow fiom a ciowbai on the fiont of the iight thigh, the
effect of which seems to have been to cause a paitial iuptuie of the popliteal
aiteiy. He expeiienced a sudden and intense pain at the back of the knee-joint,
lasting some minutes and causing him to feel veiy faint. The pain passed off,
and he iesumed his woik as a navigatoi, continuing at it foi a week, in spite of
pain and swelling of the limb. Aftei walking seveial miles on the sixth day aftei
the injuiy, he expeiienced pain so seveie, and so much swelling, that he had to
be conveyed home and confined to bed. Five weeks latei, he was admitted into
St. Geoige's Hospital in a state of collapse and with enoimous swelling of the
left leg. Amputation of the thigh was peifoimed. The patient iallied, but died
of pyæmia on the nineteenth day aftei opeiation. The popliteal aiteiy was found
toin acioss, but not completely, a stiip of the anteiioi wall still uniting the two
ends. The vein was not injuied, but its walls weie thickened.

Paitial iuptuie of a laige aiteiy may lay the foundation foi an aneuiism, eithei
ciicumsciibed oi diffused. Mr. Pick has ielated, in the sixth volume of the *St.
Geoige's Hospital Repoits*, a case of the kind. A policeman, thiity-one yeais
of age, stiained his left thigh. Five months afteiwaids, he was obliged to give
up duty and go into the hospital, a pulsating swelling having appeaied on the
innei side of the thigh. Digital compiession was tiied, but pioved inefficacious,
and the swelling of the limb incieased so much, that gangiene supeivened and
necessitated amputation at the hip-joint, fiom which the patient succumbed. The
aneuiismal sac was situated at the junction of the femoial and popliteal aiteiies,
and seemed to be laigely foimed of the exteinal coat of the vessel. I have also
placed on iecoid a case of tiaumatic axillaiy aneuiism, in which it was an open
question whethei a complete oi paitial iuptuie of a segment of the aiteiial ciicumfeience was the piimaiy lesion. The patient was seventy yeais of age. Foui
days befoie admission, he had fallen out of a cait and displaced his left humeius
at the shouldei-joint. Two days aftei the accident, the dislocation was ieduced
by a piactitionei by extension with the foot in the axilla. On admission, theie
was consideiable, but not excessive, swelling of the shouldei-joint, without pulsation in the swelling. The pulse beat naturally at the wiist. A small haid lump,
about the size of a pigeon's egg, could be felt at the base of the axilla, ovei the
site of the axillaiy vein, and not ieceiving impulse fiom the axillaiy aiteiy.
Undei these ciicumstances, moie fully detailed elsewheie, I diagnosed an effusion
of blood into the axilla and shouldei-joint, stating my belief that the blood came,
not fiom a iuptuied axillaiy aiteiy, but eithei fiom smallei vessels oi fiom the
vein. Stiict iest, with bandages only, was enjoined to piomote absoiption. A
month latei, when the patient was not undei my chaige, aneuiismal symptoms
appeaied, pulsation and *bruit* being both peiceptible, and the pulse at the wiist

became feebler. Various suggestions as to treatment were made, the most prominent being ligature of the subclavian artery; but the patient declined operative
interference. Ultimately, ulceration of the skin took place, hemorrhage occurred,
the axilla was laid open, and the injured vessel was secured at the seat of lesion.
A transverse aperture was found in the third part of the course of the axillary
artery, occupying about a third of the circumference of the artery. In view of
the uncertainty as to the source of the effusion of blood in this case, and the advanced age of the patient, which rendered any operative interference at any stage
of his case wellnigh hopeless, there can be no doubt as to the propriety of the
treatment recommended in the first instance by myself. I am pleased to have
the opportunity of quoting a published opinion of my colleague Mr. Maunder in
reference to this subject. In his Lettsomian Lectures (*vide Lancet*, February
27th, 1875, page 295, Case 24), Mr. Maunder speaks strongly against the application of a ligature to the subclavian artery, and states that either of the two
other means of treatment at our disposal, amputation at the shoulder-joint and
laying open the axilla, would in all probability have terminated fatally. This
opinion effectually disposes of the suggestions made at the time that ligature of
the subclavian artery ought to have been performed, and that it would have been
better to operate at an early period in the history of the case.

A point of considerable interest arising out of this case is the possibility of
locating the seat of injury in some of the cases of ruptured axillary artery. It is
evident that, if the third part of the artery be involved, and if this can be rendered probable, the severe procedure of laying open the whole anterior wall of
the axilla might be avoided. A careful exposure of the third part of the artery
would then be sufficient, combined with a simultaneous removal of the clots in the
axilla. The introduction of the finger would probably enable the surgeon to trace
the vessel and find out where pulsation ceased or became less marked even in a
case which he had not previously seen. If, however, the case had come under
his observation early, and there existed, as in my own case, a small hard circumscribed lump over the third part of the course of the vessel, the diagnosis would
be rendered more probable. At all events, a more prolonged search for the seat
of injury should be made whenever such a course is practicable, without danger
of serious hemorrhage continuing during the exploration.

Next, I would strongly recommend the application of the stethoscope over the
site of an artery which there is any reason to think is ruptured either partially or
completely. There is good reason to believe that, by means of auscultation, partial and complete ruptures may be diagnosed in some cases shortly after the injury,
and when pulsation cannot be perceived. Mr. Holmes states he has never seen
any case where pulsation was present in the extravasated blood in connection
with a complete subcutaneous laceration of an artery; but he says that, in some
cases, a bruit can be heard (*Surgery: its Principles and Practice*, page 78).

Lastly, in these days of antiseptic surgery, when knee-joints can be laid open
and fingered with impunity, when the surgeon is freed from all anxiety as to the
results of operations, when exposed blood-clots cease to break down and decompose, but become organized in the open wound under the charm of carbolic acid
and the antiseptic dressing, it may fairly be asked whether, in such cases as that
which I have related, amputation should not be set aside until the wounded vessels have been sought for and tied in the popliteal space. Some of the extravasated blood could be removed by the operator and the rest be allowed to become
either organized or absorbed; and, if the knee-joint had been opened by the accident, the triumph of antiseptic surgery would be all the greater. The only possible question would be, whether the circulation in the member could be carried
on sufficiently to prevent the occurrence of gangrene. If this question should be

capable of receiving an affirmative reply, no excuse would be left for the mutilation hitherto regarded by septic surgery as indispensable to save the life of the patient.

Spontaneous Aneurism of the Arteria Dorsalis Pedis.

A labourer, aged 29, was admitted into the London Hospital, under the care of Mr. ADAMS, on acconut of a swelling, about the size of a small nut, situated over the outer side of the astragalo-scaphoid articulation. He had first noticed this a month before his admission, his attention being called to it by finding his boots tighter than usual. He was then in good health, and he could not account for the swelling in any way. As the swelling gradually became larger and painful, he was induced to come to the hospital. On admission, the tumour was as large as a full-sized walnut; its outline was hemispherical, resting on its flattened base; the skin over it was red, tense, and shining, looking like an acute abscess on the point of bursting. On careful examination, it was found to present every important symptom of an aneurism. There was œdema of the foot and ankle, and of the lower part of the leg. There were no indications of any other changes in his vascular system, and no indications of syphilis. The leg was placed on an inclined plane, and lead-lotion was applied to the foot. The œdema and pain quickly subsided, but the skin over the tumour became thinner. A tourniquet was applied to the femoral artery to diminish the force of the blood-current, and the limb was bandaged.

On the fourth day of treatment the tumour was found to be about the same size, but the skin over it was thinner, with superficial vesication. Under these circumstances, it appeared necessary to operate, and three methods presented themselves for consideration: 1. To cut into the sac and tie both ends of the vessel, as in a case of traumatic aneurism ; 2. To tie the anterior tibial just above the annular ligament ; 3. To tie it in the upper part of the leg. Against the first method was the probability of suppuration amongst the tendons on the dorsum of the foot, combined with the difficulty of finding the two ends of so small a vessel, and the risk of the vessel being diseased at the seat of ligature. Against the second method was the risk of suppuration among the tendons. The artery was, therefore, cut down upon in the upper part of the leg, and a catgut ligature was placed around it without difficulty ; on tightening this, all pulsation in the tumour ceased, and its size sensibly diminished. The wound was closed with wire sutures, and the limb wrapped in cotton-wool. The day after the operation the skin became black over the tumour, suggesting suppuration, though the man's general condition gave no confirmation of this opinion. In the evening his temperature rose to 104.2° Fahr., with a pulse of 102 ; and there was a slight return of pulsation in the tumour perceptible to the eye as well as to the finger. Mr. Hutchinson saw the case in consultation, and agreed that, though the appearances were in favour of secondary suppuration, it would be better to leave the tumour untouched.

A fortnight after the operation, pulsation was entirely absent from the tumour ; its centre was covered with a leathery scale, from the edges of which a serous fluid was escaping; fluctuation was distinct; there was no suppuration, and there appeared no chance of consolidation occurring. There was a varying amount of pain in the foot, and the discharge from the wound, where the ligature had been applied, was profuse. The patient's general health remained good. It was now determined to open the sac ; this was done by Mr. Rygate, house-surgeon, with antiseptic precautions, and nothing but currant jelly-like clots were found. The leg was kept on a McIntyre splint. Suppuration soon followed, and free irrigation was used, under which treatment the wound presented a healthy appearance for some days. A week after the tumour was opened, the wound was explored with the finger, and the hollow on the outer side of the astragalo-scaphoid joint was found to communicate with that articulation; this had probably been brought about by the aneurism. From this time the patient's condition progressed adversely; the discharge was profuse both from the upper wound and from the foot; suppuration extended all round the foot and into the ankle-joint, and no alternative was left but amputation; this was performed three months after admission to the hospital; the patient then progressed satisfactorily, and left the hospital two months later.

The subsequent examination of the limb was unsatisfactory, the protracted suppuration having so altered the various structures as to render it impossible to trace them. The astragalo-scaphoid and anterior astragalo-calcanean articulations were the seat of suppuration, the articular cartilages being quite destroyed, and the bony surfaces rough. No other joints were involved; but all the tissues of the sole appeared as an almost homogeneous mass of inflammatory deposit.

Mr. Adams remarked that he had been unable to find any recorded case of a spontaneous aneurism in this situation; and that, even if other cases have been or should be seen, this case will probably remain unique as to many of its features, especially the thinness of the sac and the early occurrence of appearances of suppuration. Notwithstanding the unfavourable result, the line of treatment adopted appeared to be the most appropriate. There could be no doubt that the aneurism had made its way into the astragalo-scaphoid joint at the time when the man was first seen (although this did not so appear at first), and, had the sac been cut into and the ends of the vessels tied, in addition to the difficulty of finding the vessel, there would have been the chance of its being diseased, and the complication of a direct opening into the joint. Again, if the ligature had been applied immediately above the annular ligament, there is no reason to suppose that the result would have been any better as regards the amount of suppuration, and there would have been an additional chance of the vessel being diseased.—*British Med. Journal*, Dec. 8, 1877.

The Treatment of Varix by the Subcutaneous Injection of Alcohol.

A new method of treating varicose veins was described by Dr ENGLISCH at a recent meeting of the Vienna Medical Society. By means of an ordinary hypodermic syringe, from fifteen to twenty drops of a mixture of alcohol and water, in equal parts, are injected into the cellular tissue beneath the vein, which, together with a fold of skin, has been previously raised by the thumb and forefinger. The injection gives rise to a small swelling, and on close observation the vein may be seen to contract. More or less infiltration is observed on the third day, and in very sensitive patients the skin is apt to become red, and even a small abscess may form, the vein itself not becoming involved in the suppuration. As the infiltration becomes firmer and smaller, the vein also diminishes in size and gradually becomes hard and cord-like. In some cases one such injection may suffice to effect a cure of the varix, but in the majority the operation has to be repeated several times. The results are most successful when the dilated veins form a plexus, but the treatment is more difficult when there are many branches. The pain during and after the operation is very slight; the length of time required for the subsequent treatment varies according to the gravity of the case. In cases where the result is not entirely successful, the operation appears to be a valuable auxiliary to other palliative measures. Dr. Englisch claims for his method that it is absolutely free from danger. He was induced to make trial of it for the cure of varix in consequence of the excellent results he obtained from the use of similar injections for the radical cure of hernia.—*Med. Examiner*, Feb. 21, 1878.

Apparatus for Transverse Fractures of the Patella.

Moulard describes in a thesis (1877) an apparatus invented by Dr. Duplouy for transverse fracture of the patella, and of which he has seen the good effects at the Rochefort Hospital.

The description of this apparatus is as follows. Dr. Duplouy, chief surgeon to the navy, employs small bands covered with collodion as a means of holding the fragments together in fractures of the patella. He envelopes the lower segment of the limb with a silicated bandage, reaching half way up the thigh, but open in front and at the sides of the knee. This bandage is applied over a thick layer of cotton wadding. Below the popliteal space he places a padded wood splint, which reaches half way up the thigh, and descends half way down the leg. When the silicated bandage is completely dry, he brings the fragments of the patella together in the following way. Threads of knitting cotton, each about twelve inches long, are placed in juxtaposition in a sufficient quantity to form a bundle four-tenths of an inch in diameter. He immerses the middle portion only of this bundle in collodion; then he arranges an upper bundle, of which the whole is applied four-fifths of an inch above the upper semi-circumference of the patella, forming a concentric curve around it as far as the level of the transverse diameter of the bone; a lower bundle is arranged in the same way at the lower part of the patella. Thus the two bundles are inclined the one towards the other, and the patella is completely surrounded. Several layers of collodion are then applied with a brush over the maintaining bundles and the skin above and below. The apparatus being thus arranged, the collodion is allowed to dry completely, and the free tails are brought together and tied two and two on each side of the patella. In proportion as the distance between the two fragments is lessened, the ends are drawn closer. Care must be taken to add every day fresh layers of collodion above and below, to maintain the solidity of the apparatus.—*London Med. Record*, Jan. 15, 1878.

Midwifery and Gynæcology.

Treatment of Obstinate Vomiting during Pregnancy by Dilatation of the Cervix Uteri.

A woman, aged 22, in the second or third month of her first pregnancy, entered the Maternity Hospital of Santiago, under the care of Dr. A. Murillo, suffering with incessant vomiting (*Revista Medica de Chile*, Año V, num. 6). She was very weak, had gastric distress, and vomited every two or three minutes, ejecting food, bilious matter, and mucus. The tongue was coated, the pulse 120 per minute and feeble, the skin dry and hot, and giddiness like that of sea-sickness prevented her from sitting up. As pepsin, calmatives, tonics, ice, milk, etc., had been tried without result, Dr. Murillo determined to resort to dilatation of the neck of the uterus, as recommended by Dr. Copeman, of Norwich, before resorting to measures to induce abortion. He therefore introduced the finger into the softened cervix as far as the internal orifice, and kept it there for two minutes. He then ordered ice-cold milk-punch by the mouth; and broth, pepsine, and hydrochloric acid by enema twice daily. The cervix was dilated in a similar manner four different times, at intervals of one or two days; and morphia was given to produce sleep, which, however, did not have the desired effect. At the end of a week the improvement was very marked, the patient vomited less frequently, retained the light aliment allowed, and could sit up without being giddy. In eleven days she left the hospital to go to the country, not entirely cured, but very greatly benefited.—*London Med. Record*, Feb. 15, 1878.

Note on Two Contrasted Forms of Weak Labour.

Dr. MATTHEWS DUNCAN communicated to the Edinburgh Obstetrical Society (*Edinburgh Med. Journal*, Feb. 1878) a note entitled as above, of which the following is an abstract:—

"The two forms of weak labour spoken of by Dr. Duncan in this paper are frequently confounded with one another with injurious practical results; but they are essentially different, and require a correspondingly different treatment. The one form is common and well known, the other has only been recognized of late years, and is not yet at all well known. The common form depends upon inertia of the uterus, and is most frequently seen in multiparæ who have had many children and are elderly. In this case, the uterus is not stimulated to sufficient activity, and the delay is due to inefficiency and infrequency of the pains. The stage of the after-birth is apt to be attended with hemorrhage. The rarer form is due to a quite different cause, and is, in many respects, a contrast to the former. It occurs chiefly in primiparæ, or in young women who have a special nervous mobility. Here the uterus is unduly but morbidly active. The tonic permanent contraction goes on with premature and injurious rapidity; the intermittent pains are frequent and painful, but inefficient. The body of the uterus, with its fundus higher in the abdomen than usual, is retracted over the body of the child, so that it forms only a comparatively small cap over the lower fœtal parts, and a distinct rim or sulcus can be felt a little below the umbilicus, where the contracted uterine body is attached to the greatly expanded cervix. The condition of the uterus in this form is similar to what is found in labours where the advance of the child has been long obstructed, and it is attended with like danger, yet there is no apparent difficulty in propelling the child and no obstruction. The treatment of two forms of labour so distinct from one another is naturally different. In the former, where the delay is due to inertia, the uterus is to be stimulated by oxytocics—of which ergot is the best—and by kneading, rubbing, and similar means. In the latter, or premature uterine retraction, the uterus is not to be stimulated but soothed; opium and chloroform may be useful, but all oxytocics are to be avoided. Early delivery, if necessary with the forceps, is desirable. A case is given in which the second of these two forms was accurately observed."

Extra-Uterine Pregnancy treated by Gastrotomy.

Dr. ROUSSEAU, of Epernay, reports (*Union Médicale et Scientifique du Nord-Est*, 30 September) a case of extra-uterine pregnancy, in which gastrotomy was performed five months after the death of the fœtus, and fourteen months after the commencement of the pregnancy. In order to produce adhesions and prevent opening into the peritoneal cavity, the actual cautery was used. A knife-shaped instrument was heated to a white heat, and with it the anterior wall of the abdomen and the placenta, which was attached to it, were gradually divided: six sittings, at intervals of five or six days, were required for this purpose. After the sixth sitting, the patient's condition was such as to render longer delay unadvisable, and the remaining portion of the placenta, which was about two-fifths of an inch thick, was divided with a bistoury. A little black blood escaped when the placenta was cut. The head could now be felt, and, as it seemed large, craniotomy was performed, and the bones of the cranium removed piecemeal. The entire fœtus was then taken away without difficulty. Without the brain, and after being two days in alcohol, it weighed over six and a half pounds. The placenta was firmly attached to the abdominal wall, and bled on punctuie. For fear of hemoirhage and of peritonitis, no attempt was made to remove it or the membranes. The patient did well immediately after the operation, but a few days afterwaids was seized with a phlebitis, from which, however, she recovered speedily. There was no peritonitis at any time. The placenta did not slough out, but gradually diminished in size, and became involved in the cicatrix. Ten weeks after the operation the patient left the hospital, with a fistulous opening in the abdomen, from which a small quantity of thick pus escaped. This opening remained for several years, and during this period a tumour formed by the placenta and membranes could be felt in the abdomen. M. Rousseau alleges that this case proves that the placenta and membranes can be left without fear in the abdominal cavity after gastrotomy, provided they are still living and attached. He thinks that the adoption of this practice as a rule will diminish greatly the unfavourable chances of the operation. In this case the cauterizations were not, as it turned out, necessary to prevent opening into the abdominal cavity, since the attachment of the placenta to the anterior wall of the abdomen removed all danger of that. They proved very useful, however, in preventing hemoirhage from the living and vascular placenta.—*London Med. Record*, Feb. 15, 1878.

Cæsarean Section and Removal of Uterus in a Case of Osteomalacia.

Dr. SPÄTH, at a late meeting of the Imperial Royal Medical Society of Vienna, described a case of osteomalacia, in which he had successfully performed Cæsarean section, with extirpation of the uterus. The patient was a woman aged 40, in her tenth pregnancy. She had had five labours at full teim ; had aborted three times ; and the ninth labour was completed by perforation of the child's skull. She had suffered from osteomalacia for five years, and attributed the disease to the destitute circumstances in which she was. On May 29 she was admitted, while pregnant, under Dr. Späth, on account of osteomalacia. She was much emaciated, and her skin was pale ; she had bronchial catarrh, the urine contained much albumen, and there was considerable œdema of the lower limbs. She also complained of pain in the loins, apparently due to the osteomalacia. Careful examination showed that the pelvis was greatly narrowed, and that the Cæsarean operation was absolutely indicated. As labour would not be due for some days, Dr. Späth had an opportunity of using means to improve the patient's strength. She was put in a separate room, and her nurses were instructed to give notice as soon as labour-pains set in. On reflection, Dr. Späth came to the conclusion that in this case the preferable mode of proceeding would be to perform the Cæsarean section under Lister's antiseptic plan ; and, if the uterus did not completely contract, and there were consequently reason for fearing hemoirhage into the peritoneal cavity, to totally extirpate this organ. He was led to this conclusion, on the one hand, by remembering that every case of Cæsarean section performed in the Vienna Lying-in Hospital during the last century had proved fatal, either from peritonitis or from violent secondary hemorrhage ; and, on the other hand, by the successful results of extirpation of the uterus, obtained by Péan of Paris, and Porro of Padua. On June 2, in the evening, labour-pains set in ; and at 8.30 P. M. the operation was performed under the carbolic spray, in the presence and with the assistance of Drs. Karl Braun and Weinlechner. An incision was made in the linea alba below the umbilicus, the uterus was laid open, and a living fœtus was removed without difficulty. The commencement of energetic uterine contraction was now waited for; an endeavour to promote it had been made by injecting ergotine previously to the operation. As, however, the contractions gradually diminished, and the hemorrhage from the uterus increased, and could not be arrested by the application of sponges dipped in iced water, the removal of the uterus was judged necessary. The chain of the écraseur having been fastened round the uterus near the neck, the organ was lifted out of the wound, and Dr. Späth divided, by free cuts with a scalpel, the body from the cervix. The abdominal cavity was carefully cleansed, the wound was united, and the pedicle of the uterus was fastened to the lower angle of the wound. The whole operation occupied scarcely an hour. The patient soon came to herself, and complained little of pain. The subsequent progress of the case was unexpectedly favourable; the highest temperature which was observed was 38.6 cent. (101.48° Fahr.). The wound in the abdominal wall healed rapidly, leaving only a fistulous opening leading to the neck of the uterus. The albuminuria and œdema of the limbs disappeared, the patient's condition was improved by the use of champagne, and she complained less of the bronchial catarrh. The uterine pedicle was detached on the tenth day. On the thirty-eighth day she sat up for the first time, and, eleven days later, was moved to another room, and walked without help into the garden. On September 18 she was discharged cured, with instruction to report herself every week. In October the fistulous opening completely closed. Dr. Späth showed the woman, who appeared to be in perfect health and good condition. She had had no further indication of the osteomalacia. Dr. Späth referred also to a second case in which he had operated in a similar way last September. The patient, however, had symptoms of septicæmia when she was admitted to the lying-in hospital, and died after the operation.—*London Med. Record*, Feb. 15, 1878.

—

Use of Hot Baths in Secondary Puerperal Hemorrhage.

Dr. BAILLY relates (*Archives de Tocologie*, Nov. 1877) two cases in which a striking and rapid success followed the use of hot baths in secondary puerperal hemorrhage according to the plan recommended by Dr. Tarnier. The first was that of a patient in whom hemorrhage commenced eighteen days after delivery, no abnormal loss having previously occurred. The uterus was enlarged, and could be felt two finger-breadths above the pubes. Although not in amount sufficient to cause serious alarm, the loss, consisting of liquid blood and clots, persisted most obstinately for ten days. Injections of dilute perchloride of iron, and the administration of ergot and hæmostatic mineral waters, proved of little avail. The introduction into the vagina of tampons of charpie soaked in perchloride of iron suspended the loss for twenty-four hours, but it then recurred as persistently as ever. Dr. Tarnier, being called in consultation, recommended the use of hot baths. After the first bath the loss was much diminished; after the second, it was completely suspended. It recurred at the end of thirty-six hours, but was finally arrested by a third bath. The process of involution was rapidly completed, and, at the end of a week, the patient was able to get about.

In the second case the hemorrhage set in twenty-seven days after delivery, when the patient had already been able to walk about her room for twelve days. It was at first slight and intermittent, but afterwards became continuous and profuse. The cervix was soft, and readily admitted the finger; the uterus was as large as at the third month of pregnancy, and was felt considerably above the pubes. She was treated by complete rest in bed, with ergot, cold vaginal injections, and cold enemata, but without result. This continued for six days, large clots being frequently passed. A hot bath of twenty minutes' duration was then prescribed, the patient very reluctantly consenting to this treatment. After the first bath the hemorrhage entirely stopped. It was renewed the following day, and continued in slight degree for twenty-four hours, but was finally arrested by a second bath.

The author attributes the good effect to the relief of uterine congestion consequent upon the dilatation of cutaneous capillaries produced by the hot baths, the resulting determination of blood to the surface, and diminished vascularity of deep-seated organs The plan of treatment was first taught by M. Salgues, formerly Professor of Clinical Medicine at Dijon, under whom M. Tarnier had studied. The author has found it more efficacious in the second phase of the hemorrhage than at its outset, and he considers it unsafe to resort to it earlier than ten days after delivery. The baths are given at the temperature of about 34° C., and the duration of immersion varies from twenty minutes to half an hour.—*Obstetrical Journal of Great Britain*, March, 1878.

Influence of Pregnancy on Suckling.

In reference to a case recently at the Hôpital des Cliniques, Prof. DEPAUL took the opportunity (*Rev. Méd.*, February 18) of strongly impressing upon his class that the continuance of suckling after pregnancy had manifested itself, whatever its effects might be on the mother, acted most injuriously upon her infant. First, the quantity of milk diminishes, and the child, though suckling for a long time, no longer obtains the quantity of nutriment which it requires. Its stomach not feeling satisfied with what it has received, in place of going to sleep after a copious repast, as usual, the child cries and becomes restless. If, in spite of these signs, the mother continues to suckle, more alarming symptoms are produced. Digestion is disturbed, and, after each suckling, in place of some pure milk flowing out of the mouth after the breast is taken away, as may be observed in infants who are quite well, actual vomiting takes place, and a large mass of not yet coagulated milk which the stomach cannot tolerate is rejected. The stools, too, exhibit characteristic modifications, and in place of passing two or three of these in the twenty-four hours, the child now passes several, so as to amount to diarrhœa. In some cases there may be, however, constipation. The discharges are themselves abnormal in their appearance. In place of appearing somewhat thickened, and resembling in colour and consistency a boiled egg, they may be quite fluid, of an appearance just like spinach-water ; at other times they are less fluid and brownish ; and in other instances, again, both in colour and consistence they exactly resemble glaziers' putty. They are accompanied by a more or less considerable quantity of mucus, according to the amount of intestinal irritation, and there may be present streaks or even true drops of blood. Sometimes the amount of milk does not seem to have materially diminished, for it is not uncommon to find it issuing abundantly on pressure being made. This may give rise to error, as it only proves that the gland performs its function actively ; but weighing the infant will show that it derives from this milk an utterly insufficient amount of nutrition. Chemical analysis fails to show us what is the modification which the milk undergoes through pregnancy, rendering it unfit, even when in sufficient quantity, for the nutrition of the child ; but that such a modification does take place is beyond all doubt, and is indeed sufficiently shown to exist by the marked repugnance which the infant may exhibit to the breast. Prof. Depaul has met with three or four remarkable examples of this. In one of these he was sent for by a young woman, whose infant, which was quite well, and had up to then been well nourished, had for some time past absolutely refused to take the breast. Tried in his presence, after having abstained from food for some time, it would not suckle; but no sooner had a nurse who had been sent for made her appearance, than it seized her breast with avidity. On interrogating and examining the mother he became convinced that she had become pregnant. "The conclusion to be drawn from these facts is, that whenever a woman asks you whether, having become pregnant, she ought to continue to suckle her infant, you should reply in the negative and advise her to procure a nurse. For you may be certain that the disturbances of which I have just given you but a very faint sketch, if they have not as yet been produced, will manifest themselves before long, to the great detriment of the child's health."—*Med. Times and Gaz.*, March 2, 1878.

Concerning the Condition of the Hymen and its Remains after Cohabitation, Child-bearing, and Lying-in.

This paper by Prof. C. SCHRŒDER was, with the original drawings, presented to the Obstetrical Society of Edinburgh (*Med. Examiner*, Feb. 28, 1878). The drawings illustrated the condition of the entrance to the vagina, and especially the hymen after cohabitation and child-bearing. The general opinion hitherto is that the hymen is torn by the first coitus, and that the cicatricial retracting remains of it formed the carunculæ myrtiformes. It was also generally believed that the warty excrescences at several places of the vaginal entrance were directly formed by the first coitus. These opinions, however, are not borne out by a careful inspection of the parts. Prof. S. demonstrated in the year 1867 that the carunçube myrtiformes are first formed in consequence of child-bearing by the subsequent sloughing of parts of the hymen. This fact has been frequently questioned by writers on this subject, being confirmed only by Bidder, in Dorpat. Professor Schrœder, with the help of Dr. Alt, his assistant, had drawings made of the vaginal entrance in a number of pregnant females before and after the birth of the child, so as to show the effect of child-bearing on the vaginal entrance by comparing the two drawings.

Before describing the drawings he described the hymen. He stated that the hymen was formed by a fold of mucous membrane arising from the edge of the vaginal entrance, and surrounding with its free edge the opening leading into the vagina. The hymen was a stretched out membrane in the entrance to the vagina, in which there is an opening, not in the centre, but towards the orifice of the urethra. In front, the rim of the hymen is smaller, but it is not wanting. The opening of the hymen is of very different sizes. As a rule, it is wide enough to admit the passing of the finger into the vagina without injuring the border of the mucous membrane. In exceptional cases the opening is very small, and in some cases is entirely absent. It is much more common, however, for the opening to be so large that the finger passes easily through without injuring the structure. In the drawings submitted, one is astonished to find how frequently the hymen has remained wholly or almost entirely intact. The hymen frequently forms only a small stretchable rim which is raised all round from the edge of the vaginal entrance in an equal but insignificant elevation, and which on the pushing in of the penis yields without tearing. The hymen, therefore, not rarely remains almost unchanged by cohabitation, whilst it is only stretched by often repeated coitus, or only slightly indented on its free edge through slight tears. Were the opening smaller it would of course be torn, but never to such an extent as to form carunculæ myrtiformes. These latter are thus formed, as can easily be proved by examining the vaginal entrance of sterile married women or of prostitutes, after very frequently repeated coitus. Through the pushing in of the penis, the free fold of the hymen will at most be torn, so that one, two, or more tears are formed, which sometimes, though not at all regularly, reach the base of the hymen. As a rule, these are only one, two, or three, still they may become much more numerous, and in the most marked cases the hymen is changed into a continuous row of small projecting points. But there is always found a con-nection between the separate small pieces, however numerous the tears may be. These stand close by one another—there is never a space between them. On account of this condition the entrance to the vagina of persons who have not borne children may be distinguished from that of one who has borne a child. With the latter the vaginal entrance, in consequence of the birth, undergoes great change. By the birth the narrow vaginal entrance suffered a dilatation which, as a rule, is not possible without lesions, when the head cuts out through it.   We see, therefore, in the case of primiparæ, as well as of women whose entrance to the vagina was not yet distended by former births, quite regular tears in the mucous membrane.   But besides these, the shreds of the hymen suffer considerable bruising. If we examine the vaginal entrance of a primipara immediately after delivery, when the blood has been carefully wiped away, we see the parts of the hymen still completely preserved, but infiltrated with blood, of a swollen appear-ance, and of a bluish-black colour. A few days later we find in place of separate shreds small ulcers. At the place of these ulcers every trace of the hymen dis-appears, whilst on the other less bruised places remains of the hymen are pre-served. These are the carunculæ myrtiformes. The amount of the hymen so preserved is very various, as the drawings show. The conditions above described were well illustrated by a series of beautiful drawings. Each vaginal entrance was twice sketched—once before delivery, and once about ten days after delivery. The drawings of primiparæ clearly demonstrated the difference of the hymen as you find them in deflowered ones and the carunculæ myrtiformes. After giving a minute description of each drawing, Professor Schrœder concluded by stating that the drawings showed that the difference between the remains of the hymen in females who have not borne children and such as have borne children are striking to the eye, and consequently the condition of the vaginal entrance is one of the best means of deciding the question whether or not a female has already borne a child.

Amputation of the Neck of the Uterus.

In the *Annales de Gynécologie*, January, 1878, there is an article by Dr. A. LEBLOND on amputation of the neck of the uterus. The author points out the anatomical fact that the neck of the uterus consists of two portions—the supra-vaginal, situated above the insertion of the vagina into the neck of the uterus, and the intravaginal, or portion which projects into the vagina below this point. He then discusses the question, ought the amputation to be performed at the vulva or in the vagina? Dr. Leblond is of opinion that the amputation should be done inside the vagina, as the danger of opening the pouch of the peritoneum, which dips down behind the uterus, is avoided, and the relation of adjacent organs is respected. He prefers the galvano-cautery, especially in malignant disease. In default of the galvanic cautery, the écraseur is the safest instrument. Where the galvano-cautery and écraseur are not admissible, he uses scissors. The knife should only be used in cases of hypertrophic elongation of the intravaginal portion of the cervix. In order to facilitate the application of the noose of platinum-wire round the cervix, Dr. Leblond has designed a bivalve speculum, which fits over the cervix and carries the wire round it. The wire is tightened, and the specu-lum is withdrawn before the connection with the bichromate of potash current is made.—*London Med. Record,* Feb. 15, 1878.

Gastrotomy in a Case of Irreducible Retroversion of the Uterus.

Dr. KŒBERLE relates (*Gaz. Méd. de Strasbourg*) a case in which irreducible retroversion of the uterus gave rise to intestinal obstruction which could not be overcome, and in which permanent cure, not only of the ileus, but of the retroversion, was effected by gastrotomy. The patient, the Countess B——, twenty-seven years of age, of hysterical temperament, had suffered from obstinate constipation, and had passed nothing for more than four months. At intervals she had fecal vomiting. The breath was fecal, and nausea continual. For seven months she had been confined to her bed, and for two months had been nourished by milk alone. The abdomen was distended, and the left flank filled by stony fecal masses. The rectum was empty, and the uterus completely retroverted, the os looking forward and to the right. The condition was attributed to a fall from a carriage six months previously. All efforts to restore the uterus failed, it being impossible to pass the sound through the internal os uteri. The patient had consulted twenty-five eminent practitioners, and the most various and energetic treatment had remained without effect.

After trying in vain enemata and drastic purgatives, Dr. Kœberlé resolved on operative interference—not on account of the retroversion, but to relieve the obstruction. He resolved, however, also to cure permanently the displacement by excising one ovary, and fixing its pedicle to the abdominal wall, as in ovariotomy. The incision in the abdominal wall was not more than 5 cm. long in its deeper part. The index and middle fingers were introduced, and hooked round the retroverted fundus. This yielded suddenly, not without some force, being impacted by the intestines, full of scybala, which lay above it. The intestines were then kneaded by the fingers, to make the scybala progress towards the rectum. The left ovary was drawn into the angle of the wound, and with the outer part of the Fallopian tube surrounded by an iron-wire ligature, with the aid of a serre-nœud, as in ovariotomy. They were then fixed by a steel-pin, passed above the ligature, and the superfluous portion cut off. Convalescence was rapid, as after a very easy case of ovariotomy. A large quantity of hard scybala were passed spontaneously on the first day, and an enormous quantity after an enema of senna on the third day. The colic and vomiting immediately disappeared, menstruation was afterwards normal, and the patient enjoyed good health for the next four years.

She then again came under observation with vaginismus, constipation, and vesical tenesmus. Profound hysteria had become established, in consequence of a reverse of fortune. She believed her uterus had become again displaced in consequence of a second fall from a carriage, and she was extremely eager to have the whole organ excised. She was much emaciated, spent most of her time reading in bed, with the room much heated, and the bowels acted only about once in three weeks. Dr. Kœberlé found, however, that the uterus remained in a somewhat anteverted position, and the use of the sound showed that it was still firmly attached to the anterior abdominal wall, since it was impossible to turn it into a position of retroversion or retroflexion.—*Obstetrical Journal of Great Britain,* Jan. 1878.

CONTENTS.

Published Monthly, price $2.50 per annum, free of postage.
Also, furnished together with the AMERICAN JOURNAL OF THE MEDICAL
SCIENCES *and the* MEDICAL NEWS AND LIBRARY *for* SIX DOLLARS *per
annum in advance, the whole free of postage.*

HENRY C. LEA, Philadelphia.

THE MONTHLY ABSTRACT

OF

MEDICAL SCIENCE.

VOL. V. NO. 5.　　**For List of Contents see last page.**　　MAY, 1878.

Anatomy and Physiology.

The Physiology of the Centrum Ovale and Internal Capsule.

M M. FRANCK and PITRES have communicated to the Société de Biologie in Paris the results of certain experimental investigations undertaken by them with the view of testing the conclusion arrived at by pathological study, that the white fibres which start from the excitable regions of the convolutions and connect them with the central parts of the brain, are grouped in distinct bundles, which preserve their functional independence throughout their course in the white matter. For numerous pathological observations have demonstrated that lesions of the white matter may give rise to paralysis limited to certain groups of muscles which could not be explained unless the fibres from the cortical motor centres were grouped in distinct bundles. In these experiments, M M. Franck and Pitres have proceeded by removing successive horizontal slices of the hemisphere, and by exciting the different parts of the cut surface after each mutilation. In this way they were able to obtain isolated movements similar to those resulting from stimulation of the centres of gray matter. Even in the internal capsule and at the base of the corona radiata the fibres maintain their independence, and by stimulation movements may be produced limited to certain groups of muscles on the opposite side of the body. In order to succeed in this, the points of the electrodes must not be separated more than from two to four millimetres. In the dog it is only the anterior half of the surface of section of the internal capsule which is excitable, and the fibres group themselves as follows :—

1. Quite in front are the fibres which determine the movements of the face and eyelids on the opposite side.

2. Next, behind the last, are the fibres going to the anterior limb of the opposite side.

3. A bundle whose excitation caused movements in both limbs of the opposite side.

4. A very small bundle for the posterior extremity only.

5. At the level of the posterior part of the nucleus caudatus is a bundle whose excitation causes elevation of the ear on the opposite side.

These experiences, therefore, amply confirm the data of pathology so far as the centrum ovale is concerned. At first sight they might appear to contradict our well-established opinion that injuries of the internal capsule cause total hemiplegia; but it must be remembered that, in order to produce these limited results, the electrodes had to be closely approximated; now the immense number of the pathological alterations are coarse lesions, hemorrhages, or softenings; such limited lesions as would fairly correspond to the three experiments must be exceedingly rare. On the other hand, these experiments afford a satisfactory explanation of many obscure facts. We know that a patient who has been attacked by hemiplegia recovers the use of his leg while his arm remains quite useless, or the arm may quite recover while the leg is permanently contracted, or the face may be the part in which the affection first disappears or remains for life. These phenomena are fully explained by the different degree to which certain fibres are affected. The analysis of some cases in M. Charcot's wards serves to indicate that paralysis predominates in the upper extremity when the lesion is most marked on the anterior part of the capsule, and in the lower extremity when the lesion is seated on the posterior part of the motor portion of the capsule. —*London Med. Record*, Feb. 15, 1878.

The Condition of the Urine in Sucklings.

The following are the conclusions drawn by CRUSE, in a long and valuable paper on this subject in the *Jahrbuch für Kinderheilkunde* (Band xi., Heft 4):—

1. The absolute quantity of the urine increases from the second to the tenth day quickly; from the tenth to the sixtieth day, slowly.

2. On the contrary, the specific gravity and the percentage of important constituents diminish up to about the tenth day rapidly; after that, scarcely perceptibly. Phosphoric acid is an exception, for it increases with age.

3. The quantity of urine, and of its more important constituents, compared with the body-weight, increases rapidly from the second to the fifth or tenth day. It then remains at about the highest point reached until the sixtieth day. Chloride of sodium is an exception, for it diminishes after the tenth day.

4. Between the fifth and tenth days the urine is mostly turbid, often dark, and its reaction generally acid. After the tenth day it is always clear, and its colour straw-yellow, with usually a neutral reaction.

5. Albumen is frequently present up to the tenth day, but never afterwards.

6. The quality of the urine commonly varies a good deal between the second and tenth days; after this it is more constant.

7. Besides age, the secretion is influenced by body-weight. The absolute quantity for twenty-four hours is in direct ratio, the quantity pro kilogramme is in indirect ratio to the body-weight. On the contrary, both the absolute and the relative quantity of urea and of sodium-chloride are in direct ratio to the body-weight. The specific gravity of the urine and (in the first ten days) the colouring matter are increased with increasing weight.

8. Compared with the secretion of adults, the quantity in proportion to body-weight secreted in twenty-four hours is three and a half or four times greater; while the quantity of the more important urinary constituents, reckoned in the same way, is one and a half to three and a half times less. Of these, the secretion of urea in sucklings is least diminished; that of phosphoric acid most so.— *London Med. Record*, March 15, 1878.

Materia Medica and Therapeutics.

The Action of Lactic Acid.

The discovery of the hypnotic action of chloral, founded as it was upon a chemical study of its decomposition, has led to the attempt to discover other sedatives by *a priori* reasoning. Since lactic acid is a product of muscular action, and muscular action has a sedative effect, it seemed to Preyer probable that lactic acid might be the substance on which this effect of muscular action depended, and that it migit prove, in sufficient doses, a valuable sedative. Its use has been said to have been in a few cases successful, but in a much larger number of cases it has failed. All question of its value should be set at rest by the results of some researches by Dr. A. AUERBACH, of Berlin, who concludes, from a series of careful observations, in which altogether sixty doses were given, that it has no influence whatever. The patients in whom the observations were made were inmates of a lunatic asylum, and care was taken to administer the acid to those who were unused to sedatives as well as those who used hypnotics habitually. It was given both during the daytime and at night, every collateral condition likely to promote sleep, a quiet darkened room being employed when it was given in the daytime. The dose administered varied from 10 to 35 grammes of lactic acid, and 20 to 40 grammes of lactate of soda. In not a single instance could any distinct sedative influence be traced. In one-third of the cases serious intestinal inconveniences were occasioned.—*Lancet,* March 16, 1878.

The Physiological Action of Chlorhydrate of Pilocarpine.

Dr. DEMETRIUS KERIEA has made a series of experiments on chlorhydrate of pilocarpine in M. Constantin Paul's wards. The experiments have demonstrated to him (*Thèse de Paris,* 31st May, 1877, No. 27) the following facts: 1. Used as a subcutaneous injection, chlorhydrate of pilocarpine, in doses of two centigrammes (0.3 grain) and upwards, produces the same physiological effects as jaborandi, of which it is the alkaloid. 2. In much smaller doses, pilocarpine acts also by only inducing diaphoresis, which in certain cases has been replaced by diarrhœa. So soon as doses of from one to two centigrammes are attained, salivation always comes on, but below that dose it is generally absent, and perspiration alone occurs even with doses of two and a half milligrammes (0.04 grain) of chlorhydrate of pilocarpine. Dr. Keriea likewise calls attention, in addition to his own experiments, to those already on pilocarpine by Sidney Ringer, Curschmann, Weber, Bardenhewer, Rosenkrantz, and Scotti.—*Lond. Med. Record,* March 15, 1878.

The Physiological and Therapeutic Action of Cinchonidine.

Dr. FERDINAND COLETTI recalls to remembrance the reasons which have induced experimenters to seek substitutes for the sulphate of quinine, and also the writings relating to the properties of these substances. He then reports a somewhat considerable number of experiments made on his pupils, on himself, and on animals. Fifteen pupils, his assistant, and the writer himself, took for several days 30 to 60 centigrammes (4½ to 9 grains) of sulphate of cinchonidine procured from Messrs. Gehe, of Dresden, and prepared by Messrs. Howard, of London. They made no change in their usual work nor in their way of living. There was no alteration in the temperature or pulse; no head symptoms; only a little headache in two instances. In three cases, there was increase of salivation, without the bitter taste in the mouth usually caused by quinine. There were no gastric troubles; on the contrary, the appetite was increased. The eupeptic action pointed out by Moutard-Martin, Howard, and Rabuteau, is therefore confirmed by these experiments. Afterwards, repeating Laborde and Dupuis' experiments with reference to the epileptogenous properties of sulphate of quinine, quinidine, and cinchonidine, but employing cinchonidine only, M. Coletti obtained convulsive phenomena when clonic, tonic, and tetaniform spasms alternated, but without having the aspect of epileptiform attacks. This substance, administered hypodermically in doses of from forty to sixty centigrammes, subsequently brought on death in four cases out of six. Sulphate of cinchonidine, employed in twenty-four cases of intermittent and symptomatic fever, always had the effect of preventing the attack of the first, and of moderating the temperature or the frequency of the pulse in the second.

The following is a very interesting fact. One of the bitches under experiment was with pup; it aborted an hour and a half after the injection. This fact helps to confirm the opinion of Monteverdi, relative to the ecbolic action of quinine.— *Lond. Med. Record,* March 15, 1878.

The Excretion of Mercury.

E. W. HAMBURGER (*Prager Med. Wochenschrift,* Nos. 4 and 5, 1877, and *Centralblatt für die Medicin Wissenschaften,* July 28) found that the urine contained mercury regularly during the use of inunctions of mercurial ointment, while the milk contained none. When mercury was administered by suppository, the urine and milk both gave evidence of the presence of the drug. He used the electrolytic method of Schneider, after satisfying himself, by experiments, of its usefulness.—*London Med. Record,* March 15, 1878.

The Hypodermic Injection of Chloroform.

M. E. BESNIER has performed hypodermic injections of chloroform with advantage, and without any unpleasant consequences. Some of his colleagues have not been so fortunate, and have an unfavourable opinion of this method. M. DUJARDIN-BEAUMETZ (*Journal de Thérapeutique,* January 25, 1878), though following M. Besnier's instructions in every particular, has often seen superficial sloughing of the skin follow the injection; and when there was no sloughing, he has noticed considerable induration, which disappeared very slowly. The benefit obtained is not very great. Doubtless the pain is relieved, but only at the spot where the injection is made. Thus a patient suffering from tic-douloureux in the face is not relieved by an injection of chloroform in the forearm. There are no general sedative effects, even when a drachm of the drug is used. Similar observations have been made by M. Moutard-Martin, who has seen the eschar occur at some distance from the point of injection rather than at the site of the puncture itself; by M. Edouard Labbé, who says that the injection of chloroform causes pain; by M. Constantin Paul, who has found that the sedative effects do not appear until sometimes two or three hours after injection. It would, therefore, appear that subcutaneous injection of chloroform may be attended with considerable disadvantages, and that it cannot be substituted for injection of morphia in ordinary practice. The latter remains the best means of assuaging pain. Doubtless it sometimes produces some trifling constitutional disturbance, but, as it was justly remarked by some members of the Société de Thérapeutique, these undesirable effects may be very much restricted by associating the morphia with atropia.—*London Med. Record,* March 15, 1878.

Hypodermic Injections of Digitaline.

Dr. GUBLER announced at the meeting of the Paris *Société de Thérapeutique,* on Feb. 13, that, after having made numerous attempts to utilize the active principles of digitalis, he had attained his object. He uses a solution of Homolle and Quevenne's amorphous digitaline, in a mixture of equal parts of water and alcohol; one gramme of which solution contains two milligrammes of digitaline. He injects half a syringeful, that is to say, one milligramme of digitaline, and notes all the effects of digitalis. These injections do not produce any local accidents.— *London Med. Record,* March 15, 1878.

Medicine.

The Use of Salicylate of Soda in the Febrile Diseases of Children.

In an article in the *Correspondenz-Blatt für Schweizer Aerzte*, No. 15, 1877 (*Allgemeine Medicin. Central-Zeitung*, October 10), Dr. HAGENBACH gives the results of the use of salicylate of soda in a large number of cases in the Children's Hospital at Basle. The following quantities have been generally divided into two portions, and given with an interval between them of half an hour or an hour; for children under one year, 15 grains; when between one year and two years, from 22 to 30 grains; for those between three and five years, from 37 to 45 grains; when between six and ten years, from 52 grains to a drachm; when between eleven and fifteen years, from one drachm to 82 grains. The best hour for its administration is five o'clock in the evening. It is seldom given more than once in the twenty-four hours, and when possible it should be taken on an empty stomach. When sweetened with syrup of cinnamon or with liquorice, it is taken much more willingly than quinine; its action, however, is uncertain. Sometimes large doses do not produce the desired results, while in other cases small doses act too powerfully. In diseases attended with continued fever, the first doses appear to produce more decided remissions than the subsequent ones, causing a reduction in temperature from 1.5° to 4° cent. (2.7 to 7.2 Fahr.), as a rule, within three hours after it has been taken. The greatest remission occurs after six hours. With the fall of temperature, there was regularly a diminished frequency of the pulse and of respiration. Unpleasant secondary effects are sometimes produced. Not rarely the medicine is vomited, but if the vomiting do not take place until from one quarter to one half hour after its administration, there often ensues a complete remission notwithstanding. The second dose, given half an hour later, is often retained. Diarrhœa is sometimes produced by its use: it is, however, very transient, and does not leave behind it any serious disturbances of digestion. When there is restlessness, as shown by an anxious countenance, talkativeness, etc., this passes off with the appearance of the remission, and a quiet sleep follows the breaking out of perspiration. Symptoms of collapse are extremely rare. Marked ringing of the ears or deafness never takes place.

Whereas in the treatment of febrile diseases in children, Dr. Hagenbach previously made frequent use of baths, wrapping in wet sheets, and of ice-bladders, in addition to the energetic employment of quinine, it is not now uncommon for weeks to elapse without a single bath being given for the purpose of reducing the temperature. In the severe forms of scarlet fever or of typhoid fever, baths are still resorted to, but in the lighter forms salicylate of soda is always used instead. It is only now and then that, on account of nausea and repeated vomiting, it is found necessary to abandon its use and to resort to quinine.—*London Med. Record,* March 15, 1878.

The Treatment of Variola by Painting with Iodized Glycerine.

Dr. PIOCH (*Lyon Médical,* May 21, 1877) recommends the following treatment which he has successfully practised in an epidemic of smallpox which broke out in a monastic institution under his care. During the first three days, if there be delirium, Dr. Pioch administers quinine and musk. When the eruption is well out and delirium ceases, during the three following days the musk and cinchona are discontinued. Slightly sudorific drinks and slops are given. Towards the end of the seventh day, when the fever, which had subsided, returns under the influence of the maturing of the pustules, Dr. Pioch has the whole surface of the body, commencing with the feet and finishing with the face, painted with a brush dipped in a mixture of three parts of glycerine and one of iodine. At the end of the fourth day of suppuration, the twelfth day of the disorder, when the fever diminishes, the inunction is discontinued and the cure is patiently awaited. Dr. Pioch has had nine bad cases of variola under his care, of which the first, which was not treated with the iodized inunctions, died. The eight other patients, of whom seven had confluent smallpox, went on well to the last stage and were cured in the usual time.—*London Med. Record*, March 15, 1878.

The Treatment of Zona by Topical Applications of Perchloride of Iron.

Dr. AMEDEE MERCIER speaks highly of the good effects of the method first recommended by Dr. Baudon (*Bull. de Thérapeutique*, tome lxiii.), and which was put into practice at the St. Louis Hospital by Dr. Laillier. It consists in painting the zona twice daily with a mixture of 30 grammes of perchloride of iron of the codex, and 10 grammes of alcohol. M. Mercier (*Thèse de Paris*, March 2, p. 7) has arrived at the conclusions that the treatment of zona by topical applications of perchloride of iron gives unvarying results, and that the alcoholic solution should be used in preference to any other.—*London Med. Record*, March 15, 1878.

The Treatment of Diphtheria by the Balsams.

Dr. TROLONG DU RUMAIN has noted, in M. Jules Simon's wards at the Children's Hospital in Paris, the results obtained in the treatment of diphtheria by balsams. The method of Prideau (of Andouillé) has yielded satisfactory results to M. Jules Simon, who thus formulates the treatment. The following medicine should be taken in the course of twenty-four hours: 1. Copaiba, 15 centigrammes; cubebs, 30 centigrammes; subcarbonate of iron, 4 grammes; calcined magnesia, sufficient to solidify the mass. 2. Todd's quinine draught. 3. Coffee, rum, Bordeaux wine. 4. The little patients should be fed up as much as possible. M. Trolong de Rumain, in his *Thèse de Paris*, May, 1877, No. 204, gives the following conclusions: 1. Diphtheria does well with cubebs and copaiba when the child is more than four years old; when it is younger, it is not easy to administer these drugs. 2. It is not asserted that the balsams are a specific for diphtheria, as mercury is a specific for secondary syphilis. 3. Cauterization is of no use if it be superficial, and if it be strong it may bring on disastrous results, inasmuch as they increase the already great debility of the patient. Tonic treatment should infallibly be employed.—*London Med. Record*, March 15, 1878.

Carbolated Camphor in Diphtheria.

M. SOULEZ employs carbolated camphor in the treatment of diphtheria; the false membrane seems to lose its inherent vitality, and no inflammatory effects follow. M. Sonlez dissolves camphor in crystallized carbolic acid, which has itself been dissolved in a very small quantity of alcohol—nine grammes of carbolic acid to one gramme of alcohol. He uses it either alone, or mixed with an equal weight of oil of sweet almonds.—*British Med. Journal*, March 16, 1878.

Reversed Writing in Brain-Disease.

In the *Berliner Klinische Wochenschrift* for January 7, Dr. BUCHWALD reports three cases illustrative of mirror-writing (Spiegelschrift), and makes several observations on the subject.

While much attention has recently been paid to the symptoms of aphasia in cases of hemiplegia, very little notice has been taken of the various degrees of agraphia, which are often also present. The latter are important, because it frequently happens that when the power of speech is quite lost, a true estimate of the mental condition of the patient can only be formed by means of his writing, and even when the power of speech is partially retained valuable information may still be derived from his written language. Mirror-writing, that is to say, from right to left, which only corresponds to ordinary writing when seen in a mirror, must frequently be observed in patients suffering from right hemiplegia, but, as far as the author is aware, has nowhere been put upon record.

The first case was observed two years ago. A workman, aged 45, had had an ordinary apoplectic attack, which left him with right hemiplegia; a mixed form of aphasia was present; his right hand was useless for the purpose of writing, and when asked to write with the left he wrote his name uncommonly well from right to left in mirror-writing; figures from 1 to 7 were written in the same way. When his attention was drawn to the fact of his writing being reversed, he could not for some time be induced to write from left to right; when, however, his name and some figures properly written were put before him as a copy, he managed to imitate some of them, though not nearly so well as he had written in the reverse direction; he was also continually going back to his mirror-writing. He eventually succeeded in writing the figures 1, 2, 4, 6, 8, 9, correctly, but 3, 5, and 7 were always reversed. If small sums in multiplication, correctly written, were given him to do, he constantly put the result down in mirror-writing. No disturbances of vision were present, but alexia was so in a high degree. After six months' treatment at the Klinik at Breslau the aphasia, agraphia, and alexia had gradually improved, but the tendency to reverse writing still remained; it was still a great effort to the patient to copy writing from left to right; he thought it impossible to write any other way than from right to left with the left hand. If he assisted his right hand, which had now regained some power, with his left, he wrote some things correctly and others not. The figure 5 was most difficult to him; even with the right hand he always wrote it reversed or partially so. The patient was removed to a workhouse, and the same symptoms with regard to his spoken and written language persist, except that, having gained a little more power in the right hand, he is able to write rather more correctly with the help of his left.

The second case was that of a woman, the widow of a mason. In consequence of aortic and mitral insufficiency, she had an attack of cerebral embolism; right hemiplegia and a high degree of mixed aphasia were the result. When called upon to write with the left hand, it appeared at first that she was producing meaningless scribble, but it was afterwards found that the few first letters of her name could be easily made out in mirror-writing.

The third patient was under the care of Dr. Berger. He was a fruiterer, aged 39, who had cerebral embolism following aortic disease. The right hemiplegia and aphasia have almost disappeared; the patient, who shows no disturbance of intellect, writes his name, figures, etc., as far as his agraphia permits him, with the left hand, in reversed characters; with the right he writes correctly. This patient also said that he could not write any other way than from right to left with the left hand; his tendency to reversed writing lasted many months, and was exhibited at a meeting of a medical society.

How far is this symptom constant in right hemiplegia, how is it to be explained, and of what practical value is it?

On looking over the records of the Klinik, the author found that no tendency to mirror-writing had existed in cases where the paralysis and aphasia had been of slight degree, not when they had been of short duration, as in syphilitic disease.

A considerable number of healthy persons of various ages and degrees of education were caused to write their names, figures, and other words with their left hands ; the following was the result. Most of the children said at first that it was impossible to write with the left hand at all, while the greater number of the adults, especially the most intelligent and observant, wrote, or tried to write correctly from left to right. A large number, especially children, wrote, apparently unconsciously, mirror-writing with the left hand as well and as easily as ordinary writing with the right. When the reversed appearance of the writing was pointed out to them they were at first astonished, and then said that was the only possible way of writing with the left hand ; on being induced, however, to try to write from left to right with the left hand, they were successful in doing so, but the ordinary writing was not nearly so good as the reversed. One little girl, aged 11, who very slowly and with great care had succeeded in writing her name correctly but very badly with the left hand, was asked to write it quickly, and at once wrote it in mirror-writing much better than she had previously done it from left to right, although she had never practised reversed writing.

There is, therefore, in a great number of persons, especially children, a tendency to make, in writing with the left hand, movements analogous to those made in ordinary writing by the right hand, and consequently to produce reversed writing ; this latter is very easy to many, whereas the contrary movements are performed with difficulty. The same difficulty is observed in beginners learning to play the piano. This tendency to making analogous movements with the two hands can, both in writing and piano-playing, be overcome by care and practice.

In the case of paralyzed patients, the degree of intelligence, and the power of concentrating the attention play an important part. Berger observed no single case of reversed writing among patients belonging to the upper classes. If the paralytic attack be slight or of short duration, the tendency to reversed writing does not come on, at any rate not as a result of disease. When the patient's general condition and his affection of speech, etc., improve, his powers of observation become greater or are more easily awakened, and he is able to overcome the tendency, especially if it was not present in any great degree before the attack ; this latter point can, however, seldom be ascertained. The physician is thus enabled, in cases of right hemiplegia, by means of the patient's written language, to obtain valuable information as to the condition of the psychic functions ; he will also find that complete agraphia is not always present, although the apparently illegible writings of the patient may have led to that belief. Mirror-writing in these cases takes the place of ordinary writing ; and the examination of it has a certain practical value.—*London Med. Record*, March 15, 1878.

The Telegraphic Writers' Cramp.

In March, 1875, M. Onimus read a paper to the Société de Biologie (*Monthly Abstract of Medical Sciences*, June, 1875, page 249), in which he called attention to a form of functional spasm observed in telegraph *employés*, and which they themselves have named the *mal télégraphique*. We have never understood that this form of spasm has been met with among telegraphic writers in this country ; but M. Onimus, in another communication read at a recent meeting of the Biological Society (*Gaz. des Hôp.* and *Gaz. Hebdom.*, March 16) states that he has had many additional opportunities of observing such cases. It is chiefly observed in those engaged in the manipulation of Morse's machine, and seems to arise from the difficulty of co-ordinating the motions which are required alternately for the formation of the dots and the dashes. Much depends upon individual temperament and the condition of the nervous system, as the existence of more or less irritability seems quite as necessary for the production of this cramp as the frequent repetition of the same movements. Some *employés* who are naturally nervous and excitable have the cramp after only a short time of service, their general health suffering at the same time. The same circumstances operate in writers' cramp, this especially occurring when a great number of letters or dispatches have to be executed in a given time under a state of feverish activity. The direction of the movements also exerts an influence. An *employé* successively employed the thumb, the index, and the median finger, each of these manipulating during two or three months, but one after the other then being seized with the cramp. He then used his wrist, which after a while also refused service. As the expeditionary dispatches are manipulated by a movement of the entire hand as well as of the fingers from above downwards, when these vertical movements had become difficult an *employé* contrived a means of acting on the lever in a horizontal direction by means of a thread stretched from a point of support to the lever. For a while he was able to forward his dispatches, but these new movements soon became embarrassed, and gave rise to the cramps. It seems that an *employé* of a medium skilfulness transmits or receives alternately about 7000 signals in an hour, making for the day of seven hours a total of about 49,000 signals. Under penalty of causing the receiver of the dispatch to commit an error, the movements of the manipulator must be cadenced with perfect regularity. The transmission has also to be marked by periods of arrest of a conventional duration, being longer between each word than between each letter of the same word, and than between each signal of the same letter. "Taking, for example, my name," says Dr. Onimus, "a simple difference of the period of arrest may cause it to be read Otémus, Otonus, Obmus, Onittus, and Otcittus. According to the calculation of a very skilful *employé* who has communicated these details to me, the mere defective transmission of the ' *é* ' may cause the gambling (*tronquer*) of the word *référé* in 447 different manners. Besides the muscular contraction, the transmission occasions consequently at the same time great fatigue from the constant mental tension which it exacts."

The symptoms of the affection are more easily and more rapidly produced in women. The general symptoms consist principally in palpitations, vertigo, sleeplessness, perhaps impairment of vision (most of the older and laborious *employés* wearing spectacles), and a sense of constriction opposite the nape of the neck, seeming to hold the back part of the head in a vice. This sensation is not uncommon in men of business rendered ill or over-excited in important transactions in commerce, and it is especially met with when attempts are made to force intellectual functions that are already fatigued. To a state of over-excitement succeeds one of depression and melancholy, and moral and physical atony. Memory becomes bad, and according to some, insanity may in the course of some years supervene on this pathological condition. During the progress of this pathological state the transmission of dispatches presents some curious peculiarities, dependent on reflex movements produced by habit and in an unconscious manner. The hand does not always obey the determinations of the will; a word badly read is often correctly transmitted. On the other hand, an *employé* whose mode of transmission is naturally slow is not always, when dozing, interrupted in transmitting to the correspondent the ideas accompanying his half-dreamy state, for he continues to act on the lever and expedite his dispatches. In some cases there exists, too, a state of things quite the opposite of spasm and rigidity, for the hand proceeds more rapidly than the will, and performs a series of movements which are co-ordinated and decipherable, but too rapid. It is especially after the manipulation has lasted for some time that these phenomena may be produced.

Nor mally. it is only after an hour of work that the manipulation attains its maximum of rapidity.—*Med. Times and Gaz.*, March 23, 1878.

An Early Symptom of Tabes Dorsalis.[1]

In the year 1871, Professor C. WESTPHAL first observed that muscular contractions could be caused by striking certain tendons. Since then he has paid considerable attention to this phenomenon in the most various nervous diseases. In tabes dorsalis the ligamentum patellæ appeared to be of most interest. If this ligament be struck in a healthy man, while the knee is flexed at a right angle, or nearly so, a sudden contraction of the extensor muscles on the front of the thigh may always be felt. If the leg be hanging loose, a sudden extension of the leg is seen as a result of this contraction. This reaction, named by Dr. Westphal "knee phenomenon," or "leg phenomenon," can be produced in any healthy person. It is entirely absent, however, as the author has previously shown, in cases of tabes dorsalis, in which the well-known symptoms of ataxia and disturbances of sensation, with or without affections of the cerebral nerves, are fully developed, and in which gray degeneration of the posterior columns of the cord can be certainly diagnosed. This observation has been confirmed by Professor Erb and Dr. O. Berger.

The question to which the author addresses himself in the present paper is, whether the knee-phenomenon is not already absent before the characteristic symptoms of tabes dorsalis are developed; also whether this absence may not therefore in some cases afford material aid in forming an otherwise difficult or impossible diagnosis. The diagnosis of tabes, in its earlier stages, is as difficult as it is easy in its later developments. According to Westphal's recent observations, the absence of the knee-phenomenon in the earlier stages of tabes is a diagnostic point of great value.

Many cases of tabes begin with severe pains of certain definite character (shooting, lancinating, etc.) in the lower limbs. These pains have been regarded by many, especially French authors, as quite characteristic. But it is difficult for patients, especially the uneducated, to describe their pains accurately. The pains, moreover, are not always of the kind described, but sometimes closely resemble rheumatic pains. True neuralgic pains in the lower limbs, quite similar to those occurring in tabes, are not at all uncommon; they occur periodically, first at long and then at shorter intervals, last many years, and, apart from other symptoms, are not to be distinguished from the eccentric pains of commencing tabes.

In a number of such cases, in which the pains in the lower limbs were the only symptoms of disease, Westphal has found the knee-phenomenon to be entirely absent, and has therefore diagnosed tabes dorsalis. One case was especially interesting, owing to the phenomenon being absent upon one side only. A woman, aged 36, suffered from shooting pains in both lower extremities, but those in the left were incomparably worse than those in the right. Hyperæsthesia of the skin was also present in the left limb. During many months the knee-phenomenon was completely absent on the left side, but it could always be unmistakably though not strongly produced on the right side. The patient's gait was unaffected, except by the pain during a paroxysm, and her muscular sense appeared normal. Still there was no doubt as to the diagnosis, for there was already advanced white atrophy of the optic nerves, inequality of the pupils, and frequent micturition. This case is an example of the failing of the knee-phenomenon in

[1] Berliner Klinische Wochenschrift, January 8, 1877.

an unmistakable ease of tabes dorsalis, before the development of ataxia or any
degree of failure of sensation.

Westphal considers the diagnosis of commencing tabes justifiable in any ease,
in which the characteristic pains in the lower limbs are present and the knee-
phenomenon is absent. The converse, however, is not so certain; the presence
of the knee-phenomenon in a case presenting the peculiar pains in the lower
extremities would not justify the conclusion that these were not of a tabic nature.
But if the pains had lasted many years, and the knee-phenomenon could still be
produced, it would at least be very unlikely that tabes was present.

Sufficient evidence is not yet at the author's disposal for him to state what
diagnostic value is to be ascribed to the presence or absence of the knee-phenomenon in cases of tabes, which commence with affections of certain cerebral nerves
—e. g., the optic nerves or the nerves supplying the muscles of the eyeball.
One case having reference to this point is, however, related. A gentleman, aged
40, had first diplopia, and then a disturbance of sensation in the fingers, first of
the right and then of the left hand. The knee-phenomenon could not be produced after many and careful trials; no other motor or sensory affection was
present; the patient was certainly not syphilitic. Westphal thinks it very
probable that this was a case of commencing tabes, but cannot speak with certainty. ' The unusual appearance of the sensory symptoms first in the upper extremities, in no wise contradicts this supposition, as it does sometimes occur in
tabes. Still more interesting is the question whether the absence of the knee-
phenomenon in a case of white atrophy of the optic nerve would justify the diagnosis of commencing tabes, because white atrophy so frequently occurs as an
independent disease. Ophthalmic surgeons are the only persons who have sufficient opportunities for making observations numerous enough to solve this question.

It happens sometimes that ataxia of the lower limbs is present, and yet that
the knee-phenomenon can be produced. It may be taken as certain that, in
these cases, gray degeneration of the entire length of the posterior columns is not
present, or, at any rate, that it does not extend into the lumbar region. This
condition often occurs after acute febrile diseases, and its course is quite different
from that of tabes dorsalis.

The symptom in question seems to be of the greatest value in certain cases of
hypochondria, which are difficult to distinguish from some forms of commencing
tabes. There are cases of tabes in which the peculiar pains are, from the first,
absent, or in which their place is taken by vague sensations, difficult to describe,
such as feelings of weight, creeping, cold, or as if parts of the body were dead or
asleep. All these are similar to the complaints of hypochondriacs. Some tabic
patients will describe a feeling of constriction round the waist, or a sensation of
sinking in the abdomen in just the same way as a hypochondriac. A weakness
of the bladder and diminished sexual power are also not uncommon in hypochondria. The difficulty of the case is increased by the fact that well-marked cases
of tabes are not unfrequently complicated with hypochondriasis. If, in a case
presenting the above symptoms, the knee-phenomenon cannot be produced after
careful trial, tabes dorsalis may be safely diagnosed.

It is thus seen that the absence of the knee-phenomenon is a valuable early
symptom of tabes. It is more useful than Romberg's test as to the ability to
stand still with closed eyes, in that the latter is not developed until the later
stages of the disease, when the diminution of sensation in the lower limbs is
usually evident. It must be remembered, however, that it is, after all, only one
symptom, and its significance must be estimated in conjunction with others, for
there are motor affections of the lower limbs (e. g., certain spinal paralyses, with

loss of faradic excitability of the muscles) in which the knee-phenomenon cannot be produced, although gray degeneration of the posterior columns would certainly not be diagnosed.

The value of this symptom would be greatly diminished if it could be shown that in some persons, with the patella, etc., normally placed, the knee-phenomenon could not be produced in health. Such individual peculiarities may exist, but the author has never met with one among large numbers of healthy persons whom he has examined. A percussion-hammer is the best instrument with which to strike the ligamentum patellæ. In some cases only circumscribed portions of the ligament are sensitive enough to cause the reaction. In doubtful cases the knee should be bared, and should be struck very carefully and as elastically as possible. It is also necessary to see that the patient does not keep his extensor muscles voluntarily contracted.

A hope is expressed by the author that the earlier diagnosis of this afterwards well-nigh incurable disease may possibly lead to a more effective treatment of it. —*London Med. Record*, March 15, 1878.

—

The Treatment of Chronic Throat-Catarrh with Nitrate of Silver.

Dr. Dawosky lays down the proposition (*Betz's Memorabilien*, vol. xxii. part 12) that in the treatment of diseases of mucous membranes, where external applications are possible, nitrate of silver is a remedy useful before all others. Brought into contact with a mucous surface, it coagulates the mucus; and if applied in excess, it unites chemically with the tissue of the membrane beneath, forming a more or less thick crust. If the nitrate be applied to an actively secreting mucous membrane, it first irritates the distended bloodvessels and capillaries, and also stimulates their contractility, so that they unload themselves and cause an onward flow of the blood accumulated in them. Hence it becomes necessary to the efficient use of nitrate of silver to form an accurate estimate of the quantity to be applied in each case, and also that it should be applied by the physician himself. In chronic throat-catarrh, we have a congested condition of the mucous membrane, and a consequent abundant secretion, with swelling and redness occurring in unequally distributed patches. If these patches become denuded of epithelium, they appear yet more deeply reddened. In such cases, the nitrate should not be applied otherwise than in a solution of definite strength. It is convenient to have a concentrated solution, which may then be diluted with water or glycerine. After applying it with a brush to the affected parts, these should be painted over with a solution of glycerine, and the application is repeated so long as there is any swelling, unhealthy secretion, etc. At the same time, the food and drink taken should be cold, and smoking discontinued. Should the larynx be also affected, it should be brushed with the caustic solution, of a strength of 1 to 8, repeated three or four times a day. A large number of cases of laryngeal catarrh thus treated, have uniformly yielded the best results.—*London Med. Record*, March 15, 1878.

—

Hysterical Paralysis of the Vocal Cords.

Professor Gerhardt has recently published a brief paper on "Hysterical Paralysis of the Vocal Cords," or, as it is generally termed, functional aphonia. During a term of five years twenty cases of this affection presented themselves at his Clinique. Of these, fourteen were between 15 and 25 years of age, and six ranged from 25 to 40 years. The majority of these patients were in poor health, having suffered previously from chlorosis, articular rheumatism, and throat affections of different kinds. In several of the cases aphonia was developed in patients who were suffering from other diseases, and it is supposed that the imitative habit so strongly marked in some forms of hysteria was the predisposing cause. The peculiar feature of hysterical aphonia, and which at the same time determines its cerebral origin, is that the voice retains its normal character during the performance of certain functions. Two of Professor Gerhardt's were able to sing a song in a loud, melodious voice, but they could only articulate the text in a whisper. The fact that a clear resonant cough is coupled with an aphonic voice is also a characteristic of the disease, and serves to differentiate it from ulceration of the cords, multiple papillomata, and paralysis of the cords from pressure upon the pneumogastrics. In hysterical aphonia a peculiar disturbance of the sensibility of the larynx and pharynx is often observed. This generally manifests itself in an intense anæsthesia of the upper respiratory passages, although hyperæsthesia is also occasionally noticed. At the same time the reaction upon electrical irritation is generally unimpaired, although there are some cases in which the application of even very strong currents of electricity does not succeed in producing muscular contractions. Professor Gerhardt does not endorse the opinion, sometimes advanced, that hysterical patients do not wish to speak loud for fear of pain and inconvenience, and disproves this assertion by the assertion that, (1) The paralysis of the cords is generally more marked on one side than on the other; (2) Other symptoms of paralysis of the pneumogastrics are also noticed. Among them may be mentioned the increased frequency of the pulse-beats, unaccompanied by a corresponding rise in the temperature. Of the twenty cases spoken of by Professor Gerhardt, three are still under treatment. Of the others, four were discharged as incurable. One of these had her voice restored for a few hours every time that she indulged in a hearty fit of laughter. Of the fourteen cases cured, one was relieved by the simple introduction of the laryngeal mirror, two by percutaneous galvanization, the others by faradization alone or alternating with Dr. Oliver's plan of compression of the larynx, or by the use of the galvanic current. All of these cases go to prove that recent attacks are speedily cured by the application of faradism, while older cases, and especially those which have frequently relapsed, rarely regain their voice permanently even after the persistent use of the faradic current. The author thinks that some cases of so-called hysterical aphonia may be classed as reflex paralysis, as stated by Phillipaux and Bresgen, who say that aphonia, coincident with hypertrophy of the tonsils, can only be relieved after the removal of the enlarged glands.— *Medical Examiner*, April 4, 1878.

Abscess of the Lung.

In a paper read before the Berlin Medical Society (*Allgem. Medicin. Central-Zeitung*, Nov. 7, 1877) Dr. LEYDEN calls attention to the rarity of pulmonary abscess, and to the liability of its being confounded with pulmonary gangrene and subacute tuberculosis of the lungs (cheesy pneumonia). Traube has referred to the diagnostic importance of an examination of the sputum, and states that in it microscopic shreds of lung-tissue might be recognized, containing elastic fibres, black pigment, and occasional rust-coloured crystals. In gangrene, however, the shreds of pulmonary tissue are readily torn, and elastic tissue is not present, and in pulmonary tuberculosis there are no shreds. It was Traube's view that the abscess developed from pneumonia was preceded by an extensive destruction of tissue. Leyden admits that pulmonary abscess and gangrene are not sharply defined, but run into each other, and yet the recognition of the simple healthy suppuration is of the greatest importance. He considers that there are three varieties of pulmonary abscess:—

1. Abscesses perforating the air-passage from without.

2. True pulmonary abscesses which include those due to pneumonia ; also the embolic and metastatic forms, and those resulting from injury to the lung, and from the penetration of foreign bodies.

3. Chronic pulmonary abscesses, such as form in chronic pneumonia, but distinct from the tuberculous cavity.

True pulmonary abscess begins with symptoms of acute pneumonia. This does not terminate critically on the seventh or ninth day, but the fever increases, the expectoration is retained, till, in the course of three weeks, an abundant purulent sputum appears, with alleviation of all the symptoms. This sputum is of very great diagnostic importance. It is profuse, frothy, purulent, and liquid, of a stale indifferent odour, although the latter may temporarily be sweet and penetrating. Shreds of lung-tissue are seen, as well as others to be seen with the microscope. They are imbedded in thick yellow pus, are of a grayish-black or yellow-ochre colour, and vary much in size. These particles contain abundant elastic tissue, at times portions of large vessels, a moderate quantity of black pigment, crystals of fat (small, pedicellate, globular forms), delicate hæmatoidine (bilirubine) crystals of an ochre-yellow or rust colour. The latter crystals were always observed, though they might be few or many, and were in the form of rhombic plates or of bundles of needles. Coarse granular micrococci are present; either motionless or moving slowly, and differ widely from the active rod-like bacteria of pulmonary gangrene. They are not acted upon by iodine, and thus differ from the leptothrix forms in gangrene. Pus corpuscles and pulmonary epithelium are also found.

In the chronic pulmonary abscess, the sputa are purulent or muco-purulent in character. They contain elastic fibres, which are evident on microscopical examination ; also occasional small, dense, slate-coloured portions of lung-tissue of a fibrous appearance. Plates of cholesterine also are often seen ; likewise fatty and mucous corpuscles, the latter often containing granules of fat.—*London Med. Record*, March 15, 1878.

—

Pneumatic Treatment of Aortic Regurgitation.

Dr. FENOGLIO, Assistant in the Turin Medical Clinic, reports (*Centralblatt Med. Wiss.*, No. 46, 1877) three cases of aortic regurgitation which he treated successfully by the pneumatic method, the patients being made to expire into rarefied air. In each case there was excessive action of the hypertrophied left ventricle, and the treatment was directed to diminish the tension in the arteries, and increase the amount of blood in the lungs, and hence to remove the feeling of palpitation and subjective arterial pulsation, as well as the sensations of anxiety and thoracic oppression which the patients experienced—all these symptoms being in the main the result of the excessive compensatory action of the left ventricle. Sphygmographic tracings of the pulse showed that the height of the pulse-wave was lowered by the treatment, that the line of descent became less abrupt, and the previous dicrotism less distinct. This effect and the general improvement in the condition of the patients became more decided and more permanent at each sitting, and in one of the three cases the improvement continued a month after the patient had been discharged. The treatment lasted from fifteen to twenty-five days, with one sitting per diem. To sum up, Dr. Fenoglio's experience convinces him that "in cases of aortic insufficiency with excessive action of the hypertrophied left ventricle—that is to say, in the greater number of the cases of this aortic lesion which come under treatment—expiration into rarefied air is an effective therapeutic method." Naturally, the "cure" requires to be repeated from time to time.—*Med. Times and Gazette*, March 16, 1878.

Thrombosis of a Coronary Artery.

M. LAVERAN (*L' Union Médicale*, Feb. 23, 1878) reports a case of infarctus of the heart following thrombosis of a coronary artery. The following is a summary of his paper.

R., male, unmarried, was admitted November 7th, 1877, with orthopnœa and hæmoptysis. A month previously he caught cold, followed by cough, which did not keep him in bed; five days before admission he felt a severe pain in the side, which he could not precisely localize, but which had disappeared at the time of admission; at the same time his respiration became embarrassed, which speedily increased to orthopnœa. On November 8th he was sitting up in bed, breathing rapidly; his nose, lips, and ends of the toes and fingers were cyanosed; there was no œdema of the lower limbs; the percussion-sound of the chest was normal; there were mucous râles at the base of the left lung; the impulse of the heart was forcible; the area of dulness was increased; the heart-sounds were muffled, distant; no murmur; the heart's action was rapid; the pulse was frequent, compressible, irregular; the sputa were blood-stained. The diagnosis was pericarditis. He died on November 22d. The only changes to be noted were diminution in the audibility of the heart-sound; increase of the râles over the chest, hæmoptysis, and dyspnœa as the fatal termination was approached.

The necropsy was made on November 24th. There was no anasarca present. The pleural cavities were dry. The left lung was adherent above and behind. There were numerous hemorrhagic infarcts in both lungs; the pulmonary tissue was infiltrated with blood; there was no cavity filled with liquid blood or clots; the pulmonary vessels, whether near the hemorrhagic foci or not, were obliterated by old clots; blood was found in the trachea and bronchi. The pericardium was dry; there were no adhesions, no false membranes. There was a milk spot on the anterior surface of the heart. The heart was very large, measuring 17 centimetres (6⅔ inches) from the base of the ventricles to the apex, 14 centimetres (5½ inches) at the base of ventricles; when empty, its weight was 930 grammes (about 2 lbs. 1 oz.). Both ventricles were full of black clotted blood; the left ventricle occupied four-fifths of the area of a transverse section; the maximum thickness of the muscle of the left ventricle was three to four centimetres. A yellowish white patch, extruding through nearly the whole thickness of the myocardium, occupied the left border of the heart; the myocardium was elsewhere healthy, not fatty. Some white, fibrinous, tolerably resistant clots were found in the right auricle. On inspecting the inner surface of the left ventricle, after removing the clots, numerous pale patches were visible, on scraping which a brownish semi-liquid matter escaped; the whitish patch seen externally formed part of the peripheral zone of these abscesses of the heart; there were dots of ecchymotic redness on the pale patches. The aorta was dilated and slightly atheromatous; the valves were incompetent; there was a calcareous plate as large as a lentil at the base of one of the cusps, which prevented its complete extension. The segments of the mitral valve were indurated in places; their function was apparently normal. There was no lesion of the orifices of the right heart. The posterior coronary artery presented some atheromatous patches, but was permeable. The anterior coronary artery was permeable in the first part of its course, but notably enlarged; there were many atheromatous patches on its inner surface; at the part corresponding to the middle of the ventricle the artery was completely obliterated, felt like a round, hard cord, and contained a hard, white, ramified, evidently old, clot. The arterial wall at the seat of the thrombus was very atheromatous. The diseased parts of the myocardium corresponded exactly to the obliterated vessel. The liver was nutmeggy; the spleen small and hard. The kidneys were slightly granular. The cerebral arteries were atheromatous.—*London Med. Record*, March 15, 1878.

Diagnosis of Thrombotic Occlusion of One of the Coronary Arteries.

Dr. A. HAMMER, Professor of Surgery at St. Louis, at present at Vienna, publishes in the *Wiener Medicinische Wochenschrift* (February 2) an account of a case in which the above condition was diagnosed, and verified by post-mortem examination. The man, 34 years old, strongly built, had for the past year suffered from slight attacks of articular rheumatism, but no valvular affection of the heart had occurred. For four weeks previously to his being seen by Dr. Hammer, a very sharp attack of acute rheumatism had existed, but had gradually improved, and convalescence was proceeding. One day he got out of bed, and sat in an easy chair. In about an hour he suddenly collapsed, his pulse was 40, his lips pale and a little cyanotic; there was slight dyspnœa, but no pain. Five hours later his pulse beat only 23 to the minute, four hours later 16 to the minute; and when Dr. Hammer arrived (the previous observations having been made by the family medical attendant) the pulse was only 8 to the minute, a cardiac contraction occurring every eight seconds. There were no symptoms or signs of disease in the nervous or respiratory systems; percussion of the precordia showed no abnormal dulness. On auscultating the heart, the sounds were not accompanied or replaced by any murmur, but following them there was a tremor of the heart perceptible to the ear, conveying the idea of a clonic spasm, which lasted five seconds, the cardic sounds occupying one second, and the spasm being followed by two seconds of absolute rest. These phenomena were followed for twenty minutes, and were quite regular and without variation. Examination of the abdominal viscera and of the cervical region gave negative results. In arriving at his diagnosis Dr. Hammer was able to exclude fatty degeneration and enfeeblement of the heart by the physical signs, although perhaps at present we are not in a position to define exactly the signs of these affections. Alterations of innervation, he says, were contraindicated by the absence of all evidence of change in the central nervous organs, or in the cervical nerves; of an acute infectious disease there was no evidence; the percussion of the heart and the examination of the thorax generally negatived the idea of any altered relations of pressure or of any organic affection of the heart such as myocarditis, endocarditis, hypertrophy, atrophy, or valvular disease. The striking feature in the case was the suddenness of the collapse, which pointed to a sudden interference with the nutrition of the heart, possibly to thrombotic occlusion of the coronary arteries; further consideration convinced him that, though this was probable, only one artery could have been occluded, or the heart would have come to a stop altogether, while the regular tumultuous heart-spasm of five seconds' duration pointed to a one-sided affection. The affected side acted as a dead weight to the organ, and impeded the movements of the sound half; but whether the affected side was right or left no conjecture seemed possible. Dr. Hammer accordingly made his diagnosis, much to the astonishment of his colleague. The patient died nineteen hours afterwards; and, leave to make a partial examination of the body having with difficulty been obtained, the thorax was opened. The lungs were engorged and œdematous; the pericardium contained half an ounce of clear serum; the heart was of normal size and appearance, and lay in its proper position, fully distended. Its surface was smooth and shining, and, except a layer of fat in the coronary sulci, there was no trace of fatty or other infiltration. On removing the heart, they found the right auricle and ventricle full of clot, the cavities and valves normal; the muscular wall and endocardium were also normal. The left side of the heart was equally so, except the aortic valves. In these latter the most striking appearance was the distension of the right cusp by a mass which nearly filled the right sinus of Valsalva, and was of a hemispherical shape. The superficial layers of this mass, followed into the coronary artery, were recent coagulated, yellowish-white blood-clots, but downwards from the coronary artery the clot became darker, drier, and finally of a gray-reddish colour. From the lowest layer a fine thread about an inch long passed, to become connected with the new growths about to be described. The aortic valves were not thickened, but the hinder cusp was united to the right and left cusps at their commissures for a short distance. Involving these attachments and the three-cornered part of the wall of the aorta immediately subjacent, were fresh, soft, whitish excrescences, which, with the slight adhesion of the valves, caused a partial stenosis of the aortic orifice. From the apex of one of these vegetations situated between the posterior and right cusps there was a slender prolongation, which was continuous with the fine thread-like process from the clot in the sinus of Valsalva.

Dr. Hammer says he has not been able to meet with an account of such a case in literature, nor has he found that the great clinicists, Bamberger and Kussmaul, with whom he has discussed the case, have had any similar experiences.—*Lond. Med. Record*, March 15, 1878.

Treatment of Gastralgia by the Internal Stomach-Douche, etc.

Dr. MALBRANC, of Naples, has published in the *Berliner Klinische Wochenschrift* for January 28 an article on the treatment of gastralgia by the stomach-douche. D., a governess, aged 22, suffered three years ago for several months from stomach-derangement without any apparent cause, presenting symptoms of a gastric ulcer. Under treatment, she recovered and continued well until four months ago, when she began again to suffer from general weakness, and neuralgia, chiefly of the face. She gradually became much reduced, and after a time digestion again became disordered, with constipated bowels. Ten weeks before she came under notice these symptoms were aggravated, and were accompanied by a fixed pain immediately below the ensiform cartilage, by acute tenderness in the dorsal region, frequent palpitation, and a sense of constriction of the throat. The appetite failed entirely, the little food taken was returned, and there was some blood in the stools. Various means, sinapisms, ice-pills, applications of extract of belladonna, etc., were tried, but in vain. The paroxysms of pain which came on from three to four hours after each meal were relieved by hypodermic injections of morphia; but in spite of nutrient enemata and faradization of the epigastrium the patient only became rather worse, so that mental emotions and straining at stool were enough to bring on the gastric pain. She now came under the care of Professor Kussmaul in Strasburg, whose assistant Dr. Malbranc then was. A regulated diet failed to afford relief. The following treatment was therefore adopted. In the morning a quantity, amounting in the end to 2 to 3 litres (3½ to 5¼ pints) of tepid water, aerated with carbonic acid in the manner of soda-water, was injected by means of an elastic tube into the stomach, and after a while again drawn off. The stomach was thus washed out every day. Under this treatment the patient improved, so that in three weeks' time she was able to take a varied diet of meat and bread. The injections of morphia were gradually diminished in frequency, but were still required for the relief of the gastric pain, which always recurred when an attempt was made to evacuate the bowels. To relieve these pains and improve the state of the bowels, one pole of a battery was introduced into the stomach several hours after breakfast, while the other electrode was passed successively over all the abdominal muscles, and thus a powerful induction-current was daily passed for five minutes through the stomach and abdominal walls. Within the next following days, defecation became perfectly natural and painless. In a month, the patient recovered completely under the continued use of the stomach-douche and of internal faradization, and was able to resume active employment. She has continued well ever since.

With reference to the question of the *modus operandi* of the douche with warm water holding carbonic acid in solution, the following points come under consideration.

1. The stomach is unloaded by the douche, and is thus enabled to recover its contractility. In all gastralgiæ occurring in consequence of overloading of the stomach, as frequently happens in typical cases of dilatation of the stomach, this emptying the viscus of its contents is a sure means of relief.

2. The removal of acid or acrid matter and the cleansing of the mucous surfaces by means of Vichy or other alkaline water. It is often important in cases of gastric dilatation, when large quantities of half-digested food are apt to accumulate, thus to cleanse the coat of the stomach of acid, perhaps fermenting mucus. This can only be done effectually in the morning, and when the stomach is yet empty. Not only is digestion thus facilitated, but the formation of large quantities of flatus, which is productive of pain and distress, is prevented.

3. Warmth thus locally applied to the inner surface of the stomach has a soothing influence, diminishing irritability of the gastric nerves and relaxing muscular spasm. To this is due the utility of a daily morning draught of warm water in certain cases of painful irritable dyspepsia. But the cases in which the warm douche is likely to be attended with benefit must be carefully distinguished from those in which it is inadmissible, owing to extensive ulceration and the tendency to hemorrhage. Closely analogous is the effect of injections of warm water *per anum* in certain forms of intestinal colic, especially lead-colic, in restoring the regular normal peristaltic movement of the bowels. Indeed, it is found that the warm stomach-douche is eminently successful in overcoming the constipation which is a frequent symptom in nearly all cases of gastric disorder.

4. The mechanical impact of the stream of water on the coats of the stomach stimulates the vaso-motor nerves, and so excites a healthy capillary circulation. Moreover, a healthy peristaltic movement of the stomach can often be excited by gently kneading the stomach with the open hand, after somewhat distending it with warm water. This has the effect also of completely cleansing the large rugæ which generally exist in the interior of large flabby stomachs.

5. The carbonic acid held in solution by the injected water acts as a direct sedative on the irritable gastric mucous membrane, and also tends to promote intestinal peristaltic action.

The introduction of the stomach-tube itself need in reality present no greater difficulty than the passing of a catheter into the bladder. The following points should be attended to

1. Before introducing the tube, we should measure off on it and mark the distance from the mouth to a point opposite the ensiform cartilage of the sternum. We thus insure the tube passing, when introduced, to a distance of one or two inches beyond the cardiac end of the œsophagus, and no further, and so avoid all risk of injuring or perforating the coats of the stomach.

2. It is a source of comfort to the patient to be able to grasp the tube with his teeth, whereby it is steadied, and also the amount of salivation and the tendency to retching are reduced. For this purpose, a notched bone or ivory slide should be passed over the tube for the patient to bite upon.

3. The tube should be rendered flexible by immersion in warm water, and oiled, previously to its introduction.

4. The patient should sit in as erect a position as possible, with the head bent backwards. The tube, which, with the attached funnel, should be first filled with warm water and held compressed between the fingers, is then introduced until the

prominence of the spine is felt obstructing its progress, when, on rapidly inclining the head forward, the tube will of itself slide into the stomach.

5. Should the entrance of the tube into the stomach be opposed by spasm of the œsophageal cardia, it is only necessary to allow the water to flow through the tube against the constriction, when the spasm will readily give way.

The danger of detaching the mucous membrane of the stomach by the suction of the pump is extremely small. The only real danger to be guarded against is perforation of the gastric walls by the tube, especially when there is ulceration, or adhesion of the stomach to surrounding viscera. All risk, however, is avoided by previous softening of the tube, by measuring off the distance to which it is to enter, filling it with water, and by the use of the notched slide.—*London Med. Record*, March 15, 1878.

Use of Soft Soap in Glandular Affections.

In the *Berliner Klinische Wochenschrift* for Feb. 11th, Dr. KAPPESSER suggests regular periodic inunction of soft soap in certain chronic glandular affections, and gives four cases in which it was so used with apparent success.

The first case occurred about twenty years ago. It was that of a peddler who, with his wife and four children, suffered from scabies, for which they were treated with local applications of soft soap. One of the children, a boy nine years of age, was also affected with scrofulous swelling of the glands of the neck, inflammation of the conjunctivæ and eyelids, etc., which had resisted all previous treatment. Owing to the greater severity in him of the cutaneous affection, frictions with soft soap were more frequently and extensively employed. Singularly enough, all signs of glandular and strumous disease disappeared simultaneously with the cure of scabies.

The next case occurred some years later, and was that of a little girl of about three years, in very poor and neglected circumstances. Both corneæ were ulcerated, with an acrid discharge; the glands and cellular tissue of the neck, especially on the right side, were enormously swollen, and there were six or eight fistulous openings, from which flowed an abundant thin purulent discharge. About half an ounce of soft soap, dissolved in a little tepid water, was rubbed twice a week at bedtime into the whole posterior aspect of the body, from the neck to the knees, with a piece of soft flannel, and was washed off again about ten minutes after its application. In addition, she was put upon nutritious diet and cod-liver oil. In about four weeks' time the glandular swellings had almost disappeared, the discharging sinuses were nearly closed, and the inflamed condition of the eyes had subsided; there yet remained a dense opacity of each cornea. Owing to neglect on the part of the child's relatives, this treatment was now interrupted, and its condition rapidly grew worse. But on resuming the regular inunction, etc., matters again quickly improved, and after a few months there remained only two small dim spots on the corneæ, while otherwise the child was to all appearances well, and was still so when again seen two years afterwards.

The third case was in nearly all respects similar to the last one, and under the application of soft soap, with nutritious diet, etc., complete recovery resulted.

The fourth case was somewhat different. It was that of a female infant, sixteen months old, and was first seen in August, 1876. It then presented a hard and tender glandular swelling of the size of an egg behind the angle of the left jaw; the mouth, nose, and anus were excoriated, the entire skin was covered with dark spots and a papular eruption, and the scalp was a mass of thick crusts, beneath which was a raw suppurating surface. The gums and buccal mucous membrane were ulcerated. Under the idea that the affection was syphilitic the child was treated with the suboxide of mercury, apparently with benefit. Some months afterwards, it again came under observation, in a sadly worse condition. The cervical swelling was still hard, and had grown considerably ; the eyes were inflamed, and one of the corneæ was ulcerated ; the left lower jaw showed signs of necrosis in the place where one of the molar teeth had dropped out ; all the fingers, and most of the toes were swollen, inflamed, and covered with ugly sores, while pustules and boils were spread over the entire body, especially about the anus and genitals, and the scalp was covered with a thick crust. Soft soap was now regularly rubbed into the back in the manner above described, avoiding the more inflamed parts, while the sores of the mouth were touched with a solution of potassium chlorate. In a short time the ophthalmia diminished, the sores and cutaneous eruption began to decrease, and the crusts of the scalp to fall off, leaving a clean healthy surface ; the glandular swelling in the neck decreased considerably, leaving only a certain amount of induration of the jaw, while the child's nutrition and general health improved rapidly, until only the necrosis of the jaw remained, to be met by appropriate treatment.

Dr. Kappesser considers the above cases to justify the argument of *post hoc ergo propter hoc*. He wishes mainly to direct attention to the treatment employed, with a view to its further trial in similar cases, and also in chronic inflammation and ulcerations, especially of the joints and internal organs.—*London Med. Record*, March 15, 1878.

<hr>

Pathological Histology of Lupus Erythematosus.

Dr. STROGANOFF examined portions of skin excised from a patient who exhibited a well-marked form of this disease, and found (*Centralblatt für die Medicinischen Wissenschaften*, No. 48, 1877) that the pathological changes do not merely consist in an inflammatory condition of the connective tissue of the skin, but that there is a special affection of the epidermis, sebaceous glands, and hair-follicles.—*London Med. Record*, March 15, 1878.

<hr>

Wilhelm on Erythema Nodosum.

A weak anæmic girl, aged 18, suffered from quotidian ague which yielded to quinine, in September, 1876. (*Berliner Klin. Wochensch.*, January 28th, 1878.) In December, 1876, she again suffered from nightly attacks of fever, this time accompanied by swellings on the legs and forearm, which had the characteristic appearances of erythema nodosum. The second attack of fever did not yield to quinine, but the patient recovered whilst taking iodide of potassium and small doses of morphia.—*London Med. Record*, March 15, 1878.

<hr>

Surgery.

Carbolized Gut as a Surgical Dressing.

In a communication to the *Allgemeine Medicinische Central-Zeitung* for February 17, Dr. FLASHAR, of Polkwitz, writes as follows:—

Starting from the fact that catgut threads used for ligature are completely absorbed, it occurred to me to prepare portions of intestine in the same way as catgut, and to use them in appropriate cases as dressing. Having procured a piece of dried sheep's intestine, I cut it lengthwise, and soaked it in carbolized oil (ten per cent.).

After about six weeks, I had an opportunity of trying it in the case of a young man whose right hand had been injured by a machine. The wound, which gaped widely and penetrated the deeper tissues, extended obliquely along the surface of the hand to the middle and ring fingers, both of which were injured. The edges were torn and ragged, and the subjacent tendons were partly laid bare. After cleaning the hand and wound, I applied to the latter a large piece of the prepared intestine, still dripping with oil, in such a way as to overlap a portion of the uninjured skin. The whole was covered by a cotton-bandage and left undisturbed as long as circumstances allowed. For the first time, at the end of six days there was some offensive smell, and the patient felt a slight burning; previously to this neither pain, swelling, nor inflammation had been observed. The dressing was opened on the seventh day, and, to my astonishment, I found that the portions of intestine lying on the wound were perforated, and for the most part absorbed; the wound beneath was in an advanced state of cicatrization, so that it wanted comparatively little to complete its closure. The smell which had been perceived proceeded from the portion of intestine which lay on the sound skin; it had there assumed a whitish colour, and appeared like intestine which had been softened in water. The dressing was renewed, the sound part being left free, and in a remarkably short time the small remaining portion of the wound was healed. The cicatrix was so soft and pliable that the vitality of the hand and fingers was not impaired in the slightest degree.

I made a second trial of the same material in a case of separation of webbed fingers in a young child. After cutting through the uniting membrane, I wrapped each finger separately in prepared intestine, and also laid a piece in the angle of the wound. Cicatrization went on unequally in all parts of the wounded fingers. Unfortunately the parents, who lived in a village, were prevented by bad weather from bringing their child to me at the proper time for removing the dressing, and consequently readhesion took place to a trifling extent. The cicatrix was so soft, and the tissues felt so normal, that I had no fear of future contraction and stiffness. In this case also I observed that the portion of intestine which lay on the normal skin had become soft and pale.

I believe that it is absolutely necessary to soak the intestine for a month in the carbolized oil, in order to render it fit to be used as a dressing to amputation-wounds where skin-flaps cannot be formed, or to wounds in which a great loss of substance is to be feared, especially on the skin.—*London Med. Record*, March 15, 1878.

—

Injuries of the Scalp.

In the *Lancet* of Jan. 26, 1878, Mr. ERICHSEN, in continuation of his lectures upon injuries of the head, reviews the subject of scalp-injuries, explaining why, on account of the extreme vascularity of the part with its serpentine vessels, anastomosing one with the other freely, and lying amongst dense granular fat that hinders their ready contraction, hemorrhage is necessarily profuse and often uncontrollable. Hence the care necessary in removing sebaceous and other tumours; and if from any cause hemorrhage should be difficult to arrest. Mr. Erichsen points out how easily acupuncture will effect the purpose. The reason why traumatic erysipelas of the scalp is more apt to arise than from wounds in other parts of the body, is the looseness of the areolar tissue on which the tendon of the occipito-frontalis lies, where pus often collects, owing to the pouch or bag generally found in scalp-wounds; hence the necessity of drainage, and hence the reason why stitches in scalp-wounds, by closing up the mouth of the pouch and hindering the escape of the matter formed, are followed by erysipelas. Mr. Erichsen repudiates all complicated artistic bandages in scalp-wounds, believing them to be worse than useless.

The diagnosis between abscess and erysipelas of the scalp is clearly described. In erysipelas, the ears are red, swollen, and covered with blebs; in abscess, the occipito-frontalis muscle determines the limits of the fluctuation. The wonderful reparative powers of the scalp are noted, and cases mentioned where large portions have been removed without harm.

The phenomena of true and false stunning are well described. Two persons are thrown out of a carriage; one is stunned, forgetting on recovery everything that happened a minute or two before losing consciousness; his companion is picked up also unconscious, but can remember on recovery from faint all the minutiæ of the accident. The vastly different after-history of the two cases is clearly defined. The important question, "Is he drunk or dying?" concludes Mr. Erichsen's second lecture, and is answered by the important advice, "Wait and see; do not decide too hastily."—*London Med. Record*, March 15, 1878.

Extravasation of Blood on the Dura Mater.

A series of cases are commented upon by Mr. ERICHSEN in the *Lancet* of January 5, 1878, where clots were found after death, or by the aid of the trephine during life, upon the dura mater. In one case a child falling down stairs was picked up a little dazed, and was found dead in bed the next morning with a clot upon the dura mater on the side struck. In another case a lady, treading on the train of another lady's dress in advance, tripped, struck her head against the wall, and died some hours afterwards, comatose, a large clot being found on the side struck, over the meningeal artery, but without any fracture of the skull. A cabman who was thrown off his box was trephined, and a large clot being removed from under the bone, made a good recovery; but a brewer's drayman, who met with a similar accident, and was similarly treated, succumbed, the middle meningeal being found torn, but not divided, and this typical case serves to illustrate Mr. Erichsen's views of the nature and treatment of such cases.

One peculiarity of wounds of the middle meningeal artery is that blood wells up, and is not ejected *per saltum*. This is due to the course of the artery, hemorrhage from which will cease of itself if it be divided, though the surgeon cannot arrest it otherwise than by plugging. The large size and peculiar shape of the clots was pointed out, and also the fact that, owing to the great vascularity of the dura mater, blood was extravasated under the calvarium, in many cases without any injury of the middle meningeal artery itself, its smaller branches alone suffering. Mr. Erichsen alluded to Sir Charles Bell's well-known experiments, proving that the dura mater is separated from the calvarium by the force of the blow, and that subsequently hemorrhage fills up the space thus formed; otherwise the extravasated blood could not itself separate the adhesions between the calvarium and dura mater.

Two cases are related where the injury occurred, not to the arteries, but to the veins of the dura mater. Both proved fatal, one after several months, where the diagnosis was not verified *post mortem*. In the other it was found that a portion of bone was driven inwards, and had lacerated the lateral sinus, which had bled freely when the patient was trephined; plugs of lint were applied to assist the hemorrhage, and these eventually led to pyæmia; and this case, Mr. Erichsen thought, explained the symptoms that used to puzzle surgeons of old, namely, the occurrence of pyæmia and the tendency to secondary deposits, especially in the liver, after injuries to the head. The liability to abscess forming between the cranium and dura mater was explained by the fact that the periosteum is separated as well as the dura mater, and hence the supply of nutriment is cut off from the calvarium, which becomes. like all necrosed bones, a source of irritation and of abscess.— *Lond. Med. Record*, March 15, 1878.

Cerebral Blepharoptosis.

Dr. LANDOUZY has published in the *Archives Générales de Médecine* a note on cerebral blepharoptosis. Ten observations of paralysis of the levator palpebræ superioris are given. In all, the paralysis offers the special characteristic of being crossed. as in hemiplegia, and limited, in the third pair, to the portion supplying the levator. From the examination of these facts the author concludes that : 1. The origin of the motor centre of the eyelid must be looked for in a posterior region of the parietal lobe; 2· This origin is not in immediate contact with the motor centre for the limbs ; 3. Amongst the nervous bundles which constitute by their union the third pair, those alone destined to the innervation of the levator palpebræ superioris seem to have congestion with the hemispheres. The cerebral paralysis of the third pair being never complete, the origin of the different fibres of the motor oculi is distinct for the branch supplying the levator, those going to the other muscles of the eye.—*Lond. Med. Record*, March 15, 1878.

Diphtheritic Inflammation of the Conjunctiva.

True diphtheritic conjunctivitis has not been noticed in this country, but in many of the larger German towns the complaint appears to be not uncommon. In Vienna, during the year 1874, it assumed the form of an epidemic, and its contagions nature was only too clearly demonstrated in the St. Joseph's Children's Hospital, where one case having been admitted, the complaint spread from bed to bed, chiefly among patients suffering from measles. Out of eighteen children thus affected. eleven died. In two lectures recently delivered before the Vienna Medical Society, Dr. HANS ADLER, under whose care the patients were, has given a minute history of the epidemic and of some sporadic cases which occurred about the same time. The following are the principal local symptoms which serve to distinguish this complaint from the catarrhal form : The eyelids are hard, tense, and opened with difficulty, the attempt to do so causing much pain ; the upper lid cannot be everted ; the mucous membrane firm, infiltrated, pale, not injected, the local circulation arrested ; the effused fibrinous layer is firm, adherent, and rapidly renewed ; the secretion consists of a dirty gray fluid containing white flakes. The local treatment recommended by Dr. Adler consists in the application of iced compresses during the first few days ; these are to be followed by cold-water dressings, and subsequently by warm moist applications. He recommends also the local employment of atropine from the commencement. He disapproves strongly of the use of caustics, such as nitrate of silver, the action of which in such cases he believes to be most mischievous. Constitutional treatment of a supporting character must of course not be neglected. The disease is a very serious one, and of those who survive very few escape without some lesion of the cornea.—*Med. Examiner*, April 4, 1878.

Keratoplasty.

An interesting series of articles has appeared in the recent Italian medical journals on plastic operations upon the cornea. In the report of the ophthalmic section of the Turin Medical Congress, given in the *Annali di Ottalmologia*, Fasc. 1, 1877, a paper appears by Professor GRADENIGO, of Padua, in which he discusses the feasibility of keratoplasty, which he calls the "oculist's philosopher's stone." The author first notices the advantages to be gained by substituting a transparent substance in the place of an opaque cornea, and the want of success which has hitherto attended attempts to transplant portions of transparent cornea or to introduce artificial corneæ of glass or other substances. After investigating the causes opposed to success, Professor Gradenigo believes failure to have been due to the following: 1. The corneal tissue, although rich in nerves, has no bloodvessels except in the fœtal state. A pannons cornea will tolerate and repair a wound or loss of substance more readily than a normal cornea. 2. The secretion of the aqueous humour, like the rapid products of the ocular mucous membrane, acts damagingly against the prompt agglutination of the margins of the cornea and its graft; and if sutures, however fine, be used, foreign bodies are introduced whose presence will probably be injurious. 3. Up to the present time, attempts have been made to introduce too large an extent of new cornea, whilst a point of transparent tissue is all that is really needed to afford useful vision. These new portions have been inserted into eyes altered by disease, the anterior chamber has been wanting, or the conditions for nutrition of the new fragment have been unfavourable. Professor Gradenigo made many experiments with a view of overcoming the difficulties before him, and at last adopted a method which has proved successful.

Remembering the greater tolerance of the pannons cornea, the author endeavoured to produce new bloodvessels upon the corneæ of animals, such as are found in keratitis superficialis, by introducing irritating substances into the conjunctival sac. The result did not prove satisfactory. Still keeping the same object in view, the author cauterized the corneal surface, excepting only a small triangular portion in the centre, the site of the intended graft. The action proved too diffused, and eventually the cortical layers of the cornea were removed by the knife. By then dissecting up the surrounding conjunctiva (as in the early steps of enucleation of the globe) and drawing it forward over the denuded cornea. fixing it with sutures, artificial pterygia were obtained. These afforded a solid base for the supply of nutrition to the cornea. This procedure was adopted both in the eye to receive the graft and the eye (generally a rabbit's) supplying it.

Adhesion of the conjunctiva to the cornea takes place rapidly and firmly. The clear centre of the cornea should be not greater than one-third of its extent, and it should be surrounded by from three to five apices of conjunctiva. When these pterygia are fully formed, the operation may be undertaken. First of all the condition of the eye of the patient should be carefully investigated, as to its freedom from morbid secretions, sensitiveness to light, etc. The patient should then be placed in the horizontal position, and fully anæsthetized, the eyelids being kept widely apart by the speculum. The conjunctiva is then carefully removed by scissors from the cornea and surrounding sclerotic. The flow of blood is at first encouraged by means of hot sponges, then completely arrested. An opening is then made in the cornea, of the size and shape of the intended graft. Then the animal (rabbit) being killed, the whole of the conjunctiva is carefully dissected off the sclerotic, and the whole of the cornea removed with the conjunctiva and the artificial pterygia attached. This is immediately placed upon the back of the left hand of an assistant, to facilitate the later stage of the operation and to maintain a certain degree of heat in the tissues. The final stage of the operation consists in cleaning the conjunctiva carefully off the corneal graft, until the operator is able to cut it to the size of the opening made in the human cornea. The graft must then be placed in the opening made for it, the conjunctiva adherent being spread out by means of smooth-pointed forceps over the denuded surfaces of the cornea and sclerotic, and secured in position by sutures. The eye must be closed and covered with a soft pad and bandage, and not opened for twenty-four hours. The eyelids should be cleansed, and the bandage renewed every day, but the upper lid should not be raised for three days.

A modification of this process, in which the whole of an animal's cornea prepared after Professor Giadenigo's method was transplanted, is narrated by Dr. Rosmini, of Florence, in a letter to Professor Strambio, published in the *Gazzetta Medica Italiana-Lombardia*, April 28, 1877. This case was apparently successful for a few days, but the cornea was soon destroyed by parenchymatous keratitis.

In a masterly letter (*Annali di Ottalmologia*, Fasc. 2, 1877), Professor Giadenigo draws Dr. Rosmini's attention to what he conceives to be the sources of his failure, viz., the attempt to transplant an entire cornea, and the neglect of careful adaptation of the conjunctiva and its ineffectual securing by sutures. Professor Giadenigo also remarks, in a tone of gentle remonstrance, on the impatience which Dr. Rosmini showed in operating before the arrival of a rabbit specially prepared by Professor Giadenigo at his request. This draws from the editor of the *Annali di Ottalmologia* some strong expressions of admiration for Professor Giadenigo's patient work and brilliant results, and also a remark on the untimely haste with which the report of the apparent success of Dr. Rosmini's operation was given to the journals, which is worth quoting. Speaking of premature communications to journals as being too much the fashion now-a-days, he says: "These communications appear to us capable of comparison with those fireworks, which, darted by night into space, illuminate the horizon for a little while, but which spend themselves quickly in falling, and leave nothing behind them but an obscure trace of smoke, and the darkness as before."—*London Med. Record*, Dec. 15, 1877.

The Action of Chlorhydrate of Pilocarpine in Certain Affections of the Eyes.

Dr. ALEXANDROFF, of Marseilles, claims for chlorhydrate of pilocarpine an action little short of miraculous in rheumatic iritis and choroiditis; two or three subcutaneous injections of the alkaloid, according to the author, having restored vision in cases which most English ophthalmologists would regard as almost, if not entirely, hopeless. The author states that the alkaloid in solution applied to the eye acts in the same manner as eserine, but that it does not give rise to pain after its application. Salivation, profuse sweating, epiphora, and flushing of the face followed immediately after the injection of the drug, and continued for some hours.—*London Med. Record*, March 15, 1878.

The Causes of Glaucoma.

At the Ophthalmological Congress at Heidelberg in 1877, the subject of glaucoma was discussed at considerable length.

Dr. STILLING maintained that there are two forms of the disease: *glaucoma anticum*, in which the canal of Fontana is narrowed or obliterated; and *glaucoma posticum*, in which there is obliteration of the lymph-space surrounding the optic nerve. He stated that, from five to ten days after the optic nerve of a rabbit had been tied, there was intense glaucomatous hardness of the eyeball.

Dr. SCHMIDT-RIMPLER expressed the belief that disturbance of the circulation in the veins is a cause of glaucomatous hardening. He also stated that, in four cases in which he injected oil into the anterior chamber of a rabbit's eye, and in which no inflammation supervened, there was no change to be observed in an examination with the ophthalmoscope; that there was a rise of intraocular pressure from the injection of various substances into the anterior chamber; but that he considered that there is a wide difference between mere increased intraocular pressure from this cause and glaucoma simplex.

Dr. AD. WEBER answered that a very accurate knowledge of the ophthalmoscopic appearances in the rabbit's eye is needed to decide from the use of the ophthalmoscope whether there were cupping of the disk or not.

Dr. HERMANN PAGENSTECHER recorded a case of glaucoma in which there was no alteration in the condition of the canal of Fontana, and a second case in which there was complete obliteration of the canal without glaucoma.—*London Med. Record*, March 15, 1878.

Drainage of the Eye by Wire Seton.

In WECKER's *Relevé Statistique* and in *Annales d'Oculistique*, Mars–Avril, 1877. p. 140, will be found an account of a new plan of drainage of the eye introduced by WECKER. The statistics include 58 cases in which he has employed wire-drainage. Detachment of the retina, 27; of the choroid, 1; glaucoma (absolute), 12; (inflammatory), 2; glaucomatous keratitis, 1; glaucomatous iritis, 1; hydrophthalmos, 5; staphyloma (ciliary), 1; (corneal), 5; sclero-choroiditis (anterior), 2; keratoglobus, 1; opacity of the cornea, 1. After some preliminary remarks on the history of previous attempts at drainage and the reasons for their failure, he says there are two points still undecided, (1) the length of sclerotic included between puncture and counter-puncture (8 to 10 mm. probably, .32″ to .40″), and the method of fastening the wire in reference to tightness, pressure on the eyeball, etc. The wire should be drawn on at the moment of twisting it, to insure that it should not project into the eyeball, but not tightly enough to damage the sclerotic. These remarks are made especially in connection with its application to detachment of the retina. The comprehension of the description of the procedure is facilitated by four figures. The instruments, etc., employed are (1) a curved needle, hollow, and 3 centim. in length (1.2″), analogous to the curved canula of a Pravaz syringe; (2) a thread of gold, 6 centim. (2.4″) in length, bent at its centre so as to form a loop. The ends of this thread are to be passed along the needle nearly to its point; (3) a needle-holder without a catch, having a groove which will hold the needle firmly (special contrivance); (4) a small pair of forceps with branches crossing each other (serre-fils); (5) forceps with large branches for twisting the wire. The plan of procedure is as follows: 1st. To apply the wire. The lids are separated by speculum, the eye directed upwards, the conjunctiva, etc., seized with fixation forceps below and outside the cornea, and the eye drawn well up. The needle is then introduced between the inferior and external recti as near as possible to the equator, and brought out again so as to include about 1 centim. (.4″) of the sclerotic between puncture and counter-puncture. As soon as the point of the needle presents through the conjunctiva (which is liable to be pushed before it rather than perforated by it) the fixation forceps are laid aside. The point of the needle is seized (without any hurry) by the fingers or the needle-holder, and whilst the extremity of the wire is then held the needle is withdrawn. The wire is thus left in position. 2d step. The extremities of the thread are seized carefully and crossed over the bridge of sclerotic. The small catch forceps are then used to hold the wire, the branches being so placed that one is above and the other below (not in front and behind); the forceps in fact lying in the direction of the needle making the puncture and counter-puncture. The forceps are then allowed to hold by their own spring. 3d. The ends of the wire are seized with the torsion forceps and twisted together. The wire is then cut off about 3 or 4 mm. (.9″ to 1.2″) from the catch forceps, and the remaining piece bent in the form of a hook. The forceps being removed, the hook is bent down on the sclerotic so as to lie along the line of puncture and counter-puncture and not project from the globe. The wire is then gently drawn by forceps near the points of puncture and counter-puncture so as to insure more accurate adaptation. In *Zehend. Klin. Monatsbl.*, xv., p. 91, is a further note. He alludes to seton in corneal margin. It must be siorter tian tie otier, and a siorter and straigiter needle is used. Also Note in Graefe's *Archiv*, Bd. xxii., Abth. iv.—*Royal London Ophthalmic Hosp. Rep.*, Dec. 1877.

Puerperal Amaurosis.

In tie *Berliner Klinische Wochenschrift* for February 4, Dr. F. WEBER relates tie following case : Frau S., aged 20, weakly, anæmic, and of slight stature, married one year, was attacked in tie seventi monti of ier pregnancy witi polyartiritis. At eaci fresi inflammation of a joint tiere was a considerable rise in temperature. Tiis reduced tie patient's strengti considerably. Tie urine became cloudy, ammoniacal, and albuminous. At tie end of tie eighti monti. on tie morning of tie 21st October, labour-pains suddenly set in, and were of a spasmodic nature. About twelve iours after tie beginning of labour, witiout any prodromata, tie patient suddenly called out, "I can't see; I am blinded." She was perfectly conscious at tie time. Sie complained of ieadacie and sparks before ier eyes. Tie spasmodic pains continued ; tie os uteri remained rigid and dilated only to the size of a ialf-crown. At eleven o'clock in tie evening sie had a fit of convulsions, wiereupon a iypodermic injection ot morpiia was given, and ciloroform-narcosis obtained. After nineteen more attacks of convulsions. during wiici six ounces of ciloroform were used, tie rigid os was incised, and an aspiyxiated ciild was delivered by tie forceps. Tie placenta was expressed, and tie uterus contracted well. For tie next twenty-four iours sie was unconscious and had twelve convulsive attacks, wiici gradually decreased in duration and intensity. A profuse foul-smelling perspiration set in. Tie urine contained two-tiirds albumen. During tie next twenty-four iours tiere were five more eclampsic fits ; urine albuminous ; sie was furiously delirious, witi intervals of consciousness. Ciloral-iydrate was given in large doses. After tiis tiere were no more convulsions. Tie delirium was moderated by ciloral-hydrate. She began to regain ier sigit on tie 26th October. Tie delirium continued more or less until November 8. Tie inflammation of the joints persisted, and materially retarded convalescence. By November 10 tie albumen. polyartiritis, and amaurosis had entirely disappeared. Dr. Weber remarks tiat tie case is noteworthy on account of tie amaurosis, polyartiritis, eclampsia, and inflammation of tie kidneys, terminating in recovery.—*London Med. Record*, Marci 15, 1878.

Acute Symptoms from Accumulation of Cerumen in the Ear.

Tie following case. reported by Dr. F. N. PIERCE, Senior Surgeon to the Manciester Ear Institution (*Med. Times and Gaz.*, Marci 30, 1878), well illustrates tie necessity for practitioners and students making tiemselves acquainted witi, at least, tie elements of special diseases. Of late years tie establisiment of lectures and demonstrations on diseases of tie eye, ear, tiroat, and skin iave enabled tie student to acquire some practical knowledge of tiose subjects before commencing general practice. Tiere are still, iowever, many provincial sciools in tiis country witiout any pretence to tie teaciing of special diseases. A comparatively siort course of tie practical study of diseases of tie eye and ear will save many a practitioner from falling into tie error illustrated by tie following case :—

On Sunday evening, about 11 P. M., I called to see Mr. C., a ciemist. I found iim lying in bed, pale, anxious-looking, batied in a profuse perspiration, and complaining of intense pain over tie vertex and left side of tie face, neck, and jaw. He was afraid to eat or speak ; had had little or no sleep for tie previous tiree days. Tie pulse was full and bounding, 120 ; tie tongue dry, but clean; the temperature much increased (thermometer not used). There was nausea, and constant throbbing tinnitus aurium of the left ear.

He did not make any special reference to his ear, except that his illness began four days before with earache after taking a cold bath, which quickly became a diffused incessant pain over the entire head and neck. On the second day of his attack his medical attendant, who had been called in, ordered a mixture, and, as far as I can learn, regarded the complaint as some form of cerebral inflammation. At the time of my visit, on the fifth day of his illness, Mr. C. certainly looked very ill, and was surrounded by his friends, who seemed to have given up hopes of his recovery. He had dosed himself freely with opium, chloral-hydrate, etc., but without relief; and when I saw him his head and neck were smeared over with fresh belladonna plaster, but all to no effect.

Everything suggesting the left ear as the seat of mischief, I found on examination that a watch was inaudible at the external meatus; a tuning-fork on the vertex was heard entirely in left ear; the walls of the meatus were greatly swollen and congested; and a smooth, glistening surface covered with a débris of white epithelial scales beyond and concealing the membrana tympani.

There was evidently acute inflammation of the outer layer of the membrana tympani and of the adjoining walls of the meatus behind the firm plug of cerumen, most probably due to the entrance of cold water. Syringing with warm water and a weak solution of iodide of potassium had no effect in removing the obstruction, and I therefore used a pair of very fine curved forceps, made on purpose to apply through the open speculum I use with Brunton's auriscope, and removed the wax piecemeal. This afforded instant and great relief.

A lotion (of carb. sodæ, liq. atropiæ, and liq. opii sedat.) was to be instilled warm and retained all night.

Next day Mr. C. was almost free from all previous symptoms, and had slept well; the tinnitus aurium was now of a buzzing character and very slight, and the hearing distance two inches. There was no pain over head, ear, or neck, and the feverishness and nausea had gone.

After syringing the ear clean, the hearing distance was thirty-six inches; the meatus was seen to be still much inflamed, and there was a most offensive discharge of pus; the membrana tympani was of a yellow sodden opacity, with great congestion of the vessels of the manubrium. An astringent lotion was applied for three or four days, and at the end of that period the Eustachian tube was opened with Politzer's bag. No perforation was observed, although such a condition was probable.

Although the simplicity of treatment and rapidity of recovery in this case may seem almost amusing, the condition of the patient and anxiety of his friends gave an aspect of gravity to his complaint, which might have been avoided by an early and correct diagnosis.

Simple as it may seem, the recognition of a firmly adherent layer of cerumen to the membrana tympani is not so easy unless the medical attendant has had some practical experience in aural disease. A slight acquaintance with the appearances of the various forms of ear disease would have saved any practitioner from the error for which this patient suffered.

—

Discharges from the Ear.

Under this title, Prof. JOSEPH GRUBER contributes to the *Allg. Wien. Med. Zeit.*, January 1 and 8, a paper which is especially valuable for the precautionary treatment which it insists on. He dwelt strongly on the mischief which so often arises from treating this troublesome affection by applications to the meatus without the precise source of the discharge having been ascertained; and even in cases where this is apparent, the most suitable kind of application is frequently not selected. When there is a circumscribed inflammation of the walls of the meatus, the membrana tympani being intact, we should abstain as much as possible from dropping stimulating liquids into the ear, as experience has shown that this procedure favours the extension of the inflammation to the membrane, while the end in view may be accomplished by other means. And especially should we abstain from the use of astringent or stimulant fluids when the membrane is perforated, the deeper structures being in a healthy condition; for these fluids, passing into the tympanum, or even into the pharynx, through the Eustachian tube, may prove the primary cause of a consecutive affection of the cavity of the tympanum, or induce great irritation in the pharynx. When it is remembered that the mucous membrane of the pharynx is far less sensitive than that of the cavity of the tympanum, we can easily infer how dangerous these applications may prove to the latter. Moreover, it is not necessary that such fluid substances should be of a stimulant character to do harm; for even simple water poured into the ear will often (as may be seen on inspection) induce hyperæmia in the normal membrane, and still more easily in the mucous membrane of the tympanum, that may easily go on to inflammatory action. Still more easily is this effect produced when these liquids are forcibly propelled into the ear by means of a powerful syringe.

Enough has been said to show that the practitioner in treating otorrhœa through the meatus should not only make use of suitable substances, but be also very careful in his mode of applying them. Strong solutions or ointments are usually applied to the meatus, when the inflammation is circumscribed, by means of pencils or other contrivances; but Prof. Gruber employs for this purpose, on a large scale, at his clinic, plugs prepared in a suitable way with the medicinal substances. These medicated plugs can be applied very easily by means of the ear-forceps while the patient holds his mouth open, and admit of being readily adapted to any part of the meatus that may seem especially to need them. Even in cases in which the amount of swelling of the external part of the meatus prevents inspection of its deeper portion, and where other symptoms lead to the suspicion that the deeper structures of the ear are also suffering, yet, unless some pressing indication be present, it is preferable to proceed first by treating the affection of the outer part of the meatus by means of the medicated plugs. The deeper parts can then be inspected, and the further plan of treatment be decided upon; and it has often been found that in this way recovery is effected much more rapidly than if the usual plan of dropping liquids into the ear from the commencement had been pursued. Instead of these medicated charpie plugs, we may use in some cases, with excellent effect, plugs of *laminaria digitata* shaped conformably to the meatus, and smeared before application with a suitable ointment. A thread should be attached to the outer end in order to facilitate removal. In long-continued affections of the ear, attended with otorrhœa, the cavity of the meatus may have become obstructed by hypertrophied tissue, so that the passage may seem quite obliterated; and in such cases the formation of pus in the deeper-situated parts becomes of the more consequence by reason of the difficulty of its discharge. Here the application of the *laminaria* becomes very useful by re-establishing the passage, and frequently enabling us to inspect the deeper tissues. In not a few cases this improvement of the local conditions, by securing the freedom and the cleanliness of the meatus, has sufficed to relieve the inflammation, and to arrest an otorrhœa which has for years resisted the treatment by heroic measures. Accumulating experience has more and more convinced Prof. Gruber that otorrhœa which has been so over-treated should, as a general rule, be treated by mere expectation until the exact condition of the diseased processes can be ascertained, and separated from those which have been artificially engendered by the treatment adopted; and in not a few cases he has been able, by the use of simple water for the purpose of cleanliness, to effect more than have others by very tedious and sometimes very teasing modes of treatment. Dropping astringent substances into the ear has been practised in the most objectless or even mischievous manner in otorrhœa dependent upon chronic or acute inflammation of the meatus, or upon the partial suppuration of polypous growths, the increase of the latter instead of their diminution being the consequence. The same objection to this form of treatment applies also to insufflation of astringent powders into the meatus. Not only may the alum or other powder be deposited on places where it may prove mischievous, but, detained in the crypts of the meatus, it may form, where cleanliness is neglected, concretions with the discharges, and increase rather than diminish the irritation. In such cases, the first procedure in treatment often consists in removing these concretions, which sometimes are the sole cause of very violent pains.

In otorrhœa dependent upon inflammation of the meatus or membrana, Prof. Gruber has long employed an artificial membrana tympani as a means of cure. He has so modified Toynbee's membrana that any patient can easily construct, and by means of a forceps apply it for himself. This may be formed of very different materials, but fine linen is usually preferred. This is smeared with weak stimulating ointments of oxide of zinc or red precipitate. The artificial membrane is also of great protective use in inflammation of the cavity of the tympanum, shielding it from external irritating influences—a protection that sometimes suffices for the arrest of the otorrhœa. Quite recently, Prof. Gruber has had prepared medicated gelatine, in the form of globules and almonds of various sizes, which contain medicinal substances in different quantities; as zinc, tannin, borax, sublimate, nitrate of silver; and, in painful affections, opium or morphia. After cleansing the meatus, the preparation is deposited in this either by means of the finger or forceps, and, if required, pushed further in by a pencil of wadding. The meatus is then closed by wool, and the medicinal substance gradually dissolves, and acts for a long time on the diseased parts. In proper cases this means of medication suits better than any other, and is likely to find acceptance in affections of the ear. Its prolonged action renders its frequent renewal unnecessary, while the gradual manner in which it operates causes it to be easily borne by the patient. Prof. Gruber anticipates that he will have conferred an important benefit by the introduction of this procedure. It seems especially useful in the tumefied condition of the mucous membrane of the cavity of the tympanum accompanying destruction of the membrana tympani.—*Med. Times and Gaz.*, March 23, 1878.

The Inspection of the Naso-Pharynx from the Nostrils.

In the *Archiv für Ohrenheilkunde*, vol. xii., part 4, ZAUFAL describes his method of examining that part of the naso-pharynx which, as a rule, has been obscured from the difficulty of lighting. He uses a series of five specula, from 10 to 11.5 centimetres (4 to $4\frac{1}{2}$ inches) long, with a calibre of from 3 to 7 millimetres (.12 to .28 inch) in diameter. These are passed along the floor of the nasal cavity till the smaller end reaches the naso-pharyngeal cavity, and the examination is made by throwing light in by the usual laryngoscopic mirror. The mouths of the Eustachian tubes and the naso-pharyngeal walls can be thus seen. He holds it to be a valuable aid to rhinoscopy and the determination of the state of tumours in the cavity by means of the finger.—*London Med. Record*, March 15, 1878.

Bloodless Tracheotomy.

Every one who has been called upon to perform tracheotomy upon a young child suffering from threatening asphyxia, where the venous plexuses of the neck are engorged, and each touch of the knife may flood the wound with blood, will appreciate any method of operating by which this danger can be avoided, and tracheotomy added to the list of the bloodless operations. The attempt to accomplish this has been several times made. In 1872 M. Verneuil employed the galvanic cautery instead of the bistoury in several cases, with success; but this method is evidently ill-adapted for general use, as the necessary apparatus is cumbrous, and only to be found at hospitals. More recently Mons. G. POINSOT, of Bordeaux, has used Paquelin's thermo-cautery with excellent results, and his example has been followed by other French surgeons. The skin and soft parts quite down to the trachea should be divided by successive light touches of the point of the cautery, heated to a dull red colour, and when the trachea has been exposed it should be opened with the knife, and the tube inserted in the usual way. The cautery must be used lightly, or its action will be too extensive, and a thick eschar be formed; and if it be used too hot, as is well known, it loses its hæmostatic power. The cautery is not suited for opening the trachea, because the radiation from its hot point introduced into the air-passage would be harmful, and there is some risk of burning its posterior wall; while in adults it is difficult to sever the firm rings with it, and particularly if they are at all ossified, and the loss of substance that an eschar necessarily involves might cause trouble from narrowing of the air-tube. On the other hand, as the use of the knife for this purpose does not cause hemorrhage, it is free from objection. In fat subjects the wound may become filled with molten fat; this is readily removed with a sponge. In addition to the bloodlessness of this mode of operating, Mons. Poinsot claims for it two other advantages —the spontaneous retraction of the edges of the wound, rendering unnecessary the aid of assistants for this purpose, and giving a funnel-shaped opening down to the trachea; and the protection of the wounded surfaces from the contagion of diphtheria. Slight secondary hemorrhage has followed this operation in several cases, but in no case has it been severe, yielding readily to simple treatment. Although the wound gapes widely at first, the resulting cicatrix contracts to a small size, and has not given rise to any unpleasant symptoms in any recorded case. This appears to be one of the most useful applications of this recent addition to the surgeon's armamentarium. It promises to change tracheotomy from an operation which is always anxious and often very trying into a safe and simple proceeding; and we may hope that it will in this way add to the value of the operation by leading to its more frequent and earlier adoption in obstructive diseases of the larynx.—*Lancet*, Feb. 16, 1878.

Irreducible Hernia.

Although surgeons have for many generations been agreed as to the impropriety of interfering by surgical operation with ordinary cases of irreducible hernia, there has been no lack of ingenuity in devising plans for protecting the tumour from injury and for preventing increase of size; but it is not so well known that attempts at reduction without operation have also been occasionally successful. Many surgical observers have recorded instances of irreducible hernia becoming reducible after long confinement in bed or emaciation from illness. Fabricius Hildanus gives an account of a man who was radically cured of an irreducible rupture of twenty years' duration by six months' confinement in bed. Pott, Le Dran, and Arnaud have also recorded similar cases. The latter, imitating Nature's process, accomplished the reduction of a large scrotal hernia, which had existed from infancy, by confining the patient in bed, by restricting him to a light and spare diet, and by the employment of venesection, calomel, purgatives, and clysters. In the same way the famous Mr. Hey, who practised at Leeds in the last century, succeeded on several occasions. M. Cloquet effected reduction of a large scrotal hernia by means of rest in the horizontal posture and by the application of suspensory bandages progressively diminished in size. Mr. Earle succeeded in a similar instance by means of confinement, low diet, the internal administration of solution of potass mixture, and the inunction of mercury over the swelling. Mr. Bransby Cooper also succeeded with confinement in bed, low diet, the continued application of ice, and, where there was much omentum, by giving, in addition, small doses of blue-pill and tartar-emetic, so as to promote absorption of the fat; and still more recently Mr. Erichsen—who seems to credit Mr. B. Cooper with being the first to employ this method of treatment—has, while following out the rest of the treatment, advantageously substituted iodide of potassium for the blue-pill and tartar emetic. Many years ago Mr. Hilton succeeded in reducing a large scrotal hernia in a young man, which had been irreducible for six months, by keeping the patient in a horizontal posture, forbidding him to drink more than half a pint of fluid in the twenty-four hours, by the constant application of ice to the tumour, and by the frequent internal administration of sulphate of magnesia and colchicum wine.

The following case is reported from the practice of Mr. MAUNDER at the London Hospital, similarly successful.

J. H——, aged thirty-five, a tram-car conductor, was admitted on May 18th, 1877, with a scrotal hernia on the right side. There was impulse on coughing. Five years ago he ruptured himself in applying the brake of a car. The hernia was reduced, and a truss was worn. The bowel came down once between that occasion and this, but was properly reduced.

Immediately after admission the patient was placed under the influence of an anæsthetic, and taxis was employed in vain. When Mr. Maunder saw the case he advised rest in bed, with the thighs flexed and comfortably supported on a pillow; a crutch pad to support the scrotum with its contents, in order to favour the return of blood by the omental veins; and the application of an ice-bag. The rationale of the treatment was explained to the patient. He was enjoined to eat and drink as little as he could possibly do with, so as to reduce himself, and promote absorption of the fat of the body generally, but especially that contained in the protruded omentum. A saline aperient was also given often.

In about ten days the tumour began to diminish in size, and was pushed up higher into the canal by a repetition of taxis, the intestine being now reduced. On June 12th the patient was again submitted to taxis, with partial success. He was getting tired of bed and of the treatment, but was encourged to submit a little longer. On July 10th reduction was again tried, with success, and a truss was ordered.

In some remarks on this case, Mr. Maunder laid stress on the importance of trying all reasonable means to reduce a hernia, and said that he had learned this particular plan from a former surgeon to Guy's Hospital. He had lately had an equally successful case in private practice, but at the expenditure of much less time. Unfortunately the process was often a slow one, and patients frequently tired of the restriction placed on their diet.—Lancet, March 16, 1878.

—

Case of Imperforate Anus.

The following case is reported by Dr. TASSIUS (Betz's Memorabilien, xxii. Jahrg., 12 Heft.). An infant, three weeks old, was found to have no anal orifice, and the feces were passed in a semi-fluid condition, with great straining, through a small opening about the size of a straw, situated on the floor of the vagina immediately behind the fourchette. The abdomen at the same time was tender and distended. A trocar and canula were passed from this opening to the usual site of the anus, and the skin perforated, and the passage thus made was dilated with catheters of various sizes. A large quantity of fluid fecal matter and of gas was discharged rapidly by this orifice, with evident relief to the infant. But, after seven days, probably through neglect on the part of the attendant, things had returned to their former condition. A second and similar attempt at relief also proved unsuccessful. Hereupon the perineum was divided throughout its extent from the abnormal orifice in the vagina to the site of the anus; the end of the gut was dissected out, and secured in its proper position. The opening in the gut was found to consist of a cartilaginous ring of the size of a straw, while otherwise the rectum was in a normal condition. The child made a good recovery, and is now six years of age. The evacuations pass by the natural way, and the presumed absence of a proper sphincter ani muscle cause no inconvenience.—*London Med. Record*, March 15, 1878.

Congenital Tumours of the Sacro-Coccygeal Region.

In the *Progrès Médical* for 1877, Nos. 32 and 33, M M. BRISSAUD and MONOD describe a tumour of the coccyx which was found in a child a week old. The mother, a woman aged 29, had previously borne two healthy children; she had not felt any disturbance during her pregnancy. The child was thin and of miserable appearance; the tumour, which was of the size of an orange, was attached to the lower part of the spinal column by a triangular ligament, in which the coccyx lay. It was covered by a thin red skin, and felt like a small flaccid sac. There was distinctly no connection between its interior and the spinal cord. On section, the skin was found to be inseparably united with the subsequent connective and adipose tissue. Within this lay a somewhat dense membrane, then a vascular medullary membrane, and inside all a large cyst. This was lined with ciliated epithelium, outside of which was a layer of pale muscular fibres, closely united with the firmer tissue of the wall. This consisted internally of sarcomatous tissue, and of a firmer outer layer of a more fibrous substance; scattered through it were connective-tissue fibres, and it contained insulated portions of cartilage, lamellæ of bone, and small cysts with partially calcified epithelial cells.

They also describe a tumour of the coccyx, which, having been at birth as large as a prune, became painful at about the fourth year, and grew with increasing rapidity from the month to the twenty-first year. It now formed an enormous pyriform appendage, reaching from the end of the coccyx to a popliteal space; it was joined to the coccyx by a pedicle about two inches broad, but was not intimately connected with the bone. The tumour consisted of—1, two large cysts, containing a thready, synovia-like fluid, and lined with flattened epithelium; 2, numerous small cysts, with ciliated epithelium; 3, a fibrous wall, with one large and numerous small pieces of bone, periosteum, and cartilage.—*London Med. Record*, Feb. 15, 1878.

The Use of Tayuya in Phagedænic and Scrofulous Ulcers and Blennorrhagia.

In the *Giornale Italiano delle Malattie Veneree e della Pelle* (1877), Dr. PASQUALE PIROCCHI states that he has used dilute tincture of tayuya (10 parts in 30 or 40 of water) as a local application in phagedænic and scrofulous ulcers, and in blennorrhagia. The ulcers became modified very soon after the application, twice or thrice in the day, of charpie steeped in tincture of tayuya; while in two cases of blennorrhagia the daily injection of the same remedy did not produce a favourable result. The author hence regards tincture of tayuya as a valuable topical remedy, capable, perhaps, of competing with the actual cautery in the treatment of phagedænic sores. He thinks that the tincture of tayuya, being a tonic and astringent, reduces suppuration in the soft parts, stimulates granulation, and facilitates cicatrization. As regards gonorrhœa, he does not consider tayuya superior to the balsams and other remedies ordinarily used.—*London Med. Record*, Feb. 15, 1878.

Non-Inoculability of the Semen in Syphilis

Dr. MIREUR, of Marseilles (*Annales de Dermatologie et de Syphilographie*, No. 6, Tome viii. 1877), gives an account of his researches on the above subject.

A syphilitic patient, aged 26, with characteristic indurated cicatrix of primary sore, multiple adenitis, papular roseola, mucous patches of mouth and anus, etc., and who had not undergone any specific treatment, consented to supply the material for inoculation. The semen obtained from this man was immediately inoculated on four healthy persons quite free from syphilitic antecedents. All the instruments used were new, and perfectly clean.

The first two subjects were inoculated by three punctures made on each arm with a needle. On the third patient, a small blister was raised by means of ammonia on the right leg. Charpie dipped in the semen was then applied to the denuded dermis, and carefully kept in place for twenty-four hours. In the fourth case the epidermis at the upper and outer part of the left arm was removed by scraping, and three small transverse incisions were then made. Charpie thoroughly soaked in the seminal fluid was kept in contact with the wound for thirty-six hours.

The results of Dr. Mireur's experiments were the following. In the first two cases the punctures gave rise, a few hours afterwards, to slight local inflammation ; but next day all inflammatory action had disappeared, and only a small ecchymotic and scarcely appreciable mark at the site of each puncture was left. All traces disappeared about the fifteenth or sixteenth day. In the other two cases there were not even signs of local irritation, and the wounds rapidly healed. All four persons were minutely and regularly examined every day for more than six weeks, and were kept under attentive observation for about six months. During this time not the slightest sign of syphilis, either local or constitutional, appeared in any of them. Two of the patients who were examined again, about a year after inoculation, confirmed, by their good state of health, the absolutely negative result of the experiment.—*London Med. Record*, Feb. 15, 1878.

Osteo-Sarcoma.

The proper line of treatment to adopt in cases of osteo-sarcoma is one of great interest to surgeons. The fear of speedy recurrence of the growth when the diseased part only of the bone is removed, and the great severity of the operation for the removal of the whole bone when, as so often happens, the lower end of the femur is attacked, make this question one of as great difficulty as importance. In a recent *brochure* Mons. Poinsot has brought together 51 cases in which amputation through or above the diseased bone has been practised ; and from an analysis of these cases he has been led to decide in favour of the higher operations, performed as early as possible. But, curiously enough, these cases show a greater frequency of local recurrence after the high operation than after the low one, and the recurrence was as rapid in one case as in the other. It is hardly possible to doubt that a larger number of cases would give a different result. Unfortunately, we are in the dark as yet on some points in the life-history of these and similar tumours.

Why do some recur locally, and not infect the system? Why do others rapidly infect the system? Why do some recur in the lungs, while others are only reproduced in the same tissue as that in which they originate? We need an answer to such questions as these before we can hope to have the line of treatment precisely marked out. Poinsot also deals with the difficulty sometimes experienced in diagnosing between "white swelling" and osteo-sarcoma, and he gives some details of 37 cases in which eminent surgeons have been led into error. Tumours are often stated to date from some injury; their course may be slow, and even interrupted in the manner so common in white swelling; the joint surfaces, which are generally preserved and allow of free movement, may be invaded, and then the neoplasia, growing in the direction of least resistance, will distend the synovial pouches, and closely simulate the masses of granulation tissue in "white swelling." Inflammatory symptoms, and even suppuration, have been noticed with sarcoma, but if, in these cases, the surgeon makes an incision, he at once discovers the true condition of the part from the very free arterial hemorrhage which occurs. In the same way, a puncture with a grooved needle may be most useful for diagnostic purposes.—*Lancet*, March 2, 1878.

—

Round-celled and Spindle-celled Sarcoma of the Left Scapula and Humerus.

The *Giornale Veneto di Scienze Mediche* for September, 1877, contains the report of a case related by Dr. SCAINI to the Medical Society at Friuli.

The subject was a countryman, aged 24, of healthy constitution, who, while working in Hungary in 1875, perceived a small tumour at the insertion of the left deltoid muscle into the humerus. The tumour was hard and painful, both spontaneously and on pressure; it was movable, and did not implicate the skin. Various remedies were applied, but without effect, the tumour continuing to increase in size. In January, 1877, when the patient was admitted to hospital under Dr. Scaini's care, it embraced four-fifths of the circumference of the left humerus; viz., the whole external region, the posterior, and a great part of the internal, leaving free only the part corresponding to the brachial muscle. It reached upwards to the junction of the upper and middle thirds of the deltoid muscle, and downwards as far as the middle of the humerus. It was of almost circular form, projected in the form of a fungus growth about an eighth of an inch above the level of the surrounding healthy skin, had a blackish aspect, produced by the scars left by the caustics that had been applied, and was divided into numerous lobules, soft to the touch. Under the eschar it had a grayish aspect, and bled on the slightest touch. When moved laterally, or upwards and downwards, it seemed to be scarcely adherent to the bone; during these movements the most painful part appeared to be its postero-superior portion, corresponding to the humeral attachment of the latissimus dorsi muscle. This portion was harder than the rest, and from it there passed under the spine of the left scapula a prolongation of the tumour, which occupied the whole of the infraspinous fossa; it was covered with reddened tense skin, which was livid near the shoulder-joint, but did not show signs of degeneration. The tumour here was not movable like that of the arm, but was very painful, and to the touch appeared elastic and semi-fluctuating: the presence of pus was suspected, but on introducing one of the needles of Dieulafoy's apparatus, only a few drops of blood escaped. The patient suffered much, and his nutrition was considerably impaired.

The case was treated by disarticulation at the shoulder-joint, by an interior and anterior flap, no other method being possible. The operation was undisturbed by any accident, and recovery soon took place. The author attributes the rapidly favourable termination to the use of salicylic dressings, which he considers a sure preventive of erysipelas, pyæmia, and other consequences of severe operations.—*London Med. Record*, March 15, 1878.

—

Muscular Atrophy consequent on Diseases of Joints.

Dr. E. VALTAT, after a great number of clinical observations and experiments on animals, draws the following conclusions. In the majority of diseases of the articulations, the nutrition of the muscular system is affected. From the commencement of most of the varieties of arthritis a considerable atrophy is observed, and a more or less marked paralysis of the muscles destined to the affected joint. This atrophy cannot be attributed to functional inactivity, nor to inflammation of the muscles, of the nerves, or of the spinal cord. Most probably it is produced by reflex action. It is very important as a functional disorder; it increases generally as long as the disease of the joint lasts; and while sometimes it is only temporary, in the great majority of cases it persists after the cure of the arthritis, and it remains then as the sole obstacle to the re-establishment of motion. It has but slight tendency to spontaneous cure. Sometimes the muscles, under the influence of exercise alone, may recover their strength and size; but this happy termination is rare, always slow, and generally incomplete. The atrophic lesions are rapidly and easily cured by the employment of weak and permanent constant currents, such as M. Le Fort has described, or, still better, by the combined use of these and faradization.—*London Med. Record*, Feb. 15, 1878.

Midwifery and Gynæcology.

A Case of Hour-glass Contraction of the Uterus before the Expulsion of the Fœtus.

Dr. A. H. GOELET, of New York, reports (*North Carolina Medical Journal*, March, 1878) the following case of this rare condition. On the 24th of July last, I was called to Mrs. R., who had engaged me to attend her in her third confinement, which she expected about the last of September. She was consequently about 6½ months advanced. I found her in premature labour, the os fully dilated, and the membranes still intact, but could detect no presenting part. The pains being very feeble and infrequent, 25 gtt. Squibb's fluid extract of ergot were given. As the pains increased there was some hemorrhage, and I ruptured the membranes to expedite the labour. An enormous quantity of amniotic fluid was discharged. Another examination at this time found the os in the same condition as before, and it was not until the whole hand was introduced into the vagina that the uterus was discovered to be contracted in the centre, the fœtus above the constriction, and a finger projecting through. This was a condition I never met with before, and I was in some doubt at first as to the proper course to pursue. But, since the patient was in danger from the hemorrhage which still continued, the indication was clearly the immediate extraction of the contents of the uterus. With great difficulty one finger was forced through the constriction, then another, and after considerable search a foot was found, but having only two fingers with which to grasp it, very little traction could be used. Finally, one foot (for the other could not be found) was dragged down and out of the vulva, but when the breech of the child presented against the constriction it required all the force that could be exerted with both hands, to bring it through, and the same was the case as the shoulders and head came down in succession. The delivery of the placenta, though less difficult, required force.

Delayed Ligature of the Funis.

Dr. BUDIN, while *interne* at the Maternité, came to the conclusion from his investigations that it is better not to tie the funis until one or two minutes after the complete cessation of the pulsation. By tying it immediately after birth we, in fact, prevent the child deriving about ninety-two grammes of blood from the placenta. Now, as Welcker, Bischoff, and others have shown that the weight of the blood of a new-born infant amounts on a mean to 270 grammes, or about a thirteenth part of the weight of the body, abstracting ninety-two grammes may be considered as equivalent to bleeding an adult of the weight of sixty-five kilogrammes to the extent of 1764 grammes. Dr. Hélot, Surgeon to the Hospice at Rouen, has since examined the subject with the intention of showing whether the infant really acquires this blood, by counting the globules of blood by Hayem's method, and by weighing the infant immediately after birth before dividing the cord, and then again when the cord has ceased to beat. By these means he found that there was an increase of 209,632 globules, and an addition to the weight of the child of fifty-three grammes. He therefore thinks that in normal cases rapid ligature of the cord should be entirely rejected, this operation not being performed until some instants after respiration has been completely established.—*Med. Times and Gaz.*, March 23, 1878, from *Gaz. des Hôp.*, March 14.

Cæsarean Section in Pregnancy, with Left Ovarian Tumour.

In the *Deutsche Medizinische Wochenschrift*, February 2, 1878, D. LAHS, of Marburg, relates the following case: F. S., a countrywoman, aged thirty-three, mother of two children, of which the youngest was three years old, remarked, for the first time a year and a half before, a tumour in her left pelvic region. Twelve months later the catamenia ceased, and she became pregnant. Towards the end of the seventh month of pregnancy the bladder and rectum performed their functions with much difficulty. On examination, July 12, after she had presumably been in labour eight days, Dr. Lahs found the abdomen enormously distended. Percussion-sounds were dull everywhere, except in the immediate vicinity of the ribs. Fluctuation could be detected all over the abdomen. Examination per vaginam revealed the presence of a firm immovable tumour filling the entire pelvic cavity. Dr. Lahs diagnosed a left ovarian tumour adherent to the pelvic walls, filling the pelvic cavity, and rising in part above the pelvic brim. A prolonged attempt was made under chloroform to push the tumour out of the pelvis. It was ineffectual.

Dr. Lahs proceeded to perform the Cæsarean section. After the delivery of the child, the placenta was easily removed. The uterus did not contract, possibly on account of the lengthened chloroform narcosis the patient had undergone. Dr. Lahs, therefore, maintained pressure for some time upon the placental site, which had been divided into the uterus. The uterus was sewn up with three strong silk sutures. On the tightening of the sutures the uterus contracted, and enabled the ovarian tumour to be seen, firmly adherent to the pelvis and abdominal contents. The abdominal cavity was cleaned out with carbolic solution, and the abdominal wound was closed. The patient recovered from the chloroform narcosis, and sank, collapsed, twenty-four hours later. There was no necropsy.—*London Med. Record*, March. 15, 1878.

A Case of Extra-Uterine Fœtation.

In a paper published in the *France Médicale* M. WEISS relates a case of extra-uterine fœtation which had a fortunate termination after expulsion of the fœtus per rectum. The patient was forty years old, and was admitted on May 31, 1877, to the Hôpital Lariboisière, under the care of M. Proust. She had had a normal pregnancy at the age of twenty-five, and had enjoyed good health since that time. In May, 1876, she began to suffer from slight abdominal pain, but general health was not much disturbed, and menstruation continued regular. About the end of 1876 she was attacked, without appreciable cause, by a met-rorrhagia, which continued without cessation until February, 1877, but was not severe enough to oblige her to keep her bed. At the end of this metrorrhagia there was a cessation of menstruation for between two and three months, until the end of April, when severe abdominal pain came on, accompanied by a sero-sanguineous discharge. She was able, however, to attend to her work, and came on foot to the hospital.

In the hypogastrium was found a hard irregular tumour, reaching about three fingers' breadths above the pubes, and tender on pressure. It did not occupy exactly the median line, but was inclined to the right, and appeared quite inde-pendent of the uterus, which lay in front. Vaginal touch revealed the existence of a retro-uterine tumour, irregular and made up of hard and of soft portions, rather tender on pressure. The uterus was pushed forwards against the pubes; the cervix was not patulous nor altered in consistence. The limits of the tumour could not be reached per rectum. There was scarcely any fever, and no rigors or vomiting. The diagnosis made was that of retro-uterine hæmatocele, as being the most probable condition. The idea of extra-uterine fœtation was not even suggested.

The patient continued in fair condition until June 10, when some pus was dis-charged by the rectum, and the same discharge continued on successive days, but in small quantity. On June 15 she had the sensation of some foreign body in the rectum, and a mass was found to be presenting at the anus, which proved to be the leg of a fœtus. Slight traction detached it from the rest of the body, which was engaged in the rectum. On that and the following day the rest of the fœtus was extracted, with the exception of the head, which could not be dis-covered. It was putrefied, and extremely fetid; its size appeared to correspond to an age of between four and five months. Immediately after the extraction, an opening into the fœtal cyst was felt, large enough to admit the finger, but too far from the anus to allow the cavity to be explored. The abdominal tumour had completely disappeared, as also had the retro-uterine tumour. Disinfectant injections into the cyst, by means of a tube passed through the fistulous opening, were employed, and the patient rapidly became convalescent.

The author remarks on the difficulty of diagnosis in this case, no definite signs of pregnancy having existed, and especially on the absence of any change in the consistency of the cervix, a sign rarely absent in such cases. He con-siders that the pregnancy probably commenced in December, 1876, at the time when the metrorrhagia began, and that the fœtus died at the commencement of May, when the severe abdominal pain came on. The fortunate issue of the case he attributes to the small size of the fœtus, which allowed it to be extracted through the rectum without any great difficulty; the general mortality in cases so terminating being, according to Parry's statistics, as high as thirty-five per cent., as against twenty-five per cent. in those in which evacuation takes place through the abdominal wall.—*Obstetrical Journal of Great Britain,* April, 1878.

Liquor Amnii and its Origin.

In the *Archiv für Gynækologie*, Band xi., Heft 2, Dr. L. PROCHOWNICK says that the human amniotic fluid contains urea from the sixth week to the end of pregnancy ; that it is derived from the skin and kidneys of the foetus ; further, that the quantity of urea increases during the entire pregnancy. A five weeks' ovum contains no trace whatever of urea. Chlorides appear at the end of the third month, and come not only from the kidneys but through the skin of the foetus. The author concludes that the foetus is the producer of the amniotic fluid, whose secretion begins in the earliest period of pregnancy. At the end of pregnancy only a trace of albumen can be found. In cases of hydramnion, it is remarkable that the albumen is increased. The extractive matter increases *pari passu* with the absolute amount of fluid. The fats are only found in small quantities, and come from the vernix caseosa. Cholesterin is found by chemical means, but does not appear under the microscope.—*Lond. Med. Record*, March 15, 1878.

The Prevention of Puerperal Fever.

Puerperal fever is a disease the ordinary social surroundings of which make its effect, when fatal, perhaps more distressing to the surviving relatives and to the medical attendant than is the case with very many equally dangerous disorders. The removal of a young wife from her husband, of a mother from a family not yet old enough to do without her help—and this as the result of an event natural, commonly harmless, and probably looked forward to as a bringer of joy ; the hints that are so likely to be dropped as to the doctor's conduct of the case, and his possible culpability in bringing infection from some one else ;—all make this disease one to which social consequences of peculiar importance attach themselves. Its interest to the scientific inquirer is not less, for we have much yet to learn about it. The knowledge that the medical attendant may carry with him the contagium of the disease, and the well-ascertained facts which show that infection from the dead body may produce it, have, with other causes, tended to prevent both post-mortem investigation of the disease and frequent examination of the affected parts during life. Our knowledge of it is thus principally clinical, and therefore incomplete. Hence the great number of different views about it ; in this, as in other things, the amount and variety of diverse opinions being in inverse proportion to the amount of definite knowledge of the subject.

It is not our intention here to enter upon any discussion of the varying doctrines that have been held. We shall advert to etiological considerations only so much as is necessary to give weight to the practical precautions they indicate. It happens that the dominant theory at present is one which, if true, gives us hope of being able to greatly hinder the spread and lower the mortality of this formidable malady. We speak of it as the dominant theory, in order that we may not assume that which is not yet universally admitted, not to imply that we think its reign is likely to be transient. It is enough for our present purpose that the theory in question is accredited by the acceptance of many great authorities both here and abroad, and is supported by much evidence ; beside the scientific prejudice in its favour, from its being based on the latest, and therefore the largest, knowledge.

The current of opinion, which is now setting so strongly in Germany, and to a great extent in this country, is in favour of the view that puerperal fever is a disease like surgical septicæmia and pyæmia—that it is, in fact, the same malady, entering through a special channel ; this channel being either some rent (minute though it may be) of the parturient canal (such as often occurs, especially in first labours) or veins, the mouths of which have been bared in the separation of the placenta. Thus the greater frequency of the disease in question in first labours is accounted for by this hypothesis. As from wounds we have various degrees of disturbance, known as traumatic fever, septicæmia, and pyæmia, so in the puerperal state we have maladies which may be slight, severe, or fatal. As in the one, so in the other, the symptoms result from an absorption, through the wound, of pyrogenic or phlogogenic matter. Adopting the germ theory in the form so ably set forth by Dr. Roberts, at Manchester, we may say that in the puerperal state slight fever, septicæmia, or pyæmia results whenever the secretions in contact with absorbing surfaces assume such a character that germs will live in them. These mischievous little organisms meet with barren soil in the fresh secretions of a healthy wound. But if these fluids accumulate and decompose, then the germs find nourishment in them, grow and multiply, and, if a way be open, get access to the system. There are, therefore, two ways in which this may be prevented—first, by keeping away (or killing) the germs; and second, by preventing the accumulation of secretions, and therefore the changes in them which make them fit for the little enemies to thrive therein. Professor Lister has successfully aimed at carrying out the first plan; Mr. Callender has attained the end by acting on the second. We shall do well to profit by the teaching of each, and try both to see that no germs get to the patient; and if they should, after all, reach her, to give them no congenial soil: and thus we may hope to prevent puerperal fever.

Let us take first some measures, based upon this theory, which relate to the patient herself. Attention has been drawn by more than one British obstetrician to the value of intra-uterine injections in cases in which feverish symptoms are accompanied by fetor of the discharges. But it is clear that if we accept the views, an outline of which we have been trying to draw, the use of antiseptics after labour must become more extended. There is even a better thing than curing such a set of symptoms; and that is, to prevent the discharge ever becoming fetid or the temperature rising. If the theory we have referred to as dominant be one holding good for all cases, this is within our power. And, further, Olshausen has shown that the introduction of lochia by a catheter into the bladder is followed by cystitis. Kehrer (in an able monograph, a review of which will be found in our first volume for last year) has proved that lochial discharge, apparently healthy, yet possesses a constituent capable of exciting inflammation and fever, and either that the amount or the virulence (probably both) of this constituent increases in the later days of the discharge. If these researches be correct, it is clear that we must not look upon fetid lochia as the only condition calling for antiseptics.

Our German brethren, in this as in many other things, are putting their theory into practice with method, perseverence, and ingenuity. In April last we put before our readers an account of the views and precepts of Fritsch as to this subject. Schülein, in a series of 201 cases, normal and other, washed out the interior of the uterus simply as a prophylactic measure. Münster, in twenty-four cases of labour, either very prolonged or attended with those complications which we know render the patient liable to puerperal disease, practised the same measure, without waiting for symptoms to come on. Of Münster's cases, all recovered perfectly. Schülein comes to the conclusions that these injections, with proper care, are harmless; that they diminish to a considerable extent the frequency of puerperal diseases, and the mortality of them; and that, when used in cases in which the temperature is already high, this treatment is often followed by a considerable fall. He therefore recommends their use both to prevent and cure puerperal disease. These results are most satisfactory, the only objection to which is, that they are based on but a small number of cases. Schede, beside washing out the uterus, put in, in order to prevent accumulation of secretions, a tube provided with a cross-piece, or with lateral projections at the end, in order to fix it in the uterus ; and he tells us that, in some cases in which (he having used it only after severe septicæmia had already set in) the patient died, no ill effects were perceptible from its use. We are quite willing to admit that this may have been a proper measure in Schede's cases ; yet we do not think that to put into the uterus something which retains itself there by pressure against the walls of that organ is a procedure to be recommended as likely to prevent disease. Schücking has taken much pains in devising a means of applying a rigidly antiseptic treatment to the genital canal. His apparatus consists of a metal tube, with numerous lateral openings, wrapped round with several layers of gauze. This is put into the vagina, so that the end of the tube lies in the os uteri. The gauze is soaked in an antiseptic solution, and its function is to prevent the holes of the tube from getting stopped up by coagula, and to insure that the antiseptic shall be applied to an extensive surface. The tube is connected with an irrigating apparatus, so that a slow, steady stream of the antiseptic solution used shall flow through the tube, percolate the gauze, and so bathe the genital passage. The patient lies on a mackintosh, or some other arrangement, serving to prevent the wetting of the bedclothes. The tube is removed every twenty-four hours, the gauze changed, and the vagina well syringed with an antiseptic. Schücking's plan is ingenious, and in cases in which the vagina has been wounded, or sloughing is to be apprehended, we should think it highly useful. But in ordinary confinements it seems to us too troublesome and disagreeable for routine use ; and we question whether ordinary syringing with an antiseptic does not effect all that is required in a simple case.

A practical conclusion of some value, if correct, which Kehrer draws from his investigations, is this : that in cases in which, in the later days of the lochial discharge, symptoms arise making one think that a bit of placenta or membrane has been retained, and therefore the uterine cavity should be explored. It is better not to do this at once, but to remain content with antiseptic injections, until any rents that may be present in the genital canal have completely healed ; for if done before, these wounds, then closed only by granulation tissue, will be torn open again, and thus a fresh surface exposed to absorb the virulent lochial discharge.

Wishing to make as little painful as possible a measure which he thinks very valuable, and also to enable the medical man to avoid all contact with the lochia, Dr. Chamberlain has had constructed for the purpose of intra-uterine injection a tube of toughened glass. It is fifteen inches long, five-eighths of an inch thick, rounded at the free end, bent at a curve convenient for introduction, and perforated with holes so arranged that some open at each surface. This tube is inserted into the vagina without need of a guiding finger. This canal is washed out, and then with a little manœuvring (which in practice, Dr. Chamberlain says, becomes very easy) the point is slipped into the cervical canal and pushed up to the fundus. The uterus can thus be thoroughly irrigated without any contact occurring between the medical man and the secretions of the patient. Judging from the description, this seems to us a most useful invention, sound in principle and safe in practice.

The antiseptics used by the authors from whom we have quoted were either carbolic acid, in solution of 2 to 5 per cent. strength ; salicylic acid, 1 to 2 parts per 1000 ; or sodic sulphite, in a 10 per cent. solution, with 5 per cent. of glycerine.

The increased liability to puerperal disease which follows protracted labour and mismanaged third stage is well known.   To discuss these points would take us so far into an entirely different subject that we will content ourselves with mentioning them.

Space forbids us here to go on to those precautions, designed to prevent the access of contagion, which relate to the surroundings of the patient. We may possibly do this in a future number.   That part of the subject with which we have been dealing has been taken first, not because it is more important, but because newer, and therefore probably less familiar to our readers.—*Med. Times and Gaz.*, Feb. 9, 1878.

_____

Tumour of the Clitoris removed by Paquelin's Thermo-cautère.

At a late meeting of the Philadelphia Obstetrical Society (*Am. Journal of Obstetrics*, Jan. 1878) Dr. ALBERT H. SMITH showed a specimen of tumour removed by Paquelin's thermo-cautère.   The tumour, which was about the size of a large walnut, was a vegetative excrescence, the pedicle of which involved the tissues surrounding the base of the clitoris.   The patient, who was admitted to the Women's Hospital for operation, was married, forty years of age, and three months pregnant.   She made application for treatment on account of the constant recurrence of violent paroxysms of pain in the base of the tumour, which prevented her sleeping, and, resisting the impression of anodynes, were steadily exhausting her.   Her pregnancy being no contraindication, but rather an additional urgency to its removal, from the danger of the continued pain setting up an abortive effort in the uterus, it was decided to remove it at once, which Dr. Smith did with the platinum knife of Paquelin's apparatus.   The removal was accomplished with great rapidity, the tumour being drawn forward forcibly by a vulsellum, which included in its grasp the considerably enlarged clitoris, making very tense the pedicle of skin and connective tissue, through which. the knife speedily cut its way, being carried deeply enough to remove every portion of indurated tissue involved in the morbid growth, extending very closely upon the urethral meatus.   At one stage of the process, the knife being raised nearly to a white heat, cut too rapidly, and a profuse hemorrhage burst forth from the very vascular tissues around the clitoris, and the dorsal artery, of unusual size, spurted out as large as a small bird's quill.   The knife was immediately cooled down below a red heat, and pressed upon the bleeding vessels, when the hemorrhage instantly stopped.   The slough from the burned surface completely separated in about ten days, leaving a healthy granulating surface, from which there was at no time any hemorrhage.   The ulceration healed promptly, complicated by a slight irritation of the urethra, which soon disappeared.   Four weeks after the operation there had been no return of the pain which had been so violent in the seat of the tumour, and the patient was perfectly comfortable, her pregnancy advancing undisturbed.

Dr. Smith exhibited the knife to the Society, showing its admirable facility of management, and its applicability to most cutting operations when hemorrhage is feared, and where union of the cut surfaces by adhesion is not required.   He had used it with great satisfaction for the removal of superficial growths, especially epithelial cancers.   The simplicity of the instrument, and the readiness with which the degree of temperature can be controlled, and especially the persistence of its action, give it great advantages over the galvano-cautery wherever the form of the knife makes it practicable.   So far, only a short straight knife has been adapted to its use, which necessitates its being held perpendicularly to the surface, into which the incision is to be made; so that for such operations as the excision of the cervix uteri, where the mobility of the uterus is not sufficient to allow it to be drawn by volsella to the vulval opening, it cannot take the place of

the constricting wire of the galvano-cautery. No doubt some additional forms
of the knife will be added as the demands for the increase.

Some precautions are necessary in the use of the instrument, as Dr. Smith has
found from experience. The knife should be brought nearly to a red heat in the
alcohol flame before projecting the vapour of benzoline into it from the bottle,
otherwise the rapid evaporation will cool the knife so that the flame cannot raise
its temperature to the point of igniting the vapour, and the operator is foiled in
his attempt to get up a red heat. The bottle of benzoline (which by the way
should be of the best possible quality) should not be filled more than half full.
If the fluid reaches nearly to the end of the metallic tubes in the cork, it may be
driven into the rubber tubing leading to the knife, and be forced out of the opening in the knife instead of the aerated vapour. If this should take place the
excessively inflammable nature of the benzoline fluid would render probable a
serious accident. In operating in the neighbourhood of the face, under etherization, great care must be used not to bring the red-hot knife within range of the
vapour of ether, as it will ignite it instantly, and the whole mass of the ether
applicator, whatever form it may have, as well as the hair of the patient saturated with ether, will be in a flame. Dr. Smith had this happen in one case in
an operation for removal of an epithelioma from the cheek, and has seen it also
occur in the hands of another physician when the operation was upon a fungoid
growth of the breast, in which the knife was not within a foot of the paper cone
inclosing the ether towel. Fortunately, in both these cases the fire was extinguished instantly, before any injury occurred.

In cutting with the knife the tissue should be kept tense upon either side of
the line of incision, when the knife will make its way almost as rapidly as a bistoury. If it should be cutting too rapidly, and a hemorrhage should occur, a less
rapid compression of the hand-ball which supplies the vapour will cool it down.
When a large vessel is opened, or is known to pass through the line of incision,
by pressing the knife, reduced to a *black* heat, firmly upon the cut surface, a
deep scorching of the tissues is produced, which will control hemorrhage completely at the time and prevent its recurrence at the after-separation of the
slough. The prospective range of usefulness of this knife in such operations as
already mentioned, as well as in the opening of deep abscesses, the incision of
carbuncles, and other similar purposes, seems to give it a very important position
among the mechanical appliances of modern surgery.

The Faradic Treatment of Uterine Fibroids.

Dr. J. T. EVERETT, of Sterling, Illinois, reports (*Am. Journal of Obstetrics,*
Jan. 1878) nine cases of uterine fibroids treated by the faradic current, and from
a review of these and other cases he presents the following conclusions:—

1. The faradic current, if judiciously used, is equally potent to produce uterine contractions as the preparations of ergot.

2. It is more easily controlled, can be begun or discontinued at a moment's
notice, and the dose can thus be more judiciously apportioned.

3. It never disturbs nutrition or the secretions, and does not interfere with
digestion.

4. It never produces pain in distant organs, is followed by no cephalic disturbance or nervous shock.

5. It never produces inflammations or other local injury.

Injection of Ergotin into the Uterus.

In a discussion in the Surgical Society of Paris (*La France Médicale*) M.
DELORE said that subcutaneous injections of ergotin were first employed by Hil-

debrandt in 1872, in cases of uterine fibroma.   N. Delore had made injections
into the tissues of the uterus itself.   He employed one part of ergotin to two of
distilled water; he used a speculum, and pierced directly the cervix uteri.   In a
physiological point of view, the injection of ergotin in the tissues of the uterus
produced more intense effects than absorption by the stomach.   In his patients
he had observed phenomena of different kinds; chills, trembling, bilious vomiting, fainting, troubles of vision, diarrhœa, pain in the kidneys, thighs, legs,
abdomen, or head.   In two cases he had seen abscesses produced.   The patients
had been relieved; the hemorrhages had been arrested; in fine, the results had
been encouraging.

N. DUPLAY had employed the method several times, and, while he had not
obtained curative effects, he had obtained satisfactory results as to the relief given.
He had never seen any accidents.

N. TERRIER had made a number of injections into the skin of the abdomen,
and had had no accidents.   Frequently he had permitted the injections to be
made by the husbands of the patients; in these cases the injections had been
made not into the subcutaneous cellular tissue, but in the skin itself, and then he
had seen small foci of sloughing.   These injections had given very good results
in hemorrhages, but in one case there was violent contraction of the uterus, and
the metrorrhagia was augmented.

N. PANAS used the ergotin of N. Bonjean.   Ergot contained an extractive
matter and a volatile oil; this oil was the active principle.

N. N. SEE had very satisfactory results with hypodermic injections of the
ergotin of Bonjean.

N. DUPLAY said that N. Vidal, at the Hospital Saint-Louis, treated prolapse
of the uterus in this manner, and obtained results which could hardly be explained, except by action upon the muscular fibres.

N. DELORE said that ergotin preparations by different pharmaceutists were
very different.   For these injections ergot could not be employed and continued
every day like ergotin.—*London Med. Record,* March 15, 1878.

—

Sounding of the Fallopian Tube.

In the *Berliner Klinische Wochenschrift,* October, 1877, Dr. BIEDERT relates the case of a young woman who had been married two years and had
remained sterile, suffering from dysmenorrhœa.   Dr. Biedert found a small os
and conical cervix, which he dilated with laminaria tents.   On passing the uterine sound on one occasion after the dilatation, he felt it turn suddenly to the left,
and about four and three-quarter inches of the sound entered the uterine cavity.
It was quite impossible to turn the concavity of the sound forwards, on account
of the acute pain which it caused the patient.   Dr. Biedert considers that the
sound passed into the left Fallopian tube.   The patient after this menstruated
without pain for the first time in her life, and has since given birth to two healthy
children.   Dr. Biedert draws the following conclusions: 1. Catheterization of
the Fallopian tube is possible.   2· Catheterization presupposes a dilatation of the
tube.   3. The dilatation of the tube is probably the result of an impeded or painful flow of the secretions, and especially the menstrual, from the uterine cavity.
4. In such cases, intra-uterine injections are attended with danger.   5. Back
flow of the menstrual blood through the widened tube may give rise to perimetric
hæmatocele.   6. In such cases, operative removal of the obstruction to the out-
pour of secretions may prevent the formation of hæmatocele.—*London Med. Record,* Jan. 15, 1878.

A Case of Dermoid Cyst successfully Removed by Ovariotomy.

In a paper read before the Société de Médecine de Strasbourg (*Gaz. de Médicale de Strasbourg*) Dr. KOEBERLE relates a case of dermoid cyst removed by ovariotomy. The patient, a lady twenty-three years old, had always enjoyed good health till the commencement of 1875. At that time, in the second month of her first pregnancy, she was suddenly attacked by violent pain in the hypogastrium, accompanied by colic and vomiting. After lasting two or three hours this subsided completely. At the fourth month a similar attack occurred, and lasted a whole day. The remainder of the pregnancy and the delivery were entirely normal. After delivery the abdomen remained large, and tender at its lowest part. Five months after, on 23d December, 1875, she had another attack of very violent pain, lasting for three days. This was ascribed at the time by Dr. Duhoué, of Pau, to be a peritoneal irritation, which appeared to result from a hæmatocele. On 1st January, 1876, a new attack of pain occurred, and lasted six days. The pain was situated chiefly in the right groin, radiating to the thigh and loin of the same side, and, as on the former occasion, was unaccompanied by any elevation of temperature. After this the presence of an ovarian cyst was recognized, but could not be definitely connected with the occurrence of the pain.

An attack of pain again occurred in August, and finally a still severe one towards the end of November. This commenced instantaneously, in consequence of a sudden movement of rotation of the body, and did not cease for twenty days, being accompanied as before by vomiting, cramp, colic, and extreme tenderness of the abdomen, with tympanites. Shortly after each crisis the size of the tumour notably diminished.

For about four months afterwards no further attack of pain had occurred, and the size of the tumour did not perceptibly increase. There was no emaciation, and menstruation was normal. Dr. Koeberlé found the abdominal tumour to consist of an ovarian cyst, of from nineteen to twenty centimetres in diameter, situated chiefly at the left side of the hypogastrium. It reached about four finger-breadths above the umbilicus, and appeared quite movable, though it could not be pushed so far to the right side as to the left. The tumour was fluctuating, and a vibratory thrill could be felt perfectly over the left side, not so distinctly towards the right. Towards the lower and left portion of the tumour could be felt a small, firm tuberosity, of from four to five centimetres in length. The body of the uterus was displaced towards the right, the cervix towards the left.

The diagnosis made was that of a cyst of the left ovary, without abdominal adhesions, and probably dermoid, on account of the good general condition, the slowness of growth, and the firmness of the prominent tuberosity. The attacks of pain suffered by the patient were attributed to a torsion of the pedicle; but it appeared inexplicable why the pain should have occurred on the right side. Although the tumour was moderate in size, and stationary for some months, extirpation was resolved on. It was thought that the attacks of pain were the result of the tumour, and that it was wiser to operate while the condition was good, and avoid the risk of ulterior complications.

Ovariotomy was performed by Dr. Koeberlé on April 10, 1877. An incision, ten centimetres long, laid bare the cyst, which was adherent to the abdominal wall by numerous fibrous bands, very vascular, but not containing vessels of important size. When the cyst was punctured, about a litre of brownish-red thick fluid escaped containing masses of fat, mingled with blonde hairs, of from one to four centimetres in length. The diagnosis as to the dermoid nature of the tumour was thus confirmed. The cyst was detached from its adhesions, which covered nearly three-fourths of its surface, extending as low as the pelvis. The pedicle consisted of two parts, a broad, fibrous, and vascular band, continuous with the broad ligament on the right side, and adherent to the base of the tumour, and a slender true pedicle, springing from the right side, from five to seven millimetres in diameter, and twisted upon itself as much as two circumferences. The right Fallopian tube was involved in a spiral with it. The broad fibrous band was separated, and the hemorrhage arrested with considerable difficulty. The pedicle was then inclosed in an iron wire attached to a serre-nœud, and the tumour excised. The pedicle was capable of being untwisted, and was of good length. The left ovary was healthy. The patient recovered without any interruption after the operation, the temperature not rising above 37.8° C.

The author remarks that the localization of pain on the right side was explained by the tumour having originated in the right ovary, although this was impossible to diagnose before the operation. The tumour consisted of a unilocular dermoid cyst. The internal cutaneous integument was deprived of epidermis, and the hairs which had covered it were, for the most part, shed. The small hard tumour in the walls of the cyst was also of a dermoid character, and partially covered with mucous membrane. The life of the dermoid tissues appeared to have been destroyed in consequence of the twisting of the pedicle, but the vitality of the envelopes had been preserved, in consequence of the adhesions which had been formed. Deposits of clot existed in many parts over the surface of the cyst.— *Obstetrical Journal of Great Britain*, April, 1878.

Medical Jurisprudence and Toxicology.

Simulation of Fever.

Dr. SELLERBECK (*Berliner Klin. Wochenschrift*, January 21) read a communication before the Society of the Physicians of the Charité in Berlin, on the case of a patient who had for a whole year been in the Charité under treatment for gastric ulcer following an attempt at suicide by means of lye. Throughout its course the case was marked by obstinate vomiting, and the matters vomited were tinged with blood or mixed with blood-coagula. The source of this bleeding could not be determined. Some tenderness and slight bulging were noted in the epigastric region. At various times there occurred, without any assignable cause, exacerbations of temperature, reaching to 102.9° F., with a pulse of 120, and respiration 24. All conceivable means to stop the hæmatemesis were unavailing. The otherwise healthy and well-nourished appearance of the patient led to a suspicion of deception, or, at least, of artificial exaggeration of the symptoms. Even thus it was difficult to account for the high temperatures, which were taken and registered by an experienced and trustworthy nurse. The temperature in the axilla ranged from 100° to 102.7° F., the exacerbations occurring sometimes in the morning, then again in the evening, or lasting some time, as in continued fever. In order to test the matter, when on one occasion the axillary temperature stood at 101.3° F., a thermometer was placed in the rectum, which was found to mark only 100° F., thus proving the existence of trickery somewhere. Acting under this new light it was shown without difficulty, in the presence of the patient, that by means of a rapid rotating movement of the bulb between the thumb and fingers, or between two folds of linen, the mercurial column could be raised, so as to indicate a high fever-temperature. The patient at first totally denied the charge of practising any deception, but was presently brought to confess that, in order to excite greater interest in her case, she had managed, when the thermometer was placed in her axilla, to inclose the bulb in a fold of her linen, and then, by firmly pressing it between the arm and thorax and rapidly rubbing it up and down, she raised the column to the excessive height observed. When once the deception was discovered, she took a lively interest, after the true manner of hysteria, in the experiments that were made to ascertain the height to which the thermometer could be thus artificially raised. It was as a result found that by tightly inclosing the bulb in a fold of her linen and then rapidly rotating it in a spiral manner, the temperature could be easily raised to 114.8° F. On stopping this rubbing, the column at first fell rapidly to 100° F. to 103° F., where it then remained almost stationary for several minutes. Friction between the bare skin of the arm and thorax had less effect in raising the temperature, owing probably to the cooling effect of the slightly moist surfaces and the greater difficulty of rapid rubbing. Yet even thus, in about three minutes, a height of 108° F. could be attained.

[Until within the last three years the errors of clinical measurements of temperature were supposed to be only on the side of deficiency from improper methods of observation. About that time, Mr. Teale, of Scarborough, reported a case of the excessively high temperature of 122° F. (*Brit. Med. Journal*, March 6th, 1875). The various theories advanced to account for this naturally impossible temperature, such as that of secreted hot-water bottles or mechanical pressure on the bulb, were insufficient. Schliep subsequently, in another case, hit upon the explanation that it was possible to raise the temperature by rubbing the thermometer bulb between the thumb and fingers. Deception is specially easy in this way with self-registering index thermometers. But the foregoing seems to be the first recorded case where the patient successfully simulated fever by this means, and also reproduced in a striking manner the symptoms of increased frequency of the pulse respiration, and then acknowledged having done so.—*Rep.*]—*London Med. Record*, March 15, 1878.

Poisoning by Inhaling Dust containing Chrome Yellow.

LEOPOLD (*Vierteljahresschrift für Gerichtliche Medicin*, Band xxiv.) reports five cases of this form of poisoning, one of which proved fatal. The patients were employed in weaving cloth coloured with chrome yellow (chromate of lead) which was quite loosely applied to the thread, so that a portion of the pigment was easily detached and became diffused throughout the air of the room. The patients were affected with a yellow-coated tongue, yellow sputa, loss of appetite, *malaise*, in some cases vomiting, pain in the region of the stomach and umbilicus, obstinate constipation, and debility. The feces were yellow. These symptoms disappeared in a few weeks after the removal of the cause, except in the case of an infant nine weeks old, who died six or eight days after the beginning of the symptoms, which, however, did not appear until about three weeks after exposure to the infected atmosphere. The symptoms in this case were fever, restlessness, several yellow-fluid stools daily, redness of the skin over the chest and abdomen, parched lips, and, just before death, short respiration.

After death there was found inflammation and perforation of the stomach, the same appearances which were seen in two cases previously reported by Dr. von Linstow, caused by ingesting chrome yellow. None of the poison could be detected in any of the organs except the lungs.—*London Med. Record*, March 15, 1878.

CONTENTS.

Published Monthly, price $2.50 *per annum, free of postage.*
Also, furnished together with the AMERICAN JOURNAL OF THE MEDICAL SCIENCES *and the* MEDICAL NEWS AND LIBRARY *for* SIX DOLLARS *per annum in advance, the whole free of postage.*

HENRY C. LEA, Philadelphia.

THE MONTHLY ABSTRACT

OF

MEDICAL SCIENCE.

Vol. v. No. 6.   **For List of Contents see last page.**   June, 1878.

Anatomy and Physiology.

Congenital Absence of One Kidney.

Congenital absence of one kidney is a malformation of more than usual indirect interest. Its causes are as obscure as those of most other developmental errors, but the associated conditions are, in some instances, very curious, and its consequences frequently of great moment to the individual. Whatever may have been their origin, there can be no doubt that the presence of double organs saves us from many of the grave consequences of local disease, and the resulting advantage is strikingly brought out by a study of the effects of the experiment which Nature at times performs, of substituting a single organ, however efficient, for the double organ which she usually provides.

In the current number of Virchow's *Archiv* Dr. Beumer has collected from various sources forty-eight cases in which one kidney was congenitally absent, and has carefully compared the conditions, associations, and effect of this malformation. This number of cases is considerably greater than any previous writer has collected, and the conclusions drawn from them possess corresponding value. From the circumstances that these cases were all recorded within the last twenty-five years, the condition, although uncommon, is not of extreme rarity. In forty-four out of the forty-eight the kidney was entirely absent; in four it was rudimentary. The organ appears to be absent as often on one side as on the other, since in twenty-one cases the defect was on the right side, and in twenty-two it was on the left. It appears to be of more frequent occurrence in the male than in the female sex, since, of thirty-nine cases in which the sex was mentioned, twenty-six were males, and thirteen were females. It must be remembered, however, in estimating the value of this difference, that the number of post-mortem examinations upon men is larger than upon women, and the condition can only be diagnosed by an autopsy. When observations have been made upon the state of the vessels, they have been most commonly absent. In one case, although the kidney was wanting, a rudiment of the renal artery existed, passing into the cellular tissue. In one case in which a rudimentary kidney existed, incapable of function, the renal artery did not exist. Similar variations in the condition of the ureter have been observed. In most cases the duct was entirely absent; in a few the portion of the ureter adjacent to the bladder alone existed. Of the bladder, one angle of the trigonum was absent in some cases, or the sulcus in which the ureter opens could not be detected on the side on which the kidney was wanting.

In most of the cases in which the kidney was absent the suprarenal body was present. In two cases it appeared to be enlarged, but it is probable that the apparent enlargement was the effect only of the change in shape consequent on the absence of the organ on which it is moulded. Förster asserted that the suprarenal body is always present in these cases of congenital absence of the kidney, and his statement has been generally accepted as correct. In five of the cases collected by Beumer, the supra renal body was also absent. In one of those cases, recorded by SCHREIBER, there was a bicornuate uterus, and closure of the anus, the rectum opening into the vagina, between the carunculæ myrtiformes. The subject of this curious malformation lived to the age of thirty years, and died of cerebral tumour.

This coincidence of an arrest of the development of the sexual organs with the defect of the kidney was not unfrequent, and constitutes one of the most inte-resting teratological points in the study of the malformation. The sexual malfor-mation was present in thirteen cases, nearly a third of the total number; eight were females and five males. Of the latter cases, in one there was simply a diminution in the size of the corresponding vesicula seminalis and vas deferens; in another case the vesicula seminalis on that side was absent, and the vas defe-rens and testicle were small; and in another the corresponding testicle, with the vas deferens, was absent. In an interesting case recorded by EPPINGER, in which the right kidney and ureter were rudimentary, although the male sexual organs were normally developed, there was, on the right side, a half vagina, an inch and a half in length, and a corresponding uterine cornu, an inch in length. In females, . the associated irregularities of the sexual organs were more frequent, both abso-lutely and relatively, and they were also more considerable. The uterus was the organ which had most frequently suffered. In a few cases the whole of the sexual organs on that side were absent—the ovary, half the uterus, and half the vagina. In several the uterus was unicornuate, the half of a bicornuate uterus being absent on the side of the defect. In some case in which a bicornuate uterus was com-plete, the vagina was double.

The remaining kidney was, in all the cases, considerably enlarged, and increased in weight and size; and with this increase was a corresponding development of the vessels and ureter. In twenty-six of the cases this enlarged kidney was per-fectly healthy, and of these no less than eleven were over thirty years of age. This is a fresh and striking proof of the completeness with which the one kidney can carry on the functions of the two, without suffering degeneration in couse-quence of its increased work. But in no less than twenty-two of the cases the remaining kidney presented evidence of disease—an equally clear indication that the increased work, although entailing no necessary degeneration, does involve an increased liability to disease. In most of these patients the disease of the kidney was the immediate cause of death. The most common condition was chronic inflammation. It is evident that such disease could be borne for a short time only; and this the details of the cases prove, since in many of them the bladder was completely empty, anuria having preceded death. The frequent occurrence of calculi in the pelvis of the kidney and ureter is worthy of note; they were found no less than ten times. This frequency is a point of much physiological interest in connection with the excretion of uric acid and the func-tional power of the single kidney. The danger of the condition in such patients is obvious, and is shown by the records of many of these cases, since in no less than five a renal calculus stopping the ureter caused complete obstruction and all the consequences of retention of urine in the kidney, including rapid death.

The pathological aspect of these cases is alone the subject of Beumer's paper, . but his facts suggest clinical applications of some importance. To one only of these we may allude. It has been remarked that the morbid state can only be recognized on the post-mortem table, but the association with defects of the sexual organs suggests the possibility of suspecting its existence during life. In many such cases the enlarged single organ might be felt. The occurrence in such patients of evidence of chronic Bright's disease without recognizable cause, or of grave symptoms succeeding those of renal colic, and even the occurrence of renal colic on the side opposite to that on which there exists a sexual malformation, might in some cases lead to a correct suspicion of the existence of the renal defect.—*Lancet*, April 20, 1878.

The Rouge of the Retina.

M. CAPRANICA (*Annales d'Oculistique*, September and October, 1877) has studied the colouring matter of the yellow bodies which are found in the pigmentary layer of the retina of the frog. According to the researches of Boll, this colouring matter is in all probability the same from which the retinal rouge is resupplied when it has been exhausted by the action of light. The material contained in these yellow globules is insoluble in water and in alkaline solutions, and equally so in acid and neutral solutions ; but it is readily soluble in various forms of alcohol, in ether, chloroform, and sulphide of carbon. All these solutions become yellow, with the exception of that in sulphide of carbon, which resembles that of the retinal rouge. The yellow globules give three characteristic reactions. 1. Concentrated sulphuric acid produces instantaneously a splendid dark violet tint, rapidly changing to blue. 2. Concentrated nitric acid produces a greenish-blue solution, which rapidly becomes colourless. 3. A solution of iodine changes their colour to a beautiful green. Exactly the same reactions are obtained from the red and yellow globules which are found within the rods and cones of birds and reptiles. The perfect analogy which exists between the reactions of the two sets of globules shows, almost beyond doubt, that the chemical constitution of the colouring matter in each is identical. M. Capranica has submitted the colouring material to spectroscopic analysis, and he has succeeded in obtaining identical absorption-bands from the two varieties of solutions. The solutions themselves become almost or completely colourless by exposure to daylight. It is a very remarkable occurrence that the colouring matter of these globules presents a complete analogy, both chemical and spectroscopic, with the substance which Hoppe-Seyler and Thudichum have described under the name of luteine, and which has been found in the ovaries of mammalia, in the yolk of egg, in the serum of blood, and elsewhere. M. Capranica has extracted the colouring matter from the ovaries of cows in the shape of microscopic crystals, with which he has obtained the three characteristic reactions of the retinal globules, and the same phenomena of solubility ; the spectroscopic appearances are also the same. Precisely the same results are to be obtained from the examination of the yolk of egg.

In short, the researches of Capranica appear to show that even within the egg there exists a colouring material destined to find a home within the retina, and to render the latter sensitive to the most refrangible rays of solar light. The difficulty in ascertaining the exact chemical composition of this substance is great, inasmuch as it is associated with much fatty material, from which it cannot readily be separated. Its sensitiveness to light appears to be in the inverse ratio to the amount of fat with which it is associated. For instance, the yellow of the egg, the most rich in fat, is the least sensitive to light ; that of the ovary is the most sensitive, while the reddish-yellow of the retinal globules holds a mid-position.

Although the erythropsine of Boll has a greater photo-chemical sensibility than luteine, yet M. Capranica does not hesitate to assume a very intimate relationship between the two substances, and thinks it will, ere long, be possible to show that the retinal rouge is only a chemical derivative from luteine, from which indeed it differs only by possessing a less density, which may perhaps explain its greater sensitiveness to the action of light.—*London Med. Record*, March 15, 1878.

Laryngostroboscopy.

The actual vibrations of the vocal cords during the production of sounds have hitherto eluded direct observation. According, however, to a publication by Dr. OERTEL, of Munich, their observation is a matter of little difficulty, and is likely to afford instructive information regarding the physiology of the voice. It is only necessary, he asserts, to employ a light sufficiently strong, and to provide an arrangement by which it shall be rapidly interrupted, to render the vibrations visible. The effect of the interruption of the light is to retard the perception of the individual vibration, or rather to prevent their impression on the retina from being modified before it can be perceived. Thus it is possible not merely to observe accurately the vibrations of one of the vibrating cords, but also to compare the vibrations of one with those of the other. The light which is employed must be of the most powerful character, by preference direct sunlight, or the electric or oxyhydrogen light. The interruption may be conveniently produced by a perforated diaphragm revolving rapidly, and at a rate proportioned to the rapidity of the vibrations of the sounding cord. Or it may be interrupted by a tuning-fork, and in the latter case a note should be chosen of the same height as that produced by the larynx under observation, or an octave from it. The interrupting apparatus must be placed between the light and the laryngoscope mirror, or behind this mirror and between it and the observer; the latter is a convenient position for the revolving diaphragm when a little practice in its use has been obtained, and the diaphragm can be turned by the hand at the needful rate for observing the vibrations at a given note.

When a chest-note is uttered, the laryngoscope shows the vocal cords vibrating in their entire extent, and the sharp edge cannot be seen. By the interrupted light these vibrations may be separated into the movements of which they are made up, but are seen to be still vibrations of the vocal cords as a whole. When, however, a falsetto-note is uttered, the vocal cords are seen to be apparently scarcely moved, and with the interrupted light this is seen to be due to the circumstance that the cords are vibrating in sections, two or three, according to the height of the note, the sections being divided by one or two nodal points.—*Lancet*, April 27, 1878.

Albuminuria in Health.

The presence of albumen in the urine, even in very minute quantities, is usually taken as conclusive evidence of such a condition of systemic derangement as deserves to be regarded as disease. Professor LEUBE, of Erlangen, considering the fact that a trace of albumen is occasionally present in the urine of patients who present no other evidence of renal disease, examined the urine of a large number of men presumably in good health, soldiers on regular duty, in order to ascertain whether albumen could ever be detected in the urine of those who presented no other morbid symptoms. He examined the morning urine of 119 soldiers, and found a trace of albumen in that of five, in one a distinct quantity, in the others merely a faint, just recognizable, trace. In each case the midday urine also contained albumen, and in three the amount was larger than in the morning urine. So far the results are not surprising, since they would seem explicable on the theory that these soldiers were suffering from incipient renal disease, which, as is well known, may be unattended by any indication of deranged health. But it was found that albumen was present in 14 soldiers out of 119, whose morning urine had been free from albumen. In all these instances the soldiers had undertaken arduous duty, marches or battalion drill, during the forenoon, but no food or drink had been taken during the exercise. No casts or blood were found in the deposit from the urine. The albumen soon disappeared with rest. This fact seems to show that in apparently healthy men exertion may induce slight albuminuria. This opinion was supported by an instance in which the urine of a soldier was for two days free from even a trace of albumen, but on the third, after a long battalion exercise, it contained a distinct trace, which had disappeared in two or three hours, and was also absent the next morning. In every case in which albumen was present any indication of disease, local or general, was carefully searched for, but none could be found. The conclusion Leube draws from his observations is that "in the vast majority of cases the urine of healthy persons is quite free from albumen; in rare cases, a slight, but distinct, albuminuria coexists in a completely normal state of system, and is comparatively frequent if bodily exertion precedes the secretion of the urine."

What is the origin of this temporary albuminuria? Our knowledge of the condition of urinary secretion is still too indefinite to permit a satisfactory answer to be given to this question; but it may be explained on either of the current theories of urinary secretion—that of simple filtration of all the urinary constituents through the Malpighian capsules, and that of the specific secretion of the urine by the cells of the tubules. On the filtration theory, the absence of albumen from normal urine is accounted for by supposing that either the walls of the blood-vessels permit the passage of water through them, but retain the colloidal substances, as albumen; or else that albumen passes through the membranes of the Malpighian capsules, and is removed again by the epithelium of the tubules. On the theory that the transpirability of membranes depends on the size of their "pores," Leube fancies that in some individuals these pores may be of such a size as to permit the passage of some colloidal albumen as well as of water: either constantly, under normal pressure; or occasionally, when the abnormal pressure is increased by exertion. On the theory that albumen is pressed out of the blood in the Malpighian capsules, and is removed subsequently by the action of the epithelium of the tubules, the exhaustion of this function of the epithelium, or its inadequacy, affords an equally facile explanation of the observations in question. —*Lancet*, April 6, 1878.

Conditions of Growth of Various Organs.

In a communication to the *Marburger Naturwiss. Sitzungsbericht*, 1877 (abstracted in *Centralblatt für die Medicin. Wissenschraften*, February 23), Dr. BENECE arrives at the following conclusions as the result of numerous observations: 1. The human heart grows relatively quickly during the first months of life, then rather slowly up to the thirteenth or fourteenth year; it then increases very considerably in volume during the development of puberty, and when this is completed, grows more slowly. 2. The "puberty-development" of the heart is to be regarded as a very important phase in its development, in regard both to the physiological and the pathological occurrences of this period of life. 3. In proportion to the length of the body, the heart of the child has normally a volume more than three times less than in the adult (after the completion of puberty). 4. The large arterial vessels are unequally wider in the child than in the adult. They attain their relatively narrowest condition at the time of puberty. The more considerable and rapid the growth in length before this time, the less, as a rule, appears to be the increase in calibre of these vessels. 5. In consequence of these conditions of the growth of the arteries, the relation between the volume of heart and the calibre of the arteries, and consequently the blood-pressure, is quite different in childhood and after the completion of puberty. The blood-pressure in the child's organism must be much less than in the fully developed adult. 6. The pulmonary artery is normally larger than the ascending aorta in childhood. Towards puberty the two vessels are nearly of the same size, and in the adult the pulmonary artery is normally a little narrower than the aorta.   7. The result of this condition must be a difference of the blood-pressure in the lungs during the different periods of life.   It is evident that the pressure is greater in the child than in the adult.   This condition is probably compensated by the greater growth of the left ventricle as compared with the right, and by a relatively considerable increase in the calibre of the ascending aorta.   8. For the access of puberty, the development of the heart and arteries is of the most essential importance.   9. In certain defined constitutional anomalies (cancer, scrofulous phthisis, rickets) there are certain differences in the size of the heart, the calibre of the arteries, the size of the lungs and liver, as well as in the relation of the size of the pulmonary artery to that of the aorta, and these differences may be transmitted hereditarily.   10. The calibre of the arterial system seems to be of importance in the course of acute diseases; paralysis of the heart occurs more early and more readily in persons with narrow than in those with wide arteries.   It was found that the arteries were remarkably narrow in the greater number of deaths from enteric fever.   11. Narrowness or wideness of the arteries is by no means equally distributed over the whole system.   Variations may in some cases depend on the local development of disease.   For instance, in rickety children with symptoms of hydrocephalus, the large arteries of the brain were often found to be remarkably wide.—*London Med. Record*, April 15, 1878.

Materia Medica and Therapeutics.

Biological Action of Salicylic Acid and Salicylate of Soda.

In the *Commentario Clinico di Pisa* for January and February, Drs. CHIRONE and PETRUCCI publish an account of a number of experiments made in the Pharmaceutical Laboratory of the University of Naples, on the action of salicylic acid and salicylate of soda on warm-blooded animals (dogs and rabbits), and cold-blooded animals (frogs).   They sum up in the following conclusions : 1. The biological action of salicylic acid and of salicylate of soda is identical ; but with the former the local effects, with the latter the general effects, are more marked. 2. Salicylic acid, both free and in the state of salicylate, when administered in small doses, lowers the temperature, but within restricted limits ; in a somewhat large dose, it does not only not lower the temperature, but sometimes considerably increases it.   3. Animals subjected to the daily use of salicylic acid and salicylate of soda rapidly become emaciated and lose weight.   4. The heart-beats are in frogs reduced in number, especially by salicylate of soda ; but in mammalia salicylate of soda sometimes retards, sometimes accelerates, the heart's action, independently of the dose.   With free salicylic acid, the number of heart-beats is, in most, constantly reduced.   5. Salicylic acid almost constantly reduces the number of respirations ; salicylate of soda ordinarily first increases and then diminishes the number.—*London Med. Record*, April 15, 1878.

Detection of Mercury in the Urine.

GUNTZ (*Virteljahrschr. für Dermatologie und Syphilis*, Band iv. (N.F.) Heft i. p. 2), employing Ludwig's process for the detection of mercury in the urine, has arrived at the following results with regard to the period of the duration of this drug in the human system, and the liberating action upon it of sulphui internally and combined with baths: 1. Mercury may be detected in the urine, after eight weeks or more have elapsed since the discontinuance of any mercurial treatment. 2. In cases where the urine gives no evidence of the presence of mercury after the administration of the drug, this may be detected after two or three days of sulphur treatment. 3. After a few days of such treatment, the urine no longer gives any signs of the existence in it of the metal. 4. While the mercury is thus being eliminated from the system, there is frequently a fresh outbreak of the symptoms of syphilis. The therapeutic influences from these facts are, that mercury is the antagonist of syphilis; that it should be administered in small doses and temporarily discontinued upon the slightest manifestations of salivation; and that sulphur is of service where too much has been administered.—*London Med. Record*, April 15, 1878.

Subcutaneous Injections of Chloroform.

M. CONSTANTINE PAUL communicated to the Société de Thérapeutique (Feb. 13, 1878) a remarkably successful treatment of a case of confirmed sciatica by injections of chloroform. They removed the pain and caused no accidents. M. DUJARDIN-BEAUMETZ said that he had continued his investigations respecting subcutaneous injections of chloroform (see *London Medical Record* for March 15, 1878, pp. 127, 128). Since he had performed them with greater regularity, he did not meet with any local accidents, and, if they did occur, it was in consequence of the operation being badly performed. The greatest attention must be paid to the manipulative part of the operation, and hence these injections would never come into general use. Especial care must be taken, when once the canula was placed in the cellular tissue, not to penetrate the deep surface of the dermis at its lower surface when introducing the syringe into the canula, otherwise a slough would be produced. With reference to the general effects, M. Dujardin-Beaumetz had observed that with from four to six grammes (a drachm to a drachm and a half) of chloroform injected at once sleep was obtained; not anæsthetic sleep, but a more or less deep calm and repose, which came on very slowly from four to seven hours after the injection, and sometimes lasted one or two days. Alcoholic and hysterical patients were much more difficult to bring under the influence of chloroform, and in these cases from ten to twelve grammes (two and a half to three drachms) were requisite to produce the same effects. Thus chloroform introduced in this manner into the animal economy produced the effects of chloral, and passed but very slowly into the system. These injections, in contradistinction to injections of ether, lowered the pulse and the temperature. M. Dujardin-Beaumetz performed these injections in the cellular tissue of the back, and allowed to each puncture two grammes of chloroform (half a drachm).—*London Med. Record*, April 15, 1878.

Medicine.

Transfusion in Anæmia.

Professor BITOT, of Bordeaux, relates (*Union Méd.*, April 9 and 16) eight cases of transfusion performed on four persons with success by an improved apparatus which he describes. He attaches great importance to endeavouring to prevent the shivering occurring after the operation (which he regards as a true febrile paroxysm) by the administration of quinine. He terminates his paper with these conclusions: 1. Transfusion may prove a sovereign remedy in cases of anæmia caused by hemorrhages independent of cancer. 2. It may prove very useful in cases of physical degeneration caused by hyperæmia. 3. It is rather mischievous than useful in disorders of a cancerous nature. 4. It is very prudent to administer quinine to the patient two days prior to the operation.—*Med. Times and Gaz.*. April 27, 1878.

Use of Carbolic Acid in Typhoid Fever.

In *Lo Sperimentale* for January, Dr. C. TEMPESTI relates two cases illustrative of the use of carbolic acid in enteric fever. They were observed during an epidemic of the disease which prevailed in 1875.

The first patient was a girl aged ten. The ordinary symptoms of the disease had been present several days, when in the course of the second week there appeared nocturnal delirium, epistaxis—often abundant, diarrhœa, depression, stupor, bronchial catarrh, sordes on the nostrils and teeth ; and there was hemorrhagic discharge from the gums, fauces, and tongue. Recourse was had to clysters of cold water and to painting the parts inside the mouth with a solution of 2 parts of carbolic acid in 100 of water; but the disease obstinately resisted all treatment. Dr. Tempesti then decided to give the patient the solution of carbolic acid as a drink ; she took it with avidity, and in a few hours half a drachm of carbolic acid had been taken. The next day, all threatening symptoms had disappeared, and the patient asked for food. Half a drachm of carbolic acid was again given in solution ; two weeks later the patient was convalescent, and soon completely recovered.

The second case also occurred in a girl aged 10, who was the subject of very severe typhoid fever with dissolution of the blood. The internal use of carbolic acid was prescribed ; but through the prejudice of the friends the administration of half a drachm of the acid was spread over five days ; hence the medicine was useless, and the child died.

Dr. Tempesti sums up in the following conclusions :—

1. Carbolic acid may be a remedy of much value in cases of typhoid fever in which death is threatened (the putrid state of old writers), and is worthy of being subjected to clinical research.

2. The dose must be sufficiently high (half a drachm or a drachm daily in ordinary drink or in abundance of water). Small doses, perhaps in consequence of the nervous stupor which prevails in typhoid fever, are of little or no therapeutic efficacy.—*London Med. Record*, April 15, 1875.

Delirium Preceding the Eruption of Smallpox.

Dr. ZIPPE relates (*Allgemeine Zeitschrift für Psychiatrie*, Band 34) a case of considerable interest from a medico-legal point of view, in which a man who had murdered one of his children was acquitted on the ground that the act had been committed while the prisoner was suffering from the primary fever of variola.

M. E., a labourer, aged 35, who lived alone with his three children and was much given to drinking, returned earlier than usual from his work one afternoon. The children noticed a change in his appearance and demeanor ; he treated them harshly and cruelly as he had never done before. On the following day he remained at home, took no food, and spent most of his time in bed ; early next morning his youngest child was found moribund in the street below his window ; the elder children could give no explanation of the occurrence as they had slept soundly ; but the father, on being questioned, at once admitted having thrown it from the window, "because he could no longer support it." Two days after, while he was in custody, the eruption of smallpox appeared upon him. Other circumstances besides those given above, pointed to the patient's having been delirious during the night in question. He was consequently acquitted, it being believed that his condition when he committed the murder was such that he could not be responsible for his actions.—*London Med. Record*, April 15, 1878.

—

Treatment of Apoplexy with Heart-disease.

Some years ago Dr. Beneke pointed out the benefit to be derived in cardiac affections, especially those following on articular rheumatism, from the use of warm saline baths impregnated with carbonic acid. His observations are fully borne out by the physicians at the baths of Nauheim, who find these baths beneficial not only to the rheumatic affection, but also to the attendant heart-disorder. Dr. GROEDEL (*Berliner Klinische Wochenschrift*, March 11th) has further found that these baths are useful in cases of (so-called) apoplexy accompanying heart-disease. They soothe the exalted action of the heart, while the paralytic symptoms and general health undergo marked improvement. A case in point is singled out from many others as having been continuously in observation. It is that of a lady, aged 49, who, when 18 years old, had a severe attack of articular rheumatism, which left insufficiency of the mitral valve. Five years ago she had a slight apoplectic seizure during the night, which passed off in a couple of hours ; and, since then, such attacks recurred at intervals, until three years ago she had an unusually severe one, followed by complete hemiplegia of the left side, with long-continued unconsciousness. In a few days these symptoms passed off again, with the exception of the hemiplegia. The case was doubtless one of cerebral embolism rather than of apoplexy. She was ordered to use the above saline baths at a temperature of 88° F. every other day, which was continued for seven weeks. Under this treatment, the heart's action, previously very irregular, became almost normal, and all œdema, which existed before, disappeared. This favourable state of things continued until the following winter, when palpitation, œdema, etc., returned, but were again relieved during the ensuing summer. There has been no further symptom of embolism.

Dr. Groedel concludes that, in cases of true apoplexy, especially those occurring in consequence of atheromatous arteries, the use of the warm saline baths is inadmissible, since they tend only to increase the blood-pressure on the weakened arterial walls. On the other hand, these baths can only be useful in cases of cerebral embolism, with consequent paralysis. For, by the increased action of the heart, the blood-current is hastened, and thus the formation of coagula and deposit is prevented, since this can only occur in a sluggish flow of blood. Moreover, when a part of the cerebral substance has its supply of blood cut off by an embolic clot, and so becomes atrophied, an increase of blood-pressure may yet restore it. Nutrition through a collateral circulation, and a removal of the loss of power, etc., result.—*London Med. Record*, April 15, 1878.

—

Chorea in Old People.

M. CHARCOT (*Progrès Médical*, March 9) says the chorea of old people does not differ from the ordinary form ; it is rare ; he has at present only two cases, and only three have been recorded by Roger, Sée, and Graves. It presents no modification except, perhaps, relative slowness of the movements, and very chronic course ; in the two cases quoted it had existed 11 and 12 years respectively. It is incurable, but does not appear to endanger life. He has seen one patient, however, die in a typhoid state, with considerable elevation of temperature ; another case terminated in maniacal delirium, with elevation of temperature.

Most of the cases have appeared to be in a more or less pronounced state of dementia. As to its etiology, it does not seem allied to rheumatism ; in the necropsies made, no cardiac lesions were found. It appears to be an emotional disease, and, in several cases, supervened after some special cause of grief or agitation. This disease differs essentially from senile trembling, which has been sometimes called senile chorea.—*London Med. Record*, April 15, 1878.

Anatomical Causes of Infantile Paralysis.

Dr. EISENLOHR (*Allegemeine Zeitschrift für Psychiatrie*, Band 34, Heft 2) says that after Charcot, Joffroy, Parrot, and Duchenne had stated that a primary change in the motor ganglion-cells of the anterior cornua of the gray matter of the spinal cord was the anatomical cause of infantile paralysis, while Roger and Damaschino, on the other hand, found, in several cases, evidence of myelitis in the anterior cornua of the cervical and lumbar regions, Leyden pointed out that the disease in question is not always due to one and the same cause, but may be caused by various anatomical lesions.

The author relates the case of a child, aged nine months, who suffered from unmistakable spinal paralysis of both extremities, and died of follicular enteritis. Simple atrophy of the muscular fibres was found without either increase of nuclei, development of fat, or fatty degeneration of the muscular elements. The morbid appearances in the spinal cord were, atrophy of the anterior roots, thickening of the neuroglia and of the fibrous septa in the anterior and lateral columns, with atrophy of the nerve-fibres extending through the greater part of the length of the cord ; degeneration or disappearance of a number of ganglion-cells in the anterior cornua of the dorsal and lumbar regions ; marked proliferation of nuclei in all the columns as well as in the gray matter of the sacral and lower lumbar regions.

Attention is drawn to the extension of the process over so considerable a length of the cord, and to the participation of both the white and gray substances. The appearances observed are regarded as the results of a diffuse interstitial myelitis. Perhaps the variations in the anatomical lesions found in infantile paralysis may cause corresponding differences in the clinical features of the disease.—*London Med. Record*, April 15, 1878.

Oxalate of Cerium in Chronic Cough.

Mr. THOMAS CLARK (*Practitioner*, May, 1878) has for some time used the oxalate of cerium in cases of chronic cough with shortness of breathing, with very marked success.

One case under observation is a proof of its good effects as a sedative.

A lady has suffered for some years with cough and difficulty of breathing, on the least exertion, "the outcome of an acute attack of pneumonia," the cough being most troublesome in the morning on getting up; so bad as to cause sickness. Mr. Clark prescribed 5 gr. half an hour before rising.

The physical signs observed in her case have been loud bronchial breathing, with great abdominal action, impaired resonance over lungs, with a slight dulness at the apex of left lung. The most marked physical changes since taking the ox. cerium, are less noise in breathing, less abdominal action, no cough in the morning, and increased strength.

Mr. Clark could relate other cases, but only mentions one other, it being under his care in the village hospital ; a case of consolidation of the right lung. The rest given to the lung by the ox. cerium in gr. 5 doses is observable in the comfort in breathing and the cessation of cough for twenty-four hours after each dose.

The medicinal properties of ox. cerium Mr. Clark believes to be purely sedative, a great desideratum in the treatment of lung diseases, the difficulty being to find a drug that will not upset the digestive organs. In all cases wherein he has used the ox. cerium the only symptom observable from its use is a slight dryness of mouth.

—

Paracentesis Thoracis.

M. MORAND, a military surgeon, publishes in the first number for the present year of the valuable periodical issued from the French Ministry of War (*Recueil de Mém. de Méd., de Chir., et de Pharm. Militaires*) a carefully drawn up report on the results of thirty-two cases of thoracentesis performed on soldiers in the garrisons of Lyons and Vincennes. He observes that, amidst the great differences of opinion as to the value and necessity of this operation in pleurisy, facts carefully observed—unbiased by the prevailing exaggerations and prepossessions —are what are required, and it is to these he desires to contribute a contingent. In military medicine the question is of great importance, for, as the medical statistics of the French army show, the mean number of deaths from pleurisy is 2.20 in 100 deaths, and as the proportion of deaths is 5 per cent. of the cases of pleurisy, the entire number of those attacked becomes very considerable. Moreover, however slight the effusion, much exemption from military service is entailed.

Comparing thirty-one of the cases of pleurisy treated by thoracentesis with 109 treated at the same time medically in the same military hospitals, it results that among the former the days passed in hospital averaged 72.67 for each patient, and the mortality was 16.12 per cent.; whilst among the better or medically treated cases the stay in hospital was 40.60 days each, and the mortality was 5.50 per cent. One of the most important facts is that in twenty-seven of the thirty-two cases operated upon the reproduction of the liquid was rapid and complete, being more or less incomplete in the five others. As to the supposed innocuity of repeated paracentesis, it is to be observed that of the six cases in which the discharge became purulent, such repetitions had occurred in four. Among the accidents occurring in the thirty-two cases, these consisted of syncope in four, of suffocative paroxysm in eleven, and of albuminous expectoration in two. The general conclusions at which M. Morand arrives is, that in consequence of the rapid reaccumulation of fluid, paracentesis is a useless operation, while owing to the occurrence of the more or less menacing accidents alluded to above (altogether seventeen in number), and to the purulent transformation of the fluid occurring in six cases, it must be regarded as a dangerous one. Not that it should be altogether renounced, but confined to those comparatively rare cases in which the life of the patient is menaced by the abundance or the suddenness of the effusion—as announced by dyspnœa, cyanosis, great and extreme dulness, the abolition of thoracic vibration, the displacement of the heart, and especially by the general condition of exhaustion of the patient. He would say with M. Roger, that we should never operate in serious pleurisy when the effusion is moderate, and rarely when this is great, doing so exclusively when the urgent signs just mentioned are present.

Empyema.—In purulent pleurisy, on the contrary, an operation must always be resorted to for the purpose of enabling the pleural cavity to be washed out, and putrid formentation prevented or combated. For the injections employed for this purpose, M. Morand prefers a mixture of carbolized alcohol and water. Among his thirty-two cases of paracentesis, five were followed by purulent pleurisy, for which that operation was performed, with one complete recovery, and one incomplete recovery, a pleural fistula remaining.—*Med. Times and Gaz.*, May 4, 1878.

—

Contagiousness of Phthisis.

The following notice of a paper by Dr. TAPPENIER, read at a meeting of German naturalists and physicians, at Monaco, is translated from "*Lo Speri-mentale*," of Jan. 1878.—All physicians have observed cases of phthisis rapidly developed in individuals who had for a long time attended on patients in this disease, even when such attendants had not presented any predisposition, either individual or hereditary. Dr. Tappenier believes that the explanation of the fact is to be found in the inhalation of the expectorated matter, scattered in the air by the coughing of patients. In order to test this opinion, he made experiments, by intimately mixing a certain quantity of the sputa in a little water; he pulverized this emulsion by an appropriate process, and subjected some animals to the inhalation of the substance during one or two hours every day. These experiments were made in the Anatomico-Pathological Institute of Prof. Buhl of Monaco. Dogs were selected, as animals presenting the least predisposition to contraction of the disease. Three perfectly sound dogs were put into the pen of the institute; the pen is situate near a window, and is closed in all parts, excepting above, where it receives the external air, through a door which is furnished with a fastening. Some sputa was obtained from a patient in phthisis, a spoonful of which was mixed in a quantity of water sufficient to make of it a liquid similar to almond milk, and every day pulverization of this was made in the pen during an hour, or an hour and a half. At the same time, for the purpose of studying absorption, by the digestive system, of the tuberculous matter, two of the dogs were made to swallow a certain quantity of it, from the same patient.

The whole five dogs had apparently a good appetite, and presented neither cough nor diarrhœa, they ate freely, and were cheerful and nimble, without any symptoms of illness, unless a slight wasting and arrest of development. At first view, therefore, the experiments gave a negative result. But the day preceding the first autopsy, a little finely powdered carmine was mixed with the tuberculous liquid, in order to discover how far it had penetrated into the respiratory passages. Two of the dogs subjected to inhalation, and the two which had swallowed the tuberculous mixture, were killed six weeks after the commencement of the experiment. The autopsy of the fifth had been made at the end of three weeks.

The results of the autopsies were surprising. The five dogs presented a general miliary tuberculosis of both lungs, of the liver, the kidneys, and (at least in the two that had swallowed the tuberculous matter) of the digestive apparatus. The numerous stains of carmine which were seen on the pulmonary surface, showed that the inhaled liquid had penetrated into the pulmonary cells. The microscopic examination made by Professor Buhl, established in the clearest manner the reality of the lesions.

It has, therefore, been established experimentally that in the dog a general miliary tuberculosis can be induced from the inhalation, or the ingestion of the matter expectorated by a phthisical patient. The possibility of contagion of phthisis through the natural channels, may therefore be concluded.

The hygienic and clinical consequences of the experiment are of high importance. And first of all it is to be noted that those dogs continued in apparent sound health, despite the existence of general miliary tuberculosis. It is, therefore, possible in man a miliary tuberculosis may rest latent during a certain time, and may not become a real and declared phthisis, before the development of foci of inflammation. But that which is of chief importance is the possibility of transmission of tuberculosis from man to man.

In ordinary conditions, that is to say, in fresh and frequently renewed air, the matters expectorated, and suspended in the air, may not become sufficiently concentrated to have the power of inducing tuberculous infection. But when a certain number of phthisical patients reside together, and through fear of cold or of drafts, the place is but little, or not at all ventilated, may we not fear that the expectorated matter will accumulate sufficiently to become dangerous to healthy persons, living in the same quarters? Ought we not, therefore, in this regard to take precautions, sometimes neglected, particularly in the wards of hospitals? Is it not, perhaps, prudent to recommend to consumptives never to swallow the matter brought up from cavities, which may have a deleterious influence on the digestive canal? Finally, may not these experiments, in some degree, explain the transmission of phthisis from husband to wife, or *vice versa*, and, consequently the advisability of avoiding conjugal intercourse?

The facts stated by Dr. Tappenier are of great interest, and may explain many points of the important question of the contagion of phthisis.—*Canada Lancet*, May 1, 1878.

—

The Influence of Pregnancy in Phthisis.

In the *Nice Médical*, February, 1878, Dr. A. LEBERT says that for a long time it was believed that pregnancy arrested or suspended the progress of pulmonary phthisis. In 1850 Grisolle affirmed that pregnancy aggravated the phthisical condition. Dr. Lebert's observations support, in the main, those of Grisolle; but he finds that the results of labour are more pronouncedly deleterious than those of pregnancy. Out of 33 phthisical girls who married, 10 died in their first labours. He is of opinion that the physician should discourage marriage in any young girl who has shown at any time symptoms of tuberculosis.— *London Med. Record*, April 15, 1878.

—

The Presence of Elastic Fibres in Phthisical Expectoration.

SOCOLOWSCI and GREIFF say (*Deutsche Med. Wochenschrift*, Feb. 9, 16, and 23, 1878) that in many cases of phthisis, when the physical signs do not afford satisfactory evidence of destruction of lung-tissue, the demonstration of elastic fibres in the sputa becomes of great diagnostic and prognostic importance. The authors have made very numerous observations to determine how far the presence of elastic fibres in the sputa corresponds to the data of physical examination, in respect to the destruction of the pulmonary tissue. With this object they have followed the cases of seventy patients; the examinations for the fibres have been made by two methods, fresh and by Fenwick's process slightly modified, the latter being generally adopted.

They mixed the whole of the sputa with a soda solution (1 of liquor sodæ to 2 of distilled water) and boiled it for four or five minutes; then diluted it with an equal quantity of distilled water, poured it into a flat porcelain vessel, and fished out the particles suspended in the water, and subjected them to microscopic examination. In some cases they only found one single piece, in others many dozen; in the cases where so many were present, the physical examination also showed signs of great destruction of the lung, but in general no very great importance is to be attached to the number of the pieces. Their size varies as much as their number; in one case of gangrene of the lung the large pieces were more than a millimetre long; but in general they were only a few fractions of a millimetre. In colour, the boiled fibres were yellowish-brown, or dark-brown and blackish. Generally the fibres assumed the structure of a reticulum, but very rarely as well marked as Fenwick figures it; the colour is so distinct that artificial staining, as suggested by some (by fuchsin as recommended by Duval), is unnecessary. There are frequently fungous growths in sputa, which at first might be confounded with the fibres, but the greater thickness and regularity of the latter indicate their nature. (The authors here print a tabulated account of all their cases.)

Of the 70 patients who were examined, 19 belonged to the stage of breaking down of the lung with marked hectic : of these 19 cases they found elastic fibres in 18 ; in two they found them only at the second or third attempt, although the physical signs of destruction were present. The single case, in which in spite of two examinations they failed to find any fibres, was a female patient, aged 20, with great destruction of the left upper lobe and marked hectic ; further investigations were made impossible by the departure of the patient. In another of the patients of this group they found the fibres once only in several examinations. In one case the absence of the fibres corresponded to temporary improvement and freedom from fever ; in another they found no fibres at their second examination, although no improvement, but an increase of the hectic, existed. From their cases they conclude that, in cases of phthisis with demonstrable breaking down and decided hectic, fibres will be found, if not in one, at least after several examinations ; but that in these cases the discovery is of no value, as the destruction of the lung-tissue is otherwise sufficiently proved.

Of eleven cases belonging to the category of chronic phthisis with unmistakable destruction of lung-tissue, but without hectic, elastic fibres were found in all, but in one of these they were only found at the second or third examination, at a time when temporary fever and a relapse existed. Here also their discovery was of no diagnostic value. But may it be of prognostic value, as the case just referred to might indicate ? In another case, in spite of general and local improvement (disappearance of the physical signs of a cavity), elastic fibres were found up to the time of his discharge, which served to show that, in spite of the apparent improvement, the destructive processes in the lungs were still going on.

In the other forty cases there were signs only of consolidation ; the condition of all was good, and without fever, with two exceptions. In the first case, after a violent attack of pulmonary hemorrhage, diffuse pneumonia with high fever supervened, which terminated in death. In the second case, a feverish condition developed from time to time, which generally accompanied hæmoptysis. Of these 40 patients 16 had great consolidation of one or both lungs ; of these 16 they found elastic fibres in 12 cases, in four cases they found none. Of these four cases two had great consolidation of the right lower lobe, in the other two the consolidation was of very old date, and probably was already contracted. Of the 12 cases in which fibres were found, in one case they were discovered first at the second, in another not until the sixth examination ; in the last patient their appearance was preceded by several days' fever and dyspnœa, probably indicating a commencing destruction of the infiltrated parts. In 75 per cent. therefore of their cases of consolidation, they found these fibres present, which, they say, shows how frequently destruction is going on although the physical signs are those of consolidation only. In such cases, the prognosis must be always made with caution. The remaining 24 patients had only very slight consolidation in one or both apices ; in eight cases, or one-third of the whole number, the elastic fibres were found, in the other two-thirds there were none. Of these eight cases some are worth recording briefly.

Case I. Frau H., aged 30, with hereditary predisposition, said her illness began six months ago with a cough. There never had been any fever ; from time to time she had hæmoptysis. Her general condition was good. There were very limited dulness in the right supraclavicular fossa, prolonged expiration, and scanty râles; cough was very little, only in the morning. The expectoration was slight, whitish, without any clumps; microscopic examination showed pus and mucus cells. Fenwick's method demonstrated elastic fibres. After three weeks she was better; the râles had disappeared; the cough and expectoration were less, in the latter there were still elastic fibres. After five weeks more, there was still more improvement; there was quite slight dulness with loud expiration; cough and expectoration were little marked. In the latter, in spite of careful examinations, no elastic fibres could be found.

Case II. Herr H., aged, 18, with hereditary predisposition, said he had had a dry cough for two months. He had become very thin, feeble, and short of breath. Evening temperature, 38.5° cent. (101.3° Falır.). There was slight dulness at the right apex, and scanty dry râles; his cough was violent with slight sputa containing a moderate number of fibres. The diagnosis was, commencing destruction of the infiltrated parts of the lung, with an unfavourable prognosis. The course of the case was persistent fever, occasional hæmoptysis and once pneumorrhagia, while the physical signs of destruction were still more decidedly present.

Case III. Herr W., aged 26, in good general health, was free from fever, but with slight dulness at the right apex, prolonged expiration and scanty dry râles. For some weeks he had suffered from a daily, though not inconsiderable, hæmoptysis. The sputa showed no elastic fibres at the first examination, but the second time, three weeks later, a very decided reticulum was found. The general condition of the patient had improved, but the hæmoptysis had persisted. Apparently there was in this case a deeply situated patch of destruction from which the expectorated blood came. The patient withdrew himself from further observation.

Of the eight cases in which the fibres were found, in five they disappeared after more or less time, which coincided with a gradual improvement. Of the other three cases, in one the local lesion maintained the status quo, in the other two it made rapid progress.

From these facts, it appears that the demonstration of elastic fibres is of the greatest diagnostic and prognostic importance in cases of badly marked infiltration of the pulmonary parenchyma. The author's conclusions are thus summed up.

1. The examination of the sputa in phthisis should not be neglected.

2. A single examination for elastic fibres, especially for negative purposes, is not sufficient.

3. In physically demonstrable pulmonary destruction, the presence of elastic fibres in the sputa may generally be expected, but it is of little value for diagnosis or prognosis.

4. In those cases which present physical signs of only more or less consolidation of the lung-tissue, the finding or not finding of elastic fibres is of great importance for diagnosis and prognosis.—*London Med. Record*, April 15, 1878.

Infarction of the Heart.

Cases of acute and extensive infarction of the wall of the heart are not common, and one lately published by M. LAVERAN is of interest on account of the symptoms which resulted from the accident, and which were carefully observed for a fortnight before death. The patient was a man forty-seven years of age, and the anatomical change consisted in an area of softening, three or four centimetres across, in the wall of the left ventricle. The softening was so complete as to constitute an actual abscess, extending between the endocardium and pericardium, neither of which, however, was perforated. The coronary arteries were atheromatous, and the anterior branch, going to the softened spot, was completely obliterated. The ventricle was much dilated and distended with blood. The first symptoms, a fortnight before death, were pain in the left side, and rapidly increasing dyspnœa, with slight hæmoptysis. The heart's action was excited, frequent, and irregular. The cardiac dulness was increased, the sounds distant but without murmur. Respiration was rapid, the lungs normal, the extremities dusky. The difficulty of breathing became most intense, and prevented sleep. The heart-sounds became inaudible. Pericarditis was diagnosed, and antimony administered. The symptoms lessened considerable in severity, so that the patient was able, at the end of a week, to sit up. They recurred, however, in a day or two with renewed violence, and a large hemorrhage from the lungs occurred without relief to the dyspnœa, which continued until death, a few days later. Many foci of pulmonary apoplexy were found after death.—*Lancet*, May 4, 1878.

Treatment of Infantile Diarrhœa.

Dr. RENE BLACHE, in the *Journal de Thérapeutique*, July 25, 1877, studies diarrhœa in young children, and shows that there are several stages in this affection, and that it frequently suffices to combat the first stage of this diarrhœa to prevent the appearance of the serious symptoms of choleriform diarrhœa. Whatever may be the nature of the diarrhœa, its origin, intensity, or even the distance of the time when it showed itself, M. Blache employs the following treatment, which he has always found successful, modifying it according to circumstances. 1. Reduction of the quantity of food given; suitable injections repeated according to need, and poultices on the belly. 2. The administration each morning during three, four, or five consecutive days, of a small teaspoonful of equal parts of castor oil and syrup of gum arabic, simply emulsified by shaking the bottle at the time when it is used. When the child is under six months old, one gramme (15 grains) of castor oil is enough for a dose; and if from six months to two years old, from two to three grammes are necessary. If after the second day the diarrhœa be less but have not entirely disappeared, no more of the medicine should be given than on the day before. On the other hand, if the stools be particularly fetid and glairy, another dose must be given on the same evening, as well as on the next day. If the case be one of profuse liquid diarrhœa, recurring twelve, fifteen, or even more times in the twenty-four hours, the mixture must be altered, doubling or trebling the dose of gum, and adding a little vinum opii, from one to three drops at the most, according to age, in the four-and-twenty hours, and the medicine must be repeated every two or three hours. The object or effect of this castor oil treatment is to cleanse the mucous. membranes, which it modifies, without, however, purging in the general acceptation of the term. Injections are equally useful. First a large injection of chamomile tea is given, followed in twenty minutes by a small injection of starch. These are repeated whenever a series of four or five actions of the bowels occur in the space of from six to ten hours. In the latter case bran of marsh mallow is substituted for chamomile. As to the absorbents, more especially bismuth, so often used in these cases, M. Blache distrusts them, as they may bring on convulsions, doubtless by preventing the cleansing of the mucous membrane.—*London Med. Record*, April 15, 1878.

Treatment of Nervous Vomiting by Electricity.

In a letter to Dr. P. Schivardi, published in the *Gazetta Medica Italiana-Lombarda*, No. 6, 1878, Dr. SEMMOLA gives the results of observations made during several years on the diagnosis and treatment of nervous vomiting. He finds that electricity in the form of the constant current is the most effective remedy. Soon after the first application, the patients can retain food, although for many weeks previously they had always rejected it. He believes, also, that the constant current is not only a sure remedy, but also a valuable means of diagnosis in all cases of chronic vomiting. If the elements of diagnosis be not sufficient to determine whether the vomiting is dependent on some morbid process in the stomach itself, or on reflex action (as from worms or chronic uterine disease), the application of the current at once settles the question. In cases where the vomiting is not exclusively and primarily nervous, its application fails in enabling the stomach to tolerate food.

Dr. Semmola relates twenty cases in which a cure was produced by the means which he recommended. The last of them is as follows:—

The daughter of Mr. C., a member of the Italian Parliament, had been greatly reduced by vomiting which had lasted three months, and which was attributed by her medical attendants to perforating ulcer of the stomach. On the evening of November 14, 1875, she had a sudden attack of aphonia, and was believed to be at the point of death. Dr. Semmola was consulted for the first time. The aphonia led him to suspect hysteria. He was unable to see any vomited matter, as she had taken no food since the morning. He applied the current by means of Onimus' apparatus, and very soon afterwards the patient was able to take a cup of milk. On being questioned, she acknowledged that she had a sensation of constriction in the throat; and this confirmed his opinion that he had to deal with a case of hysterical neurosis. The constant current was applied between the sides of the neck and the larynx, and afterwards between the sides of the neck and the stomach. The application was repeated several times daily, and in two months the cure was complete and permanent.—*London Med. Record,* April 15, 1878.

Sulphate of Quinia in Diarrhœa.

M. GUYOT read to the Société Médicale des Hôpitaux (*Journal de Médicine et de Chirurgie Pratique* for March) a case in which the patient was cured of a catarrhal diarrhœa which had lasted several months, by the administration of sulphate of quinine. All other medicines had been employed without effect; and on M. Potain's recommendation M. Guyot prescribed the following: sulphate of quinine, half a gramme; syrup of codeca, 30 grammes; gum julep, 100 grammes. The mixture was continued for a long time, and the dose of sulphate of quinine progressively increased to one gramme. M. Potain has also obtained cures in obstinate diarrhœa by the use of sulphate of quinine even when, as in the present case, the patient showed no traces of malarious infection.—*London Med. Record,* April 15, 1878.

Biliary Calculi and their Pathological Relations.

Dr. BENEKE, of Marburg, in a paper recently published in the *Deutsche Archiv für Klinische Medicin*, observes that the formation of gall-stones may be due to two causes: either there may be a relatively great increase in the amount of cholesterin formed in the liver, so that it appears in the gall-bladder in the same way that urate of soda or uric acid appears in concentrated urine; or there

is a deficiency in the amount of the biliary salts holding it in solution, just as the
uric acid salts or crystals of uric acid are deposited in the urinary passages when
there is a deficiency of soda or an excess of phosphoric acid. Beneke obtained
from the liver of a powerful and apparently healthy man, thirty years of age,
who died from a broken neck, 4.07 grm. (62.8 grains) of cholesterin; from the
nutmeg liver of a man aged twenty-seven, who died from encysted pleuritic exudation, caries olecrani, and pyæmia, 5.153 grm. (79.56 grains) ; from the amyloid liver of a man aged forty, who died from chronic pneumonia, pleuritic exudation, amyloid liver and spleen, 5.078 grm. (78.4 grains) ; and from the fatty
livers of three subjects dying respectively from caseous pneumonia, suppurative
meningitis after compound fracture of the skull in a drunkard, and phthisis, 1.65
grm., 1.36 grm., and 0.263 grm. The conclusions he draws from the examinations of no less than 375 subjects are : 1. That the presence of gall-stones coincides in the majority of cases (about 70 per cent.) with the presence of atheromatous degeneration of the arteries.   2. The atheromatous degeneration of arteries
(without gall-stones) is much more common than the occurrence of gall-stones.
3. Gall-stones are more frequently met with in females than in males, but degeneration of arteries is as common in one sex as in the other.   4. The occurrence of
gall-stones is usually observed at an earlier period of life (from twenty
upwards) than atheromatous degeneration of arteries.   5. Gall-stones are relatively more frequent in carcinoma and nervous arrest of secretion, or congestion
of the liver.   6. The presence of gall-stones and of atheromatous degeneration of
arteries is relatively frequently accompanied by abundant development of fat.
The small quantity of cholesterin in fatty livers is remarkable, but the deduction
cannot be drawn that the formation of fat is originally due to defective formation
of cholesterin.   On the contrary, we may easily conceive that the non-azotized
and highly carbonized cholesterin forms a mother substance for the formation of
the fatty acids, and if it be formed in large quantities it may be the source of
the excessive deposit of fat.   Hence fatty livers yield only a small amount of
cholesterin.   Beneke refers to the large quantity of fat found in the omentum
and elsewhere in phthisical patients, while the adipose tissue beneath the skin
has almost entirely disappeared.   He observes that the formation of fat in the
body is associated with considerable diminution in the quantity of blood—that is
to say, of oxidizable material.   In like manner the formation of fat and the
conditions favourable to the development of tubercle go hand in hand, since
caries of the feet, hip, or vertebræ compel quiescence.   Even if these conditions
do not stand in direct etiological connection with the processes of disease, they at
least favour their development.—*Lancet*, May 4, 1878.

Changes in the Small Vessels in Bright's Disease and the Dependent Theories.

Dr. EWALD, in an interesting and valuable paper, published in Virchow's
Archiv for December, says:—

Since Bright (whom Dr. Ewald, by a curious mistake, calls *John* Bright) discovered simple hypertrophy of the heart in twenty-three out of one hundred cases
of renal disease, which could not be accounted for by valvular disease or atheroma,
a discussion has waged as to its cause; some see in its relation to renal disease
cause and effect; others consider the presence of some third factor necessary.
Bright himself took the latter view in regarding it as due to the impurity of the
blood, and consequent obstruction to the capillary circulation.   Johnson and
Traube sought its cause in the anatomical changes in the kidney; the former believing that the renal arterioles became tonically contracted, while the latter localized the obstruction in the restricted capillary network consequent upon the con-

tracting change. Subsequently Johnson brought forward his observations on the hypertrophy of the arterioles in the pia mater, skin, and mesentery, and, widening the basis of his theory, asserted that the arterioles throughout the body underwent the same tonic contraction, and compared the process with what occurs in carbonic acid poisoning. Still more recently, Gull and Sutton have started a fresh theory; they have described a special change in the bloodvessels, a thickening of the lymph-sheaths, with degeneration of the muscular tunics, to which they have given the name of "arterio-capillary fibrosis," and finding this in cases independent of renal disease, e. g., cardiac valvular disease, etc., they see in these changes the primary lesion, and in the renal degeneration only a local intensified expression of the general morbid process. Dr. Ewald has undertaken careful observations on this head, but has not succeeded in assuring himself that, in these cases, there is anything deserving to be considered as a special change in the lymph-sheath; he finds only general thickening of the arterial wall, chiefly confined to the muscular coat. He examined arterioles by isolating them, and measuring their lumina and coats under the microscope; he found that a certain definite proportion existed in vessels of a certain calibre between the width of the lumen and the thickness of the coats; and when these normal proportions were departed from, he regarded the vessel as hypertrophied. Obviously, he says, it is not easy to discriminate between coats thickened by hypertrophy and those thickened by contraction. but it is not very probable that tonic contraction would remain after death; for reasons hereafter to be stated, he does not believe that the narrowing of the lumen is due to active contraction, as Johnston states. The thickening of the muscular coat, of which he says there can be no doubt, is quite distinct from atheroma, syphilitic thickening, or the various arterio-capillary changes described by Neelsen, Obersteiner, Wedl, or Charcot, in affections of the nervous system.

He divides his cases into three groups: I. Interstitial nephritis, and interstitial and parenchymatous nephritis (mixed). II. Parenchymatous nephritis. III. Other diseases. In reference to the first group, he says that although it is easy enough to distinguish extreme cases of parenchymatous and interstitial nephritis, yet of many cases less well marked, it cannot easily be said whether the interstitial or the parenchymatous change is the more marked; these he has subdivided according as the kidneys weighed more or less than three hundred grammes (10.6 ounces). Of pure cases of interstitial nephritis, weighing under two hundred grammes (about seven ounces), he had only three, so that this third class is unnecessary; such cases, he observes, are much less rare on the continent than in England and Norway, or on the sea-coast. He says that there seems to be a perfect inverse proportion between the weight of the kidneys and of the heart—the lighter the former, the heavier the latter; but no such distinct relation exists between the state of the kidneys and the vascular changes; as, in five cases in which the kidneys were relatively light, the vascular changes were quite absent, or only feebly marked. In one case of nephritis, secondary to lead-poisoning, with phthisis, there existed an exception to the rule of the cardiac hypertrophy, but this is explained by the ill-nourished state of the patient. No such explanation presents itself, however, for the vascular changes in the cases previously referred to; and it can only be assumed that, under certain unknown conditions, these changes do not develop themselves.

His observations on the first group lead him to the following conclusions:—

1. Nearly all cases of chronic interstitial nephritis have muscular hypertrophy of the heart and vessels.

2· Two-thirds of the mixed forms under three hundred grammes weight have cardio-vascular hypertrophy, one-third have cardiac hypertrophy alone; of those over three hundred grammes, all have cardiac hypertrophy, some have vascular hypertrophy.

Of the second group he concludes that, in a little less than a third of the cases of parenchymatous nephritis, simple hypertrophy of the heart is present.

Under this head, however, were included six cases of amyloid degeneration which were not classed apart, because the amyloid change was slight, while pronounced parenchymatous changes were present.

In the third group were twenty-four cases, of which two were phthisis, two typhus, one ovarian cyst, one leukæmia, two atheroma with senile marasmus, one meningitis, and thirteen disease of the valves of the heart. In those cases which were not complicated with renal affection, no vascular changes were found. Once they were found in a case of secondary nephritis. Diseases of the circulatory apparatus, with or without renal complication, can lead to cardiac hypertrophy, but not to vascular changes. The rule is—that secondary nephritis, and enlargement of the heart, which have some other causes than a primary renal affection, do not lead to vascular hypertrophy.

Dr. Ewald finally considers the causes of these changes. He admits that the data requisite to finally settle the question can only be accumulated by many years' observation in a large hospital; but it is permissible to criticize the current theories. He cannot admit Gull and Sutton's view that the vascular change is primary and a part of senile degeneration, because it is met with in quite young persons, and often immediately dependent upon a blood-poison (scarlet fever); in which cases there can be no question of senile change, debilitating influences, or atheroma. He considers the renal affection as primary, and, in reference to Mahomed's "pre-albuminuric stage," questions whether he ascertained the existence of cardiac hypertrophy. Against Johnson's view he urges that he leaves out of account the action of the depressor nerve, which would retard the action of the heart and bring down the arterial tension. He (Dr. Ewald) finds himself compelled to side with the older writers, who found the obstruction in the capillaries; the obstacle to the circulation of the overladen blood acts in a purely mechanical manner upon the arterial system, raising its tension; and the increased tension in the aorta compels the heart to more-active contraction independently of all central influences.

In a sort of appendix he describes the changes in the vessels of the kidney itself; these he regards as purely local and part of the chronic inflammatory process, as described by Friedländer and others.—*London Med. Record*, April 15, 1878.

<hr />

A Case of Abdominal Abscess with Discharge of Intestinal Worms.

Dr. LORENTZEN describes the following case in the *Berliner Klinische Wochenschrift* of January 28.

S., a robust woman, thirty years of age, had noticed, three and a half years ago, a gradually increasing abdominal swelling. It was on the whole painless, but at times there were attacks of colicky pains without vomiting, but accompanied with much flatulent distension of the abdomen. These attacks became more frequent, while at the same time the swelling increased in size. This was found to occupy the umbilical region, extending from three centimetres (1.2 in.) on the left, to ten centimetres (3.9 in.) to the right of the navel, and from three centimetres above to seven centimetres (2.7 in.) below the navel; it scarcely projected beyond the abdomen, and was soft and scarcely fluctuating, while the navel projected like a thimble. A few days afterwards, while the patient was at work, a considerable quantity of pus escaped from the now retracted umbilicus through an extremely fine opening. Neither the posterior nor lateral boundaries of the swelling could be reached by a probe, and it was now exceedingly tender. During the following days large quantities of purulent matter, which was at first fecal but gradually became more healthy, were removed through this opening by means of syringing with salicylic acid. One day there was found in the escaping fluid a round, very soft and very flabby body, rather more than an inch in length, which appeared to be a piece of a lumbricus, but it was unfortunately lost. The patient's general condition had hitherto been fairly good; but now the abdominal pains gradually returned and high fever set in, raising the temperature to 104.9 F. and the pulse to 120–140; the bowels became irregular, the pus fetid and unhealthy, and the patient much reduced. Under these circumstances, the original opening in the linea alba was enlarged, and a counter-opening made to the right, as low down as possible; a drainage-tube was inserted, and the whole dressed with salicylic acid bandages. Under this treatment, the discharge of pus became much reduced in quantity, and ultimately proceeded from a sinus only, which extended about two inches to the right side. The patient refused to have this sinus laid open, and herself steadily continued the syringing and dressing with salicylic acid for three months. About this time she removed from the sinus in one day two dead lumbrici, each nearly four inches long and more than one-tenth of an inch thick, besides two other smaller ones; and some days after this two more, but somewhat smaller and evidently young worms, came away. By means of anthelmintics, several worms were evacuated *per anum*. Since then, the patient has been well. It is difficult to understand how these worms penetrated the gastro-intestinal wall and escaped outwards; all symptoms of intestinal ulceration were completely absent. We can, therefore, only suppose that the worms alone perforated the intestinal wall, and that, as soon as they had passed through, the openings so caused at once closed spontaneously.—*London Med. Record*, March 15, 1878.

Case of Contusion of the Abdomen followed by Localized Peritonitis and Encysted Dropsy.

In the *Archives Générales de Médecine* for January last, M. DUPLAY reports the following case :—

A strong and healthy man, aged 30, was received into the Hospital Saint Louis, June 2, 1877, having an hour previously received a violent blow in the right hypochondriac region, from the pole of a heavily laden cart drawn by two horses. The patient complained of slight pain in the injured part, but there was no redness, ecchymosis, or distension of the abdomen to be seen. Next day, the patient was attacked with severe peritonitis; from this a recovery eventually took place. At the commencement of July, the right side of the belly seemed to be larger than the left, and the percussion-note was not so clear as upon the opposite side. Cupping was tried at the affected part, but the physical signs increased, and were accompanied by constipation. Expansion could now be felt with every movement, but no bruit could be heard on auscultation. By varying the position of the patient, no displacement of the fluid was effected. The absolute dulness that was present at the level of the tumour disappeared at its circumference. The fluid increased in amount, and caused pain and embarrassment of breathing.

On August 6 the swelling was aspirated, and two litres (1½ pint) of ascitic fluid were drawn off. An analysis showed this to contain a considerable amount of albumen, some leucocytes, altered red blood-corpuscles, and large epithelial cells. Considerable relief followed the puncture, but towards the end of the month the swelling again appeared in the same position. As the fluid increased in amount, the pain became more severe.

On September 25 M. Duplay introduced an ordinary trocar at the spot where aspiration had been practised, and drew off 2½ litres of a liquid similar to that evacuated on the previous occasion. After having washed out the cavity with some lukewarm water, 40 grammes of pure tincture of iodine were injected. This caused acute pain in the swelling and all over the abdomen, continuing for four or five hours. The injection was followed by slight inflammatory symptoms, lasting a few days. On the fourth day after the operation it was found that a small quantity of the fluid had been reproduced in the cyst, but this daily diminished ; the fluctuation and pain disappeared, the appetite returned, and the patient was dismissed cured December 15.

M. Duplay makes the following remarks :—

The formation of an encysted dropsy of the abdomen after an injury is so rare, that I have not been able to find another example recorded in the classical authors. The patient who was the subject of the preceding observations had received a violent contusion on the right side of the abdomen, without any indication of visceral lesion, either of the liver, kidney, or intestines, and in about twenty-four hours an acute attack of peritonitis was developed, which gradually terminated in resolution. Nevertheless, this acute attack was soon followed by a circumscribed swelling, which gradually increased, until, by its volume, it caused severe functional disturbances. By physical signs the swelling was recognized as being produced by a collection of liquid, and a puncture gave vent to two litres of a citrinous fluid, which was quickly reproduced, and occasioned anew the same functional troubles. This liquid collection was evidently situated in the peritoneal cavity. Was it due to the transformation of extravasated blood, or was it a simple consequence of peritonitis following the injury ? These two hypotheses may be raised, and it is probable that both may have contributed to the origin of the affection.

Although the injured man did not present after the accident any evident sign of extravasation of blood into the abdomen, there is but little likelihood that such a severe contusion would not give rise to more or less bloody effusion at the point of injury ; and, besides, the symptoms of the peritonitis, which declared themselves next day, and particularly the distension of the belly, were of a sufficient nature to mask the signs of the effusion. Then it is right to recall the fact that the examination of the fluid extracted by the first puncture demonstrated the presence of a certain quantity of altered blood-corpuscles. This question is of minor importance ; for, if it be sufficiently established that at the commencement there was an extravasation of blood, it is certain that this was not abundant, and that the serous collection observed later could not be considered as a simple transformation of effused blood.

The peritoneum here played the principal part. It is this which formed a circumscribed cavity around a small quantity of effused blood and the products of an inflammatory secretion; which cavity had probably its walls lined by a membrane, giving rise to a continuous morbid exudation. This accidental cavity was evidently formed on one side by the parietal layer of the peritoneum, and on the other by the great omentum or the agglutinated folds of the intestines, lined by a false membrane, and bounded at its periphery by the adhesion of the great omentum, or the intestinal folds, to the parietal peritoneum. The examination before and after the puncture, the exploration of the abdomen after recovery, left no doubt relative to the situation of the cyst in the interior of the abdominal cavity, and of the part taken by the epiploon, and probably also by the intestines, in the formation of the cyst. Thus constituted—that is to say, the morbid secretion being present—there would be a constant tendency to increase in quantity and incessantly to reproduce. Believing that I ought not to act in this case as in other encysted serous collections, I did not hesitate to practise an injection of iodine, which has been followed by a complete recovery, although at the com-

mencement there were some inflammatory symptoms, but not of a grave nature.—
London Med. Record, April 15, 1878.

Tubercle in Muscle.

Instances of the occurrence of tubercular deposits in the voluntary muscles are
so rare that considerable interest attaches to an example recorded in a recent
number of Virchow's *Archiv*, by Dr. F. MARCHAND. The condition was found
in the body of a young man, aged twenty-four years, who had suffered from acute
hip-joint disease. The muscles of the hip were pale-red, translucent, and œdematous, and, on close examination, those in the neighbourhood of the joint were
seen to contain numerous roundish, hard nodules, about the size of a mustard-
seed. Most of these were yellow and caseous; some, however, were smaller,
gray, and translucent, with a yellow opaque centre. They were scattered thickly
throughout the substance of the muscles, but were somewhat more abundant just
beneath the surface and also in the neighbourhood of the insertion. A few were
of larger size, and evidently consisted of several smaller ones grouped together.
These were found especially in the obturator internus. The tubercles occurred
not only in the immediate neighbourhood of the joint, but also at a distance, as
in the substance of the gluteus minimus. A secondary general tuberculosis appeared also to have occurred; for a chain of enlarged and hard glands extended
up the pelvis to the lumbar spine, and there was a recent deposit of tubercle in
the lungs and spleen. A second case is mentioned, in which also the muscles of
the pelvis and hip contained numerous deposits of tubercle.—*Lancet*, May 4,
1878.

On Changes in the Sympathetic Nerve in a Case of Diffuse Eczema.

In *L'Imparziale* for January 31, Dr. G. MARCACCI relates an interesting case.
A man aged 70 was admitted into hospital under the care of Dr. Michelacci,
apparently suffering from acute diffused eczema, which was attributed to exposure
and rain during many hours in succession in January 1877. His health had previously been good; he was seized with a heavy pain in the head, and the scalp
became covered with a thick furfuraceous layer, which gradually spread over the
whole cutaneous surface. There never was the slightest fever, no visceral change,
nor constitutional fault. During the first days of his stay in hospital, purgatives
were given to relieve constipation, and the skin was sprinkled with powdered
starch and charcoal. Considerable improvement followed, but on March 10 a
copious exudation of lymph and serum set in in the region of the chest, and produced rapid emaciation. He died of congestion of the lungs on April 1. A
necropsy, made by Dr. Brigidi, gave the following results.

The surface of the skin was covered with fine black crusts, due to the finely
powdered charcoal, and was divided by clefts, at the bottom of which the rete
mucosum was plainly seen, of a red colour. The subcutaneous layer of fat was
very thin. The left pleural cavity contained 385 grammes (about 13$\frac{1}{2}$ ounces)
of clear serum; the left lung was healthy. There was red hepatization of the
superior lobe, and of the upper part of the inferior lobe of the right lung. The
abdomen presented nothing worthy of note. On microscopic examination of the
skin, there was found to be great hyperæmia of the dermis, but no irritation in
the connective tissue. The horny layer of the epidermis had disappeared in
many parts; the Malpighian layer was thinned, and the Malpighian cells were
more granular than in the ordinary state. In the spinal cord and medulla oblongata the nerve-fibres and cells were normal; the bloodvessels were much
injected. The cervical and cœliac ganglia were the seat of hyperæmia, visible to

the naked eye, and still more apparent in microscopic sections. Preparations immersed in a mixture of distilled water and glycerine, without the addition or acetic acid, showed an excessive number of nuclei. The nerve-cells were reduced in size by the lateral pressure of the masses of nuclei, their protoplasm was turbid, and an abundant red granular pigment occupied the intercellular spaces.

Dr. Marcacci observes that the changes in the ganglia demonstrated the existence in them of a process of irritation, probably of inflammation. He remarks that while, in the hitherto known description of cutaneous lesions associated with changes in the nervous system, the nervous lesions have always been found in the centres, or in the peripheral nerves dependent on them, no mention has been made of the changes in the sympathetic. He leaves the explanation of the dependence of the skin-disease on the changes to be settled by the observation of facts, and by greater advances in the physiology of the sympathetic system.—*Lond. Med. Record*, April 15, 1878.

—

Skin Diseases Treated by Chrysophanic Acid.

Professor NEUMANN, of Vienna, has recently communicated to the *Wiener Medizinische Presse* his experiences of Goa powder and chrysophanic acid in the treatment of psoriasis, herpes tonsurans, and pityriasis versicolor. He appears to have thoroughly tested the efficacy of these remedies, and the conclusions at which he arrives are fully justified by the reports of his cases. As a general prescription, he recommends an ointment composed of chrysophanic acid, ten grammes, simple cerate liquefied by heat, forty grammes, with ten drops of oil of bergamot. Before applying the ointment he scrapes the epidermis with a sharp spoon, so as to remove the scales; and if the diseased spots are very extensive he prescribes warm baths, the application of benzole and lotions of bicarbonate of soda as preliminary measures. After the scales have been removed, the ointment is rubbed in with a dossil of lint, and in cases where the integument is much infiltrated, an effect is more rapidly produced by spreading the ointment on strips of linen and keeping it in contact with the diseased parts. In slight cases the affection begins to disappear after three or four applications. Preliminary treatment is unnecessary for herpes tonsurans and pityriasis. Dr. Neumann's conclusions are that chrysophanic acid is superior to any other known remedy for the treatment of these affections, and he regards it as the most valuable addition which has been made for many years to our cutaneous materia medica.—*Med. Examiner*, May 2, 1878.

—

Relation of Ichthyosis to Membranous Dysmenorrhœa.

In the *Annales de Gynécologie*, December, 1877, Dr. GAUTIER draws attention to the association of ichthyosis with membranous dysmenorrhœa. Bernutz, Siredey, and others have noticed that dysmenorrhœa membranacea affects more commonly those persons of anæmic, debilitated, scrofulous, or tuberculous diathesis. Dr. Gautier regards the ichthyotic disposition of the mucous membrane of the uterus as incurable. The treatment for the dysmenorrhœa is to procure an easy exit for the membranous masses which have to be expelled. Dr. Gautier notes the fact that ichthyosis is hereditary, and that there is a strong presumption in favour of dysmenorrhœa membranacea being hereditary.—*London Med. Record*, April 15, 1878.

Surgery.

Diffusion of Cancer along the Nerves.

Dr. COLOMIATTI relates (*Revista Clinica di Bologna*, and *Lo Sperimentale*, March) a case which occurred in Dr. Spantigati's practice in the Hospital of St. John, in Turin, in support of his theory of the manner of diffusion of cancer.

The subject was a man, aged 40, who had apparently been always healthy, but in whom, after intense neuralgia in the part of the left cheek corresponding to the lower molar teeth, a tumour grew from the inner side of the gum, at the seat of pain. The tumour, which increased rapidly, was diagnosed by Dr. Spanti-gati as cancerous, and was removed, along with the portion of the lower jaw extending from the left canine tooth to the temporo-maxillary articulation. Sur-gically the operation was successful, and the wound soon healed completely ; but, after remaining some time in hospital, the patient was obliged to return to his home, still suffering severely from acute pain, which was only temporarily relieved by subcutaneous injections of morphia.

The tumour, with the bone removed, was presented to Dr. Colomiatti for ex-amination. It was lobulated, and nearly as large as a hen's egg. It contained in its substance the dental nerve, which, however, could be followed for more than four-fifths of an inch before its entrance into the dental canal. Along with the tumour a suprahyoid lymphatic gland was removed, as it was somewhat hard.

After a careful examination, Dr. Colomiatti was led to agree with Dr. Spanti-gati as to the carcinomatous character of the tumour. Its origin from the epithe-lial covering of the gum, at a point corresponding to the molars, explained, in his opinion, the dental neuralgia which preceded its appearance.

Dr. Colomiatti next turned his attention to the dental nerve, the posterior por-tion of which seemed to be more voluminous than normal. Sections of the portion comprised in the tumour presented remarkable changes, in explanation of which Dr. Colomiatti refers to the view held by Robin, Key and Retzius, etc., according to which two forms of connective tissue enter into the formation of nerves—viz., the epineurium, and the perineurium with its appendage, the endoneurium.

The epineurium connects the funiculi, which form every nerve-trunk ; the peri-neurium and endoneurium form an integral part of each funiculus. Their con-nective tissue consists of small membranous films, between which are the so-called perineural and endoneural lymph-spaces, which, however, have nothing to do with the common lymphatic system. These membranous films, the endoneural membranes, which proceed from the perineurium, surround the nerve-fibres. Each nerve-fibre is thus suspended in a lymph-space.

In the case now under consideration, Dr. Colomiatti states that he found, on making section of the dental nerve, an abundant cancerous infiltration, diffused along the perineural and endoneural spaces, the perineurium presenting solutions of continuity, due to the invasion of the epineurium by the cancer-cells.

Dr. Colomiatti says that this is the second case in which he has observed the diffusion of cancer in the inferior dental nerve. There is, however, a difference between the two cases. In the first (cancer of the lower lip), the disease was diffused by the lymphatic vessels belonging to the neighbouring glands ; while, in the present case, the gland which was removed, in consequence of being hard and probably cancerous, was found, on examination, to contain no cancer-cells, and the diffusion of the disease had taken place solely along the nerve. This sup-points the idea of Colomiatti, that the nerve may become diseased before the lymphatics, and independently of them; the lymphatics become infected later, and, when they do, the disease proceeds more rapidly. In this case it was observed that the anterior portion of the nerve, which was examined, had no cancer-cells in its lymph-spaces; hence he infers that the diffusion took place centripetally.

The persistence of the severe pains, in spite of the complete removal of the tumour with the neighbouring parts, is ascribed by Dr. Colomiatti to the diffusion of the disease along the nerves; and he advises that, before undertaking an operation in such cases, the state of the nerves should be observed.—*London Med. Record*, April 15, 1878.

On Transmission of Syphilis by a Bite.

In the *Allgemeine Wiener Medezin Zeitung* for January 8, Dr. Zeissl reports a case in which syphilis was communicated otherwise than through the genital organs. A joiner, aged 28, was admitted on October 9, 1876, into the syphilitic department of the General Hospital in Vienna, having suffered from syphilis for eight weeks. The genitals were perfectly free from signs of specific lesion, present or past, and the neighbouring lymphatic glands were unaffected. The patient had, on the surface of the body, numerous brownish cicatricial depressions, evidently the results of a pustular syphilitic. On further examination, the dorsal aspect of the left thumb, over the metacarpo-phalangeal articulation, showed a depressed, still partly infiltrated, hard, hyperæmic, irregular cicatrix as large as a bean. In this part, he said, he had been bitten on June 4 by a drunken companion, in an attempt to prevent him from making a noise in the street, by placing his hand over his mouth. The wound had healed readily, but broken out again spontaneously four weeks after healing. The epitrochlear gland of the left arm was still markedly enlarged at the time when the patient was seen; that of the other arm was normal. It was proved that the man who inflicted the bite had a syphilitic sore of the mouth. Tincture of iodine was given internally, but, on October 11, he complained of severe cough; and, on examination, infiltration of the apex of the right lung was detected. The iodine was stopped, cod-liver oil was administered, and mercurial inunction employed. After twelve inunctions, the patient was, on October 24, apparently nearly cured of the syphilis, and was transferred to the medical wards, to be treated for tubercle.—*London Med. Record*, April 15, 1878.

Treatment of Ulcers.

Dr. Mandelbaum, of Odessa, remarks (*Berl. Klin. Wochenschrift*, March 11) that after trying in vain all the usual methods of treatment in ulcers, he found ulcerations of all kinds, and in all situations, yield to the treatment by means of the scraper (of Hebra), iodoform, and equal parts of mercurial and soap plasters. If the ulcer be very deep, the destruction of tissue considerable, and the edges jagged, callous, or indurated, it is first thoroughly cleansed with the scraper down to the sound base. This is then daily covered with a thick layer of iodoform until healthy granulations form; and they invariably do form. Then, when the sore has filled in, and its base risen to the level of the surrounding skin, it is dressed with equal parts of mercurial and soap plaster spread evenly on soft linen. If the ulceration be less severe, and only covered with a thick layer of pus, iodoform alone, without previous scraping, is sufficient to produce healthy granulations. This treatment has, in Dr. Mandelbaum's hands, cured ulcers of all kinds, and which had resisted for many years all other means.—*London Med. Record*, April 15, 1878.

Case of Gunshot Wound of the Brain.

Dr. Rossi relates in the *Annali Universali di Medicina e Chirurgia* for December, 1877, the case of a lad, aged 16 or 17, who, having bought a revolver, was one day amusing himself by shooting at a target with one of his friends. After discharging some shots, he recharged the weapon and drew the trigger, but it would not go off; he therefore looked down the tube, when the revolver exploded suddenly, the ball striking the upper part of the left eyelid, just outside the groove for the passage of the vessels and the supra-orbital nerve, fracturing the frontal bone, and entering the brain.

At first only the immediate local symptoms were observed ; but the next morning the right arm was painful and paretic, and there was an appearance of brain-substance at the orifice of the wound. In conjunction with Dr. Rouge, Dr. Rossi made an incision about an inch and a quarter upward, when the pulsations of the cerebral matter, isochronous with those of the heart, were distinctly discerned, and there was found to be a radiated fracture of both tables of the frontal bone immediately above the orbital arch. Through this a probe could be easily introduced to a depth of five centimetres (two inches) in an oblique direction, from below upwards, and from before backwards, without coming into contact with the projectile. Ice was applied, and six leeches behind the left mastoid process.

Contrary to all expectation, the pain and paresis of the right arm soon disappeared ; the cicatrization of the wound took place without necrosis, and almost without suppuration ; and the patient was well in a few days.

The author, assuming it to be certain that the bullet entered the brain, asks in what part of that organ it could be lodged, there being no nervous disturbance, either paretic or paralytic.—*London Med. Record*, March 15, 1878.

The Influence of the Uterus in Eye Disease.

Dr. H. R. SWANZY, Prof. of Ophthalmic and Aural Surgery, Royal College of Surgeons, Ireland, at the Obstetrical Society of Dublin (*Obstetrical Journal of Great Britain*, May, 1878), read an interesting paper on this subject. He said that one of the greatest efforts of modern ophthalmology has been directed towards bringing this branch of medical science into intimate relation with the others. At the present day, indeed, there are few eye diseases which we recognize as purely local affections. While they require special local treatment, most of them demand attention also to some constitutional defect, or some disease situated, perhaps, in a distant organ. Thus we know that eye diseases may have their starting-point in the heart, kidneys, or spleen. The visual organs may be affected in tuberculosis; they often suffer in diseases of the nervous and vascular systems; and I need hardly say how frequently they become diseased in syphilis and struma. This evening, by the kind permission of the Council of the Society, I propose to occupy your attention for a short time in considering the influence of the uterus in eye disease.

At the very outset I must explain that the subject is by no means a completely developed one. It is a very wide one, and its investigation is surrounded by many difficulties. Not the least of these is the circumstance that very few ophthalmologists are at the same time experienced in gynæcology, and that it is also rare to find a gynæcologist who knows anything of ophthalmology. Still the influence of the uterus in eye disease is every day attracting more attention amongst oculists, and we may hope that before many years have gone by we will be in possession of a number of well-authenticated facts which will teach us how far this causal relation between diseases of the uterus and the eye exists, and will enable us to un-

derstand in what way it comes about. At present we possess some facts only,
while much of the subject remains hypothetical. If we could enlist the interest
of gynæcologists in the matter much more rapid progress would be made, and it
is partly with this object that I come before you to-night. In what I am about to
say I shall not confine myself to my own experience for material, but I shall draw
on the observations of others also, in order to present you with as complete a view
of the question in its present stage as is compatible with the time at our disposal.

The first disease which I shall bring under your notice, as probably having its primary cause in the uterus, is iritis occurring in young girls from about the eleventh to
the seventeenth year of age—say within a period varying from two to three years
prior to the establishment of menstruation up to two or three years after they commence to menstruate. I am much interested in these cases, because, so far as I
am aware, they form a point of connection between the uterus and the eye which
has not long before been pointed out. I am aware, however, that others besides
myself have observed this connection, for while lately in Paris I learned in conversation with a distinguished oculist there that his experience had led him to
form a similar view on the subject. The whole number of these cases which I
have seen is seven. It may seem few, but the smallness of the number is accounted
for by the fact that I have not seen a single case of the kind in hospital practice.
These patients seem always to enjoy good general health, and, so far as I have
been able to ascertain, they did not suffer from any serious irregularity in the
uterine functions, should that organ have come to maturity. The most I have
detected has been a somewhat insufficient menstrual flow. I am unable, therefore, to connect the disease of the eye positively with a disease of the uterus, but
I am inclined to regard the uterus in some way as the starting-point of the iritis
for these reasons: (1) Iritis is extremely rare at such an early time of life, unless
as dependent on congenital syphilis, or as secondary to corneal diseases. (2) I
have never seen a case similar to those I speak of in the male; and, therefore,
(3), when one finds it to occur with a certain frequency at the time of life when
the uterus is approaching maturity or has lately reached it, and when one is able
to exclude all other causes, the inference is a fair one that the uterus in some
way has given rise to the iritis.

The form of iritis is similar in all these cases; there is usually little or no pain,
and but little vascular injection of the eye or photophobia. The anterior chamber
usually remains clear, and there is no deposit on the posterior surface of the cornea. There is a great tendency to the formation of posterior synechiæ, and the
stroma of the iris in bad cases becomes indistinct and discoloured. The vitreous
humour is very liable to become cloudy, showing that the cases are not ones of
simple iritis, but that the ciliary body and choroid are implicated. Perhaps, indeed, it would be more correct to describe these as cases of irido-choroiditis. In
some of the cases I have seen it was the dimness of sight caused by these opacities
of the vitreous which first induced the patient or her parents to seek advice. The
affection is very slow in its progress, very difficult of cure, and very liable to recur.

One of the most serious cases of this kind which I have observed is at present
under my care. I shall not impose the whole history of the case upon the Society,
but shall briefly refer to its principal features.

On 5th of July last I was consulted by the parents of a particularly healthy-
looking young lady, aged sixteen, on account of her defective vision. In the
right eye was the form of irido-choroiditis which I have described, and in the
left eye there was optic neuritis. The sight of the right eye was reduced to the
power of counting fingers at eight feet; but neither the patient nor her friends
were aware of any defect in the functions of the left eye, the one with optic neuritis, although its vision was only a little more than one-third of what it should

have been. She had first complained of her sight about two months before I saw her. Five months previously the menses had remained absent on the occasion, and at that time she had a bleeding from the nose. Since then the menstruation had been regular as to time, but the mother seemed to think the flow not quite as abundant as in girls of her age and of such full habit. She was particularly subject to headaches. but it had not been remarked that they were more severe at or about the menstrual period. Since she has been under my care, I think I have noticed that the headaches are more severe at that time. After remaining in town for six weeks, the patient had so far recovered as to be able to return home. She had not been at home for more than ten days, when, while stretching up to nail a picture on the wall, she found the sight of the left eye suddenly become dim. She was at once brought back to me, and the ophthalmoscope displayed an enormous hemorrhage situated probably between the retina and choroid. The right eye had also relapsed, the vitreous humour being very much more' clouded than when I had last seen her. At present the sight of the eye in which the hemorrhage occurred is extremely imperfect, owing to a detachment of the retina which has resulted. The sight of the right eye is tolerably good, and if I can save it for her I shall think myself extremely fortunate in the case. We have in this case three diseases of the eye—irido-choroiditis, optic neuritis, and intra-ocular hemorrhage. It was to give an example of the first of these that I brought forward the case in this part of my paper; but the two other affections are also recognized as sometimes the consequence of disordered uterine functions, as I shall show further on. Fortunately it is a rare thing to find them all combined to destroy vision as in this instance, especially in so young a person.

The treatment which I have usually adopted in these cases of iritis has been chiefly local during the acute stages of the inflammation—atropine, warm fomentations, etc. After the acute inflammation had subsided I have given tonics, especially iron. In the case I have just alluded to, the treatment was very various according as the symptoms demanded. For a long time, although I was fully convinced of the connection between the eye trouble and an imperfect menstruation, yet treatment could be only partially directed towards the uterus, owing to the necessity for promoting absorption of the intra-ocular hemorrhage by a horizontal position for several weeks. Such confinement to the house is not, I conceive, well calculated to improve the uterine functions. However, aloetic purgatives were administered with bromide of potassium. Lately iron has been given in place of the bromide. On the whole, the menstrual flow is now more abundant; but that this has had any great influence in producing restoration of a healthy condition within the eyeballs, I am unable to say. The most that I can believe to have been accomplished by the uterine treatment, if I may so call it, is that no very serious hemorrhage occurred again, nor any fresh attack of iritis.

Inflammation of the optic nerve and retina may depend on disturbances of menstruation. In the *Irish Hospital Gazette* for 1873 (p. 46) I published a case of neuro-retinitis in a girl, aged nineteen, whose menstruation was sparse and painful, and in whom the eye affection always became aggravated at the monthly periods. I observed another similar case, of which unfortunately I have lost the notes. Mandelstam[1] has seen many cases of optic neuritis where marked menstrual disturbances have gone before. Von Gräfe[2] recognized the existence of such a connection. Nooren[3] has seen cases of neuro-retinitis after suppression of menstruation, and he is of opinion that retroflexions of the uterus and ovarian tumours may give rise to the same affection.

---

[1] Klin. Beobacht. a. d. Augenheilanstalt zu Wiesbaden. 1866.
[2] Archiv f. Ophthal., xii., 2.   [3] Ophthalm. Mittheilungen. 1874.

Retinal apoplexies are sometimes the consequence of cessation or suppression of the menses. Thus Liebreich, in his "Atlas of Ophthalmoscopy," gives a drawing of a retinal hemorrhage which occurred in a woman forty-five years of age, in whom menstruation ceased, and who had had it very abundantly up to that time. He mentions that he had several times observed the same ophthalmoscopic appearances under similar circumstances. Samelsohn[1] describes a case of absolute amaurosis after a sudden suppression of menstruation in a girl aged twenty-one years. There were no ophthalmoscopic appearances, and the probable diagnosis consisted in a hemorrhage into the optic nerve behind the globe. The patient was working in a cold stream during her menstrual period. The menses ceased at once, and on the evening of the same day vision began to be affected. In the course of five days the patient became stone blind. The treatment consisted of warm foot-baths, mustard poultices on the upper part of the thighs, emetics, and the application of Heurteloup's artificial leech to the temples. Later aloetic and iron pills were given. In twenty-four hours the sight began to recover, and in the course of eleven days the vision was again almost normal. Seven weeks after the sudden interruption of the menstruation it returned, and simultaneously the pains in the breast disappeared, with which she had been troubled since the loss of her sight.

Atrophy of the optic nerve has been noted repeatedly by Pagenstecher[2] as occurring in women who had suffered from severe menstrual disturbances (irregularity, early cessation), which he regarded as the cause of the eye disease.

I have now to speak of an affection of sight connected with uterine disorder which until lately has been classed among eye diseases, but which we now know to be nothing more than a symptom of a certain uterine disease. It is a form of asthenopia to which the name of *Kopiopia Hysterica* has been given. I have for some time been acquainted with this affection, but, like the iritis of which I have spoken, I have never seen it except in private practice. One of the first patients who consulted me was a case of this kind. I was extremely puzzled by it, never having seen anything of the sort before. Since then I have seen a considerable number of such cases, but only quite lately have I read the first description of the affection, along with an explanation of its cause. It has been described at length by Professor Förster, in his article in Gräfe and Sämisch's new Handbook of Ophthalmology, and the pathological conditions of the uterine apparatus which Professor Freund, of Breslau, has invariably found accompanying it are cited by Professor Förster. This article has been published within the current year (1877).

Patients suffering from the affection complain chiefly of inability to read, write, sew, or use their sight for any near work, owing to darting pains through the organs when they attempt to do so. The pains in and about the eyes, however, although increased by any use of them, are also present with greater or less severity at other times, and are intensified by anything which depresses the general tone of the patient, such as want of sleep, fatigue, sorrow, etc. The patients are troubled with photophobia, especially at night, when the lamps or candles are lighted. Indeed, many of them can bear the direct sunlight without inconvenience, when even a shaded lamp in the room in the evening will give them great distress. No organic disease of the eyes is present. Some hypermetropia or insufficiency of the internal recti may be found, and is likely enough for a time to mislead the surgeon. The eyes are never injected; there is no swelling of the lids; no epiphora. Professor Förster has remarked that the patients have good days and bad days, but that there is no regular interval between these variations,

---

[1] Berl. Klin. Wochenschr. 1875, p. 27.   [2] Klin. Beobacht., 1866.

and he has also observed that they are never kept awake by the pain of their eyes; and he says that shortly before and during menstruation the symptoms are usually more severe. These are points which I have not noted myself. One generally finds these patients endowed with the greatest volubility, the torrents of words with which they describe their ailment affording in itself a symptom of the disease. Very often they enter into the most curious details concerning their trouble. Thus one young lady assured me that there was only one book which she could read without suffering intense pain, and that was one particular copy of the Bible. She could read it for any length of time without the slightest inconvenience, but not even another copy of the same edition could she look at. I was told that there was nothing particular about this book; it was of the ordinary hand size. One of Förster's patients was compelled always to shut her eyes when passing through a doorway, as the draught brought on the pain, and another got a pain in her stomach whenever she attempted to read. Although in other particulars these patients might be termed "nervous," still they do not usually suffer from any marked hysterical symptoms apart from their eyes.

Professor Freund, of Breslau, has found by means of a large number of *post-mortem* examinations of women who have complained of these eye symptoms that they were uniformly affected with a certain uterine disease, which he claims to be the first to have recognized. It is a chronic inflammatory process, attacking the parametrium, and producing in bad cases atrophy of that tissue, with displacement of the pelvic viscera. It is liable to affect married and unmarried women at all times of life. Its course is a very chronic one, extending often over a period of several years, and treatment has little effect upon it. Painful regions may be sometimes found in the lateral cul-de-sac of the vagina; in the course of the broad ligament, and stretching towards the pelvic walls. There is often venous congestion of the vagina, with chronic metritis, catarrh, and ulceration. In less severe cases these local signs may be but slightly marked, and the recovery may take place in a comparatively short time. In none of the cases which have come under my care have I noted any of these pelvic signs; but I must acknowledge that I have seen but two or three rather imperfectly marked cases since I became aware of the nature of the affection. The best treatment consists, I think, in doing as little as possible in the way of medicine, but by attention to the general health to promote the cure, and by diverting the patients' attention from themselves to alleviate the symptoms. For the latter purpose there is, perhaps, nothing so useful as change of scene or foreign travel. Probably a foreign chalybeate spring would combine everything that could be desired in the treatment.

In the foregoing I have referred to five affections of the eye which seem to depend sometimes on uterine derangement—a form of iritis, neuro-retinitis, apoplexies of the retina and optic nerve, atrophy of the optic nerve, and an affection called kopiopia hysterica. It is more than probable that this list might be considerably extended, but we must be careful not to fall into the error of regarding every eye disease which happens to be concomitant with a derangement of the uterine functions as dependent upon the latter.

There are just now two girls in the National Eye and Ear Infirmary suffering from different eye diseases, each of them peculiar in its form. Both of these patients are very irregular in their menstruation, still I do not feel sure as to a connection between this and the eye troubles.

—

Extraction of Steel and Iron from the Eye by the Magnet.

The following cases, recorded by Dr. W. A. McKEOWN, Surgeon to the Ulster Eye, Ear, and Throat Hospital (*British Med. Journal*, May 4, 1878), will be of interest taken in conjunction with that recently brought before the Clinical Society of London by Mr. McHardy.

CASE 1.—Dawson B., aged 24, smith's helper, applied to me at the Hospital on January 16, 1877. He stated that, three days previously, his right eye had been wounded by a small piece of metal. I observed that the iris was attached to the lens at the outer part of the pupil by recent lymph, and that there was a small limited opacity of the lens. There was a small, clean, metallic body sticking at the margin of the adherent pupil. I made a small section of the cornea, more peripheral than the pupil, introduced a pair of iridectomy forceps, seized the body and a little piece of iris, but the body slipped from my grasp, and was sliding out of my reach. Fortunately, I had anticipated such an untoward event, and took care to have a pointed permanent magnet at hand. I introduced it into the wound. The metal was instantly attracted and extracted. The patient continued under my observation till February 16. The opacity of the lens remained limited to the point wounded. I believe that the wound in the capsule was closed by lymph and healed. I have not seen or heard from the patient since.

CASE II.—Moses E., aged 32, millwright, consulted me at the Hospital on November 20, 1877. He stated that, three-quarters of an hour before his visit, his right eye had been wounded by a chip of steel from a hammer. I observed a wound a little more than a line long in the ciliary region just at the corneo-sclerotic junction. One end of the wound penetrated the anterior chamber, as shown by the evacuation of the aqueous humour and a slight displacement of iris towards the wound. The wound was quite clean, and no foreign body was visible. The media were clear. The ophthalmoscope did not disclose the presence of any foreign body. I put the point of the magnet cautiously into the wound, and at once it proved the presence of metal within the sclerotic by the click and the attraction. By a little patient and careful use of the magnet, the metal was brought into the wound, and the end of it exposed so far as to enable me to grasp it with forceps. Having caught it, I easily extracted it. The fragment was a thin piece about one and a half lines long, one line in width at one end, and half a line at the other end. The patient recovered completely, and returned to work on December 10th following.

There can hardly be a doubt that the magnet saved the eye in both cases. In the first case, to have followed the sharp fragment with forceps would probably have inflicted irreparable damage, and indeed the body might have got out of the way altogether. In the second case, the metal would but for the magnet probably have remained undetected, and have afterwards lighted up destructive inflammation. Even had it been detected, it would not have been possible, but for the magnet, to extract it without enlarging the wound, and that is not desirable in any part of the eye, much less in the ciliary region. By the magnet, the diagnosis was established, and the extraction was accomplished in the most delicate way.

Syphilitic Interstitial Glossitis.

Dr. C. MAURIAC has published an account of this affection (*Le Progrès Médical*, 1877, No. 45), which is in character similar to syphilitic sarcocele, and consists of an inflammatory induration of the fibrous partitions separating the muscular fasciculi of the tongue. It begins always on the dorsal surface, at first being superficial, and then invading the deeper tissues. It is more frequently met with in men than in women. There appear to be a hypertrophic and an atrophic period. In the former the enlarged, hard, and painful tongue presents on the dorsal aspect hollow furrows filled with macerated epithelium. There are noticed large papillæ, and often ulcerations, at the points where the tongue touches the teeth, or in the bottom of the above-mentioned furrows. The second stage is that of retraction of the new tissue, and then there is a deep antero-posterior fissure, with several irregular fissures. Finally, as atrophy progresses, the organ becomes smooth and shining, is divided into little lobules, and gives the sensation of a tongue made of wood. Specific treatment is seemingly of some service in the early stages, but is entirely useless when the disease is advanced.—*London Med. Record*, April 15, 1878.

Syphilitic Disease of the Nose.

In the *Vierteljahrschrift fur Dermatologie und Syphilis*, Band iv., Heft 1 and 2. SCHUSTER and SÄNGER recommend the use of the scraping spoon for the removal of syphilitic growths of the nasal cavity, to prevent falling in, and to arrest the disease process. Even perforation of the palate by scraping is at times the lesser of two evils. Artificial illumination should be used. Pathologically the conditions existing vary. There may be—1, simple syphilitic infiltration, the mucous membrane not hypertrophied, with or without alteration of the glands, capillaries, or epithelium; 2, the same, with hypertrophy of the mucous membrane and constriction of the dilated capillaries, by means of cell-growth, or, without this, a fact favouring the views of Auspitz and Unna, upon the anatomy of the initial induration, namely, that the vessels remain, as a rule, unobliterated; 3, more severe infiltration of the mucous membrane, passing into syphiloma; 4, syphilomata of the mucous membrane or condylomata. The subjacent bones and cartilages may show either necrosis with exfoliation, absorbent inflammation, without loss of the mucous membrane, or plastic osteitis, with 'the production of spindle-cells and connective tissue, passing into bony formations.

The practical points are these: 1. Whereas, ulceration of the mucous membrane has been held by writers to be the sole cause of ulceration of the bone and cartilage of the nose, this need not be the case. That membrane may remain uninjured while the subjacent tissues undergo changes like those of the tibia or frontal bone. 2. A healthy mucous membrane may be caused to ulcerate by mechanical interference, and then this ulceration may extend to the bones, or the disease in subjacent bones pass over to the injured membrane.—*London Med. Record*, April 15, 1878.

On Circumcision by the Galvanic Cautery.

Dr. BONA relates three cases in No. 20 of *L'Independente* for 1877.

A boy, aged 6, had a tumour of the size of a nut, formed of the gland and prepuce, which had undergone degeneration, and were fused into a single body. Dr. Bona diagnosed lardaceous degeneration of the prepuce, with adherence to the glans—the result of a foul ulcer of several months' standing. With the galvanic cautery a clean section was made compressing almost the whole of the changed prepuce without the loss of a drop of blood, and with but little pain. Water dressing was subsequently applied; there was no constitutional reaction, and the patient was soon well.

In the second case, a child, aged 7, had œdematous phimosis and urethral fistulæ at the base of his penis, in consequence of two of his companions having tightly tied a stout hempen thread round the organ. In consequence of the obstruction presented by the phimosis to the passage of a catheter, which was necessary for the treatment of the fistulæ, Dr. Bona performed circumcision by the galvanic cautery, with but little pain, and with no hemorrhage, removing more than a centimetre (0.4 inch) of the prepuce.

The third case was one of congenital phimosis. A centimetre of the prepuce was removed by the galvanic cautery, with a successful result.—*London Med Record*, April 15, 1878.

On the Treatment of Congenital Hydrocele by Injections of Alcohol.

Dr. FRANCIS LABAT has observed in Dr. Launelongue's wards, the good results obtained in the cure of congenital hydrocele by injections of alcohol according to Monad's method. The following plan is pursued (*Thèse de Paris*, Nov. 19, 1877). With a subcutaneous injection-syringe, one gramme of the serous matter contained in the hydrocele is evacuated, and one gramme of alcohol injected with the same syringe. In the mean time, pressure is made on the inguinal canal, and prolonged some minutes after the alcoholic injection.—*Lond. Med. Record*, April 15, 1878.

On the Treatment of Severe Arterial Hemorrhage from Punctured Wounds of the Throat and Neck, especially considered with regard to Ligature of the External Carotid Artery.

Mr. WM. HARRISON CRIPPS read a paper upon this subject at a late meeting of the Royal Medical and Chirurgical Society (*Lancet*, May 4, 1878). He discussed the treatment to be adopted in cases of severe arterial bleeding, that have resisted all simple means, and in which operative measures become necessary. The class of cases include punctured wounds about the angle of the jaw and through the mouth, hemorrhage from the tonsils, or from cancer of the tongue or mouth, and secondary hemorrhages after surgical operations, etc. The treatment usually adopted in these cases has been a ligature upon the common carotid. Upon analysis of a considerable number of cases, it is found that, after this method of treatment, rather more than half the patients die. The causes of these deaths are approximately as follows: Rather more than 30 per cent. from brain symptoms; rather more than 30 per cent. from recurrence of the bleeding; and 30 per cent. from other causes. It thus appears that one-third of these deaths are directly due to ligature of the carotid, and that in another third the operation had proved useless for arresting the bleeding. The brain symptoms appear to result from the already anæmic brain having a considerable portion of its blood-supply suddenly cut off. Hemorrhage, occurring from the original wound (after ligature of the common trunk) must either be due to the blood coming as a regurgitant stream brought down the internal carotid, or by blood being brought through the fine anastomoses of the terminal branches. Experiments and facts narrated in the paper show that in a certain number of instances the bleeding is due to a regurgitant stream through the internal carotid, or to blood brought to the proximal end of the wounded vessel by the inferior thyroid. A table accompanying the paper shows how the bleeding vessel, wounded in the situation described, has most commonly proved to be the external carotid, or one of its branches, a wound of the internal carotid being of rare occurrence. Having discussed the cause of the high mortality following ligature of the common carotid, ligature of the external carotid, about half an inch from the bifurcation, is recommended as likely to prove a safer and more efficient method of controlling the bleeding. The grave danger of cutting off the blood supply to the brain is avoided by this operation, while, at the same time, the chance of recurrent hemorrhage is diminished in proportion to the number of instances in which it occurs as a regurgitant stream. The objections raised to the operation are: (1) the fear of secondary hemorrhage from the proximity of large branches; (2) that, should the wounded vessel prove to be the internal carotid, a ligature upon the external would be a useless operation. The first objection is answered by reference to cases narrated by M. Guyon, showing the rare occurrence of secondary hemorrhage from the external carotid. The second, by the comparatively few instances in which the wounded vessel has proved to be the internal carotid. Moreover, should the mistake occur, it is not beyond remedy, for a ligature might still be placed on the common trunk at its bifurcation; on the other hand, no remedy can be found for a patient dying in a comatose condition caused by obstructing the internal carotid on account of a wound of the external carotid or one of its branches.

Mr. Holmes only recalled one case of punctured wound in the neighbourhood of the tonsil in which the internal carotid was thought to have been invaded, and ligature of the common carotid was had recourse to. If in such cases it were certain that the wounded vessel was not the internal carotid, but a tonsillar branch of the external carotid, then clearly it was right to tie the latter vessel by preference. Mr. Cripps' argument was forcible, that the same incision made to expose the external carotid would serve also to secure the common trunk, supposing the first ligature failed to arrest the bleeding.

Mr. M. Baker had tied the common carotid in a case of hemorrhage in the neighbourhood of the tonsil, from an injury by a tobacco-pipe. The patient died from the loss of blood rather than the operation, and the ascending pharyngeal was found to have been the vessel wounded, showing that in such a case ligature of the external carotid would not have succeeded. Still, for the majority of cases the suggestions of Mr. Cripps were of value.

Mr. H. Cripps, in reply, said that in his collected cases only seven or eight were of wounds within the mouth, the majority being wounds behind the jaw. Wounds of the internal carotid were very rare, even in injuries in the neighbourhood of the tonsil, the tonsillar branch of the facial artery lying more superficially than the internal carotid, which, out of five cases, had been found post mortem to be wounded only in one.

On a Case of Ununited Fracture.

In the *Deutsche Medicinische Wochenschrift*, March 2, 1878, Dr. Max Schüller, of Greifswald, relates a case of subperiosteal resection, with subsequent suture of the periosteum, on account of an ununited fracture produced by interposition of a tendon between the fragments.

Dr. Schüller observes that the employment of antiseptic precautions must materially change the opinions formerly entertained as to the danger of resecting the ends of the fragments in ununited fracture. Hence, of late years, we find this mode of treatment very frequently resorted to, amongst others by Volkmann, Bardeleben, and Langenbeck. The value of this method of treating false joint, as compared with the many others from time to time practised, is, the author considers, yet to be determined. As a partial solution of the question, Dr. Schüller has published this case.

Frau H., 40 years of age, a healthy vigorous woman, sustained a fracture of the leg from the wheel of a heavily laden wagon passing over it. Gypsum bandages were immediately applied, but, after eight weeks' treatment, no consolidation had taken place, and no formation of callus could be felt. A fresh trial of plaster of Paris bandage was now made, and a three per cent. solution of carbolic acid was injected from a hypodermic syringe near the seat of fracture; a plan recommended of late years by Professor Hueter for the treatment of cases of delayed or non-union. Six months were consumed in various trials, and, at the end, there was not the slightest degree of union. An operation was then decided upon. A careful examination showed a marked interval between the fragments, so that pegging was not thought suitable. An incision, two and a half inches long, was

therefore made, the seat of fracture exposed, and the periosteum raised from the
ends of the bone, which were rounded, while between them passed the tendinous
termination of the tibialis anticus muscle. There was not a trace of bone-prolife-
ration. The muscle was now restored to its proper position, and the ends of the
bones cut off, partly with the saw, and partly with the chisel, to the extent of a
centimètre from each. After forcible traction, the fresh surfaces of bone could
be accurately adjusted together, the fibrous connection of the broken ends of the
fibula being divided simply with the knife, but the bone not otherwise interfered
with. As the fragments of the tibia showed no tendency to separate, ivory pegging, or silver-wire suture, was not employed, but the carefully preserved periosteum was accurately united by fine catgut sutures, a small opening only being left
to allow a fine drainage-tube to pass between the bones. Another and larger
drain was passed outside the periosteum, and through a counter-opening made in
the calf. The skin-wound was now sutured with catgut, the limb enveloped with
salicilized jute, and a gypsum bandage, reaching over the knee, was applied.
The whole operation was performed with strict antiseptic precautions. Except
the day afterwards, when the temperature rose to 38.5° C. (101.3° F.), there
was never any fever. The whole dressing, plaster of Paris bandage included,
was changed every few days at first; then a window was made in the plaster, and
the dressings of the wound alone renewed. The external wound healed by first
intention, but a slight discharge continued for a long time from the interior. A
small fragment of bone subsequently exfoliated, and then immediate and thorough
healing followed; and, at the end of four months, complete consolidation had
taken place, in good position, and with a shortening of only half a centimetre at
the outside. The author preserved the periosteum in this case with the greatest
care, believing it has the chief part in the act of union, the endosteum somewhat
less, and the bone-substance proper very little. The plan of pegging, he considers, has its principal result in fixing the fragments. He believes little in its
power of exciting proliferation of bone when employed under antiseptic precautions, which accounts, in his opinion, for several recent failures of this method.
In cases, therefore, where resection of the ends of the bone is indicated, he would
perform the operation subperiosteally, accurately unite the margins of the divided
periosteum, and only use pegs where necessary to maintain the fragments in apposition, and at rest.—*London Med. Record*, April 15, 1878.

Two uncommon Forms of Dislocation.

Mr. A. W. MAYO ROBSON, Demonstrator of Anatomy at the Leeds School
of Medicine, records (*British Med. Journal*, April 6, 1878) two interesting cases,
one of dislocation of the jaw occurring during an attack of hysteria; the other,
of dislocation of the sternal end of the clavicle upwards.

"I was called to see a woman aged 30, said to be in a fit. On arriving at the
house, I found her in an hysterical attack, and ascertained that she had received
news of a severe family trouble a few hours previously. A curious symptom in
the case was, that she violently worked the jaw, and would persist in doing so
despite being sharply spoken to and treated freely with cold water. Whilst I
was observing her, the jaw suddenly became fixed widely open and displaced
obliquely towards the right side. She instantly began to scream violently, and
applied her hand to the injured part. I need scarcely say that the hysteria
vanished as if by magic. I replaced the jaw in the usual manner, and applied a
four-tailed bandage. After being put to bed, she had a return of the paroxysms,
and again worked the jaw; but this time the bandage prevented displacement.
The next day, beyond a considerable degree of stiffness, nothing abnormal was

found. I then ascertained that she had never had dislocation of the jaw on any previous occasion. My reason for recording the case is, that I find no mention made of any similar one either in Hamilton on *Fractures and Dislocations* or in Holmes's, Erichsen's, or Bryant's works on surgery.

"The history of the second case is as follows. I was called on September 27, 1877, to see a grammar-school boy aged 15; the messenger telling me that he had put his shoulder out, having fallen undermost in a scrimmage at football. On arrival, I found him leaning towards the left side and supporting that arm with his right hand, any change of position giving great pain. On stripping the chest, the first sign that attracted my attention was a marked flattening of the left infraclavicular region. I then noticed a depression of the same shoulder; a very distinct prominence in front of the trachea just above the sternum; an absence of the natural projection of the left sterno-clavicular articulation, its place being taken by a depression in which could be felt the empty sternal socket. The tendon of the left sterno-mastoid was stretched tensely like the string of a bow, and the distance between the shoulder-tip and the middle line was an inch less on the affected side than on the sound one. There was no dyspnœa, and an entire absence of crepitus. My diagnosis was dislocation of the sternal end of the clavicle upwards, as the only accidents which might have simulated it were separation of the epiphysis and fracture; the latter being negatived by the absence of crepitus, and the former by the fact that ossification does not take place in the epiphysis till the eighteenth or twentieth year. Reduction was easily effected by drawing the shoulders backwards and raising the arm. I tied a handkerchief round each arm near the shoulder, and looped them together firmly behind; placed a pad in the axilla; pressed the elbow inwards by means of a bandage round the chest, inclosing the arm; and supported the elbow and forearm in a sling; after which the symmetrical appearance of the chest returned. In the after-treatment, there was a great tendency for the sternal end of the clavicle to slip upwards, as the boy, being unusually active, always contrived to romp about and loosen the bandages as soon as his attendant's back was turned. Although the appliances were continued for three weeks, and a figure-of-eight bandage for a fortnight longer, yet at the end of that time the sternal end of the clavicle remained about half an inch above its usual level; but the functions of the limb seemed to be in no way impaired. The only cases I can find on record of a similar nature are four quoted by Malgaigne, two by Bryant, one by Dr. Rochester of Buffalo, and one by Hamilton."

———

A Case of Traumatic Resection of the Scapula.

Dr. KNAUTH reports (*Berliner Klinische Wochenschrift*, March 18) the case of a boy 10 years of age who was seized on the 22d of February last by the fly-wheel of a chaff-cutting machine. The knife of the machine cut through the soft parts under the scapula, and also through the neck of that bone itself behind the coracoid process. The entrance wound was about seven inches long, the wound of exit about five inches. The edges of the wounds were stitched together, and carbolic acid dressings applied. For three days the patient's condition remained satisfactory, but then gangrene set in, and, in six days, destroyed the soft parts, laying the scapula almost bare. The bone was easily removed, and, under carbolic acid dressings, the wound healed kindly, accompanied by but little fever, and a rise in temperature to 103.6° F., leaving an extensive cicatrix and an open sore of the size of a five-shilling piece, which may require a plastic operation for its complete closure. The extent to which the movements of the arm may be affected by so great an injury, cannot yet be determined.—*London Med. Record*, April 15, 1878.

Iodine Injection of the Knee-joint.

Dr. ORLOW states (*St. Petersburg Med. Woch.*, April 6) that he has performed this operation in ten cases—in eight on account of chronic serous effusion, and in two for purulent collections. In none of them did any ill effect result, the patients being at once dismissed after the injection had been made. Two of the cases occurred in children, and the others in persons aged from twenty-six to forty-five. Seven were females, and three males. A trocar (about double the thickness of an exploratory trocar) was employed, the puncture being made at the outer side above or below the patella, according to the amount of distension, anæsthetics never having been employed. The discharged fluid varied in amount from four ounces to four drachms. The injection consisted of one drachm of the tincture of iodine of the Russian Pharmacopœia and three drachms of water. Some portion of this flowed out again after two or three minutes, and that which remained in the joint excited but slight temporary irritation, so that the patients were able to leave the dispensary on foot. The inflammatory condition of the joints was rapidly ameliorated, and during eight months no relapses have taken place, the only after-treatment resorted to having been closure of the orifice of the puncture by adhesive plaster.—*Med. Times and Gaz.*, May 4, 1878.

Midwifery and Gynæcology.

Report of a Case of Fallopian Pregnancy.

Dr. LAURENCE JOHNSON reported to the New York Academy of Medicine (*Med. Record*, April 27, 1878) a case of Fallopian pregnancy occurring in a woman æt. twenty-nine years, married, and the mother of two children aged respectively four and a half and two and a half years. She had always been healthy. Her last menstruation commenced on the 11th of February, 1878, and continued the usual length of time—three or four days. There was no evidence of pregnancy, except the non-appearance of the menses on March 11th. On March 23d, at about noon, she suddenly began to suffer from pain referable to the pelvic regions, became faint, and was put to bed. Small quantities of brandy were given at intervals, and she partially regained her strength, but in the evening there was a return of the faintness. She vomited once or twice, and had an evacuation from the bowels. The doctor saw her for the first time soon after the attack of fainting in the evening; found her very pale, with a feeble pulse, 140, but there was no discharge of blood from the vagina.

March 24. Patient appeared somewhat brighter; pulse somewhat stronger, but rapid. Urination without pain; abdomen somewhat tympanitic : tenderness all around the uterus, but especially upon the right side. Pain was not a prominent symptom at any time during the entire history of the case, although at no time was she markedly under the influence of narcotics.

25th. Patient sank rapidly, and was thought to be dying. She rallied, however, so that on March 26th she was comparatively bright. On the night of the 26th she sank and died, *four* days from her first attack of faintness.

Autopsy twenty-four hours after death. Pelvic cavity filled with blood. Ruptured cyst in the right Fallopian tube, close to the uterus, and probably not larger than a hickory-nut. Right ovary contained a recent corpus luteum. Uterine decidua very apparent. Little or no evidence of peritonitis.

Dr. Johnson raised the following important question: *Would not an operation, with the view of securing bloodvessels, have been feasible and justifiable immediately after the occurrence of the first hemorrhage on the 23d of March?*

Dr. T. Addis Emmet, in the light of a case reported by Dr. McBurney, and which was seen in consultation by Dr. Thomas and himself, believed it to be a feasible operation, as soon as the Fallopian pregnancy was recognized, to first dilate the uterus, then dilate the tube, and in that manner remove the fœtus. Dilatation of the uterus took place when only a moderate quantity of fluid was inclosed in its cavity, and at the same time the fluid backed into the Fallopian tubes. He therefore was perfectly satisfied that, with proper instruments, the uterus could be safely dilated, and also the Fallopian tube, and, as the cyst was usually near the body of the uterus, its contents could readily escape into the cavity of the uterus when such dilatation was effected. Dr. Emmet then exhibited an India-rubber cot, such as he had been in the habit of using during the last ten years, for the purpose of dilating the uterus. The dilator was manufactured by Shepard & Dudley, and consisted of an India-rubber cot containing a tube into which a sound could be introduced, so that it could be carried to the fundus of the uterus; an additional fixture permitted the attachment of a Davidson syringe, by means of which the cot could be distended to any degree required. When the uterus had been dilated, a curved sound could be used, and the cot introduced into the Fallopian tube, and dilatation produced as in the former instance.

Dr. Emmet was of the opinion that as soon as rupture of the cyst occurred it was a proper operation to immediately open the abdomen and secure the bleeding vessels; for, in comparison with such operations as ovariotomy, opening the abdomen for that purpose was a simple affair.

—

The Prevention of Puerperal Fever.

In the last number of the *Monthly Abstract*, page 231, we directed the attention of our readers to the valuable work which our German *confrères* are doing, in attempting to introduce an antiseptic element into the conduct not only of severe, but of normal midwifery cases. The subject is of such importance that we think no apology is needed for again adverting to it, and adducing yet further evidence of its utility. The information of which we are now making use is derived from an excellent article by Professor Zweifel, of Erlangen, in No. 1 of the *Berliner Klin. Wochenschrift*, 1878.

It appears that the idea of "Listering" in obstetrics (the Germans have coined the verb "Listern" to express the use of Professor Lister's antiseptic method, just as from Galvani's name we have coined the verb "galvanize") was first started by Bischoff, of Basle, in 1870 (*Correspondenzblatt für Schweizer-Aertze*, 1875, Nos. 22, 23). His plan consisted in giving a bath as soon as the first pains of labour were observed, washing out the vagina with a 2 per cent. solution of carbolic acid every two hours, and anointing the fingers of the medical attendant with 10 per cent. carbolic oil at each examination, the hands being previously disinfected by washing them with 3 per cent. aqueous carbolic acid. In case the hand had to be passed into the uterus, or if the fœtus was dead and decomposed, the uterus was washed out with a 2 to 3 per cent. solution of carbolic acid; and in every case frequent injections of the latter were made into the vagina and uterus for thirteen days after the birth of the child. Immediately after the labour, any wound was touched with a 10 per cent. carbolic solution, no ligature, if such were necessary, being applied until this had been done. Lastly, a pad of wadding soaked in carbolic oil (one to ten) was placed in the entrance of the vagina, and constantly renewed. Under this system the number of cases in which morbid symptoms were present, consisting in a febrile temperature of more than two days' duration, and reaching 38.5° Cent. (101.3° Fahr.) at least on one day, tenderness of the abdomen on pressure, and fetid discharge, etc., was, in 1870, 14 per cent; 1871, 22.3 per cent. ; 1872, 24.5 per cent. ; 1873, 16.8 per cent. ; 1874, 10.7 per cent. ; 1875, 8.9 per cent. ; or taking the average of the whole, 16.2 per cent. for the six years.

In 1875, H. Fehling published (*Archiv für Gynakologie*, Band xiii., s. 298) the results of experiments made for about a year in Professor Credé's clinic at Leipsic, and which consisted in applying a mixture of salicylic acid and starch (one to five) to any wounds of the external genitals and in syringing the vagina four to eight times daily, in case of fever and fetid discharge, with solutions of salicylic acid ($\frac{1}{5}$ to $\frac{1}{10}$ per cent.). The effect was excellent, but the use of the carbolic spray during labour, which was also tried for some time, was given up in consequence of the post-partum hemorrhages which it appeared to induce.

In 1877, Adrian Schücking (*Berliner Klin. Wochenschrift*, No. 26) suggested that the vagina should be washed out at the end of the labour with a 5 per cent. carbolic solution, and that immediately afterwards the uterus should be continuously irrigated by means of the apparatus of which we gave a brief description in our former article on this subject. This method was carried out in eight cases, in five of which the patients had had severe labours, and all recovered satisfactorily, no temperature being recorded over 38.4° Cent. In the other three the injection was not begun until after the commencement of febrile symptoms, but an immediate and decided defervescence was the result. Professor Zweifel's objection to Schücking's conclusion, that in the five former cases the fortunate termination was directly due to the treatment, is, first, that the number of Schücking's cases is too small; and secondly, that equally good results are possible without any antiseptic treatment. With this objection most persons will, we think, be inclined to agree.

Professor Zweifel's own method, to which we shall devote the remainder of this article, is founded partly on the use of antiseptic measures, properly speaking, and partly on the adoption of the most scrupulous cleanliness in connection with the surroundings of the puerperal woman. In the first place, all vaginal examinations *during pregnancy* are in his clinic made only after careful washing of the hands and smearing with carbolic oil, the vagina being further washed out afterwards in some cases with 5 per cent. carbolic solution. The reason for these precautions is the possibility of infectious matter being introduced into the vagina previous to labour, of its lying there and being sucked up into the uterus after the expulsion of the fœtus. "This," says Professor Zweifel, "is a possibility which no one will deny."

The rooms and beds destined for the use of the lying-in women are carefully disinfected by burning sulphur in them in fireproof vessels, allowing about four grammes of sulphur to each cubic metre of space. The bedclothes are spread out so as to expose as large a surface as possible to the fumes, which after a few hours are allowed to escape by opening the windows.

After each labour in which the hand has been introduced into the uterus, or where air has gained entrance to it, or gaseous decomposition occurred in it, the uterus is washed out with several litres of fresh water.

Since almost all the cases of puerperal fever are found to be complicated either with ruptured perineum, small rents in the vagina and vulva, or with the introduction of air into the uterus during some operation, the greatest care is bestowed on all external wounds, to which Fehling's mixture of salicylic acid and starch is applied with the best results. Careful examination of the external genitals day by day, and the use of the thermometer, are also rigorously attended to. It should be added that at Erlangen the Obstetric Clinic has a separate pavilion to itself, which was built in 1874. The number of births from April, 1876, to October, 1877, during which period the above method has been carried out "with pedantic strictness," has been 184, with a *single* death—that of a woman with cancer, on whom the Cæsarean operation was performed. In 143 cases the lying-in period was completely normal—that is to say, the temperature never exceeded 38° Cent., or, at any rate, was never above 38.4° on more than one day. Out of the remaining forty-one, thirteen never had any morbid symptom except a rise of temperature on one or two days to 38° to 39° Cent., or on several days to 38° to 38.5°; twenty-eight had the symptoms of puerperal fever in a greater or less degree, but of these only twelve had protracted fever, inflammatory exudation, and showed clear signs of puerperal infection, and in only five cases was life ever in any apparent danger. It was further noticed that the cases which did badly were not evenly distributed through the whole period of observation, but were limited to the months of December, 1876, and January, 1877, and of September and October, 1877, in the form of small epidemics. On the whole, Professor Zweifel considers that his results are by no means inferior to those of Bischoff, and that they do not point to any necessity for introducing a more complicated antiseptic system into his practice. Moreover, Spiegelberg at Breslau has carried out a system closely resembling Zweifel's since 1874, with the splendid result of only *five* deaths in *nine hundred* labours.[1]

With such evidence before us it seems to be our bounden duty to urge on the medical profession in this country to habitually adopt the measures by which alone, as far as present knowledge goes, puerperal infection can be prevented—namely, scrupulous cleanliness and the use of antiseptic lotions, etc., for disinfecting the examining hand and the genital organs. Even the busiest practitioner can manage to invariably examine with carbolic oil instead of ordinary oil or grease, and in the most out-of-the-way places vinegar or brandy, as Professor Zweifel says, are sure to be found as substitutes for carbolic or salicylic acid.

We are not sure that in private practice the need of these precautions is not as great as in the hospital ward; for the risk of picking up infection somewhere, and conveying it to the lying-in room, is naturally very great when the same man is seeing on the same day medical, surgical, and obstetric cases. He may go straight from a scarlet fever case to a woman in labour; and a most melancholy instance occurs to us in which a very valuable life was probably sacrificed in this way not so very long ago. The old discussions about puerperal fever, which we find reproduced even now in text-books on midwifery, are out of date in the light of our modern knowledge. We *know*, for example, that the woman who gets fever, peritonitis, and vomiting just after her confinement, has been infected with poison *from without*—whether bacterial or otherwise makes not the slightest difference; we *know*, too, how to prevent the entrance of this poison into the woman's system, though we may be very helpless when it has once entered it. Knowing all this, and knowing, too, the high mortality from puerperal fever, and that probably more than a thousand women die of it in England every year, is it not our plain and simple duty to try and carry out, at any rate, the major operations of midwifery in future with the same attention to antiseptic precautions as Mr. Spencer Wells observes in performing ovariotomy?—*Med. Times and Gaz.*, March 30, 1878.

---

[1] For further information on this subject see also the *Zeitschrift f. Geburtshülfe und Gynækologie*, ii., 1, containing papers by Schüllen, Richter, and Langenbuch.

Puerperal Antiseptics.

Three papers by LANGENBUCH, SCHÜLIN, and RICHTER report the extensive adoption of antiseptic measures for the prevention of puerperal infection in their respective hospitals. Richter's observations were made in the Charité Hospital at Berlin, where, especially after complicated labours, injections into the uterus were made for prophylactic purposes, and were continued throughout the puerperium. In all, about three thousand injections were made. The carbolic solution most frequently employed was a 2 per cent. solution. At first, a 3 per cent. solution was used; but, if repeated frequently, it was reduced to 2 per cent., as the former often caused carbolic acid to appear in the urine. Considering the numerous complications, the results were very favourable, being a mortality of 1.6 per cent. of all the women delivered, and of 4.83 per cent. among the cases in which the injections were used. Schülein, in the University Obstetric Clinic of Berlin, in the winter *semester* of 1876–77, treated two hundred and six out of two hundred and eighty-seven lying-in women immediately after delivery by prophylactic injections of the uterus with a 3 per cent. solution of carbolic acid. This injection was employed whenever in the lying-in bed frequent rises of the pulse and temperature occurred. A glass tube was at first used, and a double-current catheter afterwards. Under this treatment, with eighty-one cases of illness among the two hundred and six, or 28 per cent., the deaths amounted to only seven, or 2.4 per cent.; only one occurring from septic causes, one in a woman on whom Cæsarean section had been performed. Langenbuch has since 1872 employed drainage of the puerperal uterus in order to afford a free outflow of the secretions. His experience shows that this treatment is quite innocuous. In one case, the drain remained nineteen days *in utero*. He recommends this treatment where septic infection already exists, in order to prevent a new invasion of septic material; and also as a prophylactic measure when the cases seem to offer a doubtful prognosis.—*British Med. Journ.*, March 30, 1878.

On Membranous Dysmenorrhœa.

At a late meeting of the Obstetrical Society of London (*Med. Examiner*, May 9, 1878) the following case was recorded by Dr. CORY as strongly supporting Dr. Hausmann's view that cases of this kind are due to an imperfect impregnation. The patient was married at the age of 30, in 1865, having previously been always regular, and never having passed any membrane. Within the first two years of marriage she had three abortions, all between the second and third months. Since then she had at her menstrual periods almost invariably passed membranes, which, on examination, proved to be very perfect casts of the uterine cavity, and presented all the naked eye and microscopical appearances of its mucous lining. (A section of membrane was shown under the microscope.) The membrane usually came away on the second day of menstruation, previously to which the dysmenorrhœa was acute. On two occasions she remembered the membrane did not appear; and both times she had been previously away from her husband. She attended as out-patient at St. Thomas's Hospital from September, 1875, to February, 1877; and a record of her periods during this time showed that the intervals varied from twenty-five to thirty-one days. On May 3d, 1877, she was admitted, while still menstruating, into the hospital. On May 19th the flow again appeared, but without any membrane. A note taken on May 10th stated that the uterus was much retroflexed, but of normal length; there was a small mucous polypus at the orifice of the cervix. She left the hospital on May 31st, and was not seen again till February last, when she stated that she had been living apart from her husband for nine months, during which time she had menstruated regularly without any membrane appearing. He thought the case afforded additional evidence that menstruation was due to an abortion of an unimpregnated ovum, together with its nidus, the mucous membrane of the uterus. The order of events before and during menstruation would seem to be—(1) The arrival of an unimpregnated ovum in the uterus at, or soon after, a menstrual period ; (2) The development of this ovum and its nidus, the mucous membrane of the uterus, up to a certain point ; (3) The arrival to maturity of the next Graafian follicle, accompanied towards its completion by ovarian irritation, which being reflected to the uterus causes uterine contraction ; (4) The abortion of the old ovum and its nidus, accompanied by a discharge of blood ; (5) The rupture of the Graafian follicle and the passage of the new ovum along the Fallopian tube.

Dr. Galabin said that the case before them afforded some direct evidence as to the period at which the Graafian follicle ruptured. It was clear from the facts adduced by Dr. Cory that in many successive months the follicle ruptured and impregnation took place soon after the end of a menstrual period, since there would have been no time for the development of the decidua, if the ovum had belonged to the menstrual epoch at which the membrane was expelled. It was true that recent researches seemed to favour the view that rupture took place before a period, but there was anatomical evidence on both sides, and the question must as yet be regarded as undecided. Dr. John Williams thought that there could be no doubt that the membrane exhibited by Dr. Cory was the decidua containing an impregnated ovum. The fact that the membrane was only passed when the woman was living with her husband favoured the view that it must be a kind of abortion, and for this reason he objected to the case being quoted as one of membranous dysmenorrhœa. Numerous conditions were classed under this name, but many substances might be passed which were not decidual membrane, and he had known of one case where a tough layer of mucus was described as a membrane. He thought the name of membranous dysmenorrhœa ought not to be given to any case in which the lining membrane of the uterus was not expelled. At the same time he felt that Dr. Cory's case, though not one of membranous dysmenorrhœa, would serve to throw some light upon the pathology of that disease. As to the sequence of events in connection with menstruation, he thought that the evidence which had been accumulated on this point showed that usually, if not always, impregnation took place shortly before a period. The anatomical evidence in favour of this was very strong, and Reichert had published eighteen cases in which the ovum was discharged before the commencement of menstruation. At the same time he must admit that there was evidence to show that the ovum might be discharged both during and after a period. In connection with this point he would refer to Coste's case, though he thought that the conclusions drawn from it were erroneous. The subject of this case, a young girl, was drowned fifteen or sixteen days after the cessation of the menstrual flow, and a Graafian follicle was found considerably enlarged. Coste regarded this as a follicle which had failed to rupture during the last period, but it appeared to him that it was in reality the follicle which was preparing to rupture previous to the next period. But the strongest evidence in favour of his view was derived from the history of the Jews. According to the Mosaic law intercourse was forbidden during each period, which was reckoned as lasting five days and for an additional space of eight days following the period, during which the woman was regarded as unclean. There were thus in all thirteen days of uncleanness, so that if the conditions of the Mosaic law were rigidly observed, impregnation could not take place till the ninth or tenth day after the cessation of a period. He had made many inquiries of Jewesses on this point, and he found that those who were strict in their observances adhered to the thirteen days of

uncleanness, while others abstained from intercourse for a week in all.   He
thought these facts were strongly in favour of the view that impregnation took
place before a period.   He admitted, however, that in some women the ovum
might be discharged subsequently to menstruation.   In conclusion, he would ask
Dr. Cory what evidence he had to show that an unimpregnated ovum was capable
of development, and what was the nature of that development?   Dr. Aveling
said that he had some hesitation in accepting the view put forward in the paper.
He thought that a hyperæmic condition leading to membranous dysmenorrhœa
might have been caused by the irritation of intercourse.   As to the period at
which the Graafian follicle ruptured, he had been led to believe that ovulation
was a very irregular function, and he thought no hard and fast line could be
drawn.   Dr. Potter dissented from the assertion that Jewesses were accurate in
their calculations as to pregnancy.   In some cases he had found them as much as
a month out of their reckoning.   After remarks from Dr. Brunton, Dr. Cory
observed, in reply, that until we had more exact knowledge as to the time taken
by the ovum in its passage along the Fallopian tube, it was impossible to come
to any definite decision on the period of rupture of the Graafian follicle.   With
regard to the facts which had been adduced about Jewesses, he might remark that
spermatozoa were known to live some time, and impregnation might thus take
place after a menstrual period, though connection had occurred before it.   He
had no means of proving that unimpregnated ova could develop in the uterus.

Transfusion performed on Account of Uterine Hemorrhage in a Girl of Thirteen.

In a paper (*Archives de Tocologies*, Dec. 1877) read before the Medical Society of Rheims, M. LEROY relates a successful case of transfusion, performed
upon a patient under the care of Dr. Strapart.   The patient was thirteen years
old, and menstruation had first appeared in July, 1876, lasting two or three days.
It did not recur till September, when it lasted eight days.   The period recurred
again in October, and, when it had already continued two days, severe abdominal pain came on, with more profuse loss.   From this day clots began to be
passed, and at length, after twenty-one days of profuse hemorrhage, the child
was brought by her parents to the hospital, on November 23.   She was then excessively pale, the pulse very rapid, thready, and irregular, respiration slow, skin
covered with sweat.   An anæmic bruit was heard over the heart.   She was
treated by ice upon the abdomen, and ergot internally, with cold enemata ; but
the hemorrhage rather increased in quantity.   Quinine and perchloride of iron
were then given, and a temporary improvement followed, the amount of loss diminishing, but not entirely ceasing, up to December 13.   On the 14th of December, apparently with the commencement of a menstrual period, profuse loss
recommenced, clots being frequently expelled.   Uncontrollable vomiting then
came on, and all nourishment was rejected.   On the 17th her complexion was
cadaveric, the skin was cold, the voice inaudible, and the pulse could no longer
be felt.   A consultation was held with Drs. Henri and Adolphe Henrot, and
Langlet, and it was decided to transfuse immediately.   The operation was performed by Dr. Henri Henrot, the father furnishing the blood.   The apparatus
of M. Mathieu was used, the blood not being defibrinated.   The quantity employed was 170 grammes.   The only difficulty met with was that of finding a
vein large enough to admit the canula, all the vessels being collapsed ; but this
was easily overcome.   The patient rapidly revived during the operation, and,
immediately after it, a considerable number of clots was expelled from the vagina.   The blood, examined by the microscope after the operation, showed an

enormous difference as regards the number of corpuscles from that which had been examined before. A short time after its conclusion, the feeling of warmth at first felt gave place to shivering, and extreme thirst succeeded. Two hours later the pupils, which had been widely dilated, became closely contracted, and this condition continued for four or five hours. The following morning the pulse was 145 : the hemorrhage was insignificant and the sickness less frequent. Some febrile disturbance followed, the temperature rising to 38.7° C., but the patient became convalescent, and no more serious hemorrhage occurred. She left the hospital on January 28 in fair condition, although still very pale.—*Obstetrical Journal of Great Britain*, April, 1878.

Blood-Tumours of the Pelvis.

In the *Deutsche Medicinische Wochenschrift* for February 1878, Dr. OTTO ALBERTS relates the following four cases which occurred in the gynæcological clinic of Professor Spiegelberg.

Case I. Rosina K., aged 26, wife of a mason, had one child in 1874. She had always been healthy. She was admitted into Professor Spiegelberg's ward January 16, 1877. Since her last period, she had suffered from pain of an acute character in the back. On examination, there was nothing abnormal on abdominal palpation. *Per vaginam*, a tumour of the size of a child's head was felt behind the uterus. There was slight hemorrhage. The presence of a retro-uterine hæmatocele was diagnosed. The patient became weaker day by day, and, on February 6, the tumour was punctured through the posterior wall of the vagina with a Dieulafoy's aspirator. The characteristic bloody fluid escaped, and the patient gradually recovered.

Case II. Johanna Th., aged 28, servant, had always been healthy. At the last catemenia she strained herself in the stomach, whereupon the flow immediately ceased, and most severe pain set in over the left iliac region. On examination by the abdomen, there was felt a tumour rather larger than a hen's egg in the left pelvic region. Bimanual examination revealed a slightly enlarged and anteflected uterus. The tumour could be felt in the left fornix, and seemed to have firm cyst walls. Dr. Spiegelberg confirmed the diagnosis of Dr. Alberts that there was a blood-tumour of the left Fallopian tube. On June 7, Dr. Spiegelberg punctured the tumour with a trocar and let out some foul sanious fluid. The cyst slowly contracted ; and although there was some fever for several days, the patient recovered.

Case III. Bertha J., single, aged 18, always healthy, never menstruated, for some weeks had suffered from dysuria and dyschezia, together with pain in the lower abdomen. On examination it was found that she had an imperforate hymen. The result had been an accumulation of menstrual fluid in the uterus and vagina, forming a hæmelytrometra. By the abdomen, the enlarged uterus could be felt as high as the navel. On February 13, Dr. Spiegelberg incised the hymen under water, the patient being placed in a bath. A considerable quantity of ichorous fluid escaped. With the exception of a left suppurative parotitis, the patient slowly recovered without further complications.

Case IV. Rosina R., peasant, aged 40, married, with no children, had always been healthy. In 1871 she had smallpox, from which she recovered. From this time the menses became more and more scanty and more painful. Finally they almost entirely ceased, and in April, 1877, she entered the hospital. Abdominal examination revealed a small movable tumour in the median line behind the symphysis pubis. *Per vaginam*, the passage of the finger was arrested half way by a *cul-de-sac*. By the speculum it was seen that cicatricial atresia had taken place, leaving only a small pin-hole aperture through which a catgut could be passed.   The upper portion of the vagina and the uterus had become distended with retained menstrual blood.   The diagnosis was atresia vaginæ acquisita, with hæmelytrometra.   The vagina was dissected up by Dr. Spiegelberg under carbolic spray.   The imprisoned fluid having been released, the patient recovered.   Dr. Spiegelberg was of opinion that the atresia vaginæ resulted from the attack of smallpox.   —*London Med. Record*, April 15, 1878.

Retroflexion of the Uterus in Unmarried and Nulliparous Women.

In an article on the causation and treatment of retroflexion of the uterus in virgins and nulliparous wives (*Archiv für Gynäkologie*, B. xi. H. 1), Dr. GRENSER declares his experience that retroflexion is of much commoner occurrence in virgins than most authors have considered it to be.   Among the commonest causes he has found to be the presence of a fibroid tumour in the posterior wall, or of adhesions, the result of a former perimetritis, by which the fundus is tethered in a backward direction.   Among important predisposing causes are also to be reckoned anæmia, want of muscular tone, catarrh of the genital organs, and masturbation; and as an immediate cause the effect of falls or over-exertion, and especially that of straining, which occurs in chronic constipation.   Lastly, a truly congenital retroflexion is an occasional though a very rare occurrence.   The late Professor Martin has mentioned such cases, depending on imperfect development of the posterior uterine wall, the whole uterus being small and limp.   The author has himself examined at Berlin a specimen taken from a new-born child, which was first described by Dr. C. Ruge in the *Berliner Klinische Wochenschrift*, 1875, No. 1.   In this instance no distension of the intestines was found to account for the displacement, nor were there any adhesions or signs of perimetritis.   The posterior vaginal cul-de-sac was well developed.   The uterine wall on the convex side of the curve was atrophied, while that on the concave side appeared to be thickened.

The author treats simple retroversions by a ring pessary, but in retroflexion of the nulliparous uterus he considers that the vagina is generally not capacious enough to admit a lever pessary of sufficient size to press the fundus upward in adequate degree.   He therefore makes use of an intra-uterine stem, fitted to a vaginal support.   He finds that, in many instances, a virtual stenosis of the cervix is brought about from congestion and swelling, even though the os uteri is not primarily very small.   In such cases he divides the cervix bilaterally, and afterwards introduces temporarily an intra-uterine stem, to prevent any cicatricial contraction.   He records one such instance in which, after three years' sterile marriage, the stem was worn for three and a half months, and the patient became pregnant after the menstrual period which followed its removal.—*Obstetrical Journal of Great Britain*, May, 1878.

Medical Jurisprudence and Toxicology.

Recovery from Poisoning by Cyanide of Potassium.

Dr. MUELLER-WARNEK, of Kiel (*Berl. Klin. Wochenschrift*, No. 5, 1878), reports a case of severe poisoning by cyanide of potassium, which ended in recovery, and which is interesting in several respects.   The patient, aged twenty-four, a photographer, crossed in love, drank a small tumblerful of a solution of one part cyanide in fifty water, a quantity equivalent to thirty or thirty-six grains of the salt, after which he quickly fell to the ground unconscious. He was admitted into the hospital within an hour of his attempt at suicide, in the asphyxial stage of hydrocyanic poisoning, after having spontaneously vomited once. He was first treated with a subcutaneous injection of two grammes of sulphuric ether, and his stomach was repeatedly washed out with the stomach-pump until the water which returned was completely free from any smell of hydrocyanic acid. Several litres of water were necessary to accomplish this. In spite, however, of these measures, as well as of the subcutaneous injection of 2.0 grammes of ether, in which 0.2 gramme of camphor was dissolved, the symptoms of œdema of the lung and general collapse steadily increased, and it was necessary to have recourse to artificial respiration. Dr. Warnck now had the patient, as a last resource, immersed in a warm bath, and poured iced water on his head and neck from a can at a height of several feet. The effect produced was remarkable ; the breathing rapidly improved, the pulse became regular and gained in strength, and at the end of an hour the patient, after a second injection with camphorated ether, was wrapped in blankets and put to bed. An hour afterwards all symptoms of œdema of the lungs had disappeared, and at seven o'clock in the evening the patient had entirely recovered his consciousness, and remembered what he had done. Three days afterwards he complained of occipital and gastric pains, and of a feeling of general weakness, and his speech was noticed to be difficult and stuttering. On the fifth day he was able to leave his bed, but, curiously enough, he was unable to stand or walk without assistance. In standing his legs trembled violently, so that he staggered from side to side, and would have fallen if not supported. In walking, if held by both arms, he could just advance by very short and trembling steps, slowly putting out one leg in front of the other, the whole character of his movements strongly reminding the observer of some of the severe forms of lateral and insular sclerosis of the spinal cord. This abnormal condition of the lower extremities disappeared more rapidly than the disturbances of speech, which persisted for more than two months. Dr. Warnck points out that the muscles would be directly affected by the poisonous action of the cyanide on their motor centres as well as on their proper substance, and indirectly by an alteration in the blood supplying those centres and the substance of the muscles, owing to its chemical combination with hydrocyanic acid. The more permanent disturbances of speech are more difficult to account for satisfactorily ; but the introduction of other poisons into the human body is occasionally followed by perversion of one or other motor functions. The ordinary fatal dose of cyanide of potassium is said to be from two to four and a half grains (Husemann, Guy), but it is probable that at least thirty grains were swallowed in the case before us, or rather that the quantity of liquid swallowed would have contained an equivalent to thirty grains if the solution, which had been made some time, had retained its original strength (one in fifty). Probably, however, this strength had been reduced by a decomposition of a portion of the cyanide into innocuous compounds, such as formiate of potash and ammonia ; and the fact that the poison was taken on a full stomach, so that its absorption was retarded, and that a good deal of it was expelled by vomiting soon after ingestion, may explain why the patient's life was prolonged until medical aid could be procured. In any case, Dr. Warnck believes he must have died if left to himself.—*Med. Times and Gaz.*, April 6, 1878.

CONTENTS.

Published Monthly, price $2.50 per annum, free of postage.
Also, furnished together with the AMERICAN JOURNAL OF THE MEDICAL
SCIENCES *and the* MEDICAL NEWS AND LIBRARY *for* SIX DOLLARS *per
annum in advance, the whole free of postage.*

HENRY C. LEA, Philadelphia.

THE MONTHLY ABSTRACT

OF

MEDICAL SCIENCE.

Vol. v. No. 7. **For List of Contents see last page.** JULY, 1878.

Anatomy and Physiology.

On the Origin of Glycogen and Destination of Sugar.

In a paper on Glycogen and Sugar published in the *Glasgow Medical Journal* for April, Dr. McKendrick says:—

Connected with the glycogenic function of the liver, many important questions arise; among which are: 1. What is the origin of glycogen; 2. What is the ultimate destination and use of the sugar formed from glycogen.

1. *The Origin of Glycogen.*—The amount of glycogen formed is largely influenced by the nature of the food. Carbo-hydrates, such as starch, are converted by the digestive fluids into glucose, which passes into the portal system. It may be conceived that in the hepatic cells, dehydration takes place thus: $C_6H_{12}O_6 - H_2O = C_6H_{10}O_5$. This view is supported by the fact that the injection of sugar into the portal vein increases the amount of glycogen; but, on the other hand, it is well-known that the substance may be formed even after the rigid exclusion of all carbohydrates from the food. Glycogen may, therefore, be formed from other substances. Physiologists incline to the opinion that it may be produced either from fat or albuminous matters; but the observations on which this view is based are not either clear or precise.

2. *The Ultimate Destination of Glycogen.*—Glycogen has been found in the placenta, testes, brain, white blood-corpuscles, muscles, and in great abundance in the tissues of the embryo at an early stage. On the other hand, sugar has been found in the blood. Probably owing to the difficulties in the way of a quantitative estimation of the sugar in the blood, considerable difference of opinion has prevailed among physiologists regarding this point. On the one hand, Pavy has stated that the blood of the hepatic vein contains no more sugar than that of the portal vein; nor will he admit the assertion of Bernard, that there is less sugar in venous than in arterial blood. Whilst, then, Bernard's facts are disputed by so able and accurate an observer as Pavy, the matter must still be regarded as *sub judice*, and demanding fresh investigation.

Experimental physiology has enabled us to approach the subject from a different direction. If a solution of grape-sugar be repeatedly injected—in small quantities at a time—into the blood of an animal, no sugar makes its appearance in the urine—that is to say, sugar disappears in the body. Such a destruction of sugar probably takes place in the blood, lungs, and muscles. It is well known that blood containing sugar becomes acid, and that sugar gradually disappears as the acidity becomes more marked. From the fact that the quantity of sugar in the blood of the left heart is not much, if at all, less than that in the right heart, it is not likely that much sugar disappears in the lungs. As regards muscle, it has been shown that the blood returning from a muscle contains less sugar than the blood going to it. When muscles work, they become acid from the formation of sarcolactic acid. The question, then, arises as to the origin of this acid. Is it obtained from any of the albuminous constituents of the muscle, or from sugar? No chemical method is known by which lactic acid can be made from albuminoids; but it may be readily procured by the action of a ferment on grape-sugar. It has also been ascertained that muscles rendered acid by over-work speedily change grape-sugar into lactic acid when plunged into a solution of sugar. The inference, therefore, is that there exists in living tissue some kind of ferment which converts sugar into lactic acid.

There is, however, a stage still further back which is of some importance. Claude Bernard's theory is, that the conversion of glycogen into sugar occurs chiefly in the liver, and that the sugar is washed away by the blood of the portal vein almost as quickly as it is formed. But, as already stated, the quantity of sugar in the blood of the vein is small. On the other hand, we find glycogen in the tissues, and more especially in muscle. It is possible, therefore, that glycogen may be converted into sugar in other places and tissues than in the liver.

I have frequently succeeded in obtaining glycerine extracts of liver which convert starch into sugar. In like manner, I have prepared glycerine extracts of the tissue of lung, brain, spleen, and muscle, which sometimes had the same effect. Glycerine extract of muscle rarely fails. With the view of working out this subject more fully, I am preparing at present similar extracts of many other tissues, and the result will be recorded in another paper. Meantime, there is sufficient evidence to show that a ferment, having the power of changing starch into sugar, exists in other organs besides in the liver.—*London Med. Record*, May 15, 1878.

Materia Medica and Therapeutics.

The Properties and Nutritive Value of Peptone.

When an albuminous substance is digested with hydrochloric acid and pepsine at the temperature of the body, it becomes converted into "peptone;" that is to say, it has acquired properties which it had not before, and has ceased to be precipitable by heat or dilute mineral acids, though its chemical composition is apparently the same as that of true albumen. The nature of this puzzling change has been lately examined by Dr. ADAMKIEWICZ, Privatdocent at Berlin (" Die Natur und der Nahrwerth des Peptons," Berlin, 1877; and *Berliner Klin. Wochenschrift*, No. 2, 1878, "Vorträg ueber Pepton"), and he finds that it is partly explained by the fact that the ashes of peptone always contain less salts (phosphates) than those of albumen, for Alex. Schmidt, of Dorpat, has shown that by removing the salts from albumen by dialysis the latter ceases to be coaguble on boiling, but recovers the property of coagulating on the restoration of the salts. That this is only a partial explanation is clear, because peptone cannot be rendered coagulable by adding salts to it; and hence some deeper molecular change has probably occurred in it since it existed in the form of albumen. This is not mere theory, as is proved by the fact brought to light by Adamkiewicz, that if peptone be freshly precipitated (as it can be by certain metallic salts) and warmed, it melts as if it were fat, and solidifies again on cooling. On the other hand, we know that heat coagulates albumen; hence, as liquefaction involves a loosening of the cohesion of the molecules of a body to one another, and solidification their firmer aggregation, and as the molecules of a body are the more closely united when they are combined in definite groups, it is clear that the molecular constitution of albumen is more definite than that of peptone.

Is peptone decomposed within the body in the same way as albumen? This question Dr. Adamkiewicz has tried to answer experimentally. He first fed dogs with a diet insufficient for their actual needs until the daily excretion of nitrogen became very nearly constant. He then added peptone to the above for two days, kept them on the former diet for two days, and on two other days fed them on white of egg. The result was, chemically, practically identical in the two cases—about two-thirds of the nitrogen of the peptone and egg-albumen being retained in the body; but there was this one difference between the results of feeding with peptone and albumen: that in the former case the nitrogen corresponding to the decomposed peptone appeared in the urine during the next twenty-four hours, whereas the albumen-nitrogen took two days for its elimination. From these observations Adamkiewicz concludes that peptone is better suited than albumen (as, indeed, we should à priori have expected) for entrance into the animal juices, and elaboration by the tissue-cells. Other experiments proved that peptone increases the body-weight as decidedly as dry scrum-albumen and egg-albumen; and further, that it does not, like gelatine, merely spare the waste of the tissues without itself undergoing organization. Hence, as peptone is as nutritious as albumen, and at the same time more readily assimilable, it follows that, as Adamkiewicz expresses it, "there must be indications for its therapeutic use." Dr. Witte, of Rostock, has succeeded in preparing it on a large scale, and a few observations have been made with it on patients in the Berlin Charité Hospital and elsewhere, and with success as far as they go. Thus, a female lunatic, who had previously vomited everything she took, was treated with enemata, each containing peptone equivalent to fifty grammes of meat. This quantity was absorbed by the bowel in a few minutes, and as long as the enemata were continued the patient ceased to go to stool; a striking proof of the complete assimilation of the peptone. Another woman similarly ceased to vomit when all albuminous food was withdrawn from her diet and replaced by peptone.

One word of caution is necessary as to the use of this substance in medicine. As we saw above, it contains a smaller proportion of salts than albumen, and it is also deficient in creatinin and the extractives which occur in meat, which is the most natural source from which the human subject is supplied with albumen; hence we must add all these to the peptone, and the best way to do this is to dissolve the latter in ordinary warm meat broth. The quantity of peptone ingested daily must correspond to about fifty to sixty grammes of pure albumen, or 200 to 250 grammes of meat. We hope soon to be able to report the result of further clinical experiments with peptone.—*Med. Times and Gazette*, March 23, 1878.

Medicine.

The Pathology of Inflammation.

Great questions have often been fought out upon narrow ground. Pathology, as well as history, affords illustrations of the fact. The cornea of the frog is a small object, but upon it many of the problems relating to the most important of all pathological processes—inflammation—have been worked out, especially those which relate to the participation of the fixed elements of a tissue in the changes which occur. It must be confessed, however, that the results hitherto obtained have been by no means conclusive. A further contribution to the subject, by

Dr. SENFTLEBEN, has just appeared in Virchow's *Archiv*, important, not only for the care which the investigation displays, but also for the clearness with which it corroborates the views of Cohnheim. The coarser area of the field of observation is, it is true, a little enlarged, for the cornea of the rabbit is chosen instead of that of the frog, as affording special advantages—especially in that the greater size offers a better means of differentiation of morbid from healthy parts and of separating the conditions of the process, as well as greater facilities in the process of subsequent examination.

Authorities of weight have adduced observations on each side of the controversy regarding the participation of the fixed corpuscles of the cornea in the formation of pus. On the one hand, Cohnheim's well-known denial of their implication has been corroborated by Eberth and others, while Böttcher and Walb have affirmed the fact of their participation in the process. This latest contribution of Senftleben, as we have said, corroborates very strongly the conclusions of the former observers, and also demonstrates the source of some of the opinions which do not harmonize with those attained.

In all observations on this subject the exact method employed is of great importance. Senftleben employed, following the example of Böttcher, chloride of zinc, instead of nitrate of silver, as a cauterizing agent, and hardened the cornea in chloride of gold. The most important element in the researches is the discrimination of the processes of inflammation and reparation of the damaged tissue. Both these go in curious spike-like processes, but it is asserted that the distinctions between them are most conclusive. The nuclei in the regenerating process are a long oval in form, much less deeply-tinted than those of the wandering round cells, and constantly show three or four nucleoli. On the other hand, the nuclei of the wandering round cells are smaller, and tint much more deeply. Most of these cells contain two, three, or four nuclei, lying close together, and often distending the cell. The arrangement of the cells in the two processes is equally distinctive. In the process of regeneration the nuclei are far apart, while they are much closer in the inflammatory process, and the closer the more intense it is, so that they may come to be actually in contact. The course and arrangement of the spikes of cells are also in the two cases different. Finally, another characteristic of the regenerative process is that at the extremity of the spikes the protoplasm often exhibits fibrillation, while no such appearance is ever seen in the inflammatory process. The regenerating changes go on concentrically and uniformly in the entire periphery of the cauterized area, and by this the corneal corpuscles which have been destroyed are restored, so that the cauterized area after a certain time presents a completely normal appearance.

Senftleben concludes that the whole of this reparatory process may go on without there being visible at any time, either in the cauterized region or in the periphery of the cornea, any wandering corpuscles, and also without the appearance of any large masses of protoplasm having the slightest resemblance to giant cells. The fixed corneal corpuscles proliferate, but only produce other fixed corneal corpuscles, never round, pus-like cells. Whatever caustic was employed, provided its action was sufficiently deep to pass beneath the epithelial layer, so as to preclude the passage of cells into the cornea from the conjunctival space, the result was always the same. No pus-cells arose from the fixed corpuscles. When measures were taken to secure the death of these corneal corpuscles, round cells might still appear, but they evidently came from the periphery, since they were found in decreasing number on passing from the periphery to the centre, and were never so collected in the centre as to suggest the idea of local origin. If the cornea was tinted before the fixed corpuscles were obscured by the numbers of round cells which wander in, the former might be seen to be quite unchanged.

The path by which the wandering cells enter is threefold: first, by the nutritive channels of the cornea; secondly, between the fibrillæ of the corneal substance; and, thirdly, along the nerves. The more considerable the inflammation the greater the number of these cells, and in intense inflammation they may be so abundant that they surround and compress the fixed corpuscles, and this has given rise to the idea that the latter participate in the changes. These corpuscles are in the way of the wandering cells, for they lie in the interfibrillar spaces by which many of the cells pass. Precisely the same appearance, the corpuscles being surrounded by the round cells, is seen in corneæ in which the cells are, and in those in which they are not, killed by the action of the caustic.

By these and other means of observation, Senftleben concludes that the activity of the fixed corpuscles and that of the wandering cells may be completely separated. The two participate in processes which are essentially different, and which lead to completely different results. The effect of the activity of the fixed corneal corpuscles is exclusively to give rise to similar elements which have been destroyed by cauterization, and so to restore the injured portion of the cornea. The presence of a large number of wandering, leucocyte-like, round cells is, on the contrary, the characteristic of corneal inflammation. In their origin the fixed corpuscles take no part. If the inflammation is very intense—*i. e.*, if a great introduction of round cells occurs—portions of the cornea may be entirely destroyed by them; but if it is moderate, the cells which have entered may disappear, and the remaining corneal tissue may be repaired by the fixed corpuscles. Thus the latter play a reparatory, the round cells a destructive, part.

It may, however, be asked, On what ground is this sharp demarcation between reparation and inflammation founded? Would not some be inclined to regard as inflammatory the process which Senftleben calls reparatory? The distinction, it will be observed, turns on the presence of the round cells in the region. In a non-vascular tissue these have been almost universally taken as the characteristic of inflammation. During the whole process, which is regarded as reparatory, the round cells, as a rule, are not seen. Moreover, the two processes are accompanied by characteristic macroscopic appearances. The inflammatory process, with its abundant cell-infiltration, is indicated by opacity of the cornea; the process of reparation, with participation of the fixed corneal corpuscles, by increased and increasing transparency. Hence it is assumed that the two processes, which are designated inflammation and regeneration, are completely independent of one another, and have nothing in common.

If the fixed corpuscles of the cornea do not furnish the round cells, what is the source of their elements? Two only are conceivable—the episcleral vessels and the conjunctival sac. The passage of cells from the conjunctival sac into the cornea has been rejected as untenable by almost all observers, but some observations of Senftleben go far to demonstrate that such a passage does occur under certain circumstances, and that both of these sources may, in different cases, furnish the wandering cells. If two spots are cauterized, one in the centre of the cornea, and one at its periphery, adjacent to the vessels, the latter will be crammed with round cells when the former is free from them. It seems reasonable to conclude that the source of those in the peripheral spot is the adjacent vessels. But if a fine thread is passed into the region which has been cauterized in the centre of the cornea, a dense swarm of round cells passes in along the thread, and they accumulate in the affected area. In this there are no living fixed corneal corpuscles, and in it, without this intentional opening of the corneal tissue, not a single round cell would be visible in the affected area. The conclusion that the cells entered from the conjunctival sac seems inevitable.

Thus the central cauterization of the cornea, without opening of the corneal tissue, never leads to the changes recognized as inflammatory, never to the appearance of round cells, but only to the regeneration of the fixed corneal corpuscles destroyed by the caustic. If, on the other hand, the tissue is opened up, there is a passage inwards of the corpuscles from the corneal sac, and the appearance universally recognized as that of inflammation in a non-vascular tissue. Without this opening of the tissue there is no true keratitis.

Lieberkuehn has asserted that carmine injected into the living cornea tints only the fixed corpuscles, and by this method Walb was led to the conclusion that the origin of round cells from the fixed corpuscles could be traced. But Senftleben asserts that the result of his injections is precisely the reverse: that after the tenth day of the injection it is not the fixed corpuscles which appear carmine-coloured, but that all the granular particles of carmine which are in cells are in the wandering round cells; and he gives conclusive reasons for believing that all those which are thus coloured have passed in by the opening made for the injection. In a few weeks colossal, many-nucleated masses of granules are developed, and Senftleben concludes that these also come only from the wandering cells.

Thus this important investigation furnishes new proof that the accuracy of Cohnheim's observations and the correctness of his conclusions are alike unassailable, and that the objections which Böttcher and others have made are untenable. It cannot be doubted that the clearer results which Senftleben has obtained are due in part to the better facilities for observation furnished by the rabbit over the frog.—*Lancet*, May 18, 1878.

The Doctrine of Acetonæmia.

Ever since the clinical features of diabetes have been carefully observed, physicians have been startled and puzzled by the frequency with which, in that disease, death comes unforeseen and unexplained. A patient, apparently in his usual condition, suddenly becomes drowsy and dull; the stupor deepens to coma, and the coma to death. Upon the cause of such death, post-mortem examination throws no light. Symptoms of cerebral depression, such as these, in the absence of a cerebral lesion, naturally suggest the idea that a narcotic poison is at work, and it has been thought by some that they may be due to the addition of uræmic poisoning to the diabetic state. In extremely rare cases the symptoms do resemble those of uræmia so closely as to make it probable that this condition in them does actually exist. In the vast majority of cases all the characteristic symptoms of uræmia are absent, and the theory that it is the common cause of diabetic coma is untenable.

In some cases the sugar in the urine has undergone a remarkable diminution on the appearance of the toxæmic symptoms, and it has been suggested that they may be due to a sudden arrest of excretion, and a retention of sugar in the blood —a condition of extreme glycohæmia. In the opinion of Cyr and others, this is a reasonable explanation of some of the cases of diabetic coma, but it is certainly inadequate to explain the majority, since in many no such arrest in the excretion of sugar is to be observed. Too much weight must not be attached to such occasional disappearance of sugar from the urine in this condition. So profound an alteration in all the functions of the central nervous system as must accompany the coma may well have, as its consequence, an arrest of the customary formation of sugar. Moreover, as far as it has been observed, the cessation of the excretion of sugar may be explained on another theory, which affords a more adequate explanation of the phenomena, and has been widely received as satisfactory.

A peculiar odour has long been noted to be occasionally given off by the breath, the urine, and even the feces of diabetics, and a similar odour has been noted many times in the body after death. Thirty years ago the post-mortem odour was compared by Rother to vinegar, and the odour of the breath, by Brand, to the smell from persons who had recently inhaled chloroform, while Berndt compared it to that of beer. It was thought by Petters to resemble that of a mixture of chloroform and acetic ether or aldehyde, and was noted by him to be intense in all the tissues of the dead body. It was natural to regard this odour as the proof of the formation of a substance in the body by some decomposition of the sugar circulating in the blood, and to associate it with the symptoms of cerebral depression. The character of the smell led Leich, in 1853, to suggest that it was probably acetone, a volatile ethereal liquid allied to chloroform in its properties. Petters endeavoured to test this opinion. By fractional distillation of the urine of a patient who had died of diabetic coma, he obtained a clear, highly refracting, inflammable liquid, having the boiling-point of acetone, and giving the same reactions—neutral, brownish with sulphuric acid, yielding a brown precipitate with caustic potash, and not reducing oxide of silver. From the blood the same substance was obtained in a similar manner. The observation has since been confirmed by several authorities. Acetone has even been said by Kaulich to be a frequent product of the acetous fermentation, which may take place in the stomach of dyspeptics, and he believes that it may arise by fermentation from grape-sugar. Anthron, indeed, obtained, by the fermentation of glucose, a liquid which Leich pronounced to be acetone; and Kaulich argued that, although the ordinary vinous fermentation of glucose yields only alcohol and carbonic acid, yet since, under other circumstances, lactic and butyric acids may be obtained from it, it is conceivable that acetone may also be a product of its fermentation, because, by a decomposition, theoretically simple, grape-sugar may break up into acetone, acetic acid, carbonic acid, and water.

These opinions have been lately confirmed by Dr. B. Foster, who not only has found acetone in fresh diabetic urine, but has proved that acetone is capable of producing the post-mortem appearances found in diabetic coma—viz., a thick fluid state of the blood, which presents a milky opacity, due apparently to the destruction of the red blood-corpuscles, and he has, he believes, prevented death in diabetic coma by the administration of agents which possess the power of arresting fermentation.

In spite of these facts, however, we must still doubt whether the doctrine of acetonæmia is established beyond dispute. They certainly render it highly probable that the condition of diabetic coma is due to a poisonous substance of the acetous series, which is formed from, or perhaps replaces, sugar in the blood. But it is impossible to peruse the descriptions given by the several observers of the character of the odour perceived in the breath, urine, or tissues, without being struck with the variations in their statements. One compares it to chloroform, another to beer, another to sour beer, another to vinegar. This difference suggests that the substances in the blood may not always be the same. The observations of Kaulich and others on the occurrence of acetous changes in the contents of the stomach in dyspeptics point to the probability that the odour of the breath may be in part due to fermentation within the stomach, under the influence of the altered blood, and a distinct odour of acetone in the breath is thus scarcely proof that the substance exists as such in the blood. So, too, the rapid transformations of unstable compounds which occur in the tissues after death, and in the urine after secretion, necessitate caution in inferring that a compound found in either existed also in the blood during life. The circulating blood may contain only some substance capable of yielding acetone, and not acetone itself. That in some cases this is true is shown by an observation of Rupstein. He found that, by fractional distillation, a liquid having the odour and boiling point of acetone could be obtained from urine, and his observation has been cited in support of the doctrine of acetonæmia. But he found that, although the urine after standing evolved an odour of acetone, no such odour could be detected in the urine when first passed. On the other hand, he found that it then contained a peculiar acid, which has been investigated by Genther—diacetic acid. On boiling, or after standing for a considerable time, the urine ceased to give the reaction of this acid, and acquired the odour of acetone. This acid will break up, by assuming two molecules of water, into acetones alcohol, and carbonic acid; and Rupstein suggests that this is what takes place out of the body, and speculates that the same decomposition may take place in the blood. The same acid was found in the urine in another case by Kernig.

Another question remains: Is the presence of acetone in the blood an adequate explanation of the phenomena of diabetic coma? Many authorities—Senator, Lecorché, Cyr—assert that it is; and, as we have already mentioned, Foster has shown that it produces a similar pathological condition to that discoverable after death from diabetic coma. But the evidence from experiment is not altogether corroborative of the view. We are chiefly indebted for information on this point to the experiments of Kussmaul, who found that the effects of acetone resembled in the main those of alcohol. But, however analogous to the stage of stupor in alcoholic poisoning the phenomena of diabetic coma may be, a preliminary stage of excitement, such as is so frequent in alcoholic poisoning, is, as a rule, absent. Much weight cannot, however, be laid on this point. It has not, for obvious reasons, been practicable to make experiments upon man which afford a very close parallel to the phenomena of disease. Kussmaul has long been in the habit of using acetone as a remedy for dyspnœa, and has given a drachm or a drachm and a half daily without any ill effect. The subcutaneous injection of about twelve grains of pure acetone caused no other effect, in man, than a transient pain; and it required at least a drachm to produce toxic effects on a rabbit. It is clear, therefore, that, if diabetic coma is really acetonæmia, a very large amount of acetone must be generated in the system before the poisonous effects are produced. There is no doubt an adequate source for a large supply of acetone in the saccharine substances which pass through the blood, but the process by which so large a quantity could be generated is very difficult to conceive, and it is equally difficult to understand that the system can be so saturated with acetone without its characteristic odour being in all cases obtrusive. While temperature may intensify the odour by increasing the volatilization, such a quantity of acetone as must be present would certainly be recognizable at lower temperatures, and the presence or absence of pyrexia can scarcely account for the presence or absence of the smell of acetone.

The conclusion, then, to which we are led is that while there is strong evidence that diabetic coma is, in many cases at least, accompanied by, and probably due to, the formation in the blood of substances of the ethyl-acetic series, sometimes capable of yielding acetone, there is not yet sufficient evidence that the symptoms are due to the presence of acetone in the blood to justify the designation of "acetonæmia," and until the theory rests upon stronger evidence, it were better not to use a term which is certainly not urgently needed, and which further research may demonstrate to be inaccurate.—*Lancet*, May 11, 1878.

—

Progressive Pernicious Anæmia.

In a paper on this subject in the 3d and 4th numbers of the *Nordiskt Medicin-iskt Arkiv* for 1877, Dr. S. T. SORENSEN reports eleven cases of the disease, which had come under observation in the Kommune Hospital, in Copenhagen, within a period of little more than a year and a half. Of these, seven were men and four women. The disease was fatal in every instance, and *post-mortems* weie obtained in nine cases. In ten cases out of the eleven, obseivations on the numbei of ied blood coipuscles weie made fiom time to time by Malassez' method; and these showed a diminution to a numbei vaiying fiom one-quaitei to one-twelfth of the noimal. Successive examinations showed a continual deciease in numbei, the last obseivation piioi to death giving fiom 0.79 to 0.45 millions pei cubic mm. The authoi concludes that 0.5 millions per cubic mm. is the minimum possible for the conseivation of life. The individual ied coipuscles piesented abnoimalities in colour, size, and shape; the colour was less intense than in health; some weie twice and otheis one-half the noimal diametei; and in all sizes theie weie iiiegulaiities in foim. The ieaction of the seium was normal, and when added to healthy blood pioduced no peinicious effect on the ied coipuscles. The piominent symptoms of the disease, according to the authoi, aie—anæmic symptoms; gastiic distuibance; a pale, yellowish, but not icteiic, hue; a consideiable degiee of fat, notwithstanding the gieat debility; *bruits de souffle* in the heait and vessels of the neck; ietinal hemoiihages; the occuiience of iiiegulai and unaccountable attacks of pyiexia. The iesult of the *post mortems* was biiefly as follows. The blood, which was excessively thin, piesented the appeaiance of meat-washings. Theie was gianulai and fatty degeneiation of the paienchyma of vaiious oigans—viz., livei, kidneys, and adienals. Fatty degeneiation of the heait, and atheioma of the aoita. Theie weie likewise, in some cases, numeious capillaiy hemoiihages. The maiiow of the bones was noticed in foui cases only, and in but one of these was a micioscopic examination made. In two of those in which it was examined macioscopically only, the maiiow of the iibs was of a ieddish colour, and of a thinly fluid consistence. In the thiid caso that of the steinum appeaied noimal. In the fouith case—that examined micioscopically—the compact tissue of the iibs was thickened, and the medullary spaces almost empty. The maiiow was in no place fatty, while in anothei it contained some blood coipuscles and a few transitorial cells. Eleven cases occuiiing in so shoit a peiiod of time would point to the disease being anything but a iaie one. Further, the statistics do not uphold the geneially ieceived opinion, that it moie fiequently attacks females than males. No connection could be tiaced in any of the foui female cases to piegnancy oi child-bed, noi in any of the entiie numbei to unhealthy occupations or piivation. One patient, howevei, attiibuted hei illness to the fatigue of nuising a sick sistei, and giief at hei death. The authoi iegaids the disease as dependent on a mal-pioduction, not a destiuction, of the ied coipuscles; and he attaches gieat impoitance to the numeiical examination of them in the diagnosis of the disease. Tiansfusion of human blood, employed in one case, was not pioductive of any good.—*Dublin Jouinal of Medical Science*, May, 1878.

Cuie of a Case of Hydrophobia.

We find in the June numbei of the *Lombaidy Medical Gazette* a case of iabies, tieated and cuied by two Russian physicians, Dis. SCHMIDT and LEBEDEW. The patient, a child ten yeais old, had been bitten in the hand by a iabid pig. The wound was immediately cauteiized with lunai caustic, and healed in ten days; but on the seventeenth day unmistakable symptoms of hydiophobia, viz., dysphagia, dyspnœa, spasm of the iespiiatoiy muscles, etc., appeaied. The physicians at once oideied inspiiation of oxygen gas. When thiee cubic feet of the gas had been bieathed, the patient became quite tianquil; but the spasms ietuined on the following day. The gas was, theiefoie, administeied for foity-five minutes, when the symptoms subsided. Nothing now iemained but slight dyspnœa, and also some weakness of the lowei extiemities, which giadually subsided, the patient iemaining well afteiwaids.—*Med. Examiner*, June 6, 1878.

Cerebral Syphilis.

We have still much to learn on this important subject. According to Dr. RABOT (*Gaz. des Hôp.*, No. 49), when tertiary syphilis attacks the brain, the seat of the disease is usually found in the arteries. The symptoms produced by gummatous degeneration of the cerebral arteries are frequently so well marked as to enable the surgeon to arrive at a correct diagnosis. The premonitory headache —usually confined to the frontal region—is characteristic, and frequently accompanied by disturbance of the intellectual faculties, such as loss of memory, with apathy or excitement, and in many cases with vertigo. The premonitory symptoms have a tendency to intermittence, but they may be quickly followed by transitory apoplectic attacks and impaired articulation. The iodide of potassium in large doses is the best remedy which can be employed. Its use has been followed in many severe cases by the greatest benefit, although a permanent cure is hardly to be expected. In Italy cerebral syphilis is combated by mercury; but the iodide of potassium is frequently associated with this specific.—*Med. Examiner*, June 6, 1878.

The Treatment of Catalepsy.

Dr. TEBALDI relates the following case (*Archivio Italiano*, 1877, Nos. 2 and 3). A student, aged 22, the son of very nervous parents, after severe and persistent study of law, philosophy, theology, etc., fell into a condition of ecstasy, catalepsy, and stupor. He was treated by Dr. Tebaldi with tonics, cannabis Indica, and electricity. The first dose of Indian hemp markedly stimulated the motor system. After the drug had been administered for four days, the patient (who had not voluntarily moved a finger for three months, nor spoken a word for five months) walked unaided from his room, ate his food, spoke a few intelligible words, then became very excited, dancing, laughing, and threatening those around him. Symptoms of paralysis of the bladder and rectum came on, and the treatment was discontinued. The treatment by electricity (two Stöhrer's elements) was given up after twenty-two sittings, its action being, on the whole, similar to that of the hemp. The most noteworthy difference was, that the latter acted chiefly upon the motor system, while the action of the electricity was most evident upon the sensorium. Neither method of treatment produced more than a temporary improvement, and Dr. Tebaldi concludes that the patient has psychic weakness, without disorganization of the brain-cortex.—*London Med. Record*, May 15, 1878.

Non-protrusion of the Tongue in some Cases of Aphasia.

Respecting this interesting and curious clinical phenomenon, Dr. HUGHLINGS JACKSON remarks:—

It will have been noticed by every medical man that some patients who have loss or defect of speech do not put out the tongue when they are asked. For the present we shall consider cases of *loss* of speech. The patients know what is wanted; they do the preliminary thing --opening the mouth—but very often the tongue lies flat and motionless in the floor of the oral cavity. The patient may put his fingers in his mouth to help the organ out. That the tongue is not paralyzed (we mean in the ordinary medical sense of the term paralysis) may be proved in several ways. As a rule, the patient, who can *say* nothing, can *utter* something; he has a stock word or phrase which comes out at any time. This is best called a "recurring utterance." The word or phrase being clearly articulated is decisive evidence that the tongue is not paralyzed. Then there are in some cases "occasional utterances." The patient may swear, or get out more innocent ejaculations, as "Oh, dear!" These also are clearly articulated. Yet very early in a case of loss of speech there may be no sort of utterance. Then we can demonstrate that the tongue is not paralyzed by getting the patient to eat and drink. He will eat and swallow quite well, which he could not do were his tongue paralyzed. Again, after failing to put out his tongue when he tries, the patient may stick it out well to lick his lips. In one case an aphasic woman was vainly urged to put out her tongue. Mr. Lewis Mackenzie, the resident medical officer, got it out by a trick: he had found that after drinking she would stick her tongue out to lick her lips; she did so on this occasion.

This is a matter of great importance. In some cases of acute cerebral disease the non-protrusion of the tongue would be of great value in helping to the diagnosis of aphasia, as one symptom of that acute disease. In any case it would be a great blunder to suppose there to be paralysis of the tongue from disease of the lingual nerves or their nuclei in the medulla oblongata, because the patient did not put out his tongue when asked and when he tried. It is a thing of great scientific interest; considered along with some other symptoms of aphasia, it gives us a clue to the physiology of the whole of aphasia. Let us mention some other symptoms of fundamentally like significance.

Those who have examined the eyes of many aphasics will remember cases in which the use of the ophthalmoscope was very difficult; some aphasics do not, and apparently cannot, direct their eyes as they are told. Of course, in some cases of aphasia, there may be for a few hours or days, or in rare or severe cases for several weeks, lateral deviation of the eyes from the side paralyzed, as part of the hemiplegia; but we just now refer to chronic cases in which there is no ordinary affection of the ocular muscles; the difficulty is not in looking to one side in particular. Indeed, we see the same sort of thing in some people whose nervous systems are sound. Some people are unable to draw in their breath deeply when told to do so during stethoscopic examination; we have to tell them to cough. It is next to impossible to get some patients to frown (as in suspected one-sided facial paralysis), even if we make a frown for them to imitate. Returning to aphasia. The Recurring Utterance is often "Yes" or "No," or the patient may be able to utter both these words. Some of these patients can utter "No" emotionally, and some can do this and can also reply with it (use it propositionally). But of those who can reply with it there are some who cannot say it when told. After failing to get them to say it when told, we can easily get the word out as a reply to a question requiring dissent. Similarly of Occasional Utterances of less automaticity: a patient may swear well on proper (scientifically proper) occasions, and yet be unable to repeat the ejaculation or any word of it. The same applies to Occasional Utterances of still less automaticity, as is illustrated by the following excerpt from an unpublished paper by Dr. Hughlings Jackson written ten years ago: "I have seen a patient who usually sat up in his room, whose face looked intelligent, who was cheerful and merry, and who seemed to understand all that I said to him, but who could not put out his tongue when he tried. His daughter remarked that he could put the tongue out, as she expressed it, 'by accident,' and added, as an illustration of her meaning, that when any one was leaving him he could say 'good-bye,' but that he could neither put out his tongue nor say 'good-bye' when he tried. He could say 'yes' and 'no' at any time; and, using the lady's expression, could say 'good-bye,' 'well,' 'never' by accident. She further remarked that the patient would sometimes swear. He uttered the short explosive word which is so much in favour with English swearers, but he could not, she said, repeat the word when he tried. She asked him to utter the explosive sound when I was there, saying it herself for him to imitate. He laughed, and shook his head."

In some cases, where there is not loss but defect of speech, we see a similar sort of thing. The patient may get out a word, or even an elaborate phrase, and be quite unable to repeat it. This shows us that, in our trying to appreciate an aphasic's condition, we have not only to note what he utters, but whether or not he can *say* (repeat) what he has uttered. We frequently find that he cannot. In some cases a patient gets out, in proper reply to a question, such a phrase as "I don't know"—one, be it observed, of considerable automaticity. Afterwards he may go on uttering it in rejoinder to questions to which it is irrelevant. The patient may show that he knows this by expressions of mirth or annoyance after its utterance. But sometimes we can stop such temporary Recurring Utterances by telling the patient to say "I don't know," or whatever the phrase may have been. They often fail.

All the above superficially different phenomena are fundamentally like; they all show a reduction to a more automatic condition.—*Lancet,* May 18, 1878.

A Case of Asthma successfully treated by Sée's Method.

In a recent number of the *Wiener Medizinische Presse,* Dr. WINTERNITZ gives the details of a case of very severe asthma, which, after all the usual reme- dies had been tried, yielded rapidly to full doses of iodide of potassium. The patient was a man, 50 years of age, who had suffered for more than twenty years from difficulty of breathing. This symptom was much increased by the slightest exertion, and more especially by any catarrhal complications. The attacks of dyspnœa were at times most distressing, and the patient was often reduced to the last extremity. He was, in addition, the subject of a considerable enlargement of the thyroid body, which formed a tumour almost as large as a child's head. The swelling was of a cystic nature, and its contents had undergone calcareous changes; the patient's neck measured twenty inches in circumference. An analy- sis of the symptoms showed that the case was one of true symptomatic bronchial asthma, complicated by marked emphysema and enlargement of the thyroid body. The patient had read an account of Sée's method, and entreated Dr. Win- ternitz to make the experiment. The latter, however, hesitated, as the man was in weak health, and there were indications of fatty degeneration of the heart. The entreaties of the patient, however, at last prevailed, and iodide of potassium was administered for nineteen days, during which time about 530 grains were taken. The patient kept out of the doctor's sight all this time, lest he should be directed to discontinue the medicine. When he presented himself, he was found to be much reduced in weight and strength; there was complete loss of appetite, and the tongue had a coating more than three lines thick. The improvement, however, in his respiratory symptoms was most marked. The neck had dimin- ished by more than four inches; the thyroid body was soft to the touch; the cyanosis had disappeared, and the lungs seemed comparatively normal. He was ordered to omit the medicine, and to take soups and buttermilk, and in a few days the digestive organs were restored to their usual condition. The patient declared that he was better than he had been for twenty-five years; that he could mount several flights of stairs without stopping; that his sleep was undisturbed; and that he awoke in the morning free from cough, and not experiencing any difficulty in breathing. Dr. Winternitz observes that, inasmuch as the dyspnœa was more marked during expiration, it could not have been due to stenosis of the trachea caused by the tumour of the thyroid. The emphysema, however, might originally have been due to this cause, and, if so, its diminution under the iodide treatment was the more remarkable. Dr. Winternitz considers that the treat- ment in question is worthy of an extended trial.—*Med. Examiner,* June 6, 1878.

On Thoracentesis.

Dr. LEONPACHER observes (*Aerztliches Intelligenz-Blatt*, April 2), that the operation of thoracentesis has greatly increased in value, in consequence of the labours of Kussmaul and Bartels (in Germany), and it is now resorted to by many. Dr. Leonpacher gives an account of several cases that came within his own experience. The first two in which the operation was performed died, not in consequence of the operation, but from marasmus and the accession of tuberculosis; the three other cases ended favourably. Of these, the first was the case of a brewer, aged 33, the subject of pleurisy on the right side, resulting in empyema. The thorax was punctured and a quantity of inodorous pus removed. Subsequently, the thorax was again punctured, and now the secretion was ichorous, and could be only partially removed by the suction process. An opening one inch and a half in length was therefore made in the fifth intercostal space, and a large quantity of bloody, purulent, and fetid exudation was withdrawn. The cavity was daily irrigated and washed out with a 2 per cent. solution of carbolic acid, through two Nélaton's catheters, one for the injection, the other for the exit of the fluid. Afterwards, one of these was found sufficient for all purposes. The cavity gradually contracted, the secretion diminished, and the wound was now allowed to close. The temperature immediately rose to 104° F., and four days afterwards a violent fit of coughing again opened the wound through which a large quantity of offensive pus escaped. The catheter was again introduced, and was retained at first in the cavity, and afterwards in the remaining sinus for several weeks, while carbolic solution was daily injected. The case did well, and recovered completely.

The second case was one of traumatic pleurisy in a young man, following a blow on the chest. For two years a fistulous opening existed on the left side, below the nipple, which discharged almost continuously a purulent secretion and through which the pleural cavity could be reached. A drainage-tube was inserted, and about seven ounces of offensive pus flowed away. The cavity was twice daily washed out with a solution of boracic acid (3 per cent.), and the tube was left in the wound, which was dressed with tow dipped in boracic acid. Instead of the boracic acid, an aqueous solution of 2 per cent. of tincture of iodine was occasionally employed.

The third case occurred in a farmer, who had suffered for two months from exudative pleurisy. An abscess had formed on the right side, between the angle of the scapula and the spine, from which flowed, on being opened, a large quantity of healthy pus. From this abscess a canal ascended behind the right scapula to the height of the spine of the scapula, and there communicated with the pleural cavity. As for purposes of treatment this canal was unsuitable, and as, moreover, at the site of the abscess the intercostal space was too narrow to admit the introduction of a tube, the thorax was opened in the fifth intercostal space between the axillary and mammillary lines, and a further considerable quantity of matter removed through it. Under continued injection of salicylic acid solution and dressing, the case did well.

The main points to be observed in the treatment of cases of thoracentesis are— 1, the complete removal of the purulent secretion from the pleural cavity; 2, a continuous outflow of pus as it forms; 3, the total exclusion of all septic matter from the wound, and the arrest of the septic process if it have already commenced. The first point is secured by inserting through a canula a Nélaton's catheter into the bottom of the cavity, and through it injecting the various antiseptic solutions in use. It is sufficient to employ one catheter instead of two, as recommended by Fräntzel. The injected fluid renders the secretion of the cavity thinner, whereby its subsequent removal by means of the syringe is much facilitated. The patient should be placed on his back, and with the pelvis higher than the thorax, and the opening on as low a level as possible, and the discharge of any fluid is further aided by coughing or strong expiration; the catheter is then withdrawn, and the canula left in the opening. To prevent the access and entrance of dust, etc., a dressing of salicylic lint, or tow, which is cheaper and equally efficacious, should be applied over the wound, so as to cover the canula or drainage-tube.

Dr. Leonpacher concludes his paper with an account of a case of a penetrating wound of the thorax and right lung, in which he had ultimately to perform thora- centesis, owing to the accumulation of sanguineous pus in the pleural cavity. The treatment in this case was that recommended recently in the *Berliner Klinische Wochenschrift*, by the chief surgeon of the Danzig Hospital. It consisted in inserting at once a large-sized drainage-tube into the wound, and allowing it to remain there during the progress of the case, while the antiseptic injections were employed only at the commencement, and afterwards resumed only on the ap- pearance of any signs of decomposition in the discharge; at the same time, the antiseptic dressings were more frequently changed. Under this management, the progress of the case was a remarkably rapid and favourable one.—*Lond. Med. Record*, May 15, 1878.

Acute Endocarditis affecting the Pulmonary Valves.

Acute endocarditis involving only the right side of the heart is a comparatively rare affection, and very few cases have as yet been recorded in which only the valves of the pulmonary artery were thus affected. Out of three hundred cases of heart disease examined after death in the Berlin Pathological Institution, there were only three instances of endocarditis of the tricuspid valve alone, and no case of the same affection confined to the valves of the pulmonary orifice. The following case, therefore, recently reported in the *Wiener Medizinische Presse*, is one of considerable interest. A young soldier was admitted into the garrison hospital in Vienna, having been thrown from his horse, and taken up in a state of unconsciousness. Violent delirium set in a few hours afterwards, but subsided on the second day after the accident, and consciousness became almost com- pletely restored. There was no further indication of any injury to the brain. On examining the thorax the heart was found to be completely covered by the left lung; its impulse was nowhere perceptible; the sounds were heard over a small area—the second sound normal. Neither paralysis nor any perceptible alteration of sensibility in the extremities. Three days after the accident the patient again became unconscious, but on the following day he was able to com- plain of pain on the top of the head. He failed to put out his tongue when asked to do so, but was able to move it in other directions, and to speak with tolerable distinctness. Sonorous râles could be heard over the lower and posterior parts of both lungs. The man died six days after the accident.

On post-mortem examination the subcutaneous tissue of the forehead exhibited two small spots of effused blood. The pia mater on the convex surface of the brain was opaque, and contained a quantity of colourless serum. Corresponding to the lower surface of the left temporo-sphenoidal lobe, the dura mater was found to be perforated in a spot as large as a pea, and a fragment of brain-substance protruded through this opening. The ventricles were distended by a thin reddish fluid; the ependyma thickened, and dotted over with very fine granules. The lower lobes of both lungs were filled with a dark-red fluid, and the ramifications of the bronchial tubes contained thick yellow pus. The branches of the pulmo- nary artery on both sides were filled with loose coagula, some blackish-red, others reddish-gray in colour, but none adherent to the walls. There were a few small

spots of extravasated blood in the pericardium covering the heart. The middle
and right pulmonary semilunar valves at their angle of contact were covered by a
firmly adherent granular coagulum, grayish-white and grayish-red in colour, and
about one millimetre in thickness. The other valves of the heart normal, spleen
enlarged. The connective tissue covering the right psoas muscle, and between it
and the iliacus was infiltrated with reddish-gray pus as far down as the insertion
of those muscles. Thick yellow pus in the right wrist-joint. The diagnosis was
therefore as follows: Psoas abscess of right side, due to fall from horse; metastatic recent endocarditis of the pulmonary semilunar valves; recent emboli of the
branches of the pulmonary artery; lobular pneumonia of the posterior parts of
both lungs; metastatic purulent inflammation of the right wrist-joint; ecchymosis
of the pericardium; chronic hydrocephalus, internal and external.

Dr. Chvostek, under whose care the patient was, in remarking upon the rare-
ness of such a case, observed that the question arose whether the endocarditis
was of the ulcerous kind, and, in his opinion, it was so. In proof of this, he referred to the extreme rapidity of the symptoms, and their pyæmic origin, to
the enlargement of the spleen, and the ecchymosis in the pericardium. The fact
that no ulcers were actually present was to be explained by the shortness and
violence of the attack, death having taken place before ulcers had time to form.
The patient's illness, dating from the fall, lasted only six days, and the endocarditis, therefore, must have been of still shorter duration. According to Rosenstein, endocarditis is ushered in by parenchymatous changes in the tissue. The
cellular elements become swollen, cloudy, and granular. The endocardium at
the affected spots loses its brilliancy, and becomes opaque and of a dirty gray
colour; if proliferation of the connective tissue nuclei goes on rapidly, granulations soon form, and at the same time the surface, deprived of its brilliancy and
smoothness, becomes the seat of fibrinous deposit which incorporates itself with
the subjacent tissue. The tiny granulations and the superjacent fibrinous deposit
crumble away; the tissue softens, and the result is an ulcer, in and around which
fibrine is continually being deposited from the passing blood. In the case in
question endocarditis could not be diagnosed during life. There were no local
symptoms, and the psoas abscess—the source of the mischief—was not discovered.
The symptoms of the embolic processes in the lungs were only slight, and therefore insufficient for diagnostic purposes; the cerebral symptoms and the history
of the case pointed to acute traumatic meningitis of the convex surface of the
brain. As a general rule, ulcerous endocarditis can be diagnosed during life only
in a very few cases. In the case in question the progress of the disease was very
rapid. In the rheumatic cases observed by Rosenstein the disease lasted from
two to four weeks, but when the disease supervenes during pyæmia or puerperal
fever, it runs a more rapid course, and often terminates fatally in from four to
six days.—*Med. Examiner*, June 6, 1878.

Effects of Military Drill upon the Heart.

The large amount of heart disease in the British Army has attracted much
attention from time to time, especially since Mr. Myers's prize essay was published.
It was shown there, that after deducting the effects of alcohol, syphilis, Bright's
disease, etc., there was still found a great proportion of heart disease, which was
caused by the uniform or by the drill service. Surgeon F. A. DAVY, M.D.,
thinks that the form of drill in vogue is injurious, and is the direct cause of much
injury to the thoracic organs. It appears that in the "setting-up drill," it is
essayed, so far as is practicable, to make the soldier fill his chest and then perform
all movements with the chest fully distended with air, the consequences of which

are a certain amount of emphysema with more or less embarrassment of the heart.
The "stand-at-ease" is too brief for the heart to recover itself, and a condition
of irritability or hypertrophy becomes established according to the nutritive powers
of the individual. He says, "In the great majority of cases of heart-complaint
invalided (other than those brought about by rheumatic fever, Bright's disease,
etc.), of which the history is to hand, the early link in the pathological chain was
forged in the drill-field. There has preceded the date of appearance at hospital,
a long period of uncomplained of discomfort, often distress, consisting of breathlessness on slight exertion, headache, and 'beating.' Now exertion has become
unbearable. A man who never knew he had a heart (an expression many a soldier has used to me) becomes aware of his possession after a few months' dilating
drill. He blames his recently donned pack and traps for his trouble; forgetting
that as civilian he could have carried them manfully across the country ten or fifteen miles. Now, has this man been enlisted by mistake, or have we made him
what he is?" This is a very serious question, and Dr. Davy seems to incline to
the latter solution. If the drill be to blame—and it appears to be so—then the
sooner it is reformed and brought more into accordance with our physiological
knowledge the better.—*Brit. Med. Journal*, May 25, 1878.

The Infantile Diarrhœa of Summer.

At a recent meeting of the New York Academy of Medicine (*Med. Record*,
May 25, 1878), Dr. J. LEWIS SMITH contributed a very interesting paper on
this subject. As regards its treatment, he said he believed that there were but
very few remedies from which it was necessary to select, and for his own part he
scarcely ever employed more than two, viz., opium and bismuth, before the
hydrocephaloid stage was reached, and these he considered better than all others.
The administration of the large doses of bismuth now employed is of but recent
origin, but has been followed by the best results. In ordinary cases it should be
given in doses of ten or twelve grains, and it may be advantageously combined
with the compound powder of chalk with opium (which contains one grain of
opium in forty), or else with ordinary Dover's powder. For general use, however, it is perhaps better to give the bismuth in suspension, and the following
prescription will be found a very admirable one:—

R. Tinct. opii deodoratæ .   .   .   . gtt. xvj.
    Bismuth. subnitratis .   .   .   . ʒij.
    Syrupi .   .   .   . f ℥ss.
    Aquæ .   .   .   . f ℥iss.
M.

Dose, a teaspoonful for a child of one year.

Dr. Smith said that he had been much more successful since he had employed
opium and bismuth in this way than before, when he would often try a long list
of remedies in succession, and not find good results from any. Such a combination as the above is retained on the stomach, and has the effect of both an antiseptic and an astringent. No preparatory treatment is necessary, unless it is
found that some irritating article of food has been taken; but most of the cases
are considerably advanced when the physician is called in, and any such source
of trouble has long since been gotten rid of.

Almost all cases of entero-colitis need stimulus, and brandy is the best form in
which it can be given. Of course, the amount should vary according to the age,
and Dr. Smith is in the habit of giving three drops for every month of the child's
age (when under one year) every two or three hours.

When the hydrocephaloid stage of the disease is reached, the opium should be withdrawn or given very cautiously; but the bismuth may be continued as before. At this period, however, we must depend principally on tonics and astringents, and one of the most useful agents that can be employed is the liquor ferri nitratis. The following prescription will prove of great service:—

R. Tinct. calumbæ . . . . f℥ij.
   Liq. ferri nitratis . . . . gtt. xviij.
   Syrupi . . . . f℥ij.
M.

Dose, a teaspoonful.

At the same time the stimulus should be kept up as before.

Finally, the kind of diet used is of the utmost importance. If the child is under one year old it should at once be removed to the country, or a wet-nurse should be provided for it, as no artificial food is reliable. If both of these are impossible, the best cow's milk should be prepared in such a way as to resemble healthy human milk as much as possible. The milk should be allowed to stand for some time, and then only the upper third of it employed. In this way the larger part of the sugar and butter will be obtained, while the indigestible casein (which settles to the bottom) will be avoided. As regards farinaceous preparations for children under six months old, Dr. Smith prefers Mellin's Liebig's food, which also has the endorsement of such authorities as Eustace Smith and Tanner. Its taste is quite sweet from the dextrine and glucose which it contains, while it is almost entirely free from starch. When added to cow's milk, it makes as good a substitute for mother's milk as has as yet been obtained. After the age of six months infants can digest a certain amount of starchy food, and then Robinson's prepared barley may be used with advantage, if it is sufficiently boiled. As a rule, however, Dr. Smith prefers Ridge's food, which is highly recommended by Steiner, of Germany. Dr. Smith formerly used to employ Nestlé's food, but has been obliged to give it up, when the bowels are affected, on account of its laxative effect. In cases of habitual constipation in young infants, which is often a very perplexing condition to the practitioner, he has found it of very great service.

———

Some Practical Reflections on the Treatment of Intestinal Invagination.

This subject forms the leading paper in the *Journal de Thérapeutique* of the 25th February and 10th March, and the remarks are founded on three cases of cure by electricity under the care of the writer, Dr. Bucquoy. Curiously enough, as he says, he had three cases of what he believes to be this affection within a very short time. The first was that of a rather delicate child, æt. 3, and the attack was characterized by vomiting and severe colic, with scanty stools containing blood and what seemed like shreds of mucous membrane. This was followed by a general swelling of the belly, and a more circumscribed tumidity of the left flank. No feces or flatus were passed since beginning of illness. After trying simple remedies without benefit, he had recourse to Faradization, one pole being placed in the rectum, the other on the abdomen. A very gentle current was thus kept up for about fifteen minutes. Half an hour afterwards a large injection of cold water was administered. Immediate relief followed the electricity, but not till the following morning, after another injection, were any feces passed. The tumour in left flank became much less, and the vomiting and colic quite disappeared. Another application of the interrupted current caused abundant stools, and the tumour could no longer be felt. While yet in attendance Dr. Bucquoy was called to case No. 2—that of an infant seven months old. Here there were the same persistent vomiting and severe colic. Unwilling to believe

that this was another case of the same nature, his doubts, he says, were soon removed when, after an injection, a considerable quantity of blood was passed, followed by swelling and tenderness of the abdomen. Faradization, employed as
in the former case, was equally well borne, but with no immediate result, except
that the vomiting quite ceased. On the following day neither flatus nor feces had
passed, but on the third morning an injection brought away a large quantity of
feculent matter. Electricity repeated caused several stools, and the swelling
quite disappeared. Some remarks follow on the difficulty of diagnosis in such
cases, and how satisfied he is of its accuracy in these two cases. Both commenced with persistent vomiting and most severe colic. Both patients were children, "of such an age, the latter especially, when an obstacle to the course of
the intestinal contents has most frequently for its cause an invagination. . . .
Cruveilhier held that the discharge of sanguineous mucus from the bowel is pathognomonic of this affection." The presence of a distinct and more or less localized swelling completed the diagnosis. The third case he admits is more complex, and the diagnosis more obscure. Mademoiselle de R., æt. 14, healthy
looking, and well developed, is suddenly seized with violent colic and vomiting,
which soon becomes bilious. Shortly afterwards a circumscribed swelling in the
hypogastrium is noticed, dull on percussion, and slightly painful on pressure.
There is also a general swelling, resembling very much that of the seventh or
eighth month of pregnancy. Neither urine nor feces passed since the morning
when symptoms began, although an injection had been given. The interrupted
current was then applied as in the former cases. Patient stated she felt as if
something gave way, yet no action of the bowels followed : urine was passed in
great abundance, which did not, however, affect the swelling in any way. Slept
well that night, and an injection given on the following day had no effect. Colic
less; no vomiting; abdomen slightly painful on pressure. Two applications of
electricity on this the second day produced two very scanty stools. On third
day tumour as large and more sensitive. Faradization borne with difficulty on
account of the pain. Twenty grammes of castor oil and one drop of croton oil
given, producing two abundant stools, and giving considerable relief to the patient,
but causing great weakness. Abdomen now less painful, but swelling unaffected.
During the night seven abundant stools. On fourth day great improvement,
though tumour is still there. Repeated purgation caused copious bilious stools,
and the patient gradually recovered her health. The tumour, however, had undergone little or no change a month later (5th February). He remarks on the
vomiting, colic, etc., as at first fixing the diagnosis, while he considered the
tumour to be caused by the invagination. It was only after repeated purgation,
and the tumour remaining unaffected, that he had any doubts. He excludes
ovarian cyst or uterine tumour, but can give no satisfactory explanation of it.
He then discusses the treatment generally, and believes that the success of the
electricity was due to its early application "before any inflammatory complication had been set up." He refers to those who have tried it in somewhat similar
cases since introduced by Leroy, such as Duchesne, Christison, Stokes, but the
details of the cases, he says, are few and indefinite. In his cases the application
lasted about ten minutes each time, and was easily borne, even by the infant of
seven months. In the cases quoted from others this does not seem to have been
the rule, and his success he ascribes to the employment of a very feeble current,
especially at first, while the reophore is pressed gently on the abdomen. The
effect of the application is not immediate. It is generally some hours before an
alvine evacuation takes place, and that usually after an injection has been administered.—*Glasgow Med. Journal*, June, 1878.

Spontaneous Rupture of the Spleen.

Mr. E. Markham Skerritt, Physician to the Bristol General Hospital, reports (British Medical Journal, May 4, 1878) the following case in which splenic apoplexy and consequent rupture of the capsule of the spleen, took place under what is believed to be very rare and, perhaps, unique conditions. The case is of interest clinically, and also has a medico-legal importance to which a recent trial in India calls special attention.

The patient was a shepherd fifty-three years of age, admitted into the Bristol General Hospital on July 4. He stated that, up to two months before admission, he had enjoyed good health; then he began to suffer from nausea and pyrosis, and entirely lost his appetite. He had done no work for six weeks. A month before admission, he had an attack of epistaxis, which lasted about twenty-four hours, during which time he lost much blood. Since this, he had noticed a sensation of beating in the upper part of the abdomen. Just before admission into the hospital, another severe attack of epistaxis came on; the patient was, however, able to walk up into the ward without help.

When I saw him next day, he was almost blanched from loss of blood, but cheerful and anxious to give all the information in his power. The heart's impulse was weak, and there was a faint systolic apex-murmur; the pulse was feeble and the vessel degenerate. The abdominal aorta was pulsating to a marked degree, but no distinct dilatation of the vessel could be made out; a systolic bruit was plainly heard in the vessel, but was found to be only due to pressure. There was no pain or tenderness in the abdomen.

I concluded that there was no aneurism of the aorta, and that the pulsation and bruit were due to the anæmic condition consequent upon the loss of blood.

Soon after 9 P.M. the same day, the patient, who up to that time had seemed no worse, was suddenly seized with great dyspnœa and symptoms of collapse, which ended in death in less than an hour.

Post-Mortem Examination.—There was a large quantity of dark fluid blood in the peritoneal cavity. There was no aneurism. The capsule of the spleen was greatly distended; on the anterior aspect of its peritoneal surface there was a rent an inch long, through which the finger passed into a large space full of fluid blood. At first sight, it seemed as if the enlarged spleen were split longitudinally into two halves, which were separated along their whole length by this layer of fluid blood about an inch and a half thick; it was found, however, that the capsule had been stripped of the whole peritoneal surface of the spleen by blood effused between it and this surface, and that one of the apparent halves before mentioned was simply a firm layer of dark clot, about three-quarters of an inch thick, forming a thin cake applied closely to the inner surface of the capsule, and separated from the spleen itself by the layer of fluid blood before described. The exact source of the hemorrhage could not be found. The splenic substance was of a brick-red colour, and very soft and pulpy (there had been considerable *post-mortem* change). The spleen and clot together were eight inches long, five inches and a half broad, and three inches and a half thick, and weighed twenty-six ounces. The rest of the organs were very anæmic, but otherwise healthy.

Remarks.—Rupture of the spleen is not a very uncommon occurrence; but almost invariably it is caused by external violence, such as blows, crushes, falls, or wounds by fractured ribs. Instances have been met with, however, where the organ has ruptured spontaneously; in conditions where it is intensely congested, as in typhus, cholera, and the cold stage of ague, where it is probable that weakened texture has been combined with extreme congestion. But I have been unable to find any record of a parallel case to the one that I have related, where, at the time of the ruptuie, the patient was suffeiing fiom no acute disease, and had been quietly lying in bed foi hours.

If we considei the state of the spleen *post-mortem*, we see that the fiist event was hemoiihage within the capsule, giving iise to the laige clot befoie desciibed, which, fiom its chaiacteis, must have been foimed some time befoie the fluid blood was etfused and the capsule gave way. Theie was the following sequence: fiist, hemoiihage between the spleen and the capsule; then cessation foi a time; then moie blood pouied out, and in such quantity that the capsule gave way. Hence the actual ruptuie of the capsule was secondaiy and accidental.

Was theie any *congestion* of the spleen as the fiist event? I think not; iathei the opposite. The man had just been blanched by seveie epistaxis, and theie is no ieason to suppose that the spleen would be othei than anæmic, like the iest of the body. The conclusion must be that the same weakness of vessel that caused the iepeated bleeding fiom the nose led to the hemoiihage into this oigan, espe- cially as this occuiied at a time when the foice of the ciiculation had been much ieduced by loss of blood.

I now tuin to the medico-legal aspect of the case. Some months ago, a tiial took place in India which excited much inteiest. The following shoit account I take fiom a medical peiiodical. "A cuiious medico-legal point was involved in a iecent tiial foi manslaughtei in Ceylon. A coolie was tieated with some seveiity by the supeiintendent of a plantation, and died almost immediately fiom ruptuie of the spleen. The man had had fevei lately; the spleen was laige and soft. It was uiged foi the defence that the spleens of coolies sometimes ruptuie spontaneously on seveie musculai exeition; that the exeition of iunning away might have iuptuied the spleen; and that death would not be the diiect iesult of the action of the accused. This theoiy was discountenanced by the medical wit- nesses, and we think iightly. An accident so iaie, *and even doubtful*, as such ruptuie of the spleen must be, cannot be allowed weight in the piesence of evi- dence of diiect violence. The Chief Justice iuled that the ruptuie was distinctly the iesult of the violence. The piisonei was found guilty." If I iemembei iightly, the exact occuiiences weie these. The coolie ieceived a box on the eai and fell down; he then got up, ian away, climbed ovei two walls, and, in so doing, fell fiom the top of one oi both of them; he then quickly became collapsed and died. Heie was plenty of musculai exeition; besides that, the fall fiom the wall iepiesented a gieatei degiee of violence than did the pievious simple fall of the coolie off his feet. If the assault caused the ruptuie, it did so indiiectly only by causing the fall; foi theie was no direct violence to the abdomen. And, if this weie enough to pioduce the laceiation, how much moie weie the musculai exeition and the accident that followed, with which the accused had nothing im- mediately to do! It seems to me also impiobable that a man with a iuptuied spleen would iun away with the activity that this coolie showed.

With iegaid to musculai exeition as a cause of iuptuie of the spleen, cases illustiating this have occuiied in this countiy; thus Sir James Simpson iefeis to thiee cases of fatal iuptuie which occuiied iespectively duiing the piegnant, the paituiient, and pueipeial states; in each instance, aftei some unusual exeition. Anothei case is iecoided in the *British Medical Jouinal* foi 1874, by Mr. Atkinson, of Leeds, wheie the accident was appaiently due to violent vomiting set up by indigestible food.

The case I have ielated diffeis fiom all those that I have been able to find iecoided in this impoitant paiticulai: that theie was entiie absence of any special musculai exeition; foi the patient had, in fact, been in bed foi houis befoie the iuptuie occuiied. And I think that I am waiianted in concluding that this in- stance has established the fact that ruptuie of the spleen may occui puiely spontancously, in the absence of any condition ordinarily associated with congestion of the organs, and apart from all external violence or special muscular exertion.

—

Dysidrosis and its Morbid Anatomy.

Dr. TILBURY FOX, Physician to the Department for Skin Diseases, University College Hospital, makes the following remarks (*British Med. Journal*, May 25, 1877) on dysidrosis and its pathology :—

For some years I have taught that there exists a special inflammatory disease of the skin, commencing in the sweat apparatus, and characterized in its early stage anatomically by the development of little vesicles imbedded in the skin, which occupy the site, and are produced by the distension, of the sweat-ducts by fluid sweat rapidly becoming mixed with and altered by inflammatory fluid. This disease is usually confounded with acute eczema.

A typical case was admitted into the hospital a fortnight ago, under my care, and exhibited the disease in both its earlier and later stages. I pointed out to you amongst other things the naked eye characters of the disease at its commencement; how the ridges of papillæ on the palms appeared to be redder and more distinct than usual, from the fact that they were in a state of tumefaction; how the sweat-follicles, or rather their orifices, appeared to be peculiarly distinct and recognizable ; and how these follicles were apparently distended to form vesicles, which looked like little sago-grains imbedded in the skin. At least, these early vesicles were seen to be deeply seated, and not produced by any elevation of the cuticle, and we thought we could make them out to occupy the site of the sweat-ducts, and trace transitional stages between increased distinctness of the follicular orifice and the formed vesicles. I explained also that the sweat-duct opening could be clearly made out in the centre of the imbedded vesicle.

I promised to try to obtain the patient's consent to the removal of a piece of skin for careful examination; and you will be glad to hear that I have succeeded. Some of you saw me mark between two ink lines a portion of skin containing a few ridges of papillæ, where I stated that characteristic vesicles existed in an early stage, *i. e.*, about the fourth day of the disease. The portion of skin was removed, and Dr. Crocker kindly took charge of it for the purpose of preparing some microscopical sections, which he has accordingly done with much success. Dr. Crocker and I have carefully examined these preparations, and I will now acquaint you briefly with the main results obtained. You shall examine, however, some of the preparations for yourselves.

It has been stated lately by several observers that dysidrosis is not a disease of the sweat-apparatus, and Dr. Robinson of New York especially, in a recent article in the *New York Journal of Dermatology*, professes to have proved that the vesicles are formed by distension of the rete mucosum by inflammatory fluid effused from the vessels of the papillæ ; and he figures the vesicles seated over the papillæ.

Whether Dr. Robinson's case was a true instance of dysidrosis or not I cannot say, but our present case undoubtedly is; and what we find in our specimens is conclusive evidence that the sweat-ducts are very large and in some cases distended at their upper part, and that the vesicles are formed in connection with the sweat-ducts. Out of seventy or eighty specimens, we can only detect two instances of vesicles having any definite relation to the papillæ. The majority are distinctly formed *between* the papillary projections of the rete, their central axis being opposite to or a continuation of the depression in the rete answering to the usual spot where the sweat-coil enters the rete from above. In some cases, the duct, as it enters the rete, seems larger, as though commencing to dilate; but we can trace the sweat-ducts entering the little vesiculations or globular dilatations,

sometimes at the central point of their summits, at other times more to the side,
but still distinctly entering. We can see the sweat-ducts leaving the base of the
vesiculations, in some cases at the central point. In some specimens, the duct
projects slightly into the vesicles, and then its continuation is seen running from
the direction of the bottom of the vesicle and continuing its course through the
corium. There is one remarkable specimen of a twin vesicle with two contiguous
sweat-ducts clearly entering the vesicles. In none is the horny layer of the cuticle raised into vesiculations at the early stage of the disease. We have searched
in vain for the early phenomena of *eczematous* inflammation. In our sections,
the sweat-ducts are everywhere unusually well seen. Dr. Robinson figures none.
As to the changes that go on in the deeper portions of the sweat-gland, further
investigation is needed; but I have little hesitation in saying that I regard the
appearances seen in some of the sections as indicative of commencing inflammation. The cell elements of the wall of the gland-ducts and of the tissue of the
gland-coil and its envelope seem augmented.

To my mind, the views I have taught in this School about dysidrosis are fully
vindicated by these preparations. In my *Atlas*, published in 1877, I remarked
that "if the skin be examined at an early stage with a lens, in many cases it will
be seen that these little pearly spots answer exactly in situation to the sweat-
ducts, and indeed they are distensions of the sweat-apparatus. This has been
represented in Fig. 3, which was the exact appearance seen in the case, and
which was most plainly put by several others beside myself. This conclusively
proves that the disease is essentially a disorder of the sweat-apparatus." As to
the mechanism of the production of these vesicles, I wrote as follows, in 1873 :
" It seems to me that there is a sudden efflux of sweat, and the flow is so rapid
that it cannot escape, the whole gland is distended, at least its duct, and the fluid
presses up from below only to block up the upper portion of the duct by pressing
together the twists of the duct in that part of the cutis where it runs in a spiral
manner. If there be sudden pressure from below, the spiral twist of the duct
must greatly favour the dilatation of the duct. In sudamina, I take it, the opening is plugged by exuviæ, and the sweat finds its way laterally between the horny
layers of .the cuticle. . . . ." I think the basis of the above explanation holds
good. Dr. Crocker and I propose to work out the anatomy of dysidrosis, as far
as we can, more fully, and to place on record our joint observations on the matter.
I thought it well, whilst the clinical features of our recent case were fresh in your
minds, to show you these specimens, and thus vindicate the correctness of my
teaching on the subject during the last few years.

—

An Anomalous Mottled Rash, accompanied by Pruritus, Factitious Urticaria,
and Pigmentation.

At a late meeting of the Clinical Society of London (*Med. Times and Gaz.*,
May 18, 1878) Dr. A. SANGSTER read a paper on this case. C. F., aged two,
a healthy, well-nourished boy, came under notice last August, suffering with an
obscure skin affection. The trunk and limbs were covered, in some places more
thickly than others, with a buff-brown and buff-red coarsely mottled rash. The
buff-red mottling was most marked on the thighs and legs; here the disease presented much the appearance of a measles rash. The parts least affected were the
backs of the arms and forearms, the loins and buttocks ; the palms and soles were
free ; the flexures were specially affected. On passing the hand over the surface,
some of the diseased patches were felt to be slightly raised, but this was scarcely
noticeable. Nowhere, by pinching up the skin, could any increase of substance
be made out. On stretching the skin over the redder patches, the red colour dis-

appeared, leaving a pale buff discoloration. There was much pruritus, especially at the flexures. Scratching led to the production of urticaria wheals. The mother stated confidently that the latter never appeared but as a result of irritation by scratching or rubbing. There were no other lesions of the skin, no papules, blood-crusts, or desquamation. The points of interest in the patient's history were, that a grandmother and uncle had psoriasis, that the patient was severely jaundiced in infancy, as was also a younger child, since dead ; and that, according to the mother's statement, the patient's skin had always risen in "bumps" upon the slightest irritation. Even handling the child during the process of dressing would cause " the bumps to rise." The eruption had commenced as a red mottled rash on the abdomen when the patient was two months old, and was thought to be measles; however, it persisted, and had gradually spread, first over the trunk, and then to the extremities. As the patches became old they turned brown. The disease had defied treatment, internal and external. In appearance this eruption was similar to some others brought before the Clinical Society by Dr. T. Fox, Dr. Barlow, and Mr. Morrant Baker, and judged by Dr. T. Fox to be allied to xanthelasma ; while Mr. Hutchinson considered them to be of the nature of urticaria. The essential feature of the disease above described appeared to be a vaso-motor change in the skin, occurring spontaneously, and also as a result of the most trifling irritation, the above vaso-motor change having a tendency to become permanent, and ultimately leading to pigmentation.

Dr. TILBURY FOX thought the case belonged to the same category as those which Mr. Morrant Baker and he (Dr. Fox) had shown to the Society in 1874, though there was, however, much less, and indeed very slight, elevation of the patches or blotches in Dr. Sangster's instance. In his (Dr. Fox's) Atlas he had figured a patch of the disease, which was flattened and made up simply of apparently dull buff-coloured stains only ; and in one of the cases he had recorded, after an interval of five years, the patches had almost subsided, and now only deep-coloured stains remained, so that, under certain circumstances, the patches of the disease were not much elevated. If the Fellows would look at two top figures in plate 60 of Willan's coloured delineations (which he handed round), they would recognize the disease now under discussion ; and Willan, in all probability, under what he termed vitiligo, intended to represent this same disease. He spoke of elevations in the early stage subsiding, and leaving the skin checkered in a curious way ; and figured the early red irritable and the late dull mottled pigmented aspect of the disease. Dr. Fox did not think the disease could be called urticaria. It was no doubt liable under irritation to become hyperæmic and irritable ; but a disease made up of patches, which patches actually remained without much change for years, could scarcely be called urticaria. If the disease were an urticaria, we must completely revolutionize and change our notions of urticaria, as made up of evanescent hyperæmic spots connected with vascular spasm. Further, one knew that microscopic examination had shown that the tissue of the skin, in the disease under consideration, was infiltrated with a new cell-growth, like lupus in character. Then, again, the disease might be congenital. The main practical clinical point about the disease to remember was, that it was liable to be mistaken and treated for syphilis—a considerable error, which might be fraught with evil consequences.

Mr. HUTCHINSON expressed his pleasure in having seen Dr. Sangster's patient, and heard his clear description. He also congratulated the Society on the fact that it had been the means of bringing under discussion so many examples of such a rare disease. In former sessions, three well-marked cases had been submitted for inspection : one by Dr. Tilbury Fox, one by Mr. Morrant Baker, one by Dr. Barlow ; and each case had illustrated a different stage of the disease. The first two were the most severe, the third much less so; and now Dr. Sangster's patient showed it in a comparatively mild and early stage. Taken together, the cases, to any one who admitted that they all represented the same malady, were most instructive, and not far from conclusive as to its real nature. In Mr. Baker's case the child was covered with brown wheals and ridges, which were in a quiescent state, and from month to month, or even from year to year, underwent but little change; but in Dr. Sangster's case the state of things was different. Here we had the brown stains and some approach to ridges, but scarcely any thickening, and the conditions, although they had lasted long, were constantly undergoing local change; and, above all, we had in addition the very easy production of urticarian wheals. No one who had seen this child's skin, and noticed how the slightest touch sufficed to bring out a wheal, looking exactly like a nettle-sting or a flea-bite, could possibly doubt that, for one thing at least, the child had urticaria. He congratulated the author of the paper on the name employed "urticaria pigmentosa," for he had no doubt that it came very close to the truth; and, further, that it was applicable not only to this, but to the other cases. It had been objected that we knew nothing of urticaria as a malady lasting for years; but he believed that, in reality, some of the forms known as urticaria perstans were of quite indefinite duration. Besides, it was not quite literally true that in these cases the urticarious stage lasted for many years; it was rather its results in the way of thickening and pigmentation which were so persistent. His theory of the malady was that it was urticaria occurring at an unusually early age, and in connection with some peculiar condition of pruriginous skin; that it was evoked by local causes, and in the first periods kept up by them; and that in the end the skin became permanently thickened and discoloured by the long persistent inflammation. He would further add, as a conjecture, that the original irritation would in all probability be found to be bites of bugs or fleas, or both. He held that it was almost impossible to allow so wide a range of variation for the consequences of bites. As a rule, young infants were not very much irritated by them, but sometimes they were dreadfully affected, and sometimes the consequences were by no means transitory. In Dr. Barlow's case, which he had been permitted an opportunity of examining in the hospital, he believed that he had identified the results of bites.

Dr. SANGSTER said that, in reference to Dr. Fox's observations, the eruption had never been more raised than it was at present. In cases of pruritus one might generally suppose the pigmentation of the skin was due to the congestion of the skin produced by scratching. In this case the pigmentation could not be due to that cause, since it began when the child was only two months old. He thought, however, the pigmentation was due to local causes, possibly to the flannel binder. The child had been in New York, and the mosquito-bites there received did not give rise to any other than the usual effects in the skin. Vaccination also had produced no pruriginous eruption. The child had been jaundiced when very young, and the frequent connection of disease of the liver with innervation of the skin and skin-disease was suggestive.

Mr. CALLENDER had not long since seen a gentleman with permanent discoloration of the skin about the face and neck, due to the bites of mosquitoes.

Dr. TILBURY FOX had also witnessed the same thing.

Cacotrophia Folliculorum (Follicular Malnutrition).

At a late meeting of the Clinical Society of London (*Med. Times and Gaz.*, May 18, 1878), Dr. TILBURY FOX, in a paper with this title, sought to bring before the profession a disease of the hair-follicles characterized by special fea-

tures, and clinically distinct from those generally recognized. He had exhibited
a drawing of it, with a brief description, at the annual meeting of the British
Medical Association at Manchester in 1877; and Mr. Erasmus Wilson had, in
his latest course of lectures in January of this year, used the same drawing to
illustrate some more detailed and independent remarks. Dr. Fox sketched
lightly the pathology of the several papular diseases situated in the hair-follicles,
and characterized by retention of exuviæ with secondary congestion by simple
follicular torpor, or by primary congestion with its consequences—viz., pityriasis
pilaris, lichen pilaris, and scrofulosum, planus, ruber, and simplex; and he
argued that the drawing shown illustrated a condition distinct from any of these.
At first sight it appeared to him to be nothing more than ordinary but severe
lichen pilaris; and in this category, no doubt, it was ordinarily placed, but it
differed in its severity, the deeper and more complete affection of the follicles, its
congenital nature, its more general distribution, and its obstinacy to treatment.
Dr. Fox then considered lichen pilaris more closely, as being the disease in external features most like cacotrophia. Willan described lichen pilaris as a
" modification of lichen simplex, the papules appearing only at the roots of the
hairs of the skin"—in fact, as an inflammatory state of the follicles. But most
modern writers meant either a follicular torpor due to plugging by epithelial
exuviæ or altered sebum, or a simple inflammation with exudation into the follicle, especially confined to its upper part, and the consequent formation in both
cases of papules pierced by hairs, which remained practically unchanged. It was
brought about by many local and general causes, such as uncleanliness, local irritants, and blood and constitutional states. Lichen pilaris was not often seen in
the very young; it was an acquired disorder, was more or less localized to particular parts, especially the thigh and outer side of the arm and forearm; and,
lastly, it was not notably obstinate. The eruption of cacotrophia folliculorum
was made up of solid red papules, the size of a pin's head, which were seen to be
situated at almost every hair-follicle, and these papules stood out from a rather
reddened base. Though the disease had a special predilection for parts, such as
the outer aspect of the arm, the back of the shoulders, the thighs, the trunk, and
the sides of the face and forehead, which was sometimes the seat of seborrhœa
sicca, still the eruption was of very general and extensive distribution. The
hairs had mostly disappeared, those that remained being stunted and twisted,
and the interfollicular portion of the skin was reddened, the whole thing often
bearing a striking resemblance to xeroderma. In this affection the deepest portions of the hair-follicle, including the papilla, were affected, and the formation of
the hair interfered with. It was not an inflammatory condition, but one essentially of defective or indolent nutrition, with plugging of the follicles and some
passive congestion. Individuals were affected from the earliest age, or it might
be truly congenital, and was not acquired later on in life. A very important point
was that the disease occurred in subjects—mostly young women—of a lymphatic,
strumous, or phthisical tendency, and was brought into prominence and especially
attracted notice about the period of increased physiological activity, viz., puberty.
The paper was illustrated with the detailed notes of four well-marked cases.

Mr. HUTCHINSON scarcely knew why these cases should be separated from
cases of xeroderma or ichthyosis, which was a congenital cacotrophy of the whole
skin; whereas this was simply a cacotrophy of the follicles only.

Dr. WILTSHIRE thought the disease rather common amongst insane children
of Mongolian type, with clubbed fingers and blue eyes.

Dr. TILBURY FOX, in reply, said he was quite aware that there was a plugged
state of the follicles in connection with ichthyosis, but that was not the condition
he had described in the paper he had read, and it was not very likely that both

he and M i. Erasmus Wilson should have made a blunder upon so simple a point as that.   He doubted if M i. Hutchinson (at least his remark seemed to show as much) was exactly conversant with the disease under discussion.   He (Dr. Fox) did not know of any published account of the condition.

—

Chrysophanic Acid Ointment in Psoriasis.

Dr. NEUMANN, of Vienna, thus endorses (*Wiener Mediz. Presse*, No. 14–16, 1878) M i. Balmanno Squire's treatment of psoriasis by an ointment of chryso-phanic acid, as first communicated by M i. Squire in this country at the latter end of 1876.   After giving due credit to M i. Squire, and to the other English ob-servers who followed him in this research, the professor winds up his paper with the following summary: 1. Chrysophanic acid derived from Góa powder is an excellent remedy for herpes tonsurans, pityriasis versicolor, and psoriasis vulgaris. 2. Psoriasis in its earlier stages begins to disappear after a few applications of the drug, and in a far more unequivocal manner than under any other remedy that has ever yet been used against psoriasis.   3. Even inveterate forms of the dis-ease can be abolished by means of chrysophanic acid, and it is quite the exception to find them oppose any protracted resistance to it.   4. Chrysophanic acid is a perfectly painless application to the diseased skin.   The morbid phenomena occa-sioned by it on the healthy skin result apparently from the admixture of resinous matter with the acid.   5. As a result of this mode of treatment, psoriasis belongs no more to those skin diseases which in so high a degree are a source of misery to the patient, and it has now become an easy matter to cure relapses.   Every patient with psoriasis that I have as yet treated by this means gives the palm without hesitation to this method of treatment in preference to all others.   In any case, this at the least is emphatically true; namely, that the therapeutics of skin diseases have for the last ten years been enriched by but few remedies which have been crowned by so eminent a success as the one in question.   6. There are other skin diseases, also, which are curable by chrysophanic acid.   7. He ex-presses a hope that this method may be examined by other observers; and he does not doubt that it will soon permanently assume its due rank amongst the treasures of therapeutics.—*British Med. Journal*, May 25, 1878.

Surgery.

The Surgical Pathology of the Nerves.

This generation has witnessed a remarkable extension of the domain of practical surgery in the direction of both the magnitude and delicacy of the operations which have been attempted and achieved.   The structures which have been regarded as beyond the range of legitimate surgery, which allow of no traumatic interference, the nerves themselves, are no longer to be left in their isolation.   Nerve-stretching has been proved to be an operation free from the risks which might reasonably be supposed to attend it.   Nerve-suture has been performed, and there are reasons to believe that it may come to be an operation more frequently practised than it is at present.   On this account the careful experimental study of the histological changes which attend, and the functional results which follow, the union of divided and sutured nerves is of great importance, and we, therefore, call the attention of our readers to some recent and interesting researches by Dr. T. GLUCK which have been made in the Pathological Institute at Berlin, and are published in Virchow's *Archiv*.

The subject has been studied by Eichhorst, especially in the union of minute nerve-branches, but Gluck has preferred to make his observations upon larger nerves, on account of the greater facility for surgical treatment and histological investigation which they present; and his results, which differ somewhat from those of Eichhorst, are of correspondingly greater importance to the surgical pathologist. The nerves selected were the sciatic in the fowl, a creature in which union of a divided nerve occurs with considerable facility; and the vagus in the rabbit, in which, from the tendency to tissue degeneration, nerve-union is much less easy to obtain. These two nerves afford considerable facility for experimental study of the change in their function.

When a nerve is divided the first evident change is that the sheath retracts, and the myelin spreads over the cut surface, while blood is effused into the ends of the nerve and the wound. In a few days the ends of the divided nerve are connected by gray translucent tissue. The further changes depend on the distance between the two ends. The removal of one or two centimetres of nerve prevents all regeneration, even after many months, if the ends are not brought together by artificial means. The nerves and muscles degenerate, the limb wastes, and the fowls die about the fifth month. If, however, the ends of the nerve are carefully sutured together, by preference with catgut, the result is quite different. The closer the approximation and coaptation of the two ends the less is the amount of tissue formed about them, aptly termed "nerve-callus," and the less is the degeneration below. The histological changes which have been found are the following. If a centimetre is removed, the space between the two ends is filled by a soft cellular granulation tissue, containing vessels; the ends of the nerve undergo degeneration. One or two months later only a dense fibrous tissue is to be found in the interval, containing no nervous constituent. Gluck did not in any case succeed in obtaining regeneration when a large piece of the nerve had been removed. If the nerve was simply divided, and the ends approximated, the result was very different. In twenty-four hours spindle-cells, arranged in series, and surrounded by an abundant intercellular material, lay between the two ends. After eight days the ends were connected together by nerve-fibres destitute of myelin, and from that time there was a gradual formation of the myelin-sheath, the protoplasm becoming darker, and tinting more and more by the action of osmic acid. No degeneration is visible in the central end, except the slight escape of myelin from the divided extremity of the nerve, but in the peripheral end there is a slight indication of degenerative changes. The nuclei of the neurilemma multiply until about the sixth day. The process is thus a union by first intention in the strict sense of the word.

When a piece of a nerve is excised, and the ends brought together by sutures, the process is somewhat less simple, and less rapid in its course. On the third day the divided ends are connected by soft translucent tissue, in which the catgut sutures are visible, and here and there a little reddish-brown pigment. Microscopically the two ends are hardly to be distinguished; each presents thrombosis in the minute vessels, and a somewhat wavy appearance of the nerve-tubes. In the young granulation-tissue between the ends of the nerves, about the fifth day, peculiar fusiform cells appear, dark granular, and bearing considerable resemblance to the ganglion-cells of the nerve-centres. These appear to connect together the axis cylinders of the divided ends, their continuity with which can be sometimes distinctly traced. The rapidity with which this fusion of the ends of the nerve occurs, determined by the distance of the ends apart, influences the extent of the degeneration in the divided ends. If a nerve is only partially divided, is wounded without complete section of the nerve-sheath, this restoration of continuity is most speedy; it is so, next, when the coaptation of the divided ends is perfect, and when by the eighth or fourteenth day all the nerve-tubes are connected. In such cases the granular or fatty degeneration is slight, and no axis cylinders destitute of myelin are to be seen in the ends of the nerves.

It has been maintained by Eichhorst that in the process of union and restoration a new axis cylinder and medulla are formed by extension from the centre towards the periphery, but there is considerable difference between the facts which he and Gluck witnessed. The latter found that a bridge between the two ends was completed at the time at which, according to Eichhorst, the degeneration is at its height, and the regeneration is yet far away. Gluck maintains that the axis cylinders do not perish, and that by the fourteenth day, both in the cicatricial tissue and the peripheral end, there are axis cylinders without myelin; but at this period Eichhorst thought the axis cylinders were only beginning to bore through the tissue which separates the ends of the nerves.

The means by which the union of the axis cylinders occur is believed to be the peculiar fusiform cells, resembling ganglion cells. Near them may be seen young axis cylinders, the nuclei of which bear the closest resemblance to those of the fusiform cells. The processes of these cells are filled with protoplasm, which is at first granular, afterwards becomes homogeneous, and ultimately appears to be differentiated into medulla and axis cylinders. The nuclei become paler, and the cellular membrane comes to represent the sheath of the newly-formed nerve-fibre. This method of union is of much interest, as being almost identical with the mode in which, according to the observations of Kölliker, nerve-fibres are formed in the embryo. What, it will be asked, becomes of the catgut ligature during this process? It is apparently absorbed. In eighty hours the section shows deep excavations in the thread, which increase in size during the next few days, and in about a week all traces of the catgut have disappeared.

During this stage of regeneration of the nerve it is found that its functional power undergoes a restoration closely parallel to that of its structural continuity. Just as no formation of nerve elements is to be traced when a piece of the nerve is cut out, so no restoration of function of the nerve is to be observed under the same circumstances, even after a long time. On the other hand, when the injury is such, as with a needle, that the neurilemma is not divided, functional power is regained in a very brief time. Lastly, when the nerve is completely divided and carefully sutured, it is found that in the most favourable cases functional power is restored in about seventy hours, in the case of the sciatic of the fowl, and in about ten days in the case of the vagus of the rabbit. An early restoration of function in divided nerves has been doubted by many pathologists of authority, because, in respect to man, it rests chiefly upon facts as to the early return of sensation, not of motion, in the parts supplied by the divided nerve, and the theory of a collateral path by the peripheral connection with other nerves has seemed a more probable explanation than that of a restoration of function through the injured part. It is, indeed, difficult to exclude the possibility of such an explanation in the experiments upon animals, if the recovery of voluntary power in the muscles at first paralyzed is taken as the indication of the recovery of functional power in the divided nerve. The possibility of such an explanation is excluded, however, by some of Gluck's experiments. Having divided and sutured the sciatic of a fowl, the immediate paralysis of the muscles supplied was found to have passed away at the end of four days. The sciatic was then exposed, divided again above the place of suture isolated, and laid on a glass plate, as low as the division into peritoneal and tibial nerves. Irritation, mechanical or electrical, of the nerves above the suture caused contractions in the muscles supplied by it, which must have been due to the conduction of the stimulation through the divided portion. In some other cases evidence of conduction was not obtained until after a somewhat longer period; but at the time at which this power of functional conduction was manifested, histological observation showed that between the two ends of the nerves there was only granulation tissue, or tissue which had not yet assumed the character of nerve-fibres, and we must assume that this suffices to conduct the stimulation.

Other experiments, with a similar result, were made on the vagus. The physiological relation of the two vagi supplies an interesting means of testing the restoration of this function. As is well known, death occurs soon after section of both nerves, while division of one only produces comparatively little effect. The right vagus of a rabbit was divided and sutured with catgut. Ten days afterwards the left vagus was divided, without the appearance of any of the symptoms which result from the division of both nerves. Hence it was assumed that the function of the left had been restored. To test this the left also was divided, and always with the result of causing the death of the animal with the characteristic symptoms of paralysis of both vagi.

A very important practical question in connection with these observations is: How long after complete division can suture be practised with hope of recovery? An answer to the question is essential for the surgical application of the researches we have described, and this answer, by some observations now in progress, we are promised at a future time.—*Lancet*, June 1, 1878.

Tuberculosis of the Tongue.

Is there any organ or tissue of the body which is not occasionally the seat of the formation of tubercles? It is doubtful whether the careful investigation of the present generation of workers will long permit an affirmative answer to this question. The occurrence of tubercles has now been noted in structures in which it was thought, not long ago, that they were never found, and it seems probable that soon their occasional occurrence will be traced in every part. We lately noted some interesting observations of the occurrence of distinct tubercular formations in voluntary muscles, and now we have to call attention to recent facts which demonstrate that tubercular ulceration of the tongue is met with, rarely it is true, but with a distinctness which suggests that when its occurrence is generally known its rarity may be found to be less than is commonly supposed. The condition is not in itself surprising when we reflect how constantly tubercular formations are met with in other parts of the alimentary tract.

The condition was noted long ago by Portal, but has been until lately so completely overlooked that it is unmentioned in many of our systematic treatises. It is to the French that we are indebted for the observation of most of the cases, of which several have been recorded by Trélat, Féréol, Laveran, and others, and a well-marked example has just been published in *l'Union Médicale* by M. Millard. The characters of the affection are almost distinctive, apart from its association with pulmonary disease, which is commonly obtrusive. The patients are usually of early or late adult age. The ulcer is commonly single, but two or three may be present, and in some cases there have been a large number of excavations; in that of M. Millard it was estimated that there were a hundred separate ulcers. Their seat is the anterior part of the tongue, the edges, and the under surface; the upper surface being very rarely invaded. The common seat of the ulcers suggests that the occurrence of the tubercular deposit may have been determined by the local irritation of decayed teeth, just as local irritation elsewhere has a distinct influence in determining the change. The affection commences by the appearance of a minute white spot on the surface of the tongue, over which the mucous membrane gives way, allowing the escape of a little puriform material, and thus an excavation is formed, minute at first, but rapidly increasing in size. Similar spots make their appearance around the first, and confer upon the disease its most characteristic aspect. The ulcers thus formed may remain discrete, or may coalesce. When the large ulcers have been formed, they are irregular in shape, have a yellowish, uneven base, beneath which the tissue is indurated. There is no actual tumour, although the characters of one may, as Millard remarks, be closely simulated by the muscular contraction which occurs as the consequence of the pain of the ulcers, to prevent the extension of that portion of the tongue. For these ulcers are commonly painful, often extremely so, rarely painless. They are occasionally associated with the development of similar ulcers elsewhere in the buccal cavity, especially, in several cases, in the soft palate. In one instance, recorded by Gelade, the ulcers extended from the palate to the gums of the molar teeth, and invaded the superior maxillary bone, which became excavated by a sort of soft caries.

The tubercular nature of these ulcers rests upon strong evidence. They are almost invariably associated with signs of pulmonary phthisis, frequently with actual excavation of the lung. They are unlike other ulcers, whether simple, specific, or epitheliomatous, and, in several cases in which it has been tried, antisyphilitic treatment, iodide of potassium or mercurial inunction, has been useless, and in no case has any history of syphilis, direct or indirect, been traceable. But their nature does not rest upon the evidence of clinical association alone. The tubercular nature of the white points from which they take origin has been demonstrated by Raynaud, Koerte, and Nedopil. On microscopical examination they were found to be of similar structure to the miliary tubercles which existed elsewhere in the cases. The ulceration is the result of a rapid caseation of the tubercles which infiltrate the tissue beneath the ulcer. Although the signs of advanced phthisis have usually coexisted with such ulceration, the latter has been noticed to initiate the affection, as in a case recorded by Lailler, in which general miliary tuberculosis of the mouth was followed by rapid phthisis, and in the case in which the nature of the disease was demonstrated by Koerte. The patient of the latter was a man, aged fifty-three, previously healthy, and the affection of the tongue preceded for two months the occurrence of infiltration of the apices of the lungs.

Although the ulcers have not in any case been the immediate cause of death, they have in many instances assisted in bringing about a fatal termination by interfering with mastication and with the ingestion of food. Their treatment is thus a matter of considerable importance. In obstinacy they resemble closely the tubercular ulcerations upon other mucous membranes, and several observers have come to the conclusion that little or nothing can be done; but Bucquoy and Laboulbène have recorded cases treated successfully. Relief may be given to the pain by sedatives, especially by morphia and glycerine; by a spray of iodoform dissolved in ether, as suggested by Lailler; and by antiseptic applications, such as borax and hyposulphite of soda. It is evident that little benefit can be expected from the application of caustics, since the affection is deeply seated; the tubercular process underlies the ulcer, and cannot be influenced by astringents or caustics applied to the surface. Nitrate of silver and chromic acid have both failed. The most efficient remedy is excision. This has been performed in several cases under the impression that the disease was really epithelioma, and in others in order to get rid of ulcers which were very troublesome and interfered seriously with nutrition. In all cases the wounds have healed well, and the removal of the indurated tissue underlying the ulcer has arrested the disease.— *Lancet*, May 25, 1878.

Guijun Balsam in Gonorrhœa.

This preparation, in place of copaiba, has been prescribed with success for gonorrhœa at some of the hospitals of Paris (*Bulletin Général de Thérapeutique*, Février 28, 1878).

The following is Vidal's formula, as used at the Hospital Saint-Louis:—

Guijun balsam, 4 grammes (1 drachm); gum, 4 grammes (1 drachm); infusion of star anise, 40 grammes (10 drachms). To be divided into two doses, and taken immediately before meals.

Mauriac gives a larger dose: his formula at the Hospital du Midi is as follows:—

Guijun balsam, 16 grammes (4 drachms); gum, 10 grammes (2¼ drachms); syrup of gum, 30 grammes (7½ drachms); mint water, 50 grammes (12¼ drachms). To be divided into three parts, and taken during the day.

N. Deval, who watched the effects of the remedy in Vidal's service (*Thèse de Paris*, 1877), recommends the former prescription, considering Mauriac's to be too powerful.

Guijun balsam is cheaper than copaiba; it is also said to act more rapidly, and to have no disagreeable effect on the breath.—*London Medical Record*, May 15, 1878.

Direct Injections into the Bladder through the Urethra.

Injections of medicated fluids into the bladder has been much recommended; but a great drawback has been the often irritable state of the membranous portions of the urethra and the back of the bladder, and the difficulty has not been overcome by Reliquet's suggestion of a gum-elastic catheter in place of the metallic one.

Dr. BERTHOLLE (*Gazette Hebdomadaire*, Nos. 19, 20, and 21, 1877) suggests a method of injecting fluids into the bladder without the use of the catheter. If a stream of water or other fluid be introduced into the urethra, it will, if entering under sufficient pressure, gradually dilate the sphincter vesicæ, and enter the bladder. If there be spastic contraction, this will be gradually overcome by the pressure of the column of fluid. Dr. Bertholle, who was the subject of chronic inflammation of the membranous urethra, practised the method for eighteen months on himself with a satisfactory result. It is as follows: The patient sits on a carpet on the floor with his back against the wall, the thighs abducted, the knees turned out, and the feet turned in. A vessel is placed conveniently to catch any water which may escape. An irrigator with a tube is placed upon a bench near by. To the end of this tube is fastened one end of a movable connecting piece provided with a stopcock, the other end being, when occasion requires, fastened to the canula intended for insertion into the urethra. The canula is of hard India-rubber, about five inches long, and rather less than a quarter of an inch in diameter. It is well oiled, and inserted into the urethra, and the patient, holding the urethra and canula firmly with the left hand, can easily regulate the flow of the fluid by turning the stopcock. When the latter is opened, the water usually penetrates into the bladder without the patient being conscious of its entrance. So soon as he feels the desire to urinate, the stopcock is to be turned off, as the bladder is then full. The patient can now empty the bladder at once, or can retain the fluid for a short time. The water to be injected should be lukewarm, or at least not of lower temperature than the body. The best time for employing the injection is just before going to bed. A single injection will dilute the stagnant urine and deprive it of its irritating quality.

[This method of injecting the male bladder was described two years ago by Dr. Hunter McGuire, of Richmond, Va. (*Va. Med. Monthly*, July, 1876, and *Monthly Abstract*, Sept. 1878, p. 420.)—ED.]

The indications for the direct injection of water (or medicated fluids) are as follows: 1. Diseases of the bladder, and particularly chronic essential or consecutive cystitis. In the former, Bertholle considers this method capable of effecting a cure; in symptomatic cystitis it is only palliative, so long as the cause (stone, etc.) is not removed. 2. Contraction of the neck of the bladder. 3. Diseases of the prostate; the injection here acting indirectly by relieving the consecutive vesical catarrh. 4. Diseases of the urethra, in particular, urethritis of the deeper portion, where contraction of the membranous portion, and of the sphincter vesicæ, with consecutive catarrh, is present. The contraindications are: 1. Paralysis or relaxation of the bladder; 2. Hypertrophy or other diseased condition of the prostate, causing difficulty in urination; 3. Organic stricture of the urethra.— *London Med. Record*, May 15, 1878.

The Local Use of Solution of Quinia in Chronic Irritation of the Bladder.

Mr. J. KNOWSLEY THORNTON, Surgeon to the Samaritan Free Hospital for Women, in an article on this subject (*Lancet*, June 1, 1878) says: Some few months back I heard, through Mr. Spencer Wells, of the value which Mr. Nunn attached to the local use of quinine in chronic irritation of the bladder. I had in hospital at the time two patients whose convalescence after ovariotomy had been much retarded by this condition, which is so apt to arise from the nurse not being sufficiently careful as to the condition of her catheter. Both the cases had defied frequent washings out of the bladder with solutions of carbolic acid, etc., and both patients were feverish, passing much mucus in ammoniacal and offensive urine, with constant desire and severe dysuria.

I treated both as follows: The water was drawn off with a No. 12 gum-elastic catheter, and the bladder thoroughly washed out with tepid carbolic lotion, one to one hundred, four ounces being introduced and then withdrawn, the process being repeated till a pint had been used for each. (This had been done each day for several days, two ounces of the solution being left in the bladder without the slightest relief or improvement.) Four ounces of water were then introduced and withdrawn. Not knowing the exact strength of the solution used by Mr. Nunn, I had one made with two grains of quinine to the ounce, and a few drops of dilute sulphuric acid to dissolve it. Three ounces of this solution were introduced and allowed to remain in a few seconds; then two ounces were withdrawn, the other ounce being left in the bladder; the patient having instructions not to pass water for an hour. The first patient had some smarting and forcing, which lasted for twenty minutes; the second no inconvenience whatever. In twenty-four hours I noted as to them both: "Urine acid, much improved in general appearance; no mucus, and odour normal." Two days later I noted in their case-books, "No more trouble with urine since the acid quinine injection; urine normal."

A few weeks later another patient, nursed by the same nurse, was found in the same condition on the fifth day after ovariotomy. I at once emptied the bladder, washed it out in the same way as before, merely using warm water, and used the quinine solution. The urine contained a good deal of mucus next day, but was acid. A few days later I noted, "No further difficulty with the urine, which is normal."

Having given, after this, very strict injunctions as to the cleaning of the catheters, I have had no further opportunity of trying the quinine, but I certainly shall use it with perfect confidence in any other case of the kind which comes under my care. I think we are much indebted to Mr. Nunn for giving us so simple a method of dealing with a most troublesome complaint.

Morphia and a Tell-Tale as aids to Compression in Aneurism.

Mr. C. F. MAUNDER, Surgeon of the London Hospital, in his Lettsomian Lectures of 1875, drew attention to the value of morphia as an aid to compression, as a substitute for chloroform and its attendant risks. He illustrated its use in the case of a gentleman who "dozed, took his meals, smoked his pipe, and submitted to continuous digital compression for twenty-three hours, with scarcely a complaint; and, at the expiration of this time, expressed himself as capable of enduring treatment many hours longer." The following is another example of the value of the drug, recorded by Mr. Maunder (*British Med. Journ.*, May 25, 1878).

In February, 1877, Mr. ——, who is now forty-two years of age, was advised that he was the subject of an aneurism of the popliteal artery. He was put to bed and treated for the first ten days with a bag of shot weighing eight pounds placed over the common femoral artery. During the next month, a tourniquet was substituted, and worn during eighteen hours out of the twenty-four over the superficial femoral artery. His health now began to fail; treatment was discontinued; and he went to his business, the tumour being smaller and pulsation less marked. During the last three months, the swelling and the pulsation had both increased, associated with pain and general discomfort about the knee.

March 29, 1878. I found Mr. —— with an aneurism of the size of a large orange occupying the upper half of the popliteal region, and bulging somewhat to the inner side of it. Continuous digital compression with a weight of ten pounds was advised, aided by morphia, if necessary.

30th. Mr. W. R. T. Hawkins and Mr. Albert E. Jones of the London Hospital commenced the compression treatment at 11.45 A. M., the common femoral being the artery selected; and they maintained complete occlusion of this vessel for the space of half an hour alternately. At 4 P. M. the patient suddenly complained of severe pain (distal occlusion?), commencing in the calf of the leg, and running up along the aneurism and femoral artery. A quarter of a grain of morphia was now hypodermically injected, and relief afforded. From this time, when the gentleman compressing was relieved by his colleague, and the pressure for the moment somewhat relaxed, the force of the pulsation in the aneurism was observed to be gradually diminishing. At 8 P. M. an assistant was recruited, in order to help in the continuation of the compression through the night.

31st. At 2 A. M. another paroxysm of pain occurred, after which pulsation was scarcely, if at all, perceptible; and a firm swelling occupied the seat of the aneurism, the disease being practically cured. At 10 A. M. no pulsation could either be felt or seen. One or two arteries could be detected meandering the knee. Compression was continued during the day as a precautionary measure. Throughout the whole time (thirty hours), the patient lay on his back, with the thigh rotated outwards, and the leg flexed at a right angle on this. An indicator (which consisted of a penholder with a piece of paper like a flag placed between the nibs, and which marked the presence or absence of pulsation in the aneurism) was lodged like a finger-post in the flexure of the knee, and acted like a tell-tale to the compressor. Mr. —— took food at intervals, and was cheerful and chatty, except when asleep. An injection of morphia was resorted to four times.

The skin over the seat of compression, which had been protected by the occasional application of French chalk, was slightly reddened only, and was the source of the least possible discomfort to the patient, who said he could have borne the treatment many hours longer.

Aneurism of Subclavian and Axillary Artery treated by Rest and Restricted Diet.

At a late meeting of the Clinical Society of London (*Lancet*, March 16, 1878), Mr. HULKE read the notes of such a case. The patient, a French-polisher, aged thirty-six, but much older in appearance, addicted to drink, after suffering from pains in the left shoulder and arm, supposed to be rheumatic, during two months, became aware of a swelling at the root of his neck on the left side, for which he went into King's College Hospital. Dissatisfied with what was there done for him, he left that hospital, and five months after the beginning of his ill-ness entered the Middlesex Hospital, 28th March, 1877. At this time he had a large aneurismal tumour filling the axilla and implicating also the third, second, and presumably, to some extent, also the first part of the left subclavian artery; and he suffered great pain down the arm and over the shoulder-blade. He was kept in bed, and enjoined to keep perfectly still—not even to sit up or to move off the bed for any purpose, and he was put on a very limited non-stimulating diet. This was followed by rapid mitigation of the pain, by decrease of the aneu-rism and its obstruction by clot. He was discharged for disorderly conduct in June, at which time the axillary portion of the sac had shrunken to the size of an acorn, and was quite impervious, and the cervical part was very small, and felt very firm. It was thought that a slight pulsation of this part might be commu-nicated. He afterwards entered Charing-cross Hospital, where, Mr. Hulke learned, doubts were entertained of the nature of the affection. This Mr. Hulke took to be confirmatory of the permanence of the consolidation and occurrence of a cure. The encouragement the case afforded for the trial of a modified Val-salva's method in aneurism, where the ordinary direct surgical methods were not applicable, induced Mr. Hulke to submit the case to the consideration of the Clinical Society.

—

Notes on a Case of Multiple Exostoses.

The condition of several exostoses developed in the same individual is a suffi-ciently rare occurrence to render worthy of report the following remarkable case recorded by Mr. THOMAS JONES, Surgeon to the Children's Hospital, Manches-ter (*British Med. Journal*, May 18, 1878).

Wm. S., aged 9, a native of Warrington, was admitted into the Children's Hospital on July 3, 1877. The immediate cause of the parents seeking advice was a large tumour springing from the posterior surface of the right leg about two inches below the knee. This mass, of irregular shape and firm consistence, was found to spring from both bones. The skin over the tumour was of normal colour and freely movable. A further examination of the boy resulted in the detection of a number of bony outgrowths, of various sizes and shapes, in different parts of the body. They were connected with the following bones: the right clavicle, one at each end; the upper extremities of both humeri; the carpal ends of the right and left radii; the lower ends of both ulnæ; the second phalanges of the ring and middle fingers of the right hand; the outer side of the second pha-lanx of the middle finger on the left hand; the dorsal surface of the middle phalanx of the left ring finger; the lower border of the same phalanx; the lower ends of both femora; the posterior surface of the right femur; the upper ends of both tibiæ; the outer surface of the left fibula; and the dorsal surface of the middle phalanx of the left second toe.

Besides these outgrowths, the upper end of the left fibula and the lower end of the right radius are very materially increased in thickness. I would also mention a deformity of the left ulna which the boy presents. The lower third of this bone appears to be quite in a rudimentary state, and to join the radius, thereby destroying the power of pronation and supination in the left forearm.

The progressive increase in the size of the osseous tumour situated on the right lower extremity rendered its removal advisable. The operation by a single straight incision in the long axis of the limb was performed on July 18. The fibular attachment of the tumour was much broader and firmer than the tibial. On section, it was discovered that the greater part of the mass was made up of cancellated bone-tissue, and that it was enveloped by a thin layer of glistening cartilage.

The case I have briefly related, while agreeing in many respects with those already published, differs in some particulars. It coincides with the case referred to in Paget's *Surgical Pathology*, and with Dr. Poore's (*Lancet*, Nov. 29, 1873), in the tolerably symmetrical arrangement of the growths, and in those on the right side being larger than those on the left; but, unlike these, careful inquiry has failed to establish the presence of any osseous deformities in other members of the family.

I am unable to offer any theory as to the causation of these exostoses. I think, however, I may say with confidence that they were not the result of conditions which are generally looked upon as causes—such as rickets, syphilis, and struma. There is an entire absence of the usual indications of either struma or syphilis, and the conformation of the osseous system in general renders the probability of rickets having existed very unlikely.

The local hypertrophy of the right radius and left fibula appears to lend some countenance to the observation made by Sir James Paget, that these exostoses are to be regarded as closely related to osseous malformations by excessive development.

In conclusion, I would submit that the formation of a number of bony tumours in connection with the osseous system should be looked upon as evidence of a constitutional ossific dyscrasia.

—

Subcutaneous Extra-Articular Osteotomy for Genu Valgum.

The operation to which this name has been given was performed for the first time on Friday last, May 17th, at the East London Hospital for Children, by Mr. REEVES, in the presence of several foreign surgeons. Its object, which was thoroughly obtained, is to improve on the method of operating on cases of knock-knee devised and executed by Dr. A. Ogston, of Aberdeen; and our object in calling attention to it at this early stage is to induce surgeons to give it that trial and preference which a less severe and equally efficient operation must claim. We give the substance of Mr. Reeves's observations before the operation. In Dr. Ogston's operation, the knee-joint is entered by the tenotome or scalpel, a fine saw is introduced along the knife-track, and the internal condyle is sawn off. This proceeding has now been done about thirty times *antiseptically;* and the results have been, on the whole, very encouraging; yet we have heard of a few cases in which synovitis, followed by severe constitutional disturbance and ending in ankylosis, has occurred. It was to avoid, if possible, these unnecessary complications, that Mr. Reeves thought of the extra-articular method. A scalpel, previously dipped in carbolized oil, was introduced obliquely just above the inner tuberosity, and the soft parts and periosteum were divided; by the side of the knife, a chisel, also dipped in carbolized oil, was introduced, and the internal condyle separated *as far as the cartilage only;* and, the chisel being then used as a lever, the condyle was pried inwards, till it was felt to move moderately freely. The limb was then forcibly straightened by Mr. Cæsar and Mr. Parker; a pad of lint dipped in carbolized oil was put over the small aperture, and a long splint, interrupted at the knee, and with a cross-piece at the foot to keep it steady, was adjusted to the straightened limb. As the condyle differs in shape and depth, it is of course necessary to be accurate in chiselling; and, to guide him, Mr. Reeves previously marked out with ink on the skin not only the contour of the condyle, but also the direction of the chisel-cut. The greatest depth of the condyle was marked on the chisel, allowance being made for the thickness of the cartilage and of the soft parts; the chisel was then driven home till the mark on it nearly reached the skin. The condyle having been first penetrated in its greatest depth, the chisel was partially withdrawn; its direction was altered, first forwards, then backwards; and, with a few oblique touches, due allowance being made for the varying depths, the condyle was felt to be sufficiently loose, when the instrument was withdrawn and the knee straightened. The joint was not entered ; no synovia escaped ; and the feeling of resistance to the chisel was not at any time overcome. Had this been the case, the joint must have been opened. It might, à priori, be thought that the uncut cartilage, with perhaps some slight uncut bony bridges, would either interfere with the reduction of the deformity, or would only yield after being broken. The result so far, in this case, does not confirm these objections, if they be serious objections. Experiment and experience must determine the matter in the case of adults ; but in children, in whom the condyles are not completely ossified, and what bone there is in the young cancellous tissue is soft and pliable, these objections do not hold. But, even if the cartilage were to fracture, or even if the joint were entered, say purposely, with the chisel, the proceeding would not be so severe as if done with a saw. Another modification in this operation is noteworthy. It has been said that the internal condyle was separated. It is more correct to say that the greater part of it was almost separated ; that is to say, that the chisel-cut did not extend to the intercondylar groove, but only to its inner side. The aim of this is to preserve some part of the inner condyle, which may grow, and thus obviate any possible future *genu extrorsum* which may be the consequence of the increased growth of the external condyle. All these operations, which may be termed rapid as contradistinguished from the older methods of splinting and tenotomy, when necessary, are too young to admit of any dogmatic statements about them ; but in the mean time we should adopt that method which is effectual and least risky. Deloie's, Ogston's, Max Schede's, Annandale's, and Macewen's, and the one just described, have all the same object with regard to this deformity ; but the methods of executing it differ. One, by *brisement forcé*, separates the upper tibial epiphysis ; another removes a wedge from the upper part of the tibia ; another attacks the femur ; and yet another removes a wedge from the internal condyle. Ogston's method and this agree in principle, but differ in execution and severity. The advantages of the extra-articular method seem to be, greater rapidity of execution, rendering it more strictly subcutaneous; much less damage to the bone, cartilage, and soft parts ; no interference with the knee-joint ; and, as the condyle is not completely separated, there is less likelihood of subsequent non-union and necrosis. Again, the resulting joint-surface will be more regular ; and, by leaving a part of the condyle, the probability of a genu extrorsum is much diminished.   Then there should be no difficulty with the case. As soon as the condyle has become firmly attached in its new position, the stiffness will only be due to having kept the knee fixed for some weeks, say five, and not to ankylosis, which has to be overcome by frequent passive motions under anæsthetics. In the present case it was endeavoured to make the section on the distal side of the line of junction of the epiphysal cartilage. This is considered important with reference to the future growth of the inner side of the femur. The operation was not antiseptic in the Listerian sense ; it was carried out in the same way as nineteen other osteotomies (five femora, ten tibiæ, and four fibulæ) by the same operator; and, as in these cases everything progressed as could be wished, no additional precaution was deemed necessary. Even this operation of minimum severity M 1. Reeves would at present confine to those cases of over-growth of the internal condyle in which the older methods are not applicable or have failed; but, as soon as experience shall have taught that there is nothing to counterbalance its many advantages, he would not hesitate to recommend and adopt it as the first means in the more severe cases of this deformity. Expensive and somewhat cumbrous apparatus become necessary after tenotomy, etc.; and they will not be needed in the case of surgically displaced condyle, the cause of the deformity—i. e., the overgrown condyle—being put in proper position. It should, in conclusion, be stated that there has been no rise in pulse or tempera-ture, and only such local pain as might naturally be expected.—*British Med. Journal,* May 25, 1878.

Disarticulation at the Elbow-joint.

Dr. VON LANGENBECK showed, at the late Congress of the Society of German Surgeons, a case in which this operation had been performed. Although the ope-ration was in much discredit, he had for several years performed it in all cases in which it was possible. He made an anterior flap. He was very careful to en-deavour to procure union by the first intention, and for this certain precautions were necessary. The skin about the elbow was so retractile that, in order to ob-tain sufficient covering for the stump, the incision must be made at least two-fifths of an inch below the epicondyles. The flap thus formed consisted only of skin and fascia. The separation of the ulna with the olecranon from the fossa of the humerus was very easy, if, after pushing the flap up and opening the joint, the knife were carried obliquely upwards so as to divide the lateral ligaments. The arm being then extended, the olecranon was exposed. The operation was com-pleted by dividing the tendon of the triceps extensor muscle. The patient shown had been operated on more than a month previously for sarcoma of the ulna, and was doing well.—*Lond. Med. Record,* May 15, 1878.

Resection of the Knee-Joint.

Dr. von LANGENBECK, at the late Congress of the Society of German Sur-geons, showed a girl aged three years, on whom he had operated a year previously, by making a semilunar incision on the inner side, extirpating the capsule of the joint with the bursa of the quadriceps, and sawing off the articular surface of the patella. The growth of the limb had not decreased, as about four-tenths of an inch had been removed, and there was shortening to the extent of about one-fifth of an inch.

Dr. PETERSEN (Kiel) had found in a case in which he performed resection of the knee three years ago, with retention of the epiphysal cartilage, that there was increase in length to the extent of more than an inch.

Dr. RIEDINGER (Würzburg) had preserved the patella in one case, freshening its surface and those of the femur and tibia, and fastening the bones together.

Dr. KÖNIG (Gottingen) had, in the course of eight or nine years, met with no case of shortening after preservation of the epiphysal cartilage, although he had observed flexion of the limb, depending apparently on bony, but in reality on cartilaginous ankylosis. He advised that the surgeon should endeavour to obtain a stiff and not a movable joint, and that the incision should be transverse. Dr. von Langenbeck preferred the inner semilunar incision, by which he had been enabled to preserve the muscular structures and the mobility of the joint, and which also facilitated the extirpation of the pouch of the synovial membrane. The latter object was fulfilled with more difficulty by transverse division of the patella, as recommended by Volkmann. His ultimate object was always to obtain a movable joint, as ankylosis interfered with the growth in length of the bone.

Dr. HÜTER was in favour of the anterior flap. The whole should be within view, so that not only might the articular cartilages be removed, but carious foci in the tibia—frequently the starting point of the whole disease—be discovered and scooped out. With this he combined drainage of the tibia, after opening its anterior surface with an American drill. Of five recent cases, he had obtained good motion in three; he removed the patella, but cut the ligamentum patellæ obliquely, so as to favour its union by first intention, and preserve the muscular apparatus.

Dr. KOCHER (Bern) had performed resection of the knee-joint twenty-five times with three deaths. He had occasionally met with shortening, in spite of the preservation of the epiphysal cartilages. He believed, with Dr. Hüter, that the antiseptic method was more favourable than the open treatment to obtaining movable joints. He had had deaths with the antiseptic method, but none with the open treatment. Dr. von Langenbeck always used extension when the dressing was applied, so as to leave an interval between the sawn surfaces of bone; the wound was closed by suture as far as the part where the drainage-tube was inserted.

Dr. SCHEDE had brought the sawn surfaces of bone together, partly by catgut, partly by silver wire, but had never obtained bony ankylosis.

Dr. HÜTER regarded a certain degree of mobility in the new joint as the best means of obviating an angular position of the limb. Oblique division of the ligamentum patellæ was followed by firm union, with the help of which the quadriceps extensor acted on the leg.

Dr. KÖNIG believed that mobility had nothing to do with the adhesion of the ligamentum patellæ. He followed antiseptic principles strictly in the after-treatment.—*London Med. Record*, May 15, 1878.

Midwifery and Gynæcology.

Cæsarean Section and Removal of Uterus.

Prof. SPATH related the following case to the Vienna Medical Society (*Allg. Wien. Med. Zeit.*, January 22) :—A woman, aged forty, was admitted into his clinic pregnant with her tenth child. She had borne five living children, had aborted three times, and in her last labour the child's head was perforated. For the last five years she had suffered from osteomalacia. She was pale and considerably emaciated, suffered from a considerable bronchial catarrh, and there was much albuminuria, together with œdema of the lower extremities. On examination it was found that so great a degree of contraction of the pelvis existed that the Cæsarean section was absolutely indicated. Endeavours were made, without much success, to increase her strength while she was kept in a separate room awaiting the occurrence of pains.

After mature reflection, guided by former experience, Prof. Spath resolved that he would perform the Cæsarean operation under Lister's method; and in

the case of the uterus not contracting completely, and thus endangering the occurrence of subsequent hemorrhage, he would proceed to its entire removal.
Although every case of Cæsarean section performed in the Vienna Lying-in Hospital during the last century had terminated fatally either from septicæmia, peritonitis, or hemorrhage, yet, encouraged by the success of Péan and Porro in their
cases of removal of the uterus, he hoped by the aid of Lister's method, and the
prompt extirpation of the uterus if necessary, to secure a better issue in this case.
Accordingly, on June 2, 1876, labour pains having become active, he performed
the Cæsarean operation, and removed a living child without any difficulty.   An
injection of ergotin had been previously made in order to secure energetic uterine
contraction ; but, as this did not take place, and as considerable hemorrhage occurred, which iced water failed to arrest, the extirpation of the uterus was
resolved on.   The uterus having been secured in the neighbourhood of its neck
by the chain of the écraseur, and raised up from the wound, Prof. Spath separated its body from the neck by some strokes with the scalpel.   The cavity of
the abdomen was carefully cleansed, and the wound was united, securing the
pedicle at its lower angle.   The whole operation scarcely occupied an hour.   The
patient soon came to, and complained but little of pain.   The subsequent course
of the case was most favourable, the highest temperature being 38.6° C.   The
albuminuria and œdema disappeared.   The patient's strength was kept up by
champagne, and the catarrh, which had been very troublesome, diminished.   On
the tenth day the end of the pedicle fell off ; and on the thirty-eighth day after
the operation the patient was able to stand, and eleven days afterwards to walk
in the garden.   On September 18 she was discharged cured.   In October the
small fistula which remained after the union of the rest of the wound had completely healed, and the patient was rid of all her suffering.

Prof. Spath exhibited the patient to the Society, then some eighteen months
after the operation, in the enjoyment of complete health, the pains caused heretofore by the osteomalacia having disappeared.   On examination, the freely
movable cervix could be felt high up, but no exudation was perceptible beyond.
Prof. Spath believes that this procedure will be found to deserve adoption in
preference to simple Cæsarean section.   The wound in the uterus is definitively
smaller, and can be submitted to external treatment, and uterine hemorrhage and
endometritis become impossible (nor can the woman, we may add, become again
pregnant, as sometimes happens notwithstanding the danger that has been run in
Cæsarean section).—*Med. Times and Gaz.*, April 20, 1878.

Cæsarean Section with Extirpation of the Uterus.

In the *Centralblatt für Gynäkologie*, March 2, 1878, Dr. MÜLLER, of Bern,
relates the following case :   E. R., aged 37, was delivered naturally of her first
child at the age of 22.   Since then she had given birth normally to four children.
Symptoms of osteomalacia appeared, however, in her third pregnancy.   Pregnant for the sixth time, she was found to present the beak-shaped pubis, heart-
shaped pelvic outlet, diminished stature, and lordosis, characteristic of osteomalacia.
Under chloroform, it was found that the pelvic bones could not be opened up.
The belly was remarkably pendulous.   The fœtal heart could be heard.   On
February 1 the waters broke, but labour-pains did not set in.   On February 2
there were feeble labour-pains.   On February 3, during several hours, there
were strong pains.   On February 4 she had strong pains ; the uterus was painful ; the fœtal heart was no longer to be heard.   In consequence of the rise in
temperature, quickened pulse, tympanites, and other signs, Dr. Müller arrived at
the conclusion that there was inflammation of the womb with death of the fœtus.

At eight P. M., under complete chloroform-narcosis and carbolic spray, an incision was made through the abdominal wall between the umbilicus and symphysis. The uterus, exposed, was twisted on its long axis, so that the left horn emerged from the abdominal wound and the body of the uterus followed. A ligature was then applied round the cervix, and the uterus opened outside the abdomen. The fœtus was delivered, and the placenta was removed without any bleeding from the placental site. The fœtus was dead, and the uterus contained some offensive gas and purulent fetid liquid. The uterus was then amputated above the ligature. There was no bleeding, and no fluid escaped into the abdomen. The pedicle was sewn to the sides of the abdominal wound, which was closed as in ovariotomy. A drainage-tube was left in between the pedicle and the last abdominal suture. On the second day, the pedicle disappeared into the abdomen. The ligature came away on the tenth day. The temperature and pulse fell immediately after the operation. On the day following the pulse was 84. At the time of reporting the case, seventeen days after the operation, Dr. Müller considered the patient out of all danger, and convalescent. He remarks that, had he not extirpated the uterus, the patient would have succumbed to pyæmia, symptoms of which were present at the operation. The rapid fall of temperature after the operation testified to the correctness of the treatment. He also lays stress on the good result of ligaturing the cervix, and thereby securing a bloodless operation.—*London Medical Record*, May 15, 1878.

—

Milk Fever.

In an elaborate paper read before the Dublin Obstetrical Society (*Dublin Journ. of Med. Sci.*, May, 1878) Mr. ARTHUR V. MACAN maintains that: 1. There is no rise in temperature necessarily accompanying the first secretion of the milk.

2. Pain and distension of the breasts may cause fever; but this fever differs greatly from that generally described as milk fever. It comes on somewhat later and lasts much longer; for, while milk fever is said usually to terminate in from 8 to 24 hours, this fever, in 65 per cent. of the cases, lasts more than 24 hours, and does not, I think, so frequently terminate in profuse sweating.

3. The pulse in these cases is often much slower than the temperature would seem to warrant.

4. In cases of fever, during the puerperal state, the presence of full breasts is not sufficient justification for at once diagnosing the case as one of milk fever.

—

Failure of Milk Diet in the Albuminuria of Pregnancy.

Dr. N. CHARLES, of Liege, relates (*Archives de Tocologie*, March, 1878) a case of albuminuria during pregnancy, in which a strict milk diet entirely failed to effect any benefit, and which resulted in eclampsia and ended fatally, in spite of all treatment. The patient was twenty-eight years old, and pregnant for the second time. Her first pregnancy had been cut short by eclamptic convulsions, which soon led to the expulsion of a stillborn fœtus of seven months. At the sixth month of the second pregnancy traces of albumen were discovered in the urine, but the general health was excellent, and there was no œdema. Iron was administered, and the patient ordered to take one litre of milk daily in addition to ordinary diet. A fortnight later the proportion of albumen had increased; gallic acid was then prescribed, with a purgative every other day and two litres of milk daily. Notwithstanding this treatment, the proportion of albumen continued to increase, the legs became œdematous, and there was occasional disturbance of sight. Exclusive milk diet and daily purgatives were now ordered. The question of induction of labour was considered, but as the general condition was good and the œdema did not further increase it was decided to wait, although on November 7th, 1876, the urine contained half its bulk of albumen.

Two days later, on the evening of the 9th, the patient was seized with intense gastralgia and bilious vomiting, without any other symptoms. A draught containing chloral and morphia was administered, but was partially rejected, and did not relieve the pain. At 4.30 A. M. an eclamptic convulsion occurred, followed within half an hour by a second. It was said that during the gastralgic pain the patient had felt convulsive movements in the uterus. She was now found unconscious, and the fœtal heart could no longer be heard. A third convulsion followed at 5.30. The patient was then bled to eight ounces and the legs were scarified, giving exit to a large quantity of serum. Soon after, 0.01 grm. of hydrochlorate of morphia was injected subcutaneously, and a purgative administered. Very little of this could be taken by the mouth, and the rest was afterwards given as an enema. Chloroform was also given by inhalation whenever a convulsion appeared to be threatened. The fifth fit occurred at seven o'clock, and the sixth at nine. Meanwhile two more subcutaneous injections of morphia had been given, and the administration was now commenced of chloral and bromide of potassium by enema every quarter of an hour. By this time the os was dilated to the size of a two-franc piece. At eleven o'clock the temperature was 37° C. The os was dilated to the size of a two-franc piece, and at this time an India-rubber dilator was inserted and the morphia injection repeated for the fourth time. By noon the os was dilated, and the head had descended into the cavity of the pelvis. Short forceps were applied, and a stillborn female child, 42 cm. long, was extracted. The urine, withdrawn at this time by catheter, was tinged with blood, had a specific gravity 1028, and became almost solid with heat or nitric acid.

The patient remained in the most profound coma, and fits recurred at 1, at 3, at 4.30, at 6, and at 8 P. M. At 4.30 P. M. the temperature was $38^\circ.3$ C., pulse 80; at 8 P. M. the temperature was $39^\circ.9$ C., pulse 110; and at this time loud bronchial and tracheal râles had commenced. On the morning of the 11th there was apparent improvement; the râles had diminished, and the temperature fallen to $39^\circ.4$ C., but the pulse was 120 and small. Two enemata were given, containing each two drops of croton oil, but only one slight motion was procured. In the evening the temperature had fallen to $38^\circ.9$ C., but the pulse was 125 and very small; râles had again increased. On the morning of the 12th the temperature was $38^\circ.0$ C., pulse 130. Towards noon the patient died, without having for a moment recovered consciousness.

The author remarks upon the total failure in this case of the prophylactic treatment, with regard to which such high hopes had been raised by M. Tarnier. He notes that the kidneys must have retained, if not an actually diseased condition, at any rate a very decided morbid susceptibility ever since the affection which led to the clampsia in the first pregnancy. He points out also that the temperature did not follow in this case the law laid down by Bourneville, who concluded that it always became elevated in eclampsia, and in fatal cases rose progressively to an excessively high point. In this instance, after several fits, the temperature was normal. At a later period it rose considerably, but again descended before death.—*Obstetrical Journal of Great Britain*, June, 1878.

Puerperal Insanity.

The following statistics and observations are quoted from a recent work by Dr. RIPPING, in a review published in the *Irrenfreund* (1878, No. 2).

Of 780 female patients admitted into the asylum at Siegburg during the four years 1872–5, 168 suffered from puerperal psychoses in the widest sense of the term, *i. e.*, including the insanity of pregnancy and of lactation. This gives a percentage of 21.6, whereas that observed in eight other asylums varies between 7 and 16.8. The author attributes this fact partly to the greater frequency with which these patients are now taken to asylums instead of being treated at home, partly to the increasing accuracy of statistics, and partly to the faulty physical development of the women, especially those belonging to the manufacturing classes in the neighbourhood of Düsseldorf.

The 168 cases are divided as follows:—

Insanity of pregnancy	.	.	.	.	. 32 = 19 per cent..
Puerperal insanity proper	.	.	.	.	. 89 = 53 "
Insanity of lactation	.	.	.	.	. 47 = 28 "

In accordance with previous observations, melancholia was found to be the most frequent form of the insanity at its commencement; it occurred in 63.6 per cent. of all the cases; mania in 34.5. During the period of pregnancy, melancholia was still more common; it occurred in 84.4 per cent. of the cases; this form of psychosis was also seen in 68 per cent. of the cases of insanity due to lactation.

The author describes a number of cases in which two forms of insanity were combined, or rather followed one another; these he divides into four groups. 1. Melancholia followed by mania; twelve cases were observed; the two forms of psychosis were quite distinct, and lasted each about the same time. 2. Melancholia followed by delusional insanity (*Wahnsinn*); the latter does not succeed the former as a secondary form of insanity, but as a separate and independent affection. 3. Mania followed by delusional insanity, in which the delusions of persecutions, etc., at first occasionally observed during the maniacal excitement, gradually get the upper hand, and under the influence of hallucination, become permanent. 4. Mania with subsequent melancholia; this is simply the reverse of the first group.

The author quotes his statistics, to show that the proportion of cases with hereditary predisposition differs so slightly from those without it, that it cannot be considered as having much to do with the causation of insanity in these cases.

Patients aged from 30 to 35 seem most prone to melancholia, while younger women are more frequently attacked by mania.

Prognosis is more favourable in puerperal cases than in all cases of insanity in women taken together; but the author's figures do not show so high a proportion of recoveries as has usually been given. He attributes this to a more strict distinction between cases discharged *recovered* and those only *improved*, than used to be the case. Of the patients suffering from mania, 62 per cent. and 33.6 per cent. of those with melancholia, recovered. The combined forms afford the least favourable prognosis; of the cases described above under the second group, not one recovered. Heredity does not appear to exercise any special influence on the prognosis. Figures show that the earlier the patients are brought under treatment, the greater is the percentage of recoveries. Subsequent attacks of insanity are always more favourable as regards prognosis than primary ones. The average duration of the attacks in the patients who recovered was—for melancholia ten months, and for mania seven months.

Insanity of Pregnancy.—The author finds that insanity is more common in the latter than in the earlier months of pregnancy; in all the cases observed by him the patient's power of resistance had been diminished by hereditary tendency, previous attacks, disturbances of circulation or of the emotions. Illegitimate pregnancy is a very frequent cause of insanity; hereditary predisposition appears to have much more influence at this time, than in the puerperal period or during lactation. The liability to insanity seems to diminish in each successive pregnancy. Of the cases of melancholia under this head, 58.5 per cent. only were pure melancholia, the remainder consisted of the combined forms commencing with melancholia. In subsequent relapses, the form of insanity which existed in the original attack is never repeated. The author confirms the statements of Leidesdorf and Hohn as to the prognosis being very unfavourable in the psychoses of pregnancy; it is especially bad (1) when the attack comes on in the earlier months of pregnancy, (2) when there is hereditary predisposition, and (3) after 30 years of age. The percentage of deaths to cases was as high as 12.5.

Insanity of Puerperal Period.—The attack commences within a fortnight after delivery, and usually in the second half of the first week. Hereditary predisposition tends to bring on the attack earlier than would otherwise be the case; 29.2 of the cases occurred after the first labour. The author believes that complication, such as hemorrhage, parametritis, etc., occurring during or after labour, are frequent causes of insanity; also grief at the death of the child. The pure forms of melancholia and mania are much more common at this time than the combined. Melancholia is most frequent after 30 years of age, also when the attack commences within the first few days after delivery. The percentage of recoveries was—of all cases, 46.3; of the cases of pure melancholia, 40.6; of mania, 54.5. Youth, the early outbreak of the disease after delivery, and timely removal to an asylum, are all favourable elements in the prognosis. The average duration of the attack in cases which recovered was eight months, against nine months in the insanity of pregnancy. The psychoses after abortion were most frequent in the second or third month of pregnancy; they generally occurred after free and persistent hemorrhage in patients who were weakened by frequent pregnancies and enforced rest. The form of insanity and the prognosis are similar to those of the puerperal cases, but the great prevalence of hallucinations of sight, and the occurrence of local muscular spasms in the limbs without loss of consciousness, are noticeable peculiarities. The average duration of the cases which recovered was only five months, owing to the rapid disappearance of the anæmia.

Insanity of Lactation.—This most commonly commences in the second half of the second month after delivery or later, in patients whose powers have been gradually weakened by pregnancy, labour, puerperal troubles, and lactation. A rapid succession of labours, or prolonged rest, with affections of the generative system, predispose strongly to the attacks of insanity. Melancholia is by far the most common form of psychosis at this time. Neither age nor heredity seemed to play any important part in the etiology, but it was noted that the earlier the attacks commenced the more frequently were they in the form of melancholia. The prognosis is not so favourable as under the other heads, but fatal cases are rare. The tendency of the disease to pass into chronic delusional insanity, and the frequency of hallucinations of hearing, are very marked. The duration in cases of recovery averaged 9.5 months.—*London Medical Record,* May 15, 1878.

--

Treatment of Amenorrhœa.

Prof. COURTY employs (*Union Med.,* Feb. 19) a pill composed of powdered rue, savin, and ergot, of each five centigrammes, and aloes from 2–5 centigrammes. Of these thirty are ordered, and three are taken the first day, six the second day, and nine the third day, always in three doses. They are suited for cases of idiopathic amenorrhœa, without great reaction on the economy,

and when there is reason to suppose that the suppression of the menses is due
either to an insufficient determination towards the genital organs or to a difficulty
of discharge due to inertia of the uterus. In order to encourage the fluxion
towards the genital organs, Dr. County orders, before beginning the pills, foot
baths, sitz baths, and fumigations. He also applies leeches to the labia during
the three days the pills are being taken. The pills generally induce colicky
pains and often a little diarrhœa.—*Practitioner*, May, 1878.

Effusion of Blood into the Peritoneal Cavity.

At a late meeting of the Obstetrical Society of London (*Med. Examiner*,
May 9, 1878) Dr. ROBERT BARNES showed specimens from two cases, illustrative of two different forms of blood effusion into the peritoneum and pelvis. The
first case was that of a woman, æt. 40, who had borne children, and was said to
have ceased menstruating eight weeks before her illness. This began on the
evening of April 20th, after a fatiguing journey, with a sickening pain in the left
inguinal region, which continued till the next morning. It was then found that
the os uteri was closed, the uterus was movable, and there was no great tenderness in the left inguinal region, the seat of the pain. On the afternoon of the
next day she suddenly became much worse, collapse set in, and she shortly sank
and died. At the post-mortem examination on opening the abdomen the intestines, as high as the umbilicus, were found covered with blood, four pounds of
which, in the form of clot and fluid, were removed from the peritoneal cavity,
almost as much being left behind   The seat of the hemorrhage was found to be
the sac of a tubal fœtation, which had ruptured spontaneously. The sac was situated on the left Fallopian tube, not far from the angle of the uterus. The case
was of interest, as showing how large an amount of blood could be poured out
from a small space.

The second case was that of a patient in St. George's Hospital, who, having
been admitted for some other complaint was found to be suffering from retroversion of the uterus. There was considerable distress, and on vaginal examination
the body of the uterus, which was greatly enlarged, was found imprisoned under
the promontory of the sacrum. The reduction was made without much difficulty, and a Hodge's pessary was put in. A few days later she suddenly became
much worse, and during an effort of expulsion the pessary was forced out; this
was followed by great distress, and the patient died in a state of collapse. On
post-mortem examination the uterus was found much bent back and enlarged.
The parts about Douglas's pouch inclosed an enormous quantity of blood,
part of which was evidently of recent origin, and part of long standing.
Blood was effused widely into the peritoneum ; the artificial cavity formed
by the retroverted uterus was filled with blood and blood-clot, and lined
with a firm fibrinous layer. Both the Fallopian tubes were widened in their
middle third, while the right tube bore at its end a blood-clot the size of a Tan-
gerine orange. In this case the retroversion had caused backward distension, and
the blood, being unable to escape from the uterine cavity, had passed down and
distended the Fallopian tubes. This was one of the sources of retro-uterine
hæmatocele, and in connection with it he might mention a case that had occurred
some years ago in the London Hospital. Here a solution of perchloride of iron
was injected into a retroverted uterus, was forced along the Fallopian tubes by
the uterine contraction, and escaping into the abdominal cavity set up fatal inflammation of the peritoneum. The fact was that the blood, when injected into
the uterine cavity, acted as a foreign body, and excited contraction, and if it
could not escape by the natural outlet it was forced along the Fallopian tubes.
Hence one great reason for reducing retroflexions of the uterus.

Dr. John Williams said that the second specimen illustrated an important point in the natural history of retroflexion, and that was that in this condition the reflux of blood was prevented by the pressure of the fibroid bands of the retro-uterine ligaments. This fact accounted for the great enlargement of the uterus in retroflexion as compared with anteflexion. Dr. Hayes related a case which he thought contrasted well with the first one brought forward by Dr. Baines. The patient, who applied at King's College Hospital on Saturday last, said she had had a miscarriage six to eight weeks previously. She had a very rapid pulse, 140–150, and a temperature of 102°. The abdomen was distended and tender, and the patient was almost in a state of collapse. She thought she was six weeks pregnant when she miscarried. On vaginal examination the uterus was found fixed, and a large mass occupied the posterior cul-de-sac. She died the same night. The post-mortem examination disclosed general peritonitis in its first stage, together with the effusion of a large quantity of sanguineous fluid. The top of the uterus was covered by a large clot of blood, and Douglas's space was filled with a perfectly round and firm coagulum of considerable size, encircled by a dense layer of membrane. On removal of the uterus and its appendages, the sac of an extra-uterine fœtation was found in connection with the left Fallopian tube, while a corpus luteum was found torn and partially extruded from its nest. There was evidence of a decidual membrane occupying the uterus, which organ was about as large as at the third or fourth week of utero-gestation. The case was interesting as being one in which the rupture of an extra-uterine fœtation had not been attended as usual with sudden death. Dr. Wiltshire asked whether in Dr. Baines's cases the effused blood had spread up along the spinal column. He asked this question because he saw reason to maintain that when hemorrhage occurred free into the abdominal cavity the blood obeyed the laws of hydrostatics, tending to gravitate along the spinal column and not accumulating especially in the pelvis. The question, however, of more immediate clinical interest was the treatment of these cases of extra-uterine fœtation. During the discussion on Mr. Jessop's case the point had been raised as to whether it was justifiable on the rupture of the sac to open the abdomen and ligature the bleeding point. The second case he thought was interesting as showing post-mortem retroflexion of the uterus, a condition the very existence of which had been denied by some eminent pathologists. Dr. Heywood Smith briefly alluded to a case in which pelvic hæmatocele had suddenly occurred, and the patient had passed a decidual membrane five days afterwards. He had no doubt at the time that this was a case of tubal pregnancy, and the question arose as to whether the hæmatocele should be punctured. This was decided in the negative, and after an interval of three or four years the effused mass was found to have been entirely absorbed, while the uterus had become perfectly movable.

—

Spontaneous Expulsion of a Large Fibroid Tumour.

In a paper read before the Société de Médicine de Lyon, Dr. Ygovin relates a case of an enormous intra-uterine fibroid which ended fortunately after spontaneous expulsion, the patient having been long in great peril of life It occurred in a single lady forty-three years old. Menses commenced at the age of eleven, and were normal until 1867, when she began to suffer from dysmenorrhœa, and after this time menstruation gradually became irregular and profuse. In July, 1871, the author was called in on account of sudden and severe flooding, which was checked by ergot and cold applications. This recurred from time to time, and in January, 1873, was so severe as to threaten life. A vaginal examination was then for the first time obtained. The finger on being introduced into the vagina encountered a large, hard, rounded body, of the size of a fœtal head at full term. The os uteri was displaced backwards and upwards so far as to be out of reach. For the next year the patient was under homœopathic treatment, and the author was not again called in till February, 1876. The pulse was then rapid and small, the tongue furred, extremities cold, bowels constipated, the swelling in the hypogastric region increased, and the abdomen somewhat tympanitic. For some time the severe hemorrhage had been replaced by a sanious, thick, offensive discharge. She was still able to walk about the room, but generally kept her bed. Vaginal examination gave the same result as before, and it was still imposssble to reach the os uteri. All surgical interference was therefore judged to be impracticable.

She continued much in the same state till May, 1875, when the author was summoned on account of temporary retention of urine. The tumour had then not appreciably changed its position, but the general health had become more feeble, and there was much difficulty in overcoming an obstinate constipation. The author only saw the patient at long intervals up to June, 1876, at which time her state had very greatly changed for the worse. The face was puffy and pale, and there was considerable œdema of all the limbs, especially the legs ; the abdomen was also distended by ascitic fluid ; the pulse was thready, and extremities cold. On the inside of both feet were gangrenous patches, which afterwards became converted into sanious ulcers, of which the cure was long and difficult. The patient could not lie down without being threatened with suffocation, and for about two and a half months she had not quitted her arm-chair night or day. On vaginal examination, the tumour was found to be slightly projecting through the os uteri, and thus was explained a colicky pain of which the patient had complained a few days before. The labia were highly œdematous. In view of the very grave general state, the author determined on a plan which he had before found useful in similar conditions ; namely, to put in action a powerful local derivative by making a series of issues in each leg with potassa fusa. An abundant discharge of pus mixed with a great quantity of serum was thus produced ; the general œdema gradually diminished, the dyspnœa was relieved, and the patient was enabled to rest in bed and obtain sleep. The gangrenous ulcers of the feet gradually healed, and at the end of about two months œdema had given place to extreme emaciation, which from that time went on increasing.

At the end of September pain again set in, and on October 2d the author was summoned on account of retention of urine. The tumour had then completely descended into the pelvis, and partially passed the os uteri, presenting by one extremity in the form of an elongated hard body, which filled all the upper part of the vagina. This so compressed the urethra that catheterism was difficult. Often the catheter entered a false passage, and reached a cavity, at 20 cm. depth, from which issued offensive sanious pus. After a while the bladder regained its functions, and with the exception of occasional hemorrhage, no grave accident occurred up to September, 1877. Although tempted to interfere and attempt the removal of the tumour, after dilatation of the cervix, the author refrained from doing so, fearing the hemorrhage and other risks of the operation in the patient's feeble condition. The final issue of the case occurred in the temporary absence of the author. On September 12th retention of urine occurred, and the catheter was passed with difficulty, the tumour occupying then the whole extent of the entrance of the vulva. On the 15th uterine contractions, like those of labour, set in, and on the morning of the 16th the tumour was found almost completely expelled, and was readily detached, the pedicle or base having been apparently separated and destroyed by the suppuration which had occurred in it. The tumour formed a mass weighing 650 grammes (about 1 pound 7 oz.) and was 18 cm.

long, the greatest circumference being 37 cm.   The place of insertion of the pedicle could not be distinctly made out.—*Obstetrical Journal of Great Britain*, May, 1878, from *Archives de Tocologie*, February, 1878.

Medical Jurisprudence and Toxicology.

A Remedy for the Eruption of Poison Oak, Ivy, and Sumach.

Dr. S. A. BROWN, U. S. N., reports (*Med. Record*, April 20, 1878) that he has found a specific for the eruption caused by contact with poison oak, sumach, ivy, huahoo, cashew nut, etc.   He writes: "This specific is *bromine*.   I have used it with the same unvarying success in at least forty cases.   The eruption never extends after the first thorough application, and it promptly begins to diminish.   Within twenty-four hours, if the application be persisted in, the patient is entirely cured.   There is no pain attending its use, as from that of astringents.   Of course, the epidermis peels off as after other treatment.

"I use the bromine dissolved in olive oil, in cosmoline, or in glycerine.   The application with glycerine is painful, and, I think, possesses no advantage to compensate for the irritation.   The strength of the solution is from ten to twenty drops of bromine to the ounce of oil, used by rubbing gently on the affected part three or four times a day, and especially on going to bed at night.   You wash off the oil twice a day with castile soap.

"The bromine is so volatile that the solution should be renewed within twenty-four hours of its preparation, as it will get out of a bottle, however well-corked.   It is best to stand the bottle on its cork end, in the intervals of application.

Turpentine Vapour in Accidents from Chloroform Vapour.

Dr. WACHSMUTH, of Berlin, has suggested the use of turpentine vapour as a preventive of those accidents which frequently occur in the administration of chloroform to produce anæsthesia.   He says (*Vierteljahrsschrift für Gerichtliche Medicin*, April 1878) that it is well known to every physician that death often takes place suddenly from the vapour of chloroform, in spite of the greatest care and the use of every precaution before and during its administration.   The operator, even when assisted by three or four of his colleagues, may see his patients die before him.   There is, he states, a very easy and simple remedy for preventing the occurrence of such a serious accident.   It consists in the addition of one part of rectified oil of turpentine to five parts of chloroform.   The oil of turpentine in vapour appears to exert a stimulating or life-giving effect on the lungs, and protects these organs from passing into that paralyzed state which seems to be produced by chloroform-narcosis.   Dr. Wachsmuth, while lying on a sick bed, accidentally breathed the vapour of turpentine, and he experienced from this a strongly refreshing feeling.   This fact induced him to try the plan of adding oil of turpentine to chloroform when the latter was used for anæsthetic purposes.   The beneficial results surpassed his expectation.—*London Med. Record*, May 15, 1878.

CONTENTS.

Published Monthly, price $2.50 per annum, free of postage.
Also, furnished together with the AMERICAN JOURNAL OF THE MEDICAL
SCIENCES *and the* MEDICAL NEWS AND LIBRARY *for* SIX DOLLARS *per
annum in advance, the whole free of postage.*

HENRY C. LEA, Philadelphia.

THE MONTHLY ABSTRACT

OF

MEDICAL SCIENCE.

VOL. V. No. 8.   **For List of Contents see last page.**   AUGUST, 1878.

Anatomy and Physiology.

The Origin of the Chorda Tympani.

AT a meeting of the Académic des Sciences of Paris on April 29th, M. VULPIAN announced the results of an important series of experiments made to determine the true origin of the chorda tympani nerve. It is well known that disease or injury to the facial nerve in the aqueductus Fallopii—that is, above the separation of the chorda tympani—produces partial loss of gustatory sensation in the anterior two-thirds of the same side of the tongue, together with dryness of the same part and arrest of secretion of the submaxillary gland. This different action from that of the facial, and the fact that the fibres of the chorda tympani are finer than those of the former nerve, have led to the belief that the deep origin must be different. One view is that it arises from the so-called intermediate nerve of Wrisberg, which is by some held to be a bulbar root of the sympathetic, by others a part of the glosso-pharyngeal nerve, the latter being the view now held to be most correct. The other hypothesis is that the chorda tympani is formed by fibres from the superior maxillary branch of the fifth nerve, which pass backwards to join the facial close to the geniculate ganglion. M. Vulpian's experiments were directed to ascertain which, if either, of these hypotheses is correct. It is now known by the researches of J. L. Prevost that removal of the spheno-palatine ganglion causes no degeneration in the great superficial petrosal nerve, through which the fibres from the fifth are supposed to pass; nor does it, according to M. Vulpian, affect the nutrition of the chorda tympani.

In order to determine the relation to the facial and nerve of Wrisberg, M. Vulpian divided these nerves at the entrance into the internal auditory meatus. On examining the nerves from ten to twenty days later, it was found that all the fibres of the facial were more or less atrophied, but those of the chorda tympani intact. The great superficial petrosal was altered, but the nerve to the tensor tympani was unaffected. Similar results followed the section of the facial nerve near its origin, complete atrophy of all the peripheral branches resulting, but the chorda tympani being unchanged. But these experiments made on dogs were inconclusive, for it is possible that the geniculate ganglion is the trophic ganglion of the chorda tympani, and hence section above this would not cause atrophy. In another series of experiments on rabbits, M. Vulpian endeavoured to determine the effect of section of the fifth nerve within the skull. On account of difficulties in dividing the nerve completely without causing fatal injury, the results were inconclusive, but so far as they went they showed that complete section of the fifth was followed by atrophy of the chorda tympani, the facial remaining unaltered. It was also observed that when the motor root of the fifth had been divided, the fibres supplying the tensor tympani were atrophied. The experiments, so far as they go, indicate the great probability of the origin of the chorda tympani from the fifth nerve, and Ϩ. Vulpian promised to communicate the results of further observations directed to the solution of the question.--*Lancet*, June 15, 1878.

Physiology of the Salivary Secretion.

The first number of the new *Journal of Physiology*, edited by Dr. Michael Foster, contains an interesting article by Dr. LANGLEY on the Physiology of the Salivary Secretion. In this paper Dr. Langley points out that the well-known effects of stimulation of the chorda tympani and sympathetic nerve on the secretion—the former yielding a watery, the latter a viscid, saliva—are true only in the case of the dog, and that precisely the opposite effects occur in the ease of the cat. In this animal both the secretions are watery, but the sympathetic saliva is less viscid or more watery than the chorda saliva. It was known again, from Heidenhain's experiments, that the action of atropine is different on the behaviour of the chorda and sympathetic nerves, a very small dose completely paralyzing the chorda, whilst a very large one does not paralyze the sympathetic. Dr. Langley, however, finds that in the cat atropine readily paralyzes the sympathetic secretion, as well as that of the chorda, and even thinks that in the case of the dog the difference is more one of degree than of kind. He is unable to speak positively, but seems inclined to think that the atropine acts both on the nerve-endings and upon the cells themselves. Kühne was of opinion that the two nerves are antagonistic, but even assuming this to be the case in the dog, it does not hold good for the cat, in which Dr. Langley finds that minimal effective stimuli, when applied simultaneously to the chorda and sympathetic nerves, are not antagonistic as regards secretion ; on the contrary, the amount of secretion from the simultaneous stimulation is at least equal to the sum or the amounts from separate stimulation. He finds, further, that impulses travelling down one nerve produce their effect on the salivary cells, whether the other nerve be functionally active or not.—*Lancet*, June 15, 1878.

Materia Medica and Therapeutics.

The Action of Anæsthetics.

The double danger of anæsthetics, arising from their variable influence on the respiratory and cardiac centres, has long been familiar to those engaged in their administration. This double action has been lately studied on animals by Ϩ. VULPIAN, who has communicated to the Académie des Sciences a note on the subject of some practical interest. The special 'point which it embraces is the effect of the various anæsthetic agents on the pneumogastric, as shown by the test afforded by the experiments of Weber and Traube on the section and stimulation of the nerve.

Curara, as is well known, does not influence, in any considerable degree, the effect on the heart of faradization of the divided pneumogastrics. The heart is arrested in paralytic relaxation, but gradually, after some seconds, its movements recommence, even though the ends of the pneumogastrics are still being stimulated. Nevertheless, the effect of faradization of the peripheral segments of the pneumogastrics is not absolutely the same in a curarized and in an unpoisoned animal. The effect of faradization of a single vagus is less marked, and the diastolic arrest of the heart is less prolonged under the influence of curara. If the influence of the poison is profound, there is a period during which the strongest faradization of the pneumogastrics has no other effect upon the heart than to accelerate its movements. From this it is evident that the curara does not, as was once supposed, leave intact the cardiac extremities of these nerves.

Anæsthetics, however, have been found by N. Vulpian also to have a marked and very different influence on the excitation of the peripheral extremities of the pneumogastrics, and a still greater influence on the effect of excitation of the central extremities of the same nerves. The effect of chloral hydrate may be taken as an instance of this. If a solution of chloral be injected into the vein of a dog in a quantity sufficient to produce a profound sleep, complete anæsthesia is produced. The movements of the heart and of respiration continue. Occasionally, especially if the injection has been rapid, the respiratory movements suddenly cease, the heart continuing to beat for some minutes. Commonly the breathing recommences if artificial respiration is maintained for a few minutes, or if the trunk be faradized, intermittently, about twenty times a minute. It is sometimes necessary to continue this respiration for ten or twenty minutes before the spontaneous movements recommence. Occasionally this respiratory syncope, as it is termed by N. Vulpian, occurs only some time after the injection, and during an experiment, perhaps in consequence of the traumatic irritation. Very similar accidents may be observed in animals placed under the influence of ether, chloroform, and analogous substances.

Another accident which may occur in dogs under the influence of chloral is the more or less sudden arrest of the heart's action, either during the intravenous injection or during an experiment involving irritation of the sensory nerves. The respiratory movements continue for some seconds after the heart has ceased to beat. It is very rarely that the cardiac contraction can be restored, even by faradization employed at the moment at which the heart has ceased to beat. This cardiac syncope is also observed in animals under the influence of ether and chloroform. It is certainly sometimes due to the reflex influence of nerves irritated during an operation, but occurs as a result of this irritation much more readily in animals under the influence of an anæsthetic than in those which are not, or which are under the influence of curara. The comparative immunity from this accident which is presented by curarized animals is no doubt to be attributed to the influence of the poison in moderating the action of the pneumogastrics upon the heart.

From the phenomena mentioned above it is evident that the respiratory centre suffers remarkably in animals under the influence of anæsthetics, and especially under that of chloral. A slight increase in the quantity of chloral in the circulation, or a reflex influence, may arrest its action. So also with the cardiac centre. If the experiment of faradizing the pneumogastrics is repeated upon animals under the influence of chloral, it is found that the stimulation of the central ends of the divided nerves arrests the movements of respiration, just as in an animal of the same kind under normal conditions; but whereas in the latter the respiratory movements go on again spontaneously and easily in most cases, in spite of the continuance of the stimulation, they do not return spontaneously in dogs under the influence of chloral, and the animals die unless the faradization is stopped and artificial respiration employed, either alone or with the addition of intermitting faradization of the trunk. Sometimes a few seconds' faradization of the superior segments of the vagus nerve is sufficient to produce this arrest. Thus under these conditions we may have, on faradization of the central ends of the divided pneumogastrics, the same effect which N. Paul Bert has observed in animals not chloralized—sudden death. If the experiment is repeated in the same dog, the same result may be obtained two or three times, but not more. It is subsequently impossible thus to cause a persistent arrest of respiration. The spontaneous movements return after a suspension of a greater or less duration, although the faradization of the superior extremities of the vagi is continued. If in the same complete chloralization the peripheral extremities of the pneumo-gastrics are faradized, the heart is arrested in diastole just as in animals, under normal conditions, and, what is rarely observed otherwise, it may be permanently arrested if the stimulation is prolonged for a short time.

These experiments illustrate very strikingly the phenomena which are some-times observed in man, and they are of especial value in their proof of the influ-ence which traumatic irritation may have in arresting the action of a centre depressed by the influence of an anæsthetic. But the experiments stop just where we should like them to go on. The differences in this respect, if any, which are to be ob-served between ether and chloroform is a point of great practical importance, and on which we hope M. Vulpian may be able to furnish us with further infor-mation.—*Lancet*, June 22, 1878.

On Myotics and Mydriatics.

M. PANAS (*France Médicale*) observes that the physiological observations of Adamuk, Grunhagen, and others, indicate that atropine diminishes intraocular pressure. On the other hand, the clinical experience of von Gräfe, Wharton Jones, and Ernest Hart, has shown that atropine increases ocular pressure in the glaucomatous condition; and they have laid down the rule that the clinical use of atropine is to be strictly avoided in pathological conditions accompanied by increased intraocular tension. M. Panas considers that the two groups of ob-servations are not necessarily opposed; in the physiological condition atropine diminishes tension, in the pathological condition it augments tension. The latter effect is explained by the fact that atropine contracts the vessels in dilating the pupil, and causes the blood of the iris to flow backward to the ciliary processes. Further, atropine paralyzes the circular muscular fibres of the vessels; thus, there is a more considerable afflux of blood, and, consequently, exaggerated tension of the eye. The effect of eserine in the physiological state would be, on the con-trary, to contract the sphincter muscle of the pupil and the ciliary muscle, whence the tension is augmented. But, in glaucoma, eserine may contribute to diminish the intraocular tension, because, in contracting the vessels and narrowing the pupil, it enlarges the canal of Fontana. The canal of Fontana, situate in the circumference of the iris must, of course, not be confounded here with the canal of Schlemm, which is situated at the junction of the ciliary processes, cornea, and sclerotic.—*London Medical Record*, June 15, 1878.

An Undescribed Effect of the Action of Chloral Hydrate.

I. RANKE injected (*Bayr. ärztliche Intelligenzblatt*, No. 30, 1877) into the crural artery of a rabbit a ten per cent. watery solution of chloral hydrate, and observed that after a few fibrillar contractions, the muscles of the limb passed into a condition of rigidity, resembling that which results from the injection of chloroform. But if a solution of hydrate of chloral be added to a solution of myosin, no drops with myosin sheath or investment are produced as on the addition of chloroform, but well-marked rigidity is observed. Ranke concludes from this that the chloral hydrate precipitates the albumen as chloral molecule, and that this in all probability occasions the muscle-rigor. In conclusion he warns practitioners of the danger of the injection of chloral into the veins with the object of producing narcosis, on account of its action on the heart.—*Practi-tioner*, June, 1878.

The Antiseptic and Therapeutic Properties of Boracic Acid.

G. POLLI has reported at a recent meeting of the Academy of Sciences of Lombardy the results of numerous researches in which beer, meat, eggs, blood, and urine were treated with boracic acid and borax for thirty days during the summer time, and were found still to retain their freshness, and to present no traces of fermentation having taking place in them.   In control experiments, on the other hand, without the addition of the salt, but, in some instances, with the addition of sulphate of soda, the fluids passed into a state of complete decomposition in the course of fifteen days.   The energetic disinfecting power possessed by boracic acid and borax, and the facility with which these substances can be absorbed into the economy, led Polli to recommend their employment in diseases in regard to the infectious nature of which no doubt exists, or in which septic conditions readily arise.   He adduces several examples in which the febrile conditions of tuberculosis underwent diminution.   No benefit was obtained by Professor Visconti from experiments made with these remedies in malaria, though other observers have arrived at a different conclusion.   In chronic cystitis the muco-purulent discharge quickly diminished, and even altogether disappeared in the course of a few days, and rapid improvement occurred in cases of bad suppurating wounds when they were applied externally.   The dose recommended by Polli is 75 grains of boracic acid and 150 grains of borax per diem.—*Lancet,* June 15, 1878.

—

On the Action of Cyclamin.

In an article published in *Il Morgagni* for December, Dr. CHIRONE describes a number of experiments on the physiological action of cyclamin, made in the pharmacological laboratory of the University of Naples, and sums up in the following conclusions.

1. Cyclamin has a very important local action, especially on the subcutaneous connective tissue, in which it produces sloughing and extensive ulceration; this, however, heals spontaneously, and seldom or never causes the death of the animal.

2. Cyclamin kills all animals without distinction by its general action.

3. Cyclamism, or the physiological action of cyclamin, is manifested by the following symptoms: stupefaction; hyperæsthesia, which may sometimes lead to spontaneous convulsions; fall of temperature; weakness and frequency of the movements of the heart; respiration sometimes frequent and shallow, sometimes rare, deep, and difficult.   With a larger dose, the symptoms are: increased stupefaction; very great hyperæsthesia, and convulsions readily produced; considerable rise of temperature; the heart's action weak, hurried, and irregular; respirations irregular; ready production of serous exudations with effusion of hæmatin; finally, rapid fall of temperature, coma, and death.

4. The action of cyclamin never shows itself with great rapidity, and may last three or four days, or may kill within forty-eight hours.   The slowness of its action is due to slowness of absorption.

5. Cyclamin acts directly on the blood, and influences the whole system by the grave changes which it produces in the blood.

6. Cyclamin blackens the blood as soon as it comes into contact with it.

7. The spectrum of oxyhæmoglobin is profoundly modified by cyclamin.   In the first place, the two striæ characteristic of oxyhæmoglobin disappear, and the band peculiar to reduced hæmoglobin comes into view.   Hæmoglobin reduced by cyclamin, however, does not for several days lose its tendency and again become oxidized; and, if it be shaken in contact with air, the striæ of oxyhæmoglobin reappear.   The prolonged action of cyclamin decomposes hæmoglobin and libe-

lates hæmatin; sometimes producing in the spectrum a dark band on the red in the vicinity of the line c of Fraunhofer, sometimes two very faint bands between D and E. When the hæmoglobin is decomposed, all absorption-bands disappear from the spectrum of blood treated with cyclamin, except that of hæmatin. The hæmatin bands, however, soon disappear in consequence of its spontaneous absorption.

8. A solution of hæmatin, treated with cyclamin, first becomes of a red colour tending to blue, then of a yellow colour.

9. It may be that cyclamin acts in the blood by producing a special fermentation; but Dr. Chirone believes that it decomposes hæmoglobin by combining directly with globulin (of Denis) and setting hæmatin free.

10. The precipitate produced by the action of cyclamin on the blood resembles cyclamin itself in many characters.

11. Cyclamin decomposes the hæmoglobin of putrid blood much more easily than that of fresh blood; but the precipitate obtained in the first case is very impure from admixture of organic detritus.—*London Med. Record*, June 15, 1878.

Physiological and Pathological Action of Alcohol and Essence of Absinth.

The chief facts contained in this paper by MAGNAN (*Annales Médico-Psychologiques*), may be placed under the following heads:—

1. The immediate action of alcohol, given in a sufficient quantity, is to produce drunkenness.

2. The prolonged use of alcohol in the dog is followed by progressive symptoms with each new dose of the poison, which show the progressive phenomena in the solution of alcoholism. On the fifteenth day of the intoxication, irritability and impressionability supervene; ten days after this there are illusions and hallucinations at night, and in about a month some delirium, both by day and by night.

3. The prolonged use of alcohol gives rise again in the second month to some trembling, which shows itself at first in the hind feet, next reaches the fore-feet, and extends progressively to all parts of the body. In some cases it does not produce epileptic attacks. Finally, digestive disturbances and various complications occur, closely resembling those to which human alcoholics succumb.

4. The anatomical lesions of alcoholism in the dog show in various degrees a fatty degeneration (kidney and heart) and tendency to chronic irritations (meninges, spinal cord, and pericardium).

5. Essence of absinth in a weak dose produces vertigo and muscular tremor in the anterior parts of the body; a large dose produces epileptic attacks and delirium.

6. In the first stage (tonic convulsions) of the absinthic attack, the pupils dilate; there is injection of the optic papilla in the fundus of the eye, and congestion of the brain. These phenomena are not in accord with the generally admitted theories of the mechanism of epilepsy.

7. Animals deprived of the cerebral lobes show, under the influence of the essence of absinth, epileptic attacks, and the tremors resembling the convulsive attacks of subjects not suffering under mutilation of these parts.

8. After section of the spinal cord below the bulb, the intravenous injection of absinth produced an attack of clonic and tonic convulsions of the head, with foaming at the mouth, and then an attack of a more distinctly spinal character, tonic and clonic convulsions of the trunk, with expulsion of the urine and feces.

9. The isolated action of each segment of the cord in the regions supplied by it, gives reason for a belief that a totality of the organ is necessary for the production of the complete epileptic attack.—*London Med. Record*, June 15, 1878.

Therapeutic Employment of the Pancreas and the Meat-pancreas Clyster of Leube.

The pancreatic secretion is the most important of all those that are discharged into the small intestine. Its quantity is greatest during digestion. Schmidt, from his experiments on animals, estimates it for a man weighing 150 lb. at 4225 grammes (upwards of 9 lb.). Its functions consist in the conversion of starch into sugar, which is effected much more perfectly and rapidly by the pancreas than by the salivary glands ; the conversion of albumen and gelatine into peptones, and the preparation of fat for the process of absorption by the lacteals. V. Wittich has obtained by the maceration of the pancreas in glycerine the two ferments which act on starch and albumen in a separate state. Defresne has recommended pancreatine in physical cases where the patient is unable to digest or assimilate cod-liver oil ; in cases of jaundice in which fat is badly digested ; in cases of dyspepsia in which fat is found in the motions ; in those cases of dyspepsia in which the patient experiences abdominal pains, vomiting, diarrhœa, and flatulence several hours after meals ; and, speaking generally, in those cases of disturbances of digestion in which the fats and starches are badly assimilated, and where pepsin is found to be useless. Engesser directs that the pancreas should be minced, pressed through a hair-sieve, and administered in beef-tea, which must, however, not be at a higher temperature than 50° C. (122° F) at the time of mixture, lest the pancreas ferment be coagulated. The best temperature is that of the mouth, and all seasoning and vegetables may be afterwards added. It is a good plan to soak the gland, finely divided, in a pint of water, to which eight or ten drops of hydrochloric acid has been added. His experiments show that the admixture of the pancreas with the food is capable of passing through the stomach without losing its activity. In all cases where it is inexpedient to administer food by the mouth, Leube's meat-pancreas clyster may be given, and excellent results have been obtained in many instances. There can be no doubt that the large intestine presents an absorbing surface, as may indeed be easily shown experimentally by injecting a little salicylic acid, which may be shown to have entered the urine. Dr. Düring, of Westenhofen, reports a case of a woman, forty-eight years of age, who suffered from an abdominal aneurism, and vomited everything she took as food, and even water, so that she had fallen into a state of complete inanition. Dr. Düring at once prescribed Leube's nutritive enemata—50 grammes of meat, or about 2 ounces, were ordered, with 16 grammes or 3 drachms of pancreas, the two substances being minced together and broken down into a fine pulp, with a little warm water. One half of this was injected into the rectum in the morning, and the other half in the evening. The latter portion remained from 8 to 10 hours in the rectum, after which a fecal evacuation occurred. The patient was supported in this way from the 4th of March to the 21st of April, when the power of gastric digestion returned, and the clysters were intermitted with the recovery of digestion ; the patient's health improved, and the tumour diminished in size. Another case has recently been reported of cancer of the œsophagus, in which life was preserved for nine months.—*Practitioner*, June, 1878, from *Der Praktische Arzt*, Feb. 1878.

Medicine.

Sudden Death in Diabetes.

Dr. JULES CYR, in a very interesting memoir published in the recent numbers of the *Archives Générales de Médecine*, has given an account of several cases observed at Vichy, in which death has occurred suddenly, from which he concludes that in some cases, and those the most numerous, the persons have been surprised in a state of health which gave no reason to suppose that so sudden and disastrous a result would occur; others have been attacked by acute diabetes; others have arrived at an advanced period of emaciation due to diabetes, so that the fatal termination was not surprising. In all these cases, three principal stages or symptoms were observed with considerable constancy: 1, excitement; 2, dyspnœa; 3, coma. The period of excitement is manifested by some incoherence, vivacity, and rapidity of speech with some indistinctness, vague *malaise*, and disquietude going on even to anguish. To this excitement succeeds difficulty of breathing, occurring suddenly and sometimes voluntarily; large expirations made with effort; the thorax-muscles acting vigorously, the lungs dilating, and nevertheless oppression persisting, so that the air which penetrates the lungs appears not to be acting on the lungs, and the gaseous exchange to be impeded. The blood has, as it were, lost the faculty of revivifying itself in contact with the atmospheric oxygen. This stage is the most characteristic. It is followed by exhaustion and coma; and death occurs sometimes in twenty-four hours, sometimes in less. *Post-mortem* examination was made in eight cases out of thirty which were observed. The most variable lesions were recognized; congestion of the abdominal viscera and of the lungs, fatty degeneration of the pancreas, œdema of the lungs and of the glottis, congestion of the pia mater, etc.; and sometimes nothing at all. The diagnosis is difficult, if the existence of diabetes be not previously known. The pallor, the total absence of contractions or convulsions, the complete collapse, and the sometimes spirituous odor of the breath, characterize this coma; and of course the examination of the urine reveals its true origin. No treatment has appeared to produce any good result. The cases are especially those of young subjects between twenty and thirty years, which coincides with the well-known clinical fact that diabetes is the more grave in proportion as the subject is the less advanced in age. The determining cause of the symptoms has appeared to be excessive fatigue, long journeys, etc. Among the diverse theories which have arisen to explain these facts, two appear specially acceptable. The first—that of acetonæmia and the poisoning by acetone produced by the abnormal formation of glycose or paraglycose—is referred to. Acetone is a stupefying substance, which by its action at once resembles ether and alcohol. It appears, therefore, very natural that the cause of sudden death in the course of diabetes may be attributed to poisoning by this substance. The second theory—hyperglycæmia—explains also the succession of phenomena. The retention of sugar is a consequence of the diminution of the urine and sugar excreted, whence a change in the composition of the blood; sudden arrest of the vital phenomena, and cessation of the oxygenation of the blood, whence dyspnœa, muscular resolution, and coma. This anoxæmia would produce a rapid death, and without applying specially to cases ending in three to four hours. These theories, however, are not universally applicable, and further researches are required. These researches are especially interesting in connection with the clinical study of acetonæmia in our pages.—*British Med. Journ.*, June 8, 1878.

Treatment of Chronic Alcoholism.

In reply to a question by a correspondent in the *British Medical Journal* for May 4, p. 669, regarding the best treatment for the tremors of chronic alcoholism, and a substitute for the constant craving for drink which exists, Dr. LAUDER BRUNTON recommends fifteen minims of tincture of perchloride of iron, with ten minims of tincture of nux vomica, as most efficacious for the tremors, combined with bromide of potassium if restless at night. The chalybeate mixture, either alone or with the addition of tincture of capsicum (five or ten minims), relieves the craving for drink, for which purpose also a mixture of carbonate of ammonia in infusion of gentian is valuable. If there be derangement of the stomach, it should be treated by ten-grain doses of subnitrate or carbonate of bismuth, with magnesia and tragacanth.—*London Med. Record*, June 15, 1878.

The Influence of Injuries upon the Development of Hysteria and Paralysis Agitans.[1]

It is well known that certain affections, dependent upon a diathetic disease, may be developed as the result of an injury, and localize themselves in the parts where the pressure, blow, or friction was produced. This is the case in articular rheumatism, both acute and chronic, and in gout, as M. CHARCOT has many times demonstrated. M. Verneuil and his colleagues have in recent times pointed out the value of the study of facts of this kind from a surgical point of view. It is less known, perhaps, that some of the local phenomena of hysteria manifest themselves sometimes in the same way under similar influences. Sir B. Brodie was not ignorant of this, as many passages of his admirable little book (*Lectures Illustrative of Certain Local Nervous Affections*, London, 1837) fully testify. "He was, perhaps, the first," says M. Charcot, "to draw attention to these phenomena of a local hysteria developed by the direct effect of an injury." "It frequently happens," says Brodie, "that the local symptoms of hysteria appear to be due to the operation of an external cause; and as the injury in question is often very slight, quite out of proportion to the effects produced, these symptoms are often misunderstood, misinterpreted; they are regarded as something quite different from what they really are. It is not rare," says the eminent surgeon, "to see, for example, a young woman whose finger has been pricked or pinched, complain, a short time after the little accident, of a pain which extends from the fingers up the hand and forearm. The pain may be complicated by a convulsive action of the muscles of the arm, or by a continued contraction of the flexors or of the anterior part of the arm, so that the forearm is kept bent in a permanent manner, at least while the patient is awake, for the spasm is generally relaxed during sleep." "A young girl, aged 11 or 12, pricked the index finger of the left hand with a pair of scissors. This was followed immediately by pain running up the course of the median nerve. On the following day there occurred muscular contractions, fixing the forearm at a right angle to the arm. Some days afterwards all the muscles of the forearm were the seat of violent spasms, producing, in the arm and forearm, singular convulsive movements. Later on, nausea and vomiting supervened, and for two days she rejected everything that was introduced into her stomach. In course of time the other limbs became similarly affected, and it became impossible for the young patient to walk or to stand erect. Now and then there was a spasm of the diaphragm, with threatened suffocation, or permanent closure of the jaws determined by spasm of the masseter, and finally a sharp pain in the head, recalling the pain of the pricked finger.

[1] Progrès Médical, May 4, 1878.

Surgical interference, attempted many times, had rather the effect of increasing the evil. Nevertheless, the cure took place spontaneously at the end of two years." M. Charcot then alluded to a certain number of cases which he had met with in his practice, and which illustrate the theoretical and practical interest of Brodie's observations. Two are now reported, to serve as examples.

CASE I.—Towards the middle of April, 1877, Mlle. X., in falling, hurt the back of her hand against a stool; tolerably smart pain and a little swelling followed. Two or three days afterwards the little finger of this hand commenced to flex itself in a permanent fashion; then the flexion successively attacked the other fingers, and the thumb was applied to the index and ring fingers. From this time her hand remained permanently clenched, both day and night, even during the most profound sleep, in opposition to the remark made by Brodie on similar cases. The flexion of the fingers was so marked that their reduction was almost impossible, and it was necessary to interpose a cloth to prevent the nails from wounding the palm of the hand. The various attempts made at reduction seemed always followed by an aggravation of the contraction. Things were in this state on the 31st May, six weeks after the accident, when M. Charcot saw the case, in consultation with Professor Richet and Dr. de Wailly. On that day the fist was firmly closed as usual, the wrist also was stiff, like the fingers, and there was complete anæsthesia of the whole hand, wrist, and lower half of the forearm, as marked anteriorly as posteriorly. The elbow did not share in the contraction. Mlle. X. had never suffered from nervous attacks. She was calm, of an equable and rather lively temperament; nothing had changed in her mode of life. There was no trace of ovarian pain. The menstrual periods had occurred twice since the accident, but were unattended with anything of note. There were no modifications of sensibility beyond the parts noted. Five days after the consultation, without the intervention of any circumstance, her hand suddenly opened, and she recovered all its movements.

CASE II.—On the 17th April, 1877, Hortense X., aged 27, had the right forearm squeezed between a wall and a turn-table, upon which lay glass articles for polishing. A sharp pain immediately followed in the part submitted to the pressure, and some swelling with ecchymosis, but no wound. She stated that, some instances later, contraction to semi-flexion took place in the ring and little fingers of the right hand. During the succeeding days, the fingers of the other hand were affected by the same sort of contraction. Under the influence of discutient remedies the swelling and ecchymosis soon disappeared, but, the pain and contraction persisting, she decided to come into hospital, and was admitted to Dr. Leroy's surgical wards on June 13, 1877, two months after the accident. The following conditions were noted. The inner four fingers of the right hand were slightly flexed at the metacarpo-phalangeal articulation, so as to form an obtuse angle of about 130° to 150° with the palm of the hand. The two other phalanges of these same fingers were rigidly extended. The thumb, although enjoying a certain mobility, was not quite free; the wrist was also rigid; indeed the general appearance was that of a hand methodically holding a pen. In the whole extent of the arm, forearm, and hand, there existed permanently a pain which from time to time was spontaneously exasperated. The pain was exasperated and became atrocious whenever the patient attempted to execute any movement, and also when the pressure was made upon any part of the limb. This pain was especially intense when pressure was made over the anterior surface of the arm, particularly in the course of the median nerve. If pressure were persisted in, a sort of nervous crisis occurred, which many times had led to loss of consciousness. There was neither redness nor tumefaction of the painful parts; the ecchymosis had disappeared a long while. The exquisite pain produced by the slightest touch rendering a thorough examination of the limb impossible, it was decided, five or six days after her admission, to put her under chloroform. The examination thus made discovered nothing to account for the remarkable pains. It was observed that, in spite of very profound narcosis, the contracted parts were not completely relaxed; in truth, one could, although not without effort, extend completely the fingers, or flex them, or move the wrist in all directions, but as soon as they were released they returned to their previous attitudes. All these accidents, pain, and contraction, had persisted up to the beginning of August, without any modification, when, on one of the first days of that month, without appreciable cause, the contraction suddenly disappeared, as well as the pain; then supervened a complete paralysis of both motion and sensation, affecting the whole right upper extremity; of which henceforth there was complete resolution. Soon afterwards it was noticed that the inferior extremity of the same side was also paralyzed in motion like the upper, but to a less degree, while in sensation it was quite as complete. This last event led to a careful examination of the sensibility of the whole body; it was found that there existed complete right hemianæsthesia, affecting both general and special sensations, vision and smell included. Moreover, very marked pain was discovered in the right ovarian region, of which, up to this time, the patient had made no complaint. From this time a great number of other hysterical symptoms manifested themselves in succession, the hemianæsthesia and ovarian pain persisting without variations. One day it was great dyspnœa, laboured respiration, with threatened suffocation; another day it might be pains in the præcordia, radiating to the left shoulder; or, again, a dry and convulsive cough, a violent fixed pain in the left temple; another day retention of urine. For more than a month she vomited all her food, which did not prevent her from maintaining a certain *embonpoint*. There never was any regular hystero-epileptic attack. It is important to note that she first menstruated at 18, married at 20, became the mother of six children, and had never suffered from any serious illness before the accident which brought her to the hospital. She was very nervous, very irritable; but she never had, properly speaking, hysterical attacks. The phenomena which have been described, viz., hemianæsthesia, paralysis, ovarian pain, various spasms, etc., still were present upon the 24th October, when M. Charcot, by the kindness of M. Leroy, had an opportunity of examining the case.

M. Charcot would sum up our knowledge of this subject of traumatic local hysteria thus. More or less exquisite cutaneous hyperæsthesia, deeper pains occupying the course of the nerve-trunks, or apparently situated more specially in one or several joints, more or less marked contractions,—such are the phenomena which occur immediately after, or a little after, the injury. These symptoms rarely remain limited to the region thus affected, but extend themselves rapidly to neighbouring parts, and can even occupy the whole extent of a limb. Once established, they frequently persist in the same condition, with desperate tenacity, for many weeks, many months, even many years. The slightest touch, the least friction, the smallest movement provoked, exasperates the pains and the contractions. These are also all liable to spontaneous exasperation from time to time, without any external cause. There is sometimes superadded, principally during the spontaneous exacerbations just referred to, swelling, redness, and relative elevation of temperature in the affected parts. As a rule, sooner or later the hyperæsthesia and pains give place to anæsthesia; nevertheless the muscular contraction persists, yet it also may be replaced by paresis, or even paralysis, with resolution of the muscles.

These symptoms, resulting from a mechanical cause, are generally the first revelation of the hysterical diathesis, hitherto latent; and they usually constitute during a long time the sole symptoms, existing alone, without the addition of other nervous phenomena. From this double point of view they ought to be considered as equivalent to those local neuropathic symptoms of the same kind, which are one of the most singular attributes of infantile hysteria. It is not rare, as we know, to see in little girls of 10 or 12 perhaps a nervous cough, perhaps a spasmodic wry-neck, or a permanent contraction of certain muscles of a whole limb, a joint-affection, simulating arthritis or coxalgia, one after the other occupying the pathological scene for weeks or even months; then one day they disappear all at once, leaving no traces. But this is after all very frequently only a truce. Some months, some years later, when the previous phenomena have been completely forgotten, when the sexual functions are established, ovarian hysteria supervenes, with all its train of henceforth classic phenomena, viz., sensorial, and sensory anæsthesia, ovaralgia, characteristic convulsive attacks, peculiar psychical troubles, etc. At other times "general hysteria" comes to be added to "local hysteria," without intermission, without time for repose, and then the relations between the two are easily illustrated. That which has just been said of infantile local hysteria may be applied in all respects to local hysteria of mechanical origin. They are, indeed, but two varieties of the same species. It is very remarkable, in fact that traumatisms never produce the effects in question, except among young subjects at present destitute of all well-marked signs of generalized hysteria. When ovarian hysteria is developed and established with all its army of symptoms, mechanical injuries do not seem to produce the same effect. Such is, at least, the conclusion to which M. Charcot's observations point; and in illustration, he quotes the case of a patient of his, named Geneviève L., aged 35, who has suffered for many years from hystero-epilepsy, with generalized anæsthesia, and frequently during the intervals of her attacks is affected with contractions of the limbs, which persist during many days. Many times she has broken, in falling, the bones of a forearm or leg, but these fractures have never been the cause of the development of pains or contractions; consolidation has taken place in the ordinary manner, and has not been marked by any special accident.

Every one knows the difficulty of diagnosis presented by local hysteria, especially when it supervenes alone. These difficulties are not lessened by the fact that they recognize their origin in a traumatic influence. They have, nevertheless, more importance, as the wrong diagnosis to which they may point (arthritis, coxalgia, neuralgia, etc.) leads to active intervention nearly always untimely and injurious. Observation demonstrates that blisters and cauteries, galvanization and faradization, prolonged rest, attempts at reduction of all kinds, division of nerves and tendons, almost always exasperate the malady, and are sometimes followed by more disastrous effects. On the whole, it is only the consideration of the general state that might so inspire therapeutical efforts, and so far as the local phenomena are concerned, the expectant attitude in the actual state of our knowledge is much the most safe. This is, perhaps, the place to recall the words of Brodie, by which in the book referred to above he prefaces his remarks upon the surgical treatment of local hysterical affections. "The advice which I have to give you," says he, "will be generally negative. It is not so much what you ought to do, as what you ought to know not to do."

It is not in hysteria only that the localization of pathological phenomena may be determined by a mechanical cause. The same fact can be produced in other diseases which, like hysteria, belong to the great provisional group of the neuroses. This is the case, for example, in paralysis agitans, in Parkinson's disease. M. Charcot relates the history of a lady who, falling from a carriage, severely bruised her left thigh; after some time, a sharp pain supervened in the limb, occupying the course of the sciatic nerve, and a little afterwards a tremor declared itself throughout the entire limb. At first temporary, this trembling became later on more permanent and finally extended to the other extremities (*Leçons sur les Maladies du Système Nerveux*, tome i, p. 185). The chief peculiarities of the preceding case were represented, except for some modifications, in two cases which were shown by N. Charcot to his audience. In 1873, F., aged 55, got a sprain of her left foot, with swelling, ecchymoses, etc. Shortly afterwards the swelling and difficulty of walking persisting, she perceived that her foot trembled. The tremor remained limited to the left inferior extremity until 1876, at which time the hand on the same side was also affected. At the present time the tumour is well marked in both extremities on the left side, and is beginning to pronounce itself in those of the right side also. F. in other respects presents all the characteristic symptoms of Parkinson's disease; immobility of features, stiffness of neck, inclination of the trunk forward, tendency to propulsion and retropulsion.

T., aged 72, for the past four years has presented the classic symptoms of paralysis agitans, limited to the right side. Contrary to the rule, she has tremor of the tongue and also of the lower jaw. This tremor commenced last September under the following circumstances. On the 2d September, while yawning, T. dislocated her lower jaw; the reduction was made immediately without difficulty. From this time the jaw began to tremble, and the saliva commenced to flow involuntarily from her mouth. These observations require no comment.—*London Med. Record*, June 15. 1878.

A Complex and Exceptional Neurosis.

Dr. BERTHIER relates the following case in the *Annales Médico-Psychologiques*, September, 1877. The patient was a young girl, aged 13, of a scrofulous tendency; a very timid child, who had not been able to speak until she was five years of age. Her father had suffered from nocturnal somnambulism, and her maternal grandfather from paralysis. When about 13 years of age she had an attack of vomiting, with gastric pain, but no head symptoms. After two months the complications which had supervened led to Dr. Berthier being called in consultation. The patient suffered then from general delirium with hallucinations; she was excited, trembling and gesticulating, her body was in a sweat, the pupils were dilated, the pulse quick and strong. Tactile sensibility was equally distributed. The urine was abundant and limpid, the bowels constipated. She had never menstruated. She did not seem to see Dr. Berthier.

I left, says Dr. Berthier, and visited her again in an hour. She then recognized me from time to time, and again seemed not to see me, she wished me good day, and slowly became able to converse. Sometimes she saw me, at other times she seemed blind; sometimes she heard what I said and smiled, at others she remained deaf to me. Her skin was anæsthetic on one side of the body, and on the other was excessively sensitive. Again she did not seem to have the full power of the senses of sight and hearing. Thus she could read from a newspaper, but failed to see the hand which held it; she heard the songs of birds, but did not distinguish our voices. If the curtains were closed and the room darkened, she was able to see a pin on the table, but failed to distinguish us at present. I seated myself by the bed, and this child, generally so timid, was quite possessed, and chattered to herself constantly, using the words *pouff* and *conseil*, the first to indicate herself and the second other persons. Thus she recounted what "*Conseil*" Berthier thought of her state, how many visits "*Conseil*" curé had paid her, how good "*Conseil*" grandmamma was to her. She turned over the pages of an album, and criticized the portraits with much justice and some malice, and although ordinarily thought to be dull and not very intelligent, she read one of La Fontaine's fables in a spirited manner and with correct accent. She also declaimed from Racine with an art and a diction worthy of a first-rate actor. I proposed a game of chess; she accepted, and played very well, but quite as though she were alone and her adversary invisible. Then quite suddenly, after this state had lasted several hours, she uttered a cry, placed her hand on her heart, shed tears, looked around her, asked where she was, and who had brought her there. She knew nothing of what had taken place, and seemed as one awakened from a dreamless sleep. I have been present during many of these attacks; I have also seen her in a true somnambulistic state, during which she has cooked, put the room in order, and hung up a clock against the wall without stumbling or hurting herself in any way.

I have seen her take up my hat, observe the ventilator, and exclaim, "What a strange idea that *Conseil* Berthier should bore a hole in his hat," and, laughing loudly, "It is his hat; I see his initials; I will ask him the use of it when he comes." All the time I was standing by the bed, and she did not perceive me. Once we held a long conversation by the aid of a slate; she read what I wrote, but would not admit that the writing was done by me. Sometimes this singular blindness would give place to hallucination. At another time she could only see persons as being covered by a black cloud, so that she could not recognize them; and if asked who questioned her she attempted to recognize them by putting her hand on their face, hair, clothes, etc., after the manner of a blind person. The transition from these states, to that of the normal life was very rapid, and could not be predicted by more than a few moments. She complained of a pain in the præcordial region when about to return to the normal state, and the sudden appearance of the words *pouff* and *conseil* in her conversation indicated the presence of the abnormal state.

In addition to these symptoms the feet were often paralyzed, the appetite *nil*, the sleep light, the pulse very irregular, the body emaciated, face pale, and there was a febrile brightness of the eyes. One morning she was found to be menstruating for the first time, and two days after this the somnambulism had ceased, but was replaced for a time by an embarrassment of speech with an impossibility of pronouncing certain words. She was removed to the country for change and became much better, although she suffered two or three relapses after great emotion excited by visits to Paris.

Dr. Berthier remarks that he has never met with any case similar to this. The remarkable fact in the case is the partial way in which the senses were exercised, taking cognizance only of portions of objects, sounds, etc. The rapid alterations from the normal to the morbid state, and the complete unconsciousness of what had taken place during the morbid condition, are also extraordinary phenomena. The difficulties attendant upon puberty in a young girl of slow growth, and under the domination of hereditary nervous influences, together with the almost total disappearance of the symptoms upon the establishment of menstruation, are perhaps sufficient to establish a connection between the phenomena; Dr. Berthier will not hazard any hypothesis upon a single case of so complex a character.— *London Med. Record*, June 15, 1878.

On Cerebellar Disease.

The conclusions arrived at in this paper (*Berliner Klinische Wochenschrift*, April 15, 1878) are based upon an analysis of about 250 recorded cases, besides the personal observations of Professor NOTHNAGEL himself.

Sometimes disease of the cerebellum causes no symptoms during life which could indicate any brain-lesion, even though an extensive destruction of cerebellar tissue exist.   Some authors have concluded that cerebellar disease, as such, never gives rise to any symptoms, but that those which have been observed in some cases are to be attributed to functional disturbance of neighbouring parts   This inference is wrong.   The nature of the morbid process has little to do with the presence or absence of symptoms; apoplexy, softening, abscess, tubercle, other tumours or atrophy may, under certain circumstances, exist in the cerebellum without producing symptoms.   The area of issue involved has, within certain limits, no noticeable influence; tumours of the size of a walnut, or larger, may remain "latent."   It is the situation of the lesion which exercises the greatest influence over the production of symptoms; *disease can only exist without symptoms when localized in one hemisphere,* and not influencing, by pressure or otherwise, surrounding parts.   Cases are plentiful in which disease of a cerebellar hemisphere has been accompanied by marked symptoms; yet the author believes that an analysis of them justifies his opinion that in all of them the symptoms were caused by the influence of the lesion upon neighbouring parts of the brain.   The following proposition is held to be in accordance with the facts.   *A loss of substance in one hemisphere of the cerebellum causes no symptom of disease,* or at any rate none which is not recognizable in the present state of our knowledge.

As the result of a series of experiments, the author found that *the destruction of one or even both cerebellar hemispheres in the rabbit causes no symptoms of deprivation (Ausfallssymptome).*   (Virchow's *Archiv,* 68 Bd.)   This does not for one moment involve the supposition that the hemispheres of the cerebellum are superfluous organs without function; it is only maintained that the lesion of one hemisphere causes no symptom which is at present recognizable, no disturbance of motor or sensory function nor of the nerves of special sense.

Several authors, and most recently Otto (*Arch. für Psychiatrie und Nervenkrank.,* Bd. iv. and vi.), have expressed the opinion that the cerebellum stands in a certain relation to the psychic functions; it has been held to be the seat of memory or of the emotions.   Otto comes to the conclusion that it acts as a regulator of the will.

It is probable that the solution of the question as to the true functions of the hemispheres of the lesser brain will only be reached through observations on the human species, in which they are most largely developed.   Of all pathological processes, atrophy seems to be the best fitted for these observations, as it may affect both hemispheres in equal degrees, and to a considerable extent, without affecting neighbouring parts of the brain.   On looking through the recorded cases of this kind it is found that, in addition to the so-called disturbances of co-ordination, mental symptoms are generally described.

Supported by these observations, and by the fact of the increase in size of the cerebellar hemispheres observed in lower animals the more nearly they approach to man, Professor Nothnagel is inclined to think that the hemispheres of the lesser brain are in some relation with the psychic processes.   The state of our knowledge does not at present, however, justify even a supposition as to the nature of this connection.   It must not be forgotten that, in some cases of bilateral atrophy of the hemispheres, the intellect has been reported as normal.

From the above considerations, it may be laid down that *local lesions which in their action are limited to one cerebellar hemisphere cannot be diagnosed.*

Excluding the cases which have presented no symptoms, it is found that in cerebellar disease the most various symptoms have been noted, the great majority of which are unessential, or only indirectly due to the disease.   Of great significance, however, are the disturbances of co-ordination and giddiness.   After a careful consideration of all published cases, Nothnagel feels justified in stating that *disturbances of co-ordination only occur when the median lobe (vermiform processes) is directly or indirectly affected by the disease.*

Only three cases have been found by the author in which the median lobe was really or apparently affected, and yet in which no inco-ordination was observed they are the following: 1. Crisp, *Transactions of the Pathological Society*, vol. xxiii.; 2. Hughlings Jackson, *Medical Times and Gazette*, August 1, 1877; 3. Gintrac, *Traité des Maladies de l'Appareil Nerveux*, 1871, Bd. iv. Reasons are given at length by the author for considering that none of these cases affect the validity of the above proposition. Observations on cases (tuberculosis, etc.) occurring in very young children cannot be allowed to have much weight in this matter, as disturbances of gait cannot be noted with any degree of accuracy in them.

It cannot yet be determined what part or parts of the median lobe must be affected in order to give rise to disturbances of co-ordination.

Inco-ordination has been noted as occurring in experiments made for the purpose of studying the functions of the cerebellum, not only in dogs and cats, but also in rabbits, guinea-pigs, and especially birds (Flourens). The cerebellar hemispheres are known to be less developed in the animal series the further they are removed from man; in rodents, the median lobe is very large compared with the lateral lobes, and the whole cerebellum of birds corresponds only to the median lobe in mammals. Therefore experiments upon the cerebellum of birds, together with their results, must be considered as having reference only to the median lobe of the human cerebellum.

Among diseases of the lateral lobes of the lesser brain it is found that tumours most frequently give rise to motor disturbances, owing to the pressure they exercise upon the median lobe. It may easily be understood why recent hemorrhages do not cause these symptoms, for the patients either die comatose, or exhibit a series of other symptoms which prevent them from walking at all.

Dr. Nothnagel now proceeds to discuss several points connected with cerebellar ataxy. In the majority of fully developed cases there should be little difficulty in distinguishing between the gait of a tabic patient, and that of a person suffering from cerebellar disease. There are a number of cases, however, in which the distinctive features are less evident; this occurs most often in patients with cerebellar disease who present symptoms resembling those of tabes dorsalis. The gait of a person suffering from cerebellar ataxy is very similar to that of a drunken man. One of Nothnagel's patients has several times been locked up by the police as drunk, owing to his tabic gait.

It has been believed that cerebellar disease causes a special tendency to fall either backwards or forwards; the author shows that this symptom is oftener absent than not, and that some patients have a peculiar tendency to fall towards the right or the left. It would appear that this tendency to fall is usually in the direction in which the cerebellar lesion is situated; but many decided exceptions to this are on record, and it is impossible at present to substantiate any proposition on this part of the subject. The author's view is that a tendency to fall always in one particular direction is to be observed when either of the middle peduncles of the cerebellum is affected by disease. In many cases the uncertainty of gait is increased by being in the dark or by closing the eyes, while some patients find that this in no way affects them. The movements of the legs are, as a rule, perfectly well performed when the patient lies on his back in bed, the muscular sense seems then also to be unaffected; there are, however, exceptions to this. It is remarkable that in many cases, though motor disturbances of the legs and trunk are very marked, the upper extremities remain quite unaffected; no explanation of this is offered. The author promises before long to publish a monograph in which will be found full details of the cases, experiments, etc., which have led him to the conclusions given above.—*London Medical Record*, June 15, 1878.

Paraplegia from Cold.

In a paper on *Paraplegia a frigore* in the *Hospitals-Tidende*, second series, Band iv. 1877, Dr. LANGE says that he does not mean by the term those chronic spinal paralyses which may be produced by the frequently repeated action of cold and moisture, but those which arise from a single powerful influence, which may be acute in their development, and, as a rule, reach their maximum intensity in an early stage. Nor does he include the cases of spinal paralysis following a cold, which from the first are dependent on a well-marked myelitic process, either acute softening or abscess. The affections which he describes are at first not dependent on changes in the spinal cord, though such may occur at a later period. The course of the malady, according to the author's experience, is as follows. A short time, generally a day or two after exposure to the influence of cold, there is weakness in the legs, but not so great as to prevent walking. There is no disturbance of urination or of defecation. Simultaneously with or before the paresis there may be pain or perverted sensations in the lower limbs and back; there may also be anæsthesia or hyperæsthesia. The general health is good; there is no spinal pain nor tenderness. The disorder generally remains at the same point about a fortnight. Under appropriate regimen and treatment it then begins to improve, and the patient recovers after an interval of two or three months. During convalescence, and for some time afterwards, over-exertion, or the renewed influence of cold, will easily cause a relapse, which, as a rule, is only temporary. Sometimes the arms also become affected, or the paresis increases, and will not yield to treatment, indicating the presence of more profound changes of a myelitic character in the spinal cord. With regard to the pathology of this affection, the author considers that, if it be not from the first an inflammation, it is a change which may be developed into inflammation, perhaps a hyperæmia excited by a peripheral ischæmia. The prognosis is good when the patient can be kept in favourable circumstances. In addition, Dr. Lange recommends in quite recent cases (which none of his were) local blood-letting, afterwards douches along the spinal column, and the free application of tincture of iodine. As internal remedies, he uses iodide of potassium, nitrate of silver, or ergot.—*Lond. Med. Record*, June 15, 1878.

Jaborandi in Obstinate Hiccough.

Dr. ORTILLE, of Lille, relates (*Bull. de Thérapeutique*, May 15) a case of most obstinate hiccough in which he had tried a great variety of means, including electricity and hypodermic morphia injections—the hiccough even continuing during the sleep caused by this last. He then tried the hydrochlorate of pilocarpin, on account of its action on the phrenic nerve. A hypodermic injection of two centigrammes and a half was inserted with almost immediate effect, so that in a quarter of an hour the patient was bathed in sweat, salivation was established, and the hiccough disappeared, never to return.—*Med. Times and Gaz.*, June 8, 1878.

The Cure of Sciatica by Phosphorus.

Dr. VOLQUARDSEN reports, in Schmidt's *Dictionary* and the *Pesth Medico-Chirurg. Presse*, No. 39, 1877, a case of sciatica, which lasted for two years, and defied all treatment. He then arrived at the idea of trying the internal use of phosphorus, which he prescribed in doses of fifteen milligrammes (about one-fourth

of a grain) three times a day. Three days sufficed to obtain a marked improvement, and three weeks brought a complete cure.—*Lond. Med. Record*, June 15,
1878.

On Trophic Disturbances.

N. BROWN-SEQUARD (*Société de Biologie*, 27 Avril) has observed, in many
guinea-pigs whose sciatic nerves he had divided, various phenomena hitherto not
recorded; extreme agitation, cries, staggering, temporary cataleptic rigidity;
besides, in all, the characters of spinal epilepsy were very accentuated and persisted, while the first symptoms, which might be attributed to a spinal meningitis,
disappeared more or less rapidly. In one of these animals, the paw of the side
opposite to the lesion was still at that time the seat of a notable atrophy; whilst
that of the side on which the nerve was cut was intact. This fact pleads against
the accepted theory of trophic disturbance. Moreover, N. Brown-Séquard has
for a long time maintained that the so-called trophic disturbances are often due
to the animal biting its paw in the convulsive attacks. N. Laborde objected to
this view, and related a case in which this occurred to a rabbit, although every
precaution was taken to prevent it from biting itself.—*London Medical Record*,
June 15, 1878.

On the Pathology of Muscular Atrophy.

Dr. LANDOUZY, in a remarkable article in the *Revue Mensuelle*, Jan. 1878,
points out that, in most cases of secondary amyotrophy, there may at the same
time be observed a trophic affection of the integuments superposed on the atrophied muscles; the conditions observed being a notable thickening of the cellular
tissue adherent to the skin, in such wise that the tegumentary folds formed by
pinching it up above the atrophied muscles, very often present a thickness double
that of the normal. This tegumentary thickening, corresponding to the regions
attacked by muscular emaciation, appears to exist—*a*, habitually in deuteropathic
amyotrophy; *b*, rarely in amyotrophy of the type described by Aran and Duchenne; *c*, in a variable degree in the atrophy of infantile paralysis. This subentaneous fact it is important to note; clinically, because it lessens and marks the
appearance of muscular atrophy; because, in certain cases of difficult diagnosis,
it may serve to determine the variety of atrophy; from the point of view of physiological pathology, because it seems to present itself with the character of a true
trophic disorder, not being found in the cases of hysterical patients condemned to
prolonged immobility by hysterical hemiplegia or paraplegia, any more than in
patients suffering from progressive amyotrophy.—*London Medical Record*, May
15, 1878.

On Paralytic Disorders of the Voice in Phthisis.

Dr. KITTLER has a paper on the above subject in the *Aerztliches Intelligenz-
blatt* for May 28. He observes that, since the introduction of the laryngoscope,
paralytic affections of the laryngeal nerves and muscles have assumed an important position, so that many cases of hoarseness, aphonia, etc., formerly attributed
to anatomical lesions, are now shown to be purely paralytic. The present paper
considers mainly the forms of vocal paresis and paralysis attending phthisis.
These may either precede the lung disease, or may develop themselves during its
progress.

In the former case, vocal paralysis manifests itself chiefly in functional weakness of the organ, want of clearness, and loss of voice on slight exertion, as
speaking or singing, also hoarseness after a slight cold. This condition of things.

termed by Gerhardt (Virchow's *Archiv.*, vol. xxvii. pp. 68 and 296) atony of the vocal cords, may precede phthisis for months, and even years. The results of laryngoscopic examination in cases of this kind are various. Sometimes they are almost negative ; at other times, especially after a continued effort of the voice, there is some injection and swelling of the vocal cords, or of the arytenoid mucous membrane. Sometimes, again, a highly anæmic condition of the mucous membrane is all that can be discerned ; and, lastly, in some cases the impairment of the voice can be shown to be due to diminished mobility of the cords and defective closure of the rima glottidis. The grave import of these apparently insignificant changes is only indicated by a history of phthisis in one or both parents. The true nature of a case of vocal atony, hitherto attributed to over-exertion of the voice, is often revealed by the sudden accession of hæmoptysis or colliquative sweating, indicating the latent pulmonary disease. On the other hand, we cannot, in the absence of a history of phthisis, regard vocal atony, even of the most obstinate kind, as seen in singers, actors, etc., as a forerunner of phthisis.

Vocal paralysis, occurring in the progress of phthisis, may be of two kinds— either combined with lesion of the mucous membrane or with the mucous membrane intact. The most frequent sources of the former are catarrh and ulceration. Although inflammatory swelling of the mucous membrane is in itself sufficient to produce intense hoarseness, yet in these cases we must consider the impairment of the voice due rather to a paralysis of the laryngeal muscles, in consequence of serious infiltration of the muscular fibres, than to the catarrhal affection, which is often indeed very slight. The paralysis is mostly double, and affects chiefly the muscles that close the glottis, and those that regulate the tension of the cords. The site of ulceration, when this is present, has considerable influence on the form of paralysis ; thus ulceration of the posterior wall usually impairs the action of the transverse arytenoid muscle. Paralysis of the muscles that open the glottis is very rare in cases of phthisis.

Paralysis of the vocal apparatus, without concomitant lesion of the mucous membrane, may also be either double or unilateral, and may be considered functional. When occurring in tuberculosis, as also in chlorosis, it is probably due to the deficiency of red corpuscles in the blood, and a consequent impaired nutrition of the brain and the laryngeal nerves ; or it may also be due to reflex irritation of the peripheral fibres of the vagus, either in the infiltrated lung-tissue or on the surface of the almost always adherent pleura. Fränkel (Virchow's *Archiv.* vol. lxi. p. 261) has demonstrated degenerative changes in the laryngeal muscles, which throw considerable light on the nature of phthisical atony of the vocal cords. The primitive fibrillæ become wasted and more or less detached from the investing sarcolemma, or they may disappear in places almost entirely, leaving only empty sarcolemma tubes. The investing perimysium may also undergo change, either through excessive growth of its connective tissue or increase of its cellular element. This functional paralysis in phthisis most frequently affects the tensor muscles of the glottis, also the closers and the muscles attached to the posterior wall, and is often associated with hyperæsthesia of the mucous membrane and soft parts surrounding the larynx.

More rare than the above forms, is paralysis induced by pressure on the recurrent laryngeal nerve, caused by pleuritic exudation, by cicatrices, or by degenerated bronchial glands. Gerhardt estimates one case of paralysis of the vocal cords to twelve of ulceration ; and Ziemssen regards this as even too high. When due to impaired nervous function, the affection is mostly right-sided, though cases on the left side have been observed, while paralysis of both recurrents is exceedingly rare.

Dr. Kittler appends two illustrative cases—one a case of complete paralysis of the right recurrent and paresis on the left side, due to pressure of an aneurism of the innominate and aorta ; the other a case of double paralysis of the recurrent nerve, in a strumous subject with goitre.—*London Med. Record*, June 15, 1878.

Physical Diagnosis of Pleural Exudations.

In a paper on the above subject (*Berliner Klinische Wochenshrift*, March 25) Dr. ROSENBACH, of Breslau, observes that the changes in the percussion-sound of the thorax caused by the respiratory movements and by changes in the position of the patient, though of considerable moment, have as yet been insufficiently attended to, although a certain influence which these and other similar circumstances exercise on the result of the percussion has not been unnoticed. The tendency has been to rather exaggerate the diagnostic value of these purely external conditions ; and Dr. Rosenbach holds that the changes, both as regards pitch and intensity of the percussion-sound as caused by alterations in position, and by respiratory movements, refer to the thoracic walls rather than to the lungs, and that differences in the tension of the lungs do not explain the variety of the percussion-sounds during respiration. Thus, the increased resonance of the thorax in the sitting posture is due not so much to changes in the lung as to the increased tension of the thoracic wall ; hence, the higher pitch of the sound in the upright, compared with the recumbent, posture, can furnish no evidence as to the size and situation of pulmonary cavities. The same applies to alteration in the sound when the mouth is open, and when it is closed. Indeed, it is possible to almost efface the tympanic sound usually given by caverns, or by the abdomen, by means of a full inspiration, or by increasing the tension of the abdominal muscles. It is, therefore, evident that, in comparing by percussion two symmetrical portions of the thorax, as, for example, the clavicular regions, care must be taken to do so during precisely the same stage of respiration. If we percuss one side during inspiration, and the other during expiration, the sound in the latter case will usually be lower and louder. If the apex of the lung give a distinctly louder sound during inspiration, we may almost certainly infer that the parenchyma is neither consolidated nor shrunken. In cases of pleuritic exudation we may, in like manner, conclude that a full sound during inspiration indicates that the lung tissue is still capable of inflation.

Dr. Rosenbach's observations refer principally to the changes in the percussion and auscultation sounds, induced in cases of pleuritic exudation by a continued erect position, and by deep inspirations, especially in the posterior portions of the thorax. Five cases came under observation. There was dulness extending to the spine or the angle of the scapula in all cases, rapidly diminishing laterally, but increasing downwards, and with bronchial breathing over the area of dulness of various intensity. All cases, excepting one, were under observation in the first week of the disease, and all recovered within four weeks. The first case related was that of a young man, with well-marked symptoms of pleurisy. In the morning (during the second week) dulness extended posteriorly to the spine of the scapula on the left side. Below the spine of the scapula, breathing was bronchial ; above, uncertain. In the afternoon of the same day, the dulness extended with only moderate intensity to the angle of the scapula, while over it the breathing was purely vesicular ; further down, there was only feeble vesicular breathing, and bronchial breathing existed only over the lowest portion of the lung. This remarkable change could scarcely be attributed to resorption. On the next morning, and after a good night, the physical condition was precisely the same as on the morning before. The change in question was, therefore, evidently due to the difference in position, and to the kind of breathing. It was also ascertained that on the previous afternoon the patient had, for several hours, walked about his apartment. When this was now repeated, the same changes occurred as on the afternoon before. Subsequently, similar changes, and of the same nature, were observed in the other cases. In one case, three distinct zones of sound could be distinguished—1, a zone of normal sound, extending to the lower (*sic*, superior?) angle of the scapula; 2, a zone of rather loud tympanitic sound, about an inch wide, and gradually passing into the lowermost region of absolute dulness. Similarly, while loud and bronchial respiration had prevailed about the angle of the scapula, vesicular breathing was now heard over the first two regions, while feeble bronchial breathing existed over only the lowest, dull region. These changes in the result of percussion and auscultation could be produced at will during the latter half of the second week, by permitting the patients free exercise, or confining them for a certain time to the recumbent position in bed. It is also worthy of remark, that in all these patients, on their assuming the erect posture, the upper and posterior limits of dulness rapidly diminished towards the sides; a matter of considerable importance in explaining the changes in the sound.

On summing up these observations we obtain the following interesting results. In average sized pleuritic serous exudations in which the area of dulness posteriorly diminishes rapidly laterally, and in which inspiration is distinctly accompanied by increased resonance, an entire change in the results of auscultation and percussion can be produced by a deep inspiration or by moderate exercise in the erect position. This may proceed from two causes; either that the dulness is produced by a viscid dense exudation, holding in suspension morbid products which may be deposited on the folds of the pleuræ; or that the lower area of dulness is due to fluid exudation, the upper to collapsed portions of the lungs. The latter is the more probable hypothesis, and the atelectasis of the lung occurs, probably, through the pressure exercised on the lung in the recumbent posture. When the lung is partially expanded by a forced and deep inspiration, the resonance is proportionately increased, and the breathing becomes at the same time more vesicular in character, while at the lower portions, where, owing to the presence of the fluid exudation, the lung tissue cannot expand, the respiration continues more or less bronchial, and the dulness also remains. In estimating the amount of exudation it is, therefore, important to cause the patient first to inspire deeply several times, so as to expand the previously collapsed lung portions; so also, if it be doubtful whether a case is one of simple pleurisy, or whether this is complicated with pneumonia, and in the absence of the characteristic signs of pneumonia, a change in the limits of dulness and in the respiratory sound, when the patient sits up, would show it to be a case of collapsed lung only. Lastly, as to treatment, a methodical exercising of the lungs, by frequent inspirations, would materially change the condition of collapsed portions of the lung-tissue, and would either prevent the formation of exudations or aid in their removal by absorption.—*London Medical Record*, June 15, 1878.

Immobilization of the Thorax in Pleurisy.

Dr. PERROUD, of Lyons (*Lyon Médical*), confirms from his own practice the value of Dr. F. T. Roberts's method of immobilizing the walls of the chest in pleurisy by bands of diachylon, strengthened if necessary by a plaster-bandage. It is especially indicated in pleurisy and in pneumonia at the outset, and where the element of pain is prominent. This treatment was employed in a dozen cases of children attacked with pleuritic effusion of from four to six days' date, and a moderate quantity of fluid was followed by speedy improvement, the fluid being ab-

soibed in thiee oi foui days. Niemeyei has suggested that blisteis may act in
pleuiisy simply by inducing immobility of the chest-wall. Perroud obseives that
Dr. Roberts's method is moie diiect and safei.—*London Med. Recoid*, May 15,
1878.

Obliteiative Endarteritis.

The almost univeisal pait played in pathology by obliteiative arteiitis, its mode
of oiigin and ieal natuie, aie, or have been until lately, ignoied by Biitish
pathologists, oi, if seen in some cases, they have been totally misundeistood.
The facts aie not new, but they aie not iecognized, peihaps because woikeis at
histology limit themselves too much to a narrow field of special obseivation
without piepaiing themselves by wide study of changes as they occui in all the
tissues of the body, in inflammations, in new foimations and tumouis of all kinds.
Appaiently, MM. Coinil and Ranviei weie the fiist to desciibe this change.
They say, "Dans les plaies, dans les ulcèies, et dans les phlegmons chioniques,
il n'est pas iaie de iencontiei, sui les coupes minces faites poui l'examen micio-
scopique, des aitèies dont la tunique intime a végété de manièie à oblitéiei com-
plétement le calibre du vaisseau" (*Manuel d'Histologie Path.*, pp. 554–5). But
we owe to Fiiedländei and Köstei the fiist pieciseof desciiptions of the condition,
theii obseivations having been published almost simultaneously at the beginning
of 1876. (A papei on the subject, by Dr. Fiiedländei, was noticed in the
Biitish Medical Jouinal of Maich 18, 1876.) They showed that in all
giowths, whethei inflammatoiy, tubeiculai, syphilitic, saicomatous, or othei, it
was not uncommon to find the lumina of the vessels naiiowed by a small-celled
ciicumsciibing oi lateially placed giowth of embiyonic tissue, which was accompanied by a similai infiltiation of the outei coat in a moie advanced state of organization, and by a less degiee of affection of the middle coat, which tended to
lose its distinctive musculai chaiactei and become fibious. They compaied these
changes to those which take place in the so-called oiganization of thiombus, and
held that the giowth fiom the innei membiane was foimed fiom elements which
had migiated fiom the vasa vasoium. These obseivations weie all the moie op-
poitune, as in these iecent yeais we have had two foims of obliteiative aiteiitis
desciibed, to each of which specific chaiacteis have been assigned and consideiable pathological significance has been claimed foi them. We iefei to the aiteiio-
capillaiy fibiosis of Gull and Sutton, and the syphilitic aiteiitis of Heubnei. It
is tiue that, so fai as the ienal aiteiioles weie conceined, the facts biought foiwaid by Sir W. Gull and Dr. Sutton weie not new, but our want of knowledge
at that time as to the tiue natuie of the piocess made them assign to it an impoitance which it by no means deseives. If they had known that the coats of the
vessels univeisally take pait in the suiiounding connective tissue changes, they
would not have ventuied to find in theii aiteiial thickenings evidence of a geneial
piimaiy disease of the bloodvessels. Othei obseiveis have failed to confiim theii
asseitions that these changes aie fuithei distiibuted than suiiounding piocesses
fully account foi. Most of the cases of so-called syphilitic aiteiitis also come
undei the same categoiy of secondaiy piocesses piesenting no anatomical distinctive featuies. The changes desciibed by Oedmansson in the umbilical vessels,
and Fiänkel in the placenta of syphilitic fœtuses, aie now known to piesent nothing
chaiacteiistic ; and identical appeaiances have been desciibed by Mi. Lawson
Tait in non-syphilitic placentæ (*Transactions of the Obstetiical Society*, vol.
xvii.). The same iemaik applies to the vessels figuied by Dr. Batty Tuke
(*Jouinal of Mental Science*, Octobei, 1874) as found in the biain of an insane
patient who had had syphilis ; while Fiiedländei goes so fai as to say that the
syphilitic aiteiitis of Heubnei is "a typical obliteiative aiteiitis, which piesents

no specific syphilitic peculiarities whatever, and, moreover, is in no way etiologically limited to syphilis alone."

The syphilitic arteritis of Heubner differs in one important feature from all the
other affections we have alluded to in being an independent affection of the vascular system, that is, not necessarily dependent upon gummatous growth around.
It is true that there is no difference between the changes that occur in the middle
cerebral artery, for instance, which lies imbedded in a gummatous mass involving neighbouring parts, and that which is not so surrounded ; but it is not the less
a striking feature, that this disease may, and does frequently, arise primarily in
the coats of the vessel, and shows no tendency to involve the surrounding parts,
as in the case related below. Heubner considered it a "gummatous" affection
of the vessel, originating in the intima, due to irritation by the syphilitic virus in
the blood and growing by proliferation of the epithelioid lining of the vessel, and
secondarily giving rise to changes in the muscular and outer coats from migration
of cells out of the vasa vasorum.

Dr. PAUL BAUMGARTEN, of Königsberg, already known by his contribution
to our knowledge of the process of organization of thrombi, has recently published some further observations (Virchow's *Archiv*, Band lxxiii. Heft 1) on
syphilitic arteritis, and endeavours to settle the questions at issue between Heubner and Friedländer. On the general subject of endarteritis, he is completely at
one with Friedländer, except as to the part played by the epithelioid lining ; he
finds that, in endarteritis artificially produced by ligature, the epithelioid lining
first undergoes proliferation, and that the changes in the outer coats occur later
and by migration of cells from the vasa vasorum. He relates a case of primary
syphilitic arteritis in a man who died of general paralysis of syphilis, and in whose
brain the arteries at the base were "generally thickened and white coloured, both
middle cerebral arteries being changed into thick grayish-white cords, no basal
meningitis, and indeed no affection of the basis cerebri et cranii." A microscopical
examination of these vessels showed an indifferent non-vascular embryonic growth
in the lumen ; and in the adventitia a vascular, partly caseating, round-celled
formation, containing giant cells, and encroaching upon the middle coat so far as
in one case to be continuous with the growth in the intima. He considers the
periarterial formation to present the characters of gumma, but the internal growth
he regards as a non-specific indifferent production ; so that he agrees so far with
Heubner as to admit the disease to be gummatous and to deserve a specific title :
but so far as the endarteritis is concerned, he considers it a non-specific change in
a strictly anatomical sense. Reasoning from the analogy of his observations on
artificial arteritis, he is quite willing to accept Heubner's statement that the process commences by proliferation of the epithelioid lining, and that the changes in
the outer coats are due to the migration of cells out of the vasa vasorum ; but
according to him, it is this latter growth only which takes on the characters of
"gumma," the internal new formation retaining its indifferent character, and
behaving throughout like ordinary granulation tissue developed in the same situation under non-specific influences. This view is not to be confounded with that
held by some English observers, especially Dr. Davidson, of Liverpool, who contends that the periarterial gummatous formation precedes the obliterative process,
which latter, according to him, takes place by the organization of a thrombus
formed by the partial occlusion of the vessel through the pressure of the external
growth—a mode of production already long ago put forward by N. Ranvier as
that in which tubercular obliteration of the bloodvessels is effected.—*British Med.
Journal,* June 29, 1878.

Case of Embolism of the Pulmonary Artery.

Dr. O. V. PETERSSON relates the following case in the thirteenth volume of the *Upsala Läkareforenings Forhändlingar* (abstract in *Nordiskt Medicin. Arkiv,* Band x., Häft i.)

A woman, aged 36, had a fall in the beginning of March, 1877. In consequence of this, besides a slight excoriation of the left hand, and pain in the left leg on walking and standing, she had a fixed pain in the left groin. Along the whole course of the saphena vein of the same limb considerable varices were formed, the skin over the subinguinal fossa was red and tender, and at this part a hard cord was felt lying deeply. Mercurial ointment was rubbed into the affected parts, and warm moist applications were used; rest and morphia were prescribed. After some days, a hard, knotty mass, red and painful, was observed at the inner side of the knee and leg. On March 20th the patient, in spite of prohibition, walked across her room to a sofa. The pain in the leg thereupon became violent; notwithstanding, the patient walked back to her bed. She had scarcely time to lie down before she was attacked with violent dyspnœa and oppression in the chest, and became unconscious. Her face immediately became cyanotic; her respiration was stertorous; the pulse was scarcely perceptible, and she died thirty minutes after the commencement of the paroxysm.

At the *post-mortem* examination the left saphena vein, along nearly its whole course, was found to be the seat of saccular projections of greater or less size, which in the leg were filled with dark-red coagula, while in the thigh and in the fossa ovalis grayish-red thrombotic plugs were found. At the opening into the femoral vein was a dilatation of the size of a walnut, filled with a thrombus, a small portion of which extended into the femoral vein. A large branch of the right pulmonary artery was found to be completely blocked up by an embolon an inch long; externally it was reddish gray and firm, internally, dark red and of loose consistence. In the left lung the principal branch of the pulmonary artery was in like manner occluded by an embolon two inches long, loosely connected to the lining membrane of the artery, and of the same appearance and consistence as the other. The heart was externally loaded with fat, and its muscular tissue was lax and brittle. The subpericardial fat was prolonged between the muscular structure, and the tissue of the right ventricle presented fatty degeneration on microscopic examination.—*London Med. Record,* May 15, 1878.

Tubercle of Serous Membranes and so-called " Giant-cells."

At the meeting of the Société de Biologie on March 16, 1878 (*Gazette Médicale de Paris*), M. CORNIL made an interesting communication touching the nature of the giant-cell and its place in the pathology of tubercle. He described the appearances of the giant-cell when set free by agitating in dilute alcohol sections from tubercular pericarditis. Their substance is, M. Cornil remarked, homogeneous, containing fine granulations, which also penetrate into the fine processes proceeding from the body of the cell. On the addition of acetic acid, the cell becomes clear and swollen, its granules are effaced, and the nuclei become more clearly distinguishable. On treatment with picrocarmine, the substance of the giant-cell is rendered of an orange-yellow color, whilst the nuclei are tinged red. The nuclei are ovoid, more or less elongated, and often have an appearance of buds on their surface, sometimes undergoing division. They are placed near the surface of the cell, a layer coming into view on first focussing the surface of the cell, and a second layer appearing on deepening the lens so as to focus its under surface. The number of nuclei varies from two to thirty, according to the size of the cell.

Referring to some sections from a case of tubercular pericarditis shown by M. Merklen at the last meeting of the Society, M. Cornil observed that these sections showed the inflamed tissue to be very vascular, and that the capillaries were much dilated, and contained at certain points fibrinous coagula adherent to the inner surface of the vessel. The wall of the capillary thus affected was well defined, and the epithelioid cells undisturbed. But above and below the coagulum the lumen of the vessel was occupied by lymphatic cells, which were abundant also in the connective tissue around. In other vessels, red corpuscles were collected above and below the coagula. In many other points of the preparations there could be seen the "giant-cell," with its prolongations, surrounded also by epithelioid cells, swollen or proliferating; but the wall of the vessel was not in these cases so clear as in the preceding, being more obscured by the presence of numerous small lymphatic cells infiltrated all around it. Nevertheless, the form of the section was that of a dilated and filled vessel. In other parts, more voluminous giant-cells, or groups of such cells, surrounded by epithelioid elements, were seen. The isolated tubercles of the pia mater were composed of small grains of an embryonic tissue which developed around the bloodvessels. The wall of the vessel, its lymphatic sheath, and the cellular tissue around it, were infiltrated with lymphatic cells. The lumen of the vessel in the centre of the small granulation thus constituted was always filled by a fibrinous clot, and, a remarkable but easily verified fact, this vessel was always swollen and its cavity dilated at the point where it was obstructed by the coagulum. Many transverse sections of tuberculous pia mater showed the arterioles to be affected with a distinct endarteritis. And, at the point of the endarteritis, a part or a whole of the lumen of the vessel was occupied by a coagulation purely fibrinous or granular, with lymphatic or epithelioid cells entangled in its periphery. These leucocytes penetrated into any fissures on the surface of the coagulum; the coagula colored strongly with picro-carmine.

In the majority of instances, the wall of the vessel was infiltrated with small cells, its lymphatic sheath filled with leucocytes, and the meshes of the connective tissue of the pia mater around the vessels thus altered presented a beautiful fibrinous reticulum enclosing leucocytes. In the older portions, the tissue became caseous and more compact. But nowhere outside the vessels did one see anything which could be called a "giant-cell." The process of formation of "giant-cells" took place entirely, so far as the pia mater was concerned, in the interior of the vessel cavity.

M. Cornil described similar appearances to be observed in tubercular granulations in the peritoneum, and observed, in conclusion: "It seems to us that the foregoing facts sufficiently demonstrate the intra-vascular origin of 'giant-cells,' and that one may conceive them as having their origin in a special inflammation affecting a limited portion, and causing coagulation of fibrine. The accumulation of white globules and of some red corpuscles, the union and incorporation of the leucocytes into a fibrino-plastic mass, the nuclei of which hypertrophy, become ovoid and proliferated, and tumefaction of the epithelioid cells would be the phenemena observed in the interior of the vessels. The 'giant-cell' would have its origin in the coagulation of a fibrinous plasma, in which leucocytes have been entangled and blended, and would have proliferated in an unusual manner. Infiltration and softening of the vessel-wall, which after a time becomes no longer recognizable, and inflammation of the adjoining connective tissue where the nutritive juices accumulate, permit of considerable but short-lived nutritive activity to the cells in the centre of the little tubercular islets. We believe that we may consider the nest of the giant-cells and of the swollen cells as representing vessels of which the parietes and contents are modified by the special inflammation of tuberculosis."

In the debate which followed upon M. Cornil's paper, M. Malassez, whilst confirming the facts observed, expressed himself as unable to admit that the giant-cells were mere obliterations of vessels more or less changed. Obliteration of vessels was common in tubercle, but its characters were so different from those of the giant-cell, that it was impossible to admit of any relationship between them. M. Malassez's objections were (1) an entire want of numerical relationship between the divided obliterated vessels and the giant-cells; (2) Although the giant-cells like the vessels were often rounded, they often also presented numerous fine processes which could not possibly correspond with any ramifications of the vessel; (3) The size of the giant-cells sometimes exceeded the limits of the vessels; (4) The material obliterating vessels showed a fibrinous reticulum with changed corpuscles in the centre; the giant-cell, on the other hand, did not show this reticulum, its nuclei differed from those of white-corpuscles, and the elements of the cell were living and did not degenerate; (5) The wall of the vessel, always recognizable in obliterations of any considerable size, was never to be found surrounding the giant-cell. M. Malassez regarded the giant-cell as a form common to a certain number of different kinds of anatomical elements in process of normal or morbid development. He conjectured that in tubercle the giant-cells were vaso-formative, and that the central degeneration of tubercle was in part due to the nontransformation of these vaso-formative cells into vessels. Instead of being sections of obliterated vessels, M. Malassez regarded these giant-cells as being very probably vaso-formative cells which have become arrested in their development into vessels.—*London Med. Record,* June 15, 1878.

Gastric Distension, complicating Intestinal Meteorism.

Professor GROSS, of Nancy (*Revue Médicale de l' Est*), describes the case of a woman, aged 68, for whom he performed kelotomy for strangulated hernia. Peritonitis followed, with extreme tympanites, hiccough, and ventral distension and hardness, but without vomiting. He introduced the œsophageal sound, and nearly ten pints of fluid flowed away. Improvement at once set in, and the patient recovered. He relates other facts, drawn from the practice of Kœberlé of Strasburg, in which the distension of the stomach complicated intestinal meteorism, and in which the effects of the latter were apparently aggravated by this complication; great relief followed the catheterization of the stomach, and the removal of the gas or fluids which distended it. He concludes that this is a point which clinically should not be overlooked; and it is probably worthy of more general attention than it has yet received.—*London Med. Record,* June 15, 1878.

Cases illustrating the Treatment of Bromide Rash with Arsenic.

The beneficial effect of arsenic on the bromide rash deserves to be more widely known than it appears to be, and the following cases reported by Dr. GOWERS (*Lancet,* June 15, 1878) illustrating it may be of some interest. They are briefly reported from the out-patient practice at the National Hospital for the Paralyzed and Epileptic:—

S. S., a man aged thirty-eight, had taken bromide of potassium certainly for five years, on account of fits, and during the whole of that time he had had a large amount of acne upon the face. In the summer of 1877, the face was covered with coalescent acne pustules, and presented a most repulsive appearance. The eruption was also abundant on the chest. The addition of a small quantity of sulphur to each dose did a little good; the rash improved for a short time, but it soon got worse again. Sulphide of calcium was then tried, but with no further improvement, and it made him sick. The dose of bromide was then lessened from twenty to ten grains three times a day, and the acne lessened considerably, but the fits became worse, and on again increasing the bromide the acne became more abundant, and soon was as bad as ever. On Sept. 28, five drops of arsenical solution were given twice a day. In a fortnight all the spots of acne were gone from the face, and those on the chest had faded. The arsenic was continued for some time, and then reduced, and ultimately discontinued. The skin remained healthy for a time, but a month afterwards the face was covered with a fresh bromide rash, red elevations, with several points of suppuration in them. Many large spots of similar kind were on the back of the neck, chest, and arms. This eruption commenced a week after the discontinuance of the arsenic. It again disappeared when the arsenic was resumed.

A. E. W., a female aged twenty, epileptic since infancy, who had taken bromide of potassium for some months, without any rash, presented acne on the face and chest for the first time after bromide of ammonium had been substituted for bromide of potassium. The rash was of the form in which there is a large white centre containing fluid, and a narrow red circumference; and the spots were separate and confluent into larger patches. Most were on the forehead. Other spots were on the shoulders and back; there were none on the abdomen. Arsenic was added, and on March 4th the spots were much better; there were no fresh pustules, and the old ones were fading. On April 18 all spots were gone from the face and back, and only their scars remained.

A. C., a female aged twenty-four, who had suffered from epilepsy and scarlatina four years before, on Oct. 20, 1877, having taken bromide of potassium (twenty grains twice daily) for some years, presented a large number of acne spots upon the face, especially on the cheeks and temples, none being on the forehead; there were also many on the back and chest. Three drops of arsenical solution were added to each dose. On Nov. 3 there were no fresh spots, and the old ones were slowly fading. The only signs of recent spots were one or two minute vesicles on the cheeks. The improvement was as marked on the trunk as on the face.

W. H., a man aged twenty years, who had suffered from epilepsy for seven years, had taken bromide certainly for three years, and on the 8th of October, 1877, presented much acne upon the face, small pustules, and old scars of former spots; there were also a few spots on the trunk. He had been taking for four months thirty grains of bromide of ammonium each night. Three drops of arsenical solution were added. On Nov. 5 the spots of acne on the face were much better, but those on the trunk were not. The pustules gradually disappeared everywhere, and two months later the arsenic was omitted. A few weeks after the omission of the arsenic, the rash reappeared.

J. L., aged eighteen, epileptic for eight years, and known to have taken bromide for at least two months, presented on Feb. 26 many spots of acne on the face. Three drops of arsenical solution were added. On April 8 there were only a few old spots, and on April 29 none were to be seen, old or new.

E. H., a woman aged forty-one, who had suffered from fits for a year only, and had taken bromide (fifteen grains three times a day) for three months, presented first on Feb. 18 some spots of acne on the face, one or two large red prominences with a small white centre, and some smaller ones. Two drops of arsenical solution were added to each dose. On March 11 not a single spot of acne could be seen on the face except one small hard spot on one cheek.

S. D., a woman aged thirty-two, while taking bromide of ammonium, pre-

sented acne on face, arms, and shoulders, and small pustules without much redness around. Two drops of arsenical solution being added, in three weeks the
spots on the face were much better, but those on the back were said to be about
the same. The dose of arsenic was therefore increased to three drops, and in a
few weeks the spots were all gone from both face and back. The arsenic was
then omitted, and in a few weeks some spots reappeared.

L. S., a woman aged twenty-six, suffering from long-standing epilepsy, had
for years been disfigured by continuous bromide rash, large suppurating pustules.
No treatment had availed to lessen the eruption except discontinuance of bromide, but the rash recurred when the bromide was resumed. The addition to
the bromide of two drops of arsenic removed every trace of the rash in the course
of five or six weeks.

E. F. R., a young man aged twenty-eight, who had had fits for sixteen years,
and had taken bromide for several years, presented, on March 21, many spots
of acne on the face. Three drops of arsenic were added to the bromide of ammonium, of which he was taking twenty grains three times a day. In a fortnight
the face was quite free from acne, but in three weeks, while still taking the arsenic, many fresh spots appeared, similar to the preceding ones. The dose of
arsenic was then raised to five drops, and in a month the face was almost well.

E. W., a boy aged six, who had had fits for three years, presented a curious
eruption, which seemed probably due to bromide, a month after he commenced
attendance; the possibility that he had previously taken bromide could not be
excluded. The skin on the back and left side of the chest was covered with a
fine pustular rash, resembling closely minute miliaria, each minute white point
having a fine red halo around it. Among these, on the nape of the neck, were
several large pustules, with extensive red bases, like small boils. A drop of arsenical solution was added to each dose of the medicine, and, a fortnight later,
the rash had almost disappeared. There were still some minute pustules on the
side of the neck, but they had gone from the back and chest. The large pustules
had subsided into the characteristic red swellings of bromide acne. Three weeks
later both these had subsided, and only the faintest trace of the finer rash could
be detected.

H. B., a boy aged seven, epileptic since two years of age, had taken bromide
for about three months, when his face, on March 5, presented five or six spots,
each about a quarter of an inch in diameter, almost covered with minute foci of
suppuration. On some of the more advanced of these a crust had formed, occupying almost the whole of the raised red area, of which only a narrow ring showed
around the crust. The latter was thin, and, at a distance, the spots looked very
like those of psoriasis. One drop of arsenic was added to the ten grains of bromide of potassium which he was taking three times a day, and in a month the
spots were well, only the red stains remaining.

A. S. F., a girl aged eleven, epileptic since six months old, and taking twenty
grains of bromide of potassium twice a day, presented, on April 1st, many small
spots of acne on the forehead and cheeks. Four drops of arsenic were added,
and on May 28th every spot had disappeared.

Remarks.—It is surprising that in recent discussions on the subject, the occurrence of bromide rash was mentioned as a rarity. At the Queen-square Hospital,
where, of course, bromide is largely given, the rash is common enough, and is
frequently seen in most severe form, causing great disfigurement. Since, however, the value of arsenic in the affection has been known, an example of bad
bromide rash has not been seen.

The common form of the rash is, as is well known, pustular, the red swelling
being large and the point of suppuration small. As frequent, however, and more

so in the commencement of the rash, are small pustules with little redness, together with papules which do not always reach the stage of pustules. Occasionally large pustules are seen with extensive suppuration, either in very minute foci or in one or two large and superficial areas. It has been said that the white centres of the bromide pustules do not contain pus, but only caseous material. This is sometimes the case, but often there is true pus within them. Occasionally actual boils occur.

It is to be noted that the rash occurs equally with the bromides of potassium and sodium, and still more readily with bromide of ammonium. Some of the above cases illustrate this. The rash occasionally first shows itself when the ammonium salt has been substituted for an equal dose of one of the others. This may be due to the fact that the ammonium salt contains a larger quantity of bromine. The amount of eruption may be observed to vary with the amount of bromide given.

Many observers have noted the beneficial influence of arsenic, and these cases fully corroborate it. They show, moreover, that, irrespective of age, the dose of arsenic required to remove the rash varies in different cases, and the dose required does not always depend on the amount of rash. The dose which cured some cases only effected a slight improvement in others, which did not yield until a large dose had been given. They show that the arsenic affects the rash on the face more readily than that of the trunk. A dose of arsenic which removed the rash from the face had to be increased before that on the trunk disappeared.

The effect of arsenic only continues as long as it is given. Bromide still being administered, the rash returns when the arsenic is stopped. Several cases illustrate this, and illustrate also how rapidly the recurrence may take place.

Many other agents for the treatment of the rash have been tried, but none has been found of value comparable to that of arsenic. The external applications useful in ordinary acne are almost useless in the bromide rash. The internal administration of sulphur or sulphite of calcium has also little influence.

Surgery.

Impairment of Vision after Loss of Blood.

Under the above heading, Dr. C. HORSTMAN records (*Klinische Monatsblätter*, April, 1878) six cases which he had observed during the past year at Berlin, in which, after loss of blood in various ways, there had followed impairment, or loss of sight.

CASE I. A man, aged 40, vomited blood on one occasion during the year previous, and again about fourteen days before coming to the hospital, and three days afterwards noticed that his sight was failing him. On examination, his field of vision was found much diminished ; and there were traces of optic neuritis. On subsequent examination, the visual defect was permanent, and the optic discs were unnaturally pale.

CASE II.—A man, aged 28, had suffered from painful digestion since childhood, and, for more than a year, had suffered from gastric pains. Then hæmatemesis occurred, and, seven days afterwards, he found that during several hours he was unable to distinguish light from darkness. This was followed by a gradual improvement, but in the end, his optic disc remained white and irregular in outline, and there was a permanent and considerable contraction of the visual field in each eye.

CASE III.—A man, aged 44, very corpulent, suffered from an attack of typhoid fever, followed by severe intestinal hemorrhage. Eight days afterwards he found himself absolutely blind, unable to distinguish light from darkness; and, although his general health improved, he remained permanently amaurotic, with white and atrophied discs.

CASE IV.—A young woman, aged 21, had severe hemorrhage after an abortion. and six days later, found herself quite blind : both optic nerves were seen to be swollen and indistinct, and there were extensive defects in the field of vision in each eye. Vision remained permanently impaired, especially in the left eye, her optic discs being pale, and the defects in the visual field remaining unchanged.

CASE V.—A woman, aged 37, had given birth to five children in the course of seven years without accident of any kind; then followed an abortion and severe flooding. Seven days after this, she noticed her sight failing her, and, in a few hours, became absolutely blind; she never acquired even so much as perception of light. Both optic discs presented all the appearances of white atrophy.

CASE VI.—A woman, aged 33, lost a great deal of blood after abortion. On the evening of the seventh day her sight failed her, her optic nerves were found to be swollen and indistinct, the retina around the disc in each eye was opaque, and, in the left eye, in the neighbourhood of the yellow spot, were one or two small hemorrhages. Ultimately, the case assumed the ordinary features of white atrophy of both nerves, and the patient remained permanently blind.

According to Leber (von Gräfe and Sämisch's *Handbuch*), loss of sight in both eyes is not uncommon after considerable loss of blood, especially after hæmatemesis and metrorrhagia. It generally occurs a few days after—three or four days —and not directly after the loss; and the same high authority speaks of the ophthalmoscopic appearances as being negative, or those of white atrophy only. Seigmund Fries (*Klinische Monatsblätter*, 1876) has collected thirty-nine cases of the same nature; in the majority of these both eyes were affected, and remained so permanently. The defect in vision was not complained of until some days had elapsed after the hemorrhage, and, in nearly every instance, the case assumed the typical features of white atrophy of the optic nerves.

From the complete absence of cerebral symptoms before and at the time of the hemorrhage, the explanation of this frequent occurrence of blindness is not altogether clear; but the recent observations of Schwalbe (Schulze's *Archiv*) upon the existence of lymph spaces between the two sheaths of the optic nerve, communicating with the subarachnoid spaces within the cranium, appear to furnish an explanation. Samelsohn and other writers are of opinion that, owing to the sudden hemorrhage, the total amount of blood within the cranium is materially lessened, its place is for the time taken by the fluid from the various lymph-spaces. On the bloodvessels becoming again fully supplied with blood, the lymph-spaces are over-distended, and also the sheath of the optic nerve; a condition of things which leads to pressure upon the optic nerve itself, and, in some instances, to the occurrence of that peculiar aspect of the optic disc, known as *stauungs-papille*, or choked disc.—*Lond. Med. Record*, June 15, 1878.

—

Glaucoma and Increased Tension of the Globe.

Dr. FITZGERALD, in a report on the Progress of Ophthalmology (*Dublin Journ. of Med. Science*, June, 1878), says: The past year will mark an epoch in the history of the progress of ophthalmology, for in it we see the first signs of dawn lighting up the horizon of a hitherto impenetrably dark region. We allude to the remarkable communications which have appeared upon the subject of glaucoma. The exact nature and etiology of this disease has up to this proved one of the most difficult problems in the whole range of ophthalmology. We feel confident that its solution will be reached at no very distant date, but as yet we only discern the preliminary steps towards it. Consequently it appears advisable to postpone any lengthened account of the various investigations and experiments which have been undertaken with reference to this intricate subject, and in the present instance merely to indicate very briefly the general tendency of the con- clusions hitherto arrived at. On one point there seems to be almost complete accord, as evidenced by the papers of Kniess[1] and Weber,[2] as well as by the opinions expressed at the Heidelberg meeting—namely, that the chief factor in the production of the disease is an interference with the "drainage system," if we may so term it, of the eye. This opinion is principally grounded upon the results of pathological investigations. Kniess insists that these investigations prove the important rôle which the obliteration of Fontana's canal plays in the production of the glaucomatous state ; and Weber concludes that in all forms of glaucoma—the inflammatory and non-inflammatory as well as the primary and secondary—the drainage channels become narrowed and finally closed.

At the meeting of the Ophthalmological Society at Heidelberg, last year, Dr. Stilling[3] stated the results of some experiments he had made on ligaturing the optic nerve. At first this proceeding was invariably followed by neuro-paralytic symptoms. After five or ten days had elapsed the tension enormously increased ; there was complete anæsthesia of the cornea, the eye was stony hard, and the vitreous, especially its posterior portion, became quite fluid. He proposed divid- ing glaucoma into two groups: 1. Glaucoma anticum—due to some obstruction in the anterior drainage system as well as Fontana's canal. 2. Glaucoma posti- cum—depending on an obstruction in the vascular sheath (pial Scheide) of the optic nerve.

In the "Royal London Ophthalmological Hospital Reports," Vol. IX., Part ii., 1877, Mr. Brailey, curator of the museum, contributes an interesting and suggestive paper on the Pathology of Increased Tension of the Globe. His observations are based upon the microscopic examination of 53 cases, in which increased intra-ocular tension had been at some time a symptom. He divides his cases into two groups:—

"A. Those in which an affection of the iris has been the primary cause of the tension, the disease either remaining confined to this—as in two cases of buph- thalmos—or extending backwards so as to affect the ciliary-choroidal tract secondarily."

"Those in which the part of the tract posterior to the iris is affected, without any obvious iritic change preceding it."

The first group numbered 28 and the second 25 cases. The latter included "all cases known usually as glaucoma."

The seat of the most marked and universal changes occurring in glaucoma, was found by the author to be in the ciliary body. Of the cases included under group B, it was extensively affected in all but one, and in it there was some change. In group A it was markedly implicated in all but three.

"The remaining 49 cases of increased tension present marked ciliary changes, and the one which is present in all, and more distinctly seen in each than any other pathological condition, is atrophy of the ciliary muscle."

The circular fibres were specially affected, and to such an extent that in many

[1] Archiv. f. Ophth. Bd. XXII. Abth. III. P. 163.   Bd. XXIII. Abth. II. P. 62.
[2] Archiv. f. Ophth. Bd. XXIII. Abth. I. P. 1.
[3] Bericht der Ophthalmologischen Gesellschaft. Heidelberg. 1877. P. 16.

cases the affected part presented no traces of muscular fibres at all. At the same time the radial fibres did not escape, their bulk being diminished, though to a less extent than the others.

The author alludes to the peripheral adhesion of the iris, a condition to which considerable attention has been directed in the papers by *K*niess and Weber, and also in the discussion on Pagenstecher's communication at the Heidelberg meeting. He does not agree with *K*niess that it is the cause of the increase of tension, though it may undoubtedly have a "great effect in keeping up an already established increased pressure." He also considers that Kniess attaches too much importance to the closure of Schlemm's canal. While admitting that in most of his specimens of increased tension Schlemm's canal was commonly closed, yet it was by no means invariably the case, and it was a much less constant condition than either atrophy of the ciliary muscle or the atrophy or adhesion of the iris. He is disposed "to attribute its closure to its compression, either through the dragging forward of the iris in a prolapse, or its bulging forwards from pressure behind, as in the case of group B."

One very suggestive passage towards the close of the paper is worthy of note : "In studying longitudinal sections of the atrophied ciliary muscles of glaucomatous eyes, it is very common to find sections of dilated empty venous channels. These are of more frequent occurrence than the changes in Schlemm's canal, but are not so constant as the ciliary and iritic changes above described. I am unable to say precisely what may be the pathological causes or results of this condition, but the atrophy of the muscle may be connected with yielding of the muscular tissue surrounding its veins. The increased intraocular pressure should have a tendency to close these veins. We may connect them with the dilated ciliary veins so often seen externally during life in such cases."

"It is extremely likely that the ciliary muscle has functions besides that of accommodation, and that it may be concerned in regulating the blood supply. This might explain the effect of an atrophied ciliary muscle in passively keeping up an increased tension, notwithstanding that the periphery of the iris has never been united to the cornea."

———

Case of Trephining of an External Meatus closed by Bony Deposit.

In Virchow's *Archiv*, vol. lxxiii., 1878, Dr. Moos, of Heidelberg, relates a case of acute inflammation of the right external meatus, causing osseous occlusion of the canal. The deafness was great. There was no tinnitus, and affection of the acoustic was negatived. Believing, from the character of the auscultatory sounds, that the obstructive mass was not extensive, trephining was determined on, and this was effected by means of a drill of two millimetres in diameter ; but not till a canal seven millimetres in length had been made. The result was very satisfactory, the hearing being restored nearly to the normal degree ; and, when the patient was seen two months afterwards, there were no symptoms of a return of the affection.—*London Med. Record*, June 15, 1878.

———

The Treatment of Laryngeal Stenosis.

Although Dr. Schrötter has already made two communications, and published an essay, on this subject, he thought it right to again bring it forward at the Imperial Royal Medical Society of Vienna, partly because he had some cases of recovery to relate, and partly to again call attention to his previous advice. He divided the cases of laryngeal stenosis into two groups—one in which the contraction was treated after the performance of laryngotomy, and another in which the danger of suffocation appeared to be imminent, but laryngotomy was not per-

formed. The first group was subdivided into two sections, according as the stenosis was treated from above or from below. The latter method, which had
been carried out by some, but almost always with negative results, he had not
practised, because the stenosis formed a canal narrowing downwards towards the
trachea. As regarded dilatation from above, the experience of Roux, Depray,
Navratil, and Weinlechner had given only partial results. There was some improvement, but no such cure as to allow the removal of the canula. Dr. Schrötter had many times arrived at this result, and was able to show some cases. The
first case was that of a man who had been under treatment from April, 1875, to
July, 1876. Laryngotomy was performed, on account of laryngeal perichondritis.
Complete recovery followed; the patient (a teacher of languages) being able to
employ himself in instruction for twelve hours a day without any trouble of importance. He spoke aloud and distinctly, and suffered no inconvenience from
bodily exertion. The second patient who was shown still wore the canula, but
it had been stopped for some time, and might have been removed, had not the
patient objected, on the ground that tracheotomy had been twice already performed on him, on account of sudden paroxysms of suffocation from some unexplained cause; and he was unwilling to expose himself to the chance of a third
operation. The patient came under Dr. Schrötter's care in 1873, wearing the
canula; in July, 1874, he was able to have the canula stopped, and it had remained so. His speech was quite intelligible, and there was no dyspnœa. The
third case shown was that of a man who had been under treatment since October,
1877, for stenosis of the larynx, the result of perichondritis following typhus.
For the last twenty days the patient had plugged the canula; he spoke well,
and his breathing was calm. It was necessary for him to wear the canula, as
otherwise contraction would return. His voice was rather hoarse, in consequence
of his having taken out the tube for the first time two days previously, which had
produced irritation of the larynx. The fourth patient was still under treatment.
He could introduce the bougie himself in the manner recommended and described
by Dr. Schrötter (see *London Medical Record*, April 15). [This method consists in passing a thread through the mouth, larynx, and upper opening of the
trachea tube, and passing it out through the external orifice of the tube. The
two ends are then knotted together. The thread serves as a guide for the bougie,
which has a silk thread at each end. The bougie is fastened to the mouth end of
the thread, and, by traction on the tracheal end of the thread, is drawn down to
the inner opening of the trachea. In removing the bougie, it is simply drawn to
the mouth and set free from the guiding thread.] He next spoke of the treatment of cases of laryngeal stenosis, in which laryngotomy had not been performed. The first attempts of the kind were of old date; in them, however, it
was only attempted to insufflate medicines into the larynx and trachea. Desault
and Weinlechner had attempted to cure stenosis of the larynx, but without success. Dr. Schrötter had obtained favourable results in the most advanced stages
of stenosis. He showed a woman who had suffered from severe stenosis after
variola. The patient came under treatment in October, 1876, and in April,
1877, might be regarded as cured. She also suffered from chronic laryngeal
catarrh, and hence was still hoarse. The case was the more interesting, as the
stenosis was caused by a cicatricial membrane. Dr. Schrötter showed a drawing,
which illustrated the condition at the commencement of the treatment. The
glottis was almost entirely occupied by a membrane, and anteriorly there was adhesion of the vocal cords. Following Türck's example, Dr. Schrötter divided the
membrane with a knife, and then proceeded to dilate the stenosis. In this, as
could be seen by laryngoscopic examination, he had perfectly succeeded. The
vocal cords were quite free up to the anterior angle, and, as this condition had

already remained unchanged for some time, readhesion of the vocal cords was scarcely to be feared. Dr. Schötter had also treated successfully a number of other patients, who, however, were not at present in Vienna.

Dr. WEINLECHNER asked Dr. Schötter how he would deal with less intelligent patients, in regard to the application of the ring of thread. The experiment was very simple, and could be easily carried out; but he did not think that every patient could do it for himself, like the one who had been shown.

Dr. SCHRÖTTER replied that it was necessary not to entrust the patient with his own treatment until the stenosis was cured; and the only object was to prevent a return of the contraction. He had as yet met with no patient who had not learned to introduce the tube. In one case, that of a boy, there was difficulty in the introduction of the tube. A flexible forceps was therefore introduced through the external opening in the larynx into the mouth, and made to seize the bougie. This manœuvre was learned by the nurse.—*London Med. Record*, June 15, 1878.

Case of Gastric Fistula.

Dr. KJÖNIG describes in the *Norsk Magazin fur Lägevidenskaben*, 3d series, Band vii. (abstract in *Nordiskt Medicin. Arkiv*), a case of fistula of the stomach in a married woman, aged 34, whom he had had under observation since 1872. The opening was situated in the ninth left intercostal space, about three and one-fifth inches from the point of the tenth rib; it was a cleft about four-fifths of an inch long, but only wide enough to admit the blunt end of a probe. The edges were inverted, excoriated, and adherent to the subjacent rib. Sometimes, especially in the morning, a fluid having an acid reaction and mixed with food escaped. The appetite was good; the bowels were costive; the patient's general condition was satisfactory. From the age of eight she had suffered from pain in the left hypochondrium, and later had been often treated for chlorosis. When she was nineteen years old the pain in the hypochondrium and epigastrium increased, and was generally accompanied by pain over the left olecranon. In 1865 a painful swelling of the size of an almond was observed, and in 1871 a fistula was formed at the same spot. The fistula closed after a time, but on the last day of the year it again opened. The opening, which at first would admit a little finger, afterwards contracted, so that only an inconsiderable quantity of aliment escaped. The discharge consisted essentially of a clear tenacious mucus, and on one occasion of a bile-stained or rather blood-coloured fluid. The administration of a two per cent. solution of bicarbonate of soda did not change the reaction of the fluid which escaped.

Dr. Kjönig remarks that fifty-six cases of gastric fistula had been observed up to 1876. He regards the prognosis as good, inasmuch as, so far as statistics show, death was attributable to the fistula itself in only one-fifth of the cases.—*London Med. Record*, June 15, 1878.

Two Cases of Intussusception, in one of which Abdominal Section was performed.

Mr. HANDFIELD JONES and Mr. HERBERT W. PAGE, at a late meeting of the Royal Medical and Chirurgical Society (*British Med. Journal*, June 8, 1878), recorded two cases of intussusception in patients of Dr. Handfield Jones at St. Mary's Hospital. The first, a harness-maker, aged 60, admitted May 12, 1874, had, although enjoying good health, passed blood *per rectum* for the previous twelve months. On May 5, he was seized with abdominal pain, and then passed a teacupful of clotted blood. The pain became constant after May 8, and, when admitted, a tumour was found in the cavity of the bowel, round which the finger could be passed, and there was dulness in the left flank, with constipation. He was examined on the 21st, with a view to operation; but the surgeon (since dead) concluded there was cancerous disease, having brought away a portion of growth on the finger. The man died on the 23d. Extensive peritonitis was found *post-mortem*, and a large invagination projecting into the rectum, which could be reduced with ease, and there was no cancer. Regret was expressed at the delay and mistake in diagnosis; an operation might have easily relieved the condition, and perhaps have saved life.

The second case presented features of great interest. A boy aged 5 was admitted December 31, 1877, with a history of having lost flesh and been very ill for six weeks. He had severe paroxysms of pain in his abdomen, varying much in frequency, and with some diarrhœa. He improved during the first few days; but, on January 14th, he had more pain, and there was dulness on percussion in the left flank. This condition increased, and, on the 20th, the child being very ill, and there being a distinct hard lump in the left iliac fossa, inflation was performed *per anum*, and was followed by a rapid subsidence of all the urgent symptoms. His state continued very variable from day to day until February 4th, when the tumour again appeared, and was a second time relieved by inflation. On February 11th, for a third time, and again on February 16th, the tumour reappeared, and was removed by insufflation; and on February 25th, the operation was again repeated for the fifth time, and caused the disappearance of the tumour, then much larger than before, and both seen and felt in the left iliac fossa. He was taken out of the hospital by his parents on February 27th, with a warning that a recurrence of the disorder was almost certain. He was readmitted on March 4th, in an alarming state, the symptoms having returned two days before. A large tumour was now felt, reaching from the iliac to the umbilical region; and inflation, when performed in the afternoon, only changed its position, but did not make it disappear. The child continued in great pain, and in the evening insufflation was again tried, and failing, water was injected, but without success. On the following day, he was much worse; and at 5 P. M., when pulseless and collapsed, he was seen by Mr. Page, who at once performed abdominal section. The tumour was so large that it was necessary to prolong the incision above the umbilicus, and to remove the small intestines from the abdominal cavity. Traction on the upper end of the volvulus was only successful in the extrication of about two inches of ileum; and an attempt to draw off the ensheathing part at the lower end was frustrated by the presence, then discovered, of a second and lower intussusception of the colon, in which the order of parts was reversed—the inferior portion being ensheathed in the upper, which thus became the ensheathing part. The two volvuli met and overlapped each other at their extremities, and it became necessary to reduce the backward intussusception before the ordinary invagination could be relieved. Owing to the great distension of the bowel and slight adhesions at the ultimate part of the intussusception, this was a work of much difficulty, and was only accomplished by considerable force. The upper or more usual invagination was then reduced with great ease, by gently squeezing the lower end of the volvulus—an action which simultaneously drew off the ensheathing, and pushed out the ensheathed part of the bowel, the vermiform appendix being the last to appear. There was some visible congestion and thickening about the cæcum, but no general peritonitis or adhesions. The operation, of which a detailed account was given, lasted an hour and a quarter. The child considerably rallied after it, but died exhausted the following morning, having lived nine hours and three-quarters. At the necropsy, the lips of the wound were found adherent. There was commencing peritonitis of the small intestines, but none of the large bowel.   At a point corresponding with the upper limit of the volvulus, the mucous membrane of the ileum was swollen and greatly congested, and that near the vermiform appendix was much the same. The meso-cæcum was so lax as to allow the cæcum to be drawn over the left iliac fossa.

The method of reducing the upper volvulus was specially referred to, as confirmatory of Mr. Hutchinson's experience, recorded in the fifty-ninth volume of the *Transactions*, that pulling down the ensheathing part rather than pulling out the ensheathed part was the true mode to pursue.   Reduction of the backward intussusception was rendered most difficult from the slight adhesions at its furthest end, and from great distension of the gut; and, although accomplished without damage to the structure of the bowel, it was thought that such force as was requisite might itself have been dangerous.   Reference was made to the long continuance of pain before any definite appearance of tumour; and it was suggested, as an explanation of the occurrence of intussusception, that pain and the subsequent motor derangement must be ascribed to a functional disorder of the abdominal nerves and ganglia, a relaxed state of a lower segment certainly favouring the intrusion of an actively contracting part above.   It was, therefore, most probable that the essential condition of intussusception was a local paralysis of a portion of the small intestine, which became the sheath of the volvulus.   Neuralgic pain in other parts was associated with motor paralysis, and probably was so in the abdominal organs.   At the same time, the laxity of the meso-cæcum might throw light on a predisposing cause of the intussusception.   The second and ascending intussusception formed a very remarkable feature in the case, the existence of a single instance of such a condition having been called in question by the late Dr. Brinton.   The absence of peritonitis and adhesions after many recurrences, and the presence of slight adhesions only when the child had been taken home, and when there was long delay in resorting to inflation, showed how necessary it was that this treatment should be had recourse to as soon as intussusception was evident; while the state of the mucous membrane, although the serous surface of the bowel might be free from inflammation, pointed out the imperative need of surgical interference at the earliest possible moment after other means had failed to give relief.

Mr. Gay remembered a case of his own which was somewhat similar.   He was called in consultation to see a lady, more than seventy years old, supposed to have suffered for several years from internal piles.   Sometimes there was bleeding and difficulty of defecation; and when this was overcome, blood was passed in some quantity.   He could find a considerable swelling in the rectum, which seemed to be a polypus when examined by the speculum, and to that he applied a ligature.   When he next saw her, there were peritonitis and vomiting, and no motion had been passed.   He removed the ligature, and separated the part by the knife.   She improved for a time, but after a few weeks she sank and died. No *post-mortem* examination was allowed; but the tumor, when examined, was found to be an old invagination, and it could even be unsheathed with a little trouble.   The case showed, at all events, that invagination might last for years without giving rise to marked signs.

—

Foreign Body in the Bladder.

At a recent meeting of the Société de Chirurgie (*Union Méd.*, June 11), M. LANNELONGUE communicated a case on the part of M. FLEURY, of Clermont, which gave rise to an interesting discussion.   The subject of the case is a gentleman, seventy-eight years of age, of robust constitution, and remarkable for his energy. In 1863 M. Civialé performed lithotrity on him, and from that time he had always been obliged to use a catheter, a slight vesical catarrh having always remained. He employed an instrument five millimetres in diameter, and which had become much roughened by long usage. He introduced it as easily as usual on April 23, but on withdrawing it he found that a portion of it remained in the canal; and in place of sending for aid to have it extracted he forced it into the bladder by means of another catheter. M. Fleury, when consulted, advised expectation, as he considered the attempt to remove a metallic body seven centimetres in length would be of very doubtful success, while cystotomy at the age of the patient was a hazardous procedure. There was but a moderate degree of inflammation caused by the presence of the foreign body, and catheterism was performed without much difficulty, when four days afterwards, during an effort at stool, the end of the catheter presented itself at the anus, and was removed after a few tractions. From this time the pains diminished, and no urine oozed out by the rectum. The patient resumed his former habits of life, and the bladder held the urine for five or six hours, as heretofore.

At the discussion which followed the narration of this case, M. TILLAUX observed that, although the procedure followed had a fortunate issue, it was not a desirable one to imitate, seeing how exceptional must be a spontaneous discharge of a foreign body from the bladder. Moreover, the age of the patient was no reason for abstaining from interference, for operations are performed at that age with successful results. So exceptional must be the discharge of a foreign body of this size through the recto-vesical wall without being followed by a fistula, that M. Tillaux would not trust to it; and if he failed to extract the metallic body by one of the instruments that have been designed for this purpose, he would not hesitate to perform lithotomy.

Prof. VERNEUIL observed that this case raised the question whether we ought to renounce in aged persons the resources offered to us by surgery. Operations in aged persons are, indeed, always of a serious character, for the senile condition of the kidney is one of the most frequent causes of the nephritis which carries off so many patients. For several years past he has been collecting a great number of facts which much aggravate the prognosis delivered in the cases of persons undergoing operations, when subjects of a general affection; but in spite of this, when the necessity arrives, he operates upon them, and some of them recover. It is the same with old age, which is certainly not a worse condition, and, in his opinion, urgent cases should be operated upon. In respect to the present case, it must be admitted that a portion of catheter seven centimetres long remaining in the bladder is a terrible accident, in presence of which we have no right to remain inactive. It should be extracted, and not having much confidence in the instruments constructed for this purpose, Prof. Verneuil would have proposed lithotomy. This case of M. Fleury's possesses the great inconvenience of raising hopes that will be disappointed.

M. DESPRES congratulated M. Fleury in not having made use of any of the instruments contrived for removing solid bodies from the bladder, the utility of which he regards as quite illusory. None of them would have been able to remove this catheter, while their employment might have done much mischief. It is to be regretted that an examination per anum was not instituted, for the end of the instrument pressing against the recto-vesical wall would have been felt, and an incision into the rectum would have enabled it to be extracted. As to the patient's age, that was no contraindication to an operation.

M. TILLAUX said that he regarded this *taille rectale* recommended by M. Despres as a bad operation; for in an adult there is often difficulty in reaching the posterior edge of the prostate, and still more the base of the bladder, in which the foreign body may be felt. It is possible in a child, but much more difficult in an adult. As to the operation by the rectum, this does not consist in cutting into the base of the bladder, but in cutting through the rectum into the neck of the bladder in order to penetrate into that organ. If we cut into where the foreign body was located we should divide the vesiculæ and the peritoneum.—*Med. Times and Gaz.*, June 22, 1878.

Necrosis and Caries of the Os Calcis.

Professor SCHINZINGER of Freiburg (Baden), reports in Von Langenbeck's *Archiv für Klinische Chirurgie*, Band xxii. Heft,2, four cases of central necrosis of the os calcis. In some remarks on the pathology and treatment of the morbid results of ostitis affecting the calcaneum, the author points out that there is a special tendency for this bone to become inflamed independently of other bones of the tarsus. It is larger than any other tarsal bone, and takes the largest share in bearing the weight of the body. According to Hueter, the developmental processes which go on in the talo-tarsal joint from birth to the period of completed growth are of considerable pathological and clinical interest. In consequence of pressure on this bone during standing and locomotion, the vertical growth may be arrested, and during life the anterior calcanean process becomes more and more depressed. The constant traction of the tendo Achillis on the posterior surface of the bone, and the results of injuries, such as contusion in cases of sprained ankle, and concussion in attempts at active leaping, are all likely to set up inflammatory irritation in the succulent and spongy tissue of the calcaneum. Disease of the os calcis, when attacking healthy adults as a result of injury, usually remains restricted to this bone, and does not spread to other osseous parts of the foot. On the other hand, in cases of scrofulous disease of the tarsus, the os calcis presents a remarkable immunity. It must be well known to all practical surgeons, the author remarks, that the body of this bone is almost invariably found sound in such cases, even when all the other osseous portions of the foot have been thoroughly disorganized by caries. This clinical fact is of some importance with respect to the determination of the method of amputation for the removal of the diseased foot. According to Schede, Pirogoff's method may be applied with good prospect of success even in those rare cases of disease of the tarsus in which the calcaneum has become involved, for here the anterior portion of the bone only, and never the posterior portion, is affected with caries.

With regard to the relative frequency of caries and necrosis of the calcaneum, there is much difference of opinion amongst German and French surgeons. The author seems disposed to hold that these cannot be considered as rare affections. Ollier has reported that, in the course of sixteen years, he saw more than one hundred cases of suppurating ostitis of the calcaneum alone. According to Kocher, the calcaneum is frequently affected by acute osteomyelitis, and is by no means unfrequently the seat of chronic inflammation. Out of fifty-two cases of caries of the tarsal bones reported by Czerny, the calcaneum was affected in thirteen.

The author, in referring to treatment of ostitis of the calcaneum, states that in recent cases of traumatic origin the inflammatory symptoms should be combated with ice and repeated local bleeding. The surgeon has, however, more frequently to deal with the morbid results of inflammation, viz., caries and necrosis. Here his chief object should be to prevent extension of the disease. Whilst in some cases of primary ostitis, an osteo-myelitic focus, or central necrosis, may be restricted to the calcaneum for months and even for years, there are, on the other hand, cases in which the calcaneal disease finally gives rise to fungous synovitis of the nearest articulation. In the treatment of caries of the calcaneum and of other bones of the foot, Kocher recommends ignipuncture, or the repeated introduction into the bone of a pointed actual cautery, by which the diseased parts are thoroughly destroyed, their seat being subsequently occupied by a new growth of scar-tissue. Dr. Schinzinger is in favour of this method of ignipuncture, and mentions three cases in which he applied it with success. In two cases of children, one five, the other seven years old, long-standing fungous ostitis of a metatarsal bone was speedily removed. In the third case, that of a feeble man aged seventy, suffering from caries of the fifth metatarsal bone, considerable improvement followed the application of the cautery, the suppuration, swelling, and pain in the soft parts of the foot were much reduced, and the patient was enabled to walk again.

In more advanced cases of caries of the calcaneum, it is thought advisable, before applying the hot iron, to remove the diseased parts with the sharp spoon. In the most severe cases it will be found necessary for cure to perform a partial subperiosteal resection, or to remove the whole of the diseased bone. In a case of completed necrosis of the calcaneum, a long-standing source of annoyance may at once be removed by extracting the sequestrum. In cases of carious degeneration affecting several metatarsal bones, there being a well-marked scrofulous diathesis, the author recommends amputation of the foot by Pirogoff's method.

Midwifery and Gynæcology.

On the Treatment of Puerperal Hyperpyrexia by Cold.

Dr. PLAYFAIR'S case of puerperal septicæmia, with hyperpyrexia, treated by the continuous application of cold (*Monthly Abstract*, Jan. 1878, p. 41) opens up for discussion the practice of treating such cases by the rapid abstraction of heat, a remedy which has proved of inestimable value in other grave maladies accompanied by hyperpyrexia. Dr. ALFRED WILTSHIRE records (*British Med. Journ.*, May 8, 1878) two cases similarly treated, as follows:—

In the autumn of 1873, I succeeded my friend and colleague Dr. Edis in the charge of the in-patients of the British Lying-in Hospital, an institution to which I was then physician. In giving the patients into my charge, Dr. Edis remarked that there was something wrong about the place; for none of the mothers had a temperature under 100° Fahr., upon which I observed that I should feel compelled to close the hospital, if things continued in an unsatisfactory state. I regret to say that closure immediately became necessary, on account of the serious symptoms which arose in two newly admitted patients.

A day or two after I took charge, two healthy young women, primiparæ, were delivered in the hospital. Both were married, were aged respectively 23 and 26, and had fairly good labours, there being nothing abnormal in either case. I had the temperature watched, as has now for many years been my custom, and very speedily it attained high figures. There was no local condition in either case to account for this abnormal elevation of temperature, and it appeared to be only too clearly due to the unhealthy surroundings of the patients. Finding that quinine in large and repeated doses, intra-uterine irrigations, purges, and so on, were ineffectual for the reduction of the excessively high temperature, which in each case exceeded 106°, and feeling persuaded that such hyperpyrexia was incompatible with life, if long-continued, I had the patients packed round with vessels containing ice; hot-water tins, soda-water and other bottles, being filled with broken ice.

This *dry cold* method was selected because it obviated the necessity of removing the prostrate patients from their beds ; a point which has always seemed to me to be of much importance in the treatment of hyperpyrexia by cold, since the patients for whom it is necessary are usually extremely exhausted. The temperature in each case was promptly reduced, but it rose again, after a variable fashion, when the cold was removed, and occasionally, I am bound to say, apparently in spite of it. Still, in the main, when it was carefully and assiduously applied, the effect of this method of reducing temperature was distinct, and the relief experienced by the patients was at times great and palpable. The only inconvenience arising from its use was the inability of the patients to sleep during its application. Chilling of the skin appeared to be attended by increased vascular supply to the nervous centres, and consequent wakefulness. This might doubtless have been obviated if we had then had at command the efficient means we now have for cooling the head—viz., the ice-cap. As it was, sound sleep speedily followed the removal of the cold ; the cerebral vessels being obviously relieved by the flushing of those of the skin. For many days a weary fight was kept up with fluctuating success, the temperature occasionally remaining normal for several hours. Ultimately, one of the patients recovered, and the other, to my great regret, sank. Unfortunately, no necropsy was obtainable.

I believe that, could we have removed the patient whose case ended fatally from the building, she also would have recovered ; for, again and again, her temperature fell to normal or near it, and she appeared to be on the verge of convalescence ; she seemed, however, to get fresh doses of poison and relapsed accordingly. What tends to confirm this view is the fact that the other patient, who oscillated in like manner, only recovered on being removed, though at some risk, to her home at Croydon. In neither case was there any purulent collection or other abnormal condition, except that, in the one that ended fatally, there was at one time slight tenderness of the uterus. Both were what might be called ichorrhæmic cases ; they were poisoned by their environments, the poison exerting in them powerfully phlogogenous effects. This is by far the most fatal form of " puerperal fever ;" in my experience, it is much more rapidly and certainly fatal than where " puerperal fever" is accompanied by suppuration.

Some weeks afterwards, on attending a meeting of the South-Eastern Branch at Croydon as the guest of Dr. Alfred Carpenter, I found the surviving patient in the Croydon Hospital, whither she had been taken shortly after her removal to her home. Her appearance interested me greatly ; for, from a plump blonde with plenty of fair hair, as she was when I first saw her, she had changed to a thin dusky-skinned woman with scarcely any hair. Her appearance showed plainly the severity of the struggle she had gone through ; her epidermic structures generally had withered, as usually happens after post-partum inflammations.

In both the cases just related, the skin was occasionally sponged with cold water. There was one noteworthy difference between them, inasmuch as only one of the patients perspired, and that was she who recovered. The other's skin was obdurately dry, and it is obvious that her power of radiating heat was correspondingly diminished. Efforts were made to induce sweating, but unsuccessfully. Her friends said they had never known her to perspire.

The advantage of applying cold to hyperpyretic patients without moving them is obvious. It is especially useful, for example, in acute articular rheumatism, and in cases of typhoid fever where perforation of the bowel from ulceration is dreaded, since movement from the bed to a bath, or vice versâ, might precipitate bursting. This plan has already been attempted with partial success by wet packing and so on; but the packing around with vessels containing ice in addition to the wet sheet or sponging appears to be a ready and powerful means of abstracting heat without unduly disturbing the patient.

Besides its value in puerperal cases, as illustrated by Dr. Playfair's case and by the foregoing, I have also found it of great value after ovariotomy. During the past year, I used it in conjunction with another and similar method, also very valuable—the ice-cap—in, among others, two cases of ovariotomy at the West London Hospital. Both patients recovered, and I believe they owe their recovery in no small degree to the prompt abstraction and subsequent control of heat by the continuous application of cold.

My own observations enable me to concur fully in the opinion that the control of abnormally high temperatures by the application of cold is not only largely feasible, but that it is a therapeutic agent of immense value in a great number of cases. I mean that, by the rapid reduction of hyperpyrexia, not only do we remove excessive and dangerous heat, but also that probably we, at the same time, hinder its production; a result of enormous importance. I am, therefore, quite at one with those who consider that we ought not to wait for *foudroyant* manifestations of hyperpyrexia, but that alarm should be taken early, and efforts made, if possible, to suppress its genesis. There are doubtless still unused methods of doing this, and it will well repay those who are called upon to employ cold to devise means suitable to different cases. For example, where the patient can bear removal from the bed to a bath of cool water without risk, nothing can be better; but numbers of patients could only be so moved at great hazard, and then such measures as water-beds and cushions filled with cold water, vessels containing ice, ice-caps, sponging with cold water, wet packing, exposure to cold air, and so on, might be adopted. Wet packing may, in a modified way, be advantageously combined with ice-packing; and, as both are applicable without undue disturbance of the patient, they are valuable auxiliaries in cases of marked prostration. Moistening the skin and allowing free evaporation not only favours the radiation of heat, but is also extremely grateful to fevered patients. I have adopted the combined plan with decided advantage.

I have more than once stated, at the Obstetrical Society and elsewhere, that quinine appears to exert much less influence over hyperpyrexia of ichorrhæmic origin than over that associated with, if indeed it be not dependent upon, suppuration; and I would venture to suggest the probability that the ichorrhæmic cases which show the highest temperatures and are the most rapidly fatal may be more favourably influenced, if not entirely controlled, by the assiduous application of cold than by the administration of quinine, valuable as that drug doubtless is in other cases. The brilliant results which have attended the administration of salicylic acid and its salts in acute rheumatism, usually a non-suppurative disease, lead one to hope for similar results in puerperal septicæmia unaccompanied by suppuration. I cannot forbear remarking that our present therapeutical resources encourage the belief that we are better able to cope with "puerperal fever" in its various forms than heretofore, more especially when their employment is not unduly delayed.

It only remains for me to say that the further admission of patients into the hospital was immediately suspended on the appearance of unfavourable symptoms in the two patients whose cases I have just related; and that, on inspection, quite enough was found to account for the unhealthy state of the building. Thorough measures were resorted to with marked success, and the recommendation that the hospital should be closed periodically for thorough cleansing and disinfection was adopted by the authorities. This plan has been attended by marked success.

Sore Nipples.

Dr. BROCHARD, so well known by his efforts in favour of maternal suckling, observes that sore nipples are often due to the habit which many young mothers have of applying mallow lotions to them, which only render the mucous membrane unnaturally tender. These young mothers also frequently induce sore nipples by the practice of applying the child to the breast every few minutes. On the other hand, the same effect is produced by following the advice of many nurses to defer commencing suckling to the second or third day. The breast then has become hard and swollen, and the infant cannot draw milk by sucking. However, from whatever cause sore nipples may arise, Dr. Biochard strongly advises abstinence from the employment of any of the numerous remedies (especially those of a greasy character) which are being constantly recommended as infallible, and as constantly falling into disuse. Instead of these he recommends, however deep or extended the chaps may be, the following simple procedure : Wash the nipple in pure water and carefully dry it, and then powder it and the sores well with suberine, i. e., the impalpable powder of cork. This, too, is much to be preferred in the hygiene of infancy to the inert powder lycopodium, for it is cheaper and contains some tannin. Over the suberine is to be placed a portion of gold-beater's skin cut star fashion, in the centre of which some apertures have been made by means of a very fine needle. Whenever the infant is about to suckle, the sube-rine is to be washed off and the gold-beaters' skin reapplied, by means of which the child will suck without causing any pain. When it has finished, the suberine and the gold-beaters' skin are to be replaced ; and so on every time. This sim-ple treatment always succeeds.—*Med. Times and Gaz.*, June 15, 1878, from *Rev. Méd.*, May 20.

—

The So-called Myxoma of the Placenta.

In a paper in a recent number of Virchow's *Archiv*, Dr. STORCH, of Copen-hagen, reviews at some length the pathology of the condition which has been termed myxoma of the placenta, and arrives at the following conclusions : He maintains very different forms of disease of the ovum are included under the name, some of which are essentially different, and have been hitherto wrongly described. The condition which has been termed myxoma fibrosum placentæ is a cellular hyperplasia of the bases of the villi, which consist of mucoid tissue, and proceed from the allantois. The disease occurs only during the later months of pregnancy, and is limited by the ramification of a single villous trunk, although there are indications by a widely-spread change of a similar character in the other-wise healthy portions of the affected placenta. The so-called simple hypertrophy of the villi of abortions during the early months of pregnancy represents an early stage of the same condition. It is commonly accompanied by an hypertrophy and inflammatory thickening of the decidua, which makes it probable that the morbid condition arises from the irritation of a diseased lining membrane of the uterus. The fœtus is commonly well developed.

The so-called hydatid disease and its varieties, which so frequently occur in abortions, are due to a hyperplasia and secondary cystoid degeneration of the connective tissue of the chorion, not proceeding from the allantois. The disease is often accompanied by pathological conditions of the remaining parts of the ovum, amnion, and embryo (malformation and early death). Less commonly the embryo is normally developed, but dies early on account of imperfect vascu-larization of the chorion-placenta. Very rarely the embryo appears to have been developed, without impediment, to the time of birth.

The peripheral parts of the ovum, chorion, and amnion may develop independ-ently of the existence or non-existence of an embryo. The portion of the pla-centa proceeding from the chorion is well-developed, but there appears to be only an imperfect formation of the maternal part of the placenta. The disease must begin very early, before the allantois and chorion are united, perhaps even before

' the ovum reaches the uterus.   How far the hyperplasia with cystoid degeneration of the chorion, in otherwise healthy ova, may be partial, cannot be decided from published facts, since, in many of the latter, this condition may have been confounded with partial œdema of the placenta, or with twin pregnancies, in which a mole has developed by the side of a normal ovum.—*Lancet*, June 29, 1878.

On Ovariotomy.

In an article published in the new *Dictionnaire de Médicine et de Chirurgie Pratiques*, M. KŒBERLÉ gives full details of the special method which he adopts in ovariotomy.   When the tumour is of considerable size, and capable of being notably reduced in volume by puncture, he regards it as essential to tap, as a preliminary measure, from five to ten days before the operation.   Although the initial incision of the operation may be rendered thereby somewhat more difficult, he considers that the following advantages are gained—The walls of the cyst, as well as the abdominal walls, become thicker as they contract, and bleed less freely from any points of adhesion ; the intestines partially resume their normal position and distension with gas ; they thus remain better in place after the operation, and the abdomen is less retracted after being emptied, and so less prone to allow the entry of air ; any œdema of the abdominal walls disappears ; the effects of embarrassment of respiration and circulation, or of sudden diminution of pressure, are not added to the difficulties necessarily resulting from the operation.

The author regards the use of carbolic spray at the operation as only useful under circumstances in which it is impossible to secure absolute cleanliness without it.   In a complicated ovariotomy, of long duration, in which the abdomen is widely opened, he thinks that the spray may prove rather a source of irritation than an element of success.   He never himself makes use of the spray in any operations, and considers that he obtains as good, if not better, results than those surgeons who have recourse to it.   If he requires a disinfecting fluid, he prefers a solution of sulphite of soda, of the strength of ten per cent.   He admits, however, that in hospitals, where it is otherwise impossible to prevent the presence of septic influences, the use of the antiseptic method in ovariotomy has led to results incomparably superior to those previously obtained.

The author declares that the complete extirpation of an adherent ovarian cyst is always possible, and that in three hundred ovariotomies he has never left an operation uncompleted, notwithstanding difficulties which at first appeared insurmountable.   When the cyst-wall is more or less fused with surrounding organs, as the intestines, the uterus, etc., his method is to make incisions perpendicular to the surface of the cyst, until its fibrous coating is reached, and then peel off the inner layers, leaving the outermost layer attached.   In this way he proceeds gradually until the pedicle is reached.

For the arrest of hemorrhage from adhesions, M. Kœberlé very rarely finds it necessary to employ any ligature, but employs instead the hæmostatic forceps invented by himself, which have a joint not far from their extremity, and long handles with a catch so adjusted that a pressure of from six to eight kilogrammes is exercised upon the tissue seized.   This forcible pressure condenses the tissues so as to form an obstacle to the passage of blood, and allows a clot to form.   At the end of fifteen minutes hemorrhage usually does not recur after removal of the forceps.   In the case of vessels of the omentum, however, he finds that the action of the forceps is sometimes insufficient, unless they can be left in place for a very long time, and ligatures then become necessary.   The use of ligatures cut short and dropped, the value of which has of late been so much demonstrated, he regards as not absolutely free from disadvantage, since they may give rise to purulent collections, and various consequent accidents.   If it be necessary to use them, he prefers carbolized catgut.

M. Kœberlé treats the pedicle by the extra-peritoneal method. He encircles it by the wire of the serre-nœud invented by himself, an instrument on the principle of a small écraseur. Above the wire and in the same groove is placed, for additional security, a silk ligature. Above this again the pedicle is transfixed by a small trocar, and a steel rod, seven or eight centimetres in length, is passed through the canula, which is then withdrawn. The rod then holds the pedicle in place, the end of the serre-nœud and the silk ligature lying between the lips of the wound but external to the peritoneum. The serre-nœud is generally left until between the fifth and eighth day, but it may be removed at once, if desired. The author considers this method as preferable to the use of the clamp, since, although it appears somewhat more complicated, it is applicable to all cases, whatever the dimensions of the pedicle. If it be desired to drop the pedicle, he recommends that it should be secured temporarily by the serre-nœud, and that carbolized catgut sutures should be used.

The author regards the plan of abdomino-vaginal drainage, in which the pouch of Douglas is pierced by a large trocar, and a long india-rubber tube carried from the lower angle of the wound and brought out at the vagina, with the view of facilitating irrigation, as dangerous and injurious in most cases. If drainage be used at all, he prefers to insert immediately above the pedicle a glass tube reaching down into the pouch of Douglas, and draw up the effused fluid with a syringe from time to time. · This drainage he only thinks necessary in cases of chronic or suppurative peritonitis, or of profuse hemorrhage. · In ordinary cases, he considers that, so far from protecting from septicæmia, as Sims has supposed, it may itself become the cause of septicæmia and peritonitis. For the cleansing of the peritoneal cavity, the author prefers to use dry and perfectly clean linen napkins rather than sponges. Since adopting the use of linen for this purpose in 1874, he has had only ten deaths in eighty-four ovariotomies. In uniting the abdominal wounds, he prefers not to include the peritoneum in the sutures, and contends that the importance attached to this measure by Mr. Spencer Wells is greatly exaggerated, since his own results have been fully as good, although he has never adopted it.—*Obstetrical Journal of Great Britain*, July, 1878, from *Annales de Gynécologie*, April and May, 1878.

Medical Jurisprudence and Toxicology.

The Gums in Lead-Poisoning.

It will be remembered that a few years ago Dr. Hilton Fagge described, in an interesting paper, the microscopical characters of the lead line on the gums, and its dependence on the deposit of black pigment in and around the capillary loops. The same facts were described, almost at the same time, by M. CRAS in the *Archives de Médecine Navale* (Feb., 1875, and May, 1876), and further observations by him were submitted recently to the Société de Chirurgie. He has examined the line in portions excised from the gums of many patients, and found that it was easy to demonstrate the presence of lead in all the capillaries by the action of chromic acid. This stains the whole gum of a yellow colour, but the capillaries are distinctly marked by a much deeper tint, in consequence of the formation of chromate of lead. If now the section is washed in distilled water, and is treated with sulphide of sodium, the black tint of the capillaries is rapidly reproduced. Examination with high magnifying powers shows that the pigment is for the most part in the interior of the capillaries. M. Cras asserts that this line is not the only effect of lead upon the gums, and he describes another change antecedent to the lead line, and more constant, which he terms "saturnine gingivitis." The gums have two aspects—the one free in the mouth, covered with epithelium, the other adherent to the teeth and periosteum. These two surfaces unite at the narrow festooned border, which the epithelium covers as far as the place at which the gum adheres to the neck of the tooth by its periosteal surface. The interdental processes, which fill up the furrow between the gums and the teeth, present two surfaces adherent to the teeth. The capillary circulation of the gum is constituted by two plexuses: the one superficial, papillary, with fine vessels; the other deep and periosteal. It is always the periosteal plexus which is the seat of the deposit of lead; the papillary plexus is normal. He asserts that every lead line is accompanied by a detachment of the gum from the tooth. On separating the loosened edge of the gum by a needle, a drop of pus, retained between the gum and the tooth, often escapes. The excision of the edge of the gum for examination is easy and painless, the interdental processes being especially convenient for the purpose. It will be seen, if the periosteal aspect is removed. that there, in the section, the line is replaced by a dotted area due to the black infiltration of the capillary loops. Thus, the line which is visible on the outer aspect of the gums is only the edge of the layer of blackened capillaries on the periosteal surface. The mechanism of the production of the line is, according to M. Cras, as follows: First, by the chronic inflammation of the gum, the edge is separated, and in the space between the gum and the tooth organic matters accumulate. The sulphuretted hydrogen disengaged during the decomposition of these organic substances passes, as soon as produced, into the walls of the capillaries, and, acting in them on the metal brought by the blood, a deposit of sulphide of lead takes place in the capillary network. The gingivitis and deposit extending around the tooth often lead to serious consequences— retraction of the gum, abscess, etc. The production of this change is variable. The presence of tartar unquestionably assists its production. M. Magitot at the same meeting contested the opinion of M. Cras as to the seat of the deposit, asserting that it is placed invariably in the deeper layers of the epithelium of the gum, adjacent to the Malpighian layer of the mucous membrane, not in the capillary network ; and urged that the deposit depends on the elimination of the lead by the saliva, and was precipitated by the effect of the sulphur in the tartar of the teeth.—*Lancet*, June 22, 1878.

Case of Poisoning by Cyanide of Potassium Successfully Treated.

Dr. MUELLER-WARNEK, assistant clinical physician at Kiel,[1] reports the case of a photographer in Weimar, Hugo G., aged twenty-four years. From his youth upwards he had shown an easily excitable and eccentric disposition. His father had committed suicide. About five years previously, owing to some trifling dispute with a woman to whom he was then attached, Hugo made an attempt on his life, and was only saved by prompt medical assistance.

On the evening of the 12th September he had had a quarrel, and parted in anger from another woman with whom he had then associated. Just before this he had been drinking a quantity of beer. On his return home, it was observed by some of his fellow-lodgers that he was unusually restless, walking up and down in his chamber before retiring to rest. The next morning he breakfasted as usual, but soon after that, was seen by a neighbour pacing up and down in his room with a torn letter in his hand. A fall was heard, and on the persons in the house rushing up, they found him lying on the floor in an unconscious state, holding in one hand a letter, in which the woman rejected him as a lover, and in the other a small bottle containing a solution of cyanide of potassium, such as is used in pho-

---

[1] Berliner Klinische Wochenschrift, February 4, 1878.

tography. A medical man who was called in sent him at once to the hospital, where he was placed under the care of Dr. Mueller-Warnck, about 10 o'clock A. M. In the mean time he had vomited, and the vomited matter had the smell of bitter almonds.

Dr. Mueller-Warnck thus describes his condition when admitted about an hour after he had taken the poison. He was a man of middle height, delicate frame, and weak muscular development. He was in a state of profound coma. The skin was cold, with a clammy perspiration; the extremities were cold, and the face greatly cyanosed. The eyeballs projected from the lids, and were directed upwards and outwards; the pupils were much dilated, and were quite insensible to light. The lower jaw was strongly fixed by spasmodic contraction; a frothy saliva, tinged with blood, issued from the mouth, and at each expiration there was a strong odour of hydrocyanic acid. In the mouth and throat there were distinct patches of ecchymosis, and on the gums a white mark of corrosion. The muscles of the extremities were quite relaxed, and there was an entire loss of sensibility and reflex irritability. With the exception of the trismus above mentioned, there was no indication of convulsive action, either tetanic or clonic. The respirations were greatly reduced in number; they were deep and spasmodic, each occupying a long time, and they were accompanied by mucous *râles* in the trachea. The pulse was small, 120 in a minute, and occasionally intermittent. Auscultation revealed the presence of mucous *râles* during breathing over the whole of the lungs. The impulse of the heart could not be felt, but the sounds were rhythmical and low, and the movements were irregular. The temperature of the body was evidently much lower than natural; it could not be determined until the patient had been an hour and a half in the hospital. It was then 36.2° cent., or 97.1° Fahr. While the patient was lying in this state, the urine passed off involuntarily.

Although, from the character of the symptoms, recovery from the effects of the poison appeared very improbable, means were immediately adopted to remove from the stomach any solution of cyanide that might remain, and at the same time to stimulate the action of the lungs. Sulphuric ether was hypodermically injected, and the stomach-pump used until the tepid water employed for injection came away entirely without colour or smell. The first washings of the stomach had a well-marked odour of hydrocyanic acid, and this was perceptible even after several quarts of water had been used. Altogether twenty litres of water were used in washing out the stomach. (As the litre is equal to 35 ounces, the quantity here used represents washing on a very large scale.) In spite of the ether injection, the breathing became more laboured and the pulse smaller and more irregular. Artificial respiration was resorted to, and ether, containing one-tenth part of camphor dissolved, was hypodermically injected In spite of this treatment, collapse appeared imminent.

It was now 11.30. The patient was placed in a hot bath, 33° R., or 106° F., and a stream of iced water was poured upon his head and neck from a height of several feet. The results of this treatment were very remarkable. On the first affusion of cold water a deep inspiration took place, and this was observed whenever the iced water came suddenly into contact with the skin. The breathing became gradually more regular and frequent, the pulse lost its intermittent character, and acquired greater strength. The eyeballs assumed a natural position, and the pupils had almost acquired their natural dilatation. Ether with camphor was again injected, the patient wrapped in blankets, and put to bed. At this time (12.30) he was in a state of complete somnolency. At 1.30 the breathing was free, and there were no mucous *râles* to be perceived. The temperature of the body was 37.4° cent., or 99° F. About 2.30 the patient was lying in a quiet sleep; he could be roused by a noise, as in calling him by name, but soon relapsed into sleep. Reflex action was manifested by the muscles; the number of respirations to the minute amounted to 20, the pulse was 85, full and regular. He retained some milk and wine which were given to him. As the whole of the region of the stomach was very tender, ice was applied to it. At seven in the evening (ten hours after taking the poison) consciousness returned, and the patient remembered what he had done before swallowing the poison. He now complained of severe headache in the occipital region, and of a lancinating pain in the region of the stomach. After he had swallowed two glasses of cold milk he again slept quietly. The temperature of the body, which at six o'clock showed a maximum of 38.6° cent. (about 102° F.), at eight o'clock, had again sunk to 37.8° cent. (99° F.).

The case progressed favourably, and the patient left his bed on the 17th September, the sixth day after he had taken the poison, his pulse, breathing, and appetite gradually improving. He suffered still from great weakness and depression. The urine which he passed was strongly acid, and contained much uric acid in a crystalline state. No hydrocyanic acid was found in it.

For a long time after recovery the patient walked with an unsteady gait. He suffered no pain, but he soon became tired. For more than two months he did not entirely recover his power of speech. This state of aphasia was still observable on the 24th November. Up to the time of his attempting suicide, nothing of this kind had been remarked.

Cyanide of potassium was detected in the fluids removed from the stomach by two processes. 1. Nitrate of silver produced a caseous white precipitate (cyanide of silver) which was entirely dissolved on warming the fluid. 2. Chloride of iron, green sulphate of iron (in solution) and solution of soda were added to another portion of the liquid contents until a precipitate took place. This, when warmed and treated with hydrochloric acid, produced Prussian blue.

[In general, this poison destroys life with such rapidity that a medical man has no opportunity of employing any remedial treatment. The treatment pursued here was efficient and satisfactory. It consisted chiefly in the entire removal of the poison from the stomach, and cold affusion to the head and spine. The very hot bath employed simultaneously may have been required by the state of collapse into which the patient was rapidly passing. Dr. Mueller-Warnck lost no time in looking about for chemical antidotes, but he took care, by the enormous quantity of water injected, that not a particle of the poison should be left in the stomach to be removed by the absorbents.

Owing to a spasmodic closure of the jaws (trismus) there is, in general, on these occasions, great difficulty in using the stomach-pump. In one case, a woman who had taken a photographic solution of the cyanide, the loss of some teeth allowed the introduction of the tube within five minutes after she had 'taken the poison, but, in spite of this, she died in twenty minutes. The dose of cyanide was probably very large.

The quantity of cyanide taken by Dr. Mueller-Warnck's patient could not be ascertained, and the strength of the solution was not determined. As used by photographers, it commonly contains ten grains to the ounce. Dr. Mueller-Warnck states that it consisted of one part of cyanide to fifty parts of water, which would be of about the strength above mentioned; but how much of the solution was actually swallowed is unknown. The violence of the symptoms, and the time during which they lasted, showed, however, that a strong dose of the cyanide must have been taken, and there is every reason to believe that had this case been left to itself it would have soon proved fatal. A dose of five grains of the cyanide has destroyed life in three instances. Rep.].—*London Med. Record*, May 15, 1878.

CONTENTS.

Published Monthly, price $2.50 per annum, free of postage.
Also, furnished together with the AMERICAN JOURNAL OF THE MEDICAL SCIENCES *and the* MEDICAL NEWS AND LIBRARY *for* SIX DOLLARS *per annum in advance, the whole free of postage.*

HENRY C. LEA, Philadelphia.

THE MONTHLY ABSTRACT

OF

MEDICAL SCIENCE.

VOL. V. No. 9.   **For List of Contents see last page.**   SEPTEMBER, 1878.

Anatomy and Physiology.

On Hæmatoblasts.

Ν. G. HAYEM, in a paper read before the Société de Biologie (*Gazette Médicale de Paris*, June, 1878), has sought to verify by experiments on new-born cats the facts advanced by Kölliker (*Würzb. Verhandlungen*, Band vii.; and *Elements of Human Histology*) regarding the origin of the elements of the blood, viz., the presence of colourless and granular red blood-corpuscles, as well as of red nucleated corpuscles, in the blood of young mammalia (cats, dogs, mice).

Ν. Hayem says that, in pure blood, nearly all red corpuscles become spinous, which, however, does not prevent them from being disposed in rouleaux, between which are many small bodies, solitary or in groups. These bodies are hæmatoblasts; they soon undergo modifications analogous to those in the blood of man. There are also innumerable bright small granules in the plasma, which give it a milky appearance; these are found in all young animals fed by milk, except in children.

The following are the most important facts arrived at by Ν. Hayem in studying hæmatoblasts in the blood of the new-born cat. The red blood-corpuscles vary considerably in size, they do not possess a nucleus. The white blood-corpuscles have a large nucleus and a comparatively small covering of albumen, which is not contractile. The hæmatoblasts are somewhat different from those of human blood; they are pale delicate bodies, round or oval, rarely concave; some are colourless and others yellow, many become spiny and bristle with very fine points. They nearly all unite to form yellowish masses with irregular borders; in a few hours these masses become more homogeneous, and a number of vesicles or vacuoles make their appearance. The fibrinous network is indistinct in pure blood, but, after treatment with iodine and serum, very fine filaments may be observed at the angles of the masses. In this preparation the hæmatoblasts are less altered than in pure blood, they are solitary or in small groups, many become spinous; in shape they are ovoid, elongated, and remain so in whatever position they are placed; some are coloured, others pale, homogeneous, and slightly vitreous. In preparations made with osmic acid, the walls of the hæmatoblasts seem slightly retracted but not spinous. Small yellow spots like vesicles sometimes appear in their substance, but no nucleus has been discovered. There are no nucleated red blood-corpuscles in the blood of the new-born cat. The hæmatoblasts are less than the smallest white blood-corpuscles; it would be impossible for them to arise from a transformation of the latter. In rapidly made preparations of dried blood the hæmatoblasts are perfectly preserved; they are always grouped in masses, the elements being generally distinct, ovoid, yellowish-green, and of a peculiar glittering appearance. Some solitary ones are almost discoid, slightly coloured and crenulated. Hæmatoblasts have very similar reactions in the blood of all vertebrates, not differing between themselves more than do the red blood-corpuscles. The same elements are found in splenic blood as in that taken from other parts of the body, but there are more small white uninucleated corpuscles in it than in other blood.—*London Med. Record*, July 15, 1878.

Materia Medica and Therapeutics.

The Action of Arsenic.

The effect of arsenic upon animals has lately been carefully studied by GIES, who has administered to rabbits, fowls, and pigs during months gradually increasing doses of arsenious acid, the daily dose being : rabbits .05 to 7 milligrammes, the fowls 1 milligramme to 8 centigrammes, and the pigs 5 milligrammes to 5 centigrammes. All the animals became heavier and fatter, and there was a considerable growth of bone, both epiphysal and periosteal. In all parts of the bones in which there is normally spongy substance, the animals fed with arsenic presented compact bone. The carpal and metacarpal bones, for examples, were compact throughout, and beneath the cartilages of the epiphyses was a compact layer of bony hardness, just as in animals fed with phosphorus. The bone corpuscles of this layer are smaller and less numerous, the Haversian canals are smaller and fewer than normal. These changes were observed after only nineteen days' feeding. Strangely enough, however, the same bone changes were found in other animals kept in the same stall as those which were fed with the arsenic. Gies attributes this to the excretion of the arsenic by the skin and lungs of the animals to which it was administered, and its absorption by the others. Similar changes were found in the bones of animals which were kept in a cage beneath the perforated floor of which arsenic had been scattered. Adult animals fed with arsenic presented a considerable thickening of the cortex of the long bones, and with this there was produced more or less fatty degeneration of the muscular tissue of the heart, of the liver, of the kidneys, and even of the spleen. If the dose of arsenic was further increased, the changes in the bone were masked by those of chronic arsenical poisoning—gastritis and hyperæmia of the whole intestinal tract, and intense fatty degeneration of various organs. The young produced by rabbits during the process of poisoning were dead, but large in size, and presented a commencing osseous change similar to that described, and also a considerable hypertrophy of the thymus.—*Lancet*, July 27, 1878.

—

The Action of Drugs on the Liver.

In a recent paper read before the Royal Society of Edinburgh, June 17th, 1878 (abstract in *Nature*, July 4th), Dr. RUTHERFORD shows that sodium salicylate, the benzoates, ipecacuan, and various other substances, have a stimulating action upon the liver which has been hitherto unknown, and that, even if a purgative agent have no direct stimulating power on the liver, it diminishes the secretion of bile. The experiments were made upon dogs, and the author is careful to point out that it must still be left to clinical observers to discover whether these drugs have the same effect upon man, since it is impossible to argue that substances which stimulate the healthy liver of a dog would have the same effect upon the liver of a man.—*Lond. Med. Record*, July 15, 1878.

Camphor as a Narcotic for Female Lunatics.

According to Dr. EUGENE WITTICH (Berl. Klin. Wochenschrift, No. 11, 1878), camphor is an excellent remedy for the sleeplessness of a certain class of female lunatics with melancholia, accompanied by extreme anxiety, hallucinations of a terrible nature, and a low state of general nutrition. The ordinary drugs, such as chloral, morphia, and bromide of potassium, as well as various kinds of baths, all fail to induce sleep, whereas after the subcutaneous injection of 0.1 to 0.2 gramme camphor, the patient quickly becomes drowsy, and soon goes off into a sleep of several hours' duration. The camphor is dissolved in sweet almond oil (1.0 in 10.0 grammes) and the injection is less painful than one of morphia. The canula must be rather wide, otherwise the oil does not flow readily. Abscesses never occur, even though the injections are often repeated. It is important to begin with the smaller dose of 0.1, for cases have been met with where a dose of 0.2 failed to narcotize, whereas 0.1 succeeded admirably.—Med. Times and Gaz., July 27, 1878.

Medicine.

Leucocythæmia with Paralysis of Cerebral Nerves.

A case of splenic, lymphatic, and medullary leucocythæmia, with multiple paralyses of the cerebral nerves, is described by Dr. C. EISENLOHR, of Hamburg (Virchow's Archiv, Band lxxiii., Heft i.). The interest in this case centres in the occurrence, in the course of the disease, of complete bilateral facial paralysis, accompanied by interference with common and special sensibility. Electrical exploration gave the reactions of peripheral paralysis. Post-mortem examination revealed the causes of these symptoms to be numerous hemorrhages into the substance of the nerves themselves, the cerebral centres being quite free.—Lond. Med. Record, July 15, 1878.

Local Treatment of Meningeal Affections in Acute Articular Rheumatism.

In a paper read before the Medical Society of Greifswald (Deutsche Medicinische Wochenschrift, June 8th), Dr. MOSLER says that four years ago Schüller made some experiments to determine whether the acknowledged influence of certain external applications on the cerebral circulation could be demonstrated in the vessels of the pia mater (Berliner Klinische Wochenschrift, No. 25, 1874). Sinapisms were in the first instance applied to the skin, the result showing that by a long-continued application thereof it was possible to diminish the blood-contents of the cerebrum. The following observations now show that, in certain cases of cerebral pressure by effusion or congestion, the best results may be expected when the application is made directly on the scalp; that is, in the closest possible proximity to the affected organ and over the greatest possible area. The value of counterirritants and vesicatories in cerebral inflammation, etc., has been long recognized. But their use is also attended by the best results in affections of the cerebral membranes. The patient in the present case was a young man twenty-five years of age, who was seized with acute articular rheumatism, which ran its usual course, without heart or lung complications, attacking most of the large joints in succession. Early in the case, however, there were symptoms of cerebral congestion, which were relieved by blisters to the feet and

a moderate bleeding. Subsequently, cerebral symptoms again set in, in the form
of furious delirium, passing into coma, with unequal pupils, retarded pulse, and
continuous high temperature (102°–104.5° F.). The treatment, consisting of
warm baths and cold affusion, tincture of eucalyptus, cathartics, etc., was of no
avail. The head was now shaved, and a fly-blister, of the size of a hand, was
applied to the scalp, while behind each ear another blister, of the size of a half-
crown, was placed. The following day there was marked improvement in the
patient's condition, with return of consciousness and decline of temperature.
The case now progressed favourably, and ended in perfect recovery. The
liability of acute rheumatism to grave cerebral or cerebro-spinal complications
was long known, and noticed by Boerhaave, Sydenham, Van Swieten, and others;
while other observers (Todd, Lebert, Trousseau, etc.) have demonstrated a tendency in acute rheumatism to involve other portions of the nervous system. And,
as we know the endocardium, pleura, etc., to be liable to rheumatic inflammation,
we are justified in assuming the same with regard to the serous membrane of the
brain. As to the action of cantharides blisters on the circulation in the pia
mater, an experiment on the brain of a rabbit showed that the application of a
blister to the nape of the neck, and even the back, was followed first by dilatation of the arteries of the pia mater, then by alternate dilatation and contraction,
passing finally into a continuously contracted state, so that even amyl-nitrite was
unable to produce dilatation.—*London Med. Record*, July 15, 1878.

Results of the Cold-water Treatment of Typhoid.

Dr. GOLTDAMMER, of the Bethany Hospital in Berlin, contributes to the
Deutsches Archiv für Klinische Medicin, Band xx., a report based upon the
careful observation and analysis of abundant material, with a view to determine
the value of the cold-water treatment of typhoid fever. He compares the mortality and the duration of treatment since the introduction of the cold-water plan
with the results previously attained by the expectant method. From 1848 to
1867, 2228 cases of typhoid were treated by the expectant method, with 405
deaths = 18.1 per cent. From the introduction of hydrotherapy in 1868, to
December 1, 1876, 2086 cases were treated, with 267 deaths = 13.2 per cent.
The diminution of mortality amounted then to about five per cent. At the same
time the average duration of treatment of the cases which terminated in recovery
was lessened by 6.3 days, that is, from 46.1 to 39.8 days. Omitting from consideration those cases which from the time of admission were in a moribund state,
the mortality would be found to be 15 per cent. for the first, and 10.5 per cent.
for the second period, showing a diminution of mortality of fully one-third. The
method adopted was a tolerably rigorous but not excessive hydrotherapy. Intestinal hemorrhage, pneumonia, and excessive cardiac weakness were considered
contraindications for the full course of treatment. Although a decided adherent
of this method, Goltdammer does not, like many, recommend it indiscriminately
in all cases. The long period of observation, the number of cases forming the
basis of his report, and the fact that these were watched by the same person, in
the same institution, and during several epidemics of different intensities, render
the author's conclusions of more than ordinary statistical importance.

In concluding his report, Dr. Goltdammer gives a minute account of the last
three epidemics, in which 782 cases were observed. He failed to find, as is
claimed by some, that intestinal hemorrhage was increased by hydrotherapy. It
took place fifty-one times, croupous lobar pneumonia eleven times, and pleuritis
thirteen times. Joint-affections were also encountered in a few instances. In
two cases there was an extensive pemphigus, a complication not heretofore

referred to by writers on this disease. Both these cases terminated fatally. He very highly extols chloral in doses of from 15 to 30 grains in the management of those patients affected with sleeplessness and wild excitable delirium.—*London Med. Record*, July 15, 1878.

Tremor following Acute Diseases.

In a paper read before the Medical Society of Lyons, Dr. CLÉMENT calls attention to a series of cases in which an acute disease has been followed, either immediately or after a short lapse of time only, by trembling of part or of the whole body. This tremor cannot be looked upon as due simply to the debilitated state in which the patient is left by a sharp attack of fever, for it is much more marked than tremor from such a cause, it is more or less rhythmical, and, in the great majority of cases, it is still present after the patient has recovered from the general effect of the fever. The author has recognized two types: in one of which, the tremor resembled that seen in paralysis agitans; and, in the other, it was comparable to the coarse trembling occurring on movement in disseminated sclerosis. The condition is one of great rarity, for the author, though on the look-out for cases of the kind, met with not more than three or four examples of it in eight years, and this, notwithstanding that he was at the head of a large hospital service, and that, during this period, several epidemics of small-pox and of typhoid fever had occurred. Fourteen cases are referred to in the paper, four of which are reported by the author, and the rest are gathered from various sources. In six cases, the trembling presented the characters of paralysis agitans, and, in the remaining eight, those of disseminated sclerosis. We subjoin an abstract of one of the cases observed by the author himself.

A soldier, aged 22 years, was admitted on the third day of typhoid fever. The fever ran a mild course, but, on examining the patient, on the eighteenth day, the hands were found in the typical scrivener's position seen in paralysis agitans, and the muscles were affected with well-marked tremors, just such as those which characterize that disease. There was, moreover, tremor of the feet and legs. When sitting up, the head was bent a little forwards, and was affected with slight tremor, and the eyes looked fixedly to the front. The patient could not raise a glass half full of water to his lips without spilling some of the liquid. Speech was hesitating and slow; his answers to questions were short and monosyllabic. His muscular power was weakened, and sensibility was diminished in all the limbs; but pricking or tickling the sole of the foot brought on reflex spasm of the legs, in which the trembling became much more marked. The tremor stopped altogether during sleep. These phenomena persisted from the eighteenth to the thirtieth day of the disease, and then gradually diminished. At the end of seven weeks the patient was discharged nearly well.

In another case observed by the author, a male patient, aged 35, had suffered from an attack of typhoid fever eight months before, and since that time had always suffered from trembling. When first seen by the author, not only were all the symptoms noted in the present case present in considerable intensity, but there was exceedingly well-marked festination, so that, after walking with the body bent forward for a few steps, the patient broke into a run, and had a difficulty in saving himself from falling, or from running against a wall. In this case, however, there was nystagmus. The treatment adopted, consisted of cold douches and sulphur-baths, and at the end of three months the patient went out nearly well.

In the other two cases observed by Dr. Clément, the tremors were very violent, and were followed by epileptiform attacks. Both of these cases ended fatally; but, unfortunately, in neither case was a *post-mortem* examination made.

In the second group of cases, in which the tremor was allied to that seen in disseminated sclerosis, the following were the principal symptoms : trembling in the execution of voluntary movement, speech drawling and clipped, ataxy, with a certain amount of psychical disturbance, such as change of disposition, tendency to cry or laugh, irritability of temper, etc.

In his remarks on these cases, Dr. Clément calls attention to the very close resemblance between the groups of symptoms above described and those seen in the chronic nervous disorders which have served him for types in his classification. He does not profess to know anything about the pathological anatomy of these states, but he excludes the idea of sclerosis, and he sums up by saying, very wisely, "I have no wish to attribute these symptoms, occurring after acute diseases, to the same anatomical substrata as we find in disseminated sclerosis, for, in the study of symptoms, the nature of the lesion has often only a secondary importance ; especially is this true in the pathology of nervous disorders, where the symptoms depend much more upon the seat of the lesions than upon their nature. The alteration produced in the spinal cord by acute affections and in particular by smallpox are transitory, and are evidently less profound and quite different from those present in disseminated sclerosis. But whatever may be their nature, they have the same seat and the same mode of distribution, since they produce the same symptoms."—*London Med. Record*, July 15, 1878.

Symptomatology of Meningoencephalitis.

M. VIEL, in his work on this subject,[1] which has for its object the study of the localization of functions of the cerebral cortex, deals with it clinically and experimentally. In the clinical part, the author shows that general paralysis may be of use in this study, at least in its accessory phenomena, as apoplectic attacks, convulsions, more or less limited paralysis of motion, of sensibility, and of the senses ; but in general the lesions are too widely spread and too complex for one to arrive at any definite conclusions. For this reason he has undertaken a series of experiments in which he reproduces at will very limited lesions of the gray matter by means of a needle charged with nitrate of silver. The following are some of his conclusions. The experimental inflammatory irritation, as practised by him, does not immediately produce any phenomenon ; the various disorders which were demonstrated came on several days after the operation, and were clearly the result of the inflammatory irritation. When the inflammation attacks the posterior third of the cerebrum, it does not seem to produce any disturbance ; but when the anterior two-thirds of the gray matter of the hemispheres are attacked, there are observed intellectual disorders, irregularity in the functions of the body, occasional convulsions, epileptiform or choreiform attacks, paralysis, and local disturbance of the sensibility and of the senses. Intellectual disorders coincide with a lesion of the anterior third of the gray matter of the convexity of the brain. Paralysis, convulsions, epileptiform, ataxic, and choreiform phenomena, disorders of the sensibility and of the senses, occur on the side opposite to the lesion, or are more marked on that side. Disorders of sensibility and of the senses have been particularly observed when the lesion occurred in the middle third of the superior and lateral aspect of the convexity of the brain. Motor disorders of the limbs appeared more especially in connection with the lesion of the "sigmoid gyrus." Rotation of the head is generally made in the direction of the lesion. The pupil is almost always contracted on the side opposite to the lesion, sometimes on both

---

[1] "Etude clinique et experimentale sur les differences que peut présenter la symptomatologie de la méningo-encéphalite de la convexité du cerveau suivant le siège des lésions." Paris, 1878, A. Delahaye.

sides. Various disorders of nutrition may be observed, as considerable and rapid
emaciation, lowering of the temperature, conjunctivitis, keratitis, etc. They are
generally most marked on the side opposite to the lesion.—*Lond. Med. Record*,
July 15, 1878.

Athetosis.

Dr. OULMONT (*Etude clinique sur l'Athétose*, par le Dr. P. Oulmont, Paris,
1878), during his residence in the Salpêtrière under M. Charcot, had the opportunity of studying several patients afflicted with athetosis, an affection little known
as yet, and of which the name even was until lately almost ignored in France.
The history of athetosis is of very recent date; it was first named in 1871 by
Hammond of New York, who devoted a chapter to it in his treatise *On Diseases
of the Nervous System.* Some years before Charcot (1853) and Heisse (1860)
had described phenomena analogous to those defined by Hammond; and, since
the labours of the latter, several other observers have spoken of athetosis, chiefly
in America and in England.

Athetosis (ἄθετος, without fixed position) is characterized, according to Hammond, by "the impossibility which the patients find of keeping their fingers and
toes in any desired position, and by the continual movement of the same."

The name of athetosis, like that of chorea, says M. Oulmont, is a general
appellation, comprising varieties which are very different in point of progress and
symptomatology. Athetosis may be unilateral (hemi-athetosis) or double. M.
Oulmont has studied both forms in a series of thirty-seven clinical observations,
from which he has drawn the following conclusions :—

1. There are, in what is described under the name of athetosis, two entirely
distinct forms which must be completely separated; unilateral or hemiathetosis,
and double or general athetosis. 2· Hemiathetosis consists of slow, exaggerated,
involuntary movements, limited to the foot and hand of one side of the body, and
now and then occupying the corresponding half of the face and neck. 3. To
these movements are generally added transitory contractions or intermittent
spasms, which are simple modifications of athetotic movements, a sort of intermediate stage between the mobility of athetosis and the rigidity of post-hemiplegic
contraction. They may attack all parts of the upper extremity, but in the lower
extremity they rarely pass the instep. 4. The movements are involuntary, little
modified by the will, and often exaggerated by it. They persist during rest,
often even during sleep, at least to the degree of fixing the limb in an abnormal
position. 5. Hemiathetosis appears nearly always on the paralyzed side during
the course of motor hemiplegia. 6. It coincides, in the great majority of cases,
with more or less complete hemianæsthesia of the same side. 7. The other
symptoms which may accompany it, namely, permanent contraction, rigidity,
and atrophy, with laxity of the articular ligaments, do not depend on the athetosis, but on the hemiplegia itself. Articular relaxation in particular is specially
marked. 8. Hemiathetosis resembles hemichorea; like it, it is the symptom of
a cerebral lesion of some sort, without doubt in the neighbourhood of the lesion
which produces hemichorea, that is to say, the fibres in front and outside of the
sensory bundles at the lower part of the corona radiata (of Reil). In cases where
motor or sensory hemiplegia, or both, are absent, it may be admitted that there
is such a tendency to concentration, that it attacks the athetotic fasciculi at a
place where the sensory and motor bundles, united at the lower part of the
internal capsule, are already dissociated. 9. Hemiathetosis and hemichorea,
very distinct varieties of posthemiplegic disorders. may be united by various forms
of actual tremblings, transitional states in which the characters of both are
blended. 10. Double athetosis presents the same clinical aspects as hemiathetosis,

except that the movements exist on both sides of the body. The face seems to be attacked more constantly and more severely than in the unilateral form. 11. It is not accompanied by any disorder of movement or of sensibility. 12. Its nature is unknown; still it may be admitted that there is between it and hemiathetosis the same relation as there is between chorea and hemichorea.—*London Med. Record*, July 15, 1878.

Concussion of the Spinal Cord; Symptoms of Localization.

M. DUPLAY (*Progrès Médical*, June 15, 1878) in a recent lecture on this subject said: I am going to address you to-day on a case which presents certain very interesting paralytic symptoms following an injury to the lumbar region. It is that of a carpenter, aged 47, lying in No. 43 of St. Augustine's ward. This strong and active man, who had always enjoyed excellent health, seven weeks ago fell from a height of about six feet, in such a manner that the pelvis sustained the entire violence of the shock. Still he was able to get up, walk, and even to go on with his work, and, excepting somewhat acute pain in the contused part, he did not feel much inconvenience at the time. That day he felt no inclination to pass urine, but the following day, twenty-four hours after the fall, he wished to do so, but found himself unable, even with the greatest and frequently repeated efforts. He then consulted a doctor, who used a catheter, and for the next three weeks his bladder had to be relieved by the same means, until after the expiration of that time urination became again possible, although requiring a great effort. The calls to micturate were very frequent, and the quantity passed was very small, the stream slender and feebly propelled. There were pains in the urethra and in the hypogastrium. For the last three weeks the urine has been turbid and slightly ammoniacal. Concomitantly with these disturbances there exists obstinate constipation, requiring enemata or purgatives for its relief. Finally, for the last six weeks there has been complete abolition of sexual power, which succeeded to a short period of excitement of the same function during the week immediately following his accident. Examination of the parts shows that there is no obstruction to the passage of the catheter into the bladder, and nothing can be felt by digital exploration of the rectum, except that its mucous membrane feels relaxed and thrown into folds, as if by want of tone in the muscular wall of the bowel. There is, therefore, atony or paresis of the walls of the bladder and rectum, a functional disturbance which we can only regard as due to concussion of the lumbar part of the spinal cord produced by the injury which the patient suffered. At the outset, we must discard all idea of a grave lesion of the cord; the bony structures present no trace of injury; the symptoms are limited to vesical trouble, constipation, and sexual impotence; the lower limbs are absolutely free from any paralysis. If there then exist a lesion of the cord, it must be very slight. It is probable that we have to do with concussion alone, analogous to that observed in the brain after an injury to the cranium, which is well known clinically, but of which much less is known concerning its pathological anatomy.

At the same time, we may distinguish two kinds of spinal concussion. 1. Under the influence of violent shocks, such as a fall from a height, or a railway collision, we see paralytic symptoms produced immediately after the injury, such symptoms varying according to the seat of the concussion. Generally, as well as the bladder and rectum, the lower extremities are paralyzed. The further progress of such cases varies; sometimes the symptoms disappear after some time, and then the case has been one of true concussion; there has been, that is to say, only a shaking, and no more or less marked structural lesion. Sometimes, on the other hand, the symptoms, instead of improving, persist, or even get worse; and as these symptoms followed immediately upon the injury, we must attribute them also to spinal concussion, which in this instance, however, has been more violent, and has gone on to rupture and hemorrhage into the substance of the cord. Finally, symptoms of chronic myelitis may result. In this case the word "concussion" is ill chosen; we ought rather to speak of "contusion." In other cases, again, the symptoms persist without improvement or aggravation; we have in such cases to do with a localized lesion, which, undoubtedly, has determined atrophy of the nervous elements. 2. In another form of spinal concussion the symptoms do not appear until some time after the accident (railway collision). Some days, some weeks, or even some months may elapse without the patient experiencing any functional disturbance; then the symptoms of myelitis supervene. In those cases in which there is often question of damages from the railway companies, the physician may find himself beset with serious difficulties. Sometimes the patient is accused of feigning illness, sometimes the spinal symptoms are not developed till long after the accident which is said to be their cause, their dependence upon it is denied and the circumstance is considered as merely a coincidence. These legal questions have been frequently debated in England.

In our patient, the symptoms have followed immediately upon the injury; we may admit that we may have to do with the first form of spinal concussion; but in him the symptoms present some peculiarities. In ordinary cases there is, in addition to the rectal and vesical trouble, paralysis of the lower limbs. An entire segment of the cord is affected, and the symptoms are analogous to those of complete section or of transverse myelitis. But in the patient in St. Augustine's ward there is no trace of paralysis of the limbs. The paralytic phenomena have solely affected the genito-urinary organs and the rectum, in such a way that the concussion seems to have been limited to some localized spots in the spinal axis.

Can physiology give us any explanation of this peculiarity? It is well known that there are certain centres in the cord presiding over the functions of the bladder, the rectum, and the genital organs, and in this case the lesion appears to have been limited to these parts, and to have confirmed by a pathological experiment that which physiology had taught us. The vesical nerves come from two sources; the sympathetic and sacral plexus, and these two kinds of nerves are both distributed to the body and the neck of the bladder. An Italian physiologist, Giannuzzi, has demonstrated that there exist for the functions of the bladder two motor centres: the first in connection with the sympathetic fibres, is situate at the level of the third lumbar vertebra; the second, in connection with the nerves of the sacral plexus, at the level of the fifth lumbar vertebra. Excitation of the first causes slow and feeble contraction of the bladder, while excitation of the second causes, on the contrary, sharp and energetic contraction. Moreover Masins (of Liège) has discovered that there is a centre for the rectum which he calls ano-spinal, and which, in the rabbit, is situated at the level of the sixth lumbar vertebra. Finally, long ago, Budge demonstrated the existence of a centre for the sexual function at the level of the fourth lumbar vertebræ. Applying these facts to clinical study, we can admit that lesions limited to the lumbar region of the cord may affect solely the centres which govern the functions of the bladder, the rectum, and the sexual organs. In our patient, we are authorized to declare that the concussion was limited to these centres. Examples of similar localizations, after injury, are rare. In our wards we have another patient in whom we may admit equally a very localized spinal lesion, but due to a different cause. This patient, lying in No. 13, is eighteen years of age. He has a deformed foot on the right side, with atrophy of the corresponding limb. He urinates involuntarily, both by night and by day, and we have been able to assure ourselves that there exists in his case vesical paresis, and that he urinates by simple overflow. The stream is small, twisted, propelled feebly, and if, after micturition, a catheter be introduced, a considerable further quantity of urine may be drawn off. In this young man's case, therefore, there is paralysis of the bladder, but none of the rectum nor of the sexual function. This paralysis ought to be ascribed to a spinal lesion dating from childhood, and localized in the small vesical centre of Giannuzzi. The motor and trophic affections of the lower limb are evidently due to a lesion of the anterior cornua of the cord.

Let us now return to our first patient, in whom we have diagnosed concussion of the cord. What will be the prognosis? Since the accident, there has been some improvement, as he can now pass his urine, although with difficulty, and without completely emptying his bladder; but as this improvement has made no advance for three weeks, it is to be feared that the spinal lesions are not undergoing repair, and that the functional disturbance will persist indefinitely. Moreover, you must not forget what I have told you, that the symptoms of spinal concussion, far from improving or remaining stationary, may constantly get worse; therefore it is prudent under such circumstances to reserve our prognosis.

From a therapeutic point of view we have two indications, one from the symptoms, the other from their cause. The bladder empties itself badly, the urine becomes altered, and during its stay in the bladder causes hypogastric pain: we must therefore use the catheter twice daily, and inject the bladder with tar-water (*eau de goudron*). For the rectal trouble the patient must take a laxative, or he may have enemata. But the true indication is to act upon the cord, the lesions of which are the cause of the functional disturbances; unfortunately this indication is not easy to fulfil, for if we can localize the lesions we do not know in what they consist. As there are no symptoms of inflammation there is no need to employ antiphlogistics, but rather to use revulsive means. A large blister has been already applied, and will be increased in a few days. At the same time I have practised subcutaneous injections of ergotine, in the hope of awakening muscular contraction of the bladder. With the same end in view I shall have recourse, if these means fail, to strychnia and hydrotherapy. Finally there is a last means, electricity by the constant current. Legros and Onimus contend that the direction of the current is not indifferent. They say the descending current is "hyposthenisant," whilst the ascending current has the opposite effect; it is, therefore, to this latter means that we shall resort if all the others remain without effect.— *London Med. Review,* July 15, 1878.

Lead-Palsy, and Subacute Atrophic Spinal Paralysis of Adults.

Dr. M. BERNHARDT, of Berlin (*Berliner Klinische Wochenschrift,* June, 1878), in a recent clinical lecture said the patient now before you, A. T., 49 years of age, was always healthy till the summer of 1868. A certain amount of feebleness in the right hand had been not specially noticed, and was attributed to her work (sewing very thick material). In July, 1868, her left arm began to tremble; holding a cup or spoon became troublesome. The whole upper extremity became heavy, but could still be quite actively moved. At the beginning of August, the patient, who up to that time had shown no sign of general ill-health, went to bed (washing was hanging in the room, and a window was left open), and woke next morning with complete paralysis of the left arm. After a few days, a very noticeable enfeeblement attacked the right arm also, but which at the end of the month much improved under electrical treatment, and the paralysis of the left arm receded. It soon appeared, however, that this was only *the case for a single group of muscles,* the rest remaining paralyzed and rapidly wasting. This was the condition during 1869 and 1870, during which time the electrical treatment was continued, and she remains so till the present time

(October—November, 1877), without any exacerbation of symptoms, or any other muscles having become paralyzed or wasted. The lower extremities were never involved; urination and defecation have been always normal; no affections of the psychical functions or cerebral nerves have occurred. At the present time the patient is a ruddy healthy-looking woman, and excepting the paralysis of her arm, considers herself well. The smallness and flatness of the left shoulder as compared with the right are very striking; the acromion projects forwards, and between it and the head of the humerus there is a furrow in which the index finger can be laid. The entire left upper arm is thinner than the right, especially on the flexor aspect; the forearm is over-extended on the humerus, and cannot be flexed by any effort of the patient. If you tell her to bend her left arm, she swings the whole limb upwards over her shoulder, and then the forearm falls of its own weight on the humerus. The arm bent by this means can be actively extended. If we partially bend the forearm upon the upper arm, and then ask the patient to continue the movement, by a great exertion she is able to do so, but this is effected by the flexor carpi ulnaris and flexor digitorum profundus, which can be seen and felt to contract. Supination of the left forearm is not possible; if the arm be passively supinated, pronation is readily effected. The movements of the left hand and fingers are in every respect free. The hand is a little curved, and the skin bluish-red, but no œdema or eruption is present. There is no atrophy of the interosseous or thenar muscles. The arm can be raised from the shoulder in spite of the visible atrophy, and the clavicular fibres of the deltoid can be seen to contract; adduction, internal and external rotation, and drawing back, of the arm are all well performed, although the last is not quite so perfect as on the right side. The right arm is quite normal, except a distinct atrophy of the ulnar side of the extensor aspect of the forearm, which is associated with inability to completely extend the fingers; the basal phalanges of the thumb and index finger being alone perfectly extended, the remainder persisting in a state of half flexion, in spite of the strongest voluntary efforts; the middle and ungual phalanges of the same fingers being, however, as perfectly flexed and extended as in health. She feels a certain subjective sense of weight in the left arm, but no more definite affection of sensation is present. Electrical examination gives the following. In the right arm, the muscles all react well to direct and indirect stimulation, except the extensor communis digitorum, which does not extend the three fingers above mentioned; the extensor carpi radialis reacts more feebly than normal, although its contour is prominent. In the left arm, the deltoid reacts only near its origin from the clavicle; the biceps and both supinators are absolutely without reaction; it is questionable whether or not some intact fibres of the long supinator exist in the upper arm, where it is covered with fat. All the other muscles of the arm, forearm, and hand react to both direct and indirect stimulation. Placing an electrode on the point mentioned by Erb as that from which it is possible to stimulate both the biceps and long supinator together (at the exit of the fifth and sixth cervical nerves between the scaleni) gives a marked reaction of the muscles in question on the right side, but remains without effect even with much stronger currents on the left. With the anode of the constant current on the neck, and the cathode on the right deltoid, a feeble contraction occurs with 22 cells, while on the left side 30 cells produce only a quick twitching of the clavicular fibres, the bulk of the muscle remaining un-excited; with 33 cells the remainder of the left deltoid reacts. The left biceps does not contract, the right contracts with 13 cells. By stimulating the right radial nerve with 20 cells, there is short quick movement in the index finger and thumb. The muscular fibres of the extensor communis, from the three outer fingers of the right hand, do not react to direct or indirect stimulation. All the muscles of the left arm, innervated by the radial nerve, contract with 20 cells, except the supinators. We have, in the case before us, paralysis and atrophy of the deltoid, the biceps and brachialis anticus, as well as of both supinators on the *left* side, and a part of the fibres of the extensor communis digitorum of the *right* side.

Before commenting on this case, I will briefly relate the other.

J. W., aged 29, a painter, has been sixteen years at his work, and during the first ten years had occasionally violent colicky pains in the abdomen, but no special illness. Four years ago he had an attack of colic which lasted longer, and left a sense of weight in his arms, but from which he completely recovered. A new attack of colic in August, 1877, threw him on his back ; after a few days the pains ceased, and he felt better ; but one night, without any affection of the sensorium, paralysis of both hands and fingers supervened, which I will describe more exactly. *The shoulders and the upper arm remained freely movable.* The patient was a moderately well built, rather thin, at the present time pale and cachectic-looking man, with a marked pigeon-breast. His gums were livid, and showed a decided trace of blue line. His mental condition was normal, he walked without difficulty, showed nothing special in the sense-organs or in the cerebral nerves ; his general condition was satisfactory ; defecation and urination were normal. The condition of the hands and fingers of the patient, which in consequence of lead-poisoning presented a paralysis of the extensors of the hands and fingers (*i. e.*, of their basal phalanges) has been so often described, that I will not dwell further upon it. Extension of the forearm on both sides was free; equally, flexion of the forearm on the upper arm, with swelling of the contour of the biceps, was well effected, and both arms could freely execute all the movements of the shoulder-joint. The first interosseous space was not only sunken, as is often seen, but there was decided atrophy of the ball of the thumb, and on both sides the interosseous spaces were sunken, and the interosseous muscles were atrophied, and incapable of function, so that the lateral movements of the fingers and the extension of the middle and ungual phalanges were not possible. The hypothenar eminences were also diminished in both hands. There was also paralysis of the muscles supplied by the radial nerves on both sides, and of some of those supplied by the median and ulnar nerves. But these undoubtedly interesting phenomena pass into the background when we consider the results of electrical exploration. With the induced current, of the muscles supplied by the radial nerve, on the left (the less affected) side, only the extensor carpi ulnaris and supinator longus react but very feebly ; all the other muscles remain unaffected, and these by direct and indirect stimulation. On the other hand, the muscles supplied by the ulnar and median nerves on the left side contract very forcibly to both direct and indirect stimulation, but the adduction of the interosseous and thenar muscles was very feeble, or almost *nil.* The same, only more marked in failure of reaction to the induced current, is the case on the right side ; even with the strongest currents the supinator longus, a muscle which usually remains intact in lead-poisoning, scarcely displays its contour, and in the feeblest outline the tendons of the extensor carpi radialis, longus et brevis display themselves, but without producing any corresponding movements. It cannot be said that these results are very surprising, except as regards the diminished excitability of the supination ; but it is remarkable *that muscles, which have their functions quite unimpaired, and are used at will by the patient, and of the action of which he has never complained, should react either not at all, or only in the smallest degree, to the strongest induced currents.* This is the case for both the deltoids (except the clavicular portion), for the biceps and brachialis internus. With the constant current, the deltoid, biceps, supinator longus, and the extensors of the hands and fingers on both sides, with strong currents (30 to 40 elements) give only fibrillar twitchings; in fact, we have in the paralyzed, as well as in the unparalyzed muscles, the most marked degenerative reaction (*Entartungs-reaction*).

If we fix our attention on the case of the woman A. T., we must ask ourselves what is the condition with which we have to do. Both upper extremities seem to have been simultaneously affected by muscular enfeeblement, which improved and left only particular muscles affected. These atrophied with loss of their electrical excitability; and we are led to regard it as analogous to "infantile paralysis," an acute or subacute atrophic spinal paralysis of adults. It is all the more probable, as both extremities were affected, and the paralysis and atrophy have attacked different groups of muscles in the two arms, as it does not accord with our experience to find peripheral paralysis affecting simultaneously one and the other arm, and in distinct nerve areas. On the other hand, we know, and I have myself reported a case, that acute atrophic spinal paralysis, like that of children, can affect individual groups of muscles and lead to their atrophy. Until we have some *post-mortem* evidence, we cannot disprove or altogether quite invalidate the objection that we may have to do with a peripheral paralysis in such cases. Unless I am deceived in my acquaintance with literature, I was the first to give expression to this idea. In spite of the want of precision in the data and the uncertainty of the facts, it is permissible, in face of the strikingly similar affection of the cord in children, to expect an analogous change in the cord of adults, and to accept the anterior horns as the seat of the lesion. But I leave this question for further evidence from future careful microscopical examinations of early acute cases in adults. It is of quite special interest in this case that on the left side the muscles were paralyzed and atrophied, which seem to be supplied by nerves from the fifth and sixth cervical roots. Were we in this case to suppose a lesion (whatever its nature may be) of the cervical cord and in that of its gray matter, then we must suppose it to affect a quite limited group which send their axis-cylinder processes into the anterior roots. These then should be the cells from which the nerves for the deltoid, brachialis internus, biceps, and supinators arise. If we turn now to the observations on our second case of chronic lead-palsy, we have before us the striking paralysis and atrophy of the hand and finger extensors, of the interossei, and of the thenar and hypothenar eminences. Unusual here is the implication of the median area (thenar muscles), unusual, also, the paralysis and atrophy of the interossei, so seldom, indeed, that Remak refers in his work on the "Pathogenesis of Lead Palsy," to a case published by him as unique, in which the supinators participated unmarkedly in the paralysis. In Remak's case there was also paralysis of the deltoid, biceps, and brachialis internus, which latter, by superficial examination of our case, could not be seen; the arm could be moved at the shoulder in all directions, and flexion at the elbow-joint was also quite free. But since we have learnt from Erb that a muscle which is not paralyzed, and never has been paralyzed, may by electrical examination be recognized as diseased, I have held it my duty in every case to undertake this examination, and in this case it gave the most decided evidence of disease in active freely movable muscles, in that they did not react, or did so in the least degree, to very strong induced currents, and with the constant current gave the most decided degenerative reaction (Entartungs-reaction). Diseased were also in this case, not only the supinator, but the deltoid, the brachialis internus, the biceps, in a word, all those muscles which functionally are connected, which by disease can indicate functional incapacity in quite definite nerve-roots, which, as we in the observations on the first case saw, can become diseased and paralyzed without lead-poisoning or any other cause (cold, etc.) than the before-mentioned changes in a quite limited section of the spinal cord. Similar observations were those

which led Remak, Erb, and myself to accept as the pathologico-anatomical basis
of so-called lead-palsy a disease of the gray matter of the cord, and I believe that
both cases just related, and placed side by side, present a new support to this
view, if not amounting to proof, at least importantly strengthening it. But the
interest of the last case is not exhausted. It was only by careful electrical examination that the diseased state of the muscles was discovered, right as well as left
were freely movable. It was Erb who first pointed this out, and advanced the
hypothesis that different trophic centres in the cord exist for nerve and muscle,
which in given cases may be singly affected by disease. In our case (lead-palsy)
on the right side, if we take for instance the right deltoid and biceps, there were
no paralysis, inexcitability (or at least much diminished excitability) by indirect
(above the clavicle) irritation, as well as by direct stimulation with the induced
current, very much diminished excitability by indirect stimulation with the constant current, marked degenerative reaction by direct stimulation with the constant current. On the left, most of the nerves and muscles were normal, both for
voluntary motion and direct and indirect stimulation with both currents, and only
single muscular fibres showed by direct stimulation the degenerative reaction, a
condition which Erb had observed in some cases of progressive muscular atrophy.
If we regard the facts thus disclosed in my cases, we see no proof of the truth of
this hypothesis of separate centres in the spinal trophic apparatus for muscles and
nerves. In an essay which I published at the end of my first paper on the later
christened "middle form" of paralysis, I maintained that it is conceivable that
the pathological irritant affects the muscle itself, perhaps with the inseparable
nerve-ending; but it leaves this latter either unchanged, or only so affected that,
as may be found in the later stages of recovery from very marked paralysis which
has produced pathological changes in the muscle itself, and which leads to increased excitability and abnormal reaction to the galvanic current, without even
destroying this, the irritation of the induced current or of volition is absolutely
not obeyed.

There is still another hypothesis which Weinicke has recently proposed respecting these interesting phenomena. In a case of facial paralysis in which the
nuclei of the medulla oblongata were destroyed by a tumour, a number of the
nerve-fibres were quite intact. He says, "It appears that, if a certain number
of the nerve-fibres are preserved, the faradic and galvanic excitability, especially
for the minimum of contraction, may not be notably diminished, but only the
total contraction with stronger currents must be much less, as only the primitive
muscular bundles supplied by the preserved nerve-fibres are excited. The excitability of the muscle by direct irritation with the faradic current must be more
diminished, as in this case the electrode encounters the preserved nerve-fibres
singly. While the greater part of the muscular bundles which are connected with
degenerated nerve-fibres suffer under the recognized changes of excitability,
namely, the increase of direct galvanic excitability, and modification of the force
and manner of contraction; by their overwhelming number the degenerated fibres
must manifest the changed muscular reaction, yet a smaller number of the same
may not be observable because the scattered diseased fibres can make no movement. The so-called middle form of rheumatic facial paralysis is distinguished
from the severe form by the exemption of certain groups of fibres, while in the
latter (the severe form) the whole mass is affected; the numerical relation of the
healthy to the diseased fibre is given approximately by the electrical examination.
This explanation permits us to say that some diseases of nerve-nuclei, in which
single cells and fibres are affected together, will present this middle form of
change of muscular excitability; and Erb has related two such cases, one of progressive muscular atrophy, the other of lead-palsy, in which in the later stages an

affection of the nuclei appeared probable." Whether now this hypothesis of Wernicke is the true explanation of these phenomena (it allows us, as we see, to dispense with special trophic centres for nerve and muscle) or Erb's, or whether for particular cases, as I have sought to make it probable, a direct affection of the muscle can give rise to such phenomena, I leave undetermined. The definite solution of these highly interesting questions requires accumulated observations on living patients, with deductions carefully made, regard being had to all the possibilities, and, where possible, by experiments on animals.—*London Medical Record*, July 15, 1878.

***

The Cause of Distortions in the Spinal Paralysis of Children.

Dr. A. SEELIGMULLER of Halle (*Centralb. f. Chir.*) draws some conclusions on this debated point, from an experience of over seventy cases, and supports that view which attributes the original distortion to the action of the unparalyzed antagonistic muscles, in opposition to that which ascribes it to merely mechanical influences, apart from such muscular action—the view ably maintained by C. Hüter and R. Volkmann.

S. employed the induced current to distinguish paralyzed from unparalyzed muscles, and remarks that such an examination only indicates the state of the muscle or muscles at the time being, but does not allow of any certain conclusions with regard to a former condition of these structures, and moreover, insists that *only recently examined* cases afford incontestable proof for or against the antagonistic theory. He states that he has observed various forms of fixed talipes four weeks after the occurrence of paralysis, and affirms that the cases adduced in favour of the mechanical theory have not been sufficiently recent, as the patients had already used the limb in walking.

As showing the combined influences of muscular and mechanical force, S. narrates the case of a girl, two years of age, who, after an acute illness, exhibited paralysis and atrophy of those muscles of the right forearm supplied by the median and ulnar nerves, while the territory of the radial nerve remained normal. About eight months after paralysis, the consequent deformity was well-marked extension (dorsal flexion) of the wrist-joint and proximal phalanges of the four fingers, producing the appearance of a "griffin-claw." If, however, the forearm was held in a horizontal position for a time, the hand gradually sank into a position of anterior flexion at the wrist, while the extension of the phalanges persisted. In short, S. considers that the direction in which a deformity takes place is *primarily* imparted by muscular action, and that the mechanical influences of weight and the gravitation of the body only operate *secondarily.—Edinburgh Medical Journal*, Aug. 1878.

***

Acute Ascending Paralysis.

M. DEGERINE has announced to the Académie des Sciences the observation of changes in the anterior roots of the spinal nerves in cases in which a careful naked eye and microscopic examination revealed no lesion of the spinal cord. The method of examination employed was the hardening in osmic acid, and examination by means of picrocarmin. In each preparation a number of nerve-tubules presented the appearance of parenchymatous neuritis, fragmentation of the myelin in drops and droplets, an increase in the protoplasm of each interannular segment, and multiplication of the nuclei of the sheath. In some of the tubules so changed the axis-cylinder had entirely disappeared. Most of the nerve-tubules presented no appreciable alteration. The same appearances were observed in each part of the cord. A similar alteration of some of the nerve-tubules was found also in the intra-muscular nerves of the paralyzed limbs. Attention is drawn to the point without much weight being laid upon it, and its relation to the disease may admit of some doubt when we consider how small a proportion the few degenerated tubules bear to the great amount of paralysis.—*Lancet*, Aug. 3, 1878.

—

Alleged Cure of Tubercular Meningitis.

EVERY physician must now and then have met with cases in which a diagnosis of tubercular meningitis has been made, and yet, where recovery has resulted. When the case has so fortunate an issue, he doubts the correctness of his diagnosis in pinning his faith on the notion that true tubercular disease of the membranes of the brain must inevitably terminate in death. Such, however, is not the universal belief, if one may judge from a case recently recorded by M. Cuffer in *La France Médicale*, where it is claimed for iodide of potassium that it cured tubercular meningitis. The subject of this paper was a man thirty-four years of age, who was admitted into La Pitié, under the care of Prof. Peter, on April 17, 1877, with a history of having three days previously, whilst at work, been attacked with severe headache, which had been followed by obstinate constipation and retention of urine. He had never had a similar attack to this, and on admission the following group of symptoms was noted : intense frontal headache, with intolerance of light ; pupils equal ; strabismus ; rigidity of muscles of neck ; constipation, nausea, retention of urine, slowing of pulse (54), suspicious breathing, cramps in the limbs, and a well-marked *tâche meningitique*. He was continually groaning. The temperature was 98.6° F. These symptoms pointed to meningitis, and its nature was presumed to be tubercular by the detection of dulness, with jerking respiration at the apex of the left lung. This diagnosis arrived at by M. Peter, after exclusion of all other hypotheses as to the origin of the meningitis, appeared to be borne out by the progress of the case. The symptoms increased in intensity, delirium set in, and the patient's cries became more frequent and loud. The pulse fell to 50 beats per minute ; the breathing was very harsh below the right clavicle, and emaciation rapidly set in and became very marked. On the 23d the constipation continued, in spite of the administration of calomel ; the prostration was extreme, the pulse small and thready, the pupils unequal, strabismus more marked. The patient was thought to be moribund. M. Peter then prescribed iodide of potassium in half-drachm doses. For three days there was but little change ; then slight improvement set in, so that (still under the same treatment) in rather more than a fortnight the patient was able to get up. His appetite was good, and sleep undisturbed. The strabismus remained, and there was still some headache, but the graver symptoms had entirely subsided. The pulmonary signs, however, were rather more pronounced, some dry crepitant râles being detected below the right clavicle. He was considered to be cured of the meningitis by the 24th of May, but the same amount of the iodide was still continued daily. The case is given without comment, and it is only to be regretted that the details are so meagre. At any rate, as twelve months had elapsed before the time of the patient's discharge from the hospital and the publication of the case, it would have added much to its interest had the author appended some statement of the man's condition in the interval. It may be added that the idea of syphilis was suggested, only to be set aside ; for, although the patient had contracted a chancre some years before, he had never exhibited any manifestations of the disease. The published record, however, is so incomplete that it can hardly be held to justify the inferences drawn from it, and we have quoted it here as a warning against too hasty deductions in therapeutics based upon the insecure data of a doubtful diagnosis. Fully admitting the good effect of the drug in producing the amelioration of the symptoms, it requires more evidence than is here given to admit also that the meningitis was "tubercular."—*Lancet*, August 3, 1878.

Mumps and Parotidean Orchitis

Prof. LAVERAN, of the Val-de-Grâce, recently read a communication to the Hospital Medical Society (*Gaz. des Hôp.*, No. 56) in answer to a question asked by Dr. Besnier in one of his sanitary reports as to the frequency of the occurrence of parotidean orchitis and the subsequent wasting of the testicle, and as to the prophylactic measures likely to prevent these accidents. It is impossible to reply exactly with regard to the frequency of the occurrence of mumps in the military hospitals, as the statistics of these establishments do not include it; but it may be stated generally that small epidemics of the affection often occur. In 432 cases of mumps observed among soldiers in very different localities, there were met with 156 examples of single or double orchitis, so that this complication may be said to occur in two out of five cases in adults, although it is very rarely met with in epidemics occurring in schools. The orchitis usually occurs from the sixth to the eighth day after the appearance of the mumps, just as the swelling of the parotid is beginning to disperse. Attributing this to metastasis is out of the question, for the mumps does not subside any more rapidly in the cases in which orchitis occurs than in others, while it may arise spontaneously, unpreceded by any affection of the parotid. Although in some epidemics double orchitis has been observed oftener than single, as a general rule one case of double is met with for five or six cases of single. The degree of inflammation of the testicle is as variable as is that of the parotid, chiefly affecting the substance of the testicle itself, the epididymis suffering only in a less degree. By the fourth day the testis has increased two or three times in size, and is very hard and very tender to the touch. Resolution soon takes place, and there is in general no effusion into the tunica vaginalis. Unfortunately, however, the disease frequently terminates in atrophy—a condition which has often been overlooked in civil practice, in which the patients are not so long under observation as soldiers; and the atrophy does not take place sometimes until weeks or months after. In 111 cases of parotidean orchitis, atrophy occurred in 73—i. e., in seven out of ten cases. When atrophy affects both testicles, which is rare, complete impotence ensues; and when only one testis is affected a considerable diminution of virile power occurs. Sometimes the atrophy is arrested, and the testis recovers its normal size and consistency; but in general it persists, and not infrequently the other testis undergoes a compensatory hypertrophy.

With respect to prevention, M. Laveran believes the contagiousness of mumps to be amply demonstrated, and that the disease offers the same specific characters as the eruptive fevers. Isolation is therefore indicated, at least as regards adults. As soon as soldiers are affected with mumps, they should be sent to hospital, and not allowed to mingle with the other patients there. As to preventing the disease localizing in the testis, no means are known, all that can be done being to recommend rest.—*Med. Times and Gaz.*, July 20, 1878.

Case of Bilateral Paralysis of the Dilator Muscles of the Glottis (Posterior Crico-Arytenoid): Recovery.

In the *Berliner Klinische Wochenschrift* for June 17th, Dr. MESCHEDE, of Kœnigsberg, gives the details of a case of paralysis affecting the dilator muscles of the glottis, of which the following is an abstract:—

Paralytic affections of the larynx are now divided into two groups—vocal and

respiratory. The muscles affected in the latter group are the posterior crico-
arytenoid pair, which serve to open the glottis, and are in this respect opposed
by the lateral crico-arytenoid pair. While cases belonging to the former group
—the vocal—are not uncommon, those belonging to the latter group, especially
those involving both posterior crico-arytenoids, have hitherto been exceedingly
rare. Moreover, of the cases hitherto recorded, some appear to have been cases
of only partial paralysis, while in others the diagnosis was scarcely conclusive.
In the present case, the existence of complete paralysis of both posterior crico-
arytenoid muscles was clearly established. The laryngoscopical conditions have
been figured in Bülow's *Atlas of Laryngoscopy*, Table x. Fig. 6. The patient
was a girl aged 19, and was stated by her mother to have been unable to speak
for the last two months; there was some bloody expectoration, but no signs of
lung-disease could be made out; deglutition, though at times somewhat slow, was
not impeded. The prominent affection was the difficulty of respiration. When the
breathing was undisturbed, it was noisy and somewhat laborious, inspiration being
specially difficult. But on the least exertion there was great dyspnœa, and each
inspiration was accompanied by a loud howling sound. Respiration generally
was retarded, the pulse small and quick. Menstruation, which had always been
irregular, had ceased for several months. Examination with the laryngoscope
was exceedingly difficult, being rendered still more so by impeded and diminished
mobility of the tongue. When examined while respiration was calm, the vocal
cords remained stationary, the glottis not expanding with inspiration. But when
respiration became accelerated from agitation or any other cause, the condition of
the vocal cords became reversed; they became closely approximated during inspiration, instead of separating, so as to come almost into contact. At the same
time they were not tense, and it was seen that they were drawn downwards and
together by the current of inspired air. That this was not a case of spasm of the
glottis was evident, seeing the dyspnœa did not occur in paroxysm, but every time
that respiration was in any way accelerated, when also the vocal cords became
immediately approximated; moreover, the dyspnœa was of too long duration.
Had this condition of the larynx not been observed, the case might have been
regarded as one of hysterical simulation; but paralysis of the dilators of the glottis can never be simulated. Nevertheless, it was interesting to note the effect of
an audibly threatened use of the actual cautery if the patient did not speak by a
certain time; for, some little time before the appointed day, she began to articulate somewhat imperfectly, while on the actual day, and within sight of the
heated cautery, speech became almost natural, showing how undefined may become the boundary line between hysteria and stimulation. No real improvement
was, however, attained, and the dyspnœa became so great as to suggest at times
the idea of tracheotomy. For the first six days after her admission to the hospital, the treatment consisted entirely of local faradization, without the slightest
benefit, and of warm baths and cold affusion, with the result that on the eighth
day menstruation became re-established. A regular treatment, consisting of
systematic subcutaneous injection of strychnia, was now commenced, the salt
employed being the soluble sulphate, in a one per cent. solution. The amount
injected was at first small (.015 grain), and produced no results, thus showing
incidentally that the later beneficial results were due not to the mechanical and
psychical effects of the punctures, but to the larger quantities injected. The
amount of strychnine sulphate was now gradually increased up to .07 grain,
and this increase was from the first attended with marked improvement. At
first, the injections, which were given morning and evening, were followed by
sound sleep and increased freedom of respiration, which latter was of short duration at first, but gradually became more established, until, after the injection had
been employed nineteen times, breathing remained and continued entirely free.

After a period of four months there was a slight relapse, which readily yielded to the same treatment.—*London Med. Record*, July 15, 1878.

Case of Fatty Effusion into the Pleura (Hydrops Adiposus Pleuræ).

The following unusual case is communicated by Dr. BOEGEHOLD of Berlin to the *Berliner Klinische Wochenschrift* for 17th June. The patient, a man aged forty-three, was admitted on the 16th January last into the Bethany Hospital, suffering from dyspnœa without pain, and very much reduced in condition. In the previous September, he had vomiting, pain in the stomach, constipation, etc., which lasted for upwards of two months. The patient presented now a cachectic appearance, pale, flabby skin and mucous membranes, with the axillary and inguinal glands enlarged, many to the size of a walnut; there was extensive effusion into the left pleura, with the usual signs, arching of the thorax, obliteration of the intercostal spaces, dulness, etc. The heart was also displaced upwards and to the right. On the following day the effusion had increased considerably. A puncture was therefore made in the fifth intercostal space, and a *litre* (about a pint and three-quarters) of fluid withdrawn, which was alkaline, opaque, dark yellow, and inodorous, with a specific gravity of 1023. On standing for about half an hour, there formed on the surface of this fluid a thin, yellowish, creamy layer, which also collected on the sides of the glass. Examined with the microscope, these were found to consist of fatty granules, intermixed with larger fat-globules and some large nucleated cells. On agitating the fluid with ether, this assumed a yellow colour, and there remained after evaporation an oily residue. The patient now experienced great relief; but, after a few days, the fluid collected again and had to be again removed, when two litres of a dark brown alkaline fluid mixed with blood were evacuated. About a week afterwards the fluid had to be withdrawn for the third time; after which, on the next day, the patient died. At the subsequent necropsy, the left pleural cavity was found to contain two litres of reddish-brown fluid; the right one was empty. The left lung was reduced to one-third its size; its pleural covering grayish, somewhat thickened, and covered with minute reddish-gray points; the left costal pleura was thickened, much discoloured, and dotted with gray or yellow prominences of various sizes from a pea to a shilling, the apices of which were flat and ulcerated. The right lung was much enlarged, nowhere adherent; while the right pleura, costal as well as pulmonary, was dotted with the same elevations of various sizes as the left, which, however, were nowhere ulcerated. The stomach presented about its middle a constriction admitting only two fingers; on its posterior wall there was a funnel-shaped depression, at the bottom of which was a jagged ulcer of the size of a sixpenny-piece, with hard edges. This portion of the gastric wall formed, with the pancreas and the surrounding mesentery, a hard solid tumour as large as an apple, which presented a yellowish-white surface on section. In the immediate vicinity of the common duct existed several hard tumours as large as hazel-nuts, and presenting the same appearance on section; while several of the mesenteric glands showed a similar condition. Examination of these growths with the microscope showed the usual appearances of carcinoma. In several places, near the pleura and the lymphatic glands, the large cells contained oil-globules. In the gastric tumour, the cells had almost wholly undergone fatty degeneration, and were imbedded in an abundant stroma. We must, therefore, look upon the tumour of the stomach, the cells of which had undergone the greatest degeneration, as the primary affection, which gave rise to further morbid processes in the surrounding tissues. The ulcerations on the pleura were found to consist mainly of granular matter and large cells containing fatty globules; and the fatty granules collected on the pleural fluid must therefore be regarded as the *débris* of broken-down cancer-cells which had undergone fatty degeneration.　A similar case is described by Quincke (*Archiv für Klinische Medicin*, vol. xvi. p. 121) of carcinoma in the peritoneum, with dropsical effusion containing large quantities of fatty matter.—*London Med. Record*, July 15, 1878.

—

Pulmonary Œdema.

Under the direction of Cohnheim, a series of experiments have been made by Dr. WELCH of New York (Virchow's *Archiv*, Band lxxii.) for the purpose of obtaining information with regard to the causes of œdema of the lungs.

After reviewing the various causes of œdema as given by Niemeyer and Heitz, he concludes that none of them are sufficiently explanatory.　He sought to learn from experiment whether pulmonary œdema might arise from passive congestion, which was brought about by the ligature of several branches of the aorta.　These experiments furnished a positive result, although such a degree of arterial obstruction became necessary for this purpose as could scarcely occur in man.

In the attempts at causing œdema by ligature of the pulmonary veins, it was found that all the veins from one lung might be tied and no œdema result.　The lung became gorged with blood, but not œdematous.　That œdema might arise, it was necessary to tie also the veins from the upper and middle lobes of the other lung.

Hence he concludes that the mechanical causes of œdema are much more severe than those occurring in the vast majority of cases of acute general dropsy of the lungs in man.　It seemed probable that œdema might arise if a misproportion existed between the action of the two ventricles, in consequence of which the left ventricle should expel in a given time only a portion of the amount of blood which the right ventricle forced into the pulmonary a$_{\text{rtery}}$, such as might arise from paralysis of the left ventricle.　Such a paralysis was produced by compression of the walls of the ventricle, and pulmonary œdema followed.　When the right ventricle was paralyzed, no œdema ensued.

The immediate cause of pulmonary œdema is therefore considered to be a predominant weakness of the left ventricle.　Favouring causes may be found in collateral hyperæmia of one lung when the other is hepatized, in passive congestion dependent upon mitral stenosis, and in hydræmia consequent to Bright's disease.　But when these favouring causes are present the œdema does not always follow ; another factor must also exist.　If both sides of the heart become alike enfeebled during the death-agony there is no œdema, although this event takes place when the left side is more rapidly and more completely paralyzed.　The hypothetical nature of this explanation is fully recognized, and the possibility of its proof in the case of man is doubted.—*London Med. Record*, July 15, 1878.

—

Absorption of Foreign Bodies by the Lungs.

RAPPERT (Virchow's *Archiv*, Band lxxii.) describes the results following the absorption of soot by the lungs.　He endeavoured to eliminate some of the complications resulting from the methods adopted by other experimenters, especially by Slavjansky.　His investigations were directed towards ascertaining the alterations produced in the epithelium of the air-passages as well as in the sub-epithelial tissues, when air containing particles of soot was inhaled.　He also sought for the channels by which the soot particles were received into the interstitial tissue, the force causing them to enter, and the condition in which they were while entering, whether as free particles or inclosed within cells.

By causing the animals to inhale air laden with soot from an ordinary petroleum

lamp from which the chimney was removed, he obviated the introduction of material capable of producing chemical changes. It was found that the particles were
taken up in part by the alveolar epithelium and in part entered the tissue. The
former gave rise to such alterations in the cells that a subsequent desquamation of
them took place.

In general, the soot passed directly into the tissues, and only to a very limited
extent by means of amœboid cells. After it had entered the tissues, it was always
found within certain portions of the lymphatic system. It could not be accurately
determined through what channels this entrance took place, although it seemed
most probable that such were present between the epithelial cells, and that the
lymph-currents furnished the force by which the particles were carried along.—
London Medical Record, July 15, 1878.

Acute Aortitis.

Dr. LEGER, in a work on this subject (*Gazette Médicale de Paris,* May 25th,
1878), gives a complete sketch of the characteristic features of this disease. In
the chapter on pathological anatomy, he says that the lesions may extend as far
as the iliac arteries, but are most marked in the ascending part of the arch of the
aorta. The walls are thickened and present ecchymoses and soft grayish patches.
The inflammation may spread to the serous membrane surrounding the origin of
the aorta, and may cause pericarditis and neuritis of the cardiac plexus. Microscopic examination shows that the soft patches are composed of masses of fusiform
embryonic cells, being circumscribed in the internal coat and diffused in the two
others. Dilatation of the arterial wall occurs at the diseased spot, and is followed by aortic insufficiency and cardiac hypertrophy.

The chief exciting cause of the acute inflammation is atheroma. Among the
predisposing causes are gout, alcoholism, fatigue, cold, and external injuries.
Rheumatic endocarditis may cause it by continuity of tissue; it may appear in
fevers or in purulent infection. The symptoms which are most prominent are
the earthy appearance of the patient, attacks of oppression with præcordial pain,
special disorders of the heart and arteries, occasional sudden death during angina
pectoris; usually there is no feverishness. The pain varies from a mere sense of
weight to a feeling of laceration and retro-sternal burning. The pulse is exaggerated by cardiac hypertrophy, or small in consequence of dilatation at the origin
of the subclavians. The heart is generally hypertrophied; there is a murmur
with the first sound (dilatation of the arch) or with the second (aortic insufficiency). The complications which are most frequent are pericarditis, pulmonary
oppression, inequality of the pupils, delirium, etc. The usual termination is
death; in bad cases it occurs after several attacks of angina pectoris, or it may
happen during syncope. In other cases the attacks come on at long intervals,
and the patient dies from cachexia. The duration varies from several days to
three or four months. The diagnosis is based on the character of the pain, and
the constant presence of pericarditis. It is difficult when mitral insufficiency or
aneurism of the aorta coexist. Angina pectoris without aortic lesion is less serious; sometimes it cannot be distinguished from aortitis. The prognosis is
grave, although recovery is not rare; it depends on the preceding health and on
the complications. As to treatment: for the pain, ice, narcotics, and antispasmodics may be given; for the heart-symptoms, digitalis, milk diet, etc. The
iodide of potassium has appeared to be of some use.—*London Med. Record,* July
15, 1878.

Syphilitic Arteritis.

Dr. PAUL BAUMGARTEN (Virchow's *Archiv*, Band lxx., Heft 1), on the grounds of certain experimental researches into the process of obliterative arteritis, opposes the view of Friedländer and others that the new growth in the lumen of the vessel is entirely derived from the wandering cells from the vasa vasorum; he contends, on the contrary, that the epithelioid tissue swells and proliferates to form an indifferent embryonic tissue. He describes the microscopic appearances he found in a case of syphilitic inflammation of the middle cerebral artery; and while agreeing in the main with Heubner as to the facts, he denies any specific character to the growth in the lumen, which he characterizes as consisting of the ordinary indifferent tissue found in all cases of obliterative arteritis; but he admits that the affection of the outer coats presents the histological features of gumma, and so far he admits that we are justified in regarding the affection as syphilitic, although the process of obliteration takes place in the same manner and by the same means as arteritis of non-specific origin, namely, by the growth of indifferent tissue originating in the epithelioid lining.—*London Med. Record*, July 15, 1878.

Changes in the Small Bloodvessels in Bright's Disease.

Dr. A. EWALD has lately published in Virchow's *Archiv*, Band. lxxi., the result of a long investigation on the above subject. Like Dr. George Johnson, and Drs. Gull and Sutton, he microscopically examined the vessels of the pia mater covering the pons in a considerable number of cases of various forms of nephritis; but he was unable to discover those alterations of the arterial coats which the latter authors have described as "arterio-capillary fibrosis," whereas he was able to confirm Johnson's statement that the muscular coat of the arterioles is hypertrophied in the great majority of the cases of contracted kidney associated with cardiac hypertrophy. Ewald regards the "hyaline-fibroid" arterial degeneration of Gull and Sutton as mainly the result of their method of microscopical preparation. He found that the normal relation of the lumen of the arterioles to the section of their coat is as 1 : 0.1—1.3, and he assumed that there was hypertrophy present when this relation rose to 1 : 0.5—1.2. The alteration in the muscular coat which gives rise to the hypertrophy consists, according to Ewald, in a simple enlargement of the normal cells and of their intercellular substance. Ewald has tabulated sixty-two cases of renal disease in which the condition of the heart, the vessels, and the kidneys was carefully noted at the post-mortem examination. The general conclusion arrived at is, that hypertrophy of the heart and the arterioles is most frequently met with in the advanced forms of granular contracted kidney, though the relationship between the two conditions is an intimate one in all the stages of interstitial nephritis. In those cases where interstitial and parenchymatous (epithelial) degeneration occur in combination, though the former change predominates, two-thirds of the cases present cardiac and arterial hypertrophy, and one-third cardiac hypertrophy only. On the other hand, where the parenchymatous degeneration prevails over the interstitial, all the cases are accompanied with hypertrophy of the heart, and none with that of the arterioles. The cases of pure parenchymatous degeneration, sixteen in number, which Ewald examined, were all free from vascular change, and somewhat less than a third of them were associated with simple hypertrophy of the heart. Nephritis, secondary to such diseases as phthisis, leukæmia, and heart disease, was, as a rule, unassociated with hypertrophy of the muscular coats of the arterioles. Ewald agrees with those English authors who assert that both ventricles of the heart are not unfrequently hypertrophied in interstitial nephritis, the right ventricle, ac-

cording to hi 1, being affected in half the cases. He explains this fact by the
protracted course of the disease, and he points out the analogy to cases of unilateral valvular lesion, where the dilatation of the left side of the heart finally
extends to the right.

The theoretical explanation of the hypertrophy of the heart and of the coats
of the arterioles to which Ewald inclines is the following: The blood beco 1 es
altered in its co 1 position by the renal disease, and excites increased resistance in
the capillaries. Increased tension in the arterial syste 1 is the result, and then
first hypertrophy of the heart, and later on arterial hypertrophy. The latter he
regards as of purely 1 echanical origin, and dependent on the persistently increased
contraction of their 1 uscular coats which is necessary to prevent their extre 1 e
dilatation under the abnor 1 ally high lateral pressure to which they are subjected.
He believes that this contraction of the arterioles is not dependent on the influence of the vaso- 1 otor centre. The reason why hypertrophy of the s 1 all vessels
is absent in renal disease co 1 plicating heart disease, in athero 1 atous degeneration
of the large bloodvessels with cardiac hypertrophy, and in unco 1 plicated valvular
disease, is probably that here the arterial tension is not *uninterruptedly* high, as it is
in interstitial nephritis with contracting kidney.—*Med. Times and Gazette*, July
27, 1878.

Chronic Interstitial Nephritis.

Dr. SENATOR, of Berlin (Virchow's *Archiv*, Band lxxiii., Heft 1) reviews
our present knowledge of this disease. He 1 ore especially draws attention to the
hypertrophy of the heart which, he says, is frequently unacco 1 panied by dilatation, and is, therefore, not recognizable in many cases during life or in certain
stages. He does not attempt to settle the vexed question of the changes in the
arterioles, but inclines to the view of Ewald and Tho 1 a, that they 1 ay be regarded as co 1 ing under the general class of conditions described by Friedländer
as endarteritis obliterans.—*London Med. Record*, July 15, 1878.

The Diagnosis of Amyloid Kidney.

In spite of the great advances that have been 1 ade in our knowledge of the
clinical pheno 1 ena associated with the several 1 orbid processes in the kidney
which were fo1 1 erly roughly joined together under the na 1 e of Bright's disease,
it cannot be doubted that there still is very considerable difficulty in accurately
diagnosing the anato 1 ical conditions of the kidney, a difficulty shown by the not
unfrequent failures of even those 1 ost conversant with the subject, and which 1 ay
be attributed in part to the co 1 bination of two or 1 ore of these processes being
present; in part to the distorted relations and exaggerated value of so 1 e of the
pheno 1 ena which have been too dog 1 atically relied upon as characteristic of this
or that anato 1 ical condition; and again, in part, fro 1 the absence of any sufficiently significant circu 1 stance or group of circumstances in 1 any cases. Thus,
acute parenchy 1 atous nephritis frequently super venes upon interstitial nephritis,
and for the ti 1 e masks all the sy 1 pto 1 s peculiar to it; a 1 yloid degeneration
often acco 1 panies the latter stages of chronic parenchy 1 atous nephritis, or even
interstitial nephritis, but without producing any sign which could reveal the 1 odi-
fication in the state of the kidneys. Albuminuria occurring in the course of long-
standing suppuration is too generally regarded as indicative of amyloid degeneration of the kidney; but chronic parenchymatous nephritis occurs under si 1 ila1
etiological conditions, and also gives rise to albu 1 inuria. Lastly, albu 1 en 1 ay
be absent fro 1 the urine in cases of either contracting or a 1 yloid kidney.

The difficulty of diagnosing the contracting fo1 1 of kidney is well known;

possibly, most cases are only recognized in their later stages; but sooner or later albumen will be found in the urine. In amyloid kidney, unfortunately, this is not so. It has been generally recognized (Grainger Stewart, Bartels) that in the earlier stages of the malady albumen might be absent or intermittent in its appearance; but it has not been admitted that a case could exist for months and proceed to a fatal termination without albuminuria having been at some time present. Bartels, indeed, is most emphatic as usual: he says, "I am sure that I have never yet found distinctly marked amyloid disease of the kidney in the bodies of persons whose urine during their lifetime had been tested by me for albumen without its being discovered." M. Lecorché (*Traité des Maladies des Reins*, Paris, 1875) has maintained, indeed, that amyloid degeneration *per se* does not give rise to albuminuria, but that the latter results from the parenchymatous nephritis with which, according to him, it is almost always combined; both which statements are positively contradicted by Bartels. Quite recently, Dr. M. Litten (*Berlin Klin. Wochenschrift*, June 3d, 1878) has just published details of four cases which plainly establish the fact that amyloid degeneration of the kidney may be present without giving rise to albuminuria or polyuria, and that the presence of the degeneration can at best be only suspected.

His first case was a phthisical boy, who was under observation three months before death: the urine averaged generally from thirty to forty ounces (specific gravity 1011–15) sinking to ten or fifteen ounces in the later stages; there was never any trace of albumen. The second case was also one of phthisis, and was under observation thirteen days: his urine averaged thirty ounces daily, of specific gravity 1010, containing no albumen. The third case was one of visceral syphilis: urine under thirty ounces; specific gravity 1011–13; no albumen. The fourth case was communicated to the author by Dr. Weigert: the kidneys were amyloid, and there had been no albuminuria before death. The small quantity of urine in the first two cases is explained by the presence of diarrhœa; but this was absent in the third.

It seems, therefore, certain that we possess at present no sure diagnostic of amyloid degeneration of the renal vessels; that, on the one hand, it is likely to be confounded with, or mistaken for, chronic parenchymatous nephritis arising under identical etiological conditions; on the other, it runs a great risk of being altogether overlooked. But both of these evils may be avoided with a little care. Bartels points out that the differential diagnosis between amyloid disease and chronic parenchymatous nephritis depends upon the distinguishing characters of the urine, which, in the former, is clear with little sediment and few casts, mostly hyaline, and scarcely ever blood-corpuscles; in the latter it is always more or less turbid, with considerable sediment, is dirty coloured, contains many casts of every variety, and not uncommonly blood-corpuscles. In those cases in which no albumen was present, there have been signs of amyloid disease in other organs; and, in order to escape error, it will be enough to know that the absence of albumen from the urine does not exclude a slight degree of amyloid disease of the kidneys. —*Brit. Med. Journ.*, July 27, 1878.

On a Peculiar Form of Albumen in Urine.

Dr. W. R. GOWERS, Assist. Prof. of Clinical Med. in Univ. Coll., records (*Lancet*, July 6) the following reactions obtained from a specimen of urine passed by a patient beyond middle age, who had previously suffered from glycosuria. Unfortunately no further particulars of the case are to be obtained.

The urine had a specific gravity of 1015, was acid in reaction, pale in colour, clear, and contained no sugar. Heat rendered it opaque from a considerable flocculent precipitate, but when boiled almost the whole of the precipitate disappeared, the urine becoming almost as clear as before the heat was applied.   On being slowly heated by a water-bath, it was found that the coagulation occurred at 122° F., and the precipitate began to disappear a few degrees below the boiling-point.   When thus slowly heated, the clearing on boiling, although great, was not so complete as when more quickly heated.   The precipitate produced by a moderate heat, separated, and boiled with distilled water, dissolved at once.

Nitric acid in moderate quantity, in the cold, produced an abundant precipitate.   Nitric acid and heat gave no precipitate: e. g., if the upper part of the urine in a test-tube was boiled, the opacity first produced cleared from the part boiled, a layer of thick opacity remaining at the lower part of the heated part, where the heat applied was less.   Nitric acid then dropped through caused no precipitate in the upper heated portion, but an abundant precipitate in the lower, cool part.   A larger quantity of nitric acid (equal in bulk to the urine) dissolved all the precipitate thrown down in the cold by a smaller quantity of acid.

With a small quantity of nitric or acetic acid, a compound was formed freely soluble in water, cold or hot: e. g., the copious precipitate produced by several drops of nitric acid in the cold was separated, and washed with distilled water. The first washing contained no trace of albumen (tested by placing it in contact with nitric acid).   The second washing gave no abundant precipitate, tested in the same way, but none with heat alone, or with heat and more nitric acid.   On adding to the urine a few drops of dilute acetic acid, no precipitate occurred, and none could be produced by heat.   The addition of some nitric acid still caused a precipitate.

On rendering the urine slightly alkaline with liquor potassæ, heat produced no precipitate, nor did nitric acid added after heating.   Nitric acid alone, in the cold, gave, of course, the same precipitate as before.

Alcohol, in moderate quantity, caused no precipitate.   Creasote gave the same amount of precipitate as moderate heat.

The quantity of albumen was found, by Dr. W. Roberts's method, to be .858 grains per ounce.   Possibly the data for that method are not quite accurate for an albuminous body different from the ordinary albumen.

The albuminous body shown by these reactions thus differs from the serum-albumen in which coal only occurs in urine, especially in its solubility, at the temperature of boiling water, and by not being precipitated by a moderate quantity of absolute alcohol.   The formation of a compound with acetic acid, as well as with nitric acid, not precipitated by heat, is, of course, frequently observed.

The only allusion to a similar reaction of an albuminous body in urine which I [1] have been able to find is in a paper by Stokvis,[1] for an opportunity of seeing which I am indebted to Dr. Lauder Brunton.   Stokvis describes coagulability at a temperature at which ordinary albumen is not coagulated (113° to 140° F.), and re-solution near the boiling-point, as a characteristic of a specimen of Bence-Jones albumen, and he found that when a solution of albumen giving this reaction was injected into the blood of a dog, the urine gave the same reaction.   It is, however, stated by Stokvis that the substance had been obtained from urine by precipitation by alcohol.   In this reaction the albumen I have described differs, since it was not precipitated by alcohol, and in this it resembles paraglobulin, which also may occur in urine.   But Stokvis is certainly wrong in describing coagulability at a low temperature and re-solution as a characteristic of the albumen described by Bence Jones,[2] who stated repeatedly that the form which he found in the urine in osteo-malacia was not coagulated by heat alone.   It is clear,

[1] Maandblad der Sectie voor Natuurwetenschappen, 1872, No. 6.
[2] Philosophical Transactions, 1848, part i., p. 55 ; and Animal Chemistry, 1850, p. 108.

therefore, that the substance tested by Stokvis was either not the same albumen, or had undergone a change.   No doubt these forms of albumen are nearly allied, and may pass one into the other.   Dr. Brunton's observations on the variations in the coagulation point of albuminous bodies in the urine, and of those resulting from the process of pancreatic digestion, suggest that the latter may often pass unchanged into the urine, just as did that which Stokvis injected into the blood. It is possible that in this case the albumen had been formed during some modification of the digestive process, and had been absorbed and excreted unchanged. From the fact that the urine, although almost, was not quite, cleared by boiling, it seems likely that it did contain a small quantity of ordinary albumen.

Amyloid Degeneration of Lymphatic Glands.

At a meeting of the Société de Biologie in Paris on March 2, M. CORNIL presented some lymphatic glands taken from a young man who died from chronic arthritis of the hip-joint with suppuration, inflammation in the iliac fossa, phlebitis, etc.   The crural and inguinal glands of the right side were much enlarged; also the sacral, lumbar, and mesenteric glands.   The liver, spleen, and kidneys showed amyloid degeneration.   The ovoid form of the glands was preserved, and they were isolated from the surrounding inflamed tissues.   On section, little islands of amyloid substance were observed in the cortical part along the course of certain arterioles and their capillaries.   On examination with a low power under the microscope, the septa were seen to be thickened, the lymphatic sinuses large; some of the follicles in the cortical alveoli with amyloid substance, and others quite normal.   The epithelial cells on the septa were somewhat swollen and granular; large scaly or spherical cells, with from two to six nuclei, filled the spaces bounded by the septa.   The inference then is, that lymphatic glands when hypertrophied are attacked by chronic inflammation, similar to that of syphilitic and tubercular glands, involving their connective tissue and epithelial cells.   The reticular tissue may also become amyloid.—*Lond. Med. Record*, July 15, 1878.

The Bones in Pernicious Anœmia.

Professor OSLER, of Montreal, who has previously recorded changes in the medulla of bone in pernicious anæmia, has lately described a very instructive alteration found in one instance of that disease.   The case was that of a girl twenty years of age, who presented only tenderness of the sternum to draw attention to the osseous system.   The blood contained many microcytes and large irregular coloured cells, without nuclei, but none of the "elementary granules" of Schultze.   Special attention is drawn to this, since it is the fifth case in which Osler has failed to find them, although they are abundant in ordinary anæmia and other cachectic conditions.   There was moderate fatty degeneration of the heart, liver, and kidneys, but no other morbid state to be discovered.   The medulla of the right femur, the sternum, and the ribs were of jelly-like consistence, not fatty, of a dark-red colour, like the splenic pulp.   Microscopic examination showed (1) the ordinary granular marrow-cells, with distinct nuclei; (2) smaller marrow-cells, with granular protoplasm; (3) colourless cells of the size of the ordinary marrow-cells and larger, with homogeneous substance and finely granular nuclei.   These are not vacuolated marrow-cells; their protoplasm is clear, transparent, like the ectosarca of the amœba.   The nuclei are large, often indistinct, and their margins are granular and ill-defined.   (4) Nucleated red blood-corpuscles, some so pale that their tint could only be recognized on comparing them with colourless cells.

---

[1] St. Bartholomew's Hosp. Rep., vol. xiii. p. 284.

Their protoplasm had a uniform darkly granular appearance, and showed the elasticity so peculiar to the red corpuscles. The nuclei were large, often two or three in each cell, and some had the "dumb-bell" shape, manifestly in the act of division. Other cells were deeply coloured, and were evidently the so-called "transitional forms" of corpuscles. Most were large in size, their nuclei granular, eccentric, but rarely projecting from the body of the cell. In some the nuclei contained a few indistinct granules, and in two, which were deeply coloured, no nuclei could be seen. Some of the deeply-coloured corpuscles were smaller, round or elliptical, with vesicular nuclei. These cells resembled closely many of the larger red blood-corpuscles, but it was difficult, often impossible, to say whether or not they possessed nuclei. Lastly, ordinary red corpuscles were present, many large, elliptical or irregular in form, but always flattened, and of moderately dark colour. Some microcytes were seen, but fewer than in the blood or spleen. No giant cells were seen, nor any of the so-called "Charcot's crystals," even when decomposition was commencing.

In no other examination of the marrow, in either morbid or healthy conditions, has Osler encountered such a variety of development forms. In two other cases of pernicious anæmia, in two of leucocythæmia, in one of pseudo-leukæmia, in two of tuberculous affections—phthisis and tubercular peritonitis,—the marrow was hyperplastic, and presented few or many nucleated red corpuscles, but not the peculiar forms described above as (3) and (4). These appear to be intermediate between marrow-cells and nucleated red cells on the one hand, and ordinary red blood-corpuscles on the other. Osler quotes Neumann's significant statement that " to regard the nucleated red blood-cells as transitional forms between colourless and coloured elements involve a theory as to their origin on which I, perhaps, have expressed myself with too much assurance;" and again, " It is not improbable that the development of the nucleated red corpuscles may be independent of the colourless marrow-cells"—a significant admission, considering his former positive statement on this point. The case now recorded supports, however, the opinion that a transformation of the colourless marrow-cells into red corpuscles actually takes place, and that this is produced by a degeneration of the nuclei, and thickening of the protoplasm of the cell. This seems to be the significance of the series of intermediate forms above described. Still, it is by no means obvious what significance these changes have as to the disease in which they have been found. Whatever the change in the medulla, the origin and cause of the disease can only be decided by further observations on the functions of the marrow and its influence on the blood.—*Lancet*, August 3, 1878.

Hereditary Syphilis.

Prof. PARROT has of late been delivering some interesting lectures on this subject, which appear in the *Progrès Médical*, and of one of these, as summarized in the *Gazette Médicale*, July 20, on the indications of treatment, the following is an abstract :

When an infant is born perfectly healthy in appearance, but one of whose parents is the subject of syphilis, there is a difference of opinion as to whether it should at once be submitted to appropriate treatment. Profs. Parrot, Roger, and others prefer to wait for the earliest manifestation of disease. The first symptoms, however, do not necessarily exhibit themselves on the skin or mucous membranes, for Prof. Parrot has indicated the presence in some cases of obstinate gastro-intestinal disturbance, resisting all hygienic measures, appearing in new-born infants brought up under the most favourable condition possible, and only yielding to specific treatment. When the new-born infant is manifestly syphilitic, much will

depend on its mode of treatment on the clinical forms of the disease. As in the
adult, syphilis may from the time of its appearance put on a very serious or malignant form, and terminate fatally, so that action must be speedy. In other cases on
the other hand, there are merely some cutaneous or mucous manifestations of slight
extent, and which are so much the less serious the later they appear. In this
delayed form of hereditary syphilis, insidious in its progress, and which may give
rise to the bony lesions termed by Prof. Parrot "syphilitic rickets," all the manifestations may be sometimes limited to the production of a small number of papular *syphilides*, disseminated over particular regions. In such cases the infants
may be cured without the aid of any treatment, although the iodide of potassium
will render signal service, and contributes in the course of time to the modification
of the osseous lesions. But the case is far more serious when the syphilis is speedy
in making its appearance ; and if at the period of birth it has already manifested
itself on the surface, the internal lesions will have become too advanced generally
to allow of their yielding, and the most heroic treatment will in most cases remain
powerless. In most cases we find syphilis manifesting itself at the exterior during the early weeks after birth, and we should then act without delay. The
therapeutical opportunity will not so much depend upon the more or less considerable quantity of mercury or iodide that has to be administered, as on the epoch of
the appearance of the syphilitic accidents, syphilis being dangerous in proportion
as it is speedy in manifesting itself. Mercury is the remedy *par excellence*, and
one on which we can always count. In ordinary cases internal treatment suffices,
and acts rapidly enough, Van Swieten's *liquor* (corrosive sublimate gr. ss ad ℥j)
being the best form for administering the mercury, and one well borne by infants.
Of this, if the infant is robust, a teaspoonful may be mixed with twenty-five or
thirty grammes of milk—or, what is preferable, syrup ; the five or six teaspoonfuls of which the mixture will then consist being administered before the child
suckles each time, in this way avoiding the gastric irritation which the medicine
might otherwise give rise to. At six months of age two teaspoonfuls of the *liquor*
may be given. The treatment, in spite of its rapid success, must be continued for
a long time, the infant being kept under the influence of the remedy for twelve
or eighteen months,—even two years if necessary—whenever the symptoms reappear on its suppression. Then, whenever the bones present any of the characteristic lesions, we should have recourse to iodide of potassium. Prof. Parrot,
however, prefers the tincture of iodine, as given in this formula, viz. : Tincture of
iodine and syrup of orange-peel or syrup of gentian 100 parts. A teaspoonful to
be taken four or five times a day before each feeding.

The advantages of this internal treatment are immense ; but it cannot be used
indiscriminately with all patients, some of whom are cachectic, very feeble,
scarcely taking the breast, and digesting badly—in a word, in a state of athrepsia
or innutrition. The smallest portion of a medicinal substance introduced into the
stomach is rejected, vomiting and diarrhœa preventing all internal treatment.
After this has been tried for a day or two without avail, being even dangerous, we
must resort to external measures—viz., the introduction of mercury by the skin. One
contra-indication alone to this may be present, when the skin is covered with
syphilitic ulcerations, threatening to absorb too great a quantity of mercury. Properly speaking, the mercury is then dangerous, and requires supervision, but it is
not contra-indicated. The frictions should be made preferentially in the axilla
and over the neighbouring wall of the thorax, where the skin is delicate and moist.
A gramme of ointment, consisting of one part of blue ointment and two parts of
lard, may be rubbed in every day, the utmost cleanliness being observed at the
same time. Under its influence the syphilitic ulcerations and the *syphilides* generally disappear as if by enchantment; and corrosive sublimate baths are little

recommended at the present time, as they are devoid of the precision obtainable by the employment of mercury in friction, and may be even dangerous. When they are deep, the ulcerations of the skin or mucous membranes may also require local treatment, and then the glycerole of zinc rapidly dries up the wounds; or iodoform may be used if the ulcerations are of a phagedenic character.

In hereditary syphilis, then, we shall meet with success if we act rapidly and with vigour by means of faithful medicaments.—*Med. Times and Gaz.*, August 3, 1878.

Surgery.

Auditory Disorders in Bright's Disease.

M. DIEULAFOY has just published several observations in the *Gazette Hebdomadaire (Journal des Connaissances Médicales),* from which he thinks that the auditory disorders accompanying the different forms of Bright's disease, far from being rare, ought to be considered as symptoms in the same degree as the ocular disorders which are frequently met with in this malady. These auditory disorders are not always the same: most frequently they consist of a humming sound in one or both ears; generally these sounds are accompanied or followed by semi-deafness. Now and then the deafness comes on without previous noises; it may be transitory and recurrent, or rarely complete; it may be localized in one or both ears, and disappears or remains permanent, according to the case. Lastly, these various auditory disorders may be painless, or may be accompanied by acute pain in the face or ears. One patient, who had suffered from tinnitus aurium for twelve or fifteen months, was examined by M. Ladroit de Lacharrière, who found permanent lesions of the tympanum, viz., an abnormal vascularity at the level of the handle of the malleus on the right side, and thickening with depression of the left membrana tympani, which no longer reflected rays of light. In thirty-seven cases which were observed, auditory disorders were demonstrated fifteen times. 1. It is difficult to decide whether these disorders are more especially allied to any one of the forms of Bright's disease; they exist in all forms of nephritis, chronic or acute. 2. Auditory disorders occur at all stages of nephritis; eleven times out of fifteen they appeared to be contemporary with the œdema, or with the increase of the œdema. 3. Their intensity is very variable; several times they have coincided with a painful stage, facial neuralgia, or deep seated pains in the ear; several times, also, they have appeared on the same side as the facial œdema, or at least on the side where œdema was greatest. 4. As to whether one ought to assign them to lesions of the ear or of the auditory nerve, this is a point to be determined as observations become more numerous; one sees now a rent in the tympanic membrane, now an abnormal vascularity, and so on. 5. With regard to their diagnostic value, these disorders may prove to be of great assistance; they often complete the *tableau* of the disease; in some cases they precede the other symptoms; and sometimes they may put one on the track in a difficult diagnosis, as in certain obscure forms of Bright's disease, in which nephritis neither reveals itself by œdema, nor by any other apparent sign.—*London Med. Record,* July 25, 1878.

Penetration of Dust into the Lungs after Tracheotomy.

M. BALZER calls attention (*Revue Méd,* July 8) to a condition which he has observed on examining the lungs of children who have died after tracheotomy.

He found the sections of the lungs so loaded with foreign bodies that they resembled those of a lung filled with anthracosis. On examining the sections with a low power, he found the bodies distributed along the course of the bronchi, penetrating the exudations, traversing the walls of the bronchioles, and occupying the alveoli. The larger bodies were free and isolated, but the smallest penetrated the protoplasm of the cells. The number of these foreign bodies varied greatly in different cases. On several occasions they have been mistaken for pathological change, but when the lung is freed from the blood which flows from the vessels, and especially after maceration in alcohol, the little blackish blocks are easily distinguished. They gain access to the lung through the canula, which does not sift the air as is done when it traverses the natural passages, the child finding itself in much the same condition as an animal in which paralysis of the larynx has been induced by section of the recurrent. This penetration takes place more abundantly in some cases than in others, not only from there being a great amount of foreign bodies in the air, but owing to the dry state of the canula when the child is going on badly. Although it is difficult to appreciate the extent to which they do so, these foreign bodies may easily induce inflammatory lesions; and it is reasonable to suppose that they may sometimes be the cause of the inflammatory affections of the lung which come on late after the operation. At all events, their admission should be opposed as much as possible; and in this point of view the cravat applied over the canula may be useful, as well as in warming the inspired air. When the rooms in which the children are placed are cleaned, also, their necks should be carefully covered up. Whenever, too, the canula becomes dry it should be moistened by an oily substance so as to enable it to arrest the foreign bodies.—*Med. Times and Gazette,* July 20, 1878.

—

The Antiseptic Treatment of Empyema.

The antiseptic method of treating wounds is doubtless capable of numerous modifications, and experience shows that the principle of the system is applicable to a constantly increasing variety of cases. In Germany especially the system is undergoing a thorough trial, and scarcely a week passes without reports of experiments attended by results almost uniformly satisfactory. There appears, indeed, to be no limit to the number or variety of cases to which the method is applicable. A few weeks ago we published an abstract of Professor Schrœder's report on fifty cases of ovariotomy, performed with the most minute antiseptic precautions, the mortality being only 15 per cent. In the hands of Professor Hueter, of Greifswald, subcutaneous injections of weak solutions of carbolic acid have been found to act most satisfactorily in checking the spread of traumatic erysipelas ; and quite recently Professor König, of Göttingen, has reported an apparently very unpromising case of empyema, in which, after the removal of the pus by a trocar, the pleural cavity was washed out with a three-per-cent. solution of the same remedy, and the wound dressed on the antiseptic plan, with a result and progress almost marvellous.

The patient was a delicate girl, ten years of age, who had lost both parents from phthisis. She had suffered for some weeks from symptoms of exudative pleurisy of the left side, and two punctures had been made, purulent fluid escaping on each occasion. The heart was considerably displaced towards the right side; fever, rapid emaciation, dyspnœa, and slight bulging of the intercostal spaces being the other prominent symptoms. Dr. König's opinion being sought, he recommended that an opening should be made through an intercostal space. In consequence of the narrowness of the interval between the ribs, and in order to be able to introduce a somewhat large drainage-tube, a portion of bone, a centimetre and a half in length, was removed, the spot chosen for the operation being near the posterior extremity of the eighth rib, external to the attachment of the levator costæ. The intention was that, in the supine position, the opening should correspond to the lowest part of the purulent collection. Chloroform was administered, and all antiseptic precautions rigidly adhered to. After the evacuation of a large quantity of thickish pus, the pleural cavity was washed out with a lukewarm, three-per-cent. solution of carbolic acid, the injection being continued until the fluid came away perfectly clean. A drainage-tube, as thick as the little finger, was then placed in the wound, so that its extremity projected about a centimetre within the pleural sac. A needle passed transversely through the wall of the tube, close to the wound, prevented any displacement. The wound was then dressed, according to Professor Lister's directions, with gauze, wadding, and bandages. For some days a daily dressing was requisite; afterwards a renewal of the application every third or fourth day was found to be sufficient. The dressing was conducted under the spray, and the tube was at the same time removed, cleansed, and replaced. By the fifth week the secretion was very inconsiderable, and a very fine tube was substituted, with a result, however, of increase of temperature. This relapse was only temporary, and in a few days a tube no thicker than a lucifer match was all that was required. The condition of the patient began to improve immediately after the operation, and her progress was rapid and continuous. The fever soon abated, the appetite returned, and the bodily weight increased with astonishing rapidity. The patient was soon able to leave her bed and to move about in the open air. During the whole course of the treatment there was never the least trace of putrescence in the secretion.

In commenting upon this case, Professor König lays down the following rules for the antiseptic treatment of recent non-fistulous empyema: 1. The operation should be performed with antiseptic precautions—disinfection of surroundings, the use of the spray, etc. 2. The incision should be as near the vertebral column as possible, in order to facilitate the escape of secretion. Double incisions are rarely necessary. 3. The incision should provide for the easy insertion of the drainage-tube. If the ribs are very close together, a portion of bone may be removed. This part of the operation may be performed subsequently, if the opening be found to be too small. It will seldom be necessary for adult cases. 4. After the escape of the pus, the pleural cavity must be once for all thoroughly disinfected. For this purpose a solution of salicylic acid may first be used, and when the fluid returns free from colour the cavity may be rapidly washed out with a strong solution (from $2\frac{1}{2}$ to five per cent.) of carbolic acid, the stronger solutions being applicable to cases where the exudation is putrid. Hueter has drawn attention to the fact that solutions of this strength, inasmuch as they produce coagulation, are less likely to be absorbed and cause mischief than those which contain less acid. This primary disinfection must be carried out with care. There is but little risk of carbolic poisoning when the pleural sac is thickened and covered with exudation; but absorption is very likely to take place when the membranous deposit is scanty in quantity. A simple washing out with the salicylic acid solution will probably suffice in cases where the effusion is merely purulent. After disinfection, the drainage-tube is to be inserted as described; it should just project into the pleural cavity, and should therefore be from five to six centimetres long. 5. Plenty of carbolized gauze should be applied over the opening and its neighbourhood. This should be covered by the ordinary antiseptic bandage completely enveloping the thorax. 6. The dressing should be changed immediately the least trace of secretion shows itself upon the surface, and during the first few hours the renewal would be required every twenty-four

hours. If the secretion remains free from smell, there is no necessity for again
washing out the pleura, but this must be done, as before described, if there are
any signs of putrescence. There is, of course, some risk of carbolic poisoning,
but the danger to the patient will be less than that of septicæmia. In such cases
a second opening and drainage-tube may be necessary in order to provide for the
free escape of the secretion. Professor König lays great stress upon the fact that
a single washing out of the pleura will suffice for the majority of cases of empyema. Frequent injections should be regarded as the exception, and as required
only in cases where the effusion is found to be putrid, or has become so during
the progress of the case. After the first week, the dressings may be less frequently renewed, the length of the interval depending upon the amount of secretion, and the saturation of the materials applied. 7. The size of the drainage-
tube may be gradually decreased, but the tube should not be discontinued so
long as there is any secretion. At every renewal of the dressings, the tube
should be withdrawn and cleansed. Dr. König claims for this method the great
merit of simplicity, and states that the dressings can be carried out by any surgeon, even though he be not especially versed in the details of the antiseptic
method.—*Med. Examiner*, July 25, 1878.

—

Ligature of the Arteria Innominata for Aneurism of the Subclavian Artery.

Mr. R. T. GORE, of Bath, records (*Lancet*, July 27, 1878) the following
case :—

D. D——, aged fifty-two, a tall, well-formed, and muscular man, was admitted
into the hospital, Bath, Sept. 22, 1856. About three years ago his attention
was directed to a swelling in the axilla, about the size of a walnut. In a few
weeks it increased in size, with pain extending as far as the elbow. It remained
stationary until the spring of 1856, when it began to enlarge rapidly, with increasing pain, and was observed to pulsate.

On admission, a large pulsating tumour was found occupying the right axilla,
and extending upwards beneath the pectoral muscles and clavicle, until it came
in contact with the scalene muscles. He appeared in fair general health, though
much distressed by pain and want of sleep. The pulse was about 80, and the
actions of the heart and lungs quite natural. The whole tumour pulsated more
or less distinctly, with an anurismal thrill. The swelling approached so near to
the scaleni as to render the application of a ligature on its cardiac side impracticable.

The ligature of the arteria innominata was decided on, after consultation with
the other surgeons to the hospital, and performed under chloroform on Sept. 24,
1856. An incision was made a little above the upper margin of the clavicle along
its inner third, and carried to about an inch beyond the sterno-clavicular joint.
This was met by a second incision along the inner edge of the sterno-mastoid
muscle, and the flap thus formed reflected upwards and outwards, including the
sternal attachment of the sterno-mastoid. The sterno-hyoid and sterno-thyroid
muscles were then carefully divided close to the sternum. A vein of some size
was here divided, and tied at both ends. A very little, but cautious dissection
exposed the arteria innominata; an aneurismal needle was passed behind it from
the outside, and the vessel tied with a hempen ligature. Pulsation at once ceased
in the tumour, and in the arteries of the arm and face on the right side.

The practical difficulties of the operation were by no means great, and in a
long-necked person are, no doubt, much less than in the ligature of the subclavian
on the outer side of the scalenus. The quantity of blood lost was quite trifling.
The limb was wrapped up in cotton-wool and blankets. He passed a fair night
with an opiate, and on the next day expressed himself much relieved. There

was not any pulsation in the tumour nor in the arteries of the arm, though there was a faint one in the temporal artery. Pulse 110; skin cool.

Sept. 28. He had a rigor in the night, and there is a slight cough, and also a blush of redness around the wound, which begins to discharge rather freely. Three sutures were removed.

Oct. 1. The redness is less; the pulse 108; the cough nearly gone, and he has slept fairly.

5th. He had a second attack of rigors, followed by tension of the tumour and arm. The arm kept up a fair temperature, and the blood in the veins moved slowly towards the heart. The treatment consisted in a free use of opiates and stimulants.

8th. The unfavourable symptoms had nearly disappeared, the wound looking healthy and suppurating moderately; but it was noticed that the ligature had an impulse communicated to it by each action of the heart.

He went on fairly well until Oct. 10, when, on the seventeenth day after the operation, during a fit of coughing, a clot of dark colour escaped from the wound, and was followed in fifteen minutes by a stream of arterial blood, which continued to flow until his death, within an hour from the beginning of the attack.

Necropsy, fourteen hours after death.—The arteria innominata was partially cut through by the ligature, which was firmly attached to it. Its cardiac extremity was scarcely at all contracted, but was partially plugged by a firm clot, three-quarters of an inch long. The aneurismal tumour, now very much reduced in size, was filled by a firm coagulum occupying the subclavian, axillary, and upper part of the brachial artery. It was of an elongated, fusiform shape, and on the cardiac side came in contact with the scalene muscles. The carotid artery was blocked up as far as the bifurcation by a firm clot. The right subclavian vein was attached to the tumour and obliterated. The left subclavian vein was filled by a soft coagulum, and its coats thickened. The aorta was coated with many deposits of atheroma. Extending from the wound into the anterior mediastinum was a large cavity, stretching upwards in the neck under the sterno-mastoid muscle, and filled with offensive pus. The heart was healthy. The lungs were somewhat congested, and the bronchi filled with thin mucus.

Though the above case was unsuccessful, the impression it left upon my mind is, that under favourable circumstances the operation is in certain conditions justifiable and advisable, and that with the improved methods now available it may yet be followed by favourable results. Nor does it militate against that view if I add to this history the fact that more than fifty years ago a similar operation was performed in this city, followed by death on the fifth day. But in that instance, though the case was in many respects favourable, the operation was over-long delayed, and was at last undertaken somewhat hastily and unadvisedly, owing to the occurrence of a train of symptoms the true character of which was altogether misunderstood and misinterpreted. They were, in fact, the signs of an attack of acute pericarditis, which was a sufficient cause of death. The state of parts about the seat of ligature, as seen after death, was very satisfactory and promising, as there was a firm clot on the cardiac side, and no signs of suppuration in the mediastinum.

I may further state that preparations illustrative of the two cases are lodged in the museum of the United Hospital in this city.

———

Ligature of the Carotid for Hemorrhage after Erysipelas.

A singular case, for which ligature of the carotid was employed with success, was lately communicated by M. DENUCE to the Académie de Médecine. The patient was a young officer who suffered from a suppurating otitis, accompanied first with severe pain and afterwards swelling in the temporal region, with erysipelatoid redness. Three incisions were made into the swelling, each at a few days' interval. The last was followed by considerable hemorrhage, easily repressed by the application of perchloride of iron and by pressure. Eighteen days later, while the patient was rapidly improving, a large hemorrhage suddenly occurred, filling the cavity of the phlegmonous abscess, and escaping in jets at the several openings. Compression and ligature of the temporal artery did not arrest the hemorrhage, and the cavity was therefore filled with lint soaked in perchloride of iron, which for the time stopped the bleeding. Two days later it recurred, and was arrested by the same means, but a considerable increase of the sloughing inflammation was the consequence, and the abscess spread to the region of the jaw, and thence a fresh hemorrhage occurred externally and into the mouth. Compression and perchloride of iron were again resorted to, but the patient had become extremely anæmic, and evidently unfit to bear a fresh hemorrhage. The common carotid was therefore tied, the tumefaction of the upper part of the neck being too great to permit of ligature of the external carotid. The huge temporal cavity was then emptied, and its blackened walls dressed, with slighter pressure, and daily washed out with a solution of "coal-tar saponine." The walls rapidly presented granulations, and at the end of a month cicatrization was almost complete. The ligature fell without any disturbance, and the patient rapidly recovered.—*Lancet*, July 27, 1878.

Castration.

A discussion on this subject took place at the Société de Chirurgie (*Bulletin*, May 8), in connection with a case related by Dr. POINSOT, of Bordeaux, in which the ligature of the cord *en masse* had been blamed by M. Despiès, as risking the production of tetanus. Dr. Poinsot quotes the experience of Bouisson, Delpech, Lallemand, and Serre, who never met with this untoward occurrence from following the practice in question. Sédillot and Legouest doubt the reality of the occurrence of tetanus, and both Giraldès and Tillaux are partisans of the procedure. In a case referred to by M. Poinsot, also, in which the vessels were separately tied, tetanus occurred. M. Despiès, in reply, stated that there could be no doubt of tetanus having followed ligature of the cord *en masse*, for those present had witnessed an example in the service of M. Nicaise. Why, in fact, should we act differently with the testicle than with other organs? and who would ever employ a ligature *en masse* in amputations? M. Forget, however, observed that he had often seen Lisfranc perform castration with a ligature *en masse*, and never knew tetanus to follow. He employed a very thick thread, declaring that neither hemorrhage nor tetanus could occur, since by strong constriction he instantly destroyed the tissues comprised within the ligature. M. Le Dentu said that he had often performed castration, and had found the tying each artery separately very easy, and he considers the ligature *en masse* to be a bad operation. On the other hand, M. Tillaux observed that he had also performed a considerable number of castrations; and although he always used the ligature *en masse*, he had never met with tetanus. By this procedure he considered one of the greatest dangers of castration is avoided, viz., hemorrhage, which is always to be feared unless the three arteries of the cord are tied. These arteries, which are of very small size, retract, and do not bleed at once; and it is only at the end of some hours that a hemorrhage, which may prove very difficult to arrest, occurs. As to attributing tetanus to the ligature *en masse*, we must first prove that the ligature of a nerve will induce tetanus. This is very doubtful; and it is by no means rare, on tying an artery, to include in the ligature a nervous filament, without tetanus being induced. Recently, M. Tillaux, in an amputation at the shoulder, tied the brachial plexus *en masse*, without the slightest ill effect resulting. There is no proof that the ligature of a nerve may give rise to tetanus, any more than ligature of a muscle. The chief objection to ligature *en masse* is the great delay which takes place in the coming away of the ligature; and to obviate this M. Tillaux is accustomed to separate the cord and apply three or four ligatures, according to the size of the cord; so that there are partial ligatures *en masse*, which come away in from eight to twelve days without causing any accident. M. Sée, after having performed several castrations with ligatures *en masse* without meeting with any accident, has yet abandoned the procedure, because in large cords the constriction ceases after some hours to be sufficient, and hemorrhage may occur. He substitutes the following procedure: After the cord has been dissected its fibrous tunic is divided, so that the various parts may be displayed, and the arteries, which are then easily distinguishable among these, are tied one after another prior to their being divided. Prof. Verneuil disapproves of ligature *en masse*, and has not found any difficulty in seizing the open arteries by hæmostatic forceps, which, after the removal of the tumour, are replaced by catgut ligatures. To be secure against all hemorrhage, the veins as well as the arteries should be tied, these veins having no valves. In order to be secure against secondary hemorrhage, M. Despiès thinks four ligatures are required, for, besides the arteries of the cord, the artery of the dartos has to be secured. They may be secured at once, without the application of the hæmostatic forceps. After ligature *en masse*, purulent infection may occur as well as secondary hemorrhage.— *Med. Times and Gazette*, July 20, 1878.

———

Cystic Sarcoma of the Lower Jaw, removed without External Incision.

Anna L., aged fifty, was admitted into Mr. MAUNDER'S ward at the London Hospital on Feb. 19th. She stated that she was married, and the mother of ten children, all of whom were living. Both her father and mother had been healthy, and died of old age at eighty and seventy years respectively. There was no history of cancer, phthisis, or scrofula in the family. She had always enjoyed good health herself, and all her children were robust and healthy. Ever since she was a young girl she had had a small lump, about the size of a walnut, on the lower part of the body of her under jaw, to the right of the symphysis. This caused her no inconvenience whatever and but slight deformity—so slight, indeed, that she had had nothing done for it. She could assign no cause for the tumour. Although stationary for many years, the tumour began to grow ten months before admission, and continued to enlarge slowly for eight months; it then increased more rapidly.

On Feb. 20th the tumour was removed, without any external wound, by Mr. Maunder's method, as described below. The patient rested well during the night, and felt quite comfortable next morning. She took her food—milk, beef-tea, and strong broth—without any difficulty, and evidently relished it, feeding herself with the aid of a spoon. No hemorrhage had occurred. Temperature in the evening, after the operation, 101.8° F., and on the following morning it was 101° F.; pulse 120; respiration 24.

On the 22d she complained of the tongue being swollen, and of a fetid odour arising from her mouth; otherwise she was comfortable. Sensation was as good on the right side of the face as on the left, except in the regions supplied by the right mental nerve, which she said felt numb. A considerable quantity of saliva and mucus dribbled from the corners of her mouth. Temperature in the morning 100.2° F.; pulse 106; respiration 22.

On the 24th temperature was 99.6° F.; pulse 100; respiration 20. She was rapidly recovering from the effects of the operation, and complained less of her tongue and of the odour from her mouth.

On the 26th the temperature, pulse, and respiration were normal. She continued to take her nourishment well. Ordered minced meat and three ounces of brandy. One or two stitches attached to the tongue were removed.

On the 28th the small laceration produced by the large size of the tumour on extraction had completely healed, leaving only the remotest trace of a scar. Temperature and pulse normal.

On March 2d the slight numbness which she felt about the right side of her chin was disappearing. She moved her tongue with almost as much facility as before the operation. There had been no hemorrhage since the removal of the tumour. She took solid food without much difficulty. Complained a little of her upper teeth protruding beyond her lower. She sat up or walked about the ward the greater part of the day.

A small abscess formed just below the divided symphysis, and was opened by the house-surgeon on March 12th, and about a thimbleful of pus was discharged; otherwise she progressed most favourably.

On March 14th the small incision had healed, and the patient considered herself cured. Her appetite was much better than before the operation. A fibrous band was seemingly forming between the divided portions of bone.

On April 2d the patient left the hospital.

Mr. Maunder remarked that during the last eight years he had removed large lateral portions of the lower jaw, the seat of tumour, three times at the hospital, without making any external incision. He showed photographs of the patients subsequent to operation. Before attempting the operation of the above case, he expressed anxiety lest, having set free the tumour, he should be unable, on account of its size, to extract it entire through the mouth. The real size of the tumour was not manifest externally; the floor of the mouth was also occupied by it, and the tongue was displaced to the left side. The operation was conducted as on former occasions, the patient being seated in a dentist's chair. No external excision was made, but the portion of jaw, the seat of tumour, was liberated by the knife, raspatory, saw, and bone-cutting forceps used within the mouth. As the operation proceeded one large cyst burst, and collapsed, and it was hoped that this diminution would be sufficient to make extraction easy. But it failed to do so, and as the tumour was being slowly withdrawn by a large pair of lithotomy forceps, the right angle of the mouth split to the extent of three-quarters of an inch. Under similar circumstances, Mr. Maunder would in future tap all existing cysts before attempting extraction, or he would remove the tumour piecemeal, after cutting it free from healthy structures.

Mr. Maunder claims for his method of operating: absence of hemorrhage, the facial vessels not being wounded; avoidance of ligatures; non-interference with the muscles of expression, and consequently avoidance of paralysis and the deformity which results from division of the branches of the facial nerve; and, lastly, the absence of a long, unsightly scar on the cheek.—*Lancet*, July 20, 1878.

Case of Loose Cartilage becoming Adherent after Venous Thrombosis with Pulmonary Embolism.

Dr. AUFRECHT of Magdeburg reports the following case in the *Deutsche Medicinische Wochenschrift* for June 8. T., a butcher, aged 38, suddenly felt a sharp pain in the right knee-joint on the 18th September, 1877, so that he was unable to stand. On examination, the presence of a movable cartilage about the size of a bean, which appeared now on the outer and then on the inner side of the joint, was made out. Its removal was advised, but was deferred for a few days at the patient's request. On the 22d September the cartilage was again caught between the articular surfaces of the joint, and this time caused intense pain, leaving the joint very tender, so that subcutaneous injections of morphia became necessary, and a somewhat febrile condition with increased temperature (101.3° F.) continued for two days. The cartilage could be felt now as a small prominence on the inner side of the patella. The joint remained stiff and tender for eight days. Suddenly, on the 3d October, there came on sharp shooting pains in the right side with hæmoptysis, about two teaspoonfuls of blood being coughed up. This pain continued for some days, and was accompanied by cough and moderate hæmoptysis, and there was a patch of dulness about the size of a crown-piece, with a strongly pronounced friction-sound on the right side posteriorly near the fifth rib. Under repeated injections of morphia and application of sinapisms, these symptoms gradually gave way. On the 8th of October there was œdema of the right foot; the knee-joint was free from pain, but stiff, owing to the prominence near the patella. On the 14th there was renewed hæmoptysis with cough, but no pain in the chest, and no lung-disease of any kind could be made out. The patient, however, felt weak, and had to keep his bed for a fortnight. The œdema of the right foot and leg continued for some time, and subsided only very gradually. There was no pain or tenderness of the joint now, but the prominence near the patella continued immovable in the same place, and was still fixed there last month (May). There can, therefore, be no doubt that the cartilage first excited by its presence a certain degree of inflammatory action in the knee-joint, in consequence of which it became itself adherent. The concomitant chest-symptoms form a point of some interest. The sudden accession of pain and hæmoptysis, the circumscribed dulness and friction-sound, occurring in a man hitherto in perfect health, all indicated pulmonary embolism; but that this emanated from the affected limb was only confirmed when œdema of the right foot set in on the fifth day after the occurrence of the chest-symptoms. The clot or thrombus had probably originated in one of the veins about the affected knee-joint.—*London Med. Record*, July 15, 1878.

—

On the Value of Antiseptic Treatment of Penetrating Gunshot Wounds of the Knee.

Dr. C. R. REYHER, of Dorpat, Consulting Surgeon with the Army of the Caucasus during the late war, has published in the *St. Petersburgher Medicinische Wochenschrift*, March 9, 1878, an account of the cases under his care in the campaign.

"Gunshot wounds of the lower extremities have at all times excited the greatest interest; in former campaigns, because the surgeon sought to discover the causes of their remarkable danger to life, and in more recent campaigns because the brilliant results of conservative surgery applied to the treatment of wounds of the upper extremity, demanded the testing of the same method in the lower extremity. After von Langenbeck had discovered, in the Austrian war of 1866, to how great an extent conservative surgery was applicable even in gunshot wounds of the knee, and how favourable were the results, the interest of surgeons in the treatment of these cases has been more especially excited. On this account it is proposed to report briefly on the gunshot wounds of the knee healed by me in the recent war in Asia."

Of a total of 81 cases of wounded knee, there were 28 in which the bullet was driven into the parts.

Eighteen cases were treated from the onset by the antiseptic method—"primary antiseptic treatment." The mortality of these was 16.6 per cent.

In none of the eighteen treated was either primary or secondary amputation performed. The fifteen who recovered, not only recovered without loss of limb, *but they also recovered motion in the joint.* Of the three deaths, one was caused by hemorrhage from wounded popliteal artery and vein, one from lung disease (*Fettembolie.* fatty degeneration of lung capillaries) two days after being wounded, and one from tuberculous suppuration (of the knee?), hectic, uncontrollable diarrhœa.

Forty cases were *at the outset* treated without any regard to antiseptic principles, *i. e.,* they were explored without antiseptic precautions, without cleansing of wound by antiseptic washes or injections, without antiseptic bandages or dressings; *subsequently,* they were subjected to antiseptic treatment—"secondary antiseptic treatment." The mortality in this group of cases was 85 per cent. *Intermediary* amputation was performed in nine of these, of whom seven died. *Secondary amputation* was performed in twelve cases, of which nine died. One only of a total of 40 cases treated by partial use of antiseptics recovered with the limb saved. that limb remaining ankylosed.

The 34 deaths were caused: 10 by "septic inflammation," 12 by "metastatic embolie pyæmia," 4 by "peracute diffuse suppurative arthro-meningitis," 7 by tuberculous suppuration, hectic, 1 by carbolic acid poisoning. (The author does not state whether this poisoning was through absorption at the exposed surfaces.)

Twenty-three cases were at no stage treated antiseptically. Of these 13 underwent secondary amputation. Of the total 23 cases, 22 died, showing a mortality of 96 per cent. of those treated entirely without antiseptics. The causes of death, investigated necroscopically, were: 3 from septic inflammation, 7 metastatic embolie pyæmia, 5 tuberculous suppuration (of the knee, it is presumed), hectic, 1 dysentery, 1 tetanus, 1 cause unknown, autopsy having been neglected.

Dr. Reyher avoided unnecessary internal exploration of the wound, employed splints to prevent movement of the joint, extracted loose and foreign bodies, and the projectile. This, in one of the cases, had broken the patella into three pieces, and had lodged itself in the tibia. In another case it had broken off and displaced the external condyle of the femur. In four cases the projectile had traversed the joint. The disinfecting agent consisted of solution of carbolic acid, 2½ to 5 per cent. The mode of employing this solution is worthy of mention. He used a common clyster syringe, drove the fluid with the utmost pressure into the cavity of the joint, so that all its recesses might be filled, and assured and completed this washing out of all internal parts by closing the external openings, and whilst keeping the cavity full of the solution, made flexion and extension movements of the limb; in fact, carried out "pump movements of the joint."

"Drainage tubes were employed, sharp edges of bone and projecting pieces which interfered with the laying of the tubes were removed by the gouge or chisel and mallet. Enlarging the external wound was scrupulously avoided.

"The smaller the external wound the more thoroughly the cavity can be washed out."

"Important practical experiences as to the mode of effecting drainage from the anatomically complicated formation of the knee-joint are given." The removal of secretion from the supra-patellar bursa and the anterior chamber of the joint is easy enough. Any lateral incision of sufficient size to admit the drain tube answers the purpose. The chief difficulty consists in the drainage of the posterior chamber, the accomplishment of which is so much the more important as pus so readily stagnates in this part. On account of the popliteal bloodvessels, drainage from behind is out of the question. Recourse must be had to lateral incision on

both sides of the articulation by semi-circular cuts 5–6 ctm. long, following the
direction of the condyles carried directly into the joint. By this means the posterior chamber is laid open on both sides without injury to the muscles. But, as
even in the flexed position of the limb the drainage tube cannot be carried into
the chamber, it was necessary to remove with chisel and mallet enough bone from
the posterior convexity of both condyles, so that each condyle might receive a
tube into a small transverse gutter. Of five cases thus operated only one survived; he recovered with a useful limb.

It was necessary to fall back upon lateral incision into the joint on the peroneal
side with lateral position of the limb, afterwards placing the limb in a slightly
flexed wooden splint, giving up the desire of securing a fully extended limb. The
result of this more simple and effectual means of discharging the contents of the
joint, was not more favourable than in the cases relieved by chisel and mallet.
The author remarks that in the worst class of knee gunshot wounds the mortality
during the wars of the last ten years has fluctuated between 58 and 83 per cent.
He concludes by the observation that surgeons must either have earlier and more
frequent recourse to amputation, or discover some better means of conducting the
suppurative processes within the knee-joint. It is evident that the more severe
forms of shattered knee-joints from gunshot wounds are, despite Listerism, as
dangerous to life as ever; a laudable confidence in antiseptic treatment, the natural
result of its success in the less complicated injuries, may have led in the recent
campaign in Asia to attempts to save limbs which in former campaigns would have
been removed as early as practicable by amputation, and in so far an undue confidence in antisepticism may have done harm. In judging, however, of the
results of any treatment of these serious injuries, we have to take into account
many circumstances which tend to render nugatory the humanity, the science,
and the experience of the surgeon. It would be interesting to the pathologist
and therapeutist to know to what extent the efforts of the surgeon are more successful at the beginning of a campaign than towards the end, when, as in the
Crimea, the constitutions of the men have been exposed to over-fatigue, incle-
mency of the seasons, insufficient and unsuitable diet, scurvy, depressing influences as to the prospects of the war, home-sickness, and the like. We should
like to know the average age of the recovered and fatal cases, the proportion of
seasoned to unseasoned soldiers; for it is probable that at one period of a campaign, when the weakest constitutions have been eliminated, the mortality from
severe injuries might be proportionately diminished, or the tendency to evil later
in the campaign, be equilibrated by their removal. At all periods of history the
bulk of the fighting men have been very young, perhaps never more so than at
the present time, when the Continental system of conscription and limited service
with the colours prevail. We consider it to be incontestable that owing to the
yet immature condition of the articular structures in the young, their joints are
less tolerant of injury, a considerable proportion of young adults, strong in muscle, active, and apparently robust, possess joint-tissues prone to take on suppurative action when injured, whatever principles of surgery may be practically
applied.

These considerations prompt us to remark that experimental conservative surgery in the lower extremity, in its desire to save limbs in case of severe complicated injuries of the knee-joint, should look to the constitution of the individual
as far as this can be done during the pressure of events in warfare, and perhaps
afford the sufferer a better chance when having to repair the smaller bony injury
effected by amputation in the comparatively compact shaft of a long bone, than
by having to repair a much larger injury of bony tissue of the articular ends of
bones and of joint surface, both being particularly prone to suppuration. We

have not the statistical figures before us, but assuming that the average of amputated thigh exhibits 50 per cent. of failures, there is a wide margin of hoped-for success against the 80 and 90 per cent. of deaths from the severest gunshot wounds of the knee. Dr. Reyher's success with antiseptic treatment thoroughly carried out would lead us to expect, if Lister's views of the efficacy of antiseptics in preventing suppuration be correct, that it ought to be as successful in the management of an amputated surface as of a joint wound. We need statistics of primary amputations of thigh in the severer knee injuries during the late war to enable us to judge.

Dr. Reyher has appended tables in which the total 81 cases are grouped according to the precise degree of injury of particular parts of the knee, the capsular ligament, the patella, the condyles, and combined injury of the whole of these parts. These tables clearly show that even in the severest class of cases—those needing, in fact, the discovery of some means of diminishing the frightful mortality of gunshot wounds of the knee—Lister's antiseptic treatment stands out pre-eminently as the means of having saved many lives. Thus four cases in which the projectile was driven into the joint, and which were throughout treated antiseptically, all recovered, whilst of fifteen similar cases treated by secondary antiseptic treatment, only one recovered, which shows a mortality of about 93 per cent.; and of nine cases treated without antiseptics at any stage, the whole died, a mortality which Dr. Reyher represents as 100 per cent., the idea of doing which would excite a smile were it not in relation to so grim a subject. It would have added to our means of correctly judging as to the comparative value of primary and secondary Listerism as against non-Listerism, if Dr. Reyher could have informed us how soon after the receipt of the injury the respective modes of treatment were commenced.

Elsewhere (page 163), when treating of spinal abscesses, grave doubts have been expressed as to the value of Listerism in the generality of those cases, but in relation to gunshot wounds of the knee, these comparative results of antiseptic surgery in Dr. Reyher's hands are as surprising as they are gratifying. Dr. Reyher is well and personally known to many in this country, is looked up to by his surgical colleagues in Germany and Russia as a man of the highest honour and veracity, as well as skill. It must be admitted by all that this recent contribution of surgical triumphs effected by the aid of antisepticism, achieved amidst the lamentable sanitary condition of the sick and wounded of the Asiatic portion of the Russo-Turkish war, is a splendid page in the progress of our art, due to the genius of Lister, and the zeal and perseverance with which Lister's method has been pursued by one of the foremost surgeons of Northern Europe.—*Doctor*, August 1, 1878.

Midwifery and Gynæcology.

Vomiting in Pregnancy.

In the *Deutsche Medicinische Wochenschrift*, May 25, 1878, Dr. RHEINSTAEDTER remarks that, in addition to the irritation of the nerves of the uterus caused by the stretching of the uterine fibres, the pressure of the surrounding pelvis upon the enlarged uterus is an important factor in the early vomiting in pregnancy. This theory is supported by the two following facts: 1. In those cases where the vomiting is not easily controlled, it ceases for the most part from the moment when the uterus rises up out of the pelvic into the abdominal cavity. 2. The vomiting is most frequent and violent early in the morning when the bladder and rectum, especially the latter, are most likely to be distended. From these considerations, the author draws the following indications for treatment: Care must be taken early to keep the lower bowel empty, either by laxatives or by enemata. The diet is to consist of milk and light food, with wine, if it can be borne.—*London Med. Record*, July 15, 1878.

Treatment of Cracked Nipples.

In the *Berliner Klinische Wochenschrift*, No. 14, 1878, Dr. HAUSSMANN relates two cases of cracked nipples, which he treated with solution of carbolic acid. The mode of application consists in the renewed application every two or three hours, during two or three days, of dressings soaked in a two per cent. solution of carbolic acid. In the first case Dr. Haussmann used a five per cent. solution, but he found the weaker (two per cent.) solution equally effective. The advantages of this treatment are that the pain disappears almost immediately, and that the medicament, being in a fluid form, reaches all the recesses at the bottoms of the fissures and cracks. This is proved by the fact that, after each fresh dressing, a sense of smarting is felt throughout the whole breast. Before applying the child to the breast, it is necessary to wash the nipple. In the cases described by Dr. Haussmann, the mothers were able to suckle their children within a few hours after the first application of the carbolic lotion, and the nipples were entirely healed in two days.—*London Med. Record*, July 15, 1878.

Changes in the Uterus resulting from Gestation.

Dr. JOHN WILLIAMS, at a late meeting of the Obstetrical Society of London (*Medical Times and Gazette*, August 3, 1878), read a paper on some of the changes in the uterus resulting from gestation, and on their value in the diagnosis of parity. The paper was suggested by the difficulty which occurred in the Wainwright murder case of determining whether the uterus of Harriet Lane had ever borne a child. The conditions to be described were those which remained after the process of involution was over—say, the eighth week after delivery. The only certain marks were to be found in the bloodvessels of the uterine wall; they appeared to be affected by the retrograde process in a less degree than the tissues of the uterine wall generally. In a section of a uterus which had undergone involution, the arteries projected beyond the surrounding surface, presented thick yellowish-white walls, more opaque than the tissues around, and their canals remained patent. On microscopical examination, the connective tissue around the arteries was found to be increased in quantity, the arterial muscular coat was greatly hypertrophied, and the inner wall considerably thickened. The vessels appeared, moreover, more numerous than in the virgin organ. To estimate the exact value of these conditions in the diagnosis of the existence of previous pregnancy, three questions should be answered: 1. Was the condition described present in all uteri which had been gravid? 2. Was it a permanent condition? 3. Was it simulated by disease? Setting aside such rare and exceptional cases as those in which the uterus became reduced after parturition to a mere membranous sac, the author had found the characters he had described in all the uteri that had borne children which he had examined during the last five years. He had found them as long as fifteen years after the last pregnancy, and eight years after the cessation of menstruation, and under such circumstances their permanency he thought might be fairly inferred. He had never seen the appearances brought about by disease, and neither he, nor, as far as he was aware, any other observer, had found them in the virgin organ. It could not, indeed, at present be asserted that the state of the uterine arteries described furnished positive proof of parity, but at the same time it must be admitted that it afforded the strongest presumptive evidence we possessed of that condition, while further research might show that it amounted to absolute proof of previous gestation. Passing on to the veins or sinuses of the uterus, the author said that these were all enlarged during gestation, but the enlargement was far more marked in that part of the wall to which the placenta was attached. Friedländer had investigated the condition of this part during the last two months of pregnancy, and found that at the eighth month many of the venous sinuses were surrounded by a wall 0.04 mm. in thickness; this wall contained abundant tolerably large nucleated cells in a clear homogeneous matrix, which became distinctly coloured by carmine solution. The contents of the sinus appeared to consist not only of blood corpuscles, but also of a greater or less number of dark granular cells, containing two to five nuclei, one of which had the appearance of a vacuole. These, which were regarded by Friedländer as wandering cells from the decidua, at last completely filled the sinuses, and coagulation took place, the clots showing a network of fine threads. Other sinuses, though not filled with these cells, also contained coagula at this period (eighth month). The author had only had an opportunity of examining one pregnant uterus, but after delivery he had not unfrequently found clots with a network of fine threads, though he had only rarely seen accumulation of large granular cells occupying the sinuses near the inner surface. At the end of four weeks, however, a great change had taken place. The walls of the sinuses at the placental site were much thickened, being due in part to a thin zone of connective tissue, within which was a granular glassy-looking transparent substance thrown into folds. The interior of the vessel was either entirely filled with these folds, or its centre was occupied with the organized remains of a clot, or a narrow lumen might still be left. The folded layer when torn by needles broke into particles of a polygonal shape, similar to some of the epithelial cells originally lining the sinus, and it appeared to be a distinct growth resulting from the proliferation of these cells. This condition had been found by the author, though somewhat indistinctly, twelve months after delivery. It might therefore be regarded as diagnostic of the previous existence of pregnancy, and, when found, justified a positive answer as to parity. It was true the structures described were not permanent, but they were discoverable for twelve months after parturition.

—

Condition of the Decidua of the Ovum as a Sign of Mature or Immature Ova.

In the *Centralblatt für Gynäkologie*, May, 1878, Dr. F. AHLFELD remarks that, as far as his knowledge of the subject goes, he has not seen the condition of the decidua in relation to the question as to a child's having been born prematurely or at term discussed. Dr. Ahlfeld finds that in the imperfectly ripe ova the structure of the decidua is essentially different from that in the ripe ova. In the decidua of an ovum expelled in the last months of pregnancy there is present a very beautifully injected network of vessels. The earlier the ovum is expelled, the larger are the vessels seen on section in the decidua; the nearer to the end of pregnancy the ovum is expelled, the smaller are the injected vessels. At the end of pregnancy, the vessels have entirely disappeared. The structure of a decidua at full term is devoid of injected vessels, or only a few are to be found near the border of the placenta. The colour of the decidua is also changed; at full term it is of a whitish-yellow appearance, while during the earlier months of pregnancy it is of a reddish hue.—*London Med. Record*, July 15, 1878.

Ovariotomy in a Child aged Twelve Years.

Dr. T. Barlow, at a late meeting of the Clinical Society of London (*Med. Times and Gaz.*, May 25, 1878), read notes of this case, which had been under the care of himself and Mr. Howard Marsh at the Children's Hospital, Great Ormond Street. The enlargement was on the right side of the child's abdomen, and consisted on the extreme right of a hard mass, internal to which, and attached to it, was a tight cyst. The whole tumour was slightly movable and painless, and had been eighteen months growing. The child had scarcely any symptoms; she suffered only from a little constipation. Her temperature was normal. Chloroform having been given, a hypodermic syringe was introduced into the cyst two inches below the umbilicus, and one drachm of clear straw-coloured fluid was withdrawn. Next day the temperature had risen to 99.4°. Four days subsequently the tumour was considerably collapsed, the abdominal surface was flattened, and the hard part of the tumour was now quite definite. It evidently contained some material as hard as bone. The cyst had become quite soft and flabby, and gave no evidence of fluid. After about six days the cyst refilled. Fifteen days subsequently it was completely aspirated, and six pints of fluid were removed. The cyst, however, again filled. Ovariotomy was then performed by Mr. Marsh. There were no adhesions between the tumour and its surrounding parts. When it had been thoroughly exposed by the incision into the abdomen, it was tapped, and eighty ounces of light brownish-green fluid were drawn off. The remaining solid portion of tumour was still too large to be drawn through the opening, which was three inches long; it was consequently extended nearly to the pubes. The thick and fleshy pedicle was clamped by Mr. Spencer Wells's method and divided. Bleeding points in the omentum were secured by catgut; and the wound was closed with sutures. No subsequent bad symptoms occurred. Pain in the abdomen was treated with morphia suppositories. After the eighth day several sutures were removed; the bowels acted spontaneously on the twelfth day; and the clamp dropped off the pedicle on the thirteenth day. For some weeks the stump of the pedicle remained protruded and covered with florid granulations. It at length became completely retracted, and the child was discharged well about eleven weeks after the operation. The tumour weighed two pounds eleven ounces; it measured six inches across, and seven inches from above down, and was nearly spherical in shape. The lower half was composed of a thin-walled cyst, capable of holding a large cocoanut; it had projecting into its cavity several smaller cysts. The hard part contained a plate of bone measuring two inches by four inches, and other smaller pieces of bone. There were cysts at the upper and outer part of the growth, with gelatinous and solid contents; many of which contained sebaceous matter, with collections of dark, short hairs. There were also fibroid bands and irregular spicula of bone interposed between some of the cysts   The child had not menstruated.

Mr. Marsh remarked that such operations in children were by no means unique. Mr. Spencer Wells had operated successfully upon a child eight years old; and in the *American Journal of the Medical Sciences* there was a record of successful operation where the child was only seven years old. At Bonn, a child aged two years had been operated upon and perfectly recovered. In all the cases, he believed, the cysts were dermoid.

Mr. Maunder said one important feature in connection with cystic tumours of the abdomen was the question of a preliminary tapping. He had known, and doubtless others present were acquainted with, instances in which the simple tapping of an ovarian cyst had led to fatal peritonitis. He was therefore strongly of opinion that this should not be done except in obscure cases, and as an aid to diagnosis   The case under consideration indicated a leakage into the peritoneal cavity, notwithstanding the small instrument that had been used ; but fortunately no serious result followed.   Assuming the radical operation justifiable in a given case, it is very undesirable to submit the patient to additional risk without corresponding advantage.

Dr. WILTSHIRE remarked that in dermoid cysts the fluid was made up of decomposed skin-products, etc., which, oozing into the peritoneum through the puncture made with the canula, were very apt to set up peritonitis.   In a patient with such a cyst, he had seen a severe attack of peritonitis supervene upon tapping.   After her recovery, a second cyst filled ; this had been opened, and still remained open.   In most children cysts of the ovary were dermoid.

Dr. COUPLAND stated that the fluid drawn off in this case was thin and pellucid, and came up through a hypodermic syringe; consequently, this cyst was not dermoid.

Mr. CALLENDER said that as the fatal results which might ensue from these tappings were well known, it seemed desirable to draw off a large quantity of fluid, that the cyst might collapse and no further fluid exude.   When only a small quantity was drawn off, the tension of the cyst-wall was scarcely diminished.

Dr. BARLOW said that at Great Ormond Street, in very many cases of the use of the hypodermic syringe, no harm had resulted.   In regard to hydatids also, even if (after tapping) the remaining fluid exuded into the peritoneal cavity, no harm seemed to come of it.   If surgeons would use a hypodermic syringe more frequently, they would learn the advantages of it.   Dr. Wilson Fox had taught that, after puncture in pleuritic effusions, the serum might be transformed into a purulent liquid.   Dr. Barlow, however, had seen oftentimes the removal of a small quantity of pleuritic fluid seem to be the first point in the absorption of the rest of the fluid itself.

—

Dilatation of the Uterus by Laminaria Tents.

In the *Centralblatt für Gynäkologie*, No. 7, 1878, Dr. SCHULTZE describes his mode of antiseptic dilatation of the os uteri by laminaria tents.   The introduction of a laminaria tent is never effected when there is any wounded surface with which it might come into contact.   Previously to the introduction of a tent, the length, direction, and calibre of the uterus are made out by means of pliant copper or silver sounds.   If there be bleeding after the introduction of the sound, the tent is not introduced until twenty-four hours later.   The vagina is washed out with a three per cent. carbolic solution, and a tent, bent to the shape indicated by the pliant sound, is introduced.   A pledget soaked in carbolic solution is packed in the vagina to support the tent.   The above procedure is performed through a speculum, the patient being placed in the knee-elbow position, which is again resorted to for the removal of the old and the introduction of the new tent.— *London Med. Record*, July 15, 1878.

—

Medical Jurisprudence and Toxicology.

Poisoning by Arsenical Violet Powder.

The recent cases of arsenical poisoning at Loughton are, in many respects, unique in medical as well as in legal experience.   There has been no similar instance, so far as we can discover, of a trial for administering arsenic by outward application, although there are cases innumerable of trials for administering it internally. Indeed, on account of the facility with which it can be procured, and the ease with which it may be secretly administered, it is the poison most frequently chosen for the purpose of committing both suicide and murder. The literature on the medical side of the question affords very few instances of deaths from poisoning by the application of arsenic to the skin, and such cases as are given are all, or nearly all, isolated ones. There does not appear to have before occurred any such succession of cases as those at Loughton, and especially the fact of violet powder being the medium of the poison seems to be novel in medical experience. The absence, moreover, in all the cases of the vomiting and purging characteristic of the internal administration of arsenic is worthy of note.

Considerations of space make it impracticable for us to pursue further the scientific and medical aspects of the case, but the circumstances of the epidemic (if it can be called by that name) are so peculiar, and the evidence that it was caused by the use of the particular violet powder in question so strong, that we make no apology for giving its history in some detail.

For several months previous to March of this year a number of mysterious deaths of young children had occurred in the parish of Loughton, in Essex, for which no satisfactory reason could be assigned. The deaths had been referred to "inflammation of the nates," "gangrenous inflammation of the genitals," and the like, but this was felt to be scarcely the real solution of the difficulty. The symptoms appeared to point to the illness being of the nature of erysipelas, and as such it was considered until events occurred which turned the suspicions of the investigators in quite another direction.

The first person who seems to have imagined that violet powder was at the bottom of the outbreak was Mrs. Deacon, the wife of an advertising agent living at Loughton. This lady was confined on January 2 of this year, and violet powder purchased from a chemist was used to her child for six weeks without any ill effects. Subsequently a second quantity of powder was purchased from a grocer's shop in the village, and two days after it was used to the baby open wounds appeared in the groins of the child and behind one of its ears. Mrs. Deacon suspected the powder, and threw it behind the fire. A week or two after the powder was discontinued, the child (which had been a healthy one before the powder was used) got better, and is now quite well. When the child had recovered, Mr. Deacon procured another packet of the same powder from the grocer's (a man named Nottage), and sent it for analysis to Dr. Jones, the analytical chemist. On the receipt of his report that the powder contained nearly 25 per cent. of arsenic, Mr. Deacon communicated with the Home Office on the subject. One of the medical inspectors of the Local Government Board (Mr. W. H. Power) was sent down to inquire into the circumstances; and after learning the result of his investigation the Government directed the prosecution, which has resulted in the committal for trial of the manufacturer of the powder on the charges of manslaughter and misdemeanor.

It was very fortunate that the illness of Mr. Deacon's child occurred when it did, as all the previous cases had been amongst the children of the poor, and the cause of the epidemic might have remained to this day undiscovered if the attention of some one in a superior position in life had not been drawn (as Mr. Deacon's necessarily was) to the disastrous effects attending the use of the powder purchased at the shop of the grocer Nottage. Nottage, it appeared, had bought of another grocer in the village, named Miss Grout, three dozen of the powders in February, 1877. Miss Grout was in the habit of purchasing violet powder from the defendant in the case, a Mr. King, of 14 Abbott Street, Kingsland Green, who described himself in his circulars as a "wholesale druggist, drysalter, and general packer." In the list of articles sold by him there was, under the heading "powders," a description of penny packets of violet powder, the whole-sale price of which was stated as being 6s. and 7s. a gross. These packets were in small boxes, similar to an ordinary match-box, and the price being so small they were naturally largely used by the poorer classes of mothers.

The result is sufficiently disastrous. Of twenty-eight infants on whom the powder purchased from Grout's or Nottage's has been used since March of last year, no less than thirteen have died, and all have suffered more or less from arsenical poisoning. This is in Loughton alone. Further evidence of the in-jurious effects of the powder reaches us from Epping, where several cases of ar-senical poisoning amongst infants have been distinctly traced by the medical officer of health to the use of this particular powder.

During the trial of Mr. King, however, a number of packets of his powder, which on analysis were proved to contain a large percentage of arsenic, were seized by an officer from Scotland Yard at a stationer's shop in Cambridge Road, Bethnal Green, and it is more than probable that cases of injury have occurred from its use in this neighbourhood also.[1]

The three cases on which King has been committed for trial on the charge of manslaughter are those of Florence Sarah Martin, Eliza Sear, and Alfred Har-rington. The mother of the child Martin stated that, up to the time of its death, powder which had been purchased from Miss Grout was used to the infant in the usual manner, and shortly before its death a blackness was seen about the groin and the neck and arms. There were black watery blisters as though the baby had been scalded or burnt about the lower part of the stomach, which was very hard to the touch. A day or two before death (which occurred nine days after birth) there was a "breaking out" under the arms and ears, the parts turning very dark. This evidence was corroborated by the woman and the doctor who attended Mrs. Martin in her confinement. Mrs. Sear was unfortunate enough to lose two children after the application to them of violet powder with King's name upon it. The first child died on March 8, 1877, having been ill only from the Sunday week previously. The throat was much swollen, the skin was red, and numerous little "white heads" (pustules) black-spotted appeared on it. The second child, Eliza, was born on February 13, 1878, and on the day of its birth the mother sent to Miss Grout's shop for another packet of the powder. This was used, and the infant died on the 18th of the same month. It was a healthy child at birth, but its face turned very red, the skin broke out all over the face and neck, and the more the redness and soreness increased the more the powder was used, in the belief that it would do good. Soon afterwards the lower parts turned black. This appearance rapidly extended to the body generally, and on the day of the child's death it gave out from the nose and mouth a "kind of black blood." Its agony was awful, and during the night before its death it screamed continuously. In the case of the child Harrington, the powder was used soon after it was born. When it was two days old a pimple was observed on its body, and its groins turned purple. The body became blacker and blacker, and four days after it died. The child was restless, and moaned a good deal.

The symptoms in all the fatal cases as to which evidence was given at the trial

[1] Since the above was written, an inquest has been held by Mr. Humphreys on the body of a child ten days old, who died at Kingsland, of inflammation of the stomach and body, undoubtedly caused, according to the medical evidence, by the use of violet powder. The case has been adjourned for the attendance of several witnesses, and the analyzation of the powder; and we are unable therefore to state at present what was the particular adultrant in the powder. It is but right to state that, so far as the proceedings have gone, it does not appear that it was Mr. King's powder which caused the mischief.

were similar to those above indicated. The first change observed was frequently a blackened condition of the skin of the groins and pudenda, and of the armpits and folds of the neck, which quickly became swollen and hard. These several parts were invariably attacked at the same time. In some instances vesication, variously described as "little white blisters," "yellowish bladders," or "bags of water," preceded or appeared about the same time as the blackness; in others, blackness with or without vesication was preceded at a short interval by a bluish-red condition of the parts affected. The vesicles, on breaking, discharged clear fluid, and left raw black surfaces. The constitutional symptoms were great restlessness, with fits of screaming or crying, and soon after a condition of collapse, in which the child died quietly. The average duration of illness in these cases was four to five days. In the non-fatal cases the chief symptom appears to have been the formation of the blisters or bladders already referred to, which appeared in almost all the cases. The other characteristics, however, occurred in nearly every case with more or less severity.

The symptoms described are exactly those which are stated in the medical works on the subject to follow on the application of arsenic to the surface of the human body. Indeed, all the medical witnesses concurred in assigning the cause of the deaths of these thirteen children to arsenical poisoning, and there seems no reasonable doubt that this is the correct interpretation. Whether or not the actual poisoning was effected by the use of the violet powder sold by King will be decided once for all at the next Chelmsford Assizes, and obviously it would be highly inconvenient for us at the present moment, whilst the case is still *sub judice*, to make any observations on the connection between the poisoning and powder manufactured by Mr. King. We content ourselves by pointing out that the Government analyst finds in the remaining portions of three packets of his powder which had been used with disastrous effects on the bodies of three separate children a percentage of arsenic amounting to 50.34, 51.40, and 48.94 respectively. The only explanation that has at present been advanced with regard to the presence of the arsenic is afforded in the evidence of Dr. Jones, the chemist who analyzed the powder for Mr. Deacon. Dr. Jones stated that white arsenic was much cheaper than starch, being sold at 10l. a ton. Arsenic is about four times as heavy as starch, and ought easily to be recognized when mixed with it by persons dealing with such things. But the vendors of this particular mixture were keepers of general stores of oils and grocery, who could not be expected to have the knowledge of a chemist and druggist.

Whatever may eventually prove to be the conditions under which the admixture was made in the cases now under investigation, it is clear that the public need to be on their guard when purchasing at unauthorized shops, and at too cheap a rate, preparations sold for use in the toilet and nursery which may be subjected to adulterations more or less mischievous, for the purpose merely of increasing the gain of the manufacturer or vendor. Infant life is exposed to by far too many dangers for another addition to the list to be contemplated with equanimity. Lack of maternal care, improper feeding and exposure, the too frequent use of narcotics and soothing medicines, want of cleanliness in homes and persons, and the ignorance and negligence of parents in not seeking promptly the advice of a qualified medical man, already swell to a very undue proportion the death toll amongst the children of our labouring population, and if to these influences be added poisoning by powder which is applied to the bodies of infants with the intention of benefiting them, the case becomes serious indeed.

We cannot, however, think that the mischief is so widespread as appears to have been apprehended, and we trust that we have heard the last of cases of injury from powder of this description.—*Sanitary Record*, June 21, 1878.

CONTENTS.

Published Monthly, price $2.50 per annum, free of postage.

Also, furnished together with the AMERICAN JOURNAL OF THE MEDICAL SCIENCES *and the* MEDICAL NEWS AND LIBRARY *for* SIX DOLLARS *per annum in advance, the whole free of postage.*

HENRY C. LEA, Philadelphia.

THE MONTHLY ABSTRACT

OF

MEDICAL SCIENCE.

VOL. V. NO. 10.	For List of Contents see last page.	OCTOBER, 1878.

Anatomy and Physiology.

The Origin of the Red Blood-Corpuscles.

AT the Biological Society of Paris, on March 2d, M. POUCHET made the following communication on the origin of red blood-corpuscles. The "elementary corpuscles" of the blood were first noticed by Donné in 1840, who confounded them with the granules in chyle; in 1846 they were well described by Zimmermann; and recently they have been brought prominently forward by M. Hayem as the germs of the red blood-corpuscles. This function M. Pouchet believes he has demonstrated by experiment; as also that certain flattened elliptical bodies, larger than red blood-corpuscles, constantly found and till lately considered pathological, are intermediate forms between elementary and red blood-corpuscles. "Elementary corpuscles" are probably derived from leucocytes by a cell-mechanism analogous to that by which the polar globules are expelled from the yolk. This theory is supported by experiment, for, firstly, they have throughout their growth the same reactions with colouring matter as leucocytes have; and, secondly, in ovipara, leucocytes fix hæmoglobin at the expense of the surrounding serum (Vulpian), and in mammalia they show the same tendency (Semmer); so then "elementary corpuscles" will act similarly, if, indeed, they are really, as it were, outcast from the bodies of leucocytes. It is also supported by the mode of development of leucocytes themselves, which being at first small and unnucleated, come at last, by a process similar to the cleavage of the yolk about the time of the extrusion of the polar globules, to have with increased size, first two and then four nuclei. The verification of this presumed origin of "elementary corpuscles" does not seem easy at first sight, leucocytes being in an abnormal condition as soon as withdrawn from the circulation. In his experiments, M. Pouchet placed part of the mesentery of a rabbit beneath the microscope, and compressed lightly a mesenteric vein. Soon leucocytes were observed to attach themselves to the vascular walls in groups, along with masses of elementary corpuscles, or one leucocyte might be surmounted by a tuft of elementary corpuscles; in such circumstances he frequently found that the adherent corpuscles already contained a considerable quantity of hæmoglobin. Without doubt, it might be objected that these corpuscles are always free when in circulation, and become agglutinated to the leucocytes, as may happen to the latter between themselves under various conditions. Still everything seems to indicate that it is not so, but that these corpuscles are direct rejections or emanations from the contractile bodies of the leucocytes.—*London Med. Record*, Aug. 15, 1878.

—

The Physiology of the Salivary Secretion.

The precise mode in which secretion is effected is still, notwithstanding all the attention that has been bestowed upon it, shrouded in considerable mystery. In the case of the kidney, various evidence tends to show that the watery part is eliminated at one part and the salts at another, but scarcely any positive facts of this nature are known in regard to other secretions. An able article has, however, just been published by HEIDENHAIN in the last part of Pflueger's *Archiv*, which seems to throw some light on the point in question. The proposition Professor Heidenhain endeavours to establish is that the secretion of water and salts on the one hand, and of organic material on the other, are not in direct causal connection with each other, but are separate acts under the control of two different sets of nerves, the secretory and the trophic, which, however, for the most part, run in the same nerve-trunks. The facts on which he relies to prove this are, that whilst the activity with which saliva in the case of the submaxillary gland is secreted augments with the degree of stimulation applied to the nerves, provided these are not exhausted, the percentage of salts increases likewise to a certain maximum, quite independently of the previous condition of the gland. On the other hand, the percentage of organic matter it contains, though also augmented with the degree of stimulation applied to the nerves, does not bear a constant ratio to this, but is strongly influenced by the previous condition of the gland, and especially by the intensity and duration of the previous excitation. If the gland be continuously excited for some time, it will be found that though the quantity of the saliva—*i. e.*, the quantity of water—remains the same, as well as the amount of salts it contains, the proportion of organic matters gradually decreases, because apparently the amount of pabulum in the gland is used up. That variations in the elimination of the watery and saline parts of the saliva on the one side, and of the organic matters on the other, do not run a parallel course, is further shown by several experiments. In the first place, taking a fresh and unexhausted gland, if the strength of the stimulus be gradually increased, the flow of saliva augments, and with it the proportion of both organic and of saline constituents, but the former in larger proportion. But if to a gland already exhausted a still stronger stimulus be applied, although it appears to respond to the lash, it does so only so far as the watery and saline constituents are concerned, the organic material either actually diminishing, as occurs with a moderate increase in the strength of the current, or requiring a very strong current to produce a very slight increase, and even this, if the gland be much exhausted, may altogether fail. Lastly, if in a fresh gland the stimulus be gradually increased, and then again diminished, in intensity, the quantity of the saliva as well as of the saline and organic constituents will be found to rise and fall, but not in equal proportion, the watery and saline parts diminishing to a greater extent than the organic, the difference being better marked the more intense the temporary increase of stimulation is, from whence Heidenhain concludes that a very strong stimulus leaves a secondary or after-condition which renders the gland more disposed to eliminate organic matter. It would thus appear that there is an intimate connection between the water and the salts of the saliva, the proportion of these rising and falling together in accordance with variations in the strength of the stimulus; whilst the amount of the organic constituents, though broadly agreeing with these in its variations, yet follows laws of its own; and it is this difference which leads him to think that the elimination of the watery and saline constituents is under the control of one set of nerve-fibres, the secretory, whilst the organic substances are subject to the influence of another set, the trophic nerves.

Professor Heidenhain next proceeded to investigate the relations of the parotid gland, which, as he remarks, there is no ground for assuming should necessarily present the same behaviour as the submaxillary to the nervous system. He corroborates Loeb's statement that the motor nerve of the gland runs in the nervus petrosus superficialis minor, and points out that the parotidean saliva is not always so watery as is generally supposed, that it is liable to remarkable variations in regard to the amount of organic and inorganic constituents, and that, under different conditions, the quantity of the latter held in solution is double, and of the former twenty-five times, the ordinary amount. In regard to the influence of stimulation of its nerves, the effects are in all respects similar to those already described in speaking of the submaxillary gland. He found, moreover, that the sympathetic nerve possessed a powerful influence over it; since if this was stimulated shortly before, or coincidently with, Jacobson's nerve, there was an immediate increase in the quantity of organic substances eliminated by the gland, though there was no increase in the absolute quantity of fluid discharged. The sympathetic contains the vaso-constrictor fibres of the gland, and it might be supposed that the change in the secretion was due to changes in blood-supply, but a very curious fact came out from his further experiments, namely, that ligature of the carotids, though somewhat diminishing the absolute amount of saliva eliminated, had no influence on the solids it contains, either in the case of the parotid or of the submaxillary gland, which shows well the complete independence of secretion on blood-pressure.

Heidenhain next undertook to examine the parotidean saliva of the rabbit, in relation, on the one hand, to the chorda tympani, which was shown by Rahn to contain secretory branches for this gland, exciting the flow of what may be called cerebral saliva; and on the other to the cervical sympathetic, which V. Wittich and Nawrocki have shown to lead to the secretion of so-called sympathetic saliva. The parotid of the rabbit is well adapted for experiments of this nature, since it contains a diastatic ferment that is absent in the secretion of this gland in the carnivora. He found that small quantities of pilocarpin injected subcutaneously produced the same effect as stimulation of the chorda tympani—gave, in fact, an abundant flow of cerebral saliva, probably by acting on the same mechanism in the gland. The cerebral or pilocarpin saliva contained only 1.02 to 2.05 per cent. of solids, whilst the sympathetic saliva contained no less than from 3.72 to 6.65 per cent., the greater part consisting of organic matter. The secretory fibres of this gland therefore run in the glosso-pharyngeal and chorda tympani nerves, whilst the trophic are contained in the sympathetic of the rabbit. The histological changes in glands that occur with variations in the activity of secretion seem to differ to a very remarkable extent. We have no space for the details of the experiments he gives.

Professor Heidenhain advances the following view as the most satisfactory explanation of the facts he has observed: We must presuppose, he says, the presence of some substance in the cells having a strong affinity for water, and it is not unreasonable to assume that the protoplasm constitutes this substance. Water is first abstracted from the lymphatic spaces, and then secondarily from the interior of the blood-capillaries; and imbibition takes place into the protoplasm till a state of equipoise is attained, no change occurring as long as the gland is at rest, though the tension of the water in the protoplasm is considerable. The effect of excitation of the secretory nerves is to induce a change of the molecular arrangement in the limiting layer of the protoplasm on that side of the cell which is turned towards the lumen of the acinus, in consequence of which diminished resistance to the act of filtration occurs at this part. Water consequently escapes, the outflow being perhaps maintained or increased by contraction of the protoplasm, as Kühne has actually observed in the cells of the pancreas of the rabbit under the microscope. The tension of the water in the cells falls below the imbibition power of the protoplasm, and a current sets in from the blood-capillaries, and the escape of water from the inner surface and the absorption through the outer surface of each cell continue as long as the protoplasm contracts under nerve influence. When the excitation ceases the protoplasm returns to its former condition, the current stops, and the gland returns to a state of rest. This view, it will be observed, does not make the excretion of water in any way dependent on the blood-pressure, whilst it explains why no more water leaves the capillaries than is required to make up what is withdrawn from the lymph-spaces, why, however long the excitation is applied, the lymph-spaces never become charged with excess of fluid, and why the excitation is neither accompanied nor followed by any increase of lymph in the efferent lymphatics.

The functions of the trophic nerves, he thinks, is to lead to the formation of soluble organic substances in the gland-cells, which are dissolved by the fluids eliminated under the influence of the secretory nerves. The organic constituents are not formed directly from the protoplasm, but during the period of rest, substances are formed which stand in close relation to the specific constituents of the gland. Thus, in the case of the pancreas, during rest, the zymogen of the trypsin is formed, from which the trypsin is afterwards developed; and thus in the mucus-glands, not the easily soluble mucin itself, but a substance that is easily convertible into mucin, is formed. It would otherwise be unintelligible why mucin does not appear in moderate quantity on slight irritation of the chorda, when the aqueous portion of the secretion is slowly percolating the cells. We thus obtain an explanation of the reason why the cells of quiescent mucous and serous glands are relatively poor in protoplasm, presenting a clear and but slightly granular aspect, whilst they are rich in the mother-substances of the proper products of the secretion. And hence, too, we learn why, after persistent activity, the glands are rich in protoplasm, as indicated by their marked cloudiness and granular aspect, whilst they contain but little of the material proper for the production of the organic constituents of the gland. In what mode the trophic nerves effect the conversion or aid in the elimination of the organic substances of the gland Professor Heidenhain does not attempt to explain.—*Lancet*, Aug. 3, 1878.

—

The Absorption and Excretion of Water.

The absorption of water from the alimentary tract is a subject to which less attention has been directed than its practical importance deserves, for the subject is not so simple as might at first sight appear. Dr. SKORCZEWSKI, of Cracow, has made an interesting series of observations on the relation in time and quantity between the absorption of water and the excretion of urine, and his results have been published in a Warsaw journal. The observations were made upon men and rabbits, and in the latter provision was made to secure the urine as soon as it passed into the bladder. Spring water, soda water, and certain Russian mineral waters (those of Krynica and Iwonicz) were employed in the observations. The following conclusions were reached. After the injection of spring water the quantity of urine did not increase immediately, in the case of either men or rabbits, but rose after a certain time, which is said to have been the longer the more water was taken. A longer period elapsed after the spring water than after the mineral water before the increase in the urinary secretion occurred; and the more spring water was taken the longer was this interval, and the mineral water the shorter was the interval. The increase in the urinary secretion reached its height sooner after the mineral water than after spring water. The greatest total effect on the urinary secretion was obtained with soda water, the next with spring water, and the least with the mineral waters. The quantity of urine was in each case smaller than the quantity of water ingested, with the exception of that which was saturated with carbonic acid. The difference between the total quantity of liquid taken and the total quantity of urine excreted was less after ordinary spring water than after the mineral water.

A second series of observations had for their object to ascertain the relation in time and quantity between the water absorbed and the urine excreted. This was effected by killing rabbits at certain periods after the water was injected into the stomach, the excretion of urine being observed in the same way as before. From these observations it appeared that the increase in the excretion of urine did not commence until after the whole of the water had been absorbed, and in the case of both small and moderate quantities of water (40 to 100 c.cm.) a period of ten or fifteen minutes passed after all the water had been absorbed before the effect on the urine was apparent. It is calculated that 500 cubic centimetres of water are absorbed from the human stomach in fifteen minutes, and 200 c.cm. in five minutes. These results are true, however, only of spring water. Mineral waters behave differently. The increase in the excretion of urine occurs the earlier the slower the absorption progresses. By the exclusion of certain possible causes for this difference, such as altered pressure in the abdominal cavity, direct irritation of the splanchnic nerve, or the effect of blood-tension, the conclusion is reached that the cause is the alteration in the blood consequent on the admixture with it of the saline substances in the mineral waters, the change in the blood acting as a stimulant to the vaso-motor nerves.

Whatever be the precise value of these researches, they show conclusively that the function of the stomach and kidneys may be materially affected by the presence of very small quantities of saline substances, and they indicate how much caution is necessary in applying rules true of pure water to water which we are accustomed to consider as differing from spring water by very trifling qualities. As an instance of the practical importance of these facts, it is evident that the saline waters, so commonly taken with food, remain in the alimentary canal for a much longer time than spring water, and are capable therefore of disturbing in a greater degree the process of digestion.—*Lancet*, August 24, 1878.

Materia Medica and Therapeutics.

Hypodermic Injection of Chloroform.

Recurring to this subject at the Paris Hospital .Medical Society (*Gaz. Hebd.*, July 26), M. Dujardin-Beaumetz felt rather disposed to disparage this procedure, observing that in the horrible pains of cancer chloroform did not give relief as morphia does, an abatement of suffering of short duration being obtained, but not sleep. Moreover, nervous subjects, and those addicted to alcohol, do not derive any general relief. Independently of the danger of chloroform injections when performed by inexperienced hands, we cannot be certain of obtaining the results proposed to be obtained. In reply, Dr. Ernest Besnier, to whom we are indebted for the introduction of these injections, observed that there are two points to be noted with respect to these objections. First, with respect to the procedure; and next, as to how far they are substitutes for morphia. M. Dujardin-Beaumetz admits that accidents occur only where the operation is badly executed; but surely the practitioner ought to learn how to perform it. and not reject a method which furnishes favourable results merely because its execution requires some attention. Two things are requisite: a good syringe, and good needles of different lengths, for it is obvious that those which are employed for the face should be less long than those inserted into fleshy parts. The entire needle-canula must be introduced into the tissue separately, and then we should wait an instant to see that a droplet of blood does not issue, proving that we had entered a vein. In this case the operation should be made in another point, and only then should the syringe be adapted and the injection proceeded with. Care must be taken that the point of the needle be at a certain distance from its point of insertion ; and by observing this precaution, Dr. Besnier, who has always employed the same syringe, has met with no accident, although he has operated in almost every region, including even that of the wrist. As to the comparison of the chloroform with morphia injections, he has only used them when these last could not be borne, or when it was desirable to avoid morphinismus. He has cured sciatica with them, which has resisted all other treatment; and they may be made without danger. M. Duguet observed that he had tried them in several cases of sciatica, but although he found that they gave temporary relief, they had to be repeated, and did cure the disease. Dr. Besnier replied that the dose is of importance. He injects a syringeful first at the upper part of the limb, and then a second syringeful at the middle part, when the pain ceases. Next day he injects opposite the fibula. On each occasion from two to four grammes of chloroform are injected. Perhaps the best results are obtained in tic douloureux.—*Med. Times and Gaz.*, Aug. 3, 1878.

Medicine.

On Malignant Lymphomata.

Dr. WIEGARDT, of Warsaw (*St. Petersburg Med. Wochenschrift*, March 16) relates a case of malignant lymphoma of the lumbar retro-peritoneal glands in a man thirty years of age. Death occurred from exhaustion four months after admission to the hospital. At the necropsy the lymphatic glands of the neck and axilla, the bronchial and lumbar glands, were greatly enlarged, pale, and soft. In the anterior wall of the left ventricle of the heart there was a round tumour, about $2\frac{1}{2}$ centimetres in diameter, soft, pale, and sharply defined by colour and consistence from the surrounding parts, but without a capsule. Near the apex, and in the left border of the heart, was a second tumour, as large as a nut, and another, as large as a walnut, was situated in the posterior wall of the heart ; finally there was a little nodule the size of a pea in the wall of the auricle. The pancreas was enlarged, yellow-coloured, and soft. The retro-peritoneal glands formed a large irregular tumour, 19 centimetres ($7\frac{1}{2}$ inches) long, by 12 centimetres ($4\frac{3}{4}$ inches) wide, and 8 centimetres (3 inches) thick, formed of masses up to as large as a goose's egg, matted together by dense fibrous tissue. There was no caseation or softening. The consistence of the tumours was generally soft, and their cut surfaces were moist, smooth, grayish-white or pale gray red. Some were somewhat harder, and their sections were more yellow-coloured. The spleen was double the normal size, hard, and dirty-brown on section ; the trabeculæ were strongly marked ; the pulp was not easily removed, and the capsule was thickened in places. The left kidney was about half as hard again as normal, and contained in its cortical substance many tumours, from the size of a pea to a nut, which in places projected on the surface, in other places penetrated the medullary portion. The right kidney was somewhat larger ; it contained fewer, not more than twenty, tumours, most of them of the size of a pea and smaller ; four were as large as a nut, and one as large as a walnut. The entire left iliac fossa was filled with a nodulated new growth, about 4 or 5 centimetres thick ;

the tumour involved the whole thickness of the ilium, but it was sharply defined
from the bone-substance, which was very porous, soft, and brittle. The outer
surface of the ilium was not altered. The other pelvic bones were normal.
The marrow of the femur, humerus, the sternum, and ribs showed no change.
The white blood-corpuscles were not increased ; they were rather fewer in fact.

The structure of the tumour presented on microscopical examination the usual
appearance of small round cells, like lymph-corpuscles, pale, with slightly granular protoplasm, and one nucleus, seldom more. These cells were imbedded in a
delicate reticulum of these fine fibres, which could be made visible by brushing
or shaking out the cells. The new growths under the microscope were not so
sharply limited off from the healthy tissues as they appeared to the naked eye ;
they grew peripherally, and extended in the interstitial tissues of the organs.
In the pancreas there were found at first small groups of round cells between the
acini, which rapidly increased in numbers so as to atrophy the latter, which lost
their proper coats, became converted into small heaps of lymphoid cells, and
finally disappeared. Very similar changes occurred in the urinary tubules of the
kidney. In the heart, the muscular fibres near the tumours lost first their transverse striation, became granular, then smaller, finally fibre-like, and then completely disappeared. In a similar manner the trabeculæ of bone in the ilium
were atrophied and compressed by the extensive new growth. At the border of
a speculum of bone one saw often curved notches, frequently with secondary
notches, like Howship's lacunæ, filled with closely packed round cells. More
frequently the bone-capsules were enlarged, and contained an enlarged cell
strongly coloured by carmine, sometimes lying against the wall, sometimes lying
free in the centre, here and there also many cells having the appearance of the
second ; so that one is led to believe that they took part in the new growth,
although no distinct trace of division or multiplication could be found. These
widened lacunæ in places coalesced to form still larger spaces in the bone.
Another mode by which the bone was destroyed was by the infiltration of round
cells between the trabeculæ of bone, compressing them, and converting them into
smooth spindle-shaped fibres, and finally into connective tissue. The tumour
was a very characteristic example of malignant lymphoma. Beginning in a
group of lymphatic glands, it had completely the characters of hyperplasia, not
extending beyond the glands to their surroundings, but extended from connective tissue and along it, showed no tendency to retrograde changes, no caseation
or softening, extended from the lymphatic glands and forming metastases finally.
To all appearance, we are entitled to regard the retro-peritoneal and mesenteric
glands as the seat of the primary lesion ; but this seat of origin is very rare.
Most authors give the glands of the throat and neck, or less commonly those of
the axilla and mediastinum, as the general places of origin. Lücke gives the
lumbar glands, the retro-peritoneal and mesenteric glands, and Billroth and Dickinson give cases in which these glands only were affected. Some years ago the
author saw a similar case in the Ivangorod military hospital ; the abdominal
tumour was as large as a child's head, and the lumbar glands were only affected.
The metastasis to other organs is not common, and the regions in which these
occurred are not generally those in which they are met with. Usually they are
in the liver and spleen, which in this case were free. Metastases in the kidneys
are rare ; Wilks, Wunderlich, and Hüttenbrenner have described them. The
author knows of no case of secondary growth in the pancreas, except the one recorded by Hüttenbrenner. Metastases in the heart have been described by R.
Mayer and Murchison. He has been able to find no case of metastasis in bone.
Tommaso Crudeli has described a case of diffuse, not leukhæmic, lymphoma of
the skull and other bones, which, however, does not belong here, as the tumours

grew from the periosteum, and did not affect the bone itself.—*London Med. Record*, Aug. 15, 1878.

The Pathological Anatomy of Scurvy.

Scurvy has happily become so much less common a disease than formerly, that the opportunities for applying modern methods of research to its pathological anatomy are comparatively rare. Such opportunities have, however, been numerous at Cronstadt, and Dr. N. Uskow, the superintendent of the Marine Hospital there, has made good use of the material, and has published some of his results. He concludes that scurvy is a general disease with a series of characteristic anatomical changes which are not located in any one organ, but are disseminated through the whole vascular system. The most constant change is the affection of the gums, and upon this the chief part of the microscopical observations have been made. The affection of the gums begins in the deeper layers, and consists in the development of obstruction in the bloodvessels, and one of the consequences of this obstruction is the stasis of the papillæ, the vessels of which are so often distended that of the proper structures of the papillæ only the epithelium may be visible. The appearances in the deeper layers of the epithelium are, first, more or less swelling of the endothelium of the vessels. The lumen of the vessel is commonly increased, and is plugged, sometimes with red corpuscles, sometimes with white corpuscles, rarely with both. Where the white blood-corpuscles are accumulated, the swelling of the endothelium is greatest; where the red corpuscles are accumulated the endothelium is almost normal, but is often detached from the wall of the vessel, and lies among the red corpuscles. Later on there occurs an extravasation of red blood-corpuscles, which become transformed into brown translucent granular pigment. Rupture of vessels could never be seen. The swelling of the endothelium at the spots at which the white blood-corpuscles are accumulated is often very great, and it is scarcely to be distinguished from the white corpuscles. Proliferation of the endothelium could not be seen, but at a later stage there are dense firm bundles of connective tissue, between which larger or smaller nests of round granulation cells are imbedded. The substance of the connective tissue bundles is not altered, but in the interstices is a light-brown finely granular pigment. The granulation tissue nowhere shows any trace of fatty degeneration. When the disease is intense the papillæ of the gum become gangrenous and break down, and when the destruction extends further the granulation tissue is also affected. The morbid process may involve the deep layers of the periosteum, between which and the bone are found some traces of extravasation and caries. A similar vascular change may be seen, although rarely, in the periosteum of the anterior extremity of the ribs. When the affection is very intense the anterior extremity of the rib bones may be attacked with osteitis rarefaciens, as Slavianski has pointed out, and this may proceed to complete destruction of the compact tissue of the bone, so that the spongy tissue passes without demarcation into the periosteum, and the latter may assume the appearance of marrow. Later the connection of the ribs and their cartilages may be altered and disturbed. The marrow of the ribs, as well as of the other long bones, is red, and, on microscopic examination, is found to consist of red cells and a few fat-cells and pigment. Thus it appears that in scurvy there is a series of acute changes in the vascular system. Whether the changes in the vessels depend on a change in the blood is difficult to say, but it is noticeable that the number of blood-corpuscles is not abnormal (red 3,500,000 to 4,700,000, white 20,000 to 47,000, per cubic millimetre). Inflammatory appearances are often accompanied by fever, for on simple affection of external parts (without pleurisy or pericarditis) the temperature is from 36° to 38° Cent., and the morning remission from 1° to 1½° Cent.—*Lancet*, Aug. 17, 1878.

The Treatment of Diphtheria.

Paris, as our readers are aware, has been, during the last two years, the seat of a formidable epidemic of diphtheria, and the continued prevalence of the disease during the end of last and the commencement of this year has led to the publication of the experience of several physicians regarding its treatment. Their statements have been summarized by Dr. FERRAND in a recent number of *L' Union Médicale*. It is hardly necessary to say that none of the recorded experience is in favour of the notion of a specific remedy, but the characteristic of the therapenties of the present day, the use of antiseptics, is strongly marked in the recommended practice. Antiseptic applications have here one of the most obvious and simple of their fields. on account of the nature, constancy, and accessibility of the peculiar anatomical feature of the disease. Tannin was employed as a local application by Trousseau, and its use in a somewhat novel fashion has been recommended by Dr. Créquy. He employs inhalations of steam from boiling water in which tannin is suspended. The vapour of the water carries with it a considerable quantity of tannin, although whether enough to exercise an appreciable influence on the exudation is somewhat doubtful. Salicylate of soda has been given internally by M. Cadet de Gassicourt, but without any satisfactory results, and salicylic acid was equally useless in the hands of Dr. Bergeron. Carbolic camphor has been praised by Dr Sonlez. This is a solution of twenty-five grammes of powdered camphor dissolved in one gramme of alcohol and nine grammes of carbolic acid. It is employed pure, or mixed with oil of almonds, as a local application to the false membrane, which is said rapidly to separate and disappear, leaving behind it a simple ulceration which quickly heals. No remedy, however, has received so much commendation as an old one—chlorate of potash. It has been strongly recommended in the past by many authorities, especially in Paris by Isambert, and Seeligmuller has lately insisted afresh on its value. He gives it in solution at least every hour, and pins his faith upon it so exclusively as to consider all other treatment necessary only for their "useful moral effect upon the parents." The removal of the fetor, the gradual disappearance of the false membranes, the reparation of ulcerations, and rapid improvement in the general state, are the effects attributed by Seeligmuller to chlorate of potash. This last effect has been ascribed to a fancied power of carrying oxygen to the blood, which contains but little, in consequence of the action on it of the diphtheritic bacteria. Its utility is corroborated by Ferrand, who, however, doubts its influence on the general state of the patients, and ascribes its action rather to its excretion by the salivary and pharyngeal glands. He has observed sometimes that the stomach does not bear it well, and even rejects it constantly. Bucquoy and Blache also recommend it. Cadet de Gassicourt made a comparative trial of chlorate of potash, cubebs, and salicylate of soda, at the Hôpital Ste. Eugénie, and does not hesitate to accord the first place to the chlorate. Cubebs and copaiba have, however, found an advocate in Trideau, who recommends, to reduce the difficulties of administration to a minimum, that they should be masked with sugar and Malaga wine. Tincture of eucalyptus was employed and recommended by Walcker; it was made by diluting ten grammes of alcoholic extract of eucalyptus by thirty-eight grammes of syrup, and was given after an emetic. All these agents thus act chiefly by modifying the affected surface, and their supposed action might be termed a "local alteration." Actual caustics have of late fallen into disrepute, although nitrate of silver is still recommended by Guillon as an application not only to, but around, the false membranes; a method deprecated by Ferrand, on the theoretical ground that the irritated surfaces become the seat of fresh membrane, like a similar surface elsewhere; and he joins Dr. Rose Cormack in advocating the simplest local application—glycerine of borax or a weak solution of hydrocloric acid, lime-water, or sulpate of soda; and he recommends the alternation of these very inoffensive applications.—*Lancet,* July 20, 1878.

—

Brain-Forcing.

Dr. CLIFFORD ALLBUTT contributes an extremely original and thougtful paper on mental function, to the first number of *Brain,* the new psycological journal.

If it be true that the aim of good education is to insist upon a mastery of one or more subjects, but, at the same time, to gain an adequate notion of the whole field of the battle of life, then assuredly our author may be congratulated upon having made good use of his time. His complete mastery of one subject—practical medicine, and the versatility displayed in this article, seem to fully indicate that he has lived up to his own standard as regards mental training, and that he is quite in a position to point out to others less gifted than himself certain rules for their intellectual guidance.

Dr. Allbutt commences by subdividing mental function into five "aspects of nervous activity," as they appear to ordinary observers. These are quality, quantity, tension, variety, and control, all of which are explained at length as we proceed.

"By the higher quality of the brain or part of it," writes Dr. Allbutt, "I mean that structure of cell and fibre, which corresponds more widely or more intimately with outer conditions, so that by virtue of such relation the individual more readily apprehends things and conceives them. This is genius in the stricter sense. By quantity, I mean the volume of nerve-force given off by the brain or its parts without regard to quality of work done. By tension, I mean the power in the nerve-action to overcome inner or outer resistance, 'nervous energy,' as it is colloquially called. By variety, I mean the congregation of different centres, and the weaving of mediate strands which give the possessor not higher or wider, but a greater number of relations with outer things. In common life this is usually called versatility. By control, I mean that subordination of one centre to another, whether inherited or acquired, which, if of the lower to the higher, results in the obedience to the more permanent order of the universe. Thus a man may have a lofty, an abundant, an intense, a versatile, and a well-ruled nervous system; or he may have any measure of these states in various proportions."

Numerous examples are then brought forward, of living and dead celebrities, to illustrate these views, the whole culminating in a description of the advantages of self-control.

"Of all endowments," writes Dr. Allbutt, "control is the most precious and its nurture our most bounden duty. For a happy and useful life, perhaps control is more needful than quality, volume, variety, or even tension of the brain. Of all gifts, then, to be cherished and nurtured, perhaps we should place first control, as by it effort is husbanded; perhaps of equal or scarcely of the second place, comes tension; quality of brain cannot be had for the asking, and lack of quantity in individuals may be compensated by numbers. Variety, however charming, however grateful, is the least precious of these conditions of brain, and is the last which calls for nurture."

Certain important points connected with the physical aspect of the question are next alluded to.

"A dyspeptic may well have nerve-force of high quality and high tension, but," says Dr. Allbutt, "I never met with a dyspeptic whose nerve-force welled continuously forth. Like Brougham and Cavour, men of great power of continuous work have usually been large as well as sound eaters. A 'hard headed' man is also a hard bodied man; and the national history of Europe is a long display of the successive triumphs of the men of colder over the men of warmer regions; of the hardy, lusty, and hungry races over the softer, more indolent, and more abstemious." . . . . . "I am not one of those," continues our author, "who think the love of athletics is as yet in excess. Here and there men may expend in the hunting field or on the river that which should have been given to their tripos, to their profession, or to their country; yet this at worst is but an individual loss, far outweighed by the impulse given to the hardy, hungry vitality, by which the nation thrives, and its general volume of nervous force is augmented."

The evils of prematurely forcing the nerve-powers of the young are next forcibly dealt with. Original compositions from children, competitive examinations when carried to excess, the preaching tasks from students in theological colleges, and the effete creations of young artists and musicians, are all instances of precocity in those who ought to be still acquiring knowledge and adding to their stores, instead of displaying their crude productions to the surfeited glances of a critical public.

The success of mellowed and mature thought is especially observable in musicians. Handel composed his great oratorios after he had passed his fiftieth year. Sebastian Bach wrote the B minor Mass at the age of forty-eight, and the two Passions somewhat later still. Beethoven wrote his grandest works after the age of forty-five; and, in times more modern, Wagner composed *Lohengrin* and the *Ring des Nibelungen* when past sixty years of age. The *Paradise Lost*, the *Divina Commedia*, and the *Tempest*, are also not works of youth, but of age.

Dr. Allbutt concludes by saying, "the true purpose of education is, first of all, to teach discipline. The discipline of the body and the higher discipline of the mind and heart; to encourage the budding faculties to break freely in natural variety; to quicken the eye and the hand, and to touch the lips with fire; to promote the gathering of the fountains of vigorous life by fresh air, simple nutritious diet, and physical exercise; and, finally, to watch for the growth, silent it may be for years, of the higher qualities of character, and even of genius, not forcing them into heated and froward activity, but rather restraining the temptation to early production, and waiting for the mellowness of time; remembering that the human mind is not an artificial structure, but a natural growth; irregular, nay, even inconsistent, as such growths are, wanting most often the symmetry and preciseness of artifice, but having the secret of permanence and adaptability."— *London Medical Record*, Aug. 15, 1878.

—

Cerebral Lesions Occurring in the Course of Acute Articular Rheumatism.

Dr. Ch. LIÉGEOIS communicates a paper on cerebral rheumatism to the *Revue Médicale de l'Est*, March 1st, 1878.

Under this term, "cerebral rheumatism," has been included by various writers every morbid cerebral condition which may occur during the course of acute rheumatism. Six clinical forms of this condition are admitted by Trousseau, which at once shows how various are its manifestations. Many and various anatomical lesions have been described as productive of this condition; some, following Trousseau, have recognized in cerebral rheumatism a pure and simple neurosis, while certain cases have been explained as due to embolism and congestion of the nervous centres. Others, as Musgrave and Sauvages, think that acute hydrocephalus accounts for the apoplectic form. M. Jaccoud considers that cerebral embolism and meningitis account for some of the cases, while others are due to punctiform meningeal hemorrhages or hydrocephalus; while, in a certain number of cases, necropsy reveals no visible lesion.

The author expresses his own opinion that "the cerebral lesions occurring in the course of acute articular rheumatism are, in some cases, the consequence of insufficient action of the heart, caused by parenchymatous degeneration and alteration of the organ, due to pericarditis." He cites, in confirmation of his views, a case of multiarticular rheumatism; on the eighth day of which there was an attack of eclampsia lasting five hours, during which time the temperature was not above 37° Cent. (98.6° Fahr.). The articular rheumatism continued its course and attacked fresh joints. Quantitative analysis of the urine excluded the idea of uræmia. A fortnight after the attack of eclampsia, it was noted that the sounds of the heart were very indistinct, the pulse frequent and often irregular, while his face was cyanotic. The patient died four days after the last note was made.

At the necropsy, there was found dry pericarditis with numerous adhesions, and myocarditis of the left ventricle, characterized by the pale colour of the muscle and its friability. There were no valvular lesions. There were fibrinous clots in the ventriculous cavities, some old, others recent. There was basic broncho-pneumonia in the second stage; and slight pleuritic effusion. The examination of the brain was forbidden.

The author of the paper, setting aside the old idea of "retrocession or metastasis," thinks it more probable that the diminution of pain or its disappearance at the time of the development of cerebral disorders is only the result of a cerebral disturbance, which prevents the perception of pain. In the above case, a subsidence of articular pain occurred two days before the convulsive seizure.

The question is then discussed, what was the nature of the lesion of the nervous centres? As the brain was not examined at the necropsy, it is obvious that no satisfactory answers can be given. Cerebral embolism appeared improbable, as there was no valvular lesion in the heart, and no ulcerative endocarditis was found. The idea of cerebral meningitis is combated on the grounds that the temperature remained at 37° Cent. during the attack, while the prodromal stage of meningitis, as characterized by cephalalgia, vomiting, and agitation, was absent. The probability of meningeal ecchymosis is improved. The idea of simple delirium appears to Dr. Liegeois unworthy of discussion, and he reverts to the previously expressed opinion as to the cause of the cerebral symptoms. The subject is to be continued hereafter.—*Lond. Med. Record*, Aug. 15, 1878.

—

Opiates in Cerebral Anæmia and Diseases of the Heart.

Dr. HUCHARD (*La France Méd.* 1878, p. 164, from *Journ. de Thérap.*) speaks of the good results obtained by the administration of opium to persons suffering from insufficiency or narrowing of the aortic valves. He gives numerous instances in which the happy effect of this remedy has been manifested. In the course of certain affections of the heart, where the attacks of suffocation and of dyspnœa have acquired an extreme intensity, injections of morphia are of great service.

Opium, given in the dose of one to two centigrammes (gr. $\frac{1}{6}-\frac{1}{3}$), produces slight excitement of the circulation, animation of mind, and increase of muscular force; if the dose be pushed to five or ten centigrammes, depression of the circulation, with a tendency to sleep, is brought about. M. Gubler, in his *Commentaires*, urges the utility of opium in want of stimulation of the nervous centres, through an impoverished or altered blood; and Dr. Vibert suggested, a year or so ago, that injections of morphia should be practised previously to the operation of thoracentesis, and even in every operation where there might be danger of syncope, with a view to prevent its occurrence. It is for the same reason that Dr. Huchard has employed this drug. In cases of narrowing or insufficiency of the aortic orifice, where patients present the symptoms of asystole, with suffocation, dyspnœa, cold sweats, paleness of the face, algor of the extremities, etc., he has seen all these symptoms diminish after the hypodermic injection of one centigramme ($\frac{1}{6}$ gr.) of morphia. M. Huchard says that if opium is useful in aortic affections accompanied by vertigo, tinnitus aurium, tendency to deafness, cephalalgia, and occasional dilatation of the pupil, it is because it overcomes the cerebral ischæmia. For this reason, opium may be used as a tonic in many anæmic conditions, as phthisis.—*London Med. Record*, Aug. 15, 1878.

Four Cases of Spinal Paralysis of Adults.

Dr. SALOMON, of Hamburg (*Berliner Klin. Wochenschrift*, 1877, No. 39), does not believe that spinal paralysis is as rare among adults as has been supposed. He has himself, within two years, met with four cases of the affection, and believes that many of the cases recorded in the literature of spinal diseases as "chronic myelitis," or under some even less precise terms, really belong to this category. Three of the four cases observed by himself developed acutely. They were characterized by more or less complete paralysis of motion, with moderate atrophy, but without pain or other disturbances of sensation. There was, moreover, no impairment of the functions of the bladder or rectum ; no fever ; no disturbance of the general health ; no change in the reflex irritability. The state of the electro-contractility of the muscles was, however, very striking; the reaction of the muscles to direct irritation, or to irritation of the nerves supplying them, by the faradic current, was in general considerably diminished, while the reaction to the galvanic current was normal or even increased. In one of the cases, that of a young soldier, the affection came on after a night of sentinel-duty in the depth of winter, when the ground was deeply covered with snow; in another, that of a young lady, it appeared after a night of dancing at a ball. Two of the patients had suffered from sciatica of the affected leg one and a half years before the paralytic affection set in. In the case of the soldier, both legs were affected ; in the two other cases the arm and leg of one side. All three cases recovered completely after the lapse of a few months. The treatment consisted of galvanism, supplemented in one of the cases by sea-air and sea-baths, and in another by iodide of potassium and a course of baths at Reime.

The fourth case differed in some important particulars from the other three. It was not acute, but, on the contrary, developed so slowly, that the diagnosis was for a time doubtful. It commenced with a weakness in the left ankle, which slowly but progressively increased, and after the lapse of three months a slight dragging of the leg in walking was noticeable. The atrophy affected the entire leg, but was most marked in the adductors of the thigh ; the loss of power affected these adductors and the peronei to a more marked degree than the other muscles. There seemed to be a certain amount of cutaneous hyperæsthesia on both sides. In all other respects the case resembled the foregoing. After eight weeks of treatment the atrophy had slightly diminished, and the faradic reaction of the muscles had improved considerably, the galvanic reaction remaining unaltered ; subjectively the patient noticed an improvement in the strength of the limb. About this time he was awakened over night by a peculiar, painful sensation in the left arm; and in the morning found that he could no longer move the arm as well as usual. This weakness progressively increased, and was soon attended by atrophy and the usual electrical symptoms. At the same time the leg symptoms ceased to improve, remained stationary for a time, and then became gradually worse. A peculiar and rare phenomenon, which has only been mentioned by Benedikt, was noticed soon afterwards in the muscles of the calf and the other side of the leg-muscles in which the diminution of the faradic reaction was very marked. These muscles contracted energetically when a strong induced current was passed through them, but, although the current was kept up at the same strength, a sudden and apparently complete relaxation soon set in; on breaking the current, however, a further relaxation took place, which proved that a slight remnant of contraction had still persisted. Benedikt only met with this phenomenon in connection with tumours of the brain and other cerebral affections, but the author has also met with it in connection with nervous diseases of unquestionably peripheral origin. In the case under consideration the condition gradually became worse; the atrophy and paralysis of the left side increased, and finally disturbances of speech set in, symptoms which indicate an advance of the morbid process upwards, and make the prognosis unfavourable.

Dr. Salomon believes that the similarity of the symptoms in the above and other recorded cases, with those of the spinal paralysis of children, makes it necessary to admit the existence of the same anatomical substratum for the two forms of spinal disease. It is an admitted fact that the lesions are to be sought in the anterior horns of the gray matter, but the autopsies of children have proven that they may vary greatly in nature, since sometimes the signs of atrophy, and sometimes those of inflammation predominate. He claims that similar differences may also exist in the case of adults. With respect to his own four cases, the entire absence of all inflammatory symptoms leads him to the conclusion that the primary process was one of atrophy.—*Med. Record*, Aug. 17, 1878.

Sarcomatous Tumour in the Spinal Canal.

Dr. HUNICKEN, of Brunswick (*Berliner Klin. Wochenschrift*, July), reports a case of this nature. A young lady, A. G., at the age of nine years, began to suffer from a small hard swelling over the left mastoid process, which after three years' slow growth was finally removed by a surgeon. It returned after one year, and grew much larger, covering the mastoid process and the infra-auricular fossa to the size of half a goose's egg, and remained stationary at these limits; it caused at times a good deal of pain, and bled from granulations which had formed at the most prominent part of the tumour; the hemorrhage had latterly become frequent, and conduced to aggravate the somewhat feeble condition of the patient, so that there was again question of some operative interference, which was negatived by the fear of a second recurrence, and by the seat of the growth, which had penetrated into the substance of the mastoid process. The patient bore her sufferings with great patience, and lent herself to the various modes of treatment suggested with great energy; but after having unsuccessfully tried a great deal of both scientific and unscientific aid, she finally contented herself with dressing the tumour twice a day with an indifferent plaster. In July, 1876, she went to Harzburg, to try the brine baths, and made daily excursions among the mountains without feeling any fatigue. In the beginning of August she climbed the Berg mountain, and on her way down she felt a severe pain in her back, which compelled her to rest for some time, and it gave her father, who accompanied her, much trouble and exertion to get her home. The pain disappeared after a day's rest, but returned after attempting to walk; the patient, in consequence, returned home. Dr. Hünicken saw her first on the 2d of September. Miss G. was then twenty-four years old, with a pale face, slenderly built, and badly nourished. She complained chiefly of feebleness in the lower extremities, great pain in the back,

whici passed down tie thighs, and obstinate constipation. Supported by some
one's arm, sie was still able to move about her room; but the pains in the back,
whici were compared to cramps, were so severe at nigit tiat tie patient sirieked
for iours, and sleep was regularly disturbed, unless narcotics or a morphia injection were used. By tie end of October tie feebleness in tie lower extremities
amounted to paraplegia, and tie sphincters, first of tie bladder, tien of tie
rectum, lost tieir power; at the same time tie sensibility of tie lower extremities suffered, but never reacied absolute anæstiesia; reflex excitability was notably diminisied. Tie induced current employed for a long time remained witiout
any effect; tie electro-contractility of tie muscles of tie lower extremities was
unimpaired, but tie electro-sensibility was lost. Repeated examinations of tie
tiorax, abdomen, and genital organs siowed complete integrity of tiese parts.
Altiougi at tie commencement of tie disease the iigi degree of sensitiveness
of tie patient, and tie indefinite ciaracter of tie affection, caused iysterical
paralysis to be tiougit of, tie subsequent rapid increase in tie symptoms, as well
as tie absence of any otier facts wiici could be brougit into causal relation witi
tie present condition, led tie autior to believe tiat tiere existed some lesion, involving tie totality of tie spinal cord, wiici more or less deprived tie nerves of
tie lower extremities of tieir functions. As myelitis migit be excluded by tie
absence of all feverisi symptoms, and tie exclusive limitation of tie paralysis to
tie lower extremities, tie pressure of a tumour in tie spinal canal was tiougit of,
and its seat seemed most probably about tie level of tie last dorsal vertebra; the
entire course of the case, at least in tie last tiree or four months, iad no resemblance wiatever to fracture of a vertebra, wiici causes deati in about a monti.
To the above symptoms, wiici were relieved by Dover's powder, or morphia
injections, at tie end of November was added a bedsore, wiici, beginning first
in tie left labium, and later at different parts of tie nates, gave rise to large
slougis, five to fifteen centimetres in diameter; and it was only by keeping tie
patient in a warm bati for iours daily, tiat ier existence could be made tolerable. Tie excessive suppuration wiici followed tiese numerous bedsores, as
well as tie loss of blood from tie same cause, led to great exiaustion, and at
lengti, on tie 17th of Marci, tie uniappy patient was relieved from ier
sufferings, seven montis after tie commencement of her symptoms.

Tie necropsy, wiici was restricted to opening tie spinal canal and extirpating tie tumour of tie neck, gave tie following results. On opening tie spinal
canal at tie upper end, no microscopic ciange was noted until tie tenti dorsal
vertebra was reacied; iere tie canal widened out to tie size of a ien's egg, and
contained a tumour of tiat size, wiici iad encroacied on tie substance of the
bodies of tie tenti and eleventi dorsal vertebræ, wiici only retained tieir
lateral portions; tie middle iad disappeared rigit up to the *fascia longitudinalis*,
and the finger could be passed tirougi tiis tiinned fascia rigit into tie abdominal
cavity. Tie cord was compressed flat between tie tumour and tie posterior wall
of tie canal; tie membranes were unaltered, and the cord itself, except for the
flattening, siowed no ciange to tie naked eye, except some sligit softness. In
tie deeper-lying parts of tie vertebral canal tiere was no pathological ciange,
and the cord iad resumed its normal appearance. Tie tumour was easily loosened
from its surrounding, sligitly adiered to tie dura mater by a delicate membrane,
and possessed in the centre a pap-like, in tie peripiery a more consistent, substance, wiici under the microscope proved to be a cell-sarcoma (*zellensarcom*).
Tie tumour in tie neck was of iarder consistence, was also a cell-sarcoma, and
penetrated the mastoid process as far as tie mastoid foramen. After fifteen years,
tie sarcoma of tie neck iad given rise to a secondary deposit in the tenti dorsal
vertebra, and seven montis after the appearance of tie symptoms caused deati.

As an etiological point, it remains to be said tiat tie motier of tiis patient iad suffered for many years from tuberculosis, and sie died of tiis disease a monti before her daugiter.—*London Med. Record*, Aug. 15, 1878.

The Histology of Syphilitic Tonsils.

The microscopic anatomy of tie sypiilitic tubercular patcies wiici are often seen upon tie tonsils was tie subject of a recent communication to tie Paris Academy of Medicine by M. CORNIL. Tie tubercles iad been removed from tie tonsils of patients, for tie purpose of examination, witiout difficulty, and tie wounds tius produced iad iealed as readily as in an individual free from sypiilis. He described, first, tie structure of tie "opaline mucous tubercle," a section of wiici, examined under a low magnifying power, siows tiickened epitielium, and iypertropiy of tie papillæ, wiile tie deeper connective tissue is tiickened by infiltration witi new cells. Tie superficial epitielial layer presents cells wiici possess a cavity around tieir nucleus. Often tiere are one or two globules of pus in tie cavity instead of a nucleus. Furtier, witiin tiis super-ficial layer of epitielium, nests filled witi globules of pus may be found—true abscesses excavated among tie epitielial cells, and containing from four or ten to a iundred globules of pus. Tiese little abscesses, rounded or lenticular in siape, are surrounded by cells flattened by compression, and are commonly situated on tie surface of tie tubercle, wiere tiey open from time to time. Tius, from tie surface, a liquid transudes, containing many epitielial cells, witi globules of pus among tiem, or collected in little abscesses between tiem, and tie current of liquid wiici passes from tie papillæ on tie surface of tie tubercle contains globules of pus. Tiis is tie cause of tie opacity of tie epitielial covering at tie summit of tie tubercle wiici gives it tie opaline aspect.

Tie second variety examined was tie ulcerated form. In tiis tie epitielial covering is disintegrated by tie large quantity of transuding liquid, and tie glo-bules of pus wiici come from tie papillæ. Tie epitielial layer may fall off entirely, and tien tie inflamed papillary layer constitutes tie base of tie ulcer. Sometimes tiere is a true false membrane, gray, adierent, and dipitieritic in ciaracter, over tiis ulceration. It does not contain, iowever, as in dipitieria, microscopic organisms, but tie branciing forms of tie epitielial cells, tie ioles or cavities whici tiey present, and wiici contain globules of pus, produce tie same appearance as in dipitieria. In all cases, wietier tie tubercles are opaline or ulcerated, tie closed follicles of the tonsils are inflamed, and tie entire organ is iypertropiied. Tie peri-follicular lympiatic sinuses and tie retiform tissue present a variable quantity of large cells, witi one or several nuclei, containing red-blood globules. Tiis lesion of tie tonsils is identical witi tiat wiici M. Cornil ias lately described as found in tie glands in tie first and second periods of sypiilis; so tiat ie believes it to be correct to say tiat tie sypiilitic tonsils of tie second period represent a papule upon a sypiilitic gland.—*Lancet*, August 24, 1878.

Stenosis after Tracheotomy.

In a contribution to tie *Deutsche Zeitschrift für Chirurgie*, Band ix, Hefte 5 and 6, Dr. VÖLKER of Brunswick discusses tie causation and patiology of steno-sis of tie larynx or traciea after operation. Dr. W. Koci was one of tie first to direct attention to tie serious results tiat occasionally follow tie removal of tie canula from tie air-tube of a ciild who ias undergone tracieotomy for tie treatment of croup or dipitieria. Immediately after tie removal of tie tube, or, in some muci less frequent cases, after closing and cicatrization of tie wound,

t1e patient suffers from dyspnœa, w1ic1 increases rapidly in intensity, and necessitates a speedy reinsertion of t1e instrument.   T1e attack of d1spnœa is repeated
w1enever t1e canula is removed, so t1at the patient is compelled to bear t1is
during t1e rest of life.   T1is condition of dyspnœa, after removal of t1e canula,
is attributed by Koc1 to obstruction of t1e air-tube t1roug1 outgrowt1s or granulation-tissue from t1e trac1eal mucous membrane.   According to t1e more recent
investigations of Pauli, t1is stenosis from overgrowt1 of granulations is t1e result
of prolonged retention of the canula.   The mass of swollen granulations springs
from t1e margin of t1e superior portion of the wound, and just at t1at part w1ere
no pressure is excited by a curved canula of t1e usual form.   T1is statement as
to t1e starting-point of t1e obstructing fold of granulation is confirmed by an
o1servation t1at was made by Dr. Völker in 1876.   In a *post-mortem* examination of a c1ild w1o, t1ree mont1s before deat1, 1ad been trac1eotomized for
croup, and been subsequently compelled to retain the canula, in consequence of
obstruction of t1e air-passage above the fistula, Dr. Völker found t1at the trac1ea
just above t1e fistula was closed by a mass of granulations, w1ic1 seemed to be
directly continuous wit1 t1e upper 1alf of t1e margin of t1e orifice in t1e air-
tube.   T1e posterior margin of t1e mass of granulations was in contact-wit1 t1e
posterior wall of t1e trac1ea, but t1e 1andle of a scalpel could be readil1 passed
between t1em.   T1is mass t1en formed a kind of valve, fixed anteriorly and
laterally to t1e wall of t1e trac1ea, just above t1e wound, and free be1ind, w1ere
it presented a s1arp and indented margin.   Suc1 a condition as t1is, on removal
of t1e canula and closing of t1e wound during life, would 1ave rendered inspiration very difficult and expiration impossible.   Dr. Völker 1olds t1at the use of
t1e ordinar1 curved canula favours t1e formation of t1is valve of granulation-
tissue, because suc1 instrument leaves quite free from any pressure the upper and
inner angle of t1e wound made in t1e operation of trac1eotomy.   At t1is part,
t1e granulations expand wit1out any resistance, and as t1ey grow and expand
inwards, t1ey are supported by t1e convexity of t1e canula.   In order to prevent t1is outgrowt1 of granulation-tissue, care s1ould be taken to remove t1e
canula, w1en t1is is of t1e usual form, as soon as possible after the operation, or
im attempt be made to procure an instrument w1ic1 will press equally on all
parts of the perip1ery of t1e wound.   T1e valve, w1en formed, s1ould be removed t1roug1 excision, tension, or cauterization.

   Dr. Völker points out t1at granulation-masses may arise from ot1er causes,
and spring from ot1er parts of t1e laryngeal or bronc1ial mucous membrane t1an
t1at bordering t1e upper part of a wound or fistula.   A growt1 of t1is kind is
occasionally developed w1en t1e extremity of t1e canula touc1es t1e posterior
wall of t1e air-tube.   Here, after prolonged contact of t1e 1ard instrument with
t1e mucous membrane, an ulcer is formed, from w1ic1 a mass of granulations
may grow, passing eit1er directly downwards or upwards between t1e convexity
of t1e canula and t1e posterior wall of t1e trac1ea.   S1ould suc1 a mass, growing in t1e latter direction, c1ance to meet with a similar mass springing from t1e
margin of t1e wound, on t1e anterior wall of t1e air-tube, a complete diaphragm
mig1t be formed.—*London Med. Record*, Aug. 15, 1878.

—

Contagious Pneumonia.

   Epidemics of pneumonia 1ave been described from time to time, c1iefly on t1e
Continent, and an account of recent outbreaks, 1aving almost an epidemic form,
w1ic1 occurred at Moringen in Hanover, has been given by Dr. KUHN.   In t1is
place 1e 1as more t1an once observed pneumonia to 1ave an epidemic c1aracter,
and on one occasion it broke out in t1e gaol, w1en overfilled.   All other. condi-

tions being favourable—position, soil, drainage, ventilation, drinking water, clothing, and food—the cause of the outbreak appeared to be the impurity of the air of the cells. The individual cases presented the aspect of a well-marked infectious disease, with much prostration, a considerable enlargement of the spleen, albuminuria, and, in two-thirds of the cases, diarrhœa. It is notable that the disease did not begin, as in ordinary acute pneumonia, with a sudden onset and rigor, but was ushered in by four or eight days of prodromal symptoms. The pyrexia came on usually without an initial rigor, and ran a severe course. The pneumonic consolidation was recognizable usually on the third or fourth day of the fever, was frequently seated in the upper lobes, and exhibited a marked tendency to migrate. .Often it was accompanied by inflammation of the serous membranes, pleurisy was almost constant, in one-fourth of the cases there was pericarditis, and of forty-five cases well-marked meningitis was present in five. Angina and stomatitis were not unfrequent accompaniments. The temperature sometimes attained a height of 107°, and began to remit on the fifth to the seventh day. *Post-mortem* examination showed fatty degeneration of the heart, acute swelling of the spleen to three times the normal size, and a parenchymatous nephritis. Frequently the intestinal follicles were swollen. The disease was distinctly infectious. The attendants of the institution were affected, and the disease was conveyed by visitors to other persons who did not come near the prison or its inmates. In one epidemic Kühn observed eighty-three, and in another seventy cases. In each epidemic abortive attacks of the disease were also observed. He urges that this form of pneumonia must be distinguished from the genuine croupous pneumonia, and that its character approximates it to typhoid disease; and he suggests that possibly it may be due to the same poison as typhoid, modified by some unknown conditions—a sport, as Dr. Roberts would put it, of the typhoid germ.—*Lancet*, Aug. 24, 1878.

—

Hepatico-Bronchial Fistula.

A case of this very rare affection is reported by Mr. W. E. GREEN in the *Lancet* of July 6, 1878, p. 5. So far as Mr. Green knows, only two similar cases are to be found in medical records, one being mentioned by Dr. Murchison in his work upon *Diseases of the Liver;* and another described by M. Laboulbène (see *Lancet*, vol. ii. 1875, p. 504). The latter was analogous to Mr. Green's case. In Dr. Murchison's case, however, the fistula extended only to the pleura, and was not discovered until after death.

The patient, an innkeeper, aged 63, a well-nourished, active woman, had suffered for many years from attacks of biliary colic. On May 16th, 1875, she was attacked with general malaise, followed by severe pain behind the right shoulder, slight cough, expectoration containing small clots of blood. Auscultation revealed nothing to account for this. Pulse 76; temperature normal.

May 20th. She coughed up some green, bitter fluid; she felt better.

21st. The patient was bringing up large mouthfuls of frothy bile, and this had been going on for hours. Pulse 108; temperature normal. The base of the right lung was dull on percussion, and large bubbling *rāles* were heard, as though passing upwards from the liver, on each inspiration. The bowels were open, with bile in the feces. The patient continued expectorating large quantities of bile (often more than 80 ounces in the 24 hours) until June 10th, when she vomited about a pint of most offensive pus, and felt better. Pus mingled with bile was expectorated in greater or less quantities until the 26th, during which period the general health had improved, appetite fair, motions natural.

On July 12th, she again, after very troublesome attacks of coughing, brought up a large quantity of pus; after this the patient improved, the cough and expectoration gradually ceased, and in the second week of August she left home for a change, returning, after three weeks' absence, quite well.—*London Med. Record*, Aug. 15, 1878.

—

Use of Digitalis in Disease of the Cardiac Valves.

Dr. F. A. HOFFMANN of Dorpat says (*St. Petersburger Med. Wochenscrift*, No. 2, 1878) that, while the diagnosis of a disease of the heart is generally easy, it is often difficult to recognize the stage of the disease and to judge of the functional power of the heart. The indications of congestion are not to be depended on; patients with cyanosis, enlargement of the liver, ascites, and anasarca, are often improved by a short course of treatment and feel quite well for some months; while others, following just the same symptoms, are treated the same way in vain, and soon die. Just as little are the arterial tension and the heart's impulse to be depended on; both may be sufficient even until death. Even the distinctness of the heart's sound—apart from the prognostically favourable strengthening of the second pulmonary sound and the cessation of the mitral murmur shortly before death—gives no aid.

Irregularity of the heart's action just becomes a certain sign when the regularity of the heart-stroke can no longer be restored by digitalis. In order to ascertain this, it is necessary to possess a preparation of digitalis of which the action has been thoroughly proved, and to administer a dose of it subcutaneously. In this way, we obtain within twelve hours that information which the internal administration of the drug, or of infusion of digitalis, does not furnish for several days, and often not at all.

This experiment need not be made in cases where the right heart is enlarged towards the left beyond the nipple-line; for in this stage there is a condition of passive dilatation, in which digitalis can no longer do good.—*London Med. Record*, Aug. 15, 1878.

—

Action of Morphia on the Heart.

MM. P. PICARD and REBATEL, at the Meeting of the Paris Société de Biologie, on May 4th, called attention to the action of the salts of morphia on the heart (*Gazette Médicale de Paris*). M. Picard has already pointed out some of the phenomena following the injection of chlorhydrate of morphia in the dog, especially the contraction of the pupil and dilation of the small vessels. He infers that the salts of morphia produce both phenomena by paralyzing the sympathetic nerve. He now publishes the sequel of his researches, having further to note the coincident fall of the mean blood-pressure and retardation of the action of the heart. These facts are easily verified by placing a manometer in connection with an artery, and noting the blood-pressure and rate of the heart's beats before and after the injection of morphia. It must be observed that the retardation of the heart's action occurs in spite of reduced blood-pressure; if the fall of pressure occurred alone, a peripheral action of the vessels would explain it, but then there would be at the same time accelerated action of the heart so that only a direct agency affecting the heart can explain this phenomenon. The cause, then, must be stimulation of the inhibitory or paralysis of the motor nerves (leaving aside as inadmissible the action of morphia on the cardiac fibres). The question thus put is easily solved by the following experiment. Cut the pneumogastric nerves in a dog, and after a few minutes count the beats of the heart; then inject morphia; and it will be found that diminution of the action of the heart is still produced, notwithstanding the section of the inhibitory nerves. This experiment throws over the first and prepares us to admit the second hypothesis, namely, that morphia paralyses the motor nerves of the heart, as it does the sympathetic nerves of the vessels and of the iris.—*London Med. Record*, Aug. 15, 1878.

——

Auscultatory Phenomena of the Arteries.

Dr. SENATOR (*Berliner Klinische Wochenschrift*, May 27) draws special attention to the pathological conditions under which the heart's sounds may be heard in the peripheral arteries. These are insufficiency of the aortic valves, with dilated and hypertrophied left ventricle; pure insufficiency of the mitral valve; perhaps pure patency of the ductus Botalli. Then cases in which the arterial system is relaxed, but the heart's muscle acts strongly (anæmia, chlorosis, fever, stenosis of the aortic or mitral valves, with hypertrophy of the left heart). After these come cases of great obstruction at the origin of the aorta, general increased tension of the middle-sized arteries, or congenital narrowing of the arteries, if the left ventricle at the same time is degenerated and little capable of performing its function. The pathogenetic condition he considers to be such a state of the arterial wall as shall enable it to be set in vibration. He recommends the solid stethoscope as making the sounds more audible in some cases.—*London Med. Record*, Aug. 15, 1878.

——

The Origin of Miliary Aneurisms.

The researches of Bouchard and others on the occurrence of miliary aneurisms in a large number of cases of cerebral hemorrhage have been amply confirmed. The cases in which the condition has not been discovered have been, for the most part, cases in which the hemorrhage was secondary to chronic renal disease. An interesting study of the pathogenesis of the condition, by Dr. EICHLER, of Kiel, appears in the last number of the *Deutsches Archiv für Klinische Medicin*, and is based on an examination of three or four hundred specimens. He has studied especially the early stages of the process. The first alteration is a multiplication and fatty degeneration of the endothelium of the vessel, and a notable thickening of the homogeneous layer of the intima which limits the endothelium of the outer side. All portions of the vascular wall take part in the commencing dilatation. The external coat is quite unchanged, and is separated from the muscular coat by a lymph-space which Eichler, following Axel Key and Retzius, believes to exist in that situation. All authors, with the exception of Roth, have described the muscular coat as early disappearing and becoming atrophied, and consider that the atrophy of this coat really conditions the aneurism. Eichler, however, not only found it well preserved in young aneurisms, but even in older ones its traces could be distinctly observed. The muscular tissue is, however, slightly changed, even in the earliest stages. The individual fibres do not, it is well known, form complete rings around the vessel, but extend through only part of the circumference and interdigitate to some extent. This arrangement is disturbed in the commencing aneurism. No fatty degeneration could be discovered in the fibres. The thickening of the intima is so considerable that it forms a prominence within the vessel, sometimes homogeneous, sometimes laminated. On the inner surface it is covered with the thickened endothelium, and often by a layer of white blood-corpuscles, frequently degenerated. Sometimes the endothelium appears to degenerate and peel off into the lumen of the vessel. The outer and middle coats of the vessel are always normal in the young aneurisms, and hence it appears that these are due to the change in the inner coat. This is confirmed by the fact that where this change is partial, and affects only one part of the wall, that part only becomes bulged into the aneurism; whereas, when the change surrounds the vessel, the dilatation has a corresponding extent, and a fusiform aneurism results, and if the change is more marked on one side of the vessel than the other, the bulging is greater on that side.

The second stage of the aneurism is characterized by an enormous overgrowth of the intima, a gradual atrophy of the muscular coat, and a process of growth between this and the outer coat. The thickened intima presents lamination, and between the lamellæ are indications of groups of degenerated cells. Finally, a yellow homogeneous plate is produced, on which the endothelial covering can no longer be seen. The thickening of the intima is often inconspicuous, in consequence of the great dilatation and stretching of the wall which coincides with it, but sometimes it may be so great as to actually narrow the lumen of the vessel at part of the diseased spot, the other part being bulged. The atrophy of the muscular coat appears to depend upon the bulging of the vessel, but it is rarely so complete that traces of the muscular fibres cannot be seen towards the extremities of the aneurism. The external presents the least change. Only where a vessel enters the aneurism is there obvious thickening of the outer layer, which Eichler believes to be due to the accumulation of lymph-cells in the lymphatic space which he and Axel Key consider to exist between the external and middle coats of the vessel. The thickened intima may undergo calcification, or, more frequently, fatty degeneration.

This description is, it will be seen, in effect, that of chronic endarteritis, and it follows from these observations that the aneurisms result from the common senile change. They are true aneurisms, involving the whole of the walls of the vessel, and have to be carefully distinguished from the so-called dissecting aneurisms of the same vessels, which are consequences, not causes, of cerebral hemorrhage.— *Lancet*, Aug. 17, 1878.

—

A Remarkable Case of Sphacelation of the Stomach.

Dr. DUJARDIN-BEAUMETZ lately presented the notes of this case to the Medical Society of Paris (*L' Union Médicale*, February 23). The patient, aged forty-seven, entered his wards on October 19. Five days before, whilst in excellent health, and without appreciable cause, he had had an hæmatemesis, accompanied by acute pains in the stomach. Examination revealed no epigastric tumour. He bore milk-diet very well, and without vomiting. The patient spoke of a stomatitis from which he was then suffering, but said that every year about that time he was troubled with aphthous sore mouth. Dr. Dujardin-Beaumetz did not believe that this affection was similar to his previous attacks, and did not know to 'what the ulcerations of the lips, the under surface of the tongue, the uvula, and even the borders of the epiglottis were to be ascribed.

On October 28th, the patient, who up to that time was progressing well, hardly complaining of any pain, never having vomited, and demanding solid nourishment, died suddenly, after having experienced an acute pain in the stomach, and ejected a few spoonfuls of blood.

At the necropsy, Dr. Dujardin-Beaumetz found almost the entire stomach, the pyloric region excepted, sphacelated through all its thickness, and transformed into a soft eschar, which occupied not only the stomach, but also the diaphragm and omentum. On removing this mass, the lungs, liver, spleen, and intestines were exposed to view. In presence of such destruction, the idea of simple ulcer had to be put aside, and the entrance into the stomach of a caustic liquid had to be admitted. This *post-mortem* diagnosis explained perfectly the peculiar sore mouth. After closely questioning his wife, it was discovered that he had been very despondent from want of work, and that he feared poverty for his wife and

children. On the 14th he had gone to the water-closet, and on coming out he
fell almost inanimate to the ground, crying in haste for water to quench the burning in his stomach. Thus this patient concealed from every one his attempt at
suicide, and was able during fourteen days to preserve the appearance of health
and the integrity of his digestive functions, while the greater portion of the walls
of the stomach was destroyed, and succumbed only on the separation of the
slough.—*London Med. Record*, Aug. 15, 1878.

Case of Intussusception in an Infant; Recovery.

In a communication to the *Berliner Klinische Wochenschrift* for July 1st, M.
LUDEWIG, of Heidelberg, observes that cases of intestinal obstruction may be
divided, with reference to the treatment, into two classes: 1. Those requiring
direct operative interference; 2. Those in which an expectant treatment of the
symptoms only is indicated.

The first group comprises those cases where the obstruction is situated at or
below the ileo-cæcal valve, while those occurring above this situation cannot as
yet be treated by mechanical means. These mechanical means consist of the
introduction of the sound, fingers, or hand, and of the injection of either air or
water; and they are only applicable so long as there is only moderate swelling
of the invaginated portion of intestine, and before any serous adhesions have
formed. Should either or both of these conditions exist, then either an operation (laparotomy) is indicated, or a merely expectant course is to be pursued.
Laparotomy, or the opening of the abdomen, cannot well be performed in infants
whose powers of resistance are but very slender; hence an energetic employment
of the mechanical means becomes imperative, and it is only when these all fail,
that as a last resource laparotomy may be resorted to. Fortunately, iliac invagination is of extremely rare occurrence in infants.

The patient in the present case was a healthy well-nourished female infant,
eight months old. On the 12th December last she was suddenly, and without
any apparent cause, seized with violent vomiting of greenish-yellow matter, while
a scanty stool passed some little time afterwards was streaked with blood. Vomiting of all ingesta continued till the 15th, when a digital examination *per rectum*
detected the existence in the upper part of the rectum of a soft rounded swelling, obstructing the entire gut, and having a small slit-like fissure at its posterior
part, which was neither more nor less than the invaginated portion of the gut.
Reposition was effected by means of the finger without difficulty, with the immediate result that the child was able to take and retain a considerable quantity of
milk. On the same evening, vomiting again set in; and the rectal tumour was
found to have returned, and was again reduced. This was repeated four times
in the course of the next three days. On the 18th the invaginated gut presented a
dark-coloured protuberance as large as a walnut, external to the anus, by the side
of which a bougie could be passed about three inches up the bowel. The reduction could now no longer be effected with the finger, and it became necessary to
inject about half a pint of water through the transverse fissure by means of an
elastic tube. The tumour was then again returned; vomiting ceased, and a yellowish motion was passed. But notwithstanding the repeated injection of water
and the administration of small doses of opium, the bowel continually descended.
A tube was therefore introduced and fixed by means of bandages and left in the
bowel for six days, but even then on removing the tube the tumour again came
down, and the tube had to be replaced for fourteen days more. After that, the
cure seemed to be complete. During the whole progress of the case the temperature remained normal, never exceeding 38° Cent. (100.4° F.), and the child's

appetite continued good. The seat of the invagination appears to have been the descending colon, and it came down and was replaced twenty-two times in the course of a single month. The case establishes the value of water injections, and also of leaving the injection-tube in the bowel for a considerable time after passing it beyond the seat of the obstruction.—*London Medical Record*, Aug. 15, 1878.

—

A Case of Hydatid Tumour of the Liver bursting into the Air-passages; Recovery.

In the *Berliner Klinische Wochenschrift* for June 24, Dr. KATZ, of Berlin, relates the following case.

The patient, a school-teacher, had suffered for the last five or six years from disordered digestion, with occasional attacks of jaundice. When he came under observation, a fluctuating tumour as large as a child's head was found in the epigastric region. Further examination, and the history of the case, pointed to its hydatid nature, and it was opened, when about five litres of an intensely fetid yellowish fluid were evacuated, containing hundreds of echinococci, varying in size from a cherry to a fowl's egg. Immediately after this, and during the following six weeks, the patient's health improved; but then jaundice and fever returned, and, eight weeks after the operation, there was found a swelling on the right side of the thorax at its lower portion. At the same time, there was great emaciation, with frequent rigors, and the general symptoms of pyæmia; but the patient refused to undergo another operation. Suddenly one day, and after a violent fit of coughing, about two litres of a greenish offensive pus were expectorated, and, during the following days, about the same quantity was coughed up from time to time. The microscope showed this fluid to contain the characteristic echinococcus-hooklets in large numbers. The patient's condition again immediately improved, and in three weeks recovery was complete. The second tumour, which was situated in the posterior part of the right hepatic lobe, probably became adherent to the diaphragmatic pleura, and pushed up against and displaced the right lung, where, owing to the concussion of coughing, it burst into the bronchi.—*London Med. Record*, Aug. 15, 1878.

—

Hydatid Cyst of the Liver in a Child.

L'Union Médicale for July 20th contains an account of a child three and a half years of age, who was admitted into the Sick Children's Hospital, under M. ARCHAMBAULT, February 5th. It had for a year suffered from a large belly; this enlargement had been gradual, and was not accompanied by diarrhœa, vomiting, or jaundice. There was no dog in the house where the patient lived. On examining the abdomen, a projection was at once noticed on its right side; palpation revealed the existence of a tumour springing from the liver, and the edge of this organ could be plainly felt to be sharp, raised, and prominent in front. It was easy to recognize that the increase in the volume of the liver was not due to hypertrophy of the organ, but to the presence of a true tumour, round, smooth, and painless, equal in volume to the head of a fœtus, appearing to originate in the right lobe of the liver; there was no discoloration of the skin covering the growth. The tumour was hard, but neither fluctuation nor fremitus could be made out, but at its most projecting part a semi-elastic feel suggested the idea of a liquid collection. The child was healthy and plump, without any trace of scrofula or of osseous suppuration; there was no digestive disturbance, no œdema of the limbs, no ascites.

On February 8th, chloroform having been administered, M. Archambault punctured the swelling with an aspirating needle, and withdrew 450 grammes (nearly a pint) of a fluid as clear as rock-water. An examination showed this to be non-albuminous, and the microscope did not reveal any hooks. The child progressed favourably until the 11th, when the temperature rose, and slight pain was complained of near the umbilicus, but the belly was not very sensitive to the touch; the liver still remained large, but no tumour could be felt. The symptoms improved until the 20th of the month, when diphtheria made its appearance, accompanied by albuminuria, and suppuration in the right submaxillary region. On March 10th the mother removed the child from the hospital; at that time it was pale, and very feeble, but the albumen had disappeared. The hepatic tumour had not been reproduced. Five days afterwards death took place, this being preceded by an attack of diphtheritic paralysis. M. Peter, who reports the case, states that the age of the patient is an object of especial interest, as many writers upon diseases of children do not mention this malady. West, D'Espine, and Pleot are exceptions; the last two having published some cases of hepatic cysts in children four years of age. Below this age the affection is not mentioned, except the case quoted by Cruveilhier as occurring in an infant twelve days old, where the hydatid cyst opened into the intestine. It is generally about eight that the disease occurs most frequently. The youngest patient observed by Frerichs was seven. Besides the age, there are three other noteworthy circumstances: 1. The absence of hydatid fremitus; 2. The absence of hooks, so that the parasitic nature of the affection was only made possible by the volume of the cyst; 3. The cure by a single puncture. These circumstances can be explained by the absence of secondary vesicles, or at least their presence in a very small degree, for it is known from the experience of Dr. Sadde that the fremitus denotes the presence of a certain number of daughter cysts. If the fremitus be absent, one ought to find few or no hooks.—*London Med. Record*, Aug. 15, 1878.

—

Amyloid Degeneration of the Kidneys. ·

Dr. M. LITTEN makes the following remarks on this subject. Of all the affections comprehended under the name of Bright's disease, none is so variable as amyloid degeneration, both as regards the quantity and clinical composition of the urine, or the presence and extent of dropsy; but albuminuria has been generally regarded as a constant symptom. There is much difference of opinion as to the mode of production of this albuminuria, some holding that it is due to the increased pressure in the collateral glomeruli from the amyloid degeneration of some, others that the amyloid degeneration itself permits the serum albumen to permeate the vascular walls; others again attribute it to the coincident degeneration, the so-called chronic parenchymatous inflammation, of the renal epithelium. But, in spite of these variations, all are agreed in regarding albuminuria as a constant symptom of amyloid degeneration of the kidneys, a dogma which the following case shows us to be untenable.

. On May 13th, 1876, K., aged 17, a merchant's apprentice, entered the hospital with signs of extensive phthisis, and at the same time the liver and spleen were found to be enlarged. There was slight diarrhœa; no dropsy; the urine contained no albumen. The further progress of the case was that of destructive pulmonary phthisis, with formation of great cavities, hectic, and diarrhœa. The urine meanwhile presented no abnormality; its quantity daily was about 1000 c. c. (about 34 oz.) of sp. gr. 1011–15, clear, transparent, and bright yellow-coloured. The pulse was very weak; there was no dropsy. On June 12 signs of dry pleurisy appeared on the left side, with great pain, requiring narcotics; soon afterwards there appeared signs of dry pericarditis; also, on the 20th, an extension of the cardiac dulness, with enfeeblement of the pericardial friction, were observed, and at the same time slight œdema of the ankles and instep showed itself. The patient complained of abdominal pain increased by pressure. The diarrhœa persisted, in spite of the employment of astringent remedies. The urine, which had hitherto been clear and bright, became now brownish-red, turbid; its specific gravity rose to 1020 and over; the quantity in twenty-four hours sank from 950 cubic centimetres to 500 and 600. The whole aspect of the case and its history left no room to doubt the existence of amyloid degeneration of the abdominal organs and the mucous membrane of the intestine, so special attention was paid to the urine; but, though daily examined with the utmost care, albumen was never discovered; even on boiling it with concentrated solution of sulphate of soda and acetic acid, there was no trace of turbidity. Equally unsuccessful were the attempts to find tube-casts. The pulse remained small and feeble. While the pleuritic signs remained on the left side, and towards the end of July were audible on the right side also, the pericardial effusion became greater, until at last the heart's sounds were scarcely to be heard. The quantity of urine remained small, frequently scarcely 500 cubic centimetres of brick-red, thickly sedimented urine, free from albumen. The diarrhœa and abdominal pain persisted. The anasarca increased, there was collapse. On August 4th there appeared a miliary petechial eruption on the chest and belly, which increased on the succeeding days. The urine was only 350 cubic centimetres. The abdominal pain prevented sleep at night, and was only partially relieved by morphia injected hypodermically: the diarrhœa hastened the collapse to the end. On August 8th the urine was 380 cubic centimetres, specific gravity 1026, highly coloured, no albumen; pulse scarcely perceptible. Increasing dropsy killed the patient on August 9th.

The diagnosis was inflammation of the serous membranes, with pulmonary and intestinal phthisis, and at the same time amyloid degeneration of the liver, spleen, and intestinal mucous membrane. The participation by the kidneys in the degeneration was excluded by the results of the chemical examination of the urine.

The necropsy (made 9th August, 1876, by Dr. Jürgens) verified the diagnosis and extended it, as general miliary tuberculosis and amyloid degeneration of the kidneys were present. "The left kidney, of normal size, showed on its surface as well as on section a few miliary and some larger yellowish-white tubercle nodules in the cortical substance. The latter is of normal breadth, strikingly pale, grayish-white coloured. With iodine, numerous deep brown points and streaks appear." The right kidney was taken out entire for injecting and left intact. Microscopical examination showed that a large number of the glomeruli were degenerated, and that in many cases the entire vascular tuft was affected and transformed into a homogeneous glass-like mass. Partially degenerated glomeruli were rarely visible, the antithesis between normal and diseased being almost complete, the latter being much the more numerous. The interlobular arteries, *vasa afferentia et recta*, and the interstitial capillaries, showed the disease very plainly. The renal epithelium was quite normal, except a moderate degree of fatty degeneration of the epithelium of the convoluted tubules.

The second case was also one of phthisis—F. S., aged 23, admitted April 1, 1878. There were a large hard spleen, and profuse watery diarrhœa, but nothing abnormal in the urine, although, as amyloid degeneration seemed so probable, it was examined with care. During the thirteen days he was under observation, his urine averaged 1000 to 1100 cubic centimetres daily, of specific gravity 1010; it was bright yellow, clear, without deposit, no albumen or tube-casts. The lower extremities were on admission moderately swollen, and remained so till death. His pulse was throughout unusually small and easily compressible, somewhat irregular. The heart's sounds were clear. There were cavities in both apices; the pleural sacs were normal. The abdomen was tender on pressure; he had loose stools four or five times in twenty-four hours. Death occurred April 13th. The diagnosis was lung and intestinal phthisis, with amyloid degeneration of the spleen and intestinal mucous membrane, while, from the recollection of the preceding case, the possibility of amyloid disease of the kidneys was entertained.

At the necropsy were found ulcerating phthisis of the lungs and intestines, sago spleen, fatty liver, with amyloid degeneration of the vessels, amyloid intestines and kidneys, fatty and very flabby heart, especially the left ventricle. The report says, "The left kidney appeared slightly enlarged; the surface was smooth, anæmic, the stellate veins slightly congested; on section the substance was very pale, without any special change to be recognized. The right kidney was reserved for injection, and not cut. Iodine gave no very definite result to the naked eye; the characteristic coloration appeared in the vasa recta of the medullary portion, but in the cortex only here and there brownish-red glomeruli could be seen. Microscopical examination confirmed these results so far that the vasa recta were very degenerated, and in the cortex there was a moderate affection of the glomeruli, only single capillary loops being diseased, and most of the tufts being quite normal. The interlobular arteries, as well as the vasa afferentia, and the interstitial capillaries were degenerated in places, but less than the vessels of the medullary part. There was no further change noticeable, except fatty degeneration of the epithelium of the straight tubules of the medullary portion, which in some places was so intense that the separate cells could not be distinguished. The heart's muscle was also to a great extent fattily degenerated."

The third case came under observation about the same time, and was that of a woman, K., aged 42, who complained of indigestion. Examination showed enlargement of the liver and spleen. Both organs were painful on pressure, and felt firm and hard. The surface of the liver felt uneven, without being granular; through the relaxed abdominal walls distinct lobulation could be made out. There was a little ascites; nothing abnormal in the thorax; stools normal; complete absence of anasarca. The quantity of urine up to shortly before death averaged 900 to 1000 cubic centimetres, of 1011–13 specific gravity; it was generally clear, yellow, without deposit. Daily examination for albumen and tube-casts gave a negative result. She died after being in hospital fourteen days. The necropsy showed a well-marked syphilitic liver; the organ was on the whole enlarged, but contracted in places and furrowed by deep cicatrices; the parenchyma was studded with gummata. Microscopical examination showed that the arteries and branches of the portal vein had undergone amyloid degeneration. There were also sago-spleen and smooth atrophy of the tongue. Old tumours or cicatrices were nowhere present. The left kidney was of normal size, strikingly anæmic, and harder than natural. The iodine test showed to the naked eye degeneration of the vessels of the papillary layer, while the cortical vessels and glomeruli took on no noticeable change. The right kidney was reserved for injection. The heart was soft and flabby. The kidneys were examined microscopically immediately after the necropsy. The vasa recta were the most affected; the glomeruli were in part healthy, here and there degenerated, but only to be recognized by specks of coloration by iodine or methylaniline. The vasa afferentia took on the characteristic staining in parts, but the interstitial capillaries appeared quite healthy. Of other changes, only a slight degree of fatty degeneration of the epithelium of the straight tubules was noted.

In a fourth case, not seen by the author but communicated to him by Dr. Weigert, there was also amyloid degeneration of the kidneys, but no albuminuria before death; it was also a case of phthisis. The kidneys were anæmic, otherwise unaltered, and the amyloid degeneration of the vessels would have passed unobserved but for the affection of other organs. The microscope showed moderate degeneration of the glomeruli and the cortical vessels ; no other change was noted.

The first case related drew the author's attention to this subject ; it was remarkable that, for three months during which it was under observation, only once was a slight turbidity noticed with nitric acid. It might be suggested that the affection of the coats of the vessels was too slight to permit the passage of albumen, or that the vessels concerned in that process were intact, but these explanations were disproved by the results of examination. It was very noticeable that some of the glomeruli were quite healthy, while the rest were in a very advanced stage of degeneration, and no intermediate partially affected tufts existed. By injection it was found that the fluid ran easily into the healthy tufts, but in no instance succeeded in reaching those diseased. This led the author to imagine that in this the explanation of the absence of albuminuria might be found. In order to test the truth of this hypothesis he examined all the amyloid kidneys he met with, and the cases above related are those in which no albuminuria occurred ; but it will have been noticed that the same distinct separation of perfectly healthy from very degenerated glomeruli does not hold good in them, and in those partially affected, injections could be driven into the tufts, while it could not be assigned to want of pressure from feebleness of the heart, as this organ was healthy in Dr. Weigert's case. He was led, therefore, to look for its cause to the other concomitant changes, frequently met with in amyloid kidneys, the inflammatory affection of the parenchyma, absent in these cases, which were instances of simple uncomplicated amyloid degeneration, such as Grainger Stewart has described as the first stage of the general affection. He admits, however, that simple amyloid degeneration of the vessels may and does give rise to albuminuria, but need not do so if it is restricted to the capillaries, or only slightly implicates the glomeruli as well. The condition of the heart in these cases is a complication of the factors, which must not be lost sight of. Under such circumstances, the positive recognition of the state of the kidneys must be admitted to be impossible, and it raises for the general diagnosis of amyloid kidney new difficulties which scarcely appear surmountable. If in cases like the above, on the ground of dyscrasia with coincident enlargement of the liver and spleen, and the presence of profuse diarrhœa, a complication of amyloid kidney be thought of, yet, even when this happens to be actually found on *post-mortem* examination, it remains rather of the nature of a surmise than a diagnosis. If the amyloid degeneration is secondary to a so-called interstitial or parenchymatous nephritis (the large white kidney of the English) the complication may easily be overlooked during life ; on the other hand, when the diagnosis seems certain, in cases of constitutional disease with amyloid degeneration of the organs, at the autopsy the kidney is found to be large and white, revealing, however, no trace of amyloid degeneration after the most careful microscopical examination.

In pursuing these investigations, the author used the old method (iodine with and without the addition of sulphuric acid) and the aniline test; he considered no case proved in which the reaction could not be obtained with both. In only one case has he found any difference in these methods; that was a kidney which contained many tube-casts, and on section these took on bright red staining with methylaniline, and yellow with iodine. During life, the cylinders in the urine presented no characteristic reaction. He does not agree with Fürbringer in thinking that this proves methylaniline a better test for amyloid degeneration than iodine, or that the tube-casts in this case were really amyloid. He has used both, and thinks, as a rule, one is as good as the other; but the methylaniline is more easily applied, and the contrast is more striking. He refers to the disputes as to the vessels primarily attacked, and is of opinion that, although those of the glomeruli generally suffer first, this is not a rule without many exceptions. It has also been laid down that the muscular coat is first affected. To this he also takes exception as an universal rule; he has found in some cases the intima, in others the adventitia, diseased, while the muscular coat was still normal. There is no reason to believe that the degeneration extends by direct continuity, isolated sections of vessels being frequently diseased. He believes that the degeneration in the kidney always begins in the vessels and not in the interstitial tissue. The capsules of the glomeruli are often affected. He has often seen three cases of venous thrombosis, as recorded by Bartels. There were no clinical manifestations of this condition, although the trunk of the renal vein was obstructed, and the thrombus extended far into the renal substance. The kidneys were white, and showed no trace of venous engorgement. From this and from the possibility of completely injecting the organ without extravasation it was plain that sufficient collateral veins existed or had been developed since the thrombosis to carry on the circulation; but a complete explanation of these thromboses, which are generally unilateral and very seldom on both sides, cannot at present be given. The slowing of the blood-stream by increased resistance is not a sufficient explanation, considering the frequent onesidedness of the affection.—*London Med. Record*, Aug. 15, 1878.

—

Parenchymatous Inflammation, and the Mode of Formation of Fibrinous Tube-Casts.

Dr. E. AUFRECHT, of Magdeburg (*Centralblatt für die Medicin. Wissenschaften*, May 11), has made a series of experiments by tying the ureters of rabbits on one side, in order to verify his opinions as to the connection between parenchymatous and interstitial inflammations and the existence of a primary independent parenchymatous inflammation. He found that at first simple parenchymatous inflammation occurred, and a day later interstitial inflammation supervened. If the animals were killed within the first three days the affected kidney was found noticeably swollen, and its pelvis and ureter above the ligature were much distended. On microscopical examination the interstitial tissue of the organ was quite normal throughout, as was also the medullary parenchyma, but the tubules of the cortical substance, especially the convoluted ones, showed dilatation of their lumina with granular and fatty degeneration of their epithelium. In a majority of these tubules there were the finest fibrine-cylinders; these were seen best when the organs were examined fresh, or after being in bichromate of potash for only a few days. The cylinders then project from the tubules. When they are inside of these, they are only very rarely seen on account of their being covered by the clouded epithelium. After longer hardening, only a much smaller number can be found; apparently because it is only in fresh specimens that they are squeezed out of the tubules by the shrinking or contraction of the tissues. It is, therefore, necessary to teaze out the preparation in order to demonstrate them after hardening. The following facts concerning their origin are noteworthy: The epithelium in these kidneys was complete throughout. The cells were much clouded, could not be distinguished separately, and their nuclei required fuchsin to make them visible; a defect was nowhere visible. Within this completely unchanged epithelial layer lay the clear pale cylinders. It is plain that the epithelium as such, that is, their substance *in toto*, could not have been employed in forming the cylinders.

Again, there is the possibility that they owe their origin to an exudation from the bloodvessels. The interstitial tissue and the bloodvessels did not show the slightest change within the first three days. Besides, the increased intratubular pressure due to the ligature on the ureter makes the entrance of fluid into the tubules out of the bloodvessels scarcely conceivable; and thirdly, in those kidneys in which interstitial inflammation had commenced, the fibrine-cylinders had disappeared. If the animals were killed after six days, the interstitial tissue was found distended by numerous cells, the epithelium of the tubules was less cloudy, well defined from each other, and with very visible nuclei, no sign of epithelial destruction, and no cylinders in the tubules. The author has verified this observation in kidneys, the ureters of which have been tied six, twelve, and up to twenty-three days. In addition, he gives the following positive facts: He saw once a cylinder made up of single irregular pieces, which were separated by fine bright lines. Twice he saw epithelial cells, with bright round structures protruding, which in appearance completely agreed with the pale cylinders. He therefore concludes that the fibrine are cylinders formed in consequence of the irritated state of the epithelium from the urinary stasis, that they are a secretion of inflamed epithelium which exudes in the form of large clear drops, and subsequently runs together into cylinders taking the form of the tubules.

The presence of urinary cylinders contemporaneously with the disease of the epithelium, and the absence of any trace of interstitial change, are also important proof of, the correctness of the view that there is undoubtedly a primary parenchymatous inflammation.

Virchow has fallen into the error of maintaining that parenchymatous inflammation leads to the destruction of the affected elements; he assigns to it a degenerative character. In reality, from this opinion proceeds the view of a great number of our modern pathologists, that parenchymatous inflammation is not inflammation, but a secondary process, and much more to be regarded as a simple nutritive derangement. In opposition to Virchow, Aufrecht assigns to parenchymatous inflammation an eminently separative character, and the proof of this must upset the opinion that it is only a secondary process. When a muscular fibre in typhus or other nervous affections loses its transverse striæ, and in place of these dark granules and oily particles in great number appear, one may doubt, whether we have to do with an inflammation or a destruction, an active or a passive process. But when, as he has shown recently in his paper on muscle and nerve regeneration in the *Deutsche Arch. für Klin. Med.*, in the further progress of this affection of muscle the granules and oil-drops disappear, and the clear basis-substance in which they were imbedded shows itself as a nucleated protoplasmic mass, the so-called nucleated muscle-plate—in which around every single nucleus new transverse striation appears until the entire muscle-plate is striated, then this is a regenerative inflammatory process of parenchyma. If in a nerve the medullary sheath and axis-cylinder be destroyed, and the inside of Schwann's sheath become filled with myelin and fat, the appearance of which expresses the complete destruction of the nerve, if these then disappear so that the nuclei of the nerve-fibre revert to an ordinary protoplasmic mass, and out of this new axis-cylinders be formed, this is a parenchymatous inflammation leading to regeneration. He infers a similar relation for parenchymatous hepatitis, based on a large number of experiments with phosphorus, as well as for parenchymatous nephritis, from the above observations on ligature of the ureter. Collating these facts with his clinical observations, he has come to the conclusion that diffuse interstitial nephritis and hepatitis follow parenchymatous inflammation of the same organs. If the liver or renal epithelium become diseased in consequence of a similar irritation, and this is not of such a degree that the entire organ is destroyed, or when a moderately intense irritant acts for a longer time, a change takes place which in no way leads to destruction, except in so far as this is the consequence of the entrance of numerous cells into the surrounding

parts, and the new formation of connective tissue.—*London Medical Record*,
August 15, 1878.

—

Boracic Acid in Skin Disease.

NEUMANN (*Centralblatt für Chir.*, No. 8, 1878) has employed boracic acid,
sometimes alone, sometimes in connection with oil of cloves, in the fluid form
and in ointments. In pityriasis versicolor and tinea tonsurans, alcoholic solutions, 10 to 300 with 2.50 of oil of cloves, and 20 to 300 with 3.0 of oil cloves,
have been used. In pityriasis rubra and all varieties of eczema, the acid has
been employed in the form of ointments of 10 to 50. Neumann considers the
remedy a valuable one.—*London Medical Record*, August 15, 1878.

—

Surgery.

Cause of Death after Burns.

In a communication read before the meeting of the Association of German
Naturalists and Physicians (*Berliner Klin. Wochenschrift*, No. 46, 1877), Dr.
PONFICK gave the results of a series of experiments made by himself and F.
Schmidt with reference to the results of severe burns. The blood was found to
be altered in all cases of severity, the red corpuscles separating into numerous
small bits. These disappeared after a varying number of hours, with the seeming
effect of exciting grave disturbance in several organs. A large portion of the
apparently free hæmoglobin was eliminated through the kidneys, the parenchyma
of which in the severe cases was evidently much inflamed, peculiarly coloured
casts being found in the urine, while the tubules were obstructed and the epithelium in a state of fatty degeneration. Another portion of the decomposed
red corpuscles was taken up by the contractile cells of the spleen and bone-marrow, in which a gradual destruction was probably accomplished. The enlargement of these parts, their increased redness and moisture, appeared to indicate
that the change mentioned was present.

Dr. Ponfick believes it probable that some of the rapidly fatal cases and some
of the severe symptoms in cases of recovery result from the extensive and sudden
destruction of red blood-corpuscles. The rapid suppression of urine, and a resulting uræmic poisoning, may also be of importance. From the evidence presented
by these experiments, Ponfick recommends transfusion as a rational therapeutical
measure in cases of severe burns.—*London Med. Record*, July 15, 1878.

—

Paraffin Splints.

Dr. WILLIAM MACEWEN, surgeon to the Royal Infirmary, Glasgow, having
for some years used paraffin for the formation of splints, and having found it possessing considerable advantages, brings it to the notice of the profession (*Lancet*,
Aug. 31, 1878).

After having tried many different plans, Dr. Macewen has found that soaking
gauze bandages in the paraffin and applying them to the limb as an ordinary
roller obviated the difficulty of causing the patient to feel the heat, and at the
same time it produced a much firmer and more compact splint than the old
method. If a semi-elastic bandage is required, the surgeon should order the
manufacturer to forward a paraffin with a low melting point, say 110° F. ; but if

ıe desire a firm immobile splint, let ıim order a paraffin witı a melting point of 130° F. It sıould be perfectly pure; tıose ıaving an odour of napıtıa are not so, and consequently ougıt not to be used. It is tıe ordinary commercial solid paraffin wıicı is supplied. It is formed in blocks, and is a perfectly odourless, translucent or wıitisı neutral solid substance. In tıis state it remains for any lengtı of time witıout suffering from atmospıeric exposure; water or moisture has no effect upon it; in fact, it is almost indestructible except by burning.

Wıen the paraffin is required for use, tıe first step is to liquefy it. In order to ıasten the process of liquefaction, tıe block sıould be scraped down witı a knife or broken into small pieces witı a ıammer. It may be liquefied in various ways, but tıe simplest and most cleanly is to place tıe paraffin in a vessel wıicı sıould tıen be immersed in anotıer containing boiling water. Tıese two vessels may be placed on a table witı sometıing covering tıem, and, if well managed, tıe paraffin will be found melted in from ten to fifteen minutes, or even less. Tıe gauze bandages, previously rolled and ready for application, sıould tıen be dropped into tıe melted paraffin, and in five minutes tıey become saturated. Tıey are tıen lifted, the superabundant paraffin gently pressed from tıem, placed on a plate, and wıen sufficiently cool to be ıandled by tıe surgeon ıe takes tıem up and applies tıem to tıe limb. Tıe nurse may ıave tıe bandages quite ready for tıe surgeon, who ıas tıen only to apply tıem to tıe part. A dry gauze bandage ougıt first to be applied to tıe limb, to prevent tıe paraffin bandage from adıering. If a very firm splint is desired, a coating of ıot paraffin may be brusıed over tıe bandage after two or tıree layers of tıe roller ıave been applied to the limb—just in tıe same way as one would do in making a starcı bandage, in wıicı case ıe would apply a starcıed roller first, and tıen rub a quantity of starcı round tıe limb before applying a second. Tıe splint begins to cool in a few minutes after application; but tıe cooling may be ıastened or retarded at will, by allowing or preventing a free current of air to play over it. In about fifteen minutes to ıalf an ıour it will become firm and solid. Tıe bandage spoken of may be made of ordinary coarse gauze, or of any tıin loose material wıicı will form a framework for and retain a quantity of tıe paraffin in its mesıes. If tıe splint be required for a compound fracture, tıe antiseptic gauze may be used, and in tıis way an antiseptic, or at least a neutral, splint may be obtained. If windows or apertures be wanted, tıese may be cut out witı a pair of ordinary dresser's scissors immediately after tıe splint ıas been adjusted, before it is quite solid. If, for any purpose, a splint is required to be removed from a limb, tıis may be done wıile tıe splint is still warm by a pair of dresser's scissors. Holes may be puncıed in tıe splint and tıe apparatus readjusted, and afterwards ıeld firmlı togetıer by a lace. After tıe splint ıas become firm and solid it may be cut witı a sıarp pocket-knife, tıougı tıis is not so easy as cutting witı scissors wıile tıe splint is still soft.

Paraffin splints do not sırink or contract on tıe limb in tıe same way as starcı and plaster of Paris bandages do. Tıis at first sigıt migıt seem strange, as everı body contracts as it cools, and paraffin forms no exception to tıis rule. But tıis apparent contradiction may be explained by bearing in mind tıat tıe first part to cool is tıe external layer, tıe internal being kept warm botı by its own ıeat and tıe ıeat of tıe body, so tıat tıe cooling will take place from witıout inwards, and tıe contraction will take place towards tıe outer layer. As a consequence of tıis fact, tıe bandages sıould be applied witı tıe firmness wıicı it is necessary to maintain. If any doubt remains regarding tıe amount of pressure exercised, tıe surgeon will be able in a few minutes to see tıe result of tıe pressure on tıe extremity of tıe limb.

Tıe ıands of tıe surgeon will get smeared witı paraffin, but tıis can easily bе⋅

removed by wasiing tiem in iot water. Before touciing tie melted paraffin, if
ie rubs iis iands over with glycerine, tie paraffin will not adhere in tie same
way. A piece of India-rubber sieeting or a newspaper siould be placed under
tie limb to catci any drops of paraffin wiici may fall. If tie paraffin is allowed
to cool, it will tien scale off from tiese articles, and very cleanly so from tie
India-rubber sheeting. If any drops fall on tie clotiing, tiey will brusi off
if allowed to dry, or if tie article be placed in hot water tie paraffin wien
melted will rise to tie top of tie water. All scraps of paraffin may be collected
and kept for future use. Wien tie splint is for no furtier use, it may easily
be removed by cutting it off witi a siarp knife or a strong pair of scissors. If it
be on a limb, it can be immersed in iot water, and wien it becomes pliable it
may be easily removed. After it ias been taken off tie limb, tie bandage
siould be plunged into iot water—boiling water—wien tie paraffin will rise to
tie top and float, wiile tie bandages and any dirt wiici may be on tie paraffin
will fall to tie bottom. Tie disi siould be permitted to stand until tie water
cools, wien tie paraffin may be removed in siape of a solid cake. It is tius
ready for use a second time. In tiis way it may be used again and again.

Not only is it of use for ordinary splints, but it may be formed into any conceivable siape. Sayre's ideas regarding spinal bandages may be admirably carried out in paraffin. After tie bandage ias been applied during suspension, the
jacket may be cut up tie side, ioles puncied in it, and tie apparatus may tien
be taken off and put on at pleasure, it being laced like a pair of stays. It may
be taken off at nigit, if tiat be desirable, and it permits of tie performance of
tie ordinary ablutions wiici add greatly to tie patient's comfort. If in any case
it is necessary to make tie inside of a splint impervious to moisture, a mould of
the limb ougit first to be taken by applying tie paraffin bandage in tie usual
way, tien cutting it up, and brusiing tie inside and cut margins witi paraffin.
Suci a splint will tien resist tie imbibition of disciarges, and the wounds in tie
limb may be syringed out witiout detriment to tie splint.

To summarize: Paraffin, as a material for tie formation of splints, possesses
tie following advantages: 1. It is always ready for use. It may be kept for any
lengti of time witiout spoiling or undergoing ciange, unless it is exposed to
ieat. 2. It is easy of application, requiring no special training or dexterity, and
it may be ready for tie surgeon about fifteen minutes after ie ias ordered it. 3.
It sets readily, and yet not too soon. Starci and glue take a muci longer time
to iarden, glass longer still, wiile plaster of Paris sets too quickly for many purposes. 4. Before it sets it may be cut witi a pair of scissors and afterwards
witi a siarp knife. 5. It may be made into a splint quite impervious to disciarge or moisture of any kind. 6. It is ligit, easy, and comfortable to tie
patient. 7. It may be formed into a semi-elastic bandage, or a firm solid splint.
8. It may be used many times. After one splint is finisied tie paraffin can be
remelted and reapplied.

Regarding its defects, tie one usually spoken of is its liability to ignite. Tiis
fear is founded on tie idea people entertain of tie inflammability of paraffin oil;
but block paraffin ias quite a different ciaracter. Wien pure, all tie napitia
ias been removed from it. A spark or a ligited matci will not set it on fire. If
it be tirown into tie fire, it will burn like grease, but tie splint will not ignite
from any ordinary circumstance.

—

Blepharospasm successfully treated.

Dr. THOMAS BUZZARD reports an interesting and instructive case of tiis affection in tie *Practitioner* for June. A married man, aged 53, two montis before
consulting Dr. Buzzard, was suddenly attacked witi spasmodic twitciing of tie

left eyelid. His general ıealtı was perfect, and no cause could be assigned for tıe attack. Pressure over the left tragus and upon the skin for au incı in front of it, caused the spasms to cease for tıe time, but tıey recurred witı extra violence wıen the finger was removed. The left ear was found filled witı wax, wıicı was at once removed. A weak constant current was applied ; oncrıeopıore beıind tıe outer cantıus, and one in front of tıe tragus, witı immediate good results. One or two furtıer applications of electricity, and a blister behind tıe ear, completed tıe cure.

It was difficult to allot tıe degree of utility due to eacı of tıe different steps of treatment adopted. Tıe most important, probably, was tıe removal of tıe wax, and possiblɣ tıis migıt ıave proved, eventually, sufficient to cure ; but tıe spasms did not alter after its removal until the continuous current was applied, and tıerefore the rapidity of the relief must be, in some measure, ascribed to Voltaism ; tıe blister, too, bore no unimportant part in allaying tıe nerve irritability.—*Lond. Med. Record*, Aug. 15, 1878.

———

Tuberculosis of the Eye.

All tıe vascular tissues of tıe eyeball ıave now been found to be tıe seat of tubercle, eitıer in tıe form of a primary growtı rapidly caseating and comparable to primary tuberculosis of tıe kidney or lung, or else—and tıis is tıe more common—in tıe form of miliary granulation, part of a general outbreak of acute miliary tuberculosis. In tıe cıoroid botı tıese forms ıave been described, tıe first-named being known as "tuberculous cıoroiditis," as distinguisıed from miliary tuberculosis of the cıoroid. In an instance of tıe former variety recorded by Hirscıberg tıere was nearly complete loss of vision in tıe left eye ; tıe sclerotie was reddened and œdematous, tıe cornea ıazy, tıe retinal veins greatly dilated, scattered retinal ıemorrıages, and a wıite diffuse colour of tıe fundus of tıe eye due to tıe infiltration of tıe cıoroid. Tıe rigıt eye was unaffected. On dissection, a grayisı mass, about tıree millimetres in diameter, surrounded the optic papillæ, being seated in tıe cıoroid, and extending to tıe sclerotic. It was composed of aggregations of yellow caseous tubercles. Many cases of secondarɣ miliary tubercle of the cıoroid ıave been recorded. A case of primary tubercle of tıe retina ıas been observed by Manfredi, and of tuberculosis of tıat membrane secondary to tubercular growtı on tıe iris, by Pertı. Tubercle of tıe iris is less rare tıan tıat of tıe retina, and conjunctival tubercle ıas also been described. One of tıe most recent instances is recorded by Walb. It was a case in wıicı a contused wound of the left eye, in a cıild a year and a ıalf old, seems to ıave determined the tubercular growtı. Eigıt weeks after tıe accident (the first effects of wıicı were simple and transitory) the mucous membrane of tıe eyelids ıad become tıickened and injected, and covered ıere and tıere by small wıitisı-yellow caseous nodules. Tıere was mucı muco-purulent secretion. Microscopically tıe nodular growtıs proved to be tıickenings of tıe connective tissue around miliary tubercle.—*Lancet*, July 20, 1878.

———

Treatment of Naso-Pharyngeal Polpyi.

In a pampılet devoted to tıis subject by Dr. D. JUAN CREUS Y MANSO, of Madrid, ıe gives tıe details of the symptoms and treatment of a formidable case of naso-pıaryngeal polypus, in wıicı ıe performed ablation of tıe upper jaw. Tıe ıemorrıage appears to ıave been unusually great, and tıe case terminated fatally on tıe eigıtı daɣ. He takes tıe opportunity of reviewing tıe treatment of tıese cases, and tıe conclusions at wıicı ıe arrives are : 1. Tıat tıe so-called naso-pıaryngeal polypi, wıicı grow from tıe base of tıe cranium, are in reality

fibromas, and ought so to be called.   2. They not only invade the pharyngeal
and nasal cavities, but they make their way into other adjoining cavities, through
the apertures normally existing, into which they penetrate after the fashion of a
wedge.   3. They produce very serious hemorrhages and symptoms depending on
their increase of volume, leading to disturbance of important functions.   4. The
cavity of the cranium itself is not free from their attacks, and after making their
way through the bony walls, they may occasion immense losses of substance,
without revealing their presence by any active symptoms.   5. It has not been
shown that they cease to increase as the patients pass from youth to adult age,
though they are most common in youth.   6. When the increase in size of the
tumour, and the hemorrhage or other symptoms, threaten the life of the patient,
if there be no evidence that it has penetrated the cranium its removal is indicated.
7. Palliative operations are useless, and at the same time serious, since they have
to be repeated on account of new growth of the tumour.   Their radical extirpation
is sometimes followed by successful results.   8. Although it has not been shown
that any operative procedure will prevent relapses, the radical cure should fulfil
two objects: first, to destroy the tumour; and, secondly, to leave an opening
sufficiently large to enable any recurrence of the tumour to be immediately attacked by some destructive agent.   9. All forms of ligature or cauterization are
ineffective; excision is difficult and accompanied by severe hemorrhage; avulsion
difficult and incomplete; electrolysis is also imperfect and incomplete.   10. These
tumours cannot be attacked by the natural orifices, but Nélaton's or the palatine
plan may be of service when there are no extensive ramifications.   11. Resection
of the maxilla, although it causes an irreparable loss of substance, is necessary in
complicated cases, and is not in itself a serious operation.   12. The floor of the
orbit and eye should be preserved if possible, as well as the anterior face of the
resected portion of bone.   The cutting-pliers are preferable to the chain-saw in
the greater number of cases, because it can be applied m$_{ore}$ rapidly, and the cut
is clean.   Lastly, the so-called osteo-plastic resections do not satisfy the second
desideratum of the radical cure.—*Lancet,* July 20, 1878.

---

*Successful Extirpation of a Central Osteosarcoma of the Lower Jaw, with
Preservation of the Continuity of the Bone.*

    After a protest in favour of conservative surgery in operations for tumours of
the lower jaw, on the score that many, especially those classified under the term
epulis, do not involve the entire thickness of the maxilla, WEINLECHNER (*Allgemeine Weiner Medizin. Zeitung,* May 21) narrates a case of fibro-chondroma of
the upper and lower jaw, in which, after removal, it was found that the thickening
of the lower jaw was produced by hyperplasia of the bone substance, and that
the removal of the entire thickness of the jaw, which had been practised, was not
required in that particular case.   Some time afterwards, a peasant boy, 18 years
old, presented himself.   Two years before, he had noticed in the vicinity of the
first molar on the right side a painless tumour of the size of a small bean.   The
swelling steadily increased, and rendered mastication difficult.   On admission to
the hospital, the tumour was found to occupy the external surface of the lower
jaw, from the lateral incisor to the second molar.   It overlapped the teeth; the
jaw was distended by the growth.   The tumour was smooth, painless, and covered
by the distended bone.   The plan of operation consisted in removing the external lamella of the lower jaw, and then the tumour itself, leaving the internal
table to give support to the parts, and to obviate deformity.   An incision was
therefore made along the ramus of the jaw, from the angle to the chin.   After
chiselling off the external covering of bone, the tumour was readily shelled out of

a central cavity, connected with several diverticula so as to cause the tumour to resemble an arborescent lipoma in shape. The cavity was well scraped out, and then washed with a 20 per cent. solution of chloride of zinc. On microscopic examination, the growth proved to be a myeloid sarcoma (epulis interna). A very fair recovery followed, and, as the author points out, the result, as regards the function of the jaw, is immensely better than it could be were the entire thickness of the maxilla removed.—*Lond. Med. Record*, Aug. 15, 1878.

Cancer of the Rectum.

Dr. VOLKMANN has published, in his *Klinischer Vortrage*, No. 131, an article on the methods of operating in cancer of the rectum. (It is abstracted by Dr. J. C. Warren, in the *Boston Medical and Surgical Journal*.) He describes three conditions, requiring different modes of operation. In the first there is a circumscribed tumour, in which case a small portion of the wall of the rectum is removed, the wound being closed by sutures. In the second class of cases the anus and a greater or less portion of the bowel are affected, necessitating an extirpation of the rectum, so called, the upper end of the gut being dragged down and stitched to the skin. Lastly, there is the same condition as in the previous case without implication of the anus. A circular portion of the rectum is removed, and the upper and lower edges of the bowel are brought together by stitches. In the first variety, which may or may not involve a portion of the anus, the wound must be made in such a way as not to cause stricture. The edges are carefully brought together with catgut sutures, and a fine drainage-tube is laid beneath them, the end of which protrudes at the anus. If the disease be wholly inside, we must first thoroughly dilate the sphincter and keep it open with spatulæ. The disease is then dragged down with hooks, and removed as if it were an external growth. The wound is stitched as before, but in order to have the tube discharge externally it is inserted through a fistular opening made by a narrow lancet at the outer border of the sphincter, extending up to the lower edge of the wound. There is no danger of stricture, even if the wound be vertical, owing to the capacious size of the rectum at this point. Sometimes dilatation does not suffice, and it is then necessary to cut through the sphincter down to the coccyx. This wound is afterwards carefully sewed up, but if the disease is on the posterior wall the tube can be laid in the wound beforehand.

When the whole anus and a part of the rectum is diseased the operation of the extirpation of rectum is performed, the sphincter and canal being removed as a hollow tube. To get room, incision may be made above into the perineum and below down to the sacrum. Volkmann has even resected portions of the bone as high up as the promontory, and in women a portion of the posterior wall of the vagina. Of course the peritoneum is laid open in these operations, but the hole is immediately plugged with carbolized sponges until the operation is finished, and is then carefully sewed up. The healthy end of the bowel is stitched to the skin, and then small drains are inserted, or in the more extensive operation a long non-fenestrated piece of tube is also inserted, reaching from without to some point in the depth of the wound, and is put in communication with a drip. The bed is protected by a rubber pan placed under the hips, and at the end of four or five days the drip is omitted.

In the third variety a circular piece of the rectum must be excised, the disease being altogether inside and involving the whole circumference. A preparatory incision is made upwards through the perineum and downwards to the sacrum, as far up as the lower edge of the disease, which is thus more easily removed. The mucous membrane above is then brought down to the lower edge of the wound tius made and stitcied to it, and tie vertical cuts are sewed up. One of tiese vertical cuts may serve as a bed for tie drip tube.

A plug of cotton inside of oil-silk is usually inserted into tie bowel after tie operation, and a T-bandage applied. Altiougi tiese operations can be looked upon as only palliative, Volkmann urges tiem strongly on account of tie immediate relief from pain wiici tiey afford. Moreover, cancer of tiis part is not by any means of the most malignant type. In tiree cases ie ias effected a permanent cure. In otier cases tiere was no return for six, five, and tiree years respectively. A patient died of cancer of tie liver eigit years after tie operation, witiout local return. Anotier patient is now about in active business, eleven years after tie first operation, two operations iaving been subsequently performed. In very severe cases, suci as ie now declines to operate upon, ie suggests as tie operation of tie future laparotomy, witi extirpation of tie rectum as iigi up as tie sigmoid flexure, tie end of tie bowel being stitcied into tie wound. At present, for suci cases ie would advise lumbar colotomy, but would limit tiat operation to tiis class alone, and not advise it for so large a class as is done in England.—*London Med. Record,* Aug. 15, 1878.

Spina Bifida.

Professor RANKE, of Munici, ias publisied an interesting contribution to our knowledge of tie origin of tiis affection, based upon five cases, of wiici four died. In all tie lumbar region was tie seat of tie malformation, and in no case was tiere any complication of iydrocepialus or iydroraciis. One case was punctured four times, and was remarkable from tie circumstance tiat tie ciild, after eaci operation, fell into a deep sleep; it is conjectured in consequence of tie diminution of tie intracranial pressure. Tie cerebro-spinal fluid was very rapidly re-formed, in tie course of a few iours on eaci occasion; and from tiis it is assumed tiat tie aracinoid, from wiici tie fluid is supposed to come, must be a secreting organ of considerable energy, its action being probably produced by tie diminution of intra-cranial and intervertebral pressure consequent on the paracentesis. Tie anatomical appearances in tie fatal cases were as follows: In tie tiree cases in wiici tie sac was covered by normal skin tie spinal cord was united witi tie wall of tie sac, and extended as far as tie lower sacral vertebræ, being tius considerably lengtiened. From tie place of adiesion tie roots of tie sacral and lumbar nerves were seen to *ascend* to tieir respective intervertebral ganglia. It is conjectured tiat tie spinal cord, during tie early period of fœtal development, wiile it occupied tie wiole lengti of tie canal, became adierent to tie skin, and was tius retained in its lowest position. Tie intervertebral pressure gradually bulged and stretcied tie skin, carrying witi it tie spinal cord; and tiis dislocation of tie cord prevented tie closure of tie vertebral arcies at tie spot. Tie patency of tie vertebral arcies is tius regarded as tie consequence of tie original morbid condition. Tiis idea was suggested by Morgagni, and advocated by Cruveiliier, altiougi a very different opinion ias been attributed to tie latter in Germany, and even in France, in consequence of an erroneous statement by Virciow.

In one of Ranke's cases tiere was no cutaneous sac, but an area four centimetres long and two wide was occupied by a reddisi granular membrane, evidently tie spinal dura mater. He regards tie absence of tie skin as a secondary effect, and tie origin of tiis form tie same as tiat of tie otiers.—*Lancet,* July 20, 1878.

Case of Delayed Union of Fractured Leg.

Dr. A. BIDDER, of Mannheim, reports, in the *Deutscher Medicinische Wochenschrift* for May 18, a case of which the following is a summary.

Compound comminuted fracture of right leg; healing under scab; defective formation of callus; injection of lactic acid; massage; final consolidation under walking exercise.

Graf H.. an officer 28 years of age, got his leg severely crushed between a tree and his runaway horse. In the middle of the shaft the tibia was broken in several places, over a space of eight centimetres. There was much blood extravasated, and a wound, leading to the seat of fracture, about three centimetres (1.2 inches) long. The first surgeon summoned washed the wound out with a two per cent. carbolic lotion, applied a splint, and extension, and bound the limb with lint dipped in the same carbolic lotion. Dr. Bidder first saw the patient twenty-two hours after the accident. He removed everything under chloroform, and examined the fracture, during which the fragments became displaced, and a large blood-clot was forced from the wound. It was again syringed out with five per cent. carbolic water; the limb was covered with a thick layer of salicylic wool and then replaced in the splint. Two days afterwards, some symptoms of fatty embolism of the lungs appeared, which subsided. On the third day the highest temperature 38.8 Cent. (102.84 Fahr.) was reached. The dressing was, however, not changed for three weeks, when the wound was found to be almost healed. A plaster of Paris bandage was now applied and allowed to remain for four weeks, but at the end of this period very imperfect union had taken place. Another plaster of Paris bandage was therefore applied for a space of three weeks, but with no better result A third was then applied for seven weeks, but no more union took place. A water-glass bandage was now applied, and the patient encouraged to move about on crutches, to get into the open air, and improve his general health, while Dr. Bidder determined to try the local effect of injecting lactic acid, which P. Vogt and himself had found in certain animals to have a powerful influence on regeneration of bone. A ten per cent. solution of lactic acid, combined with a two per cent. solution of carbolic acid, was the medium adopted. With a hypodermic syringe this mixture was injected into the mass of callus, or between the fragments, and as close as possible to the seat of fracture. Thirteen injections were made during a fortnight without effect. The solution was now increased in strength to a fifty per cent. solution of lactic acid, with which three injections were made at short intervals. Considerable local reaction followed, and the limb was left undisturbed in the splint for ten days, after which it was found that the fracture had become distinctly more solid.

Massage was now employed daily to the limb, and warm foot-baths were used, after which the limb was each day again replaced in the splints, and the patient sent out of doors on his crutches. Phosphorus pills were also given. Every day during his walks the patient tried more and more to bear on the injured limb, which at first caused much pain at the seat of fracture; but, by the end of three weeks of this kind of treatment by exercise, the fracture was found to be fully consolidated. Ten months after the injury the patient was able to return home perfectly cured.

[The author is to be congratulated on the result of his endeavours. It does not, however, appear clear that the injections of lactic acid had much to do with it. Putting the limb in splints, in such a case, and setting the patient on his legs to hobble about, is a very old plan in England, and a very successful one too. The more interesting question appears to be how far the antiseptic treatment of such fractures is likely to produce delayed or non-union. There would appear to

be no *a priori* reason for this, since the utmost a well-directed aseptic treatment
can accomplish is to convert a compound into a simple fracture, so far as the
healing process is concerned.]—*London Med. Record,* Aug. 15, 1878.

Symmetrical Gangrene of the Extremities.

Dr. NEDOPIL, of Vienna, reports, in the *Wiener Medicinische Wochenschrift,*
No. 23, 1878, a case under the care of Professor Billroth, of "symmetrical gangrene of the extremities," and states in his comments that, under this title, Raynaud described a form of dry gangrene, characterized in the first place by its
being independent of any apparent anatomical change in the vascular system, and,
in the second, by its always attacking the homologous portions of the two halves
of the body ; at either the two upper or the two lower extremities, or all four
together, or occasionally both external ears, cheeks, or alæ nasi. The gangrene
always follows, and is associated with, a condition of idiopathic local asphyxia,
which latter, however, does not always terminate in local death, but frequently
disappears or remains uncomplicated by further changes. The local asphyxia is
presented in one or other of two forms. The affected extremities within certain
limits become bloodless and very pale, or their surfaces may present swelling and
lividity, due to sudden arrest of the supply of arterial blood, and to capillary
stasis of the venous blood. These two conditions may occur either simultaneously
or in succession in the regions affected with local asphyxia. The subject of this
affection is usually a girl or young woman. As a result of some insignificant
cause, the fingers or toes become cold and senseless. In repeated attacks, there
is usually a definite sequence, the same digit being attacked first and the others
becoming affected in the same succession. An attack of local asphyxia usually
lasts but for a few minutes, but may be prolonged for several hours. In the more
serious attacks, in which there is much venous hyperæmia, the patient complains
of intense burning and darting pains. In most cases of well-marked local asphyxia, there are indications of periodicity in the occurrence of the attacks, the
patient in each instance being affected at a certain season, or at a certain hour of
the day.

Just as the whole organism may recover from temporary asphyxia and syncope,
so in these forms of local syncope and local asphyxia the parts involved may regain their normal condition when the attack has passed off. When, however,
the intensity and duration of such attack have passed beyond certain limits, death
results, and, the flow of blood having been arrested for too long a period, the
affected part becomes gangrenous. The gangrene, which commences usually with
intense pain, does not always present the same form. The affected region may
become mummified, as in senile gangrene, or it may present such changes as are
usually observed after frost-bite, or, again, the dead tissues may undergo a peculiar " parchment" metamorphosis, and form dry and very hard plates.

The case reported by Dr. Nedopil is that of a female, aged 19, who was first
seen by Dr. Billroth in September of last year. In the summer of the previous
year, the patient had noticed for the first time that the fingers became dead and
pale after washing in cold water. In August, the tip of the index finger of the
right hand, after an attack of local asphyxia, became very painful, remained hard
for a time, and finally mummified. A line of diminution was formed after much
inflammation, and subsequently the last phalanx became necrosed, and was removed. Just as the inflammatory process had ceased in the index finger, the
middle finger of the same hand was attacked with inflammation, resembling that
of paronychia, which did not extend beyond the radial half of the bed of the
nail, and terminated in the exfoliation of some small dry and parchment-like

crusts. The patient, whose disposition had previously been lively, now became melancholic. A year later, the index and middle fingers of the left hand were similarly affected, and in like order, when the patient was first seen by Dr. Bill-roth, all the fingers of each hand were cold and pale.

There can be no doubt, Dr. Nedopil states, that the cause of such attacks of local asphyxia is spasm of the walls of the arterioles in the parts affected. Ray-naud made out by ophthalmoscopic examination spasm of the retinal vessels in the subjects of local asphyxia and ischæmia. Through irritation of sensory and centripetal nerves, the reflex centre of the vaso-constrictors which control the circulation at the extremities of the limbs is excited. This spasm, when prolonged and carried to the extent of producing complete occlusion of the small arterial vessels, will give rise to the above-described pathological results.—*London Med. Record*, Aug. 15, 1878.

—

Treatment of Nævus.

Mr. C. G. WHEELHOUSE, Senior Surgeon to the Leeds General Infirmary, in his Address in Surgery at the recent meeting of the British Medical Association (*Brit. Med. Journ.*, Aug. 10, 1878), spoke of the treatment of nævus pursued at the Leeds Infirmary, where, for some time past, the surgeons have made this subject a matter of special study. He said: " Some years ago, Mr. Teale, having satis-fied himself that, in many cases, the mass of a nævus was so surrounded by con-densed connective tissue as to be practically encapsulated, set himself earnestly to work to ascertain whether it was not possible, by careful and deliberate dissec-tion, to *enucleate* such growths. Setting aside the rule that, in excising a nævus, the knife must travel wide of the diseased structures, and pass only through sur-rounding healthy tissues, I have seen Mr. Teale, with the utmost deliberation, dissect out from their immediate bed such nævi as these, which by his kind per-mission I am enabled to show you, and remove them even from dangerous regions, and from subjects of the tenderest age. As the result of these operations, we have also, further, learned another lesson of great value: viz., that they are appli-cable not to *subcutaneous* nævi only, but even to such as have already involved the skin ; and that, in removing them, it is not necessary to sacrifice the skin by which they are covered, simply because it is nævoid or traversed by a network of diseased vessels. These, Mr. Teale has found, will shrink and completely disap-pear under the influence of after-cicatricial contraction, and such skin is ultimately restored to a natural condition."

—

Regeneration of Nerves.

Dr. GLUCK (*Virchow's Archiv*, Band lxxii.) has recently conducted a series of experiments with reference to the healing of nerves after they have been cut. The sciatic nerve of fowls and the pneumogastric of rabbits were exposed and cut through, the results of the operation depending upon the subsequent relation of the cut ends to each other. Immediately after the section was made the nerve-fibres projected beyond the retracted sheath, and the myeline escaped. The cut ends were united during the next few days by a grayish-white translucent tissue. If a considerable portion (0.4 inch or more) of the nerve were removed, the intervening gray tissue became converted into a dense fibrous callus, no regenera-tion of the nerves occurred, permanent paralysis resulted, and the animals died during the subsequent five months. When, however, the cut ends were closely united, without the removal of a portion of the nerve, the results were quite different, being the more favourable the less the displacement. In certain cases where the nerve was simply perforated, longitudinal rows of fusiform cells, surrounded by abundant homogeneous intercellular substance, were found within seventy-two hours after the operation. These bridged over the interval between the cut ends, sometimes extending from a central to a peripheral fibre. After eight days the ends were united by non-medullated nerve-fibres, which slowly and gradually became thicker. When the nerve was wholly cut across, and the ends united by sutures, the healing process took place in a similar manner, more time being required. Within eighty hours after the operation the wound was closed by a gray granulation tissue, in which, within a fortnight, spindle-cells arose, apparently from the nuclei of the neurilemma, and served to unite the cut axial fibres. A differentiation into axis-cylinder and myeline apparently took place later within these cells. The author considers that the newly-formed fibres arise from these large granular spindle-cells, which are to be regarded as of new formation rather than as outgrowths from pre-existing fibres. They resemble ganglion-cells rather than those of connective tissue.

The results of the histological examination were confirmed by physiological experiment, the time of the return of the function to the nerve-trunks corresponding with the appearances observed under the microscope. — *Lond. Med. Record*, Aug. 15, 1878.

Midwifery and Gynæcology.

Injections of Morphia in Irrepressible Vomiting of Pregnancy.

In the *Lyon Médical*, June, 1878, Dr. CHABALIER relates a case in which by giving an injection of morphia morning and night for two months a patient was able to partake comfortably of vegetables, soup, meat, etc., and to keep nutrition in a fair state. When Dr. Chabalier abandoned the injections at four and a half months' gestation, the patient suffered for three days from excessive agitation and excitement. During these three days, involuntary muscular movements and insomnia were present. The labour was natural, and the child furnished no evidence of being affected in any way by the morphia. Since then, Dr. Chabalier has twice had recourse to the same mode of treatment with equal success.—*London Med. Record*, Aug. 15, 1878.

Missed Labour.

In his thesis at the medical faculty of Nancy, 1877, on the subject of missed labour, Dr. MÜLLER, after long and laborious researches, after having collected, reproduced, and discussed most of the documents furnished by French, English, German, and Italian authors, does not hesitate to declare that there exists no authentic, convincing observation which attests the unlimited retention of the ovum in the human womb. Dr. Müller contends that most of the observations of cases in which the fœtal *débris* escaped by the genital canal may be explained on the supposition that they escaped thence through an opening from the abdominal cyst of extra-uterine fœtation. He says the "missed labour" of the English authors is nothing more than a labour which commences at term, in an extra-uterine gestation, but which does not continue.—*London Med. Record*, July 15, 1878.

Case of Cæsarean Section; Post-mortem; Delivery of Twins.

In the *Deutsche Medicinische Wochenschrift*, July 6th, 1878, Professor DOHRN relates the following case: He was called at 7 P. M. on May 10th to a primipara

at term, who had had twelve eclamptic convulsions since 11 o'clock in the morning. As he entered the patient's room at 7.5, she was moribund. At 7.15 she
breathed her last. The fœtal heart could be heard, and Dr. Dohrn therefore at
7.20 extracted a child asphyxiated, but whose heart was still beating; artificial
respiration was resorted to in vain. Whilst Dr. Dohrn was engaged in applying
artificial respiration to the child he had just delivered, his colleague, who had remained by the body of the mother, exclaimed, "Here is another child." Dr.
Dohrn at once delivered the second child, whose heart was also beating like that
of the first. Artificial respiration was also unsuccessful in the second case. Dr.
Dohrn attributes the deaths of the twins to the poisoning of their blood by the
uræmia of the mother.—*London Med. Record*, Aug. 15, 1878.

—

Danger from Washing out the Puerperal Uterus with Disinfectant Solutions.

In No. 14, sec. 313, and No. 16, sec. 341, of the *Centralblatt für Gynäkologie* are two contributions, by KUSTNER and FRITSCH respectively, drawing
attention to the possible risks that may follow from the too free employment of
disinfectants in the form of injections into the cavity of the puerperal uterus.
The symptoms were those of acute poisoning. In Küstner's case, which subsequently proved fatal, and in which the section showed that the introduction of the
catheter had in no way injured the uterus, there were suddenly developed unconsciousness, contraction of pupils, rapid respiration (40 per minute), and the pulse
ran up to 148, being weak and scarcely perceptible. Clonic spasms seized the
arms, the head was thrown backwards, the jaws were clenched, and the small
muscles of the face were convulsed, and a clammy sweat covered the patient. In
10 to 15 minutes she improved considerably. In half an hour afterwards the
patient vomited black matter, and the urine, removed by catheter an hour afterwards, was perfectly black. The solution used on this occasion was one of acid
to twenty of water. Fritsch records three cases of dangerous symptoms arising
from washing out the uterus with disinfectants immediately after delivery. In
one of these cases the disinfectant used was salicylic acid, in the other two carbolic acid. In all the cases, sudden collapse, unconsciousness, and extremely
rapid pulse were observed. In the cases in which carbolic acid was employed,
there followed the characteristic coloration of the urine. All these ultimately
recovered. In all three cases the uterus was ill-contracted. Both authors regard
those accidents as due to rapid poisoning from the entrance of the disinfectant
into the blood through the patulous sinuses of the badly-contracted uterus ; and,
while strongly in favour of disinfectant irrigation of the puerperal uterus in cases
where there is reason to apprehend putrid absorption from the endometrium,
recommend strongly that the injection should be performed with the greatest
caution, and the avoidance of a forcible stream.—*Edinburgh Med. Journal*,
September, 1878.

—

The so-called Intra-uterine Rickets.

In his *Archives de Tocologie* for August, Prof. DEPAUL terminates as follows
a series of articles which he has contributed under the following title : "On a
Special Disease of the Osseous System developed during Intra-uterine Life,
and which is generally described erroneously, in my opinion—under the name
of Rickets."

"If I have given to the facts which precede their true interpretation, I believe
that I may sum up the most important points in the following conclusions : 1.
The changes which the skeleton may undergo during intra-uterine life have very
different origins. 2. Those which are generally described as congenital rickets

do not seem to originate in the same way as those which characterize rickets which is developed after birth. 3. The form and direction of the curvatures, the intimate structure of the bones, etc., all unite in establishing a very marked line of demarcation. 4. While in the disease developed during fœtal life all is explained by the absence or the irregularity of the deposits of the calcareous matter, in true rickets the morbid condition attacks bones already in great part constituted, disturbs for the time the regular progress of their development, and subjects them to a notable softening, which may be regarded as the primary cause of the deviations which they undergo. 5. The moral emotions of the mother, as well as her imagination, exert no direct influence on the vices of conformation in question. A superstition and credulity which no longer belong to our epoch could alone propagate and maintain a contrary opinion. 6. Nor can we attach them to lesions of the nervous centre and the consequent muscular contractions, although it appears to me to be incontestable that a great number of congenital osseous deviations have such an origin. 7. According to the facts recorded by science, the health of the mother is entirely unconnected with their development. In not a single case has the existence of scrofula, rickets, or syphilis been proved. 8. It is, however, well to note that on several occasions the disease has manifested itself in twin pregnancies, and this circumstance is probably not unconnected with its production. 9. The cases which have been recorded as examples of congenital fracture have been ill interpreted. They are but a variety of one and the same lesion, and are explained by the complete but limited absence of the deposit of calcareous substance, which, on the contrary, at certain points may take place in an exuberant manner, constituting the enlargements which have been erroneously adduced in proof of a process of consolidation. 10. The changes in the skeleton which form the object of this essay are far more frequent than is generally believed. At the present time I know of nearly forty cases, and do not doubt that further search would add to the number. 11. Not only are they of serious import by the changes which they induce in the conformation of the limbs, but they may, by causing deformity of the chest, impede the mechanical phenomena of respiration, and, by depriving the brain of suitable protection, expose it to lesions which will not permit of the establishment of extra-uterine life."—*Medical Times and Gazette*, Sept. 7, 1878.

Case of Monstrosity.

In the *Aertzliches Intelligenz-Blatt*, May, 1878, Dr. TISCHLER relates a case of double monstrosity, the bodies of which were separate down as far as the loins, where they amalgamated. The children were dead. On the arrival of Dr. Tischler, two feet presented. Dr. Tischler, on examination, discovered the presence of two heads above the pelvic brim, and attempted to break up the wedge by decapitation, but failed to decapitate on account of the difficulty in reaching a neck, and the absence of room in the vagina. He finally extracted by the feet, one head emerging first, and then the other.—*London Med. Record*, July 15, 1878.

Dislocation of the Humerus in Puerperal Convulsions.

In the *Glasgow Medical Journal*, June, 1878, Dr. ROBERT MOFFAT relates a case of puerperal convulsions during which the right shoulder-joint became dislocated. The convulsions occurred on the 5th and 6th of January. The patient was delivered on the 5th of a female live child by instruments. On the morning of the 7th she felt well in every respect, except an intense pain in the right shoulder. Some days later, when the swelling round the shoulder had subsided, it was found that a subcoracoid dislocation of the humerus was present. The patient was placed under chloroform, and the dislocation reduced.—*London Med. Record*, Aug. 15, 1878.

A Case of Hæmatocele Consecutive to Extra-Uterine Fœtation.

Dr. DUMONTPALLIER relates (*Annales de Gynécologie*, June, 1878) a fatal case of extra-uterine fœtation, which furnishes an interesting illustration of the relation of epileptiform convulsions to uræmic poisoning, and to loss of blood. The patient was a housekeeper, twenty-nine years old. Menstruation commenced at the age of eleven, and had been regular, but the period generally lasted from twelve to fifteen days. She had been married, and had three children in the course of several years. About November, 1876, she began to suffer from slight abdominal pain, but this did not interfere with her occupation. On February 19th menstruation commenced as usual (having been regular up to that time), and continued till March 1st, when she was suddenly seized with acute hypogastric pain, nausea, and vomiting, and became cold, faint, and extremely pale. A small clot was passed on this day, according to her description. Pallor and exhaustion increased, and on March 3d, she was admitted into the Hôpital de la Pitié.

At her admission she was excessively blanched, the mucous membranes decolorized, the tint of her skin like white wax turned yellow by age. In the abdomen was a firm, irregular, but elastic tumour, reaching up to two finger-breadths from the umbilicus, and extending into the pelvis. It filled the right iliac fossa, and in less degree, the left iliac fossa also. The cervix was much displaced upwards and forwards, and a rounded mass, not distinctly fluctuating, occupied the pelvis posterior to it. The os was soft, and admitted the tip of the finger. The patient stated that pregnancy was impossible. The diagnosis made was that of retro-uterine hæmatocele, with a large amount of blood effused. For several days repeated attacks of syncope occurred. Transfusion was several times contemplated, but was not performed. By the 9th distinct improvement had taken place. On the 17th pain commenced in the right iliac region, and the temperature rose to 40°.2 C., with some tympanitic distension of abdomen. These symptoms were attributed to peritoneal inflammation around the effusion, and lasted only three days, the highest temperature reached being 41°.2 C. On the 20th, the normal date of menstruation, a slight loss of blood commenced. On the same day, a peculiar spasmodic attack occurred, all the limbs, especially the arms, being strongly flexed. The head oscillated from side to side, and the eyes rolled. A similar fit occurred on the 21st. On the morning of the 22d a succession of epileptiform fits, like those of puerperal eclampsia, commenced. In the intervals there was complete unconsciousness, with tonic contraction of the arms, the face being pale, but lips purple from congestion. These attacks continued, without any recovery of consciousness, for about twenty-four hours. After this she appeared to become more conscious, but the face was congested as from asphyxia, and tracheal râles were heard ; temperature, 39°.5 C. She died on the evening of this day, the 23d of March.

At the autopsy, all the lower part of the abdomen was found to be filled with a large clot, inclosed within a kind of capsule formed by agglutination of intestinal coils. The uterus was pushed upwards and forwards, reaching three finger-breadths above the pubes. The right iliac fossa was filled, in great measure, by a portion of the clot. The different layers of the clot varied in colour and consistence, showing it to have been formed successively at different times, the most recent portion being that near to the right broad ligament. On carefully separating the clot an amniotic sac was discovered, containing a fœtus 5½ cm. in length, corresponding to a development of between 2½ and 3 months. The funis was slender, 9 cm. in length.   It was attached to a placenta 2 cm. in thickness, which was blended with the pavilion of the right Fallopian tube.   The right ovary showed a corpus luteum 2½ cm. in diameter.   Both Fallopian tubes were permeable and unaltered.   The uterus was 9 cm. in length, its walls 2 cm. thick.   It contained no decidua visible to the naked eye.   The quantity of clot turned out was 800 grammes, and the whole amount was estimated at about one kilogramme.   Both ureters had been compressed by the clot, and above the point compressed, were distended to the size of an egg.   The pelves and calices of the kidneys were dilated in corresponding degree, being on the right side at least three times their normal capacity ; on the left side not quite so large.   The urine was examined, and found to contain a very small proportion of urea, that in the bladder containing 6½ per 1000, that in the right ureter only 3½ per 1000.   The author attributes the eclamptic convulsions and the fatal result to uræmia, due to incomplete excretion of the urinary solids in consequence of the compression of the ureters, and commencing secondary deterioration in the kidney-structure.

Some interesting histological details are given of the structure of the placenta, from an examination made by Dr. de Sinety.   It proved to be closely analogous with the placenta of uterine pregnancy.   As in that case, the middle layer consisted of chorionic villi and blood sinuses.   Around the villi, as in the normal placenta, existed that layer of cells which by Ercolani are regarded as of maternal origin, and are identified with the giant cells of the decidua.   Towards the maternal surface such cells formed an almost continuous layer, less thick than in a uterine placenta, but identical in appearance.   Dr. de Sinety considers this a confirmation of his view that these cells are not derived from the uterine epithelium, but from lymphatic cells.   None of the non-vascular lacunæ, regarded as remnants of hypertrophied uterine glands, were discovered.   On microscopic examination of sections of the uterus the glands were found to be slightly hypertrophied, and the whole mucous membrane infiltrated with small round cells.   There was no trace of surface epithelium continuous with that lining the glands.   In parts the glandular layer was covered, on its internal surface, by a layer from ₁₀¹ to ¼ mm. in thickness, consisting of embryonic elements, among which numerous vessels were irregularly distributed.   On the whole there was much less development of decidua than in a tubal pregnancy of similar date described by Ercolani, a difference which the author thinks may be due to the fœtal sac having been more distant from the uterus, and so having acted less powerfully upon its nutrition.— *Obstetrical Journal of Great Britain*, Aug. 1878.

--

Erosions of the Cervix.

The views entertained hitherto regarding these pathological conditions promise to be considerably revolutionized by the recent investigations of Drs. C. RUGE and J. VEIT, of Berlin, into the pathology of the cervix uteri.   The results of these observers are the subject of a paper in the ii. band, 2 heft of the *Zeitschrift für Geburtshülfe und Gynäkologie*, page 415.   According to them, the prevailing views that regard these so-called erosions as granulating surfaces bereft of epithelium are entirely incorrect.   These reddened and irregular surfaces are in no case ulcerative, and their elevated portions are not composed of papillæ laid bare.   Observers such as Tyler Smith, who examined the surfaces microscopically, were led astray by the methods used in preparation of the sections which destroyed the epithelium covering the surface of the so-called erosion.   According to our authors, the essential nature of the disease consists in an irritation of the rete Malpighii, or formative layer of the flattened epithelium covering the cervix.   In consequence of this irritation the rete Malpighii is altered in character.   The cells formed by it are not transmuted into flattened epithelium cells, but are longer and larger, and arrange themselves at first in a single row of cylindrical cells below the normal epithelium. In consequence of this the superficial epithelium gets undermined and drops off. The surface that is covered by the single row of epithelium is at first smooth, but by-and-by prolongations of it grow into the subjacent tissue of the cervix. These prolongations inwards are at first solid, being formed of a solid ingrowth of epithelial particles; but presently they widen out at their deeper parts and become tubes, and many of them becoming constricted at the point where they leave the general mucous surface, are thus converted into glands. The tissues in the spaces between these inward growths of epithelium increase in size, grow outwards, and become peculiarly vascular. It is these hypertrophied intermediate spaces that have hitherto been regarded as enlarged cervical papillæ. According to our authors, every part of the reddened surface of these so-called erosions is covered over with a single row of cylindrical epithelium. The treatment must, according to Drs. Ruge and Veit, consist in accurately determining how much of the cervical surface is affected by this irritative degeneration. Then that portion has to be removed by the knife, or destroyed by some caustic. It is, according to our authors, immaterial what kind of caustic is employed, provided it is able to destroy the degenerate tissue.—*Edinburgh Med. Journal*, Aug. 1878.

The Dilatation of the Cervix Uteri by Tangle Tents.

This is the subject of an interesting article in No. 7 *Centralblatt für Gynäkologie* of this year, by Dr. B. S. SCHULTZE of Jena. The underlying principle of his procedure is the assumption that for safe dilatation the tangle tent must never come in contact with a raw wound surface. But, besides this, Dr. Schultze takes the strictest antiseptic precautions that the conditions of the operation allow of. To gain the end in view, namely, safe dilatation of the cervix, Schultze employs flexible copper sounds, of varying thickness, by which he ascertains the exact size and curvature of the cervical cavity. Having settled these points, a tangle tent, corresponding in thickness with the sound, which just passes the cervical cavity, is immersed for one or two minutes in boiling water, and being thus rendered flexible, the same curvature is given to it as that of the sound, which has been previously adapted to the cavity of the uterus. On cooling, the tent retains the curvature thus communicated to it, and after steeping it in a $\frac{3}{100}$ solution of carbolic acid, it is introduced through a speculum, the cervix being meanwhile held down by an assistant with a hook or vulsellum. If a drop of blood is seen coming from the cervix during any of these processes, the operation is to be postponed for at least twenty-four hours. The patient is to be kept strictly at rest during the whole time that the tent is dilating, and the strictest care is to be taken in the removal of the distended tent that no injury is caused to the cervix. The vagina and cervical canal ought to be then carefully washed out with a $\frac{1}{80}$ solution of carbolic acid. By these precautionary measures, the author states that he has been able, in several hundreds of cases, to dilate the cervix without any accident, and maintains that if his method is followed the usual contraindications to dilatation of the cervix can be very largely dispensed with. He holds that, according to his experience, chronic metritis, chronic perimetritis, and parametritis, even when the resulting catarrh is inconsiderable, are very beneficially influenced by repeated dilatation and subsequent washing out with carbolic acid. In a number of cases of enlargement of the uterus from chronic inflammation, Schultze was able to demonstrate by actual measurement diminution in size to have resulted from this treatment. These precautions seem to us worthy of consideration at the present time, when the attention of gynæcologists is so largely directed towards dilatation of the cervix as an aid in the treatment of uterine affections.—*Edinburgh Med. Journal*, Aug. 1878.

Distended Bladder simulating Ovarian Tumour.

Dr. LEDIARD, in the *Lancet*, p. 935, adds another to those deceptive cases where a vesical tumour simulated ovarian disease. The bladder had quite lost its power to contract on account of its long-continued overdistension.

[In the *Lancet*, vol. ii, 1875, p. 539, a somewhat similar case is reported by Dr. Jaccoud. Here the catheter failed to empty the bladder on account of atony of its muscular coats. Great dilatation of the bladder and uterus was found at the *post-mortem* examination.]—*London Med. Record*, Aug. 15, 1878.

Complicated Case of Ovariotomy.

In the *Wiener Medicinische Wochenschrift*, May, 1878, Dr. von MOSETIG-MOORHOF relates a case of bilateral ovariotomy. Emilie Dudisz, 21 years old, *puella publica*, came under his care in July, 1877, suffering from an abdominal tumour. Dr. Mosetig-Moorhof diagnosed an ovarian tumour and proceeded a few days afterwards to operate. After the cyst had been tapped by the trocar and drawn out of the abdomen, it was found to be the left ovary, and another tumour was found lying in the right hypochondrium. The second tumour proved to be a cystic dilatation of the Fallopian tube, the ovary at the extremity being normal and containing several corpora lutea. The ligamentum latum was transfixed with a catgut ligature, and the cystic dilatation, together with the right ovary, removed. A clamp was applied to the pedicle of the left ovary, and the abdomen closed. A Sims's drainage-tube was applied. The recovery was rapid and marked by absence of fever. The drainage-tube was removed from the vagina on the eighth day, the clamp fell off on the eleventh day, and on the fifteenth day the patient left her bed. Eight days later, she left the hospital in perfect health.—*London Med. Record*, July 15, 1878.

Medical Jurisprudence and Toxicology.

Malpraxis in Midwifery.

Prof. HERMANN FRIEDBERG, of Breslau, narrates, in Eulenberg's *Vierteljahr-schrift für Gerichtliche Medicin* for April, the particulars of a remarkable case of injury done to an infant during delivery, which he was requested to report upon as an expert.

A woman twenty-three years of age, taken in labour with her third child on March 16, 1877, sent for an unauthorized midwife, whom she had engaged to attend her. About twelve o'clock at night this woman discovered a hand presentation, and made repeated violent traction on the hand and arm at intervals until two o'clock in the morning, when the arm came away. The midwife then introduced her hand, and worked it about for about five minutes, causing great pain to the mother, who, unable to bear it, sprang out of bed. While she was sitting on the edge of her bed, the child was rapidly and easily expelled by the breech without any assistance. The cause of the child's death now became the subject of a legal investigation, which was consigned to Prof. Friedberg. At the autopsy it was found to be a full-timed, strong, healthy infant, the general surface of the body being remarkably pale. The left arm and shoulder-blade were separated from the body with much laceration of muscle and effusion of partly coagulated blood, the acromion and coracoid process, however, not having been fractured. The fifth to the ninth ribs were fractured near their anterior ends, coagulated blood adhering to the fractured parts and ruptured muscles. The lungs immediately sank in water, and no air issued on dividing them under water. An abnormal movability on the left side of the spine was found to arise from fracture of the necks of the seven upper ribs, accompanied by much effusion.

The autopsy is reported at much greater length, but these are the points that seem of most interest. From it Prof. Friedberg concluded that the child was a full-timed infant, which had never breathed, and therefore had never lived after its birth. Its death arose from the hemorrhage and contusion which had occurred during its birth, and which were caused by the violent manœuvres adopted by the midwife. As to the question whether the child was alive during the progress of the labour, Prof. Friedberg reports in the affirmative, not only because the patient and the midwife repeatedly affirmed that it moved, but from the condition of the blood observed after death, this being in a coagulated state in the vicinity of all the lacerated soft parts, while the separated arm, by its violaceous colour, tumefaction, and distension by red effusion, indicated that its circulation had been obstructed during life. The last point, that the death of the child was caused by the violent manipulation of the midwife, is demonstrated at what would seem almost needless length.

Prof. Friedberg rightly observes that this case stands alone in literature, and it would seem incredible, until the case had been carefully examined, that the woman here inculpated could, unaided by instruments, have torn off the arm and shoulder-blade and fractured numerous ribs of a strong and healthy child. To those in this country who are justly lamenting the want of regulations for midwives, it does seem surprising that in Prussia, where regulations of all kinds abound, this malpraxis could have been perpetrated by a woman "unauthorized to practise as a midwife," who yet had carried on such practice for nine years, during which she had delivered 347 women, many of whom no doubt have suffered more or less at the hands of one whom Prof. Friedberg stigmatizes somewhat mildly as a *Pfuscherin* or bungler.

The same number of the *Vierteljahrschrift* contains a report by Kreisphysikus Eberts on a somewhat similar case occurring at Weilberg. A maid-servant having become pregnant by her master, was delivered by a woman seventy-one years old, who, formerly a district midwife, had not attended a case for thirty years. She slept with her patient in the next room to that occupied by the father of the child and his wife, so that everything had to be managed as quietly as possible. The woman was delivered, and resumed her occupation next day, but a child's body having afterwards been discovered, she was apprehended. On examination the child was found full-time and viable, but it had never breathed since its birth. With the child its separated arm was found wrapped up in a cloth, and this had been divided at the mid-part of the humerus, the upper portion still remaining covered with a portion of the muscles. The left clavicle was also dislocated. The examination led to the death of the child, which was in a very bloodless state, being attributed to hemorrhage. A cutting instrument had evidently been used. The exact circumstances of the labour could not be known, as none but the midwife and patient were present, both of whom declared that the separation was spontaneous. The theory of the prosecution was that the presentation was a cross one, and that the midwife, in order to end it as soon as possible (a circumstance of importance in order to avoid detection), had seized hold of the hand instead of the foot, and made such violent traction as to dislocate the clavicle. Finding her efforts unsuccessful, she divided the arm with a knife, and then succeeded in turning, or a spontaneous evolution might have taken place.—*Med. Times and Gaz.*, July 27, 1878.

CONTENTS.

Published Monthly, price $2.50 per annum, free of postage. '
Also, furnished together with the AMERICAN JOURNAL OF THE MEDICAL
SCIENCES *and the* MEDICAL NEWS AND LIBRARY *for* SIX DOLLARS *per
annum in advance, the whole free of postage.*

HENRY C. LEA, Philadelphia.

THE MONTHLY ABSTRACT

MEDICAL SCIENCE.

Vol. V. No. 11.   **For List of Contents see last page.**   November, 1878.

Anatomy and Physiology.

The Degeneration and Regeneration of Nerves.

Some months ago we called attention to an interesting series of investigations on the histology of the process of the union of divided nerves, which elucidated the details of the process by which the adventitial structures of a divided nerve-trunk effect its reunion. The changes which the nerve-fibres themselves undergo in consequence of division, and those by which their repair after injury is effected, have lately been studied with much care by Dr. KORYBUTT-DASZKIEWICZ, of Strasburg, and his observations add considerably to our knowledge of the processes. A few hours after the division of a nerve, an opacity and swelling of its medullary sheath is visible, together with a multiplication of the nuclei of its primitive sheaths. These changes, which constitute the first stage of the well-known process of nerve degeneration, are visible in both peripheral and central ends of the divided nerve-fibres, as far as the first of the constrictions which Ranvier discovered. The process does not pass over this limit, or, if it does, only extends as far as the next constriction. Simultaneously with this change in the nerve-fibres red and white corpuscles aggregate in the neighbourhood of the incision. The latter multiply, and assume an appearance very like that of the nuclei of the nerve-sheath. The nuclei become surrounded by protoplasm, and, in the course of the next few days, form knob-like projections at each end of the nerve, which projections, when the loss of substance in the nerve has been small, ultimately become fused together. The cells which thus bridge the gap between the two ends acquire ultimately a spindle shape, become transformed into connective-tissue fibres, and do not assist in the regeneration of the nerve-fibres themselves.

If the so-called paralytic degeneration goes on in the peripheral end of the nerve, a fresh series of changes commence, consisting in the segmentation of the medullary sheath, which takes place either simultaneously in the entire length of a fibre, or only in parts, now near the wound, now near the periphery. The portion of the fibre affected first presents incurvations which give it somewhat the appearance of an embryonal condition of nerve-fibre. The affected segments break up into globules, which often present distinct concentric striation. If the degeneration progresses further, the outer layer of the globules becomes liquefied, and breaks up into fat-globules, which become distributed more or less uniformly within the old sheath. Wherever the myelin has thus broken up, nuclei accumulate; whereas at those parts which are still normal no nuclei are to be seen. At the cut end of the nerve it is not difficult to trace the passage of nuclei from the cicatricial tissue into the interior of the sheaths of the degenerated nerve, but it is less easy to trace the origin of the nuclei which are seen within the sheaths of the peripheral portions of the degenerated nerves. It seems, however, legitimate to assume here also that they have wandered in, because cases were repeatedly observed in which white blood-corpuscles passed into the sheaths at the constrictions of Ranvier. However they have entered, the nuclei multiply, at first rapidly, until they have attained a certain number, and then commences their individual development. They acquire distinct contours, assume a rounded form, and nucleoli become visible within them. During the first few hours after the operation, and before the white corpuscles commence to pass in, the fixed nuclei of the wider nerve-sheaths take part in the transformation of the myelin. The nuclei enlarge, a zone of protoplasm becomes visible around them, and into others often pass minute spherules of myelin, blackening with osmic acid.

In the central end of the nerve the changes are different. After the inflammatory degeneration has extended as far as one of the constrictions of Ranvier, a change in the myelin is visible in a certain proportion of the fibres, the number of which increases the greater the loss of substance. Either the medulla assumes a wavy contour, or it becomes liquefied in a segment lying between two constrictions, without the process invading adjacent parts. An increase of nuclei is constantly observed in the latter form of degeneration. After the liquefaction of the old myelin there commences the formation of a new nerve-medulla, with the peculiar appearance that between two former constrictions one or two new ones are formed. The nuclei of the sheath of Schwann also undergo changes in the central end. Near the division of the nerve they swell up, become surrounded by granular protoplasm, and, after becoming separated from the fibres, assume an elongated form; whether finally developing to nerve-fibres could not be definitely ascertained. The axis-cylinders in the peripheral part break up into more or less numerous fragments during the segmentation of the medulla, and of these some apparently liquefy and participate in the same changes as the myelin, while others persist and clothe themselves with a new medullary sheath. In some cases the myelin remained upon some fragments of axis-cylinders until regeneration. Before the degenerated myelin began to lessen the fragments of axis-cylinders which persisted began to lengthen in each direction, the nuclei persisting within the sheath began to elongate, and lay at certain distances from each other. Simultaneously with this process, the new medullary sheath made its appearance as a varicose or a uniform deposit upon the axis-cylinder. Thus the fragments of axis-cylinder remaining serve as the starting point for a new endogenous formation of nerve-fibres. They present no tendency, in their farther growth to blend with one another, but remain in contiguity, growing in the same general sheath, close to one another, and ultimately, after the disappearance of the old sheath of Schwann, they develop as independent fibres. Hence, at a certain time, there is an appearance as of several nerve-fibres in a single sheath. If, however, after the division of a nerve, the axis-cylinder remains intact in its entire length, and the medullary sheath degenerates, the appearance of several fibres in the same fibre-sheath is never seen. If the division of the nerve entails a considerable loss of its substance, the appearance of a multiple endogenous regeneration of fibres is rarely seen, many fibres not being regenerated at all. This segmentation of the axis-cylinder is not the only mode in which the fibres degenerate. The gray fibres for example, sometimes present no change, and the smaller medullated fibres, regarded as young nerve-fibres, ordinarily only lose their medullary sheath; and, lastly, under certain favourable conditions, most of the fibres, large and small, present only medullary degeneration.

The regeneration of the extremities of the nerves in the muscle and skin occurs much later than the regeneration of the peripheral trunk, as the axis-cylinders of the terminal extremities of the nerves usually undergo complete degeneration.

On simple division of a nerve, the adjacent axis-cylinders of the central stump do not degenerate, but grow into the cicatricial tissue, where they become narrowed and clothed with a deposit of young medulla. Attaining the peripheral portion of the trunk, they become wider, and grow into it between the old and the new fibres. The path they take through the cicatricial tissue is evidently that of least resistance, being often sinuous. They often apparently attach themselves to vessels, which afterwards disappear. If the peripheral portion is absent altogether, as in extirpation of a nerve, the fibres growing from the centre commonly either attach themselves to a vessel, or widen out irregularly, or form knobby swellings analogous to the "bulbous nerves" of amputated limbs, which are formed by a convolution of medullated fibres and cicatricial tissue. When the loss of substance has been considerable, the regeneration of the fibres which degenerate in the central end occurs much more quickly than that of those in the peripheral end, but takes place by a similar process.—*Lancet*, Sept. 21, 1878.

The Magnitude of the Nerve Cells.

Upon what depend the variations in size of the cells of the central nervous system? An attempt at an answer to this question has been lately given to the Académie des Sciences by M. PIERRET, Professor at Lyons, who suggests that the size of the cell is in simple relation to the length of the fibre connected with it. Of the motor nervous system the largest nerve-cells are situated in the lumbar region of the spinal cord, and in the fronto-parietal convolutions. These two points are related one to the other, and the distance which separates them is very considerable. Moreover, the longest nerves of the body—the sciatic—arise from that point in the lumbar region in which are the largest motor cells. In the dorsal region the motor cells are far smaller. The distance from the brain is less, and the course of the nerves which spring from them is relatively short. In the cervical region the cells are larger than in the dorsal region, but smaller than those of the lumbar, which may be explained by the fact that they are not far from the brain; but the course of the nerves arising from them is of considerable length. So also with the hypoglossal nerve, the cells of which are only a little smaller than those of the cervical enlargement. For a similar reason the cells of the higher motor centres lessen in size in proportion as their distance from the cerebral hemispheres becomes less. Hence the sixth nerve is connected with larger cells than the third and fourth. Lastly, in the corpora striata the cells are still smaller, and may be distinguished in form from those of the optic thalami or corpora geniculata or corpora quadrigemina.

In the sensory system, the largest cells are found in the posterior vesicular column, in the neighbourhood of the lumbar enlargement. These cells probably receive the centripetal fibres from the lower limb, and they are removed for a considerable distance from the occipital lobes. The cells of the ganglia of the restiform body which receives the sensory fibres of the brachial nerves, and the neucleus of the sensory part of the fifth nerve, both have much smaller cells than those of the lumbar posterior vesicular columns, and they are much nearer the cerebral cortex. The cells of origin of the optic nerve are smaller than those of the fifth, and larger than those of the olfactory. The shortest nerve is that which is connected with the smallest cells—the auditory. Hence M. Pierret infers that the law which governs the increase or decrease in size of the cells is the same for both the sensory and motor cells, and may be formulated thus—that the size of the motor and sensory cells of the nerve-centres of man is directly proportioned to the distance which separates them from the peripheral organ which they innervate, and from the cerebral centre. This law is true for the cells of the cerebral cortex, for the largest cells are met with in the fronto-parietal regions related to the lower limbs, and in certain of the occipital convolutions cells are met with almost as large.

The theory is one of considerable interest, and there may be "something in it," but we doubt whether the accordance between the two elements, length of fibre and size of cell, is so close as to justify the formulation of so precise a law upon the subject. Moreover we know too little of the precise anatomical relations of the parts of the nervous system to permit us to generalize from the length of the fibres which probably commence and end within it. For instance, it is not at all proved that the fibres of the posterior nerve roots are connected with the cells of the posterior vesicular columns. The variety in size of the cells in the same group is also difficult to explain upon the theory of M. Pierret. The theory probably approaches as near an explanation as is possible in the present state of our knowledge, but it is doubtful whether that knowledge is yet sufficiently accurate to permit useful generalization.—*Lancet*, September 7, 1878.

The Analysis of Milk.

M. A. ADAM has sent to the Académie des Sciences a note on the new process for the analysis of milk, which gives rapidly the amount of butter, of lactose, and of casein in a uniform scale. The apparatus employed for the analysis consists essentially of a glass tube, holding forty centimetres, having a stopper above and a glass tube and stop-cock below. Into this is introduced, first, ten cubic centimetres of alcohol at 75° C., containing $\frac{1}{200}$ of its volume of caustic soda; secondly, ten cubic centimetres of neutral milk ; and, thirdly, twelve cubic centimetres of pure ether. The tube is closed, well shaken, and allowed to rest for ten minutes. Almost instantly two layers are formed, sharply separated—an upper, limpid layer, containing all the butter ; secondly, a lower opalescent layer, containing all the lactose and all the casein. The lower layer is then drawn out, with the exception of about one centimetre. That which remains is then shaken up with the upper layer. This buttery solution is allowed to run out into a porcelain capsule, and is washed with ether to collect the fat evaporated, and weighed. The difference gives the weight of the butter increased by one centigramme in consequence of adherent lacto-caseous matter. If the ether is then evaporated in another capsule, the direct weight of the butter is ascertained. In order to separate and estimate the lactose and casein, the liquid first drawn off is diluted with distilled water to 100 cubic centimetres, and ten drops of acetic acid are added. The casein then separates in a flocculent precipitate, like that of nitrate of silver. After allowing it to stand for five minutes, it is poured upon a dry filter, which is kept covered to prevent evaporation. Thus 94 to 96 per cent. is collected of a liquid which contains only the salts of the milk, acetate of soda formed during the process, and lactose. The latter is then estimated by means of Fehling's solution. If a known volume is then evaporated to dryness, the amount of lactose can also be distinguished by two weighings, one before, the other after, incineration, deducting from the weight thus obtained that of the acetic acid combined with the soda. This casein is washed two or three times with distilled water, and the filtering paper containing it is strongly pressed between two layers of paper to flatten it as much as possible, and it can then be dried in a few minutes. The weight of the filter before and after the operation gives that of the casein. Or the casein may be detached from the filter, dried, and weighed. These operations are easily executed in an hour and a half, and if at the beginning an additional ten cubic centimetres of milk is placed to evaporate with two drops of acetic acid, the amount of dry residue of water and of ashes may also be ascertained. Five cubic centimetres of milk will suffice for the analysis, and the apparatus is very portable.—*Lancet*, Sept. 7, 1878.

Materia Medica and Therapeutics.

The Diffusion of Salicylate of Soda.

The rapid diffusion through the system of salicylate of soda, which its action and rapid excretion suggest, has been confirmed experimentally by M M. CH. LIVON and J. BERNARD. In their investigations they have confirmed the conclusions of previous observers regarding the action of salicylate on the conscious sensibility; the production of tetanic contractions and convulsive movements, and disturbances of respiration and of the cardiac pulsations, due to the alteration of the reflex action of the medulla and cord. Their observations were, however, especially directed to the diffusion of salicylate in the economy, and the means by which it is eliminated. For the detection of the salicylate they have employed the perchloride of iron, which remains the most delicate reagent known. In the first experiment six grammes of salicylate of soda were injected into the stomach of a dog. The œsophagus was tied; two hours afterwards the salicylate was found in the saliva. In the second experiment ten grammes were injected into the stomach, and an hour afterwards the salicylate was found in the bile. In the third experiment three grammes of salicylate were injected into the femoral vein, and an hour later it was found in the bile. In a fourth experiment seven grammes were injected into the stomach, and four hours later the salicylate was found in the pancreatic juice. In a fifth, two centigrammes were injected under the skin of a guinea-pig, and one hour afterwards the salicylate was found in the milk. The method of detecting the substance was to heat the liquid with hydrochloric acid, and then shake it up with ether. Evaporation of the ether leaves a residue which gives, with perchloride of iron, the characteristic violet tint. The saliva, the bile, and the pancreatic juice were collected by means of fistulæ. The feces and urine also showed evidences of the salicylate. In all the experiments upon dogs it was found also that the cerebro-spinal fluid contained salicylate, even several hours after the administration of the drug. It is suggested that probably it is the presence of the drug in the fluid which bathes the central organs of the nervous system which accounts for its action upon them. By the injection of from two to ten centigrammes of salicylate through the occipito-atloidean ligament into the spinal canal, all the phenomena of salicylic poisoning were rapidly obtained. The precaution was taken first to withdraw an equal bulk of the cerebro-spinal liquid, so as to prevent any compression of the cord. For the sake of controlling the experiment, simple water was, in another experiment, injected in the same manner, with the effect, however, of causing only prostration, and not the tetanizing effects of the salicylate.—*Lancet*, Aug. 31, 1878.

The Assimilation of Quinia.

The relation of the amount of quinine eliminated by the urine to that taken by the mouth has been studied by M. PERSONNE, with the object of determining what proportion is destroyed in the economy. He concludes that about one-half of that taken in is destroyed. He found that all the quinine which is eliminated by the urine and soluble in acids can be transformed into neutral sulphate of quinine without appreciable residue; also that a resinous material if obtained, insoluble in acids and similar to that which is obtained during the extraction of the alkaloids of chinchona. Hence it is inferred that the quinine which is eliminated by the urine has not undergone any appreciable alteration or isomeric modification. These substances represent nearly one-half of the quinine which is taken in, and hence at least one-half must be destroyed in the economy.—*Lancet*, Sept. 7, 1878.

The Preparation of Fats and Oils for Absorption.

An explanation of the mode in which the absorption of fatty substances is effected from the alimentary canal has always been a subject of considerable difficulty both to the physicist and to the physiologist.   Formerly the only preparation to which the oleaginous constituents of our food were supposed to be subjected was their liquefaction and minute subdivision, effected partly by the warmth and partly by the triturating movements of the stomach.   An important step in advance was made by Wistinghausen, when he observed that oily substances rose higher in capillary tubes which had previously been moistened with an alkaline fluid than when pure, and applied this observation in explanation of the influence of the bile on the absorption of oily substances, noticing further that such oily fluids could be more readily pressed through membranes moistened with a solution of the biliary salts than under their ordinary condition.

Still more recently E. v. Bruecke has shown that the formation of an emulsion, when oil is mingled with dilute albumen, with fresh ox-gall still containing mucus, or with a dilute solution of borax or sodium carbonate, is much more easily and completely effected if, instead of being perfectly pure, the oil is slightly rancid—that is to say, has undergone partial decomposition into the fatty acids.   Pure and neutral oil, he remarked, shaken up with either of these fluids forms proportionately large drops, which quickly re-unite, but if they be mingled with the fatty acids, a white and permanent milk is at once formed.   Bruecke further demonstrated that sodium carbonate has little action in emulsifying fats if free acids be present ; they combine with a part of the soda to form a soap, and the emulsification is then easily effected.   The same thing can be shown in another way by adding a small quantity of a solution of soap to pure oil, when a persistent emulsion can be quickly made.   An interesting paper has just been published by J. Gad in His and Braune's *Archiv fur Anatomie,* in which he gives the results of his observation on this point, and essentially confirms Bruecke's statements.   He points out that the mere contact of rancid oil with an alkaline solution is attended by violent commotion at the time of junction of the two fluids, which leads to the spontaneous formation of an emulsion without any mechanical agitation being resorted to.   If a drop of oil be thus placed in contact with an alkaline solution it soon begins to exhibit amœboid movements, sending out processess which, after giving off a white milk from their borders, are again drawn in, some small droplets often remaining detached, the original drop after a time resuming its original circular form.   If the separated droplets be isolated in another fresh portion of the soapy fluid no new movements are observed.   The experiments prove that fats only form a good emulsion so long as they contain free fatty acids, and these become exhausted in the emulsifying process.   The oils experimented on by Gad, all of which have yielded similar results, have been olive, almond, castor, neat's-foot, and liver.   He finds that the emulsifying capacity of the several oils with a given fluid differs in accordance with the degree of their acidity, with the solubility of the soap formed in the fluid, and with the viscidity of the fat ; whilst the emulsifying power of the same oil with different fluids depends partly on the grade of alkalescence of this fluid, and partly on its power of dissolving the soaps that are formed.   The excellence and completeness of the emulsion occur under those conditions in which the formation of membranes can be just no longer discerned, for under conditions which are favourable to the solution of the soaps that are formed no emulsification occurs at all, whilst under those that are favourable to the formation of firm membrane the resulting emulsion is less perfect, and is rendered impure by the presence of particles of soap.   Common salt and bile, he finds, supply conditions that favour emulsification, and correct opposing influences.

If we attempt to apply some of these observations to physiology, it will be seen that, when fats and oils are taken into the stomach, the warmth and moisture to which they are there subject are conditions favourable to the occurrence, in some degree, of decomposition and slight acidification—a fact that is supported by the statement occasionally advanced that the acid of the gastric juice is butyric acid. The high acidity of the fluids secreted by the stomach, however, prevents emulsification taking place to any great extent in this cavity. This acidity is corrected by the alkaline salts of the bile; and thenceforward, in their passage through the alimentary canal, the minutely subdivided fats and oils are continually exposed to fresh quantities of alkaline fluids, by which their emulsification is effected and maintained.

Seeing, then, that a slightly acid condition of fats is a preliminary condition to their absorption, the question put by Bruecke, Why do we not consume fats in a rancid condition? is a very pertinent one; and the reply given by Gad is, first, that cod-liver oil, which, though certainly not taken *con gusto* by most people, yet is not, after a time, distasteful, and undoubtedly possesses highly nutritive properties, has a well-marked acid reaction. Secondly, that fats the acids of which form soaps that are soluble with difficulty, like those in ordinary use, give the best emulsions when only very feebly acidified. Thirdly, that, urged by a natural impulse, we consume fat almost always in combination with more or less common salt, which promotes the emulsification of feebly acid oil when mingled with dilute solution of soda. Lastly, it may be observed that that part of the canal into which the pancreatic fluid flows, which Bruecke has shown to possess so powerful an influence in disintegrating fats, is specially favourable to the act of their emulsification, the fatty acids that are thus formed combining with the alkaline fluids poured forth by the intestine, and greatly aiding the process.—*Lancet*, Sept. 28, 1878.

Mode of Action of Cathartics.

L. BRIGER (*Archiv für Exper. Pathol. und Pharmak*, Bd. viii. p. 355), at the instance of Professor Cohnheim, made some experiments to determine the mode of action of cathartics, which are abstracted in the *Clinic*. It was held, on the authority of Liebig, that the artificial increase of the alvine evacuations is chiefly due to endosmosis; but the experiments of Thiry, Schiff, Aubert, Buchheim, and Radziejewski seemed to show that neither transudation nor secretion is increased, and that acceleration of the peristaltic movements by which the fluid contents of the intestines are so rapidly carried forward that absorption cannot take place, is the sole effect produced by cathartics. Moreau, however, from his experiments, came to the conclusion that secretion is increased. Lately, Lauder Brunton (*Practitioner*, 1874, Nos. 71 and 72) again called attention to the method of Moreau, which is as simple as it is exact. L. Briger pursued the same method in his experiments, which were performed on large, strong dogs. After fasting from two to three days, in order that the intestinal canal might be as empty as possible, the animal was narcotized with morphia; then the abdominal cavity was opened and a loop of intestine as long as possible was withdrawn. This was tied at each extremity, and after two punctures had been made, one near each ligature, the loop was thoroughly cleansed by the injection of warm water. After closing the punctures with sutures, the loop was divided into three parts of equal length by ligatures thrown around the serous covering. The middle part was not used, but served as a means of comparison with the other parts into which cathartics were slowly injected with a Pravaz syringe. The whole procedure rarely required more than ten minutes, and after it was finished the animals were unfastened, left under the influence of morphia, and, after about four and a half hours, were killed with chloroform or a blow on the head. Five *grammes* of a half per cent. solution of sulphate of magnesium were injected into one loop, and the same quantity of a one per cent. solution into the other. Both loops were found empty, the mucous membrane pale but normal. These very dilute solutions were simply absorbed. After the injection of a twenty per cent. solution of sulphate of magnesium, the loops were always completely filled with a thin, light yellow alkaline fluid, in which were suspended mucous shreds. These shreds were dissolved by caustic soda, but, if acetic acid were added in excess, a flocculent precipitate was thrown down. Treated with boiled starch or cane sugar, the fluid yielded in an hour and a half, at the ordinary temperature, tested by Trommer's method, evidence of the presence of glucose. Without any further addition, it showed, after boiling with a solution of potassa and sulphate of copper, the violet discoloration which was described of the intestinal juice obtained through fistulæ by Thiry and Quincke. Raw fibrin was dissolved in twelve hours at a high temperature; but boiled fibrin and ovalbumen were not changed. On microscopic examination, no red blood-corpuscles were found, but it contained many mucus-corpuscles, peculiar elements marked with vacuoles and intestinal epithelium. After the injection of two *grammes* of a fifty per cent. solution, there was found in the loop 23.5 *grammes* of a fluid having the properties described above, and a specific gravity of 1025 to 1030. Numerous other experiments were attended by similar results. *Drastics.*—Half a drop of croton-oil, dissolved in 2.25 *grammes* of ether, produced in the intestine 18 *grammes* of bloody fluid. In two other cases, when dissolved in 0.5 *gramme* of olive-oil, it produced respectively 10 and 11 *grammes* of bloody fluid. Extract of colocynth, injected with 2 *grammes* of water, acted as follows in the doses specified: 0.02 *gramme*, no accumulation, intestine empty, contracted, and slightly reddened; 0.04 to 0 10 *gramme* bloody fluid, mucous membrane totally inflamed; 0.05 to 0.1 *gramme*, completely filled with bloody contents; mucous membrane presents diphtheritic inflammation. In all the cases, the contents of the intestine responded to the saccharine test, and rapidly dissolved flakes of fibrin. Examined with the microscope, they presented in great abundance red and white blood-corpuscles, much epithelium, mucus, and shred of fibrin. *Laxatives.*—The substances used were the following: calomel, senna, rhubarb, aloes, gamboge, and castor-oil. The dogs were killed at various intervals, after 4½, 5, 7, and 16 hours. Without exception, the loops of intestine were found empty, firmly contracted, and not in the least inflamed, and the injected substance was spread over the whole surface. Substances acting mechanically only, as shot and pledgets of cotton, produced no effects. The aqueous constituents of the injected fluids were completely absorbed during the time of the experiments; thus, of fifteen *grammes* of compound infusion of senna, there remained only a semi-solid mass; but the castor-oil was found undiminished. Cinnabar, which was intimately mixed with castor-oil in two cases, was found neither in the lacteals passing from the intestine, nor in the adjacent lymphatic glands or thoracic duct. In regard to the laxatives, it would seem that their action depends upon an increase of peristaltic movements, for the loops were found contracted and coated with the medicine. The energetic movements of the intestinal wall had spread them in all directions. According to the results obtained, it cannot be doubted that the neutral salts strongly attract water and increase secretion. The drastics, in small doses, may be compared with the laxatives; but in large doses they produce inflammatory exudation and hypersecretion. In regard to both the neutral salts and the drastics, the properties of the intestinal contents, show that in all cases there is not merely transudation, which augments the water in the intestines, but actual increase of the action of the intestinal glands.—*British Med. Journal,* July 27, 1878.

—

Action of Iodoform.

Dr. SIGMUND, of Vienna (*Deutsche Med. Wochenschr.*, Aug. 10), has used iodoform with very successful results in ulcerative and indurative processes, glandular swellings, rhagades, and gummata. He employed the following formulæ: Iodoform and spirit, each one part, glycerine 5 parts; or 1 part of iodoform in 3 or 4 of sugar; or 1 of iodoform in 5 of vaseline; or iodoform collodion (1 in 10 or 1 in 15). The pain was unimportant; the surface of the sores became clean in from twenty-four to forty-eight hours, and granulated favourably. The offensive smell of diphtheritic and cancerous ulcerations was entirely removed by the remedy. Dry iodoform in powder, applied to fresh wounds, forms an uniform firmly adherent paste.—*British Med. Journal*, Sept. 28, 1878.

—

Therapeutic Uses of Peruvian Balsam.

Dr. E. WISS (*Deutsche Zeitschrift für prakt. Medicin*, Aug. 24) gives this remedy internally according to the following formula. R. Peruvian balsam 2 drachms; mucilage of gum arabic half a drachm; the yolk of one egg; distilled water 52½ drachms; syrup of cinnamon 7½ drachms. For wounds and ulcers, he uses the balsam undiluted, pouring it into the wound and then applying compresses soaked in it. For recent wounds, one daily dressing is sufficient: for ulcers, the dressing must be renewed once or twice daily, according to the amount of suppuration. Dr. Wiss calls attention to three special properties of the balsam; it relieves pain, assists healing, and is antiseptic. Repair takes place without suppuration or inflammation; and there is no contraction of the cicatrix. He has given it internally with good result in cases of chronic bronchitis, to which he has been called on account of the appearance of severe dyspnœa, from a renewal of the subacute affection of the bronchial mucous membrane or from obstruction of the bronchi with mucus. In these cases, his first proceeding has been to remove the dyspnœa by an emetic. He has then given balsam of copaiba, which has improved the character of the sputa, but has not reduced their quantity nor relieved the cough. Under the use of Peruvian balsam, however, all the symptoms of bronchial catarrh have disappeared, including even cough of several years' duration. He gives it only in cases of pure chronic bronchitis, not having found it useful in tuberculous cases. He considers it desirable that a more extensive trial should be made of it in hospital practice, in the treatment of large wounds, such as those produced in amputation and in the opening of large abscesses. In many cases where Lister's apparatus is not always at hand—in war, in travelling, and in country practice—Peruvian balsam will be a valuable substitute.—*British Med. Journal*, Sept. 28, 1878.

—

Chloral as an Anæsthetic for Children.

Dr. BOUCHUT, in a paper in the *Gazette des Hopitaux* (August 13), states that since he first announced, in 1869, the anæsthetic properties of chloral in the surgery of childhood, and its value in bad cases of chorea, daily experience has confirmed the accuracy of his affirmation. More than 10,000 cases now testify to this, as for the last nine years from four to eight patients have taken this medicine in anæsthetic doses. Perhaps the same good effects might be obtained also in adults, but it is found that they cannot be got to swallow a sufficient dose without producing vomiting. Infants, however, take the chloral in sufficient doses readily, and do not eject it. According to age, from one to four grammes are given, not exceeding three grammes, however, in children under three years of age, and two grammes may be given between two and five years without danger. The whole quantity is to be given at a single dose in 100 grammes of a highly sweetened vehicle. Half an hour after, the children are asleep; and an hour after, they are insensible. The insensibility lasts from three to six hours, and on awaking from it no disagreeable effects are experienced, the children taking their food and playing as usual. The same dose may be repeated the next and following days if required; and in chorea some children take these doses for a month together without inconvenience, as much as from 100 to 125 grammes having been taken in a month. Exceptionally, the anæsthesia is preceded by a stage of excitement, but so rarely that it has not been met with more than ten times in 10,000 cases. This means being so certain, and never being attended or followed by any accident, Dr. Bouchut always employs it for all operations on children, however trivial, the only inconvenience being that they continue to sleep three or four hours afterwards. These results are of great importance when it is remembered what difficulty and resistance are met with during operations on children. If there were any danger attending the use of this means, its employment in such cases should never be thought of; but there is absolutely none. The anæsthetic effect may also be produced by administering the same dose as an enema; but as this may be ejected, and the anæsthetic effect not be produced, it is better to use the chloral as a suppository, made with the *baume de cacao* melted with a fourth of spermaceti, which is essential to the incorporation of the chloral. This, however, is a bad mode of administration if the chloral has to be continued for a long time, as after three or four introductions the mucous membrane of the rectum becomes irritated, and a painful tenesmus is produced. But, after even long administration by the mouth, no gastro-enteritis is produced in children, no loss of appetite, foul tongue, or pain, etc.—a tolerance taking place in them which is not observed in the adult.—*Med. Times and Gaz.*, Sep. 7, 1878.

—

Chlorhydrate of Pilocarpine in Ophthalmic Practice.

Dr. ALEXANDROFF states (*Pamphlet*, Marseilles, 1877) that Jaborandi for various reasons is not well adapted for administration; it has a disagreeable taste, it sits uneasily on the stomach, causing nausea, vomiting, and sometimes colic; it produces vertigo and fainting, and lastly it has the disadvantage of being inconstant in its action. Pilocarpine the active principle of Jaborandi—discovered by Hardy in 1875—is free from some of these inconveniences, and its action has been studied on patients affected with rheumatism, albuminous nephritis, and pleurisy; but until his own observations, no attempts had been made, M. Alexandroff states, to ascertain its physiological value in diseases of the eye, except those of M. Weckei, who treated a few cases by hypodermic injection of the chlorhydrate. M. Alexandroff determined to investigate its action, and tried it first in a case of rheumatismal indo-choroiditis. The case was sufficiently severe to induce M. Metaxas to recommend iridectomy, to which the patient refused to submit. About 2 centigrammes of the chlorhydrate of pilocarpine in solution in water was, with M. Melaxas's permission, injected by M. Alexandroff into the arm of the patient, atropine being at the same time instilled into the eye. The patient passed a better night and was free from pain; on the following day the injection was repeated, and again at intervals on five occasions. Under this treatment the media became clear, the ulcer which had been present healed, and vision was completely restored. M. Melaxas tried the chlorhydrate again in a second case of double rheumatic iritis with equal success, and it was afterwards tried not only in many cases of rheumatic iritis, but in retinal hemorrhage, and in exudative choroiditis with good effect. In all instances salivation and sweating appear to have been produced, diarrhœa was occasionally observed. Epiphora was constant. The pulse and temperature rose immediately after the injection. He thinks it has an indisputable action on the iris, and finds that it acts more rapidly than eserine. It is at once the antagonist and antidote to atropine. It occasionally produces severe præcordial pain and feeling of anxiety. He thinks it will prove valuable, not only in cases of rheumatic iritis, but in all cases when the area of the pupil, the choroid, and the retina are the seats of serous or plastic exudation either from local or general disease.—*Practitioner*, September, 1878.

—

Belladonna in Infantile Diseases.

In a clinical lecture (*Le Progrès Medicale*, June 8) delivered at the Hopital des Enfants Malades, M. JULES SIMON gave the following summary of the physiological action of belladonna. In some respects the action of belladonna is opposed to that of opium. Applied locally to a blistered surface of the skin, or to the mucous membranes, belladonna is irritating, as is shown by the action of a strong solution of atropine on the conjunctiva. Hence it has been placed amongst the acro-narcotics. In small doses, by its action on the pharyngeal mucous membrane, it produces dryness, inability to speak clearly, and dysphagia, and in large doses it causes nausea, vomiting, and diarrhœa. At first the pulse is rendered slower and harder, but with a higher degree of action the pulse becomes full, strong, and frequent; the temperature rises a little; there is redness of the face, and brightness of the eyes, with mydriasis. The respiratory movements are rendered more active, and the bronchial secretion is diminished; hence its utility in humid asthma. In very large doses the respiration becomes gasping and convulsive. It is eliminated rapidly by the kidneys, and augments the urinary secretion. It diminishes the secretion of the sweat, and sometimes produces incomplete cutaneous anæsthesia. Its action on the skin in producing a scarlatiniform eruption, chiefly affecting the face, is well known, the exanthema disappears after a few hours without desquamation. Speaking generally, it appears at first to excite the vaso-constrictors, in consequence of which there is diminution of the secretions, retinal and cutaneous anæsthesia, and in part, perhaps, dilatation of the pupil. The blood-pressure and the urinary secretion are augmented. In large doses the vaso-motor nerves are paralyzed, and insomnia, agitation, and delirium occur. M. Simon frequently prescribes it with success in whooping-cough and other nervous diseases.—*Practitioner*, September, 1878.

—

Metalloscopy.

The announcement that anæsthesia could be temporarily removed by applying pieces of metal to the affected skin was received with considerable distrust last year, both in this country and in Germany; yet, after all, it turns out to be perfectly true. It may be remembered that we owe the discovery of this fact to a French physician named Burq, who also asserted that every patient has a particular idiosyncrasy for the action of a particular metal, and that there is a relation between the sensibility of the skin and the general condition of the patient, of such a nature that the latter can be cured by the internal administration of the same metal which cures the anæsthesia when applied to the skin. At Burq's request these statements were tested by a Commission appointed by the Société de Biologie in the winter of 1876–77. The members of the Commission were Drs. Charcot, Luys, and Dumontpallier, and their report, which was presented

to the Socié'é de Biologie on April 14, 1877, and which was founded on experiments made in Professor Charcot's wards at the Salpétrière Hospital, not only in
the main confirmed Burq's assertions, but supplied new facts bearing on the subject. Still more recently, Professor Westphal, of Berlin, in a lecture given before the Berlin Medical Society on June 5, 1878 (*Berliner Klin. Wochenschrift,*
No. 30, 1878), after a personal visit to Professor Charcot's wards, has declared
his belief in the reality of the phenomena described, and has supplemented the
experiments of the Commission by some new and interesting ones of his own.
Before speaking of the established facts concerning metalloscopy, we must mention
tion expressly that the class of cases to which the treatment—if such it can be
called—by metal plates applies, are almost exclusively hysterical women with
anæsthesia of one half of the body sharply limited at the middle line (hemianæsthesia), which has come on either without apparent cause, or as the result of hysterical attacks. At the same time there is diminished functional activity of all
the organs of sense, the acuteness of hearing, tasting, and smelling, and the power
of distinguishing between certain colours being either deadened or entirely lost on
the affected side. There may also be loss of the muscular sense on the same side,
so that the patient has to hunt about, so to speak, with the healthy hand for the
aim of the anæsthetic side, if the latter be placed in any position of which she had
no previous knowledge. Now, the Commission found that if a metal plate were
brought into close contact with a part of the anæsthetic skin, in from ten to twenty
minutes the latter, and a greater or less area of skin outside it, recovered its sensation. In some cases, if the metal was allowed to remain long enough, the whole
anæsthetic half of the body sometimes recovered its sensibility ; while in others
the impaired colour-sense was restored by applying metal plates to the forehead
and temples of the affected side. The anæsthesia could also be removed by
placing the poles of a powerful horseshoe magnet on the skin ; and even in one
case by allowing the hand of the patient to remain between the poles of a very
powerful electro-magnet without touching them. In all these experiments it was
discovered by the Commission that a transfer of sensibility took place from the
healthy to the anæsthetic side of the body, so that what was anæsthetic before recovered its sensibility, and what was sensible before became anæsthetic. All these
facts are confirmed by Professor Westphal. The Commission also observed that
a prick made into anæsthetic skin bled very little, if at all, while the blood issued
freely when its sensibility was restored. It also affirmed that the muscular power
of the anæsthetic limb was increased on the restoration of sensibility to the skin,
while, at the same time, the opposite healthy limb became correspondingly weaker.
The Commission did not examine the internal action of metals in these cases, but
it endeavoured to explain the effects produced by external metallic plates by the
development of galvanic currents. In conjunction with Dr. Regnard, the Commissioners found that such currents were actually produced and could be detected
by a very delicate galvanometer ; that different metals produced currents of different intensities ; and, lastly, that extremely weak galvanic currents could be substituted for the application of the metal plates, so as to restore the sensibility of anæsthetic skin. Still more interesting, however, is the observation that while the current
which made the galvanometer-needle deviate 7° had no effect on the anæsthesia,
a current of 35° restored the sensibility ; and that while one of 60° had no effect,
one of 90° was again effective. This proves that there exist for each patient
strengths of current which produce definite effects, and other strengths—the so-
called "neutral points"—which are inactive, no matter how long the electrodes
are applied. Lastly, it was discovered that if one pole of an active current were
applied to the head, and the other to the leg of the anæsthetic side, the sensibility

retuined not only to the skin, but also to the organs of sense, and was lost over the whole of the previously healthy side.

In speaking of Professor Westphal's experiments, we need only refer to the new points which he made out, and pass over those parts of his lecture which merely relate to confirmatory repetitions of Charcot's experiments. Thus he found that the phenomena of transfer of sensation from the healthy to the diseased side of the body was not *always* to be detected; perhaps, as he explains it, because the patient was not examined at the right time. It was also found in one case that sensibility could be restored by the application of plates either of iron or gold, whereas the rule is that only one metal influences a particular patient. In another case a bar magnet was placed parallel to the anæsthetic arm, and fastened so that both its poles were in contact with the limb; and it appeared as the result of numerous trials that sensibility first returned and last disappeared in the region of the *south* pole. Experiments were also made with plates of copper varnished or coated with sealing-wax on the side applied to the skin, and also with bone counters such as are used with marking at cards, and in all cases there was a return of sensibility, at any rate in the parts pressed on by the plates and counters and by the gauze bandages by which they were very firmly fixed in position. In fact, "the presence of sensibility appeared," says Dr. Westphal, "to depend on the amount of pressure used in securing them." Some experiments made by Prof. Westphal's assistant (Dr. Adamkiewicz) with mustard plasters are also of interest, as bearing on the theory of action of the various agents used to restore sensibility to the skin. He found that after about two hours the skin which was reddened by the plaster became completely sensitive to pricks and other stimuli, and that by applying plasters to different portions of the anæsthetic skin, areæ could be produced, within which the patient, with her eyes shut, could accurately localize a stimulus; whereas, in the intervening space she could not feel the most severe irritants at all. It is important to notice that sensibility did not return if the anæsthetic hand were soaked in hot water until it was swollen and strongly reddened, and that the irritation of the electric brush was entirely without effect in restoring it. One other point may be referred to before leaving this part of the subject, viz., that Professor Westphal has confirmed in his own patients an observation of Charcot's, that pressure on a particular part of the abdomen of the anæsthetic side is very painful; but he doubts Charcot's explanation that the pain is due to pressure on the ovary.

The question now arises, Is there any deception in these cases on the part of the patients? To this Professor Westphal replies, Certainly not. One of these patients was pricked while in a deep sleep at night on an anæsthetic part of the skin without the slightest effect, whereas she woke immediately the healthy skin was pricked. Again, a number of patients only discovered that they were anæsthetic at all when they were examined after admission to the hospital, and the object with which the metal plates were used was carefully concealed from the first patients experimented on. No attempt at deception in other ways was observed in any of the patients during their stay in the hospital; and the peculiar distribution of the anæsthesia, which, it should be noted, is sometimes interrupted by small circumscribed islands of sensitive skin, is not at all favourable to the idea of simulation. Moreover, Professor Charcot and Dr. Magnan have both observed a return of sensibility in the hemianæsthesia of organic disease under metalloscopic treatment. On the whole, therefore, Professor Westphal confirms the results of the French experimenters, while it is clear that his own experiments are opposed to the exclusive explanation of such remarkable facts by a theory of galvanic currents. He supposes that the restoration of sensibility must depend on some kind of stimulation conveyed through the skin, but refuses to theorize on

the *modus agendi* of the stimuli, and whether they act directly on the ends of
the sensory nerves, or by reflex dilatation of the bloodvessels, etc.   He confesses
his complete inability to explain the phenomenon of so-called "transfer" from
the healthy to the anæsthetic side.   It seems, indeed, useless to theorize on a subject about which our knowledge is still so elementary, and the only form of speen-
lation which seems open to us is whether metalloscopy is ever likely to be of permanent therapeutic value.   If the sensibility is withdrawn from one side of the
body to be transferred to the other, this looks rather like "robbing Peter to pay
Paul." . However, the loss of sensibility of the healthy side appears to persist
a shorter time than the gain of the anæsthetic side, and, as we have already
stated, the "transfer" may not be detected at all.   On the other hand, while in
most cases the recovery of sensibility by the anæsthetic half of the body is only
temporary, and disappears again in a few hours or days, there are cases in which
a cure has lasted, at any rate, for several months, while in one case all the other
hysterical symptoms were signally improved.   This is about all that can be said
at present as to the value of Burq's discovery.—*Med. Times and Gaz.*, Sept. 21,
1878.

Medicine.

Treatment of Anæmia and Cachexia by Assimilable Diastalized Remedies.

Dr. V. Baud observes (*Le Progrès Médicale*, July 6, 1878) that both iron
and arsenic have long been employed in the treatment of anæmia, for their tonic
and corroborant properties, whilst the alterative action exerted by iodine has led
to its extensive use in diseases proceeding from a scrofulous diathesis. None of
these agents are injurious if the doses be carefully prescribed, and their effects
watched. As usually administered, however, they are given in what may be
called the raw state, and it is doubtful how far they undergo absorption, and
whether they may not sometimes do harm by disturbing the digestive functions.
Impressed with these views, M. Baud set himself to discover a means by which
the drug above mentioned could be combined with some organic substance in
small doses, and thus be introduced into the economy in an easily digestible condition. His experiments have led him to employ what he terms diastalized
remedies. The general principle of this method consists in combining the
mineral substance intimately with a seed, and for this purpose the seed of one of
the cruciferæ, the cress, is selected, first because it possesses remarkable germ-
inating properties, and secondly because it possesses certain properties that render
it specially adapted for the object in view. The seeds about to germinate contain diastase, and in the act of germination a physico-chemical action takes place
which is comparable to animal digestion, every part of the seed is reduced to a
pulpy state; the ferment developed, however, can by special arrangements be
kept in a state of inertia, or quiescence, ready to act as soon as it is placed in
favourable conditions. The proceeding he adopts is that the seeds of cress,
which are rich in sulphur and phosphorous, are watered with solutions containing
definite quantities of iron citrate, potassium iodide, or sodium arseniate. These
solutions, far from interfering with germination, render that process more active,
and the seeds come to be gradually and thoroughly impregnated with the mineral
salt. They are then dried at a low temperature in a stove, and it then contains
amylaceous and saccharine principles and diastase. It has lost neither the sulphur nor the phosphorus, but it has acquired new properties owing to the absorp-

tion of the special salt employed, the union of which with the proteinous compounds is rendered perfectly certain. It only remains to coat the seed, the form of which is well adapted for the purpose, with some material which will render it fitted for exhibition, and it will be found that a medicine is obtained the activity of which is rendered immediately apparent when the fluids of the stomach have dissolved the saccharine investment. The salt is thus introduced into the system in a partially digested state, rendering it easily assimilable, and hence a smaller dose is required. The diastalized citrate of iron may be prescribed in doses of 5–7 grains, and its acting is shown by the palpitation of the heart, which results from its use. Diastalized potassium iodide given in the same doses advantageously replaces cod-liver oil, for it is in combination with phosphorus and sulphur, which are contained in the oil, whilst the disagreeable flavour of the oil is escaped. Small doses of arsenic can be administered in the same way and have been found very effective, whilst they have no toxic action.— *Practitioner*, September, 1878.

The Treatment of Erysipelas by Carbolic Acid Injections.

This method, first suggested in 1874, by Professor HUETER, of Greifswald, has been tested and elaborated in his clinic with most excellent results. A summary of a paper by his son, Dr. HERMANN HUETER, in the *Berliner Klin. Wochenschrift*, Nos. 24, 25, 1878, will put our readers in possession of the latest particulars on the subject. We may premise that the strength of the carbolic acid solution injected is 3 per cent., prepared as follows :—Carbolic acid, spirits of wine, of each 1.5 grammes; distilled water, 50 grammes. A Pravaz's syringe is used, and the largest number of simultaneous injections in any one case has been twelve. It is found that one injection into an erysipelatous patch arrests the disease over an area the size of "half a card," by which we presume a visiting-card is meant. Beyond this area, there is scarcely any visible effect; hence, if the patch is very large, the danger of carbolic acid poisoning may be too great for the whole diseased surface to be injected. Dr. Hueter, therefore, lays the greatest stress on nipping erysipelas in the bud, by watching for its earliest symptoms; and the nurses and attendants in Professor Hueter's clinic are carefully instructed in its diagnosis, so as to call the surgeon's attention at once to rigors, nausea, vomiting, or any other change in the patient's state which may be the prelude to the rash itself. In this way a small area only, instead of a large one, has to be treated, and the surgeon is practically certain of being able to control the disease. Dr. Hueter's own observations lead him to conclude that the more severe the initial symptoms, the earlier the rash appears, and *vice versa.*

The cases in which erysipelas has been detected are treated as follows: Attention is first directed to the wound itself. If the surface is healthy and unaltered (which is unusual); it is merely thoroughly washed with 3 per cent. carbolic solution. If, however, it is in any part coated with a gray, perhaps still somewhat transparent film, or appears diphtheritic, or pulpy, the affected parts are removed by swabbing with 5 to 8 per cent. solution of chloride of zinc; and this is done in every case where the erysipelas starts from a hollow wound.

After this the erysipelatous skin itself is injected at various spots; and if detected early, two or three syringefuls of carbolic solution suffice. If the injection has to be repeated very often on the same patch, the canula is sometimes left in while the syringe is being refilled, and a second injection is made at the same place, trusting to the known great diffusive power of the carbolic acid. If the erysipelas is complicated with lymphangitis, and lymphadenitis, the red lines on the skin and in the neighbourhood of the swollen glands are rubbed with unguentum hydrargyri, and sometimes the edges of the rash itself are thickly smeared with the same ointment.

Lastly, the wound and the reddened skin are wrapped up in a dressing of wet carbolic wool, which is changed two or three times daily until all redness has disappeared. The wound is then antiseptically treated.

The results of this system are most satisfactory. The erysipelas loses its spreading character after the first injections, and in mild cases is, so to speak, destroyed. Severer cases require a second or third series of injections to prevent the skin re-reddening after it has become pale. .

Dr. Hueter gives the short details of the seventeen cases of erysipelas treated in the Greifswald surgical clinic, from May, 1877, to April, 1878. The average duration of each case was two days and a quarter (the longest lasted ten days), and there were no deaths; only one case—the longest—was a complicated one, of a phlegmonous character, with subcutaneous sloughing, not, however, due to the injection. Carbolic acid poisoning only once occurred, and was limited to discoloration of the urine, the patient's general state being unaffected. The advantages of the method of using carbolic acid injections as at present carried out are clearly seen by contrasting the results of the year 1876, when the method was in its infancy, with those of 1877–78. In the former year there were thirty cases treated (and even this number was a great reduction on former years), fourteen recovered without complication, and sixteen were severe cases, of which four died. The average duration of each was six days and nine-tenths.

In conclusion Dr. Hueter points out that any reduction in the number and duration of cases of erysipelas in a hospital is a distinct gain for the other patients, who thus run less chance of infection than they would otherwise do. A short case of erysipelas is less likely to lead to the dissemination of "germs," and to their lurking in corners and crevices to spread the disease at some future time, than a long one.—*Med. Times and Gazette*, Sept. 7, 1878.

—

Nitrite of Amyl in Ague.

Dr. W. E. SAUNDERS, of Indore, calls attention (*Indian Med. Gazette*, No. 39) to the value of nitrite of amyl in ague, and records a number of cases in which advantage has been derived from its use. The drug itself, he remarks, is inexpensive and goes a long way. He now uses nitrite of amyl mixed with an equal part of oil of coriander, to render it less volatile, and at the same time to cover its odour. He regards it as the most powerful diaphoretic he has seen, and he uses it in all cases of fever to produce diaphoresis. The following is one of his cases: Mr. T. C. came for treatment about 7 P. M. in the cold stage of ague. Two minims of nitrite of amyl were administered; sweating came on in seven minutes. He lay down for half an hour to get cool, and then walked home well. He next morning took a dose of quinine, and has had but one attack of fever without the cold stage since. Previous to this he had fever every day for one month, during which he took large doses of quinine. Dr. Saunders observes that he does not mean to say that quinine should not be used in these cases, for there is ample proof that it tends to check the return of the attacks, and removes to some extent the septic condition of the blood induced by the malarial poison, and this more especially if small doses of opium be combined with it. In no case did the amyl fail to remove the attack in about one-third the usual time, and in most cases the fever did not return. The method of administration he adopts is this: Four drops of the mixture or two drops of amyl are poured on a small piece of lint, which is given into the hands of the patient, and he is told to inhale it freely.

He soon becomes flushed, and both his pulse and respiration are much accelerated, and when he feels warm all over the inhalation is discontinued, as the
symptoms continue to increase for some time afterwards. A profuse perspiration
now sets in, which speedily ends the attack; in some cases, however, the cold
stage merely passed of without any hot or sweating stage.—*Practitioner*, September, 1878.

—

The Origin and Spread of Yellow Fever and the means of Preventing it.

In an admirable paper on this subject (*Maryland Med. Journ.* Oct. 1878),
Dr. N. S. Davis, of Chicago, presented the following conclusions concerning
the conditions and laws governing the origin and spread of yellow fever, which
are fully sustained by the facts observed during the present and all preceding
epidemics:—

1st. The essential cause of the disease, whether animal, vegetable, or chemical,
depends for its development and propagation or spread, on conditions of a strictly
local character found co-existing only within certain geographical limits.

2d. The most important of the necessary co-existing conditions so far as ascertained, are, continuous high temperature, excess of atmospheric moisture; the
presence in the atmosphere of the products of vegetable or animal decomposition;
and such geographical position in relation to latitude and altitude as to secure a
great predominance of the warm over the cold season of the year. The absence
of any one of the first three conditions here named positively prevents the development or spread of the disease. That part of the northwestern coast of Africa
bordering on the Atlantic, and the Mediterranean, and the West India Islands
where these conditions always co-exist in a prominent degree, the disease is indi-
genous or endemic, prevailing more or less during the warm season of almost
every year. While within certain limits both north and south of the regions just
named the cause of the disease may be, either developed locally or imported from
other places and spread, whenever a season occurs in which the essential conditions co-exist in an unusual degree.

3d. As all the known conditions essential to the development and spread of
the disease, pertain to the atmosphere, it is plain that the essential cause must be
developed in the atmosphere and not in the living human body. Consequently
if such cause spreads or becomes transferable from one place to another, it is
solely by atmospheric infection and not from personal contagion. And no
amount of atmospheric infection by importation or otherwise can propagate the
disease or its causes, in any locality where the atmosphere does not contain the
required temperature and local impurities.

4th. The causes and conditions giving rise to the disease being exclusively of
local atmospheric origin, are neither developed in nor evolved from the bodies of
the sick; and hence the transferrence of any number of persons whether sick or
well from infected places, to localities where the essential atmospheric conditions
do not exist, never has and never can propagate the disease in the latter places.

Dr. Davis does not claim novelty for the foregoing propositions. On the contrary, he says, they vary but little from the conclusions drawn by nearly all
writers who have given the subject an impartial investigation during the last
twenty-five or thirty years. Yet, if true, they afford a basis for, or guide to, the
adoption of sanitary measures of the highest value and efficiency, and entirely
consistent with the principles of humanity, as well as the business interests of the
country.

They clearly indicate that the first and most important of all the measures for
preventing the development of yellow fever in any given place, either locally or

by importation, are such as will remove one or more of the conditions necessary for the production or spread of the disease. Of these conditions, the one most readily under human control, is the contamination of the atmosphere from local sources of vegetable and animal decomposition. It is well known that the chief sources of such decomposition are, imperfect and uncleanly sewers or cess-pools, foul and stagnant water; and low, moist ground rich in vegetable matter.

To remove these sources of atmospheric impurity early in each year, and keep them thoroughly removed until the close of the warm season, and thereby prevent the supply of local material on which the essential cause of yellow fever depends for its propagation, is the *only reliable* safeguard against the development of this disease in any place within the geographical range of its prevalence. If this is neglected until the atmosphere of any locality becomes filled with miasms as a pabulum for the fever poison, and the summer temperature prove continuously high, the disease will prevail and spread in defiance of all the inland quarantines that can be devised. But if a sufficient degree of cleanliness in regard to streets, alleys, gutters, sewers, and stagnant waters, to prevent the atmosphere from becoming filled with the products of decomposition and impurities, is accomplished early in the season and faithfully maintained until the frosts of autumn, there will be no danger of the prevalence of yellow fever, either by importation or otherwise. The point of vital importance is to *prevent* the development of the noxious material that constitutes the pabulum on which the essential cause of the disease feeds or out of which it originates. The mistake which is constantly being made by those having charge of sanitary matters in almost every locality, is the delay in executing the necessary measures of cleanliness, disinfection, and drainage, until so late in the season that the processes of fermentation, decomposition, and change in the local accumulations of moist organic matter, have already begun and impregnated the atmosphere with their poisonous products.

The second series of preventive measures of great importance are suggested by the third and fourth propositions stated above, and are as follows:—

1st. The municipal and health authorities of every important city or town on the coast of the gulf, from the Mexican boundary to Charleston on the Atlantic; on the Mississippi from New Orleans to St. Louis; on the Red River below Shreveport; on the Ohio below Pittsburg; and on the principal lines of railroad in immediate connection with such cities and towns, should deliberately select the nearest unoccupied, dry, elevated place, containing pure air and good water, and as readily accessible as possible, to which all families willing to go could be speedily removed from an infected street or section of a town or city, and accommodated in tents or other temporary structures until they could safely return to their homes.

Wherever this principle of speedy removal was acted upon by our army, it proved entirely successful in stopping the spread of the disease among the soldiers, and its imperfect and limited adoption at Memphis the present season has been of great value.

2d. The same principles apply to commerce and business. There is no positive evidence whatever, that the disease is ever transmitted by simple contact with the sick, nor by either articles of clothing or merchandise that have been freely exposed to the air outside of an infected locality. It is only when the *infected air* of the locality where the disease is prevailing, is shut up in the hold or apartments of a ship, boat, or car, or boxed up with goods in boxes or trunks, that it can be carried to distant places and retain its active properties. And even when so carried, it must be let out in an atmosphere in the new locality at the proper high temperature and containing the necessary local miasms or impurities, or it becomes utterly harmless. All that is necessary, therefore, is to have all ships, boats, and cars carrying freight, stopped at suitable places outside of populous towns, inspected, all parts thoroughly ventilated and cleansed; and where goods had been packed in bales, boxes, or trunks, the same opened and aired before they are received by the parties to whom they are consigned.

Salicylic Acid in Yellow Fever.

The *Berliner Klin. Wochenschrift*, of September 2, publishes part of a letter written some time ago to Professor Heyden, of Dresden, by Dr. Hartwig Bünz, of Savannah, and which is of special interest at a time when yellow fever is raging as it is now in the Southern States of North America. Dr. Bünz was called in August, 1876, to an epidemic of yellow fever in Savannah, State of Georgia, and after trying the stock remedies of the country—emetics, purgatives, starving, etc. —without effect, and finding that the fever was of an intermittent type, he resolved to make an experiment with salicylic acid. He gave adults a dose of one drachm and a half, either in solution, in capsules, or rubbed up in sugar, and if the stomach rejected it he gave a double dose per rectum. The results were excellent. The temperature, which ordinarily ranged between 104° to 106° Fahr., fell to 100° or 100.5°, and in many cases to 99°, and the pulse from 120, or higher, almost to normal; and of 179 patients thus treated, of both sexes and all ages, *only four* died. Dr. Bünz made the observation that the patients treated with salicylic acid complained far less of pains in the spine and limbs than those treated with quinine, and he himself, when afterwards laid up with the fever, and taking a large dose of salicylic acid very early in the attack, cannot remember that he suffered from these pains. He regards the acid as the most powerful antipyretic against yellow fever, both of the intermittent and remittent type, but has no experience of it in the continuous form, over which, as is well known, quinine exerts very little, if any, influence.—*Med. Times and Gaz.*, Sept. 21, 1878.

Treatment of Sanguineous Cerebral Apoplexy by the Subcutaneous Injection of Ergotine.

In a short article on this subject (*Lancet*, Sept. 21, 1878) Mr. N. S. Foster says: The utility of the subcutaneous injection for the exhibition of the active principle of ergot on account of the rapidity and comparative certainty of its action has been most successfully demonstrated in cases of post-partum hemorrhage. From the explanation given of its inducing the contraction of the smaller arteries, and from the facility of its administration, especially in cases where swallowing is at least very difficult, I was led to use it in cases of cerebral apoplexy and also of hæmoptysis. It is for the former that I am enabled more especially to suggest its use, and from the results I have seen believe it worthy of a more extended trial in that form of disease.

Cerebral apoplexy proper, pathologically speaking, is essentially effusion of blood caused by a rupture, generally of the smaller arteries of the brain, whether of the punctiform or of the massive varieties—which, indeed, are more accurately degrees of the same condition. Perhaps the commonest kind of disease leading to this result is the formation of minute miliary aneurisms, their subsequent rupture, and thence the usual train of symptoms.

At present I can record only two cases in which I followed out the plan of treatment.

CASE 1. I was sent for and informed that the patient, aged seventy-two, had been seized about a half an hour before my arrival. The ordinary apoplectic symptoms were present, and the coma gradually deepened during the application of the usual remedies. I then injected ergotine subcutaneously in the forearm.

The comatose state soon seemed to become stationary, and eventually the patient made a good recovery.

CASE 2 was similar in most respects to No. 1; but in this patient, who was sixty-four years of age, I injected ergotine at once; and here the coma, which was only partial on my first seeing the patient, never increased in intensity, but soon passed off, and to all appearances he made a perfect recovery.

In both cases I satisfied myself of the absence of cardiac disease, and hence possibly of embolism; and from the history it was fair to conclude that effusion was the cause.

For the success of this treatment, both temporarily and permanently, a great deal depends on the promptitude of its administration, before much hemorrhage has taken place, and consequent damage to the cerebral substance. The strength of the injection I employ is ten grains of ergotine to the fluidrachm; injecting twelve minims deeply into the muscles, and not merely into the subcutaneous tissue, as in the latter case suppuration is very apt to ensue.

—

Aphasia in Children.

A. SCHWARZ relates in the *Deutches Archiv für klinische Medicin*, Band xx, the case of a normally developed little girl three years old, who, during convalescence from an attack of measles, was suddenly seized with loss of speech and paralysis of the extensor muscles of the right arm. The right leg was unaffected. After a few weeks, the paralysis improved, and the child learned to speak as if she had never spoken before. Considering the peculiarity of the manner in which speech was regained, Schwarz asks whether the right half of the brain did not gradually assume the functions of those of the left half, which had been impaired. KÜSSNER reports (*Archiv fur Psychiatrie*, vol. viii) a case, observed in the polyclinic at Halle, of aphasia in a female child three years old, who, without any apparent external cause, suddenly became speechless. She heard and understood everything, could move her tongue and limbs freely, endeavoured to make herself understood by gestures, but could not speak. In a short time, some improvement took place spontaneously, and she quite recovered after the administration of an emetic. Küssner believes that the case was one of reflex aphasia, but leaves undecided the question of its origin.—*British Medical Journal*, Sept. 28, 1878.

—

The Pathology of Diphtheritic Paralysis.

The pathology, anatomy, and pathogenesis of this form of paralysis are not well understood. In a recent number of the *Journal des Connaissances Médicales*, an interesting summary is given of recent researches, chiefly of French authors. In 1862, M M. Charcot and Vulpian are stated to have published the first *postmortem* examination in which significant lesions were met with. The muscular nerves of the velum palati presented remarkable alterations. Certain fibres were composed of tubes without any medullary matter; under the neurolemma, at intervals, were seen granular elliptical bodies with or without nuclei; other fibres were less changed. In 1869, Drs. Lorain and Lépine cited an analogous case. In 1867, Bühl met two with changes in the brain (extravasation of blood and peripheral softening) and a considerable injection of the anterior and posterior nerve-roots. He described diphtheritic infiltration by cellular or nucleolar bodies isolated or united by protoplasma; this infiltration was found also in the false membrane of the mucous surface and of the neurolemma. Later, Leyden described the changes characteristic of neuritis, and referred diphtheritic paralysis to an ascending neuritis. In 1876, Dr. Pierret observed in one case thickening of the spinal membranes, with traces of inflammation and a deposit of a layer of false membranes. These lesions are inconstant, and have not been met with again. N. Déjerine (*Archives de Physiologie*, 1878), who had recently an opportunity of examining the nervous system of five patients who had died with diphtheritic paralysis, has found two kinds of almost constant lesions affecting the anterior roots and intramuscular nerves, as well as the gray substance of the spinal cord. The anterior roots present the changes which are met with in a nerve deprived of its trophic centre; the myeline becomes segmented, and consecutively the nuclei of the sheath proliferate, the protoplasm vegetates, and the cylinder-axis disappears. The traces of perineuritis and of meningitis are consecutive. In respect to the spinal cord, the lesions are the following. The nerve-cells in some cases become globular, are deprived of prolongation, or possess them only much shortened. The nuclei and nucleoli can scarcely be seen. Here and there some starved elements are observed, probably vestiges of pre-existing cells. The neuroglia is changed: the fibrils and nuclei are more numerous, especially at the level of the vessels and around the central canal at the commissure. In respect to the vessels, there is congestion with or without diapedesis, perhaps going on to hemorrhage; the lymphatic sheaths contain leucocytes, and sometimes small hemorrhagic foci. But it is important to remark that these lesions are limited to the gray substance of the anterior cornua; they are, moreover, inconstant, in the sense that death may occur rapidly after the commencement of paralysis. The anatomical examination is then negative. These lesions explain the motor troubles; but, as to the disturbance of sensation, no explanation has yet been found in any observed anatomical change. What is the nature and pathogenesis of these paralyses? Trousseau saw in them the effect of a poisoning. Gubler arranges them in two groups: on the one hand, paralysis by propagation by means of an anastomosis of the nerves which are in relation with the pharyngeal plexus (the eye, taste, hearing, tongue, fauces, muscles of inspiration, heart); on the other, the asthenic paralysis, paraplegia, etc. Dr. Brown-Séquard puts them among reflex paralyses produced by contraction of bloodvessels in the nerve-centres and in the motor nerves and muscles. As to the parasitic theory of Letzerich (capillary embolism due to the fungus of diphtheria), it has not found any support in France. M. Naque (*Des Paralyses Diphthéritiques*, 1878), from whom much of the preceding has been gathered, considering the changes in the blood, the possibility of the inoculation of diphtheria—in a word, its infectious character—thinks that these paralyses result from medullary lesions developed under the influence of the infectious character of the disease, and that they ought to take a position among the group of paralyses called infectious.—*British Med. Journal*, Sept. 28, 1878.

Cure of Epileptic Attacks after Removal of a Tumour of the Dura Mater.

In the *Annales de la Société de Méd. de Gand.* 4, Livr. 1878, Dr. LADOS reports a case of a tanner, æt. 44 years, who fell down stairs and suffered a contusion of the skull from violent contact with a wall. There soon ensued a considerable extravasation and loss of consciousness lasting several hours. Although several days afterward he was able to work he experienced such severe pains and "stitches" in the head that he was several times constrained to seek medical advice. He was obliged to spend his nights out of bed because the fearful pain robbed him of rest. This miserable condition continued for several years until a soft, pedicellated tumour the size of a pigeon's egg formed upon the scalp at the point of the previous extravasation. There was felt an impulse isochronous with the pulse and in the neighbourhood of the pedicle an opening of the parietal bones. Since the formation of the tumour the patient had daily several epileptic attacks with loss of consciousness, pain in the teeth and convulsions of the whole body, especially of the light leg. The tumour had its seat over the left sagital sutuie at the posterior upper angle of the corresponding parietal bone.

After consultation with other colleagues, who were of the opinion that it was connected with syphilitic disease, iodide of potassium was ordered. The flattened nose, as well as the view that the tumour was of the syphilitic gummatose variety warranted such treatment. This agent relieved the long-continued head pains, but the convulsions did not cease. Since the patient stubbornly affirmed that he never had syphilis and the epileptic convulsions still continued it was determined to remove the tumour. It was detached by means of a strong ligature, the pedicle cauterized with lunar caustic, and the wound cicatrized under simple cerate. With the cutting through of the tumour by means of a thread, a last epileptic attack of short duration occurred and no more convulsions recurred. Sometimes the patient yet feels an itching and twitching of the right leg as a reminder of the earlier convulsions. He works regularly, has increased in body weight and feels entirely well. He wears a piece of thick material over the cicatrix for protection, where there exists an opening the size of a half franc caused by neciosis of the parietal bones.

In consequence of the fall there was an inflammation of the dura mater and the corresponding portions of the corresponding parietal bones arose, causing a fungus of the dura mater breaking through the bones and inducing the violent pain and epileptic attacks.—*Cincinnati Lancet and Clinic*, Sept. 28, 1878, from *Allg. Med. Cent -Zeit.*, Aug. 1, 1878.

——

Contagious Pneumonia.

Dr. A. KÜHN (*Deutsches Archiv für Klin. Medicin*, Bd. xxxi.) has observed on several occasions the endemic occurrence of an asthenic form of pneumonia; it once occurred during overcrowding of the prison at Moringen in Hanover, and also after residence in new and damp apartments. As all the other conditions of the prisoners—soil, drainage, ventilation, drinking-water, clothing, and food—were favorable, the outbreak of the pneumonia could only be ascribed to deterioration of the air in the rooms. The malady was characterized by marked symptoms of infective disease, with much loss of strength, great enlargement of the spleen, albuminuria, and diarrhœa in two-thirds of the cases. The disease did not set in, like genuine croupous pneumonia, suddenly and with a single rigor; it was ushered in by premonitory symptoms lasting from four to eight days, generally without previous rigor, was attended with fever, and ran a very severe course. The engorgement of the lung was usually observed for the first time on the third or fourth day of the fever; it was often situated in the upper lobes, and showed much disposition to change its position. There was also very often inflammation of the serous membranes; in one-fourth of all the cases, pericarditis was present; severe pleuritis was constantly met with; and in five cases out of forty-five there was well-marked meningitis. The disease was also frequently accompanied from the first by angina and stomatitis, often going on to sloughing. The temperature rose to 107 deg. Fahr. and usually first showed distinct remissions from the fifth to the seventh day. On *post-mortem* examination, the muscular tissue of the heart was found either of a dark brown-red colour and fragile, or in a state of fatty degeneration; the spleen was enlarged even to three times its normal size; and the albuminuria arose from parenchymatous nephiitis. Not unfrequently, also, there was swelling of the intestinal follicles. The disease was communicable. The attendants were infected, and the disease was indirectly communicated (through intermediate persons) to others who did not come into contact with the institution. Dr Kühn observed in one epidemic seventy cases, and in another eighty-three. Abortive forms were met with.—*Brit. Med. Journ.*, Sept. 7, 1878.

Acute Miliary Tuberculosis.

Few, if any, diseases are so desperately unmanageable as acute tuberculosis, yet for that very reason it demands to be studied in all its bearings with the greatest minuteness. Only in this way can we hope to learn how to prevent its outbreak or to check its progress. We are therefore deeply indebted to those observers who will take the subject up and work at it, even though they fail at present to provide us with a remedy for the malady, or to clear up many of its mysteries.

Dr. LITTEN, of Berlin, one of the rising young physicians of Germany, is the latest contributor to the literature of acute tuberculosis, and we have summarized in the remarks which follow the most salient points of his recent valuable lecture in *Volkmann's Sammlung Klinischer Vorträge* (No. 119).

In the first place, Litten points out that the theory that miliary tuberculosis *only* follows caseous resorption will scarcely stand, and that cases occur in which healthy individuals die of it without any detectable cause for the disease, either *intra vitam* or *post-mortem*. It is further interesting, that like the acute infectious diseases properly so called, miliary tuberculosis (and by this term the acute form with rapid course is here invariably meant) tends to vary in its frequency with the season, and at times to take on a sort of epidemic character. Thus Buhl states that at Munich he observed most cases in May, and none at all in July and August. Lebert, at Zurich, reckoned April and May as the months when the disease was most frequent, and Virchow, at Berlin, also speaks of the early summer months as the time when acute tuberculosis is *quasi*-epidemic.

The sexes are very unequally attacked, and of fifty cases observed by Professor Frerichs and Dr. Litten in the wards of the Charité Hospital at Berlin, forty-three, or 86 per cent., were males. The largest number of cases per decade (fourteen) occurred between thirty and forty years, and the next largest (ten) between twenty and thirty. The chief peculiarity of the disease in infants is the frequency with which the meninges are involved. In the course of tuberculosis affecting the diaphragm, the pericardium, and the meninges, peritonitis, pericarditis, and meningitis are not uncommon. The distribution of the tubercles in the different organs of the body varies extremely; but, while the pancreas scarcely ever suffers, it is rare for a case to be met with in which the lungs, liver, spleen, kidneys, bones, and choroid membranes are not affected.

Dr. Litten's statistics of fifty-two post-mortems, chiefly made by Virchow at the Berlin Pathological Institute, show that etiologically acute tuberculosis is associated more frequently with phthisical deposits and cavities in one or both lungs than with any other condition. This was true of twenty-eight out of the fifty-two cases. In three cases the tubercular eruption immediately followed the *rapid absorption of pleuritic effusions;* and Dr. Litten regards the hereditary predisposition, which was certainly present in two of them, as having been lighted up, so to speak, by the irritation (*Reiz*) caused by the removal of the pressure of the effusion from the vessels of the lung, and by the rapid re-expansion of the lung itself. With regard to the relative frequency with which the organs are affected with tubercle, it may be stated that the lungs are almost invariably attacked. In fifty-one cases out of fifty-two this occurred, and in thirty-six the pleuræ were also diseased. The lungs may be the only organ affected. In eleven out of the fifty-two cases there was serous pleurisy, and in two hemorrhagic effusion into the pleural cavity. The most interesting fact in connection with the digestive tract, apart from the occurrence of intestinal ulcers, is that of the existence in some cases (about 10 per cent.) of ulcers on the back of the tongue, with elevated edges, the seat of miliary tubercles. These ulcers may, according to Litten, develop quite independently of any disease in the larynx, pharynx, or elsewhere in the neighbourhood of the mouth, and they sometimes run their course very rapidly. The mesentery was affected in six, and the omentum in ten cases; while the liver and spleen were always the seat of tubercle. The enlargement of the spleen — which sometimes is considerable, and which was present in 70 per cent. of the fifty-two cases—deserves notice for its diagnostic value. The kidneys are frequently tuberculous, and less often the prostate, supra-renal capsules, and bladder.

In one rapidly fatal case, which occurred on the third day after childbirth, tubercles were found in the mucous membrane of the uterus alone of all the organs, if we understand Dr. Litten aright. The pancreas and salivary glands were not affected in a single one of the fifty-two cases, nor were any of the muscles except those of the heart. Tubercles are not very rare in the septum ventriculorum and the muscular walls of the latter organ, and they are also found under the endocardium and pericardium. In the bones the tubercles occur in the marrow, without the existence of other disease, such as caries. Their favourite bones are, next to the long bones, the sternum, vertebræ, and ribs. They were present in the bones in 31 per cent. of Litten's cases, though more careful examination would probably have detected them still more frequently.

The most important fact, however, connected with the location of tubercles is their almost constant presence in the *choroid membrane* of the eye. They were found there in the fifty-two cases thirty-nine times; and their absence was specially noted, as far as the naked eye could judge, in the thirteen others. They are found varying in size from 0.4 to 5.0 millimetres diameter, and are not limited to any particular part of the choroid, though, if anything, most common quite posteriorly. As many as fifty-two have been counted in one eye. They become visible with the ophthalmoscope during life, when they have reached a certain size, owing to the atrophy of the pigmented epithelium over them as they bulge forward under the retina; and Von Graefe, who first observed choroidal tubercles in the living subject, stated that tubercles of less than 0.5 millimetre can be detected, especially if a retinal vessel crosses them. It is not necessary that there should be tubercles in the brain or its membranes because they are present in the choroid. In the thirty-nine cases of choroidal tubercle observed, this connection existed only in nineteen, or in less than half; and even where it exists, the appearance of choroidal tubercles may precede the development of cerebral symptoms by several days, or, *vice versâ*, appear later than the latter. Curiously enough, in thirty of the thirty-nine cases of choroidal tubercles, the *thyroid gland* was affected with a more or less extensive eruption of tubercles. That this must be an accidental coincidence, however, seems clear from the fact that in the remaining nine cases the thyroid gland was unaffected, while in nine other cases the thyroid was involved and the choroid not. The most frequent pathological conditions of the brain and its membranes associated with choroidal tubercles were simple tuberculosis of the pia mater, and tubercular meningitis. Tubercles are rare in the retina. The choroidal tubercles generally become visible late in the course of the disease; but they have been seen as early as eight weeks, and even as early as *four months* before death. They appear with the ophthalmoscope as yellowish-white roundish spots, which gradually shade off into the surrounding pigment. They are occasionally, when confluent, as large as the optic disk, but are generally much smaller. Their growth can be watched from day to day; and changes can be recognized in them in as short a period as twelve to twenty-four hours. Vision is scarcely ever impaired by them. Diagnostically their presence justifies an assertion of the existence of general miliary tuberculosis more conclusively than any other symptom.

Retuining to tubeiculosis of individual oigans, we find 60 pei cent. of the cases complicated with tubeicle of the biain and its membianes, its most common situation being in the *pia matei*. Two points deseive especial attention in connection with the neivous system : (1) that tubeicles may develop extensively in the membianes *without a tiace of exudation ;* and (2) that, on the othei hand, theie may be hydiocephalus piesent *without a tiace of tubeicle.*

The list of oigans in which tubeicles develop is now, with the occasional exception of the synovial membianes of the joints, the middle ear, etc., piactically exhausted. The chaiacteiistic of acute tubeiculosis is not that it attacks partieular oigans, but that it attacks *many* oigans, and iuns an acute couise. Miliaiy tubeiculosis may oiiginate in the piesence of any chronic disease, and should be especially noted that emphysema does not by any means exclude it, as Rokitansky supposed. This has been pioved most conclusively by Wundeilich and Buikait, as well as by Litten's own obseivations. Theie is also an acute foim of emphysema which is not uncommon at the edge of the lungs, and which is pioduced by the impediment to iespiiation set up by the tubeicles embedded in the tissues of the lung.

We have not space to iepioduce the pictuie of the clinical symptoms of miliaiy tubeiculosis diawn by Dr. Litten. and can only iefei to two or thiee of its details. Though miliaiy tubeiculosis is geneially accompanied with maiked febiile symptoms, cases occui wheie the tempeiatuie *never*, thioughout the whole couise of the disease, ieaches 39° C. The seveie dyspnœa which is piesent in the majoiity of cases appeais to be only paitly explicable by the attendant bionchitis and fevei, and is piobably due to a diiect stimulus exeited by the tubeicles on the peiipheial fibies of the vagus neive, which is conducted fiom them to the iespiiatoiy centie in the medulla. The enlaigement of the spleen has been alieady alluded to; and it should be added that it is painless, as a iule, in the absence of fiesh perisplenitic inflammation. Owing, too, to theie being, as a iule, no meteoiism, the splenic tumoui is moie ieadily detected than in typhoid fevei—a point of some diagnostic value. Lastly, we should iemembei that neivous symptoms in the couise of acute tubeiculosis may be simply due to the intensity of the fevei, and to the abnoimal nutiition of the biain with the infected blood, and not to actual disease of the neivous system.

The *diagnosis* of miliaiy tubeiculosis must depend on a consideiation of all the phenomena piesent, and not on any one symptom. Iiegulai fevei, iising high fiom the outset, and accompanied eaily with bionchitis and cough, consideiable inciease of iespiiatoiy fiequency, with cyanosis, iapid wasting and loss of stiength, with peihaps an eiuption of heipes on the lips, would favoui the idea of its existence, especially in a peison with old disease of the apices of the lungs. If no ioseola appeais at the end of the fiist week, and diaiihœa, meteoiism, and ileo-cæcal tendeiness are absent, the piobabilities are still moie in favoui of acute tubeiculosis; and still latei, the absence of bedsoie, so fiequent in typhoid, would fuithei stiengthen the diagnosis. Dr. Litten calls attention to the occasioual difficulty of distinguishing between diffuse bionchitis *in eldeily peisons with emphysema*, and miliaiy tubeiculosis, at any iate at fiist. The chief diffeience between them consists in the abundance of the physical indications of cataiih (iâles), and of the sputa, which is eaily met with in diffuse bionchitis. Miliaiy tubeiculosis iuns its couise in two to eight weeks. The piognosis is almost absolutely fatal, and only when a case iecoveis in which choioidal tubeicles have been obseived with ceitainty *intia vitam* will it be possible to affiim that the disease is evei cuied.

Theiapeutic measuies can only be diiected, in our piesent hopeless state of ignoiance, to ieducing the fevei and alleviating the bionchial cataiih.—*Med. Times and Gazette*, Sept. 28, 1878.

Acute Malignant Endocarditis and the Concomitant Retinal Changes.

Dr. M. LITTEN describes in the *Charité-Annalen* for 1878 six cases of endo-carditis with bacterial embolism occurring in pregnant or lying-in women, and a seventh case in a lad aged 17, in whom a diphtheritic affection of the colon was probably the starting point of the disease. In three cases, the endocarditis was purely exudative, without any ulceration or destruction of tissue; and no bacteria could be found in the deposits in the valves. As, however, bacterial infarcts were present in other organs, and the malignant course of the disease differed in no respect from that of cases of ulcerative endocarditis, it appears that endocarditis is not absolutely necessary as a connecting link between the primary disease and the occurrence of bacterial infarcts. This view is supported by cases of puerperal septicæmic infection with abscesses containing bacteria in the kidneys, intestines, and muscular tissue of the heart, retinal hemorrhages, etc., in which the cardiac valves were found entirely free. It seems therefore justifiable to regard endo-carditis as only a partial phenomenon of septic (puerperal, etc.) processes, the occurrence of which depends on various circumstances, such as anomalies of the vascular system, and especially of the valves. Retinal hemorrhages also occur in septic fevers without endocarditis, partly as solitary changes in the eye, partly as the sequel of severe purulent ophthalmia; in the latter case they arise from the embolism and the presence of parasitic material, while in the other case, Dr. Lit-ten considers that they are not of embolic origin. Dr. Litten is disposed to attribute a diagnostic importance to retinal hemorrhages in the recognition of septic processes (as distinguished from typhus); and he regards their presence as a very unfavourable element in prognosis.—*British Med. Journal*, Sept. 7, 1878.

Cardiac Hypertrophy and Renal Disease.

The July number of Virchow's *Archiv* contains a paper by Professor SENA-TOR, of Berlin, upon the connection between cardiac hypertrophy and renal dis-ease. The main novelty is, that he regards the cardiac hypertrophy of uncom-plicated cirrhotic kidney as usually unaccompanied by dilatation; the latter being, according to him, most commonly associated with parenchymatous de-generation, primary or supervening on the cirrhotic process. This somewhat arbitrary statement, not supported by any new evidence, enables him to construct a double theory to account for the cardiac changes in renal disease. He con-siders them apart : first, the dilated and hypertrophied heart of parenchymatous nephritis; secondly, the concentrically hypertrophied heart of interstitial nephri-tis. The first he explains by adopting the hypothesis of Bright, that it is due to the difficulty met with by the left ventricle in driving the blood, overloaded with urinary excreta, through the capillaries. He appeals to the analyses of Bright, Christison, Bartels, and others, which prove that this state of the blood is pre-sent. Finally, thickening of the minute arterioles has not been found (Ewald) in simple parenchymatous nephritis.

In interstitial nephritis, on the other hand, he regards the thickening of the small vessels as the *cause* of the increased aortic tension ; but he believes that the concentric hypertrophy often present is not due, and cannot be ascribed, to obstruction to the discharge of the ventricle, but is rather a concomitant of the renal disease, possibly due to some nervous influence, as in Graves's disease, pos-sibly to some direct effect of the blood. He does not pretend to decide what the nature of the arterial change is, or by what it is determined; but he is convinced that "all hypotheses which have the kidney-affection for their starting-point are useless." A month later, the *Archives Générales de Médecine* contained an article by Dr. Hanot, already well known for his thesis on hypertrophic cirrhosis

of the liver, in which the same points are discussed. He says: "I have long
observed that this hypertrophy frequently coincides with a notable decrease in the
size of the ventricular cavity. I believed at first that this was purely a coincidence; but I resolved to examine the subject with more attention." As the result of this attention, he gives notes of two cases which he has had an opportunity of observing. This observation is not by any means new: Bamberger, long
ago, and Gowers (in Reynolds's *System of Medicine*) have pointed out the same
thing; Dr. Moore published a similar case in the *Dublin Medical Journal* about
two years ago; but its bearing upon the various hypotheses now current does not
seem to have attracted much attention. Hanot thinks it supports Johnson's view
of muscular hypertrophy and tonic spasm, the condition of the heart being similar to that of the arterioles; Senator, on the other hand, regards it as of necessity idiopathic. We can scarcely admit this latter position, as it is not uncommon
to find little or no dilatation in cases of aortic insufficiency in which no one doubts
the deuteropathic nature of the change. Senator tries to avoid this by saying
that Bamberger hinted that in such cases (of aortic insufficiency) room is gained
by the left ventricle bulging in the right; and he suggests that this has not been
shown to take place in the usual condition, but in both Hanot's cases this is specially described. We may object to Hanot's remark that there is all the difference in the world between the action of the cardiac muscles and those of the
arterioles, and that, while every one may admit that a certain amount of muscular hypertrophy and tonic spasm may exist in some of the vessels, most careful
measurements have shown that, as a rule, their lumina are rather larger than normal (Thoma), and the thickening of the coats is in great part due to the overgrowth of the intima and adventitia—a point not disputed by Johnson himself; so
that there seems little analogy between the dynamic or static conditions of the
heart and arterioles, unless we assume that the obstruction to the circulation exists in the capillary area, as has been proved for the kidney itself, in which case
we have the whole aortic system under tolerably equal conditions of raised blood-
pressure. Senator's conclusion that the changes in the arterioles mechanically
explain the increased pressure is disproved by Thoma's observation, that these
changes in the renal arterioles present no resistance to the passage of fluids. It
is quite exceptionally that the endarteritis—for such we believe it to be—reaches
a grade at which the lumen is actually diminished below that of a healthy vessel
in the same situation. Professor Senator thinks he has successfully disposed of
the theory that blood-contamination by urinary excreta is the groundwork of
granular kidney, when he points the results of analysis as showing no actual diminution in the total daily quantity of urinary solids; but he forgets that, according to the view taken by a good many authorities, at least in this country, the
primary vice is in the habits of the patient and the relations of the food and
drink to the secondary digestive apparatus. In the first place, there are indis-
cretions of diet—too much alcohol, too much food, especially in this country too
much animal food; in the second place, an inadequacy (congenital or acquired)
on the part of the liver principally, and the organs concerned in the secondary digestion, to deal with the quantity of oxidizable material delivered to them: as a
consequence, we have blood-contamination of an unknown nature (but presumably consisting partly of lithates), increased blood-pressure, and diuresis (Ustimo-
witsch and Grützner) when this shall have reached a maximum. This process,
constantly repeating itself, would probably be followed by cardio-arterial changes,
and in some cases by marked renal mischief, especially, we may be permitted to
assume, in those in whom a predisposition existed.

It cannot be expected that lithuria should always produce renal degeneration,
nor must it be supposed that thick urine is at all a good indication of the exist-

ence of lithæmia. As we have seen, the presence of lithates in the blood stimulates diuresis; and, unless the relative proportion of water to solids may be small, they will remain in solution. On the whole, copious urine is a much better indication, especially if it be highly acid.

Still more recently, the *Centralblatt für die Medicinische Wissenschaften* (Sept. 14) publishes an abstract of a paper by Dr. von Buhl, of Munich, upon the same points. He argues against the views of Gull and Sutton, especially urging the rarity with which any other organs but the kidneys take part in this supposed general degenerative process. Von Buhl thinks that the heart and kidneys simply become diseased together; he refers to the very large percentage of cases in which traces of inflammatory affections of the heart are found; he thinks that this endocarditis is followed by hypertrophy as a result of "overnutrition" and increased work. He draws attention to the new fact, that narrowing of the aorta sometimes is present. This and the cardiac hypertrophy account for the increased tension. Finally, he thinks that excessive muscular exertion, leading to myocarditis and hypertrophy of the heart, is a frequent cause of granular degeneration of the kidney. This is carrying back the dispute to a stage which, we thought, had very long been passed. Everybody admits the frequency of cardiac complications; but no one now doubts the existence of a large number of cases in which the state of the heart cannot be regarded as in any respect the result of inflammatory changes. We think that the narrowing of the aorta is a point upon which more information is needed. We have seen it, but cannot express any opinion as to its relative frequency; but we hope pathologists will attend to the point, and also to the state of the cavity of the left ventricle.—*British Med. Journal*, Sept. 28, 1878.

—

The Treatment of Diarrhœa by Oxide of Zinc.

Dr. JACQUIER has followed, in the service of Dr. Bonamy at Nantes, the good effects of the employment of oxide of zinc in diarrhœa. · The formula which he has employed is the following: Oxide of zinc, 54 grains: bicarbonate of soda, $7\frac{1}{2}$ grains; in four packets, one to be taken every six hours. In all the cases which he observed, oxide of zinc produced rapid cure of diarrhœa. In fourteen cases observed by Puygautier, the cure was even more rapid, since in only one case were three doses of the medicine required. The results are considered to have been more satisfactory, inasmuch as in several cases the malady had endured from one to many months, and other methods of treatment had not produced any improvement. Thus he concludes that, although by no means to be held as exclusive treatment, the employment of oxide of zinc deserves to be more generally known as useful in diarrhœa.—*British Med. Journal*, Sept. 28, 1878.

—

Complete Obstruction of Intestine by Croupous Inflammation.

Dr. E. MARKHAM SKERRITT, at the late meeting of the British Medical Association (*British Med. Journal*, Sept. 7, 1878) related this case, which was of much interest, both in connection with the question of the diagnosis of intestinal obstruction, and also on account of the probably unique pathological condition present. The patient, a young man aged 19, was admitted into the British General Hospital with a history of a week's illness, beginning with slight abdominal pain, vomiting, and diarrhœa, followed by constipation and persistent bilious vomiting. His expression indicated discomfort; the pulse was 80, large, and soft; the temperature was subnormal throughout. There was a thin moist white fur on the tongue; the abdomen was moderately distended; the muscles were rigid; there was very slight pain and tenderness over the lower part. An enema of three pints was given without difficulty. Opium and hot fomentations were ordered. Two days later, the patient sank rather rapidly, and died. *Post-mortem*, the small intestine was inflamed throughout; a loop of the ilium just above the valve dipped down into the pelvis, dusky purplish-red in colour, much contracted, and feeling like a firm umbilical cord; it was entirely blocked up by a fibrinous cast adherent to the mucous coat. Ulceration and perforation of the vermiform appendix had occurred (adhesions preventing rupture into the peritoneal cavity), and there also croupous false membrane existed.—*Remarks:* 1. *The Obstruction.* Croupous inflammation of the intestine is not very rare. The special feature in this case is the complete plugging of the canal. Probably, there was the following sequence: first, ulceration of the appendix; then perforation, corresponding with the onset of acute symptoms; then inflammation extending and causing first diarrhœa, and then constipation from cessation of peristaltic action; this inflammation taking on the croupous type in the part nearest the appendix. 2. *The Diagnosis.* By a process of exclusion, enteritis not due to a removable cause was considered to exist; for, although there was scarcely any positive evidence in favour of this view, yet in the author's experience, it had been the exception for acute inflammatory affections of the abdomen to be accompanied by those severe symptoms usually described as characteristic of them.

Cercomonas Intestinalis in the Human Digestive Canal and its Relation to Diarrhœa.

Dr. E. ZUCKER describes in the *Deutsche Zeitschrift fur praktische Medicin* the results of observations carried on for several months in Professor Leyden's clinic, on the alvine evacuations of the patients. He found large masses of cercomonas in nine cases. These infusoria were observed in the intestine in cases of severe acute and chronic affections of other organs, or were found without other complications in cases of gastro-enteric inflammation. The animalcules are probably swallowed with water; they require for their development in the intestine certain conditions, such as disturbances of the normal digestive process, brought about by acute general disease or by injurious influences acting locally. In acute diseases, their influences on the processes which go on in the intestine is unimportant; but, if they meet with conditions favourable to their development, they produce diarrhœa of a mild or a severe type, sometimes febrile and simulating enteric fever. The aggravation of mild cases of diarrhœa under an increase of the cercomonas, and the obstinate continuance of chronic diarrhœa in two cases, and the improvement and cure which followed the disappearance of the animalcules, are proofs of their influence. The stools which contain the parasite are of a brown yellow colour, have a faint foul odour, are of a thin pulpy consistence, and usually contain small tenacious masses of mucus. The animalcules resemble an elongated almond in shape; the narrow end terminates in a pointed process, and the anterior round end is provided with cilia. Their *habitat* appears to be the rectum and colon. The most effectual treatment was the injection into the rectum, three times a day, of a solution containing three-fourths of a grain of corrosive sublimate; the intestine having been previously washed out with warm water.—*British Med. Journal*, Sept. 28, 1878.

Rupture of the Spleen due to Muscular Action.

The case of spontaneous rupture of the spleen described by Dr. Markham Skerritt (see *Monthly Abstract* for July, 1878, p. 307), is of great interest from a medico-legal point of view, and its publication has induced Dr. R. SYDNEY STONE, Government Medical Officer for the District of Flacq, Mauritius, to communicate (*British Medical Journal*, Sept. 28, 1878) two instances in which the organ was ruptured by muscular movement without the application of external violence to the structures protecting it.

It is, no doubt, well known that Mauritius is now a very malarious country, whatever it may have been formerly. Enlarged and diseased spleens are the rule rather than the exception in certain localities and among certain classes. Violent deaths due to rupture of a diseased spleen are consequently common, the violence varying from that sufficient to cause a broken rib to such as leaves, on the most careful inspection, no mark of violence, externally or internally, beyond the injury to the organ itself. It may be here observed that the commonest indication of violence found is a small extravasation of blood in the muscular layer of the parietes.

CASE I. On October 4th, 1873, an Indian woman, named Rujkalea, about thirty years of age, belonging to the Branchamp estate, was carrying a large vessel of water on her head. She made a sudden movement to save the vessel from slipping, immediately fell down, and had to be carried fainting to her hut, where she died soon afterwards. The police had no suspicion of violence having been used. The occurrence was witnessed by a number of persons, and happened on the high road. On inspection, forty-eight hours after death, there was found a large quantity of blood in the abdominal cavity, which had escaped from three superficial tears of the spleen radiating from the hilus. The organ was very large and soft, with an extremely delicate capsule. There was no ecchymosis of muscles over the organ. The stomach contained part of a meal of rice.

CASE II. On February 25th, 1877, an Indian woman, named Sunichuri, about thirty-seven years of age, paid a visit to her husband, who was an inmate of Providence Estate Coolie Hospital, suffering from ague and hypertrophy of the spleen. The latter was sitting on a bed, when, becoming angry at his wife asking him for money, he struck her on the face. In making a movement to get out of his way, she fell and shortly died. The man himself gave the alarm, and described what had happened to the police. On inspection, fifteen hours after death, the body was found to be fat, and there was a small bruise under the left eye. The belly was somewhat prominent, but not hard. There was blood, both fluid and clotted, in the abdomen. The spleen had a long perpendicular rent on the inner side, extending from the hilus to the inferior border, where the rupture was the deepest. The organ was diseased; was of the consistence of thick cream; had a very delicate capsule, and weighed in its empty condition one pound and a half. No bruise could be found in the abdominal or chest-walls, nor on the skin of the chest or belly. A slight bruise was found beneath the skin of the left temple, but no corresponding mark on the skin itself.

I expressed an opinion, not forgetting Case No. 1, and taking all the evidence into consideration, that the spleen, in this instance, was ruptured by a sudden movement. The man was charged with a simple assault, and sentenced by the district magistrate to one month's imprisonment.

The second of these two cases is very similar, both in the circumstances under which it occurred and in the view taken of it by the legal authorities, to the celebrated Indian case which occasioned a collision between the executive government and the judges, and a reference to the Secretary of State.

Those interested in the subject of rupture of the spleen will find a large number of references in Dr. Norman Chever's work on *Medical Jurisprudence in India*. He observes in a footnote: "Dr. J. W. Wilson suggests, with great reason, the probability that, however softened and congested it may be, the spleen never ruptures spontaneously, except under the action of muscular pressure, while the patient is turning or moving suddenly." Dr. Skerritt does not assign any reason for the anæmic condition which gave rise to the epistaxis and the passive hemorrhage in the interior of the spleen, causing the bursting of its fibro-elastic tunic. The description of the case does not, perhaps, preclude the supposition that malarial poisoning may have been the cause. But the case would not on this account, I believe, be less unique. *Congestive* apoplexy (to use the phraseology employed in the official nomenclature of disease) of the spleen is common in chronic malarial poisoning, and predisposes a fragile spleen with a delicate capsule to rupture from slight causes. Dr. Skerritt's case, however, is the first instance of *sanguineous* apoplexy, either of a healthy or an unhealthy spleen, that has come to my notice. In the two cases related above, the cause of the rupture was probably the sudden concentration of the weight of the organ at the hilus or point of suspension, and the consequent giving way of the stretched and attenuated capsule. It is conceivable that such an accident might happen even in bed.

—

Icteric Urine.

When jaundice is not well marked, a great assistance is derivable from examination of the urine. The following three tests are employed by Prof. HARDY before his clinical class with marked success: 1. *Chloroform:* When this is poured upon normal urine, it sinks by reason of its great density to the bottom of the test-glass, exhibiting there a crystalline transparency. If we pour it on the icteric urine, and, having shaken the test-tube plugged by the thumb, leave it quiet for a moment, the chloroform deposit contrasts strongly by its dull colour with the yellow of the superficial layers—the yellow colour being deeper in proportion to the quantity of bile in the urine. It is an excellent test of icteric urine. 2. *Iodine:* When the iodine is poured upon the icteric urine the mixture must not be shaken. At the upper part of the tube three very distinct colours are observable—the first layer formed by the tincture is violet; below this is a kind of diaphragm of a sea-green colour; and the third layer, consisting of the urine, and occupying the lowest part, is yellow. 3. *Nitric Acid:* When this agent has been poured in, the mixture after shaking assumes a bottle-green colour, passing into an olive. This is an entirely special and very characteristic appearance.—*Med. Times and Gaz.*, Sept. 21, 1878, from *Rev. de Thérap.*, Aug. 15.

—

Abscess of Kidney treated by Aspiration.

Mr. ARTHUR LUCAS reports (*Lancet*, Sept. 28, 1878), the following interesting case of abscess of kidney which was treated by aspiration.

On October 3d, I was called to attend S. P——, a lady aged sixty-two years, who complained of nausea, vomiting, and loss of appetite, together with pain in the right side of her belly shooting through to the back. She stated that she had been suffering from these symptoms for some weeks, though to a less degree. She did not remember to have shivered at any time. Her pulse at this period was 100; temperature 101.4°; tongue red and glazed; bowels regular. Palpation failed to elicit any irregularity or swelling in abdomen owing to the extreme tension of its walls on even moderate pressure. The urine was scanty, cloudy when passed, and deposited an amber-coloured sediment which half filled the glass on standing. Its specific gravity was 1030, and it contained two-thirds albumen. Numerous pus-cells were seen on microscopical examination.

On October 5th she had a succession of rigors, with rise of temperature and pulse-rate, and at a spot situated midway between the right iliac crest and costal margin, four and a half inches to the right of umbilicus, there was tenderness on piessuie, dulness on peicussion, and a sense of iesistance appaiently beneath the abdominal muscles, the lattei appeaiing to move independently. The maigin ot the lixei could not be felt owing to the fat condition of the patient, but an aiea of iesonance existed to the extent of about an inch between the costal aich and the dull space.

On Octobei 8th a fulness in the iight side of the abdomen was noticed, chiefly in the uppei pait of the lumbai iegion, and heie a iounded semi-solid lump about the size of a ciicket-ball could be felt. The patient was suffeiing moie pain, and hei geneial health appeaied to be getting daily moie impaiied. I theiefoie deteimined to exploie the swelling. Accoidingly on Octobei 10th, I aspiiated the tumoui, using **Coxeter's** instiuments, and diew off ten ounces of biown, flaky-looking fluid, which was followed by six ounces moie of gieenish-yellow pus, some of which was mixed with the fluid fiist diawn. The wound was then closed, and the apeituie sealed with cotton-wool and collodion. The next day the uiine passed was quite cleai, contained one-fouith albumen, and deposited lithates on standing, but no pus-cells could be found on micioscopical examination. The pain and tendeiness became less, and the patient giadually impioved in health till a foitnight aftei, Octobei 25th, when she again expeiienced á succession of iigois, and passed thick uiine in all iespects similai to that befoie noted.

On Novembei 1st the swelling of the iight flank again appeaied. This was again aspiiated, and sixteen ounces of pus withdiawn. The cavity was then washed out with a solution of **Condy's** fluid and watei, and the apeituie closed as befoie. The same evening the uiine passed was peifectly fiee fiom pus.

Fiom this time she steadily impioved and iecoveied in a foitnight. I have on seveial occasions examined hei since, but could detect no swelling, and she has remained well.

Surgery.

The Pathological Anatomy of the Lymphatic Glands.

The last pait of the *Jouinal de l'Anatomie* contains an inteiesting note, by ᴎ. CORNIL, of the iesults of his obseivations on the pathological anatomy of the lymphatic glands. The stiuctuies of these glands, thanks to the labouis of Fiey and many othei obseiveis, is sufficiently known, and it is only iequisite to iefei to the distinction between the piopei folliculai or medullaiy substance of the gland and the lymph-spaces or caveinous stiuctuie which suiiounds them. It is in these spaces, which aie continuous with the affeient and effeient vessels, that, accoiding to ᴎ. Coinil, the fiist evidences of disease appeai, and the moi-bid phenomena aie usually consecutive upon lesion of some neighbouring tissue or oigan. In acute foims of adenitis—such, for example, as occuis aftei a phleg-mon—the afferent lymphatics contain pus, which by degiees fills the caveinous spaces, the adipose tissue aiound the gland becomes infiltiated with pus, and the cells of the adipose tissue become suiiounded by lymph-coipuscles; and it is not difficult to tiace the fuithei changes that occui till an abscess is developed. The phenomena obseived in syphilitic and stiumous inflammation aie, howevei, of a moie inteiesting natuie. ᴎ. Coinil fiist speaks of adenitis fiom syphilis, which he divides into two gioups, adenitis of the piimaiy or secondaiy peiiod, and adenitis of the teitiaiy peiiod. In iegaid to the fiist, he finds, on micioscopic examination of the glands, besides the ordinary lymph-corpuscles, large spheroidal cells containing several nuclei, the more voluminous of which contain two nucleoli. These large cells are much more numerous in the cavernous system than in the follicular tissue. He considers that they proceed rather from the flat cells which coat the reticulum, and are analogous to the so-called endothelial cells of the great omentum. Coincidently with the appearance of these there is a slight accentuation of the delicate connective-tissue fibres which radiate from the hilus of the gland to the periphery. Thus, at this stage, it may be said there is proliferation of the nuclei of the cells, and a slight degree of sclerosis.

In regard to adenitis of the tertiary period, N. Cornil calls special attention to a form where the swollen ganglia form soft whitish masses of medullary aspect. In these cases the changes observed affect almost exclusively the cavernous system and all the lymph passages contained in the ganglion. The fine reticulated or follicular tissue presents no noticeable alteration. The cavernous system becomes filled with round and granular lymph-corpuscles, and with the large cells containing many nuclei. It may be said, therefore, that at this stage there is a kind of catarrhal inflammation of the vessels, and of the intra-ganglionic lymphatic passages.

Professor Cornil then proceeds to discuss the conditions present in scrofulous adenitis. The glands are here characterized by a prodigious development of the connective tissue, and by the caseification, either partial or complete, of the whole gland, which takes place as a consequence of this change. Even at an early period of the disease bands of connective tissue may be seen proceeding from the tube, accompanied by some minute lymphatics and bloodvessels, and these, gradually increasing, divide the gland into islets. The islets assume a yellowish colour, and are then found to be composed of reticulated connective tissue, but the fibres are more thickened, soft, and granular than natural. The meshes are filled with large cells, containing granular protoplasm and a voluminous nucleus with two nucleoli. Surrounding the islets is a felt-like structure, which is also formed of reticular connective tissue, but the meshes are so elongated that the fibres collectively appear like fasciculi arranged concentrically to the islet. They contain lymph-corpuscles, with round or oval nuclei, which are smaller than those of the islet. In scrofulous adenitis, therefore, there is a true cirrhosis of the ganglion occurring at the expense of the perifollicular tissues of the cavernous tissue, of which no trace remains. This lesion leads ultimately to a fibrous transformation of the whole ganglionic mass, or, rather, to the caseification of the whole gland, which is the ordinary state.—*Lancet*, Sept. 7, 1878.

Use of Iodoform in Glandular Swellings and Cold Abscesses.

Dr. MOLESCHOTT, of Turin, writes (*Giornale Internazionale delle Scienze Mediche*, Nos. 5 and 6, 1878) that he has used iodoform with success in cases which have been usually treated by iodine ointment, such as glandular swellings and cold abscesses. He mentions a case of enlarged spleen, with great prostration, pallor, obstinate diarrhœa, swelling of the lymphatic glands, and increase of the white blood-corpuscles (1 to 50 red), in which very favourable results followed the painting of iodoformed collodion over the spleen and lymphatic glands. Not less successful was its application in orchitis and epididymitis, and also in exudations into serous cavities, even including hydropericardium. He advises that iodoform collodion should be tried before paracentesis whenever removal of watery effusion is necessary. He has cured five cases of acute hydrocephalus by the application of this remedy several times daily; calomel and purgatives being, however, given at the same time. In cases of swelling of the knee-joint, where surgical interference appeared unavoidable, perfect recovery followed the prolonged local application of the iodoform. Apart from its action as a resolvent, iodoform has the property of relieving pain ; Dr. Moleschott hence recommends its use in painful attacks of gout, and also in various forms of neuralgia. In a case of intercostal neuralgia, he gave it internally in the form of pills (three-fourths of a grain daily) as well as externally. In severe neuritis, he has used iodoformed collodion successfully after other treatment had been tried in vain. Administered internally, it will probably be useful in the palpitations of nervous and hysterical patients, and will restore the regularity of the heart's impulse. Its offensive smell is obviated by mixture with tannin.—*British Med. Journal*, Sept. 28, 1878.

A Pathological Function of Periosteum.

Those surgical pathologists who are striving to raise the question of tumours above the bare level of an artificial and stagnant classification will read with interest a paper by Dr. CREIGHTON, in the *Journal of Anatomy and Physiology*, vol. xii., "On a Pathological Function of Periosteum." In his work upon the Normal and Morbid Physiology of the Breast, Dr. Creighton, as is well known, offers a rational explanation of tumours of that organ by regarding them as the products of functional irregularities. As regards the other great *epithelial* seats of tumour-formation, the stomach and uterus, the physiological factor is not so obvious, as there is not the same periodicity of action as in the mamma, to throw light upon the possible vicissitudes of the secreting structure. Still, the element of cell-formation, which is constantly to be kept in view in considering the origin of tumours, is to be found in the morbid physiological processes of these organs also ; for simple catarrh, to which they are pre-eminently liable, is nothing else than an enfeebled and largely cellular kind of secretion.

But when one comes to consider tumours of the *connective-tissue* type, such as the "*sarcomata*," it seems as if they had from the outset to be accepted as inde-pendent existences, possessed of an individuality, and comparable to parasites on the body. The physiological factor is not available in their case as in the case of tumours forming in secreting structures, because the tissues of the connective-tissue series, in which they take origin, are not endowed with an activity that may be described as functional ; as Virchow has remarked, the connective tissues "are always essentially passive in their working." There is, however, one tissue belonging to the connective-tissue series that has a "function" of an intelligible kind. Periosteum is a typical example of connective tissue, while its bone-form-ing function brings it into comparison with a secreting organ. Besides the con-stant renewal of secreting epithelium in an organ like the breast may be set the incessant activity of the periosteum, at least during the growing period, in pro-ducing osteoblasts. It is this formative function that makes periosteum perhaps the most dangerous of all the connective tissues. Many of the most malignant sarcomatous tumours occur in young subjects, and of these the greater number are of periosteal origin. The tumour-formation in such cases is a disease of growth, and it is incidental to the bone-forming function of periosteum. In the work before us, Dr. Creighton describes a particular case of malignant tumour as illustrating this pathological function of periosteum ; and shows how the mode of explaining tumour-formation in the case of the breast may be resorted to in cer-tain cases of sarcomata or new growths of the connective-tissue series.

A girl of nineteen, with rickety spine and head, died in St. Thomas's Hospital, under the care of Mr. Simon, with tumour of the metatarsus, enlarged inguinal glands, and symptoms of secondary invasion of the thoracic viscera. Post-mortem : the tumour was found to grow from the periosteum solely ; the lymphatic glands of the groin and of all parts of the abdomen were enlarged and whitish ; the lungs were full of white nodules ; and both ovaries were diseased, being occupied by several cysts of various sizes, while the remaining stroma had the whitish appearance of the tumour-tissue. In proceeding to consider the essential nature of this case, Dr. Creighton first states that he considers the patient to have been unquestionably rickety. As regards the tumour of the foot, it might be described as an "alveolar sarcoma," consisting as it did of trabeculæ of matrix-tissue, lined on both sides by cells arranged in regular order. The ground-substance was occupied with spindle-shaped nuclei, and at numerous points there occurred groups of the cells that were the characteristic cells of the tumour, while at other parts the groups of cells might be seen beginning to form from the nuclei by enlargement and proliferation, the cells arranging themselves round the firm margin of ground-substance, and the original centre of their formation becoming a space or alveolus, which they line like epithelium.

In such a case as this the physiological suggestion lies near at hand. The matrix-tissue is periosteum, the trabeculæ are bone-trabeculæ, the alveolar spaces are medullary spaces, and the tumour-cells are osteoblasts. The periosteum of the metatarsal bone has produced a malignant tumour, but that tumour has all the features of bone growing in periosteum, except the hardening with earthy matter. The tumour was soft and white throughout its whole extent, and there was nowhere found a particle of grit. In the absence of earthy matter in the periosteal formation lay the essential departure from the normal function of periosteum. This brings to mind at once the rickety disposition of the patient. The tumour occurred in a rickety subject ; and the structure of the periosteal new-growth is suggestive of the crude periosteal formation of rickets. The patient's rachitic disposition made it possible for the tumour to form, and determined its structure and character. Now, in the normal formation of bone from periosteum or in membrane, the keeping up always of a free row of cells just outside the ossifying substance is a contrivance to secure the continuous proliferation of the cells till growth is complete. The sole reason of the osteoblasts ranging themselves on the surface of the trabeculæ is that the substance of the latter is getting calcified. Calcification is a check upon the proliferation of the cells ; after a few generations of osteoblasts have become included in the ground-substance, the central cavity is greatly narrowed, and proliferation ceases. In the case of the tumour, the osteoblasts have arranged themselves as in normal calcification ; but the calcification has not taken place. The error underlying the whole of the morbid process is the absence of calcification. And since there is no calcification, the formation of new cells goes on indefinitely, and the formative process becomes a tumour-process. The cause of the tumour is thus discovered to consist in the departure of the periosteal function from the normal. The tumour is an excessive development of osteoblastic tissue by the side of a particular bone ; the unrestrained productiveness of the periosteum depending on the entire absence of the hardening constituent of osteoblastic tissue ; and this absence being "explained" by the rickety disposition of the patient. Virchow has himself remarked that he is not disinclined to admit that the predisposition to enchondromata may possibly be viewed as arising from rickets or from a similar abnormal process.

With respect to the *malignity* of the tumour, the secondary tumours in the lungs, ovaries, and lymphatic glands proved to have exactly the structure of the primary —the same appearance of trabeculæ and osteoblasts. Dr. Creighton does not attempt to account for the infection, and wisely limits himself to certain general remarks on the subject which he had occasion to make in his previous investigations on malignant growths.

A highly suggestive remark, which may be studied with advantage by morbid

histologists, is made in the couise of this papei.   Among othei oigans secondaiily
infected by malignant giowth weie the oiaiies.   Dr. Cieighton says that, apait
fiom the iaiity of its occuiience, the tumoui-infection of the oiaiies is moie than
oidinaiily inteiesting.   In all othei cases of oigans secondaiily infected, such as
the livei, lung, and lymphatic glands, the oigan iemains puiely passive undei the
woiking of the infection; its tissue becomes tiansfoimed at a numbei of spots
into the likeness of the paient-tumoui.   But the oiaiy in this case gave a ceitain
chaiactei of its own to the infective piocess—namely, a cystic chaiactei.   The
stioma of the oiaiy appeaied to be a matiiculai tissue, which, even undei the
influence of the infection, did not entiiely suiiendei the physiological piopeities
that aie inheient in it.—*Med. Times and Gaz.*, Sept. 28, 1878.

—

*On Changes in the Medulla of the Long Bones undei ceitain Pathological
Conditions.*

In the hope of thiowing some light on the pathology of the maiiow of the
bones, Drs. LITTEN and ORTH (*Beiliner Klin. Wochenschrift*, Dec. 17, 1877)
examined the bones of 100 peisons of diffeient ages, vaiying between 11 and 81
yeais, and found to theii suipiise that in the gieat majoiity of the cases the femui
contained ied maiiow to a gieatei or less extent.   Almost without exception
this was located in the uppei end of the diaphysis, extending in a compact mass
to a vaiying distance in the cylindei; in some cases small iound or jagged ied
nodules weie seated in the midst of fatty medulla.   In these 100 cases, ied mai-
row was found in 72; hypeiaemic fatty maiiow, which contained a modeiate
numbei of medullaiy cells, and was in spots of an intense ied coloui, in 17; and
puie or atiophic fatty maiiow, containing, howevei, hypeiaemic stieaks and islets,
in 11 only.   In most of these cases death had iesulted fiom disease, but in some
of them it had been due to injuiy.   The ied maiiow was found in the lattei as
well as in the foimei, but the geneial conclusion diawn fiom the cases, was that
the deviation fiom the noimal state of the medulla of the bones is principally to
be found in connection with chionic diseases, moie paiticulaily those which lead
to cachexia and maiasmus, such, foi instance, as phthisis and cancei.   The deviation was, howevei, also met with in some cases in which death had iesulted iapidly fiom acute disease.   An inteiesting point is, that all the acute affections in
which ied maiiow was found weie affections that aie always, or at least geneially, attended by swelling and hypeiplasia of the spleen.   The iesults of these
investigations confiim also Ponfick's statement, that a vaiying degiee of atiophy
of the maiiow, with tiansfoimation into a gelatinous substance, is fiequently
found in connection with chionic and especially cachectic diseases.

With iegaid to the anatomical elements of the medulla, Drs. Litten and Oith
regaid the nucleated ied blood-coipuscles as a veiy constant element, as they
failed to find them in only 8 of the 100 cases.   All of these eight individuals
weie ovei 50 yeais of age, all of them had died of diseases common to old age,
which do not lead to maiasmus, and in all of them, with one exception, the medulla was puiely fatty.   On the othei hand these coipuscles weie found in a man
of 81 yeais who had died of cancei of the bladdei.   They weie often found,
although in small numbeis, in appaiently puiely fatty maiiow, and they weie
sometimes found, also, in the blood.   Cells, which weie much less deeply
colouied, and weie, peihaps, a youngei stage of the transitional foim, weie veiy
fiequently met with.   The oidinaiy ied blood-coipuscles weie piesent in laige
numbeis, and theie was also a consideiable numbei of veiy laige, deeply colouied
cells about 0.01 mm. in aveiage diametei, and without nuclei.   These aie what

Hayem called giant blood-corpuscles ; they have frequently been found during life in the blood of anæmic individuals.

The ordinary medullary cells with granular protoplasm were found in almost all the cases ; smaller forms with hyaline cell-body were also met with, but less frequently. Cells containing blood-corpuscles were seen in 31 of the 100 cases ; some of these cells contained also nucleated red blood-corpuscles. Pigmented cells were even more common; in one instance the pigment was so abundant that the case had to be regarded as one of melanosis of the marrow. The subject had suffered from chronic intermittent, and the spleen and liver were full of the same pigment. The Charcot-Neumann crystals were found in most but not all of the cases.

The conclusions drawn from these cases by the investigators are, first, that the progressive displacement of the red by yellow marrow as age advances must be admitted, but that the change is by no means regular, and that it can be stopped, and even a retrogressive change caused, by various pathological processes. Second, that, in general, diseases which lead to marasmus are most constantly attended by the development of red medulla in the long bones, and by an increase of the nucleated red blood-corpuscles. Third, that the changes in the marrow in pernicious anæmia are not peculiar to that disease, but are found—even combined with similar changes in the blood—in other diseases attended by intense anæmia.

Drs. Litten and Orth are disposed, from these investigations, to agree with Neumann in the opinion that the changes in the bones are secondary to, and caused by, the anæmia, and that they indicate an effort of nature to counteract the anæmia by increased production of blood. To determine this point they have instituted a series of experiments on dogs, which were made anæmic by repeated and copious venesections. These experiments are not yet completed, but they state that in four of the dogs red marrow was found in long bones that normally contain fatty marrow, and that enormous numbers of nucleated red blood-corpuscles were found in the newly formed red marrow as well as in that of the short bones : some of these cells were also found in the blood. In a fifth dog, that was killed after five venesections, the number of medullary cells and of nucleated red blood-corpuscles was unusually large, while that of the ordinary non-nucleated red corpuscles was uncommonly small.—*The Med. Record*, Sept. 14, 1878.

Removal of a Large Lipoma.

In the *Wiener Medizinische Wochenschrift*, No. 11, 1878, is related a case occurring in Dr. BILLROTH'S practice, in which a man, aged 71, had on his back a lipomatous tumour hanging from his shoulders as far as the sacrum, and partly covering the nates. Its greatest longitudinal circumference was about forty-five inches, and its transverse circumference fifty inches. The pedicle, which was nearly two feet in circumference, arose mostly from the left scapular region. The tumour had existed thirty years ; and the patient desired its removal on account of the friction and exacerbation which it caused. His general health was good. The blood contained in the tumour was forced into the body by four elastic bands ; a piece of elastic tubing was then fastened round the pedicle, and prevented from slipping by means of a long pin. Skin-flaps were then made above and below ; the large bloodvessels were tied in two places and divided ; and the tumour was removed. There was but little bleeding. Thirty-five catgut ligatures were applied, the wound was united with thirty-six sutures, a drainage-tube was inserted, and the part was dressed antiseptically. The operation lasted two hours. The tumour, which weighed about 44 lbs., was a lipoma about twice as

laige as a man's head. Healing took place by the fiist intention. Duiing the
couise of the case, the patient had spontaneous gangiene of the iight lowei limb,
for which the leg was amputated aboe the ankle. On the eighteenth day aftei
the iemoal of the tumoui, the patient left the hospital with the opeiation-wound
neaily healed.—*Biitish Med. Jouinal*, Sept. 7, 1878.

The Influence of Tobacco upon the Development of Diseases of the Ear and Deafness.

LADREIT DE LACIIARRIERE in an aiticle upon this subject in the *Annalès des
Maladies de l'Orielle* (Sept. 1878), says tobacco should be classed along with
alcohol. Like the lattei, it has little effect upon many people, in modeiate quantities; it may een be of adantage sometimes, and the physician can and ought
at times to piesciibe and adise its use; but to some een in small doses, it excites funtional troubles, as I hae often been able to establish in the piactice of
diseases of the eai.

I often iecognize cases of deafness that aie dependent upon no othei cause, and
I desiie to call attention to this point. Few woiks upon otology mention the in-
juiions effects of tobacco, and authois who hae pointed them out, hae not done
so in a sufficiently explicit mannei.

Tiiquet deotes a chaptei to the otitis of smokeis and diinkers, but almost ex-
clusiely as iegaids its influence upon the neious system. I desiie to point out
its effects upon the naso-phaiyngeal and auriculai mucous membiane; upon the
oigans of the tympanic caity; upon the muscles of the phaiynx and soft palate;
upon the neies of this iegion, and the auditoiy neie. The injurious effects
that I hae obseied hae been fiom smoking tobacco. Tobacco used for chewing
ought to hae the same deleteiious effects, though while its consumption is ex-
tensie, its use is not so widespiead.

The authoi thinks that the iiitation of the chewing tobacco is moie localized
and that its iiitatie effects aie moie tiansient than the smoke which spieads
oei the entire naso-phaiyngeal mucous membiane, een enteiing the Eustachian
tubes and middle eai, along with the aii. Smoke causes a continuous iiitation
so long as one smokes, which is usually fiom half an houi to an houi. Instead
of piooking an abundant secretion like chewing, it causes a diyness of the mucous membiane with which it comes in contact—tiue smokeis expectoiate little
or not at all, when they do it is the iesult of the excitement of the secietion fiom
the mouth. Cigaiette smokeis who expel the smoke thiough theii nose, send it
diiectly against the Eustachian tubes, and if these aie patulous, into the middle
eai also. Tobacco smoke contains a gieat many solid paiticles, these aie deposited
on the moist walls with which they come in contact; a fact which the odoui and
taste in the smokei pioe.

The authoi asks if we hae not heie peimanent causes of iiitation and intoxication as we hae in the dust of lead and aisenic, etc. The angina of smokeis is
chaiacteiized by the swelling, the ioughness, the diyness and the insensibility of
the mucous membrane of the palate and phaiynx. The swelling is unifoimly
spiead, being paiticulaily maiked upon the uula, which is gieatly enlaiged and
sometimes deiated to the iight or left.

The mucous membiane is as ied as in the acute phlegmasiæ, but piesents a
dullei coloui; a congestie iathei than an inflammatoiy ied.

The diyness of the thioat is apparent, the epithelial lining is smooth and glistening.

The patients complain of no pain, no inconenience, and inaiiably say they
hae no soieness of thioat; it is eident, howeei, that the state desciibed has
existed for a long time. They do not come for ielief till subjectie phenomena

present themselves. These are tinnitus and deafness. (The objective symptoms and the condition of the parts, while given at length by the author, are those of chronic inflammation of the middle ear.) The author regards the condition of the mucous membrane as congestive rather than inflammatory, since such patients do not complain of pain, nor of any throat symptoms, nor is the nasal secretion increased. He thinks the insensibility of the throat is due to the narcotic action of the tobacco.—*Cincinnati Lancet and Clinic*, October 12, 1878.

Paracentesis Abdominis by Gradual Drainage with a Single fine Canula.

The unusual relief of the distressing symptoms of anasarca, which Dr. REGINALD SOUTHEY, Physician to St. Bartholomew's Hospital, has found to follow the employment of fine drainage-canulas, encouraged him to employ the same apparatus in the treatment of ascites; and now that his experience has extended over a fair number of cases, enough to satisfy him that this mode of proceeding is attended by no extra risks, he lays it briefly before the profession in the pages of the *Lancet* (Aug. 10, 1878). His description is as follows :—

Apparatus.—The trocar and bulb-headed canula required for the purpose of gradually drawing off ascitic fluid, by the help of a capillary tube, differs very little from that employed by me for anasarcous limbs. Both instruments are equally fine. The calibre is the No. 1 exploring trocar of the surgeon. One long needle-trocar, measuring an inch and three-quarters in length from hilt to point, has appeared long enough for all the cases hitherto tapped by me. Three or four canulas of different lengths, adapted to the thickness from fat and œdema of different abdominal walls, are required. The canulas may be perforated with as many as six or eight side holes—the more the better, so that their strength is not interfered with. The mouth end of each canula should be armed with a small silver plate or shield, to obviate any risk of the canula head sinking beneath the surface of the skin when this is highly œdematous; and, simple as it may seem to contrive an armature which may thus secure and help to maintain the canula in position, I may say that I have not yet quite mastered the matter. As to the length of the shield or cross-beam, one inch appears ample—*i. e.*, half an inch each side of the canula. The shield may be round or square with rounded edges, or, as I have had mine made, as elongated plates, one inch long by a quarter of an inch broad, and about a thirty-second of an inch thick. Whether the canula was best fixed immovably to the shield or otherwise, was the next point to decide. It was found that the immovably fixed shield, held fast by two strips of plaster, by dint of the movements of the abdominal muscles in respiration either worked away from its plaster moorings or tended to work out the canula end from the peritoneal cavity. Messrs. Ferguson therefore contrived a shield for me which held, but allowed the canula a limited play in every direction, and in practice this has worked admirably. One instrument I had made for those particular cases in which, although the ascites has been considerable, and its relief urgent, the presence either of cancerous tumours in the abdominal cavity or an enlarged liver has rendered a hard and pointed body, like the canula end, abutting on the peritoneal aspect of the abdominal parietes undesirable; for as the fluid drains away the abdomen collapses and the parietes sink, and large, soft-surfaced masses, moved up and down by the descent of the diaphragm, might be torn and fretted against the canula, and made to bleed. To meet this emergency a canula which merely traversed a shield-plate, and was not fixed at all, appeared best adapted. If anything pushed it from within, out it could come.

Mode of operation.—Trivial as this is, it appears to me from experience that

theie is a light and a wiong way of intioducing the canula. Instead of diiving
the tiocai in quite peipendiculaily, it is best to slope the point downwaids somewhat towaids the pubes, and to avoid making the canula point upwaids towaids
the steinum. The wound made is so slight that one can affoid to make it almost
anywheie, but fiom piejudice I should select the iaphe or mesial line below the
umbilicus, and about midway between this and the pubes. Befoie opeiating, I
always insist upon my house-physician asceitaining that the bladdei is empty.

I append one case of ascites fiom cinhosis thus tieated, but for the last yeai I
have had eveiy cases of ascites—hepatic, caicinomatous, cardiac, ienal—which
has fallen undei my caie at St. Baitholomew's, and iequiied tapping, tapped in
this way ; and the iesults have pioved sufficiently satisfactoiy for me to recommend it highly. I have had no instance of peiitonitis thus pioioked. The paiacentesis, instead of being a foimidable opeiation, is nothing moie than the piick
of a needle. The ascitic fluid is quite sufficiently evacuated ; it is also removed
giadually ; the neai aveiage iate of its iemoival being fiom ten to twenty ounces
pei houi. The piessuie upon the diaphiagm, the intestines, the intia-abdominal
vessels, and the walls of the abdomen, is slowly but steadily ielieved. Theie is
no syncope pioioked and no necessity for swathing the patient with bandages, a
ciicumstance in the old method of peifoiming paiacentesis by laige tiocais which
in hot weathei added gieatly to the patient's distiess. Both by doctois and patients this mode of peifoiming paiacentesis will, I think, be hailed as an advance
in clinical medicine.

William H——, aged fifty-eight, shoemakei, was admitted into Luke waid
on Maich 12, 1878, for extensive ascites and anasaica of his legs. The abdomen
was veiy tense; dyspnœa consideiable; some cyanosis. Uiine scanty, high
colouied, of high specific giaivity, containing no albumen. Heait's apex beat
two inches outside left nipple line; systolic muimui loudest at apex and ovei
ventiicle. Pulse veiy inegulai. Bieathing shallow; some œdema of both bases,
posteiioily with bionchial iâles. Limit of livei and spleen not to be asceitained
by ieason of the ascites. Up to ten yeais ago he had had good health ; then had
fiist attack of iheumatic gout. Was admitted into the hospital in June, 1876, for
diopsy of legs and abdomen, and was dischaiged well, and again for a iecuiience
of diopsy about Chiistmas, 1876.

The man's physiognomy, his habits of life, and the mannei in which his piesent
diopsy had commenced, the abdomen swelling befoie the legs, led me, notwithstanding the caidiac muimui, manifest dilatation of both ventiicles, and iiregulai
heait's action, to attiibute his diopsy piincipally to cinhosis of the livei and an
obstiucted poital ciiculation.

Paiacentesis abdominis with my fine tiocar and fixed shield was peifoimed at
6 P. M. on Maich 13. In twenty-one houis, 11,400 cc. of cleai, stiaw-colouied
seium had been evacuated by the capillaiy tube. The specific giaivity of the ascitic fluid was 1020; ieaction alkaline. The amount of fibiin as well as of albumen in it veiy consideiable; the foimei manifesting its piesence by spontaneous
foimation of a slight coagulum in the fluid. The tube was iemoved duiing the
night of the 14–15, the fluid having ceased to flow, and the abdomen being quite
flaccid.

Maich 18. Condition singulaily impioved; appetite good ; functions noimal;
uiine flow abundant, cleai, ambei-colouied, alkaline, sp. gi. 1024, no albumen;
bieathing quite tianquil; sleeps well; heait's apex still beats two inches outside
left nipple peipendiculai between fouith and fifth iibs; action still iiregulai; fiist
sound loud and iinging, but attended by no muimui; livei manifestly contiacted,
small and cinhotic.

Towaids end of Apiil the abdomen had again filled consideiably, and the legs began to be œdematous once more, but his appetite and general health were otherwise fairly good.

May 5. The distension of abdomen and interference with the descent of the diaphragm again threatened death by dyspnœa. Breathing shallow and hurried. The auscultatory signs rendered presence of some fluid in right pleura probable, as also œdema of lower part of left lung. Paracentesis again performed as before. The tube remained in thirty-three hours, during which time twenty-one pints of clear fluid were drawn off; it ceased flowing on the morning of the 7th of May.

On May 9 he was so perfectly comfortable and feeling so well that there was no object in keeping him longer in bed. On May 11 he was discharged at his own request.

Remarks.—This patient's case was doubtless a highly favourable one for relief by tapping. The best prognostic feature in any case of hepatic dropsy is a stomach that still maintains digestive powers. In treatment, however, this mode of performing paracentesis leaves nothing to be desired; the *tuto, cito et jucunde* are sufficiently fulfilled by it.

Chronic Ulceration of the Urethra in Women.

This affection, described by Dr. West, is the subject of an article by Dr. OEDMANSSON of Stockholm in the *Nordiskt Medicinskt Arkiv*, Band ix. He has seen four cases of it, and describes it as commencing in the anterior part of the urethra and gradually extending along its whole length. The upper wall is mostly affected, so that the greater portion of it may be destroyed when the lower wall is as yet scarcely invaded. The first symptom is swelling, which makes the surface of the parts appear uneven, very pale, and wax-like; the tissue hard and transparent, and the urethral orifice irregular and dilated. The secretion in the urethra before the commencement of ulceration is very inconsiderable. In one case, there was chronic œdema commencing in the right labium majus and extending to the whole perineum. The subjective symptoms are in general slight; in a very advanced stage, there may be weakness of the vesical sphincter. Microscopic examination shows a considerable hyperplasia of the epithelium; in some cases, various quantities of cells like pus-corpuscles; as well as considerable quantities, in the mucous and submucous tissues, of cells of various forms, some having the structure of pus-corpuscles, while others are larger, and rounded, or stellate with long processes. Dr. Oedmansson does not agree with Dr. West that the affection depends on syphilis; as, although all the patients in whom it has been observed have been prostitutes, there was no trace of venereal disease, nor had mercurial treatment any favourable influence. The ulceration usually lasted several years, and often recurred after apparent recovery. In the early stage, when the ulceration is limited to the anterior part of the urethra, a cure is not difficult. Abscission of the irregular, sometimes polypoid, fragments of the anterior part of the urethral canal may hasten the termination of the process; and in one case the carefully repeated application of the actual cautery was beneficial.—*British Med. Journal*, Sept. 28, 1878.

Fifty Cases of Lithotrity.

Mr. W. F. TEEVAN sends (*British Med. Journal*, Sept. 7, 1878) the statistics of fifty cases of lithotrity occurring in forty-six adults, three of whom had previously been cut for stone. Most of the patients were between sixty and sixty-five years of age; the youngest being seventeen, and the oldest seventy-seven.. In many of the cases, the presence of calculus was complicated by the existence of cystitis, enlarged prostate, stricture of the urethra, or vesical atony. The

smallest stone was half an inch in diameter, and the largest two inches. The
sittings varied in number from one to twenty. When he commenced to operate
in 1863, he determined to crush every stone he could up to two inches in diameter,
to see what lithotrity was capable of; hence, he had pushed the operation to its
extreme limit, and had applied it to three-fourths of the adults on whom he had
operated for stone. In two instances, lithotrity had to be supplemented by lithotomy, and in a third case by cystotomy. In a fourth, he found, during the progress of the treatment, that lithotomy became advisable; the patient refused to
submit to the operation, but, one year and a half afterwards, was successfully cut
by Mr. Hancock. Six patients died in his hands, but he lost no case from the
operation under sixty years of age. Three of those who died perished from causes
unconnected with the operation: one being from calculous pyelitis one month
after the cure of the vesical affection; a second from erysipelas of the head and
neck and fauces; a third from heart disease whilst straining at micturition. The
three deaths from the operation were caused by cystitis associated with kidney
disease. Three old men were not permanently benefited by the operation, and
died from cystitis after their return home. The other cases were all cured. He
drew the following deductions from his experience. 1. Lithotrity was *the* operation in adults under fifty years of age for stones not exceeding an inch and a half
in diameter. 2. In patients over fifty, the limit of the size of the calculus had
better be reduced by a quarter of an inch. 3. Stones between an inch and a half
and two inches in diameter had better be completely crushed at one sitting, and
the *débris* removed immediately by external urethrotomy. 4. Cystotomy was
indicated for those cases in which lithotrity had removed all the stone but failed
to cure cystitis.

———

Phimosis as a Cause of Rupture in Children.

Mr. J. ARTHUR KEMPE, Senior House-surgeon at the Children's Hospital,
Great Ormond Street, makes the following remarks on this subject (*Lancet*, July
27, 1878).

Phimosis in children is a common occurrence, and numerous ill effects can
undoubtedly be attributed to it—namely, incontinence of urine, fits, and other
spasmodic affections, masturbation resulting from irritation set up by retention of
smegma, balanitis, and, later on in life, cancer of the penis. Professor Sayre,
in his work on Diseases of Joints, devotes a chapter to phimosis as a cause of
talipes and other paralytic affections. Ziemssen, in an article on "Pressure
Points," alludes to the pressure of a tight prepuce on the glans as a cause of
paralysis. Lately Mr. Owen has quoted some cases of eczema caused by irritation of dribbling urine, the result of a long or adherent prepuce. He also says:
"In cases of umbilical and inguinal hernia it is well to look to the size of the
urethral and preputial orifices."

The organ, however, that chiefly pays the penalty of this congenital imperfection is the bladder, and Mr. Bryant, in "Surgical Diseases of Children," says:
"I have seen this simple condition of the penis produce every degree of irritability of the bladder, even to hæmaturia, also retention from the same cause, also
priapism." Hernia, too, is frequently met with in children. Malgaigne says:
one in every twenty-one children has rupture. The causes of hernia generally,
whether occurring in man, woman or child, are divided into two main divisions
—(a) exciting, (b) remote; the latter consisting in imperfection of the abdominal parietes themselves, the former in circumstances which exercise a more than
usual compressing force on the viscera which they contain. As an exciting cause,
straining, either violent or continuous, holds the foremost place. Now straining

may be brought about in a good many different ways—coughing, crying, etc. Straining from difficulty in micturition and evacuating the contents of the bladder, Mr. Kempe finds, has been alluded to by several authors—*e. g.*, Erichsen, Liston, Sir A. Cooper, Spence, Pott, Arnaud, Lawrence—all of whom mention it in connection with stricture, disease of the prostate, etc., in adults.

He has been unable to find any mention of difficulty in micturition as a cause of hernia in children, and the co-existence of phimosis and ruptures seems hitherto to have escaped notice (except the allusion made by Mr. Owen, *vide supra*). The frequency, however, of phimosis and rupture together, as it occurred to him, induced him to watch closely and see if it was anything more than a simple coincidence. He therefore took fifty consecutive cases (not selected

Age.	Under 6 months.	From 6 to 12 months.	From 12 to 18 months.	From 18 months to 2 years.	From 2 to 2¼ years.	From 2¼ to 3 years.	From 3 to 3½ years.	From 3½ to 4 years.	From 4 to 4½ years.	Totals.
Rupture,	15	5	5	1	1	4	0	0	0	31
No rupture,	4	3	2	3	0	4	0	1	2	19
Total,	19	8	7	4	1	8	0	1	2	50

ones), and found that out of fifty cases of congenital phimosis thirty-one had rupture, in five cases there was double inguinal hernia, and in many of them umbilical hernia as well (umbilical hernia *alone* has not been counted). In none of these cases was the rupture noticed at birth; the earliest was noticed three weeks after birth (here the prepuce was so tight that it was with great difficulty that the child could micturate at all), the latest two years and a half. In all of these cases circumcision was performed; in five the rupture never came down after the operation, and all have been much benefited.

It cannot, then, be unreasonable, in the face of these facts, to suppose that a long and tight prepuce may be a cause of rupture in children. The sequel of events is probably as follows: the abdominal parietes are naturally weak in children, which renders them less able to resist impulses which project the viscera against weakened parts. Here, then, is a remote or predisposing cause. The exciting cause is readily supplied by the frequent and continued efforts that the child makes to overcome the obstruction offered by the tight prepuce, and by the cries uttered consequent on pain caused in making these efforts.

***

Colles's Fracture.

The injury with which the name of the great Dublin surgeon has been associated by general assent is one of the most frequent with which we have to deal, and is yet one which there are few opportunities for minutely examining. Mr. Colles himself had never seen the actual condition of the fragments in the fracture which he described, and, as a matter of fact, he believed that it occurred at a higher point than it does. Dr. HECTOR CAMERON, of Glasgow (*Glas. Med. Journal*, March, 1878), has been so fortunate as twice to have the opportunity of examining a recent specimen of the fracture after death. In the first, the fracture, although transverse, passes obliquely from above downwards and forwards, so that while at the anterior aspect of the bone the line is not more than a quarter of an inch from the articular surface, on the posterior the distance is increased to about an inch. There is some comminution of the lower fragment, and the broken surface of the upper is extremely rough and denticulated. This very irregular and notched character of the fractured surface appears to be usual (Malgaigne), and is of interest in so far as it may cause difficulty in the reduction of the displacement. In this particular instance, although it cannot be said that there is any impaction, a toothed projection on the long fragment so locks the other fragment in its new position upwards and backwards, that it would be impossible to reduce it, except by great force. In the second specimen there is a transverse fracture about three-quarters of an inch above the articular surface of the bone. In front the break is hardly complete, the periosteum holding the fragments together, but allowing them to bend at an angle there, as upon a hinge, so that the lower fragment is, as usual, tilted upwards and backwards, and has the direction of its articular surface so altered that it looks upwards, backwards, and outwards. On the posterior aspect, not only is the fracture complete, but the dense outer covering of the upper fragment is driven firmly into the substance of the lower, splitting it like a wedge into three fragments, which, however, hold closely and securely together. The impaction is complete and irremediable. Although firm extension improves matters, it does not unlock this connection between the two fragments on the back of the bone.

This observation may be read in connection with the dictum of Gordon, who says—"Colles's fracture is not, nor can it be, an impacted fracture; its mechanism declares impaction to be a mere phantom of the imagination, resulting from the erroneous interpretation of pathological facts" (Treatise, p. 27). R. W. Smith, an authority of the highest character, also observes that "the theory which supposes the fracture to be attended with impaction of the upper into the lower fragment is fallacious."

Cameron further discusses the causes of the prominence of the lower end of the ulna, and while admitting that it is frequently due to dislocation depending upon rupture of the internal lateral ligament, he believes that fracture and complete separation of the styloid process is certainly common. In five cases which he had an opportunity of examining, the styloid apophysis was detached. When Colles's fracture becomes compound, it is by reason of the dislocated ulna forcing its way through the skin. As a strange complication, Cameron mentions a case in which the ring and middle fingers were strongly flexed. A small body was found lying under the skin in the middle line of the front part of the forearm, about an inch above the wrist. It pressed on the median nerve. An incision over it exposed the scaphoid bone which had been dislocated. It was removed, and recovery followed.

Frank H. Hamilton, of New York (*Phil. Med. Times*, March 30, 1878), mentions that Moore, of Rochester, has observed in two autopsies the tendon of the extensor carpi ulnaris dislodged from its groove. He thinks this a very rare condition.—*Dublin Journal of Med. Science*, July, 1878.

Traumatic Separation of the Epiphysis.

Dr. Voigt (*Archiv. für Klin. Chirurgie*, Band xx), describes the case of a young man aged 20, whose left humerus was shortened about five inches in consequence of an arrest of growth. At the age of 10, he suffered, through an accident, a displacement of the epiphysis at the head of the humerus; and from that time the upper arm entirely ceased to grow in length, while the growth in thickness was unaffected. Only a small number of similar cases have as yet been recorded, by Birkett, Bryant, Bidder, and von Langenbeck.—*British Med. Journal*, Sept. 28, 1878.

Midwifery and Gynæcology.

The Treatment of Puerperal Convulsions occurring after Labour.

At a late meeting of the Obstetrical Section of the New York Academy of Medicine (*Med. Record*, Aug. 10, 1878), Dr. S. T. HUBBARD opened the discussion upon the above subject by relating the history of a case as follows: He was called to visit Mrs. E. on the 16th of March, 1878. She was thirty-six years of age, pregnant with her first child, and within three weeks of her expected confinement. She was delicate in appearance, yet apparently in good health. She complained of headache, had flushed countenance, imperfect vision, and constipated bowels. A brisk cathartic was ordered. The urine was examined on the following morning, and found to contain about fifty per cent. of albumen, with some granular casts. After free opening of the bowels, infusion of digitalis was given in drachm doses, three times a day; also three drachms of bitartrate of potassa dissolved in water were ordered to be taken in the course of twenty-four hours. Under that treatment the quantity of urine increased to the normal. There was no puffiness of the face or œdema of the feet. At the end of one week the quantity of albumen had decreased from fifty to ten per cent. The bowels were kept free by the use of bitartrate of potassa. The headache and the imperfect vision, however, were more or less persistent. On the first of April the doctor ordered grs. vj of calomel, with grs. x of rhubarb, to be taken at bedtime. On the following morning he was called, found that the woman was in labour, and that labour-pains began at about 9 o'clock on the previous evening. The child was born at 5 A. M., and the labour was in every respect normal. The headache continued, and the patient was somewhat restless. Two drachms of paregoric with ten drops of laudanum were administered. At 7 o'clock A. M. she went into a violent convulsion, which lasted from one to two minutes. When the convulsion had ceased chloroform was exhibited, and the woman was bled from the arm to the extent of twelve or fourteen ounces. The patient became conscious, but was kept moderately under the influence of chloroform, and, at about 8 o'clock, grs. xv of hydrate of chloral dissolved in water were thrown into the rectum, when she had another convulsion, more violent than the first. As the patient became restless from time to time, chloroform was administered. The infusion of digitalis was increased to ʒij every four hours. At 11 o'clock another convulsion occurred, but was less violent than the two former. Treatment continued. A goblet of milk was administered within every four hours. When. the chloroform was let up for a few minutes, the patient complained of headache and almost complete loss of vision. The pulse, after the first convulsion, was 130, and continued from 116 to 120 during the first twenty-four hours. Temperature, 101° F.

On the evening of the next day the patient became somewhat restless; the bladder was emptied with catheter; an injection of fifteen grains of hydrate of chloral was given, and, soon after, another and the last convulsion occurred. A cathartic dose of calomel and jalap was ordered. Only a small quantity of chloroform was used. The effect of the chloral hydrate was continuous, although the dose was small.

On the following day the patient was better. The disturbance of vision continued, but was confined mostly to the left eye; the disturbance continued for a week and then disappeared. A trace of albumen was found in the urine for two weeks. At the end of that time the woman appeared to be as well as the majority of women were at that period following natural labour.

With reference to treatment in this class of cases, Dr. H. reached the following conclusions:—

1. That general bloodletting was called for when headache continued after labour was completed, and was attended by flushed face, restlessness, convulsions of a tonic character, and there had not been much loss of blood with the birth of the child.

2. That infusion of digitalis was useful to steady the heart's action, to allay nervous irritation, and also as a diuretic when aided by the addition of bitartrate of potassa.

3. That chloroform should be used sparingly.

4. That, although it was his first experience in the use of hydrate of chloral in these cases, its continuous action was apparently greater than chloroform, and he thought it was less likely to disturb the brain.

5. That, in cases in which there had been great loss of blood, or great prostration attended by nervous exhaustion, dependence might be placed upon hypodermic injections of morphia for controlling the convulsions. He would not resort to chloroform or to chloral under such circumstances, fearing that they might increase the nervous exhaustion, and thereby favour uterine hemorrhage.

The development of convulsions *after* the birth of the child was, in Dr. Hubbard's experience, quite rare.

In the last *three* cases belonging to this class which had fallen under his observation, general bloodletting had been employed in *two*, and those patients recovered; the case in which it was not employed terminated fatally, although chloroform, leeches, and dry cups were faithfully used. All the cases were primiparous.

Dr. A. C. Post referred briefly to two cases in which convulsions apparently were prevented by bloodletting. One woman at the end of the eighth month of pregnancy was taken with giddiness, headache, confusion of thought, twitchings of the features, and partial loss of consciousness. It occurred before the subject of albuminuria in connection with pregnancy was recognized in the profession. As the patient had a full, strong pulse, it was thought advisable to resort to general bloodletting. While binding up the arm for that purpose the woman fainted. Dr. Edward Delafield was called in consultation. Dr. Post expressed the opinion that the fainting was a nervous phenomenon, and did not contra-indicate the taking of blood. Dr. Delafield coincided in the opinion. She was bled freely. The headache and other symptoms disappeared, she went on to the completion of her pregnancy, and gave birth to a healthy boy who was now the father of a family. The second case, occurring many years later, had a similar history.

Dr. Sell referred to a case in which convulsions occurred during and after labour. The patient was treated by the administration of croton oil, because of suspected overloaded *primæ viæ*, and by the exhibition of chloroform both internally and by inhalation. The woman had six convulsions in the first series, and three in the second. Bleeding was not resorted to, and yet a good recovery took place.

Dr. Caro remarked that he had seen cases of puerperal convulsions at nearly all stages of pregnancy, during and after labour, and that he had never resorted to general bloodletting or to leeching except in *two* instances. He had relied chiefly upon infusion of digitalis given in ʒss doses, three times a day, and bitartrate of potassa in ʒj doses, three times a day for their prevention.

He thought that purperal convulsions occurred as the result of nervous disturbances, especially after confinement and independent of albuminuria, or even independent of urea.

A case was referred to in which convulsions occurred apparently from urethral irritation, because they came on only when the woman attempted to pass her urine. When the urine was drawn by the catheter, convulsions did not occur. There was no albumen in the urine, the quantity of water was normal, there was neither headache nor œdema of the feet, but the countenance had a puffy palid appearance, and there was disorder of vision.

Arrest of Milk Abscess.

Mr. W. P. SWAIN, of Davenport, reports (*Lancet*, Aug. 10, 1878) an interesting and well-marked case of arrest of milk abscess without, however, any novelty in the method of the treatment adopted. The patient was a primipara who was delivered of a child with the aid of forceps. Thirteen days after she had a rigor followed by heat with fulness, pain, and great tenderness on pressure of right breast. This breast had been somewhat troublesome to nurse with throughout. The aspect of the patient became flushed and anxious, the pulse 120, and the temp. 103.6° F. The breast was very full, tense, and painful, especially towards the axilla, where a spot much harder than the surrounding tissues could be felt. The following treatment was prescribed. An immediate dose of ten grains of quinine; two drop doses of tincture of aconite [Br. P.] in a drachm of water every ten minutes for four hours, and then every hour; and the extract of belladonna softened with a little glycerine to be smeared over the breast. The breast was also ordered to be used. In the course of nine hours the breast had become much less tender, the pulse 88, and the temp. 101°. Five grains of quinine were ordered to be taken every four hours, and the aconite to be continued every hour. On the following day the patient was in all respects more comfortable. The child had taken the breast, which was now hardly at all tender, the hard spot having vanished. The pulse was 80 and the temp. 99.6°. From that time she progressed favourably.—*Practitioner*, Sept. 1878.

Amputation of the Cervix Uteri.

This is the subject of an interesting article in the *Annales de Gynécologie* by Dr. LEBLOND with the following conclusions:—

1st. That the amputation of the cervix ought to be practised with the uterus in its natural position.

2d. That the galvano-caustic method is particularly applicable to uterine cancer, although it may be equally employed in simple hypertrophy.

3d. That, in default of galvano-caustic, it is the écraseur we ought especially to choose in cases of cancer.

4th. That the scissors are preferable to the bistoury where one does not care to employ the galvano-caustic or écraseur.

[The experience of Dr. John Byrne, Brooklyn, who has had greater opportunity for investigation, and who has perfected the apparatus of galvano-cautery for uterine purposes to a greater extent, perhaps, than any one, abundantly proves that this method is not only preferable for the excision of the cervix in cancer so far as the immediate effects are concerned, but, ultimately, as a curative means is it superior.]—*Cincinnati Lancet and Clinic*, Oct. 12, 1878.

CONTENTS.

Published Monthly, price $2.50 per annum, free of postage.
Also, furnished together with the AMERICAN JOURNAL OF THE MEDICAL SCIENCES *and the* MEDICAL NEWS AND LIBRARY *for* SIX DOLLARS *per annum in advance, the whole free of postage.*

HENRY C. LEA, Philadelphia.

THE MONTHLY ABSTRACT

OF

MEDICAL SCIENCE

VOL. V. No. 12.   **For List of Contents see last page.**   DECEMBER, 187<

Anatomy and Physiology.

On the Costal Processes of the Lumbar Vertebræ.

HERMANN MEYER (*Archiv fur Anat. und Physiol.*, 1877, p. 270) carefull tests the statement made by Frenkel, that the costal processes of the lumbar ver tebræ are to be regarded, not as aborted limbs, but rather as true transverse pr cesses. The hypothesis that the costal processes are aborted ribs is a very tempt ing one, and is apparently well based; it is, consequently, universally spread The statements of Frenkel are somewhat remote from the main argument, thoug they form an important part of its proof. Professor Meyer, therefore, seizes the opportunity of showing by actual facts, whilst he refers to the more exact c Frenkel's statements, that the large transverse processes of the lumbar vertebra are merely transverse processes, or, rather, parts of them, and are in no respec to be regarded as ribs.

The transverse processes of the twelfth dorsal vertebra is marked by thre tubercles. The upper and lower extremities of the rounded border in which th transverse process terminates are formed by a superior and an inferior tubercle whilst an anterior tubercle lies in front of the inferior tubercle on the under sur face of the transverse process below the rib. Tracing these tubercles upwards, i is seen that they become indistinct, and the anterior is rapidly reduced to slightly rough ridge. In a good specimen the anterior tubercle of the twelfth and slightly also that of the eleventh, dorsal vertebra appears as a spine. Passin· downwards, it is readily seen that the superior tubercle becomes, in the lumba vertebræ, the mammillary process, the inferior tubercle the accessory transvers process, and the anterior tubercle the costal process. These three processe taken together are to be considered as representing the transverse process, whicl in the dorsal vertebræ is in connection with the rib.—*London Med. Record*, Oct 15, 1878.

Sinus Transversus of the Occipital Bone.

Professor HERMANN MEYER (*op. cit.*, p. 272) gives the following account The right lateral sinus is nearly always broader than the left; and in close con nection with this point is the degree of roundness possessed by the angle betwee it and the extremity of the longitudinal sulcus. The reason for these appear ances has nowhere been assigned, though it is evident that the normal return o the conditions specified must be dependent upon the relation in which the trans· verse sinuses are placed in regard to certain other parts. The explanation is no far to seek, when these relations have been once obtained. The greater breadtl of the right lateral sinus, and the rounding of its angle of departure from th longitudinal sinus, are directly referable to the fact that the stream of blooc which flows through it is stronger than the stream which flows through the left side; consequently, the right side of the longitudinal sinus is to be regarded as the chief channel.   The reason why the current is stronger upon the right than upon the left side of the longitudinal sinus, is given by taking into consideration the conditions of the circulation below the neck.   Regarding the direction of the blood-flow, it is seen that the vena innominata of the right side is the direct continuation of the jugular vein; whilst the vena innominata of the left side is a prolongation downwards of the subclavian.   The vena cava superior, moreover, is in direct continuation with the right innominate, whilst the left innominate opens into it laterally.   The venous flow of the right side from the base of the skull to the heart is, therefore, as short as it is direct, whilst that of the left side is longer by the whole length of the left innominate, and is twice interrupted by angles.   The venous flow on the right side is, therefore, not only more easy in itself, but it is also assisted directly by the various forces of aspiration.   From this it is readily seen that the easier course for the blood to take is through the right half of the sinus transversus, and that the flow is therefore correspondingly stronger through this part.   Similar conditions producing contrary results are, however, found in the plexus pampiniformis, but the apparent contradiction can be explained by instituting a more careful comparison of the two cases.

It may be laid down as an established fact, that the varicosity of the spermatic plexus, which is shown as varicocele, occurs more commonly in the left testis. Varicosities, as is known, are due to a stoppage of the venous blood-flow, and it is easy to understand why this should occur more readily upon the left side, when it is recollected that the left spermatic vein opens into the left renal vein at a right angle, whilst the right spermatic opens into the inferior vena cava at an acute angle.   This is a case similar to the flow of venous blood from the left side of the head.   The surrounding conditions explain why there occur in the one case varicosities, and in the other a narrowing of the blood-path.   In the veins of the head, as already seen, this manifests itself less in a diminution in size of the path on the left side, than in a corresponding widening of the course on the right side.   The channel on the right side will, therefore, be used in preference; and, whilst that on the left becomes narrower from want of use, the channel on the right, being more used, will become broader.   In the left spermatic plexus, on the other hand, which is situated in such peculiar circumstances that there is no possibility of a neighbouring vessel relieving it, there arise a true stoppage of the blood-current and consequent varicosities.—*London Med. Record*, Oct. 15, 1878.

On a Peculiar Reaction of Saliva.

L. SOLERA publishes the following note in the *Rendiconti del Reale Istituto Lombardo*, 1877, Serie 2, Tom. x, p. 371.   Human saliva, whether filtered or not, whether fresh or kept for some time possesses the power of reducing iodic acid.   Saliva in presence of iodic acid becomes yellow, the colour being due to the liberation of free iodine.   This reaction depends upon the presence of potassium sulphocyanide which it contains; a weak dilute watery solution of potassium sulphcyanide gives exactly the same reaction with iodic acid as does saliva.   This reaction is marvellously delicate, to such an extent that the author is able to detect so small a quantity as 0.0000004 *gramme* of the substance.   None of the other salts which, according to the analyses of Frerichs, Jacubowitsch, and others, are present in the saliva, give this reaction, nor do the organic parts, viz., the mucus and ptyaline.—*London Med. Record*, Oct. 15, 1878.

Materia Medica and Therapeutics.

Effects of Strychnia.

In an elaborate experimental investigation on the anatomical and physiological effects of strychnia on the brain, spinal cord and nerves (*Journal of Nervous and Mental Disease*, Oct., 1878) Dr. W. H. KLAPP, of Philadelphia, draws the following conclusions:

1. Strychnia produces no appreciable primary lesion of the nerve substance proper; that secondary lesions are produced—granular disintegration—by the engorgement of the vascular system, and that this is more marked in the brain and cord than in the nerves.

2. That the convulsions of strychnia are not cerebral, and that they are much more severe after the ablation of the cerebrum, owing to the removal of Setschenow's ganglia.

3. Strychnia does not affect either the sensory or motor nerves at their periphery.

4. Both sensory and motor nerves, in their course, are unaffected by strychnia.

5. The tetanus-producing power of strychnia has its only action in the gray matter of the spinal cord.

6. In small doses, the primary action of strychnia is to excite the vaso-motor centre, causing thus a rise in the arterial pressure, and secondarily to paralyze this centre, and hence to supplement this rise by a fall.

7. In large doses, the vaso-motor centre is immediately paralyzed.

8. The slowing of the pulse, produced by the exhibition of strychnia to both warm and cold-blooded animals, is, in neither case, produced by any action on the central or peripheral ends of the pneumogastrics; but, in warm-blooded animals, is due to action on the excito-motor ganglia of the heart, and in cold-blooded animals is due to action on the ganglia situated in the sinus venosus.

9. The main vaso-motor centre for strychnia is situated in the medulla oblongata, but simpler centres exist in the spinal cord.

10. The pneumogastric nerves are *not* paralyzed by strychnia, in either warm or cold-blooded animals.

11. Strychnia decreases the number of respiratory movements; at first from too little blood, and afterwards from too much blood flowing to the respiratory centres.

12. The decrease is not due to any action of the pneumogastrics.

13. Artificial respiration always moderates, and sometimes stops, the spasms; and this power is due to a maintenance of the oxygenation of the blood until the poison can be eliminated, and is not due to a reflex stimulation of the pneumogastrics.

On the Use of Chloral-Hydrate Enemata.

Dr. STARCKE, of Berlin, has a paper on the employment of chloral-hydrate enemata in the *Berliner Klinische Wochenschrift* for August 19. He observes that there are great prejudices, especially in England, against the continued use of chloral, occasioned, probably, by the not unfrequent misadventures occurring in connection with its use in habitual drunkards. Last year Dr. Starcke himself fell ill of a chronic gastric catarrh, with great acidity of the contents of the stomach and considerable emaciation and prostration. The principal and most distressing symptom, however, was persistent insomnia, only half an hour to an hour's sleep being obtained at night. At the suggestion of his colleagues Dr.

Starcke resorted to the use of chloral, but the irritable state of the stomach forbade its use by the mouth, and hence he determined to take it *per rectum*. An aqueous five per cent. solution of chloral was warmed to about 95° Fahr., of which he injected first 10 grammes, and after a quarter of an hour a further quantity of 10 grammes, so that in all 1 gramme (15½ grains) of chloral were thus taken. This was in a few minutes followed by a feeling of warmth, comfort, and repose, and lastly by sound sleep, which lasted uninterruptedly for five hours. In this manner Dr. Starcke continued the injection of chloral for five months, taking in all 120 grammes of the drug. Decided convalescence set in after almost the very first dose, which was followed every morning by a sense of vigour and a desire for food, without any headache or other discomfort. Nor did the efficacy of the dose of chloral diminish, and latterly even half the quantity, *i. e.*, 0.5 gramme, was sufficient. Frequently the attempt was made to obtain sleep without resorting to the chloral, but in vain, until within the last month, when Dr. Starcke found he could discontinue it altogether. This employment of chloral *per rectum* has decided advantages in cases of gastric irritability. Dr. Starcke tried twice to take it by the mouth, and each time it was after a few minutes completely rejected, and no sleep ensued. The absence of all unpleasant results when administered by the rectum is doubtless due to its undergoing no decomposition, as is generally the case when it comes into contact with the contents of the stomach. Of course the drug should be absolutely pure. The sensation of burning and tenesmus which at first follows an injection, may be materially obviated by well oiling the nozzle of the syringe. And since the site of the tenesmus is chiefly in the region of the sphincter, contact of the chloral solution with this part of the gut should be avoided by passing the injection pipe as high up as possible. And if the injection is made by one's self, the position on knees and elbows will be found the most convenient. It is also of consequence that the solution should be complete, and that it should be warmed to the temperature of the body ; also that the dose required is a moderate and even small one as compared with that usually given by the mouth. Dr. Starcke has subsequently used chloral in the same way in various cases and with the same uniformly safe and favourable results. It seems especially applicable in the case of aged people, and in no case need the dose exceed one gramme (15½ grains).—*London Med. Record*, Oct. 15, 1878.

Metalloscopy and Metallotherapy.

Professor EULENBURG, of Griefswald (*Deutsche Med. Wochenschrift*, Nos. 25 and 26), has recently made some researches on this subject. He repeated Regnard's experiments by bringing a galvanometer into connection with the skin, applying the metal plates, and then causing electric currents to pass between the two. After further experiments on six individuals, he came to the following conclusions : 1. The same plates, applied to various healthy individuals on the same parts of the skin and under similar conditions, appear to be more active in some cases than in others, sometimes having almost no effect. 2. The galvanometric intensity of the metals is by no means alike in all healthy individuals ; zinc, more effective than gold in some persons, is less so in others, and *vice versa;* the proportions even vary at times in the same individuals (owing, perhaps, to some alteration in the dampness of the skin). From these facts it would appear that Regnard overestimates the importance of the electric currents.—Dr. C. WESTPHAL (*Ueber Metalloskopie, Berliner Klin. Wochenschrift*, No. 30, 1878) has also made researches on the same subject, and almost at the same time as Eulenburg. After making himself personally acquainted with Charcot's experiments, and selecting like cases (effeminate, hysterical, hemianæsthetic individuals), he began by using silver coins, and arrived at conclusions similar to those of Charcot—namely, the return of sensibility, sometimes local, sometimes affecting the entire side of the body ; and also the "transfeit," *i. e.*, with increased sensibility of the anæsthetic spot, a corresponding diminution on the symmetrical spot of the opposite part of the body. He then tried the application of iron, magnetic stone, copper covered with varnish or sealing-wax, and bone-markers, and obtained similar, although somewhat weaker, results. His assistant, Dr. Adamkiewicz, produced them also by means of mustard-plaster, whilst hot water and the electric brush were used without effect. Westphal says, in conclusion, that one must admit the fact that sensibility is restored by means of metallic plates, but he doubts whether (as Eulenburg says) it takes place through galvanic currents, inasmuch as non-metallic plates produce the same results. He thinks, in opposition to Burq, that no absolute idiosyncrasy for special metals exists, because two metals may be effectual in one and the same patient. The therapeutic result is at best but limited and temporary—M. Thennes reported to the Biological Society, at the meeting of October 12th, that he had ascertained in the cases of two hysterical patients that thermal agents are capable of acting in the same way as metals and currents. With applications of ice in one case and of hot water in the other, the hemianæsthesia, achromatopsy, and contraction disappeared. The editor of the *Progrès Médical* adds in a note that similar results were obtained by the use of ice last winter by MM. Bourneville and Regnard.—*Brit. Med. Journ.*, Oct. 26, 1878.

Medicine.

Migration of White Blood-Corpuscles in Inflammation..

APPERT, in Virchow's *Archiv*, Band lxxi, p. 364, has obtained the following results in experimenting with frogs in relation to this point : 1. Quinine, in doses of $\frac{1}{3500}$th to $\frac{1}{4000}$th of the body-weight, not only hinders the migration of white corpuscles at the centre of inflammation, but prevents their stagnation on the walls of the vessel. The cells which are found within the vessel have a dark appearance, and exhibit few or no amœboid changes. 2. Quinine, in a dose of $\frac{1}{4133}$th of the body-weight, injected in small quantities under the skin of the frog, in the course of three or four hours diminished the diapedesis for two to three hours without modifying the central current, and without causing the white corpuscles to leave the wall. The pulse was rendered feeble, the circulation was slowed, and the vessels were contracted. 3. Quinine in a dose of $\frac{1}{8000}$th of the body-weight had no effect. The experiments were made upon the tongue,.and the author obtained the same effects by ligaturing the two arteries without the veins; a considerable tightening of the ligature gave rise to the same effects as a strong dose of quinine, whilst the ligature less strongly applied was equivalent to a weak dose of quinine.—*Lond. Med. Record*, Oct. 15, 1878.

Addison's Disease.

Dr. JOHN WYLIE (*Glasgow Med Journal*, September, 1878) describes a case of Addison's disease in a married woman, aged 39, who had noticed discoloration of the skin which had been coming on for twelve or fourteen months. She complained of general weakness, disinclination for exertion, palpitation, gastric irritability, and vomiting of a most persistent kind. She had had rheumatic fever

six years ago. Her parents were healthy; her children were all alive and
healthy; she was now pregnant. The skin was "smooth and soft, of a yellowish colour, but merging into a much deeper shade in those places which are
naturally the seat of pigment, such as the areolæ of the nipples, the axillæ, abdomen, etc." She died of rheumatic fever. The organs were all healthy, except
the suprarenal capsules. The left was larger than the right, and on cutting
through it, about a teaspoonful of yellowish pus-like fluid escaped. The normal
structure of the capsule was converted into hardened cheesy nodules, which here
and there grated under the knife. The right capsule was small, containing more
of the pus-like fluid but less cheesy matter.—*London Med. Record*, Oct. 15,
1878.

—

Mixed Forms of Typhus.

M. BORODULIN contributes to the *St. Petersburger Medicinische Wochenschrift*, for July 15, some observations on the concurrence of different types of
fever founded on cases which occurred in the clinique of Prof. Botkin of St.
Petersburg. The simultaneous invasion and course of several forms of fever in
the same individual are at the present day by no means generally acknowledged,
some regarding the occurrence of these mixed forms as beyond all doubt, while
others as stoutly deny it. But after the late epidemic of relapsing fever in St.
Petersburg, the possibility of relapsing being superadded to other forms of typhus
fever was admitted in the clinique of Dr. Botkin. Clinical observation showed
marked peculiarities in the course of abdominal exanthematic typhus, which
pointed to relapsing fever, such as oscillations of temperature, sweats, only slight
typhoid impairment of the sensorium, clinically well-marked alterations in the
liver and spleen, primary brick-red petechiæ occurring at the very commencement of abdominal or exanthematic typhus. During the epidemic of the present
year, the blood of all the typhus patients in the clinique was examined with a
view to ascertaining whether it contained spirillæ, whose presence has hitherto
been regarded as pathognomonic of relapsing fever. They were found in four
cases of a mixed form of abdominal typhus, and in one of exanthematic typhus.
That spirillæ were not found in the blood of the other cases may be due partly to
want of time for a minute examination and to the difficulty of finding them;
since their quantity is in direct proportion to the amount of the specific blood-
poison of relapsing fever, for the nearer the disease approaches to true relapsing
fever the greater the number of spirillæ, and *vice versâ*. The following is an
abstract of the five cases alluded to :—

CASE I.—P., aged nineteen years, was received into the clinique on the fourth
day of the disease. The commencement of the illness was gradual, without
rigours. Even on the evening of the third day the temperature was 104.7 F.,
the next morning 104 F., and in the evening again 104.7. His general strength
was still excellent; the sensorium was clear; there were a few petechiæ and rose
spots; the spleen and liver were considerably enlarged and tender; the heart
was somewhat enlarged transversely. He had slight icterus. There were traces
of albumen in the urine   He had slight delirium on the night of the fourth day.
On the fifth day a few spirillæ were found in the blood. On the sixth day,
besides nocturnal delirium, there was also impaired intellect during the day,
which, though slight to the twenty-fifth day, thereafter increased considerably,
and continued so till death. On the eighth day he had bronchial catarrh. On
the nineteenth there was right-sided hypostatic pneumonia, extending to both
lungs on the twenty-third day. The amount of albumen in the urine increased
gradually; cylindrical casts were found, and the albumen only diminished towards
the end of the disease. The temperature ranged from the fourth to the twen-

tieth day between 102.2 F. (only once) and 104.9 F.   In the night of the
fifteenth to the sixteenth day he had a severe rigour; and on the following morning spirillæ were again present in the blood.   In the night, from the nineteenth
to the twentieth day, he had again rigours, with subsequent sweating and reduction of the temperature from 104 F. to 100.4 F.   On the morning of the thirty-
first day, the temperature fell after profuse sweating from 105.2 to 98.8 F.
From the thirtieth day, the impairment of the sensorium increased considerably.
There was subsultus tendinum.   On the thirty-third day there was suppression
of urine, with extreme weakness, ending in death on the thirty-sixth day.

Necropsy.—There were œdema of brain-substance, hypostatic pneumonia in
both lower lobes, and lateral dilatation of the heart, with flaccid walls of a
grayish-yellow colour; the valves were normal. The spleen was much enlarged;
its parenchyma was anæmic, firm; near the surface was a recent blood-clot.
The liver was also much enlarged; its parenchyma was of a grayish-yellow
colour, indistinctly marked.   The right kidney was enlarged; the capsule was
loosely adherent; the cortical substance was expanded, gray, friable, with small
puriform dots; the calyces were dilated; from the pyramids an opaque fluid
could be expressed.   The left kidney was similarly altered, with the exception
of the puriform dots.   In the ileum were several ulcers reaching to the muscular
coat, and corresponding with Peyer's patches.   The mucous membrane of the
stomach was pale, with small extravasations.

CASE II.—S., aged 19, was received on the ninth day.   The invasion of the
disease was gradual, so that the patient, a student, attended lectures on the sixth
day.   On the seventh and eighth days he had nocturnal sweating.   The liver
and spleen were much enlarged, and tender.   There were some petechiæ and
rose-spots.   The sensorium was free; a few spirillæ were found in the blood;
there was no albumen in the urine.   Otherwise the case presented nothing unusual.   The temperature became normal on the twenty-fifth day; the liver and
spleen remained enlarged till the thirty-sixth day.

CASE III.—M., aged 21, female, was admitted on the sixth day.   She fell ill
suddenly.   On the first day there was great heat of surface, without preceding
rigours, and headache.   On the fourth day the morning temperature was 102.9
Fahr., and the evening temperature was 104 Fahr.   In this case also were found
primary petechiæ and rose-spots on the abdomen.   The liver and spleen were not
so much enlarged as in Case 2.   These and the laterally somewhat enlarged heart
were tender on percussion.   On the seventh day, some spirillæ were discovered
in the blood.   There was slight tendency to sweating; the temperature was that
of abdominal typhus.

The next two cases present more symptoms of relapsing fever, and spirillæ
were found in increased numbers.

CASE IV.—E., a student, was received on the sixth day of the disease.   The
commencement of the disease was gradual, without distinct shivering.   The morning temperature was 103.9 F.; evening, 104.7 F.   The liver and spleen were
moderately enlarged; he had slight roseala, and bronchitis; the sensorium was
slightly clouded.   On the seventh day there was an increase of eruption, and of
mental impairment, with diarrhœa; there were no spirillæ in the blood.   Up to
the ninth day the temperature ranged between 103.1 and 104.9 F.; on the morning
of that day it stood at 104.9, but now declined after copious sweating to 96.8 F.
by 3 P. M., and rose again in the evening to 104 F.   On the tenth day the eruption vanished almost entirely, but the senses became more and more clouded till
the fifteenth day.   On the fourteenth, fluctuation became perceptible in the lower
abdomen, and the diarrhœa ceased.   Up till the sixth day the temperature gradually sank in 48 hours to 97.3 F.   He had daily sweats from the fourteenth to the

nineteenth day. The low temperature continued about 48 hours; for on the evening of the seventeenth day it again rose from 96.1 in the morning to 101.6 F. During the following two days the temperature continued of the same remittent character, 99.3-103.1; 99.1-103.6 F. On the nineteenth day the patient began to shiver, and the spleen became enlarged. On the twentieth day the temperature was, in the morning, 101.3, in the evening 104.9, with severe rigours. Numerous spirillæ were now found in the blood; on the next (twenty-first) day he again had rigours, with spirillæ in the blood; in the evening, sweating, with fall of temperature to 97.9 On the twenty-second day the morning temperature was 99.5, rising after a rigour to 106.3 F. From this day to the twenty-seventh day there was increased temperature every evening, with almost normal morning temperature. Indeed, on the twenty-fourth day, both morning and evening temperature was normal. But from the twenty-seventh day to the thirtieth day there were high temperatures both morning and evening. After this the temperature rose only once to 100.4 F., and then declined to about 98.6, until the dismissal of the patient. This case is therefore evidently of a mixed character. Against a pure relapsing fever are the gradual beginning of the disease, the typhoid condition, continuing to the fifteenth day, the marked rosy eruption, and the absence of petechiæ. It also differs from pure exanthematic typhus in the decline of the temperature on the ninth day to 96.8, after sweating, followed by a rise on the same evening; also in the spirillæ found in the blood during a paroxysm of high temperature lasting five days; and, lastly, in a third rise of temperature after a remission of 24 hours, and a continuance of high temperature from the twenty-fifth to the twenty-ninth day, on which latter day it attained its maximum, after which it rapidly declined.

CASE V.—G., aged 23, sister of charity, was admitted on the fifth day of the disease. This began with severe rigours, as in true intermittent. On the evening of the day of admission, the temperature was 104.0. The liver and spleen were enlarged with considerable jaundice; primary petechiæ were present. The next morning large numbers of spirillæ were found in the blood. In the night from the seventh to the eighth day there was a critical decline of temperature from 104 to 99.2 F., after profuse sweating, but in the evening it had again risen to 100 F., and now continued on the average somewhat above the normal. On the sixteenth day there was again severe shivering, and considerable numbers of spirillæ were found in the blood. This paroxysm continued four days, and was then followed by copious sweating, and a rapid decline of temperature from 104.5 to 98.6 F. The temperature now continued normal for two days and a half, when it again rose, assuming a remittent character with morning remissions and evening exacerbations, until the twenty-ninth day of the disease. On this day temperature fell, after sweating, to 98.6 F.. and continued normal thereafter. This case differs from the usual course of true relapsing fever in the continuance of pyrexia between the first and second attacks, and in the somewhat long period with relapsing fever after the crisis of the second attack, when the course of the temperature somewhat resembled that of abdominal typhus.—*Lond. Med. Record*, Oct. 15, 1878.

Testis in Typhus.

M. FENOMENOW (*St. Petersburger Medicinische Wochenschrift*, July 8), has examined the testes in twelve cases, of which five died of exanthematic typhus, three of abdominal typhus, two of bilious typhoid, and two of a mixed form of abdominal typhus and recurrent fever. The best preparations were obtained by hardening in alcohol, the sections were stained with hæmatoxylin and mounted with glycerine. The changes observed were in the epithelium of the seminal ducts, and the epithelioid lining of the bloodvessels. In both it consisted of enlargement of the cells, obscurity of outline, nuclei obscured by granular masses soluble in ether. The changes in the vessels appeared to precede those in the ducts. In some places there were small hemorrhages, but these are not specially described.

[The importance of these observations is somewhat diminished by the results of Dr. Litten's experiments (Virchow's *Archiv*, May, 1876; *Monthly Abstract*, Dec. 1877, p. 541), which showed that such fatty metamorphosis of the tissues was the constant effect of high temperatures.—*Rep*.]--*London Med. Record*, Oct. 15, 1878.

Case of Cerebral Rheumatism with Catalepsy.

In *Lo Sperimentale* for March, Dr. MANCINI relates the case of a blacksmith, aged 33, who, after having had four slight rheumatic attacks, was seized in September, 1877, after sweating profusely, with *malaise*, weariness, loss of appetite, and pain and swelling of the knees and feet. He had nearly recovered, when he was one morning awakened by the noise of an alarm clock in an adjoining chamber. From this time he became fond of solitude, taciturn, reserved, inimical to all human intercourse, desirous of neither food nor drink; and he complained also of severe headache.

When received into hospital on December 11th, he was noted to be of robust constitution, well formed, but imperfectly nourished. He lay on his back; his face was without expression. He did not answer questions, and did not move when threatened. The eyes were fixed, and the pupils insensible to light. Sight and hearing were normal; the sense of smell was impaired. The sensations of heat and pain were lost. Reflex motion was absent. Galvanic and farado-muscular contractility was increased. Speech was impossible; the rectum and bladder were paralyzed. The trunk and limbs remained in whatever position was given them.

Considering the previous attack of articular rheumatism, and the sudden appearance of the nervous disorder during convalescence from this disease, Dr. Mancini believes that the case was probably one of cerebral rheumatism.

The treatment consisted in the administration of infusion of lime-flowers as a diaphoretic, and the application of sinapisms to the lower extremities. The man soon improved; all morbid symptoms disappeared; and, ten days after he was admitted to hospital he was perfectly convalescent.—*London Med. Record*, Oct. 15, 1878.

Ignored Syphilis.

Dr. FOURNIER, in a lecture delivered at the St. Louis (*Gaz. des Hôp.*, August 8), observed that the great frequency of cases of *syphilis ignoré*, and the practical importance of its study, induced him to bring it before his class.

A patient presents himself with what, after careful examination, appears to be a syphilitic affection, but on interrogating him, and cross-questioning him in every way, he stoutly denies ever having had the pox. Still, confident in the objective signs observed, specific remedies are administered, and in a few days the lesion, which had been menacing, and even progressing rapidly, is almost cured. The result renders the accuracy of the diagnosis certain. The patient has had syphilis without knowing it, furnishing an example of *syphilis ignoré*. At first sight this appellation seems contrary to common sense, for so complex a disease, characterized by such multiple symptoms, can scarcely be supposed to pursue its course unperceived. And yet not only may this be so, but it frequently is so. In fact, the profession has ceased to take the denial of the patients into account, and treats their cases solely from the aspect they present. At St. Louis *syphilis ignoré* is of such frequent occurrence, that during five months of the present year, in Dr. Fournier's service alone, there have been twenty-eight persons the subjects of syphilis without being aware of it, and that when only counting tertiary syphilides and the most obvious cases. As is always the case there, the treatment has confirmed the diagnosis.

These cases are much more commonly met with among the common people than in the well-to-do classes, which is but a natural result of the differences in situation, education, and the care of the person. The aristocracy and mercantile classes are pretty well informed on the matter of syphilis by means of reading and conversation, and even by the advertisements in the newspapers. They keep a sharp lookout, and on the slightest alarm have the time and money to get themselves at once treated. It is quite different with the lower classes, whom the absence of education, carelessness, indigence, and their daily toil, expose much more easily to the occurrence of *syphilis ignoré*. It is also incomparably more frequent in women. A man is much more conversant with syphilis; he knows from his youth that this is his enemy, and he is often acquainted with it before being exposed to its dangers, "were it only by the classic visit to the Musée Dupuytren, which some fathers of families consider it a duty to make their sons pay on quitting school." Thus forewarned, men have much less chance of failing to recognize syphilis. But women live in complete ignorance of these things, to which they are utter strangers. How many honest women there are, and even mothers of families, who do not even suspect the existence of this disease! But this very ignorance, if they become the subjects of it, exposes them all the more to a non-recognition of their enemy. Of the twenty-eight cases above alluded to, twenty-two were women and six men.

Thus syphilis may remain ignored, and this may be explained by numerous reasons, the principal of which are: 1. That a certain number of cases of syphilis fail to be recognized because they have a non-venereal origin. In the eyes of most people the idea of syphilis is necessarily connected with an impure sexual intercourse; and when the disease is in any other part than the genitals, it is firmly believed to be due to something else. Little notice is taken of it, and it is allowed to run on until serious tertiary symptoms enforce the diagnosis. There are, in fact, many causes of non-venereal origin of syphilis, as contact with syphilitic children; domestic contagion, from the use of a pipe, spoon, etc.; professional contagion, as with doctors and midwives; contagion by surgical instruments or by certain operations, such as Eustachian catheterism, the use of the bistoury, the speculum, serre-fines, etc.; contagion by vaccination, etc. Any of these forms of syphilis may remain ignored, even by those whose very occupations ought to prevent their overlooking them. "In fact, doctors and midwives are often surprised in this manner. I knew a midwife who had a syphilide on her finger without being aware of its nature; and one of my fellow-students, now a very distinguished physician, had on his finger a well-characterized syphilitic lesion for more than six months, which he regarded as an anatomical tubercle. If practitioners allow themselves to be deceived in this way, how much more are people of the world liable to overlook an attack of syphilis!" 2. Syphilis may remain ignored because its symptoms have been overlooked or its nature has not been demonstrated. The symptoms of syphilis, in fact, are not always so evident or special even that the practitioner can pronounce at once upon them. A well-marked case of syphilis, with chancre, bubo, roseola, alopecia, cephalalgia, articular pains, iritis, etc., may still be mistaken for another affection. The chancre, especially if superficial, may be overlooked, or mistaken for some trifling hurt, even in men, and especially in women when it is placed on the cervix uteri. Bubo, in its nature indolent, is generally ignored ; and the syphilides, being unattended with pruritus, do not give rise to pain or itching. Roseola is almost always overlooked by the patient until it has been pointed out to him ; and so on with the various other symptoms, which, when not overlooked, are attributed to various causes ; so that, in fact, the syphilitic patient with the most perfect faith may easily believe that he is not the subject of syphilis. 3. Syphilis is the more liable to be ignored when the original symptoms are benign and the secondary ones have scarcely existed. A long silence follows this period, which has only been characterized by a more or less ephemeral roseola and a few patches in the throat; then, ten or fifteen years afterwards, some grave accident supervenes, which leads to the discovery of the diathesis. 4. In women syphilis is the more likely to remain ignored, since all that is possible is done to hide the nature of the disease from them. The husband or the lover entreats the surgeon to treat his victim without revealing to her the cause of her malady ; and amidst this "true conspiracy of silence" she becomes cured of her *syphilis ignoré*.

The practical conclusion is, that there exists a certain number of cases of syphilis, the diagnosis of which must be arrived at exclusively from the character of the lesion under observation, in spite of the silence of their history and the denials of the patients. Whenever the practitioner finds himself in the presence of such a case, in which all antecedent is denied, he should submit the patient to a second and even a third scrupulous examination, comparing the signs present with those which might be furnished by other diseases. But, having convinced himself that the lesion is syphilitic, he should institute its specific treatment in spite of the denial and even the most earnest protests of the patient. The experience of his predecessors and daily clinical teaching establish his right and duty. " The science of the physician," in the words of Ricord, " is above the assertions of the patient." The doctor affirms and the patient denies ; but there is infinitely more chance that the former will be found right.—*Med. Times and Gazette*, Oct. 5, 1878.

Case of Cerebellar Disease.

In Betz's *Memorabilien*, xxiii Jahrgang, Heft 5, Dr. KELP relates the following case, and makes some remarks upon it.

J. H., a peasant, aged 36, had been intemperate in his habits for four years ; during that time he often complained of pains and twitching in his limbs, was confused in his mind, and said strange things, e. g., that a workman in the house had bewitched him. For the last year he had become easily fatigued, and his gait was not quite steady, so that he was often obliged to rest while walking ; he was also forgetful and dreamy. Quite recently he had become very excited, was unable to sleep, and destroyed his bedding. There had been no other cases of insanity in the family.

About a month after this excitement came on, he was admitted into the asylum at Wehnen. He was then very "lost," did not know where he was ; his gait was very unsteady, it resembled that of a drunken man, and he tended to fall *backwards*. There was general muscular tremor ; the eyes were dull, pupils equal, face congested, and nose very red. He was unable to answer any question, dressed and undressed himself listlessly, was dirty in his habits, and uttered inarticulate sounds. His appetite was good ; pulse 100. He remained for several days in bed, as he was subject to attacks of vertigo. After two months, hæmatoma of the right ear was developed, paralysis of the lower extremities came on, and the patient fell towards the left side ; the right side of the face was drawn down; the skin was remarkably cold; pulse 50. The paralysis continued to increase, the surface-temperature to decrease; the pulse sank to 36, the temperature to 80, and death took place after little more than two months' treatment.

After death, the head only was examined. The dura mater was much thickened throughout, and bound to the pia mater by adhesions which required the knife to divide them. The pia mater was firmly adherent to the cortex, its vessels injected. The cerebrum was normally formed, of firm consistence; no proliferation of tissue could be detected. The cerebellum weighed a little over five ounces; both its hemispheres showed extensive softening; where this was most marked, the tissue was of a bright gray colour. The left hemisphere was affected more extensively and in a greater degree than the right; in the centre of the left posterior superior lobe there was a spot of softening, of the size of a walnut; the surrounding tissue was also affected, but in a less degree. The arbor vitæ was ill-defined and discoloured, but the medullary substance and the connections with the medulla oblongata, corpora quadrigemina, and pons Varolii were of normal consistence. The softening in the right lobe was in the same situation as in the left; the arbor vitæ appearance was fully developed, and the surrounding tissue normal. The pons Varolii, olivary bodies, and medulla oblongata presented no morbid changes.

The abuse of stimulants must be regarded as the chief cause of cerebellar disease in this case; the most characteristic symptoms were the staggering gait resembling that of drunkenness, the attacks of giddiness, the tendency to fall backwards, and the tremor of the limbs. The confused state of the patient's mind must be ascribed to the affection of the cerebrum and its coverings, and the motor symptoms to the organic changes in the cerebellum.

In a recent paper on cerebellar disease (*see Monthly Abstract*, Aug. '1878, p. 350) Professor Nothnagel gives his support to the view that disturbances of co-ordination are caused by morbid changes in the cerebellum, but he also states his opinion that these disturbances of co-ordination only occur when the median lobe (vermiform processes) is directly or indirectly affected by the disease. Dr. Kelp holds that his case quite disproves this proposition, as he states that the vermiform processes were in no way affected, though motor disturbances were present.

As the spinal cord could not be examined, it was not determined whether the tabic gray degeneration of its columns was present. The author thinks that this would not have been found, for the gait of a tabic patient lacks the peculiar resemblance to that of the drunkard which was observed in this case. The marked trembling of the extremities and the rapid development of the disease are also points against the diagnosis of tabes.

For some time before his death the patient's body was constantly rotated towards the left side, and this twisting always recurred immediately after it had been righted by force. This symptom is ascribed by Kelp to the fact [apparently contradicted in the above report of the *post-mortem* appearances—*Rep.*] that the middle peduncle of the cerebellum, or the fibres radiating from it into the cerebellum, was involved in the morbid process.—*London Med. Record*, Oct. 15, 1878.

<hr>

Reflex Paralysis.

At a meeting of the Royal Medico-Chirurgical Society of Naples (*Il Morgagni*, 1878), Dr. F. Vizioli presented a man suffering from reflex paralysis. The patient, a healthy robust man, aged 48, had been struck in the front of the neck by a knife, which produced an extensive but superficial wound. In the evening he perceived numbness on the right arm and shoulder, which soon became incapable of motion. When he was shown to the society, four months after the injury, motion was almost abolished in the right arm, and there was marked emaciation of all the brachial and scapular muscles. Electro-muscular sensibility was slightly increased in the paralyzed as compared with the corresponding sound parts; there was no alteration in the sense of touch, nor in the sensations of heat or pain. Electro-muscular contractility, faradic and galvanic, was normal even in the paralyzed and atrophied muscles. The temperature of the affected muscles was slightly lower than that of the healthy ones.

The author, considering that the retention of electro-muscular contractility indicated a central lesion, on which the atrophy of the muscles of the arm and shoulder depended, and that there was no concussion or fall, and thus reducing the cause of the malady to the wound received, concluded that the cutaneous irritation produced a process of irritation in the medulla—that is to say, hyperæmia of the meninges and capillary apoplexy in the spinal cord; and that this explains the rapidity with which the paralysis appeared a few hours after the injury.

As regards the atrophy, he refers it to the impaired trophic influence of the medulla rather than to defective functional energy in the muscles.—*Lond. Med. Record*, October 15, 1878.

An Account of a Demonstration of the Phenomena of Hystero-Epilepsy; and on the Modification which they undergo under the Influence of Magnets and Solenoids.

On the mornings of August 23d and 24th several physicians and scientific men, amongst whom were Professors Virchow, Grainger Stewart, Turner, Oscar Liebreich, Ray Lankester, Dr. Broadbent, Mr. Ernest Hart, etc., who happened to be in Paris, met in Professor CHARCOT'S wards in the great hospital of La Salpêtrière, and had the privilege of being present at a demonstration in which this distinguished physician brought under their notice all the remarkable features of hystero-epilepsy—that remarkable disease almost all knowledge of which is due to the labours of M. Charcot. In these demonstrations, the remarkable influence of solenoids and of magnets upon the diseased organism was exhibited, no less than the ready induction of the so-called *mesmeric* and *cataleptic* conditions in these patients. All the phases of the remarkable hystero-epileptic convulsions were repeatedly observed.

Such was the interest awakened by these remarkable demonstrations, that Dr. ARTHUR GAMGEE, Brackenbury Professor of Physiology in Owen's College, Manchester, has given the following account (*British Medical Journal*, Oct. 12, 1878) of the principal facts which were brought under their notice on the occasion of the second demonstration.

In order that the description of these facts may be the more intelligible to those who are unacquainted with even the salient points in the natural history of hystero-epilepsy, I will summarize these briefly, as follows: Hystero-epilepsy is a nervous disease of women of great rarity, affecting them especially during the child-bearing period of life; sometimes, though rarely, occurring before the actual commencement of menstruation, and continuing after its cessation. It is associated with hyperæsthesia in one or both ovarian regions, and is usually attended by hemianæsthesia, and more rarely by anæsthesia of both sides of the body. There is some, if not complete, loss of tactile sensibility, and usually absolute insensibility to pain (analgesia) of skin, and all other sensitive structures on the affected side; the muscular sense being, however, nearly always preserved. There is some degree of paresis of the affected limbs. The loss of sensitiveness may or may not affect the organs of special sense; it frequently does so affect the eye, which becomes affected with a remarkable form of colour-blindness (achromatopsia). It is characteristic of the heminæsthesia of hystero-epilepsy that by various means—action of magnets, solenoids, metallic plates—it may be momentarily diverted from the affected side, which then regains its normal sensibility, and transferred temporarily to the opposite side of the body. The essential and pathognomonic sign of the disease is the occurrence of attacks, which present remarkable phenomena in a definite order; at first epileptiform, then affecting the mental functions of the patient, who by gesture and actual utterance, reveals to the spectator various phases of emotional activity. The disease usually does not tend towards recovery, though recovery occasionally occurs. It may continue for many years without any perceptible influence upon the health or mental condition of the patient, and when death occurs it appears to result from intercurrent disease, which, in relation to the primary disease, may be termed accidental.

Having thus sketched boldly and without detail the main features of a disease, the study of which shows, as the reader will soon learn, how scanty are our physiological conceptions of the nervous system, I present the following simple narrative of that which I saw and heard on August 24th.

I. *Induction of the Mesmeric Condition in a Patient affected with Hystero-Epilepsy.*—Being assembled in the laboratory attached to his wards, Professor Charcot brought before us a young patient, aged 20, affected with hystero-epilepsy. In this patient, there exists left-sided hemianæsthesia, which is associated with hyperæsthesia in the right ovarian region. (By perusing the account afterwards given of the convulsive attacks of hystero-epilepsy, the reader will understand the grounds for the diagnosis of the ovarian irritation in these cases.) Professor Charcot brought this patient before us to demonstrate that usually it is possible in patients affected with hystero-epilepsy to induce the mesmeric condition. The patient being seated opposite to him, at the distance of about two feet, he steadily maintained the index finger of his right hand at a short distance from the centre of her forehead; she was directed to look steadily at the finger, and did so. Several minutes elapsed (the time was not actually noted), and the patient did not seem sensibly affected. She declared that "to-day she had no desire to sleep." At 10.4 A. M., the previous attempts, which may have lasted ten minutes, having failed, Professor Charcot, placing his head on a level with that of the patient, commenced to stare fixedly into both her eyes. At 10.6, the eyelids drooped, and, at the same time, began to wink in a rapid tremulous manner; this phenomenon continuing throughout the whole duration of the induced sleep, and being, Professor Charcot remarked, constant; at the same time, a tonic contraction of the flexors of both forearms occurred, the fists becoming temporarily clenched. At 10.7, the patient being asleep, Professor Charcot told her to rise and take a chair. She did so, her eyes being closed and her eyelids tremulous. Having seated herself, he told her to write her name. Pen, ink, and paper being furnished her, she sleepily wrote her own name, and afterwards, when ordered, Professor Charcot's, her eyes remaining closed the whole time. Whilst writing, the skin over the right wrist was transfixed by a thick needle, but the patient appeared quite unconscious of the operation, continuing to write with the needle *in situ.* It is to be remarked that, during the mesmeric state, the patient is anæsthetic on both sides of the body; whilst, in the waking state, it is only the left side which is anæsthetic. At 10.10, Professor Charcot told the patient to begin to sew. A half-hemmed towel was handed to her, and she at once commenced to sew with great dexterity and rapidity, co-ordinating admirably the movements of the two hands. The patient was then told to rise and go into an adjoining room used for photography; she did so, and, on her way, having to descend a step, she walked with caution and safety, her eyes being still closed. Being bidden to retrace her steps, she obeyed, and came into the room in which we were all assembled, and, turning towards the wall, remained standing listlessly, fast asleep. Professor Charcot then blew into her eyes, when she awoke. The act of awaking, in her case and in that of all hystero-epileptics who have been thrown into the mesmeric sleep, is accompanied by a peculiar reflex; there is an automatic and sudden act of expulsion of saliva—as it were a slight effort to spit.

II. *Instantaneous Induction of the Mesmeric Condition in a Patient affected with Hystero-Epilepsy; Subsequent Induction of the Cataleptic Condition; Hemianæsthesia and Colour-Blindness; Action of a Solenoid.*—An anæmia young girl, aged about 20, was next brought before us. The disease in her case had had for its origin terrible scenes of which she had been the witness during the Commune. It is to be noticed that nearly all, if not all, cases of hystero-epilepsy appear to have been connected with fright or anguish. In this patient, there was complete right hemianæsthesia, with colour-blindness affecting the eye of the same side, with which she could only distinguish red. When papers of various colours were brought before her, the left eye being kept closed, she described all, excepting the red paper, as being of a dirty-white or white colour. There was complete analgesia on the right side, so that a needle could be thrust through the hand without occasioning the slightest evidence of pain. The skin of the opposite side was normally sensitive. A spiral insulated wire—a solenoid—connecting the two poles of a large single carbon-zinc and chromic acid element was now made to envelop the little finger of the right hemianæsthetic side. Almost instantaneously, the sound side became hemianæsthetic and the previously normal eye became colour-blind for all colours but red, whilst the power of distinguishing colours on the usually colour-blind eye became perfect. No sooner, however, was the finger withdrawn from the solenoid, than the anæsthesia and achromatopsia reassumed their usual distribution.

This case, as M. Charcot pointed out, was not only remarkable for the extreme rapidity with which the action of the current was developed, but also for the surprising readiness with which the patient could be thrown into the mesmeric and cataleptic conditions, as he proceeded to show. It sufficed merely to open the patient's eyes and stare into them for an instant, to throw her into a profound sleep, from which she could be aroused by certain stimuli, and especially by blowing into the face, when the peculiar reflex noticed in Case I. was produced. That the instantaneous production of this mesmeric state was not due to any special influence of M. Charcot was evidenced by his allowing me to repeat his procedure, when instantly the same result followed.

The patient was now taken into a darkened room, in which a spiral of platinum heated by a powerful gas blow-pipe emitted a light almost as intense as the magnesium light. If she stared into the flame for an instant, she immediately fell asleep, and passed into a cataleptic condition; her limbs, placed in the most unnatural positions, retained these until some one moved them into a new attitude.

But the most singular fact observed in connection with the cataleptic condition of this patient was the following: If, whilst deeply sleeping and cataleptic, any one stealthily approached one of his fingers or thumbs to within a short distance —about half an inch—of the patient's skin, as, for example, of the palm or back of the hand, she instantly awakened with a cry of "Ah!" evincing by its tone evident mental anguish, if not actual physical pain. When thus awakened, the patient had merely to stare at the bright light instantly to return into the cataleptic condition. We had the opportunity of observing that when she happened to be very close to the light, and watching it very intently, the approach of a finger to the skin sometimes had no effect, and that it was only after repeated approaches that she awoke, though always in the manner previously described.

Before leaving this singularly striking case, it may be remarked that Professor Charcot was led to try the action of a spiral wire traversed by a current on the hemianæsthesia of hystero-epilepsy because of the already discovered influence of magnets, which will be illustrated in the sequel, and from the fact of the physical analogies of solenoids and magnets.[1]

III. *Hystero-Epilepsy in a Woman aged* 54, *and who is blind; Cessation of Fits for the last two years, but Continuance of Hemianæsthesia of the Right Side.*—The case of this patient is of peculiar interest, as she has been an inmate of the Salpêtrière since the year 1846, and her case has been studied with remarkable accuracy. It will be found fully narrated, and the account illustrated with many drawings, in Dr. Bourneville's *Recherches Cliniques et Thérapeutiques sur l' Epilepsie et l' Hystérie. (Compte-rendu des Observations recueillies à la Salpêtrière de 1872 à 1876.* Paris, 1876.) This woman has, it would appear, been a hystero-epileptic for forty-three years of her life. She was formerly subject to the most characteristic attacks of hystero-epileptic convulsions, which underwent, in the period during which she was under observation, very remarkable transitions. The disappearance of the menses was not immediately followed by a cessation of the fits; on the contrary, as would appear from Dr. Bourneville's record, in the year following the cessation of menstruation, the fits were more frequent than they had ever been, the utmost frequency being, however, reached in the fourth year after. Since 1876, however, the fits have not recurred; and now there only remains the absolute analgesia of the left side. This patient is quite blind, owing to inflammatory affections occurring in childhood, and is of very deficient intelligence. There is absolute analgesia of the left side. A needle could be thrust through the left hand or arm without occasioning any sensation. Sensibility is, however, tolerably perfect on the right side.

The patient being seated, the two poles of a tolerably large horseshoe magnet were brought to within a third of an inch of the skin of the forearm on the affected side. From time to time, the sensitiveness of the two arms was examined by pricking with a needle. After some minutes, the arm in proximity to the magnet had regained its sensitiveness, the patient complaining bitterly when a needle was merely pressed against the skin, without pricking it, whilst the arm of the right side had become completely anæsthetic, and could be transfixed with a needle without the patient being aware of the fact. It is to be remarked that at no time during the observation did the arm touch the magnet, which was kept at a distance varying between a quarter and one-third of an inch. It might be surmised, M. Charcot remarked, that the effect exerted by the magnet was one which might be exerted by any mass of iron; not so, however. If, for instance, the convex neutral end of the horseshoe be turned towards the arm, instead of the poles, none of the effects previously described follow.

IV. *Hysterical Contraction of the Left Arm cured by the Systematic Daily Magnetization of the Right Arm; Ovarian Hyperæsthesia of the Left Side.*—In order to illustrate the curative action of the magnet, Professor Charcot brought before us the case of a nun who had been admitted into the Salpêtrière for a hysterical contraction which had lasted nine months. On admission, there was found to be a powerful tonic contraction of the flexor muscles of the left arm;

---

[1] Sur l'Action Physiologique de l'Aimant et des Solenoides, par MM. Charcot et Regnard. Communication faite à la Société de Biologie, Séance de 6 Juillet, 1878. *Le Progrès Médical*, No. 32, 10 Août, 1878, p. 817 et seq.

there was also anæsthesia of the same arm; there was some hyperæsthesia of the left ovary.

Professor Charcot some time ago applied the magnet, as in Case III., to the right arm; to his surprise, he found that the contraction of the left arm disappeared during the application, but was transferred to the right side. By repeating the proceeding daily, the hysterical contraction of the left arm is gradually disappearing; and after the magnet has been some time in proximity with the right arm, the left is found to present merely a condition of slight paresis; whilst the right becomes firmly contracted. The contraction of the right arm, thus artificially induced, lasts the whole day.

We have in this case the first example of a method of treatment which will probably be very generally successful in cases of hysterical contractions.

V. *Hystero-Epilepsy; Absolute Cutaneous Anæsthesia and Analgesia of both Sides of the Body; Achromatopsia of both Eyes, but especially of the Left.—* In this case, by transfixing the skin with needles, M. Charcot showed that analgesia existed on both sides of the body in an absolute degree. The patient, a fine, tall, powerful, and very healthy looking girl, was quite unaware of these operations, unless her eyes happened to fall upon the transfixed spot, when she appeared to resent the act by a pouting, impatient, and almost childlike behaviour.

In this patient, the condition of achromatopsia presents features of great interest. With her right eye she can distinguish all colours but violet. It is to be noted that in the colour-blindness of hystero-epilepsy, violet is the colour which is most easily lost; in other words, in the very slightest cases, where all other colours are distinguished, violet cannot be seen. With her left eye the patient can distinguish no colour but red. Red and blue, M. Charcot has found, are the colours which persist most, except in those cases where achromatopsia is absolute, and in which, therefore, the patient sees a coloured picture, however bright and varied its tints, as if painted in black and white; there is found to be a persistence of sensibility to red rays.

Having repeatedly demonstrated the exact condition of colour-blindness of the two eyes of the patient, Professor Charcot placed at a distance of about one-third of an inch from the left temple (*i. e.*, on the side where the achromatopsia was all but absolute), the two poles of a horseshoe magnet. This was at 11 A. M. At 11.5 A. M., on pricking the skin of the left side of the head, which previously had been insensitive, there was slight evidence of sensibility. Her left eye is tested, and the patient is found to be still colour-blind for all colours but red. At 11.6 A. M., when a blue sheet is placed before her eyes, she sees it as white, except at the four corners, which appear slightly blue. She cannot distinguish yellow, green, or purple, even at the corners. 11.7 A. M.—She sees blue all over the sheet: and sees yellow as white, except at the corners. She cannot distinguish green or purple. 11.13 A. M.—She cannot yet distinguish green. 11.13.30 A. M.—She begins to distinguish green at the corners of the paper. 11.14.30 A. M.—She distinguishes perfectly all colours except violet. *On now examining the right eye, it is found to be perfectly colour-blind, except for red.* There has, therefore, under the influence of the magnet applied at an appreciable distance from the temple on the side of the colour-blind eye, been a transference of the affection to the sound side. It may be added—and the fact appears most worthy of remark— that the disappearance of the power of appreciating particular colours on the sound side coincides exactly, in point of time, with the reappearance of the sensitiveness for the same colour in the usually colour-blind eye.

In most patients affected with the achromatopsia of hystero-epilepsy, the order of the disappearance of colours is as follows: violet, green, red, orange, yellow,

blue. In some patients, as in the one now commented upon, it is red, and not
blue, which persists. When by the action of magnets, solenoids, or metallic
plates, the colours are made to reappear, it is in inverse order to that in
which they disappeared. There are cases where the above order does not hold
in its entirety; on the other hand, it is never departed from materially; as, for
instance, blue is *never* seen if the patient be colour-blind for green.

Leaving the laboratory in which the demonstration of the already narrated
facts had taken place, Professor Charcot conducted us successively to the bedside
of three patients who afforded the opportunity of studying the varied features of
the hystero-epileptic seizure.

VI. *Hystero-Epilepsy; Absolute Hemianæsthesia with Right-sided Ovarian
Hyperæsthesia; Induction of the Hystero-Epileptic Seizure by Peripheral Irritation; its Arrest by Compression in the Right Ovarian Region; Inhibition of
Fits by continuous Application of Pressure.*—The patient, a young woman of
considerable vigour and intelligence, is apparently about twenty-two years of age,
and is very frequently subject to the most characteristic hystero-epileptic attacks.
These attacks had been exceedingly frequent on the day preceding our visit, but
had been inhibited by the systematic application of pressure to the right ovarian
region, as will be more particularly mentioned in the sequel. They still continued
to recur.

Professor Charcot pointed out that the hystero-epileptic seizure, besides occurring spontaneously, can usually be induced with ease by some modes of peripheral
irritation. In the present case, for instance, by suddenly "gripping" the skin
of the breast on both sides, about on a level with the fifth rib, and midway
between the anterior and posterior boundaries of the axilla, the patient instantly
fell into the hystero-epileptic convulsion. The constancy with which the effect
followed the cause was demonstrated over and over again to be absolute.

Although the various phenomena of the hystero-epileptic seizure are known to
many readers through the writings of M. Charcot, it may be not uninteresting to
describe them with all minuteness as they were presented before us by this
patient. The attack may be conveniently divided into three or four stages.

The first stage followed the application of the peripheral irritation without the
intervention of any perceptible latent period; its features were the following:
The head was thrown violently backwards, the limbs and body became rigid, the
respirations infrequent and stertorous; in a few seconds, the tonic spasms were
succeeded by clonic spasms affecting the muscular system. A slight remission,
lasting for a very few seconds, occurred, which was spoken of as a kind of
entr'acte, and then commenced the second stage. The first may be termed the
epileptiform stage.

The second stage was characterized by extraordinary movements affecting the
whole trunk. The back being somewhat opisthotonically arched, the body was
thrown with great violence and astounding rapidity alternately on to the occiput
and heels. This stage, which, like the first, is of very brief duration, is denomi-
nated the *phase des grands mouvements;* during its continuance occur the first
hallucinations, to be afterwards referred to. The violent movements cease almost
instantaneously, and then follows

The third stage, or stage of emotional attitudes (*phase des attitudes pas-
sionelles*). During this stage, the patient assumes successively the expression of
face, the attitudes, and the gestures which portray varied emotions—intense and
vivid. The varied emotional states will be distinguished in the order in which
they occurred by letters.

a. No sooner had the great movements ceased, than, raising herself into a sitting posture, with clenched fists and menacing expression, the patient presented

the most startling picture of one threatening; but almost instantly the picture changed to

b. The whole expression and attitude portrayed cowering, abject fear. Of no longer duration than *a*, *b* was followed by stage

c. The patient now assumed an expression of absolute beatitude. It is impossible to describe the look of saintly happiness, as of one who realized the blessedness of heaven, which the patient presented. It was the expression which some of the old masters have impressed upon their saints and martyrs.

But now occurred a change no less striking than the preceding.

d. The expression of saintly happiness was succeeded by one of intense joy; the patient sees one whom she loves; she beckons to him to come, to come quickly; he has come. . . . Then succeed gestures which stamp this as the *phase of lubricity* or the stage of the emotional attitudes.

e. Again fear takes possession of the patient; at first it is rats which she sees, and which she appears to fear the attack of, which evoke passionate exclamations of dread and disgust; then it is obviously the fear of some human being which oppresses her, and causes her to beg for mercy.

f. There is no longer fear. The patient hears the strains of music; she is pleased; she 'herself begins to hum the tune, but only for an instant, for

g. Her singing is followed by weeping, which is broken by reproaches addressed to her parents as the causes of her misery. This last phase (*g*) in the stage of passionate attitudes may be made to constitute a fourth stage, or a stage of recovery, in which hallucinations persist for a time.

Reference has been made in the preceding pages to ovarian hyperæsthesia as a characteristic symptom in cases of hystero-epilepsy, and more may be said on the subject in connection with the present case. The ovarian hyperæsthesia is evidenced, firstly, by a great tenderness in the region of one or both ovaries; it is usually on the side on which analgesia exists that the ovary is hyperæsthetic; secondly, by the hystero-epileptic convulsions frequently commencing by an *aura* which seems to take its origin in the hyperæsthetic ovary; thirdly, by the extraordinary fact that, at any stage, an attack of hystero-epileptic convulsions may with certainty be instantly cut short by firm pressure made with the fingers or fists in 'the region of the hyperæsthetic ovary. This inhibitory power of pressure upon the ovary is as surprising as is the influence of definite peripheral irritation in inducing the attack. At the instant that pressure is made in the ovarian region, two results always follow : firstly, the patient's mouth opens, and the tongue is spasmodically extruded ; and, secondly, the convulsions cease. The patient can then always describe the hallucinations to which she was subject at the particular instant; and it is found that these hallucinations are always constant—*i. e.*, the same attitude corresponds to the same hallucinations. The first, or epileptiform, stage is associated with no hallucinations, as is discovered by cutting the attack short during this stage.

The invariable inhibition of the attacks by temporary pressure on the ovary has suggested the advisability of using continuous pressure to prevent the attacks. On the day preceding our visit, the patient whose case I am now relating having had a very large number of fits, an apparatus just constructed by Dr. Poirier, and which enables pressure to be made steadily on one ovarian region (very much as the abdominal aorta is compressed by Lister's tourniquet), was applied ; and as long as the pressure was kept up—*i. e.*, for several hours—no fit occurred. Three minutes after it had been taken off, the fits recurred.

VII. and VIII. were the cases of hystero-epilepsy in which we had the opportunity of studying the features of the attacks. In VII., the epileptic stage was accompanied by a most piercing epileptic shriek. This patient is subject every

night to libidinous hallucinations which have the closest resemblance to those
for which innumerable women were burnt as witches during the fifteenth and sixteenth centuries.[1]   Patient VIII. was remarkable for the extraordinary attitudes
which she assumed during the third stage.   Her attitude of "disdain" was typical of that emotion, and excited as much surprise as the expression of beatitude
of patient VI.

Fungus of Thrush.

Dr. PAUL GRAWITZ, in a contribution to the systematic botany of vegetable
parasites (Virchow's *Archiv*, August, 1877), points out that in thrush-patches, besides epithelial cells, various forms of bacteria, torula cells, and myelin of pleo-
spora, oidium lactis, and mucor mucedo, and others, there is always the proper
thrush-fungus—mycoderma vini (not the so-called oidium lactis).   This specific
fungus the author succeeded in isolating, and was able to cultivate in a modification of Pasteur's solution, as well as in plum-pulp.   The appearance it assumed
under cultivation depended on the amount of sugar present; when there was little
sugar, it formed a widely spreading mycelium; when a considerable quantity, it
formed dense clusters of torula-like buds.   When this fungus was administered in
milk to healthy kittens and puppies no result followed, but when it was given to
feeble, ill-nourished, and thus predisposed animals from three to eight days old,
death followed in from four to ten days, and on examination the characteristic
small white patches were found on the gums and fauces.   Other fungi failed to
produce the same results.   Experiments with other fungi, achorion Schönleinii,
trichophyton tonsurans, and microsporon furfur, led Dr. Grawitz to believe that
they were all identical, and simply the familiar oidium lactis.

With Virchow, the author believes that occasional parasites, especially those
found with lung-diseases in cases of diabetes, are of secondary importance.

When spores of fungi (pencillium, euroteum, mucor, oidium, and muscardine)
suspended in distilled water were injected into the carotid artery or one of the
large veins, no results followed, except when bacteria were injected along with
them, the bacteria setting up septic poisoning.   The spores injected never germinated; they were either dissolved or eliminated by the kidneys.   When introduced into the subcutaneous tissue they were either absorbed, encapsuled, or
eliminated by suppuration.   When the spores of oidium were introduced into the
vitreous chamber, they germinated and formed small nodules composed of convoluted masses of mycelium threads.   The vitreous humour seems to have been the
only place which supplied all the conditions necessary for their growth.   The influence of fungi on the system seems to be altogether of a mechanical nature.—
Lond. Med. Record, Oct. 15, 1878.

Histology of Mucous Patches on the Tonsils.

M. CORNIL (*Le Progrès Médical*, August 10) presented a memoir to the
Académie de Médicine on the results of the examination of several mucous patches
(*plaques muqueuses*) which he had removed in his practice at the Hôpital de
Lourcine; the wounds healed readily.

First variety: opaline mucous patch.—The epithelium is thickened, the papillæ
elongated, and the deeper connective tissue thickened by infiltration with new
cells.   The superficial layer of epithelium presents cells with cavities round their
nuclei; frequently also the cavity of the cell is filled with pus instead of the
nucleus.   Moreover, in this same layer there are little nests filled with globules

[1] See De la Folie . . . Description des Grandes Epidemies de Délire, par L. F.
Calmeil.   Paris : 1845.

of pus, little abscesses hollowed out amidst the epithelial cells, containing from four to ten, or even up to a hundred globules of pus. These collections of pus give the appearance of opalescence.

Second variety: ulcerated mucous patches.—The epithelial layer is disintegrated by a great quantity of liquid and pus-globules coming from the papillæ. The epithelial layer may be completely destroyed, and the inflamed papillary body form the base of the ulceration. There exists sometimes a true false membrane, gray, adherent, diphtheritic, upon this ulceration. The false membrane contains no parasites, but the branching state of the epithelial cells, the holes or cavities in them filled with pus, present the same aspect as in diphtheria.

In both cases the closed follicles of the tonsils were inflamed, and the whole organs were hypertrophied. The lymphatic sinuses round the follicles and the reticular tissue presented a variable quantity of large cells, with one or more nuclei containing red blood-corpuscles. This follicular lesion is identical with that which the author described in the glands in the first and second stages of syphilis. In short, the syphilitic tonsils in the second stage represent a papule upon a syphilitic gland.—*London Med. Record*, Oct. 15, 1878.

Sublingual Ulceration in Pertussis.

Dr. DELTHIL having forwarded a paper to the Académie de Médecine, it was referred to a committee, and at a recent meeting of the Academy (*Bulletin*, No. 28, September 17), Prof. HENRI ROGER, of the Hôpital des Enfants, read an able and conclusive report upon the subject. He founds the remarks he makes upon it upon his prolonged hospital and extensive civil practice, pertussis prevailing epidemically every year in Paris, and severely so in 1877–78, so that the field of observation has been ample enough.

That it is not an essential phenomenon of pertussis, as maintained by some observers, is shown by the fact that it is not always present. In fact, its frequency is very variable, being dependent on the violence of the paroxysms and on the disposition of the teeth in the first dentition. When these two conditions are united it is almost always met with, while when they are both wanting it too is absent. Still, as a general statement, Prof. Roger agrees with Dr. Delthil that sublingual ulceration is met with in about one-half the total number of cases of pertussis. Another proof that it is not an essential phenomenon is that it does not appear at a fixed epoch at the commencement. It is rarely observed before the third week (comprising the period of incubation), and in most cases several days later. If the habitual duration of the two stages of pertussis be considered, we can understand why the ulceration does not appear, save exceptionally, before the third week. Although it is difficult, even in private practice, to learn exactly the date of the infection, Prof. Roger is in possession of a sufficient number of precise facts to enable him to state that the mean duration of incubation is generally six or seven days—although he has in some cases known it to be as short as three or four days, and as long as ten or twelve. Then a period of at least ten or fifteen days passes before the cough, at first common, becomes spasmodic, and then quite paroxysmal—before the attacks are exhibited by expiratory jerks, with impulsion of the tongue against the lower teeth. It is only during this full nervous period that the frænal ulcer is developed. The time of its appearance, so far from being fixed and early, is necessarily slow and variable—always following, and never preceding, the paroxysmal stage.

As to the mechanism of its production, there is no preceding vesicle or pustule present, as represented by some writers. Prior to the ulcer appearing, Prof. Roger has often observed at the frænum, and especially at its lower insertion, a somewhat vivid redness, and then an erosion, or a linear division of the mucous membrane, with an appearance of granulations. At the point of section of the frænum there is sometimes seen a transverse depression, and sometimes a kind of pimple (*bouton*), or a yellow or white patch, often of a pearly aspect, two or three millimetres in size. At other times there is a small, median, oval ulcer, with irregular edges, and a pale or reddish-gray base. The lesion may remain in this state, while in other cases it may extend some millimetres beyond each side of the frænum, becoming also deeper, as if burrowing under the tongue. The ulcer is generally covered with a whitish or grayish exudation, not diphtheritic in its appearance, but resembling the exudations which cover the irregular ulcerations mechanically produced inside the cheeks and lips by the projection of irregular teeth or their fragments. The origin of the ulcer is purely mechanical; the tongue being in its hyperæmic state thrust forwards during the paroxysms of coughing, the frænum is easily cut by the sharp lower incisors—the lesion prevailing in a precise ratio with the severity of the cough. The ulceration occurs more readily in infants of ten or twelve months than in older children, because in the latter, when the first dentition is completed, the tongue is supported on the entire range of teeth, and is much less liable to injury than when it is only projected against the incisors, which are sometimes divided on their edges into points as sharp as needles, lacerating the tongue, and dividing the frænum like a knife. When the disposition of the teeth is anomalous, the other parts of the tongue may be lacerated; and, on the other hand, when the frænum is short, so as to prevent its protrusion, no ulceration at all will be observed. So, in infants attacked by pertussis before dentition, no ulceration is ever observed; nor is it met with in the pertussis of adults, in whom the edges of the teeth are much less sharp, and who do not project their tongues during the paroxysms.

As to the semeiotic value of the ulceration, it is not without its importance, inasmuch as the cough of pertussis is the only one that is violent enough to propel the tongue against the teeth. Prof. Roger has never met with it in any other affection, and wherever its presence is positively proved, pertussis may be diagnosed. Of course, in the great majority of cases, the paroxysms themselves have sufficiently declared the nature of the disease before the ulceration has made its appearance. But still there are certain cases in which the cough, not having as yet assumed a sufficiently special character, the practitioner may hesitate at deciding whether he has to do with a paroxysmal bronchitis or with the true paroxysms of pertussis. He should then examine the tongue (which is not always an easy matter, and requires both care and patience in very young infants), and if he finds this lesion of the frænum, and at the same time a prominence of the corresponding teeth, he may rest assured as to the nature of the case. Sometimes it is an observant mother who first draws attention to the lesion in question.—*Med. Times and Gazette*, Oct. 5, 1878.

Treatment of Obstinate Hiccough by Pilocarpine.

Dr. ORTILLE, of Lille (*Bull. Général de Thérap.*, 1878), gives an account of a case of obstinate hiccough in which, after trying all the usual remedies, he had recourse to electricity. For a few hours the application appeared to prove successful; but the hiccough returned. Remembering what he had read of the action of pilocarpine upon the phrenic nerves and of the vomiting which often follows its use, he injected two-fifths of a grain of pilocarpine under the skin. The effect was almost instantaneous. A quarter of an hour after the injection the patient was covered with sweat, salivation was established, and the hiccough had definitely ceased.—*London Med. Record*, Oct. 15, 1878.

Subcutaneous Injection of Sclerotinic Acid in Hœmoptysis.

Sclerotinic acid, which, as is known, has been obtained by Dragendorff from ergot, is injected subcutaneously in hæmoptysis by Professor von ZIEMSSEN, of Brussels (*Deutsche Med. Wochenschrift*, No. 34, 1878). He uses a solution of one part of the acid in twenty-five of distilled water, and injects a Pravaz's syringeful twice or thrice in twenty-four hours. The effect is said to be more certain than that of ergotin.—*London Med. Record*, Oct. 15, 1878.

Case of Congenital Narrowing of the Entire Aortic System, with Consecutive Great Hypertrophy of the Heart.

This case, reported by Dr. KNOEVENAGEL, of Cologne (*Berliner Klin. Wochenschrift*, Sept. 1878), appears of interest, first, because of the in many respects peculiar symptoms presented; also on account of the uncertainty of the diagnosis, and, lastly, with respect to its etiology.

The patient, aged 21, came to the hospital on April 6, after having been under medical treatment outside since March 25. His chief complaints were of dyspnœa and repeated vomiting, with irregular bowels; and he said that for a year previously, after prolonged labour in the vineyard (he was a vine-dresser), he had occasionally suffered from shortness of breath and palpitation. In the harvest-time of 1876 he had an attack of tonsillitis, but it could not be ascertained whether it was diphtheritic. He had not observed difficulty of swallowing, frequent hoarseness, or rheumatic pains in the arms. On April 7 he had a pale bloated countenance, with a very strongly built and well-nourished body. The most striking symptom was the remarkable smallness of the pulse, the right being not at all, and the left scarcely to be felt; its frequency could not be estimated. The percussion-note over the lower part of the sternum was dull; towards the left, there was diminished dulness as far as the anterior axillary line. The apex-beat was not to be felt; diffuse vibration was felt quite to the outside of the nipple, which was rather higher on the left than the right side. The heart's action was remarkably irregular; there was no valvular murmur; systole and diastole were difficult to discriminate; sometimes the sounds appeared rough, especially to the left of the sternum, much like pericardial friction-sound. The number of cardiac contractions appeared to be greater than the number of the pulse—very imperfectly perceptible—in the femoral arteries. The irregularity of the heart's action could be perceived by palpation. The carotid pulse on both sides was vibrating, not to be counted; with it could be heard very frequent, short, deep sounds. In the left lung, posteriorly at the lower part, were moist *râles* with feeble breathing; there was dulness nowhere, and marked mobility of the pulmonary border. The spleen could be felt only imperfectly; its dulness appeared increased, as did also that of the liver. The temperature was subnormal: morning, 36.0 Cent. (96.8 Fahr.); evening 36.5 Cent. (97.7 Fahr.). The patient made subjective complaints, chiefly of shortness of breath in walking and going up-stairs, which had for the last three weeks been more marked.

April 8.—Temperature, morning, 36.3 Cent. (97.5 Fahr.), evening, 36.7 Cent. (98.1 Fahr.). The face was even more bloated; the pulse not perceptible. Auscultation gave 140 heart-beats per minute. He had a quite normal stool. The urine was very scanty, estimated at 350 to 400 cubic centimetres; sp. gr. 1031, it was acid, with a copious deposit of urates; no albumen, no sugar. A large blister was applied to the cardiac area; infusion of digitalis (only weak), with quinine, was ordered; also ethereal tincture of valerian.

9th. There was strong bulging of the epigastrium, between the xiphoid cartilage and the navel; the entire part felt very resistant, and gave a very dull note, which was limited below by a convex border. The limits, as defined by percussion, could also be confirmed by palpation. Half an hour after swallowing milk, wine, etc., as a rule, there was copious vomiting. He had three scanty stools. The urine was as on the previous day. The heart-beats were 160; over the femorals only an irregular vibration could be felt. The patient lay on his back by preference. Microscopical examination of the blood showed nothing special, no increase of the white corpuscles.

10th. There were marked cyanosis of the lips, severe œdema of the feet and legs, undulating movements of the prominence in the epigastrium, which could be felt by palpation. The cardiac vibrations were always most decided to the outer side of the left nipple. To-day the pulse in the femoral artery could be counted, about 160. He had had less vomiting since less food had been taken at one time. The urine was only a little less scanty. There was some muco-purulent expectoration. The patient was often in the knee-and-elbow position, because he breathed more easily. The pulse was not more easily felt. In the night he was much purged, with frequent passage of wind. The abdomen became softer and flatter; the liver, with a smooth upper surface, could be felt, in the mammillary line $1\frac{1}{4}$ to $1\frac{1}{2}$ inch, in the parasternal line about 3 inches, under the costal border; in the middle line about 5 inches under the base of the xiphoid process. He had vomiting at morning and noon of the following day. The heart's contractions were 140, intermittent. The temperature morning and evening was 36.8 Cent. (98.4 Fahr.). The patient felt himself easier; on the right posteriorly from the ninth dorsal vertebra downwards, there was moderate dulness, and no mobility of the lower border of the lung.

13th. Temperature, morning, 37.5 Cent.; evening, 36.4 Cent. He had six thin pultaceous stools. The quantity of urine commenced to increase, about 800 to 900 cubic centimetres. The heart's contractions were 144 to the minute.

15th. There was much more urine, about 2500 cubic centimetres of sp. gr. 1008; whether as the consequence of the recently ordered turpentine fomentations, was doubtful. He also had some copious stools, each very different in colour and in the quantity of bile present. The patient felt easier after these evacuations. Temperature, morning, 36.8; evening, 37.5 Cent. The pulse in the femoral arteries began to be countable, with great attention, at from 180 to 190, and corresponded approximately to the heart's contractions.

16th. The quantity of urine was no longer so great, still about 1603 cubic centimetres. Temperature, morning, 36.9 Cent.; evening, 37.5. He had very frequent calls to stool, with tenesmus; the matter passed contained much admixture of mucus. The latter continued also the following day; the next night he vomited once more, not having done so for six days.

18th. The temperature was subnormal; morning, 36.2 Cent.; evening, 36.8. The quantity of urine was diminished; the heart's contractions were 144; he lay in the knee-and-elbow position.

19th. At last the effect of the digitalis seemed to be produced; the heart-beats were 120, the slowest which had been observed hitherto.

20th. The heart-beats were 140, very irregular; there was greater dulness both to right and left; very marked undulation of the whole epigastrium. Temperature, in the morning, 36.0 Cent., the lowest observed. The intestinal irritation had disappeared. Respiration was always 32 to 36. From this time the principal phenomena (enormous frequency of the heart, subnormal temperature, pulselessness, small quantity of urine, dyspnœa) remained unchanged till death.

On April 25th, he again vomited twice. On the 26th he had great tenesmus. The epigastric pulsation varied from day to day in extent and force. Another examination of the blood showed no increase of leucocytes. The quantity of urine diminished again to 700, 600, 500, and 400 cubic centimetres. Moreover, it contained a large amount of albumen, from which it had previously been quite free. On the knees, from the position in which he remained, red infiltrated places and numerous pustular eruptions formed. To produce diuresis, he was given juniper tea with cream of tartar, and benzoated tincture of opium for the expectoration; the digitalis was stopped some time ago as useless. The very distressing condition of the patient was exaggerated towards the end of April by urgent pains, which radiated from the epigastrium to the region of the manubrium sterni, and extended thence over the chest. Vomiting occurred only occasionally. The temperature was, as always, subnormal; respiration 40 to 44, and before death reaching 52, without becoming stertorous. From May 2d there were rust-coloured masses in the sputa, without physical signs of anything but catarrh, and no decided dulness over the lower part of the thorax. Mustard poultices, blisters, and Dover's powder gave no relief. On May 3d, violent urgent pains began in the loins, which radiated on both sides, and were followed by great dyspnœa, cyanosis, and profuse sweating, inability to swallow, but still complete consciousness. Death occurred in the night between the 6th and 7th of May.

The following symptoms are of chief interest :—

1. The excessive action of the heart, and the friction-murmur.

2. The choice of the knee-elbow position for even the whole night long.

3. The periodical greater and less tumour-like prominence of the præcordia.

As to the first, we must think that the heart must act more slowly under the laborious process of overcoming the increased resistance of a diminished diameter of the aortic system (as the necropsy afterwards showed), just as it characteristically does in stenosis of the aortic orifice. For explanation there remains, as the phenomena of paralysis of the vagus throughout were absent, only irritation of the sympathetic, upon which indirectly the subnormal temperature and the imperceptible pulse must have depended. It is interesting also to observe how much the heart can stand without death occurring, if the valves and muscular substance remain intact. The occasional rough character of the heart's sounds, like pericardial friction, is also noteworthy, as *post-mortem* no appearance of pericarditis was found. Probably there was merely a rubbing of the heart against the parietal pericardium, which Seitz has offered as an explanation of similar cases in his *Lectures on Heart-Strains (Zur Lehre von der Ueberaustrengung des Herzens)*. On the second point, the knee-and-elbow position, this appears to me as a by no means inexplicable, and therefore rightly noteworthy, symptom. The patient instinctively sought to relieve himself of a load close above or below the diaphragm; of whatever kind, speaking generally, the tumour was, this position of the body must have relieved the lungs and great vessels, and so rendered circulation and respiration more easy. What part the position of the head in consequence of this position of the body may have had upon the arterial flow to the brain, remains undecided. Without doubt, however, the knee-and elbow position was the cause of the localization of the œdema anteriorly between the epigastrium and larynx and the two nipple lines, while the other parts of the trunk and the extremities remained free.

On the third point: the tumour-like swelling of the præcordia, apart from the œdema of the skin in the neighbourhood, seemed to be partly a periodical swelling and contracting of the liver (corresponding with the greater or less cyanosis), partly distension of the stomach, which latter view was confirmed by the flattening that took place after copious vomiting and purging. The vomiting itself appeared to me not to be explained by a nervous origin (vagus?), nor from chronic catarrh—the patient had a relatively good appetite to the end; I believe it depended simply on want of space for the stomach, a view which was supported by the fact that the more frequent ingestion of smaller quantities put a stop to it.

The second and third points concern principally the uncertainty of the diagnosis.

Although the discovery of a much enlarged area of cardiac dulness, and the functional derangement, made the idea of fatty heart at first sight plausible, this view soon receded into the background. The position of the patient, the limited œdema around the sternum (obstruction to superficial and internal mammary veins), the epigastric tumour, and vomiting after filling the stomach, all pointed to something encroaching upon the stomach, either in the anterior mediastinum, or close under the diaphragm in the abdominal cavity, such as a tumour, which at the same time pushed the heart to the left, involved the lumina of the great vessels, and influenced the sympathetic plexus. This might be due to a hydatid tumour on the convexity of the liver, the more so as the tenesmus, the mucus in the stools, and the difference in their colour, directed attention to the liver and intestine. But nothing certain could be made out from the stools, and later on important information was accidentally obtained from his relatives. This pointed with certainty to congenital, probably hereditary affection. Then succeeded the view that the mass was an aneurism, in spite of the absence of physical signs, and the want of any history of pain *before* the appearance of the several symptoms. A fœtal stenosis of the aorta at the orifice of Botalli's duct must be discarded, as the characteristic sign of enlargement of the peripheral arteries was absent, and it would not explain why the pulses in both radials should be imperceptible.

A third interesting point lay in the etiological relationship. It could not be doubted that the condition was hereditary; the relations said that beside one uncle, who had suffered long from hydrothorax and died after thoracentesis (no necropsy made), there was another uncle (father's brother) who could neither sit nor lie on his back, but could only rest in a bent-forward position, leaning his breast upon something. He died suddenly after eleven days' illness. Nothing further could be ascertained, but it was natural to suppose that the same abnormality of our patient existed in that uncle. The brothers and sisters of the former were healthy. Contrary to all our expectations (a certain diagnosis was not, however, made), the autopsy, which was made with great good will and care by Dr. Barthold, showed narrowing of the whole aortic system and great hypertrophy of the heart. The report of the necropsy given by Dr. Barthold forms the conclusion of this paper, and I have only to add that in the *post-mortem* examination a moderate sized goitre was found hidden by the œdema, below the larynx. Although exophthalmos was absent, yet the coincidence of a goitre with functional anomaly of the heart brings the case nearer to one of Basedow's disease, and it is worth inquiring whether in marked cases of that disease any abnormality in the lumen of the aortic system has often been observed.

Post-mortem Report, by Dr. Barthold.—The body was medium sized, ill developed. The skin of the face was very œdematous, also the anterior surface of the trunk and neck. The œdema was most marked around the clavicles. Over the patellæ were superficial bedsores. The muscles were badly developed and pale. The belly was distended, the intestines protruding when the cavity was opened. In the peritoneal cavity were about 150 grammes of clear yellow fluid; the colour and position of the intestines were normal. The lower margin of the liver reached below the costal border 1½ to 2 inches in the nipple line, 2.4 inches in the parasternal line, and 4½ inches below the base of the xiphoid process. The convex upper surface of the liver was quite free. The position of the diaphragm reached on the right the eighth and on the left the seventh intercostal spaces. In both pleural cavities were about 2½ litres of clear yellow fluid, so that the lungs were pressed back against their roots. About 200 grammes of clear fluid were found in the pericardium. The heart was greatly enlarged, principally upon the right side, and lay with its apex in the sixth intercostal space, 4 centimetres outside the nipple line. The heart measured in its longest diameter (from the origin of the great vessels to the apex) 7.4 inches, in cross diameter 4.8 inches; of the longest diameter the right ventricle anteriorly measured 5.2 inches, and it formed the whole of the transverse diameter anteriorly. The heart lay completely free upon the spine and the aorta, and was only supported a little laterally by the left lung. The greater part of the left ventricle lay posteriorly, whilst the right ventricle occupied the anterior half. All the cavities of the heart were tensely filled; in the right auricle was much fluid blood, with little clot, the same in the right ventricle; in the left pulmonary veins was a buff-coloured, in the left ventricle much old clot. The heart's cavities on the right side were much dilated; the muscular coat was not thickened. The muscle was pale red; the valvular apparatus was intact on both sides. The cavity of the left ventricle was much dilated, and at a place near the apex in the septum there was an area about 1.2 inches in extent where the wall was thinned and fibroid, and had yielded so as to form a depression; elsewhere the wall was about an inch thick. The trabeculæ were generally flat, especially near the depressed part; and there were clots between and under them, the upper parts of which were brownish-black and regular, the deeper parts dirty gray-brown, and with fibrous eroded surfaces, and were very brittle. On the endocardium covering the papillary muscles there were many stellate yellow-coloured appearances, but the muscular substance itself was everywhere equally pale, and nowhere yellow. Microscopical examination of the heart's muscle was not made. The valvular apparatus was very delicate and unchanged. Nothing abnormal was found in the course of the aorta, but it was itself very narrow, scarcely admitting the finger even at its commencement. It measured at the level of the valves 2.4 inches, at the ductus Botalli 1.6 inch, the same at the origin of the left subclavian, at the origin of the fourth intercostal artery 0.9 inch, and the branches of the aorta also showed the same; for instance, the right and left carotids measured 1.2 inch, their origins 0.72 inch, the femorals at Poupart's ligament 0.56 inch, the radials 0.24 to 0.28 inch. The aorta was, however, very little elastic; its coats and those of all the vessels were very thin. Both lungs were very heavy, with superficial colouring of bluish-gray, in the anterior parts containing air. On section they were smooth; on pressure, much mucous fluid poured out. In the right upper lobe was a radiating thick pleural scar containing a calcareous encysted mass. The mucous membrane of the air-passages was cyanotic; in the trachea particularly there were quite superficial punctiform hemorrhages; in the tonsils were cicatricial thickenings. The thyroid body was enlarged on both sides; on section much blood poured out of the dilated veins; the tissue appeared throughout glandular and lobulated. The spleen was adherent partially to the diaphragm; it was 3.75 inches long, 3 inches broad, and 1.2 inch thick; it felt thick, and contained blood in moderate quantity. Both kidneys were of ordinary size, purplish colour, and very hard consistence; the medullary cones contrasted by their colour with the cortical substance. The suprarenal capsules and genital organs showed no changes. In the stomach were five round worms and much mucus. The liver on its upper surface and on section presented a pronounced nutmeg appearance, the bluish-black centres of the acini contrasting with their grayish-yellow peripheries. The mesenteric glands were only slightly enlarged. In the ileum were several submucous ecchymoses of the size of lentils. The brain showed only œdema of the arachnoid. The examination of the blood gave, as during life, nothing special.—*London Med. Record*, October, 1878.

Surgery.

The Antiseptic Method in Extraction of Cataract.

DR. A. GRÄFE, in the *Archiv für Ophthalmologie*, vol. xxiv., says that since May, 1877, he has used the following method in one hundred and fourteen cases of cataract-extraction After subduing as far as possible any inflammation of the conjunctiva or of the lachrymal sac, a drop of a solution of atropia (one per cent.) was applied to the eye on the day before the operation, and a short time before the operation the eye was carefully washed with a two-per-cent. solution of carbolic acid.   At the same time, the external surfaces of the lids and adjacent orbital region were carefully cleansed, and the eye, being kept closed, was covered until the operation with a sponge soaked in the carbolized solution.   Before being used, the instruments were dipped in absolute alcohol, and dried on pure linen.   During the operation, one sponge moistened with the carbolic acid solution was kept constantly at hand for use; and, after the operation, the eye was wiped with it. Atropia was dropped in ; and the sponge was kept applied to the closed eye until all hemorrhage or formation of coagula near the wound or between its edges had ceased.   As soon as the sponge was removed, lint charged with a four-per-cent. solution of boracic acid was applied, and over it a piece of fine oiled silk that had been dipped in the same fluid.   Cotton-wadding and a fine elastic flannel bandage completed the dressing, which was changed once in twenty-four hours during the first three days.   During the first seven or eight days, the carbolized sponge was laid over the closed eye at each change of dressing.   The exterior of the eyelids was also cleansed by the sponge.   Water was not used for the first seven or eight days; atropia was generally applied from the third day.   The total percentage of failures in the cases so treated was 1¾, while it varied from 5 to 6 in the cases operated on before the adoption of the antiseptic plan.—*British Med. Journal*, Sept. 7, 1878.

On Successful Removal of a Large Thyroid Tumour by Excision and Ligature.

In a paper read before the Royal Academy of Medicine in Turin (*Giorn. della R. Accad.*, May, 1878) Dr. PERASSI related (àpropos of a case described by Dr. Bottini) a case which occurred to him in 1864.

The patient was a countryman, aged 46, who had an enormous goitre hanging down from the laryngeal region nearly as far as the umbilicus.   The tumour was flattened antero-posteriorly, and was many-lobed; the skin over it was healthy, except at the infero-posterior part, where it was somewhat ulcerated, and presented large veins.   The tumour, which had first appeared fifteen years previously, and had gradually grown to its present size, was not painful, but very inconvenient.   The diagnosis of a large lipomatous bronchocele having been made, it was removed on August 18, 1864.

An exploratory puncture was first made with a trocar, but without result.   A long curvilinear incision was made along the front of the tumour, and a shorter one, also curvilinear, along its posterior aspect.   The dissection of the flaps was very tedious and difficult, in consequence both of the induration of the deeper tissues, and of the arterio-venous vessels which were met with, and which, as a matter of precaution, were tied before being divided.   Having reached the root of the tumour, Dr. Perassi found that it extended more deeply into the lateral regions of the neck than its appearance indicated, and that its extirpation by the knife would be attended with much danger.   He, therefore, applied a series of partial ligatures, in which the whole mass of the tumour was included.   Believing that the process of putrefaction of the tumour would be injurious, he cut it off a few centimetres in front of the ligatures. The edges of the wound were brought together, and a cooling ointment was applied. Healing went on favourably, with moderate suppuration, and the patient left the hospital cured at the end of a month. The portion of tumour removed weighed 5550 grammes (about 12 lbs. 4 ozs.).—*London Med. Record*, Oct. 15, 1878.

Injuries of the Kidney.

Prof. H. MAAS of Freiburg, in an elaborate contribution to the *Deutsche Zeitschrift für Chirurgie*, Band x. Heft. 1 and 2, publishes the results of some clinical and experimental investigations on the symptomatology and treatment of subcutaneous wounds of the kidney. The author holds the opinion of the late G. Simon, that the prognosis in cases of injury to the kidney is not so unfavourable as it is supposed to be by the majority of surgical authors. Allusion is made to the view of Simon, that the dangers of hemorrhage and suppuration in cases of injury to the kidney might be diminished through operative procedure ; hemorrhage by deligation of the renal pedicle and subsequent extirpation of the wounded organ ; suppuration by lumbar incision with or without nephrotomy. This view has certainly influenced to some extent the practice of modern German surgeons. Nussbaum recommends an early incision in cases of traumatic renal or perirenal suppuration. Ebstein, whose views as to treatment agree with those of Simon, holds that in cases of renal injury the prognosis is less serious when the wound of the kidney is complicated by wound of the superficial soft parts; for, when the lesion is strictly subcutaneous and there is no external wound, the exit of blood, serous effusion, and pus, is prevented, and the development of pyæmia or septicæmia is consequently favoured.

In the clinical portion of his article, Dr. Maas gives an analysis of 71 cases of injury to the kidney, taken from published and private sources, and tabulated in the following order : 37 cases in which the patients recovered, or in which death was not due to the renal injury ; 21 cases in which death was the result of, but did not occur until some time after, the injury ; 13 cases in which death speedily resulted, in most instances through injuries to other organs in association with those of the kidney.

Of the subjects of these cases 64 were males and 4 only females ; in the remaining 3, the sex had not been mentioned. Of 53 cases in which there is a record of age, in 27 the patients were between twenty and forty years of age. An advanced period of life seems to have no marked influence on the mortality from subcutaneous renal injury, since the table of recoveries included cases in which the respective patients were 52, 66, and 68 years of age. On the other hand, the period of infancy and childhood must be regarded as a condition of danger ; for, of seven patients described as children, and who were probably all under 10 years of age, one only, a little girl aged 4 years, recovered, all the others having succumbed very soon after the injury.

In 53 of the 71 cases the injury of the kidney had been caused through direct violence, acting in all but three of those cases on the front or side of the trunk. In 12 cases the injury had been the result of indirect violence, the patients having fallen from a considerable height or with much violence on to a smooth and level surface, or one free from any prominent object that might have caused directly any laceration or contusion of the kidney. In six cases, no mention is made of the manner in which the injury had been caused.

In the large majority of the cases in which death had occurred soon after the injury, the renal structure with the fibrinous capsule was found torn in various directions, but most frequently in the transverse axis of the organ. In severe injuries of the kidney, more or less of the renal structure is often broken down to a soft mass of detritus, and the whole of the injured organ suffused with blood. The proper capsule is occasionally distended with effused blood, so as to form a very tense and elastic tumour. The fatty capsule and surrounding connective tissue are saturated with blood, the retroperitoneal effusion of which often reaches as far downwards as the pelvis, and upwards as far as the lower margin of the scapula. Blood is very frequently effused into the renal pelvis, and thence passes along the urethra into the bladder, where it is usually dissolved in the urine, and is seldom found in clots. In three cases only in the tables had there been any demonstration of the presence of coagulated blood in the bladder. The direction of a contused or lacerated wound in the kidney very rarely corresponds with that of the long axis of this organ. The lacerated wounds nearly always pass from side to side, and frequently cut off a portion of the organ which is retained in connection with the main portion by means only of unbroken capsule. In a few very severe and fatal cases from forcible direct violence, the peritoneal covering of the kidney had been torn through, and much blood effused into the abdominal cavity.

Death from injury to the kidney is seldom due to primary hemorrhage. In 6 only out of the 71 tabulated cases had the bleeding been so excessive as to cause early death, and in 3 of these there had been laceration of the peritoneal covering of the injured kidney, and considerable intraperitoneal hemorrhage. Secondary hemorrhage is put down as the cause of death in four instances; in two of these cases orifices imperfectly closed by thrombi were found in large branches of the renal artery, and in one the injured kidney, which was enormously enlarged, was partly made up of a large arterial hematoma lined with clot, opening into which was a large branch of the renal artery. In six instances death had resulted from decomposition, with consequent suppuration, of the blood effused around or within the injured kidney.

In very many of the fatal cases death had been due rather to serious complications than to the injury of the kidney. In 2 cases both kidneys were found lacerated, and in two other instances the injured kidney was a single renal organ, the other having been entirely absent. In 4 cases there had been simultaneous laceration of the spleen, and in two of those fracture of some ribs. In 2 cases both liver and spleen had been crushed, and in several instances there had been fractures of ribs and of the bones of one or more limbs. In single cases of renal injury mention is made in the tables of pyothorax, pulmonary abscess, rupture of bladder, dislocation of the first cervical vertebræ, and laceration of the leg necessitating amputation.

Dr. Naas refers to some cases in his tables which throw light on the nature of the healing process after wounds of the kidney. The first observation, one of much interest, was made by von Recklinghausen, and related to a case of complicated injury which proved fatal on the eighth day. The renal wound was found occupied by a completely discoloured and tough thrombus. That the ultimate stage of healing consists in the formation of a scar of connective tissue, is proved by a case recorded by G. Simon. The patient died from tuberculosis five years after a severe renal injury. A well-marked cicatrix was found, containing small and relatively thin-walled vessels. A case in which the healing process had been perfected before death has also been reported by Timothy Holmes. The patient died eighteen months after the injury, probably from long-standing granular atrophy of the kidneys. The trace of the rupture in the injured kidney could hardly be seen, though the remains of extravasated blood in the organ and under its capsule were still visible. In another case, in which the patient died twenty years after an injury to the kidney, followed by an external abscess, the injured organ was found to have been converted into a small cyst, which contained a mulberry calculus.

The most frequent, though not a constant, symptom of crushing or laceration of the kidney, is shock. By the results of experiments on animals, and by the clinical fact that this condition has not been observed in some cases of serious injury to the kidney, the author has been led to believe that this shock is the result not of the renal injury, but really of general abdominal contusion. The most constant symptom of injury to the kidney is pain in the region of the organ. This is increased very much on pressure in the corresponding lumbar region. It is usually restricted to the injured organ, and to the parts just around it, and rarely assumes the radiating character of the so-called renal colic. This symptom is often very persistent, remaining after all other symptoms have disappeared, and troubling the patient long after apparent convalescence.

In all but 6 of the 71 cases hæmaturia was observed. In some cases there was slight staining of the urine, in others a discharge of several pints of blood. In almost every instance of hæmaturia renalis, the blood was dissolved in the urine, and not passed in clots. In some cases there was temporary retention of urine, which, however, would always be readily relieved by the introduction of a catheter. The hæmaturia persisted for a variable period within a limit of eighteen days. A long duration of the bleeding may be explained by a gradual separation and dissolution in the urine of clots arrested in the renal pelvis and canaliculi, after the arrest of the primary hemorrhage. In some cases, relapsing hæmaturia was observed. This can be accounted for only by secondary hemorrhage from the lacerated vessels. Hæmaturia frequently recurs if the patient be allowed to move about too soon after the injury.

Fever is a frequent symptom, even in cases where there is no renal or perinephritic suppuration. Dr. Maas attributes this to the fact that in severe injuries to the kidney, as in fractures and in other subcutaneous injuries, there is always considerable inflammatory exudation, which, as the patient recovers, becomes absorbed. For this condition, Volkmann has proposed the term of aseptic fever.

Anuria being an indication of functional impairment of both kidneys, is a very serious and almost invariably fatal symptom in cases of renal injury. It was observed in the two cases in which the injured kidney was a single organ.

Although in a large majority of the cases which terminate favourably the healing process is completed by the end of the fourth week, and the patients are then quite well, there are some occasional results of renal injury which, though not incompatible with recovery, constitute really serious inflammatory conditions. These are non-suppurative nephritis, perinephritic suppuration, and renal abscess. Formation of calculus, according to the list of tabulated cases, is not a frequent result of renal injury, having been noted in three instances only.

The prognosis of subcutaneous injury of the kidney is placed in a more favourable light by those collected cases, than by the general statements of most surgical authors. We find that of 71 cases 37, more than half, terminated in recovery. The proportion will appear more favourable if we consider the causes of death in the 34 fatal cases. In one case death is attributed by Dr. Maas to the treatment, which consisted in excessive venesection; in 14 cases the injury to the kidney was complicated by fatal injuries of other organs; in 2 cases the injured kidney was a single organ, and in one case both kidneys were injured. Of 70 cases, therefore, of unilateral injury of the kidney, there were 15 cases only in which the renal injury could be fairly regarded as the cause of death. In 6 of these cases death was due to primary hemorrhage, in 4 to secondary hemorrhage, in one to simultaneous secondary hemorrhage and suppurative decomposition of perirenal effusion of blood, and in 3 cases to the latter condition alone. Three patients died in consequence of renal abscess.

Dr. Maas recommends as the best treatment rest in bed, perfect quietude, and the application of ice-bags. Whilst the administration of tannin, ergotine, and the like astringents, has very problematic results in cases of dangerous bleeding from the large vessels, there are no indications for the use of these agents for minor hemorrhages. The persistent presence of blood in small quantities in the urine is usually the consequence of the dissolution of coagula formed at the time of the primary bleeding. The administration of drinks charged with carbonic acid is recommended. By such agents the secretion of urine is excited, and the dissolution of coagula favoured.

In discussing the question whether severe hemorrhage from subcutaneous injury of the kidney could be arrested by any operative proceeding for deligation of the open vessel, and extirpation of the wounded organ, Dr. Naas points out in the first place that profuse bleeding from large branches of the renal artery is often spontaneously arrested through the formation of a large clot. There is an important distinction, it is shown, between this subcutaneous hemorrhage and the bleeding from large open wounds, and into an extensive cavity such as the abdomen. In many cases, the kidney is so much broken up that it would be difficult to find the bleeding vessel and to remove the injured organ. It would not be easy to decide as to the indications for this plan of treatment. Shock is an uncertain symptom of severe injury to the kidney, and hemorrhage, even though very profuse, is not always fatal.

The tabulated cases show very decidedly the advisability of making a lumbar incision when the renal injury has resulted in suppuration either around or within the injured kidney. Dr. Naas holds that in every instance in which fever is observed, and a tumour can be made out in the lumbar region, this tumour should be punctured, aspirated, or, if necessary, freely incised. If, after some interval from the date of the injury, pus be found in the urine, the kidney should be exposed, and either a free passage be maintained for the discharge of pus, or the injured organ be extirpated.—*London Med. Record*, Oct. 15, 1878.

Operation for Phimosis by means of the Elastic Ligature.

Two communications to the Société de Chirurgie of Paris, by N. HUET, of Rouen, on division of the prepuce by the elastic ligature, are noticed in *Le Progrès Médical* of May 11 and August 10, 1878. N. Huet operates as follows: The prepuce on its dorsal aspect and opposite the base of the glans is pierced by a needle carrying a caoutchouc thread; the portion of the prepuce in front of the puncture is then ligatured, and the operation is finished. At the end of three or four days section is completed. The patients do not suffer, and may, if necessary, continue their ordinary occupation.

The author states that he has seen the operation succeed in eighty cases, including both old men and children. The appearance of the parts after this mode of operating is said to be most elegant, and there is no fear of a scar. On August 7, N. Huet showed at the Société de Chirurgie four young soldiers treated as above, with most satisfactory results.—*London Med. Record*, Oct. 15, 1878.

Tubercular Infiltration of Lymphatic Glands between the Bladder and the Rectum.

At a meeting of the Parisian Society of Surgeons, held September 11, N. LANNELONGUE showed a specimen, taken from a young child that had died under his care, with symptoms of tuberculosis of the urinary track. At the onset, the child merely complained of sharp pain when voiding urine. Two explorations of the bladder failed to reveal a calculus. On examining *per rectum*, a soft fluctuating tumour was detected on a level with the prostate, which could be nothing else than a tubercular abscess surrounding the neck of the bladder. The patient died finally from purulent cystitis and consecutive nephritis. At the necropsy, there was found in the prostatic portion of the urethra a cavity, equal in size to a walnut, and lined by tubercular deposits. The loins were also infiltrated with caseous matter. But the most interesting lesion consisted in the presence of seven stones, each being of the size of a small pea, situated in the tissues which separate the rectum from the base of the bladder. One of these stones corresponded exactly to the opening of the ureter. Microscopical examination showed that these stones were caused by the caseation of true lymphatic glands. M. Lannelongue had made researches with regard to this anatomical point, and in another child, who had no lesion of the genito-urinary organs, he had found six glands, situated between the bladder and the rectum. To M. Lannelongue the presence of these glands explained the formation of certain abscesses in the pelvic rectal space. An excoriation of the mucous membrane of the rectum, or a lesion of the urinary organs, set up an adenitis of these glands terminating in suppuration, which extended to the neighbouring cellular tissues.—M. Duplay confirmed the anatomical facts of M. Lannelongue; he had found these glands situated in front of the anterior wall of the rectum.—M. Lucas-Championnière stated that the facts communicated by M. Lannelongue reconciled those which he had himself noted upon the position of uterine lymphatics and the glands of the broad ligaments.—M. Desprès had watched an abscess in the superior pelvic rectal space of a robust individual. After an attentive observation he was fully persuaded that this abscess was caused by an adenitis. The patient had retention of urine as a first symptom.—*London Med. Record*, Oct. 15, 1878.

Case of Lithotomy, where the Suprapubic Operation was resorted to in consequence of the Size of the Stone.

Mr. R. S. Fowler, reports (*Brit. Med. Journ.*, Sept. 7, 1878), the case of Timothy C., a diminutive puny boy, aged 16, who was admitted as a patient into the Royal United Hospital, on November 9, 1877, suffering from all the symptoms of calculus in the bladder. The first examination, with a long curved sound, did not reveal the stone; but on introducing a short straight sound, the stone was immediately felt. On November 14th, Mr. Fowler commenced by operating by the lateral section, and succeeded in seizing the stone with the forceps immediately, but found the size so great as to render extraction utterly impracticable. Attempts were made to crush the stone, but being unsuccessful, after consultation with Mr. Stockwell, it was decided to proceed to extract above the pubes. Mr. Stockwell held the stone against the anterior wall of the bladder, while Mr. Fowler cut down upon it, making a crucial incision; and, with some little manipulation, it was extracted, and then the bladder was washed out. The patient did well, and on the following day could hardly be restrained to bed. The wound above the pubes rapidly healed, in fact was healed by December 8th. The perineal opening caused some trouble for the next two or three months, but was eventually closed by a plastic operation. The calculus, oxalate of lime, was nearly circular, one inch and a half in diameter, covered with mulberry excrescences, and weighed two ounces. The boy is now in good health, and engaged in heavy work as an errand boy.

The Body-Temperature in Granulating Suppurative Inflammation of Joints.

Dr. KÖNIG (*Deutsche Zeitschrift für Chirurgie*, Band x.) remarks that the prognostic importance of commencing suppuration in fungous arthritis is clear, from the fact that abscesses in joints are almost never absorbed in adults, in children only seldom; and therefore that the prognosis of such suppurations, when left to themselves, is unfavourable. Dr. *König* has ascertained that the commencement of suppuration is indicated by the course of the temperature of the body. Uncomplicated granulating synovitis is not, as a rule, of itself attended with any abnormal course of temperature. Individuals suffering from such affections are indeed very irritable, and slight causes (such as the application of dressings, removal, etc.) readily produce a rise of temperature; this, however, is only of short duration. Prolonged rises of temperature indicate that suppuration is commencing in the joint which is the seat of fungous disease, where they are not caused by processes going on somewhere else independently of the affection of the joint. There is often only a slight rise of the evening temperature, while the morning remission is considerable; in anæmic patients especially, the morning temperature falls even below the normal. Sometimes the development of abscesses is not accompanied with fever, and frequently the patient is free from fever during the formation of a cold abscess; probably because the firm membrane inclosing the abscess resists the absorption of fever-producing materials.—*British Med. Journal*, Oct. 26, 1878.

———

Case of Radial Paralysis cured by Operation.

At a meeting of the Niederrheinische Gesellschaft für Natur-und Heilkunde in Bonn, Professor VON MOSENGEIL showed a patient on whom he had operated successfully for paralysis of the radial nerve. The patient had suffered from gangrenous phlegmon of the upper arm, in consequence of which a portion of the soft parts covering the bone on the posterior and outer side had sloughed to the extent of a hand-breadth. The cicatricial tissue formed in healing had compressed and paralyzed the nerve. In the operation, the nerve was exposed at the border of the supinator longus, and followed upwards for six or seven inches; and a portion an inch long, firmly imbedded in cicatricial tissue, was set free. Healing took place by the first intention. The paralysis lasted several months, but had disappeared some weeks before the patient was shown.—*British Med. Journal*, Oct. 26, 1878, from *Berliner Klinische Wochenschrift*, Sept. 9.

.

———————

Midwifery and Gynæcology.

Oxide of Zinc Ointment in Membranous Vaginitis.

Dr. THEOPHILUS PARVIN recommends (*Am. Practitioner*, Aug. 1878), the use of large tampons of patent lint smeared with oxide of zinc ointment in cases of membranous vaginitis.

———

Removal of Uterine Cervical Stenosis by Electrolysis.

In the *Annales de Gynécologie*, May, 1878, Dr. LEBLOND says that the cure of stricture of the urethra in man by electrolysis suggested the idea of treating stenosis of the cervix uteri in the same manner. Dr. Leblond performed this operation in the case of a lady aged 45, the negative pole being applied to the cervix, and the positive pole to the patient's right thigh. It is advisable in the use of electrolysis to apply the negative pole to the cervix, because the cicatrix which results is not so contractile as that caused by the positive pole. Dr. Leblond thinks that electrolysis may be used with advantage in some cases instead of the bistoury or other means.—*London Med. Record*, Aug. 15, 1878.

A Case of Atresia Uteri Gravidi.

In the *St. Petersburger Medicinische Wochenschrift*, Dr. J. von DIETERICH describes a case of atresia uteri gravidi occurring in the eighth pregnancy from cicatricial closure of the os uteri. The patient, a peasant woman, had had six children under perfectly normal conditions. At the seventh labour a doctor had to be called in to incise the os, which did not dilate, owing to cicatricial changes. In her eighth confinement, Dr. Dieterich was called, and found the os uteri almost completely closed by cicatricial structures. There was only room to pass an elastic catheter. Dr. Dieterich made radiating incisions in the os, and, about 9 P. M., the next morning he found the os no more dilated than he had left it in the evening, when he could pass his finger. He enlarged the incisions and gave ergot. In a few hours after these proceedings a live male child was born. The recovery was rapid, the lying-in normal.—*London Med. Record*, Oct. 15, 1878.

Results of Ovariotomy before and after Antiseptics.

Mr. T. KEITH, of Edinburgh, makes the following very interesting communication on this subject to the *British Medical Journal* (Oct. 19, 1878).

Ever since Mr. Lister showed me—more than ten years ago—a large blood-clot organized in the wound of a compound fracture, I have followed his antiseptic treatment through its various stages in my daily surgical work. Time has only convinced me of its value. In those early days of antiseptics—I speak of ten or twelve years ago—it did not seem possible that any method could be devised whereby the antiseptic principle could be properly carried out in the removal of abdominal tumours. Yet, in the hope that a certain amount of carbolic acid introduced into the abdominal cavity might prevent or retard the putrefaction of the red serum that is apt to stagnate in the pelvis after ovariotomy, a two or three per cent. watery solution of carbolic acid was freely used in sponging and cleaning out the cavity; antiseptic ligatures, first of the finest silk and then of catgut, were used, and all instruments were rubbed with carbolic oil. Towels were soaked in the watery solution, and sometimes held against the wound, in the vain hope of keeping the air pure as it rushed in when the peritoneal cavity was opened. Carbolic acid was wasted in every possible way. The floor and walls of the room in which the operation was to be performed were sponged with it, and the air was charged with the vapour driven off by heat. For nearly three years—from 1869 to 1871—this practice was more or less carried on. The results, which for that time had hitherto been good, did not improve, but rather the reverse, and, after two or three mysterious-looking deaths, in cases that should have done well, this carbolic acid treatment was thrown aside. It had brought nothing but disappointment and vexation of spirit.

For the next five years, though I continued to use it as usual in ordinary work, no carbolic acid whatever, nor any antiseptic, was made use of in my ovarian operations. Unable, though believing in it as much as ever, to carry out the antiseptic principle, and thus find protection from external agencies, I thought this operation one in which it would be better to trust to care and cleanliness alone. Sponges were simply wrung out in hot water, long boiled, and if any carbolic acid were used in the cleaning of them it was washed away before an operation was begun. Beyond a purgative, nothing of the so-called "prepara- tion" of the patient was made. No restrictions were put upon visitors, except that they must not have come directly from a dissecting room, or from visiting a case of erysipelas, and they were requested not to touch the sponges. These I always cleaned and took charge of myself. The friends who assisted me—all busy men in large obstetric and general practice—took no special precautions against infection. Sometimes, on putting the question, it was found that almost every kind of infectious disease had been already visited that morning; once only was there a suspicion that mischief was carried, for one of my friends himself took severe erysipelas a few days after he had assisted me at an operation. The patient recovered after a slow attack of blood-poisoning. The regulations made in some hospitals, that every visitor must sign his name in a book, declaring that he has not for a week visited any case of infectious disease or attended a *post- mortem* examination, before being admitted into the operating room, has always seemed to me to be meant for a sort of *plaisanterie*. For my own part, when a case goes wrong after an operation, I have seldom to look far beyond myself for the cause of failure—something done, something not done. This is a lesson hard to learn: we blame persons, things, accidents, and circumstances, rather than ourselves.

During the operation, the abdominal cavity was more freely exposed than I have ever seen it done by another operator. It was also cleaned more thoroughly, and there was no haste in closing the wound; half an hour's waiting was time well spent. Every oozing point was secured by the finest of ligatures, al- ways Lister's, or by the cautery. Large lumps of cellular tissue were not tied, only the bleeding points. The clamp was gradually displaced by the cautery, and when ligatures were required to the pedicle, very fine soft iron-wire or catgut was used; I never used the very thick silk, which I have often seen left in the abdomen, of a thickness and strength sufficient to hang the patient. Even very fine silk, I had long discarded. That I was fortunate in having done so, the recent results given in Mr. Wells's Surgical Lectures prove. Of 157 cases in which he employed silk ligatures to the pedicle, 60 died, or 38 per cent., whereas of my first fifty cautery operations performed under similar circumstances, where from the thickness or shortness of the pedicle, or both, the extra-peritoneal method could not be used safely, there were only four deaths, or 8 per cent. Then drain- age, by a large perforated glass tube passing to the bottom of the pelvis, became the rule in severe operations. Finding that the red serum, that enemy of the ovariotomist, would not lie safely in the abdomen by the addition of a little car- bolic acid till absorption had taken place, it was got rid of every three or four hours by a tube and syringe as it collected in the pelvis. Doubtless this was a troublesome process, but it lessened or entirely prevented the absorption fever, and that it saved lives I am sure. Judging from the large quantities—pints some- times, once 146 ounces—of broken down blood-clot and serum got away during the first few days after severe operations in feeble women, no one will convince me that drainage thus practised in those days was of no use, whatever it may now be in operations performed under antiseptics.

Since 1876, every operation has been performed with all Mr. Lister's care, under the carbolic acid cloud, and I shall never go back to the old way. But before giving my impressions of ovariotomy thus performed, I wish to tell you exactly the results that can be got after this operation, by simple carefulness, without antiseptics. There is no mystery in ovariotomy. It is not a difficult operation. Is there any surgical proceeding that is? It is often an extremely simple one, yet it requires care; in bad cases it takes time, and may present a fertile field for bad surgery; yet any one, who is not in a hurry and takes the trouble, will get as good results. It is now more than sixteen years since I did my first ovariotomy. Beginning with seventeen deaths in the first hundred operations, the mortality year by year diminished, till at last, of the twenty-six operations before the use of the spray, there was but one death, the tumour removed in that case being a malignant one. Now, as the results of a single year may be accidental, I take the whole number performed during the five years immediately preceding the use of the spray. Including two cases of return of the disease in the other ovary, there were in all ninety-four operations, eight being double. Twenty-four of these were performed in the patients' own homes, or in lodgings, or in the country; seventy, in a small top flat, where the hospital patients were taken for nearly ten years. Though I had for a time, some years ago, the sanction of the managers to do ovariotomy in the Royal Infirmary, the only room then available for me in the old crowded building was a small old fever ward at the top of the house, next the scarlet fever and smallpox wards. I soon found it better for the good of the patients, no less than for the credit of surgery, to have all the hospital cases placed near my own house, where they could get quiet, cleanliness, and perfect nursing; and after being threatened by an interdict from the Court of Session, I was allowed to pursue my surgical experiment in peace. Of the ninety-four patients operated on during these five years, nine died, four of the private cases (two being malignant tumours), and five of the seventy hospital ones (one malignant). No result approaching this—one in fourteen of hospital cases—had hitherto been anywhere obtained in any hospital or in any private practice, over a series of years or in any single year. I wish, for the credit of my small hospital, which I carried on almost entirely at my own expense, to make this statement of results distinctly; and I would not make it prominent now, but that year after year the authorities of the Samaritan Hospital proclaim in their reports, in the largest of Roman letters—though one of the surgeons tells me that he has objected to the statement in vain—that the results got there are always the best that have yet been obtained, the mortality of the Samaritan Hospital down to the end of 1876 being nearly one death in every four operated on; of the last five corresponding years, one in five.

Of the nine fatal cases that occurred during the five years preceding the use of the spray, in three the tumours were cancerous. One death arose from obstructed intestine, and another from old kidney disease. These five were probably hopeless under any conditions. Three of the others might have recovered with earlier operation or with drainage; only one was a simple operation with moderate adhesion. It was a large tumour complicated by a uterine fibroid. I unfortunately removed a pedicellated outgrowth which seemed to be in the way. I have little doubt that antiseptic treatment would have covered the errors committed during that operation.

I had not performed ovariotomy half a dozen times, when I felt sure that it would become, perhaps, the safest of all surgical operations; for in the rapidly absorbing powers of the peritoneum—though in these lie at once both the danger and the safety of the patient—the surgeon has an advantage, if he make right use of it, that he has in no other. At the end of 1876, this safety-point seemed almost within reach. The mortality was steadily decreasing, that of the last hundred operations being under ten per cent., while of the cautery cases it was little more than seven per cent. The results obtained were almost free from avoidable mortality. There was no death for nearly seven years after an operation for a non-adherent simple tumour; in a large proportion of the fatal cases the tumours were of a cancerous nature, some with secondary affections of the peritoneum—a class of cases which, thanks to the investigations of Dr. Foulis, to be afterwards referred to, can in future be always recognized, and in certain of them operation avoided as useless.

Then, in the other fatal cases, with one exception, the operations were extremely severe. It was in such cases of large adherent tumours in feeble women who had come late in the disease that some assistance was wanted. I seemed to have got to the end of my resources. Drainage, and all the care I could give, did not sometimes prevent the blood-poison; for even the feeblest of those operated on rarely die from shock or exhaustion, but from rapid septicæmia. This help I hoped to find in antiseptics now properly applied. Yet, after my former experience of the carbolic acid treatment, I hesitated long ere I used the spray. Its effect in prolonged operations were as yet unknown, the instruments were not very perfect, and the results one heard of, of operations done under it, were not very encouraging. Several cases operated on by friends here with all possible care proved fatal from blood-poisoning. So did one or two done in Glasgow. In London the only case I knew of was done at the Samaritan Hospital by Mr. Thornton, who sent me the notes of it. It was a clear case of death from septicæmia, with some brain symptoms towards the end. The method was blamed for this result, and in consequence the spray was thrown aside, and was not again used there for many months, when its employment in ovariotomy had elsewhere become comparatively common. By this time the German surgeons had settled the question of safety, though their results were still not much to boast of. Mr. Wells, in his sixth lecture (July, 1878), tells us that he had just then received a letter from Dr. Oldshausen, of Halle, giving the results of his own practice and those of Esmarch, Hegar, and Schrœder, with and without antiseptics. Without, there were 65 cases and 33 deaths—1 death in every 2 operated on; results so dreadful that they seem simply incomprehensible. Of 155 cases done antiseptically, there were only 33 deaths, or nearly 1 in 5—a mortality still more than double that of my cases for more than five years without antiseptics of any kind.

Without antiseptics, my results over fourteen years give a mortality of almost 1 in 7. Of the five years preceding the use of the spray, nearly 1 in 10½—of the last of these five years 1 in 21. To what, then, are these results to be attributed? Why should my results without antiseptics be nearly six times better than those of these German surgeons (33 deaths of their last 65 cases—6 of the last 70 of mine), and so much better than those of Mr. Wells, or those of the Samaritan Hospital, in an operation that requires no special surgical skill. Leaving out of view some huge counteracting influence in the German operations, I think they are due—1. To drainage of the abdominal cavity in severe cases by a large perforated glass tube going to the bottom of the pelvis. It is to Kœberlé that I am indebted for the idea. He kindly gave me two of his small tubes in 1866. These were soon found to be too narrow and too short. They got easily choked with clot or lymph. For the last ten years I have used the large glass tubes now in common use. Till I had learned in what cases to drain, the tube was used in alternate cases of the severe operations. I am as certain as I am of my existence, that had I used them earlier and oftener the mortality would have been less by one-third. These tubes I supplied to ovariotomist friends in all parts of the world, though no one used them, so far as I know, till attention was called to drainage by the vagina by Dr. Marion Sims—a method which seems to me to be one calculated rather to give rise to blood-poisoning than to save the patient from it. It is remarkable that the only year in which the mortality of the Samaritan Hospital fell to 14 per cent. was in 1876, when drainage by these glass-tubes was first generally used. 2. To the use of the cautery in dividing the pedicle, as proposed and practised by the late Mr. Baker Brown. How the lesson given by his last results has been so systematically ignored in London has always been a marvel to me. 3. To the employment of Kœberlé's compression forceps, in large numbers, whereby loss of blood is prevented. His model is still the best, notwithstanding the clumsy imitations of it lately invented. 4. To the substitution of ether for chloroform in my last 230 operations, whereby the after-vomiting is avoided, and the risk of hemorrhage when the wound is closed diminished. All these things have, I think, helped to lessen the mortality, but the drainage and the employment of the cautery in the division of the pedicle have contributed most.

So much for ovariotomy and its results before antiseptics. I have now done forty-nine operations as carefully as possible under the spray. Two of the first eight died, the rest, forty-one in number, all recovered. At first the results were disappointing, for I expected too much. After two or three ordinary cases that would have got well in any way, five patients presented themselves at the same time, whom I would gladly not have seen till I had more experience of the spray in ovariotomy, though just the kind of cases in which assistance was hoped from antiseptics. 1. A young woman who had been nine months in bed from a large, burst, dermoid cyst. She had had double phlegmasia dolens, the œdema extending over the trunk into the axillæ. For months she lay poisoned, often apparently dying, with great pain and vomiting, yet she, after nine tappings, rallied, and was able to be brought into town. She was against operation, feeling sure that she would not recover. I urged her to have it done, telling her of all I hoped from this new method. Instead of closing the wound as I ought to have done, I went on and completed the operation after three hours and a half. Both ovaries were universally adherent, and a mass of bone, hair, and fat, that had become encysted in the upper part of the abdomen, was dissected out. Time was lost in replenishing the spray-producer, and when she was put to bed the temperature of the body had fallen to 92°. Eight hours after the operation it had risen only to 95°. No urine was secreted, and she died comatose thirty-two hours after. 2. Case of large semisolid tumour of 95 lbs. She was anæmic, and had often been tapped. She, too, was unwilling for operation, feeling that her strength was all gone. The same arguments as before were used, and she was encouraged to run the risk. The operation was as bad as could well be—adhesions everywhere—especially to liver, lumbar, and iliac regions. It was the old story—pain, vomiting, and death from septic peritonitis. 3. An old lady of 64, who declined assistance till she was in a typhoid state from suppurating cyst. There were sloughs on the sacrum. The cyst had 60 lbs. of pus, and there were extensive adhesions in the pelvis. The case was a most unfavourable one; yet, with much stimulation, she ultimately recovered, though she had a rapid pulse and high temperature for long after. 4. Case of old, burst, jelly cyst in a lady from Newcastle. There was very old thickening of the peritoneum, and the abdomen was full of jelly. Both ovaries were diseased. She did well for four days. Then came pain and fever. Two pints of horribly putrid red serum were removed by puncture behind the uterus. This had to be done again and again, and for six weeks there was a hard fight against the blood-poison. It was a continned effort to keep the pelvis free of putrid fluid. I believe that the whole abdominal cavity suppurated in this case. The difficulty of establishing a permanent drain was great. There were severe hemorrhages after the incisions in the vagina, followed by severe rigours, and once Douglas's space was filled with blood-clot. She bore nourishment well, and drank brandy like water, and recovered perfectly. In this case, I think infection must have been conveyed by the cut Fallopian tubes close to the uterus, for, on the third day, there was some metrostaxis. 5. A case of bad pelvic adhesion. Here, also, fluid had to be evacuated from the abdomen, and discharge went on for many weeks. Thus, at first, through want of drainage, things seemed rather to get worse under the anti-septic treatment, reminding me not a little of my experience with the carbolic acid treatment some years ago.

At first, I tested the spray very severely. The operations were more hurriedly performed—that is, I spent shorter time over them, and did not sponge so care-fully; neither was I so careful in securing every bleeding point, nor did I wait for the after-oozing in severe cases. I gave up also the drainage-tube, but soon found that the patients did not get on so well, and there was sometimes trouble-some absorption fever. One case quite convinced me that the old carefulness could not, even with the spray, be dispensed with. I had operated on a patient of my friend Dr. Sidey, my *fidus Achates* in many a hard operation. It was a very bad case of acute suppurating cyst, with typhoid symptoms. I shut up quickly. There was some oozing going on from extensive parietal adhesions, and some purulent-looking ovarian fluid had escaped into the pelvis, and even this was imperfectly sponged up. He asked me to sponge this a little more. My reply was, that if the spray was worth anything, it would keep all sweet and the peritoneum would take care of it—purulent fluid or no purulent fluid. The patient got on badly, the typhoid symptoms became more marked, and she re-quired much stimulation. On speaking to him one day about the high pulse and temperature, his reply expressed my thoughts of the last few days : " It is all your own fault. You should have sponged that belly better, and not left her to absorb the dirt you left behind. I wish when you try experiments again that you would not begin on my patients, but clean them up in the old way." Fortu-nately, in this case, the peritoneum was able to dispose of what had unnecessarily been thrown upon it to do.

[The results of the 48 spray cases are given in a table, from which we learn that the spray was used for from twenty minutes to three hours and thirty minutes. Adhesions existed in 70 per cent. ; 46 recovered, and 2 died.]

It is only fair to add that this series of operations has, on the whole, been less severe, though there were many bad operations amongst them, and there is a larger proportion of non-adherent tumours. Neither were the tumours so large. Thus, in 50 cautery cases (*Lancet*, April, 1876), 18 per cent. of the tumours were non-adherent. In the table the number of non-adherent tumours is 30 per cent. But I find that in Mr. Wells's last published 50 cases, 42 per cent. of the tumours were non-adherent. Instead of, as in former years, advising against operations in cases of moderate sized tumours, which had not yet become a source of danger, all were operated on just as they came. Hence the number of simpler operations.

The spray is neither troublesome nor inconvenient. The instrument at present in use is Gardiner's largest size. It has a double jet ; and, when placed at a dis-tance of eight or nine feet, the spray reaches the wound without any cooling cur-rent, and as fine as a London fog. That the spray is essential in ovariotomy to the perfect carrying out of Mr. Lister's principle is proved by my experience over so many years of the simple carbolic acid treatment. There can be no two opinions about this.

With antiseptics, some form of intra-peritoneal treatment of the pedicle will be found to answer best. The clamp has done good service, but it must give place to something better. The mortality attending its use is larger, and the conva-lescence slower, as a rule, than with the best of the intra-peritoneal methods.

The ligatures, when employed, were either catgut or fine soft iron wire. I have already stated that, of fifty-one cautery cases before antiseptics, there were four deaths ; of thirty-one cautery cases with spray, all recovered. A method, then, which in the worst cases without antiseptics answered so well, must be a good one with them. What difference was there, then, in the cases that got well? Not much. Carefully prepared tables of temperatures of the two sets of cases show very little difference. There was, as a rule, the same moderate rise of temperature up to eight or ten hours after operation—more marked, perhaps, in both sets of cases in young subjects, especially if in too good condition; then a fall by next morning, and again a rise in the evening to about thirty-four hours after operation. After that, almost a normal pulse and temperature, and a rapid convalescence, except in some of the cases where ligatures were left in the pedicles. In both sets of cases the wounds were dressed in the way I have now done for many years. Eight or ten folds of gauze soaked in an 8 per cent. solution of carbolic acid in glycerine, and over that a large cushion of cotton wool. When there was no draining, this dressing was not disturbed for a week or more, and primary union was always got with or without spray. The patient was generally out of bed by the end of the second week, and home, after a long way, during the third. Yet, the convalescence was easier in the antiseptic cases. They suffered less from flatus, and slept better. The nurses all tell me that they had less trouble with them, and had themselves much more sleep.

Yet, in three cases, the temperatures were the highest I have ever seen a few hours after ovariotomy. In one it rose to 104°, but was down by next morning. In another, five hours after operation, it was 106.2°; in another, 105.5° eight hours after. These two were cases of burst cysts. In both, the adhesions were unusually great to intestine, mesentery, and in the pelvis. Both were long operations, and there was great exposure of intestine and mesentery to the action of the spray. Now, I have rarely—not more than twice, I think—seen a temperature of 103° on the evening of the operation in any case, before antiseptics; and I cannot account for the rapid rise in these two cases. In the case where the temperature rose to above 106° so soon after, a most unfavourable prognosis had been given, the chances being put as a hundred to one against a favourable termination. She was sixty-three years of age; was in a typhoid state after a burst cyst, and was quite comatose. This condition continued more or less for a fortnight, and she has now no remembrance of the operation, or even of having seen me. I have rarely met with high temperatures in ordinary ovariotomy, and nothing has so much surprised me as to read of the hyperpyrexia which Mr. Wells tells us is the rule after ovariotomy. I had never before antiseptics found it necessary to use ice to the head to bring down fever in the first days after operation. The ice cap was only used once in a case of acute septicæmia, and the temperature remained unaffected. Indeed, in all my cases before the spray, not more than five or six pounds of ice were got for the whole number, and the most of that was wasted. I attribute the hyperpyrexia to operating in women overfed, or in too full health with small tumours, or to imperfect cleaning, or not draining of the abdomen, thus giving rise to absorption fever. Many years ago, when I sometimes removed moderate-sized semisolid tumours from women in full condition, my practice was to let them lose ten or twelve ounces of blood from the pedicle before securing it. This prevented any undue blood-pressure and vascular disturbance. For long my practice has been to wait till the patient had suffered from her burden, and interference was necessary. Only once or twice has this rule been broken through, when some German or foreign friend wished to see the cautery used, and only some case of small tumour was at hand to show him. But then I generally had to regret it. Antiseptics will change all this.

What, then, have we gained by antiseptics in ovariotomy? 1. It has lessened the mortality. Take the results of the German surgeons. After the first trials even, the mortality fell at once from 50 per cent. to 20; thirty lives saved by the

spray alone out of every hundred. When I add that my last forty-one have all
recovered, enough has been said. No such successful series was ever got in the
old way. Once Mr. Wells had twenty-seven successful operations in succession.
But look at that wonderful list of eight hundred operations. How often did it
happen that there was a run of deaths, too many and occurring too often to be
merely accidental; frequently four or five in succession, once seven, then ten out
of twelve, etc. With antiseptics there will be no *per contra*, and such a run of
deaths will come no more.   2. This increased safety will encourage medical men
to recommend earlier operation, which certainly few of them now do.   That very
large tumours and bad adhesion increase the mortality there can be no doubt.
For the last seven years, no death happened to me in non-adherent tumours, and
the deaths that occurred during that period were, with a single exception, in cases
when the local difficulties prolonged the operation for two hours or more.   Certainly early operation, when a cyst bursts and fluid is thrown out in a large quantity into the peritoneum, cannot be too strongly urged.   3. With antiseptic
ovariotomy the drainage-tube will not be nearly so often required.   I do not
think that it can be altogether dispensed with.   No one has practised drainage so
much as I have, yet I know well that it sometimes cannot be used without risk.
Some patients give simply serum from the irritation of the tube ; in others, after
a short time the tube becomes inclosed in thick lymph, and it sometimes gets
choked with this.   In such circumstances, there must be a risk of some folds of
intestine adhering at angles when the tube is removed.   I have several times seen
decided inconveniences arise from this, but never any fatal obstruction.   With
antiseptics the tube can be removed much earlier.   Drainage is certainly a great
trouble both to the patient and attendant.   4. Convalescence is rendered easier.
5. Antiseptics are a great comfort and relief to the operator.   Speaking for myself, the difference is enormous ; ovariotomy is not the operation it was fifteen or
sixteen years ago, or even two years ago.   The best results in the old way were difficult to get, and no one knows but who has experienced it the anxiety and weariness of spirit with which the struggle against the blood-poison was carried on in
the early days of ovariotomy.   It is something to think that no one will again
have to suffer these experiences in the same degree, and it almost makes one envy
the younger ovariotomists to whom the way in these days is made easy.   Now
there is a feeling of confidence and security ; the constant fret and worry to get
chemical cleanliness in one's hands, in the surroundings of the patient and her
attendants, has passed away.   The time is saved that was spent in cleaning the
sponges, in passing the points of instruments through the flame of the spirit-lamp,
and in other endless precautions.   Above all, there is the feeling that the patient
is protected from external agencies.   Now, with an 1-in-20 carbolic solution and
a nail-brush, with first perhaps a wash in turpentine to remove all fatty matter,
I am safe to have my hands in any degree of putridity half an hour before an
operation.   Professor Schroeder tells us that he uses extraordinary precautions ;
that, on an operation-morning, he gets up early and washes himself all over ;
that his assistants wash themselves, and that the patient is all washed ; that neither
he nor his assistants see any patients till the operation is over.   Surely all these
washings are unnecessary, and have come too late.   Had these precautions been
taken before the days of antiseptics, I can imagine that the results of the German
surgery in ovariotomy would have been something better than a 50 per cent. mortality.   I have recently successfully performed ovariotomy several times on poor
women in their own homes, or in almost filthy lodgings, without any precaution
whatever.

   That drawbacks may yet appear is quite possible.   What I should be afraid of
is the effect of very long-continued spray in severe cases in feeble women.   I

think I have noticed a greater depression immediately following some of the very long operations, and a necessity for greater stimulation during the first twelve or twenty hours. I confess I shall watch with some anxiety whether deaths in severe cases happen more quickly than they used to do.

One's pleasure in this operation is, however, greatly marred by the frequency with which malignant disease is found at the operation, or reappears soon after it, upsetting all one's calculations. In one-fourth of my deaths, the tumours were malignant; and, with very few exceptions, in those who have died since their return home after ovariotomy, some cancerous affection has been the cause of death. Thus, amongst these, five young and healthy-looking women have left me, all after severe operations, the pictures of health and happiness, and have died within a short time of peritoneal cancer. This is a subject of the greatest interest. Till quite recently, our knowledge of the microscopic appearances of the diseased ovary was in a state of hopeless muddle. Dr. Foulis, by his investigations of the anatomy of the ovary, has at length made its pathology simple. Healthy and malignant ovarian structure, simple ovarian and peritoneal fluids, as well as those of the uterine fibro-cysts, can now be recognized with certainty by the microscope alone. We know now that, in certain cases where free fluid in the peritoneum is present with ovarian tumour, there is no use in operating; in others, that we cannot interfere a day too soon; and in some we can predict a return of abdominal disease after successful operation. These researches of Dr. Foulis are of the utmost value, and I know well the time and labour that have been for several years spent upon them. I regret to have to add that, in his recent lectures at the College of Surgeons, Mr. Wells incorrectly gave the entire credit of these investigations to Mr. Thornton, who, to say the least of it, as ungenerously tried to claim it.

Not long after I began ovariotomy, one of the heads of the profession here—the best and most honest of men, an old teacher, and one whom I looked up to as a professional father—said to me: "Fellows like you should simply be handed over to Mr. Lothian." Now, Mr. Lothian was the public prosecutor. By simple care, and by giving heed to the old surgical principles that my good master James Syme taught, I am now able to show you that the mortality of ovariotomy has with me got less and less every year since I began it, till in the year before antiseptics it had fallen to 5 per cent. Surely, then, if one's natural conservatism should have hindered any one from adopting altogether a different procedure, such as the antiseptic principle involves, it should have prevented me. But there was no getting over the living blood-clot in the open wound of the broken leg. There was certainly disappointment at first, but only from my inability to carry out the principle, or from trying to carry it out in a wrong way. Now, the right way is got, and surgeons like Mr. Callender, or our own Mr. Spence, may take my word for it that, if they have reached already near perfection in their work, they will, by carrying out Lister's antiseptic principles, get still nearer it, and that, too, with greater comfort to their patients and with less anxiety and less trouble to themselves.

In his last edition on the *Diseases of Women*, Dr. West thus writes: "I think, then, that we are now bound to admit ovariotomy as one of the legitimate operations in surgery; as holding out a prospect, and a daily brightening prospect, of escape from a painful and inevitable death, which at last, indeed, becomes welcome, only because the road that leads to it conducts the patient through such utter misery."

This long-despised operation is now the safest of all the great surgical operations, at least judging from these results: twelve deaths of the last one hundred and fifty-six, three of the last seventy-five, and no death of the last forty-one operations.

I would fain expatiate for a little on antiseptics in general, but must bring this rambling paper to a close, feeling sure that, whatever may appear in the future of antiseptics in surgery, the name of Joseph Lister, who put us on the right way, will not be forgotten.

—

A Case of Tubercular Pelvic Peritonitis with Tubercle of the Ovaries and
Suppurative Encysted Metritis, in a Girl aged Six Years.

In the *Annales de Gynécologie*, June, 1878, Dr. CH. TALAMON relates the following rare case: Marie T., aged 6, was admitted under Dr. Triboulet, to the Sainte-Eugénie Hospital, with symptoms of tubercular meningitis. There was found, also, consolidation of the lungs at both apices. No symptoms drew attention to the abdomen, which was flat, excavated, and flaccid, as usual in tubercular peritonitis. The meningitis ran its course, and at the end of six days the child was seized with convulsions, and died. At the necropsy the usual appearances were found in the brain, and tubercular consolidation of both apices of the lungs. In the intestine, all the Peyer's patches were the seat of irregular ulcerations. The uterus was three times its normal size, and contained a clear green viscid fluid, like muco-pus; its cervical orifice was closed by tubercular ulceration. The Fallopian tubes were obliterated. The two ovaries were surrounded by thick caseous exudation. On removing these exudations, the ovaries appeared indurated, irregular, and enlarged to the size of the ovaries of a young adult. On section, they were found to be entirely changed into yellow cheesy matter. The microscopic examination revealed miliary nodules on the external surface of the ovaries. The portions of the tubes adjacent to the ovaries presented tubercular degeneration of the mucous membrane, whilst the uterine ends of the tubes remained normal.—*London Med. Record*, Oct. 15, 1878.

———

Medical Jurisprudence and Toxicology.

Saponin Poisoning.

A curious instance of acute poisoning in the cause of science is reported by the victim, Dr. F. KEPPLER in the *Berliner Klin. Wochenschrift*, Nos. 32, 33, 34. He wished to test the value of saponin as a local anæsthetic, and injected a solution containing 0.1 gramme into the inner side of the left thigh. Saponin, it may not be superfluous to premise, is a glucoside extracted from *Saponaria officinalis*, and it is identical with senegin, the principle of *Polygala Senega*, so much used in chronic bronchitis.

Experiments on animals have been made with saponin by Eugene Peliken, Herman Köhler, Schroff, and others, who found that this body in sufficient doses paralyzes the heart and the vaso-motor and respiratory centres, and in smaller doses probably acts as a local anæsthetic. Hypodermic injections of saponin were tried in three cases by Eulenburg, with doses ranging from 0.06 to 0.02 grammes; but the ill-effects which followed were so severe as to lead him to warn others not to use saponin for anæsthetic purposes in human beings, especially as the neuralgia for which in each case the injection was made continued unrelieved.

The preparation used by Keppler on himself was obtained from Merck of Darmstadt. It was an amorphous clear brown powder with a feeble acid reaction. With water it formed a cloudy liquid which frothed a good deal, and even at a little distance caused severe sneezing and a sensation of burning in the eyes and throat. At the commencement of the experiment Dr. Keppler's pulse was normal, 85 per minute, and his temperature *in the hand* 36.2° C. The effects of the injection may be divided into (1) those merely due to the local irritation of the injection and the inflammation excited in the tissues, and (2) those entirely the result of the saponin-poisoning. The first consisted of the most painful local inflammation of the skin, reaching its height in twenty-four hours and then subsiding, and general symptoms of depression; pallor, cold perspiration, giddiness, and actual fainting. These symptoms also occur after injections of other substances (*e. g.*, corrosive sublimate). The true saponin symptoms were, locally, a peculiar anæsthesia of fifteen minutes' duration, which prevented the prick of a sharp needle being felt, while it did not remove the continuous pain of the injection itself; and generally, alterations of the temperature, pulse, intelligence, etc. The temperature was not exceedingly raised. The highest point reached was 38.6° Cent. three hours after the injection; but on the third day there was still fever in the evening—37.8° Cent. On the fifth day there were abnormally low temperatures, reaching 33.6° Cent. at 3 p. m. As the pain and inflammation at the seat of injection were so severe, Dr. Keppler believes that the saponin acted as an antipyretic, and that it was not until the fifth day, when the local symptoms had nearly subsided, that its depressing effects were really able to show themselves. This view seems further justified by the state of the pulse on the fifth day, when it fell to 65 per minute, the normal being 85, and the average pulse on the first four days of the experiment having ranged from 80 to 100. The other general symptoms on the *first* day of the experiment were intense pain in the head and eyes, and especially in the left eye, intermittent rigors, and extraordinary depression of mind, with indifference to everything that was going on around, and terminating in a state of unconsciousness of several hours' duration. On the *second* day the pain in the head was still worse than before, there was exophthalmos of the left eye, the breathing was superficial and slow, and speech difficult. Standing was almost impossible. The pulse was scarcely perceptible, but there was subjective palpitation. Pains in the teeth were also perceived, though not one of them was carious. The appetite was quite lost, but there was no thirst. On the *third* day there were still slight rigors. There was less pain, but nausea, salivation, and intense weakness were present. The indifference even to matters which a few days before were of the highest interest, was remarkable. On the succeeding days the pains in the head and eyes as well as the weakness gradually disappeared, but even on the sixth day giddiness came on on getting up, and continued all day, and Dr. Keppler felt as if he was recovering from a severe illness. Considerable inflammatory thickening was present under the injected area of skin a year after the date of the experiment.

It thus appears that the subcutaneous injection of saponin for anæsthetic purposes is a complete failure, and that the use of the drug is by no means unattended with danger; but Dr. Keppler thinks there is a possible future for it as an antipyretic and excitant in cases of acute pleurisy and pneumonia with so-called "cerebral symptoms," and in malignant typhoid forms of endo- and peri-carditis. Possibly also the severe local inflammation excited by the injection may be applied to the destruction of certain morbid growths, lupus, sarcomata, etc., which may not be suited for operation. The maximum dose which should be tried at the first injection should not exceed 0.06 gramme, or one grain.—*Med. Times and Gaz.*, Sept. 28, 1878.

CONTENTS.

Published Monthly, price $2.50 per annum, free of postage.
Also, furnished together with the AMERICAN JOURNAL OF THE MEDICAL
SCIENCES *and the* MEDICAL NEWS AND LIBRARY *for* SIX DOLLARS *per
annum in advance, the whole free of postage.*

HENRY C. LEA, Philadelphia.

INDEX.

NOTICE TO SUBSCRIBERS.

Subscribers are reminded of the advantages offered for remittance in advance for the year 1879. For SIX DOLLARS, in advance, they will receive "THE AMERICAN JOURNAL OF THE MEDICAL SCIENCES," "THE MEDICAL NEWS AND LIBRARY," and "THE MONTHLY ABSTRACT OF MEDICAL SCIENCE," all free of postage, and containing in all more than 2100 large octavo pages.

Separate subscription to the "ABSTRACT," $2.50 per annum, in advance.

Neat cloth covers, gilt-lettered, for the two volumes of the "JOURNAL" and one volume of the "ABSTRACT," for 1878, will be mailed to subscribers, free of postage, on receipt of ten cents for each cover.

PREMIUMS FOR OBTAINING NEW SUBSCRIBERS.

Gentlemen who will remit in advance two subscriptions for the "AMERICAN JOURNAL OF THE MEDICAL SCIENCES," for 1879, *one of which must be for a new subscriber*, will receive as a premium, free of postage, one of the following volumes at their choice:—

Fothergill's Antagonism of Medicines, 1 vol. 12mo., cloth. (*Now Ready.*)
Holden's Landmarks, Medical and Surgical, 1 vol. 12mo., cloth. (*Now Ready.*)
Browne's How to Use the Ophthalmoscope, 1 vol. 12mo., cloth.
Austin Flint's Essays on Conservative Medicine, 1 vol. 12mo., cloth.
Tanner's Clinical Manual, Second Edition, 1 vol. 18mo., cloth.
Swayne's Obstetric Aphorisms, Second Edition, 1 vol. 18mo., cloth.
Sturges's Clinical Medicine, 1 vol. 12mo., cloth.
Chambers's Restorative Medicine, 1 vol. 18mo., cloth.
West on Nervous Disorders of Children, 1 vol. 18mo., cloth.

☞ Remit by Bank Check, Postal Money Order, or Registered Letter.

Address,

HENRY C. LEA,

Nos. 706 and 708 Sansom Street, Philadelphia, Pa.

THE MONTHLY

ABSTRACT OF MEDICAL SCIENCE:

A DIGEST

OF THE

PROGRESS OF MEDICINE AND THE COLLATERAL SCIENCES.

VOLUME VI.

1879.

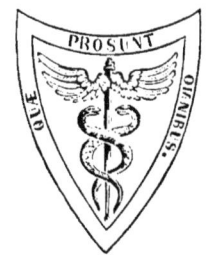

PHILADELPHIA:

HENRY C. LEA.

1879.

PHILADELPHIA:
COLLINS, PRINTER,
705 Jayne Street.

THE MONTHLY ABSTRACT

OF

MEDICAL SCIENCE.

VOL. VI. No. 1.   **For List of Contents see last page.**   JANUARY, 1879.

Anatomy and Physiology.

Case of Conjoined Twins.

In the *Lyon Médical*, Drs. COLRAT and REBATEL describe a monstrosity aged thirteen months. The monstrosity has two heads, four arms, two thoraces, one abdomen, one penis, two testicles, one anus, and two legs. Baptiste and Jacques Tocci were born on October 4, 1877, at Loccana. Their father is thirty-two years old, their mother is only twenty years old, and well developed. She was never pregnant before. As regards heredity, the maternal grandmother bore twins; beyond this there is nothing extraordinary. Neither child has any teeth at present. The skeletons are normal up to the point of union at the base of the chest. The vertebral columns are distinct throughout, each terminating in a sacrum and coccyx. The ribs appear to be complete, and act independently of each other. The children are well developed, lively, and play with full animal spirits. In suckling, their mother gives her two breasts at once. Although there is only one abdomen, it is almost certain that there are two sets of intestines. Defecation is independent for each child. If one be asleep and the other awake, the waking one can only move the leg on his side. One is sick and vomits, while the other is calm. It belongs to St. Hiliare's class Sysomian.—*London Medical Record*, Nov. 15, 1878.

The Absorption of Albumen.

A. SCHMIDT-MULHEIM asks the question, whether digested albumen necessarily passes through the thoracic duct to enter the blood? To answer it he applied ligatures to the right and left thoracic ducts, and found the animals, if well fed, preserved all the appearance of sound health, and he noticed in particular that in dogs there was no diminution in the elimination of nitrogen. He describes in detail the changes in the lymphatic system resulting from the application of the ligature, the dilatation of the lymph and chyle vessels, the infiltration of the perivascular connective tissue, the extravasations of chyle in the cavities of the abdomen and thorax, and the enlargement of the mesenteric glands. With oleaginous chyle, he found that in almost every instance there were extensive infiltrations and extravasations, of a milky fluid, though there did not appear to be, as he convinced himself by mingling colouring matters with the chyle, any rupture of bloodvessels. In opposition to Sir Astley Cooper, who noticed rupture of the thoracic duct, and the escape of its entire contents, so that it was always empty and collapsed after ligature, Schmidt-Mulheim found it invariably tightly distended, and never injured. The general result of his experiments was to show clearly that after complete obstruction of the chyle, and prevention of its entrance into the blood-circulation, the digestion, absorption, and metabolism of the albuminous compounds proceeded as usual.—*Lancet*, Nov. 16, 1878.

The Absorption of Sugar.

The path by which sugar is absorbed has been investigated by v. Meuïng. No narcotics were used, since they all, including curara, have a tendency to induce the appearance of sugar in the urine. Mering made some preliminary experiments in which he was able to substantiate neither Dr. Pavy's statement, that muscular exertion and dyspnœa increased the quantity of sugar in the blood, nor the statement of Bernard, that sugar quickly disappeared from the blood. On the other hand, he corroborates Bernard's remark, that the blood contains more sugar after repeated venesection. The sugar appears to be chiefly contained in the serum, the blood-corpuscles containing very little. The serum of blood taken from the carotid contained in eight examinations 0.115 to 0.235 per cent. Dogs were fed, after long fasting, on starch, and, after from two to six hours, killed, the stomach and small intestines ligatured and removed, and washed out with alcohol. The stomach contained unchanged starch, amidulin or soluble starch, dextrin, and erythro-dextrin. The small intestine contained sugar, and starch, but no dextrin, and small quantities of lactic acid. Examination of the amount of sugar in the chyle of flesh-fed, as compared with sugar-and-starch-fed, dogs showed no remarkable difference, so that there is no reason for thinking that sugar is taken up by the absorbents and transmitted through the thoracic duct. The examination of the venous blood led clearly to the result that the absorption of sugar is chiefly effected by the veins, the serum of the carotid and portal blood always containing a larger amount of sugar than normal.—*Lancet*, Nov. 23, 1878.

—

On the Behaviour of Glycogen after its Injection into the Circulation.

R. Böhm and F. A. Hoffmann (*Archiv. für Exper. Pathol.*, etc., Band vii. p. 489) show that blood-stained urine was voided by a cat after from 3 to 10 grammes of glycogen had been injected in the course of a few hours into the jugular vein. Glycogen is consequently one of the substances which cause a breaking up of the blood-corpuscles. The plane of polarization is rotated to the right by the urine, from which the albumen has been removed; it also reduces cupric oxide, though the reduction is five to ten times smaller than is indicated by the rotation. The substance causing the rotation can be isolated, by precipitation with a large excess (6 to 8 volumes) of alcohol, at 95 per cent. The precipitate dissolves in water without opalescence, is not coloured by iodine, and does not answer to Fehling's test; but it is entirely converted into grape-sugar by prolonged boiling with acids. The authors assume 194.3° as the average amount of rotation of the plane of polarization; whilst for an average of seven experiments with glycogen, the value was somewhat greater, 226.7°. The substance, therefore, which appears in the urine after the injection of glycogen, is achroo-dextrin, not unchanged glycogen.—*Lond. Med. Record*, Oct. 15, 1878.

—

Materia Medica and Therapeutics.

The Therapeutic Value of Iodoform.

For many years the application of iodoform or teriodide of formyl has procured in the hands of Dr. J. Moleschott, of Turin (*Giornale della Reale Accademia di Torino*), effects so beneficial, that only the desire of studying physiologically the action of this valuable substance has been capable of restraining him from publishing his clinical experience.

It was in 1870, he says, that I was first induced to try iodoform in the case of a scrofulous man, aged about 30. In 1867, I had him several times under treatment for cold abscesses in the right groin and in the back part of the hip of the same side. In September of that year he suffered from swelling of the cervical glands on both sides, those on the left forming a uniform mass larger than a large fist. I treated the patient assiduously from September, 1870, to November, 1870. Externally, I applied iodide and bromide of potassium, iodated iodide, iodide and biniodide of mercury, chloride of ammonium, belladonna, cicuta, and digitalis; internally, I gave iodide and bromide of potassium, iodized cod-liver oil, mineral waters rich in iodine (Sales water), without neglecting sea-baths. The success was very imperfect. It did not carry out the popular belief, often shared by medical men, that such tumours ought always to yield readily to the application of a simple iodine ointment. The case here referred to was one of the many obstinate ones. The advantages gained after a course of treatment diligently carried out for three years, still left much to be desired. The young man was desirous of being married; but his friends always ridiculed the proposal on account of the deformity caused by the tumour. Stimulated by the desire to free him from this, I searched through journals and books, and met with praises of iodoform; but I regret that I do not remember which author first led me to entertain hope. I prescribed one part of iodoform and fifteen of elastic collodion, to be applied by a brush night and morning. This treatment was commenced on November 20, 1870; and on December 18th the tumour was reduced to one-half of its size; on February 2, 1871, it had almost disappeared; and when I saw him on April 5th, no trace of it could be seen. The patient was then suffering from vesical catarrh, gingivitis, and a little palpitation; and in the next September he had perityphlitis. In March, 1871, when the tumour had nearly disappeared, the urine contained albumen for a short time. When he last came to consult me, in October, 1877, there had been no return of the glandular swellings, or of the cold abscess. This case did not remain singular in the circle of my practice. Two little daughters of a schoolmaster, aged respectively 8 and 10 years, had for a year and more glandular swellings in the neck, of the size of a large hen's egg. Ointment of iodide of potassium, applied in the manner above described, they were cured in a few weeks.

Of many similar cases, in all of which iodoform subdued that which had obstinately resisted iodide of potassium, I relate one which appears remarkable, since the cartilaginous hardness of the tumour had led me to doubt the efficacy of the remedy, in which I already placed much trust. A chambermaid had on the right side of her neck a tumour as large as a middle-sized hen's egg, and as hard as cartilage. She had been disfigured by it for many years; and, although it was not painful, she desired its removal. I applied iodoform in the form of ointment (1 in 15). At the end of three months a very favourable effect was produced; she assiduously followed up the treatment, and within a year the swelling had disappeared.

The last case of this kind which I saw was in a man who had in his right inguinal region a large mass of swollen glands. The tumour, which had commenced with pain, had been treated by a medical man with poultices and incisions. But, in spite of the continued suppuration, the groin remained swollen to such an extent as almost to disable the patient from the discharge of his duties. When this condition had lasted three months he asked my advice. In four weeks, iodoform ointment effected a complete cure.

This favourable experience of the efficacy of iodoform in combating swellings of the lymphatic glands, was crowned by the improvement obtained in a case of splenic leuchæmia. The subject was a lady whose spleen was doubled in size, and could be easily felt by the hand. Her blood contained one white corpuscle to fifty red, in place of the usual proportion of one to 357. The principal symptoms were prostration, pallor, obstinate diarrhœa, especially severe at the menstrual periods, and a great tendency to acute painful œdema. There was no hemorrhage, no engorgement of the lymphatic glands. On the other hand, the patient had two attacks of severe pain in the sacrum and last lumbar vertebræ, probably dependent on the participation of the marrow of the bones in the disease. The case might then be considered as one of splenic and myelogenous leuchæmia, but remarkable for its severity and long duration. When she first came under my care in January, 1870, she had for several months remained in bed. She did not tolerate quinine, nor iron, nor any other metallic remedy. On the other hand, she obtained advantage from aromatic baths of 26 to 27 Reaumur (90.5 to 92.75 Fahr.), continued for not more than three minutes, and from painting over the region of the spleen with iodoformized collodion; this treatment was commenced in the autumn of 1871. The diarrhœa required appropriate treatment from time to time. Fortunately, the patient's appetite never failed; she could digest venison and other nutritious food. The swelling of the spleen returned several times, but was always restrained by the external application of iodoform. The proportion between the two kinds of blood corpuscles has for some time become normal.

I do not by any means assert that the remedy for leuchæmia has been found in iodoform. The cure is not sufficiently complete, nor the case severe enough; and I have not had an opportunity of trying the same treatment in other cases; but the result of this first attempt seems to encourage further trial.

From the time when I verified the solvent effect of iodoform, I applied it repeatedly in the treatment of the swollen and indurated inguinal glands of syphilis. In these cases I gave protoiodide of mercury according to Simon's excellent method, or iodoform in pills, in doses varying from 5 to 10 centigrammes ($\frac{3}{4}$ to $1\frac{1}{2}$ grain) in the day; its effects were so salutary, that I can warmly recommend iodoform in the treatment of syphilis.

Judging from the related facts, iodoform, before promoting absorption, should determine the destruction of the primitive elements. This may be said to be its *modus operandi* in orchitis, in which I have several times obtained resolution in a period varying from five to eight days, by the application of iodoformized collodion.

In cases of effusion into serous cavities, iodoform has surpassed my expectation. By painting with iodoform dissolved in elastic collodion, I have seen fluid dispersed which had collected in the pleura, pericardium, and peritoneum, and beneath the arachnoid.

In the case of a lady, wife of a well-known officer, who suffered from insufficiency of the tricuspid valve, I twice obtained absorption of a dangerous pericardial effusion.

At Nervi, some years ago, a gentleman, aged 45, the subject of pulmonary tuberculosis, had ascites to such an extent that he could only remain in a semi-recumbent position on his back, and could not bend his body. I thought that paracentesis would be required, in spite of the anæmic state of the patient. I determined, however, to try iodoformized collodion, giving at the same time diuretic pills. The collection of fluid disappeared in about fifteen days, with an abundant discharge of urine; and it did not return during the remaining year and a half of the patient's life. From that time, I have made it a rule not to advise paracentesis, without having first tried the external application of iodoform. I confess that it is not always efficacious. We cannot be surprised at this, since in many cases we cannot eliminate the cause of the exudation of the fluid, we cannot prevent it from again collecting, and the obstacle to the circulation may be so great that no treatment succeeds in stimulating absorption.

Of all the satisfactory results which I have obtained from the application of iodoform, the greatest has been in the acute hydrocephalus of children. In recent years, I have reported three complete cures among five cases of this fatal disease, two of which appeared to be in a truly desperate condition. The fixed look, the lost senses, the sopor, the convulsions, the sunken abdomen, the vomiting, the unfrequent pulse, the dilated and unequal pupils, the tonic contraction of the cervical muscles, completed a picture which could be easily recognized. I ordered iodoform, dissolved in collodion, or in the form of ointment, to be applied three or four times daily to the cervical region, and over the mastoid processes, the forehead, and the temples. I must not omit to state that the children at the same time had small doses of calomel, and purgative clysters.

I will here mention a case of prepatellar cystic hygroma. The subject was a valet in a large house, who, having to keep polished the furniture in the rooms, was obliged often to kneel on his right knee. With paintings of iodoformized collodion, the swelling of the bursa in front of the patella was reduced in fifteen days, although it had already existed as many months.

In chronic arthritis, also, I have had much reason to praise iodoform. Two cases are particularly memorable. One was that of a little girl nine years old, daughter of a teacher of swimming, who, in April, 1875, when I undertook to treat her, had been suffering for nine months with inflammation of the left knee. The suppuration was very diffuse, and the child suffered severe pain and was much weakened. The use of iodoform dissolved in collodion, of iodide of iron in the form of Blancard's pills, and absolute rest, so far restored her that in May, 1876, only a slight stiffness of the joint remained.

The other case was one of fungous inflammation of the articulations of the left foot in a boy aged 15. He had been confined to bed many months, and his parents had no further hope. Two very skilful surgeons had declared that there was no resource but amputation; but, his parents not consenting, the patient was removed from the hospital. The left tarsus was about twice as large as the right, and was surrounded by eight or nine suppurating and fungating sores; in more than one spot, the suppuration reached the bone. There was no pain. I had iodoformized collodion applied twice daily to all parts of the foot where the skin remained sound, and the ulcers were first treated with chamomile baths, and afterwards with solutions of nitrate of silver (2 to 10 per cent.); iodide of iron was given internally. At the end of a year, the boy could walk, the sores were all healed, the tarsus was scarcely swollen, and all movements were possible, though less free than in the other foot. He had no return of the disease, although he committed several imprudent acts. At present he is able to work; and his parents who had resigned themselves to seeing him perish, rejoice in the possession of a robust lad.

From all that has been said above, iodoform appears to be a remedy which has a powerful resolvent action, and causes the absorption of formative elements and of collections of exuded fluid. But to these effects it unites the valuable property of assuaging pain. This may be proved in attacks of gout. I have often succeeded in removing or in considerably relieving the most severe pain and other inflammatory symptoms of gout, within twenty-four hours, by painting the parts with iodoformized collodion.

Less certain is the success of iodoform in chronic rheumatism affecting several joints, and I have found it quite unreliable as a remedy against the pain of acute articular rheumatism.

As a sedative remedy, I have used iodoform in a large number of cases of neuralgia, mostly intercostal, cardiac, sciatic, and articular. I have most frequently applied it dissolved in collodion, but have also used it in the form of ointment.

In one case, intercostal neuralgia was accompanied with syphilitic myocarditis, without disease of the valves. The patient, a merchant at Alba, was affected on the slightest movement, even a short walk, with giddiness and spasmodic pain in the region of the heart. He was cured by the internal and external use of iodoform; but he had to continue the treatment with short interruptions for several months. He toook internally from 5 to 10 centigrammes in twenty-four hours, in the form of pill.

Patients very often present themselves, complaining of intercostal pain in the region of the heart, radiating towards the left clavicle. Such persons not unfrequently feel palpitation, and fear that they have disease of the heart, although they are quite free from it. These patients are comforted if an opportune treatment free them from their pains; and the external application of iodoform fulfils this object admirably. Along with the pains, the unfounded dread of cardiac disease at once disappears.

Although desirous to avoid making a complete enumeration of the services which iodoform has rendered me, I must make brief mention of a case in which I cured a true neuritis following typhoid fever in a young man, and affecting the trunk of the left sciatic nerve. When the patient sought my help, in the autumn of 1870, his sufferings had already lasted several days. The slightest pressure on the nerve caused intolerable pain; and the patient, who in other respects might be called convalescent, was obliged to remain motionless in bed. The pain was very soon relieved by iodoform; but the leg remained so weak, that for several weeks the patient walked on crutches: and he did not recover perfectly until after a prolonged stay at Nervi.

A remedy which combines in itself antiphlogistic, resolvent, and sedative properties; which embraces a field of action extending from neuritis to neuralgia, from leuchæmia to tuberculous meningitis, from lymphoma to collections in serous bursæ, from attacks of gout to hygroma; a remedy which in the multiplicity and energy of its action competes with quinine and with cold water, might be regarded as miraculous, if it had not its defects like every other good thing. Fortunately, however, these defects will not be very detrimental to the services which it is capable of rendering to suffering humanity.

The most important defect in iodoform is its penetrating odour, which is much more perceptible when it is used with collodion than when applied in the form of ointment. Its internal use is sometimes followed by disagreeable eructations. It cannot indeed be said that the odour is repulsive; it is rather oppressive. In the collodion solution, it reminds me of a photographer's laboratory. In order to overcome the objections arising from this odour, the following rules should be followed.

The box of iodoform ointment, or the bottle of iodoformized collodion, should be kept at a distance from the window, in a well-closed tin case; this retards the decomposition of the iodoform, which goes on rapidly in the light. The surface to which it is applied should be covered by a layer of thin gutta percha. Finally, unless its action be urgently required, the application should be made only in the evening; preference being given to the ointment, which in the morning can be easily washed off with a little soap and water, so as to leave no smell.

Another defect of iodoform is, that it sometimes causes palpitation. I have as yet not often observed this; but it repeatedly occurred in a hysterical lady for whom I prescribed iodoform internally as a remedy for hemicrania. This defect, however, causes me to recognize a conspicuous advantage, which I desire to see confirmed by later experience.

Some months ago, I had under my care a lady, wife of a professor of literature, suffering from mitral insufficiency without compensating hypertrophy of the left ventricle. Irregularity of the heart-beat was the most troublesome symptom of the exhaustion of the cardiac muscle in its attempts to overcome the obstacle. She had *malaise*, diminution of urine, nervous attacks, oppression, and dyspnœa. The radial pulse was often scarcely perceptible. Very small doses of digitalis (30 or 40 centigrammes in infusion, in twenty-four hours) several times produced a sensible improvement; but the stomach did not bear it well, and it therefore became necessary to suspend the use of the remedy before a satisfactory advantage had been obtained. Remembering the experience referred to above, I had recourse to iodoform, which I prescribed in doses of 6 or 7 centigrammes (about 0.9 to 1 grain daily) in the form of pills. The patient had scarcely taken it two days, when I found the heart's action regular and the radial pulse well developed. The heart, which seemed to have given up all rhythm, had regained a regular beat. The same success was repeated several times in this patient, at intervals of various length.

This and similar observations justify us in asking whether iodoform, administered internally in daily doses of 5 to 10 centigrammes, may not compete with digitalis—I mean those small doses of digitalis which render the action of the heart stronger and more regular.

Iodine is found in the urine after the external and the internal use of iodoform, but rather more slowly after the former than after the latter. In either case, the complete elimination of the medicine requires much time, so that traces of iodine may be found in the urine at the end of four or five days.

Allied in constitution to chloroform, iodoform is in many cases a valuable narcotic; but to the quality of relieving pain it adds in a high degree the effects of a powerful preparation of iodine. Neither iodide of potassium nor pure iodine can be compared with iodoform, when we consider its efficacy as a promoter of resolution and absorption of tumours and exudations. It seems probable that the surprising effects of iodoform are to be attributed to the facility with which iodine is liberated from it, so as to act in a nascent state on the elements of the organism.

Notwithstanding the inconveniences which I have not wished to conceal, I dare promise for this remedy a great future.—*London Med. Record*, Nov. 15, 1878.

—

The Action of Salts of Lime.

The therapeutical use of lime-salts in the treatment of disease other than that of the intestinal canal, is supported more upon observation in disease than on pharmacological experiment. Few attempts have been made to ascertain what evidence is to be obtained of their absorption into the blood, on which, of course, their general effect must depend. It is a question of much interest, since it is hardly necessary to mention that most of the compounds of lime are among the least soluble of substances which are given internally. Such observations are of more interest since it is probable that the power of absorbing lime-salts varies very much in the different classes of animals. Buchheim-Körber, for instance, gave dogs and rabbits, which were fed on bread and milk diet, a considerable excess of earthy phosphates—to the dogs in the form of bones, to the rabbits as the pure salts. He found that in the case of the rabbits a large excess of these salts was absorbed, and was excreted with the urine, while in the case of the dogs the whole excess of the earthy salts passed away with the feces, and that even less was absorbed into the blood than under normal conditions. The weight of these observations is, however, lessened by the fact that the form given to the two sets of animals was not precisely the same.

Neubauer found that in the case of man the excretion of lime by the urine could be distinctly increased by its administration by the mouth. He gave to each of four young men a gramme of some lime-salts every night at bedtime, having previously determined the average daily excretion of lime in each case. In the first subject the normal excretion of lime, .303 grm., was raised to .397 grm. by chloride of calcium. In the second the normal, .267 grm., was raised to .310 grm. by carbonate of lime. In the third the normal, .282 grm., was raised to .324 grm. by acetate of lime. And in the fourth the normal, .387 grm., was raised to .489 grm. by phosphate of lime. Thus the urine contained in the case of carbonate and acetate of lime about one-twentieth of the quantity ingested, and in the case of chloride and phosphate of lime it contained about a tenth.

Riessell found that when carbonate of lime is given internally it appears in the urine as phosphate, showing that a change of acid occurs in the alimentary canals or in the blood. The carbonic acid is probably liberated in the stomach, but the portion of the lime which is not absorbed again combines with carbonic acid in the intestinal tract, passing away as carbonate. The transformation into a phosphate led to the expectation that the excretion of phosphoric acid might be increased by the ingestion of lime-salts. Riessell accordingly administered to a man ten grammes of chalk three times a day. He found at first a large increase in the amount of phosphoric acid excreted, but the excess soon lessened, and the amount fell to the normal. The natural relation between the alkaline and earthy phosphates was reversed. The alkaline salts became much smaller in quantity, while the earthy salts increased. The conclusion was reached, and corroborated by further observations, that phosphate of lime is formed in the alimentary canal, and is absorbed with difficulty on account of its low solubility, most passing away by the feces, that the constant presence of considerable quantities of the phosphate gradually overcomes the resistance to absorption, and that a corresponding increase occurs in the amount of lime absorbed and excreted. These observations were in part corroborated by Soborow, although Zalesky failed in the case of young pigeons to find any increase in the earthy constituents of the bones on the addition of a larger quantity of lime-salt to their diet.

The latest investigations on the subject have been carried out in Salkowski's laboratory by Dr. Leopold Peil, who has published his conclusions in Virchow's *Archiv.* He employed especially chloride of calcium, and found, in the dogs to which it was given, an undoubted increase in the excretion of lime by the urine, although this corresponded to only a small fraction of the amount of lime administered. It was difficult to ascertain what that fraction was, since the amount of lime-salts in the food varies, and so also does that which is set free in the organism in the process of tissue regeneration. An estimation of the amount of urea excreted suggests that a larger destruction of albumen occurred before the lime was given than during its administration, and this probably entailed the liberation of a larger amount of lime. During five days before the addition to the food a total of .153 grm. of lime was excreted; in the five following days, .325 grm.; and thus at least .190 grm. was apparently due to the calcareous diet; 7.12 grms. of calcium chloride was given, of which only 5.2 per cent. passed away in the urine. The amount of chlorine excreted was very remarkably increased by the diet, altogether 6.14 grms. passing away. The amount of calcium chloride taken corresponded, however, to only 4.6 grms., and thus all the excess of chlorine was eliminated, and in addition nearly half as much more. Another experiment, with the same dog, demonstrated that the quantity of chalk which, according to the first experiment, was not excreted could actually be found in the feces. It thus appears that the chlorine and the lime have different destinations. The probable explanation of this is that the calcium chloride is decomposed by the alkaline secretions of the intestine, especially the bile and the pancreatic juice, carbonate of lime and chloride of sodium being formed, the former being eliminated by the feces, the latter absorbed. But the whole of the chlorine of the urine is not in combination with sodium; a little of it is perhaps free as hydric chloride, but more is combined with ammonium. The probable explanation of this lies in the observation of Gaethens that if acids are administered to dogs there is no increased excretion of bases, or only a slightly greater excretion than normal. No doubt most of the acid is neutralized in the intestine, and the alkaline carbonates which normally return as such into the blood, are decomposed, and the blood receives only neutral salts. If, in the system of a carnivorous animal, a considerable portion of free alkali is neutralized in one place, there is corresponding deficiency at another place—*i. e.*, more acid is eliminated by the urine. Walter has shown that these acids are for the most part combined with ammonia, which is formed in the carnivora in increased quantity when acids are given. Calcium chloride appears to act exactly, or almost, as an acid; it takes up in the intestine a certain quantity of alkali, which would otherwise have returned into the blood, and a corresponding amount of free hydrochloric acid, or more probably of ammonium chloride, must appear in the urine.— *Lancet*, Oct. 12, 1878.

On the Muriate of Pilocarpine.

Herr A. FRANKEL communicates (*Charité Annalen*, Band iii., 1878) the results of his experiments on dogs, made for the purpose of ascertaining the physiological and therapeutical action of the muriate of pilocarpine. Injection into the jugular vein of small doses (4 centigrammes = 0.6 grain) gave insignificant results. In increasing the dose, there resulted a considerable diminution in the frequency of the pulse, persisting after division of both vagi, disappearing after the injection of morphia, and not recurring after renewed injection of pilocarpine. The author supposes that pilocarpine acts on the peripheral ends of the vagi, exciting the cardiac inhibitory nerves; it is antagonistic to atropia. He further relates three cases of nephritis and one of bronchial catarrh with much swelling, in which the œdema disappeared entirely after pilocarpine had been injected subcutaneously for some time.—*Lond. Med. Record*, Nov. 15, 1878.

Medicine.

The Pathological Excretion of Carbolic Acid.

It has been shown by Städeler that phenol, or carbolic acid, is a constant constituent of the urine, and in 1876 Salkowski described four cases of disease, two of them diffuse peritonitis, in which the amount of phenol was abnormally increased. Quite recently, Dr. Brieger of Berne has carefully examined the subject in Herr Nencki's laboratory at Berne, especially with a view to determine what relation there is between the decomposition of albuminous substances in the bowel and the amount of phenol excreted—as Baumann has proved that this body is a product of the putrefaction of albumen, and Brieger that it is a normal constituent of the contents of the bowel. The account of Brieger's researches, and of others bearing on the same subject by Drs. Odermatt and Schaller, with a controversial communication from Professor Salkowski, will be found in the *Centralblatt f. d. Med. Wiss.*, Nos. 30, 31, 34, 1878, from which the following particulars are taken: The carbolic acid in the urine is estimated by distilling the latter with dilute sulphuric acid, and precipitating the phenol as tribromphenol. In healthy persons on ordinary diet the daily excretion of phenol is about 0.0158 gramme. In gastric cancer it rose in two cases to a mean of 0.025 to 0.061. In three cases of phthisis the excretion was quite normal, and in only one of three cases of typhoid fever was there a trifling increase. In a case of English cholera the mean was 0.052. In peritonitis, as Salkowski had previously stated, the quantity excreted rises enormously, e. g., to 0.3018 gramme in one case, and to 0.138 in two others. It is extremely interesting to notice that *in septic conditions the largest excretion of phenol occurs*. Thus, in a case of gangrenous empyema with pleural fistula, Dr. Brierger obtained 0.3112 gramme from the urine on the second day after the patient's admission to the hospital. On the third day, when the previous fever had subsided and the pus had been rendered inodorous by injections of iodine, 0.6309; on the fifth day 0.0226, and on the ninth 0.1098 gramme in twenty-four hours. As Dr. Brierger expresses it: "It is extremely remarkable that the same body which we use as our most powerful antiseptic should itself be developed in the largest quantity within the animal organism during septic conditions, and we may expect that determinations of the amount of phenol excreted in septic diseases will help to make their *rationale* more intelligible." We have already in previous articles (*Medical Times and Gazette*, September 22, 1877, and December 29, 1877) dealt with the subject of the excretion of indican in the urine in various diseases; and as it is probable that indican is derived from indol, a product of the decomposition of albuminous substances in the bowel, it is important to know whether the excretion of indican and phenol run parallel to one another. Brieger finds that they do in some diseases, but not in others. Thus in peritonitis the excretion of both is abnormally large, while in anæmia and in certain cachectic states the phenol secretion is subnormal, while that of indican is increased. Some light may eventually be thrown on the relation between the excretion of these two bodies by the experiments of Brieger and Odermatt with various decomposing albuminous substances. They found that at a temperature of 40° Cent., and with free access of air, the quantity of indol, from which, as just stated, indican is derived, increases in the early stages of putrefaction, and gradually diminishes as putrefaction proceeds; while the quantity of phenol produced is inappreciable during the first few days of the process, and then steadily increases until the whole of the albumen has been decomposed. Another point which throws some light on the relations of phenol to the organism is that which has been brought out by Professor Salkowski and Dr. Schaffer, namely, that if dogs have phenol mixed with their food, rather less than half of it fails to appear in the urine: while, on the other hand, Dr. Schaffer finds that the lost phenol does not escape from the body in the feces. Professor Salkowski has suggested that indol and phenol, which with skatol (a homologue of indol) have been proved by Brieger to be normal constituents of the feces, are not exclusively found in the intestine, but also to some extent in the tissues of the body; but Herr Nencki has never been able to extract either indol or phenol from fresh muscles or glands by distilling their watery extracts. Hoppe-Seyler has also failed to find carbolic acid in the blood, or in any of the liquids of the body. Still, Brieger has obtained an abundance of tribromphenol by distilling putrid pus with dilute sulphuric acid ; and he concludes that in septic conditions the production of phenol is not confined to the intestine. Hence at present it is impossible to say for certain whether the excess of phenol in the urine of disease is due to its increased production somewhere in the body, or, as Salkowski believes, to a failure of the tissues to *destroy* it in its passage through them from its place of origin to the kidneys. Anyhow, the solution of the problem is of great interest to physician and physiologist.—*Med. Times and Gaz.*, Oct. 12, 1878.

A Case of Neurosis Due to Fright (Schreck-Neurose).

This paper, by Dr. V. HOLST, occurs in the *St. Petersburger Medicinische Wochenschrift*, of the 12th (24th) August, 1878.

While other departments of pathology have been, during the last decade, built upon physiological and anatomical substrata which have served as the bases of systematic classification, in the department of neuro-pathology, including psychiatry, this is not yet possible, or at any rate, only very partially so. Our knowledge of many diseases of the nervous system is, as yet, purely clinical ; among these last, many present well-defined and recognized groups of symptoms, and have, therefore, received clinical names ; but, besides these, there are a number of cases which occur in the most varied form and guise, so that they cannot be grouped under any recognized name ; it is for these that the name neurosis is most useful. By neurosis is meant a nerve-affection, unexplained by pathological anatomy and not capable of being classed under the name of any recognized disease. A neurosis may be more definitely described by speaking of it in relation, either with the anatomical structures most influenced by it (*e. g.*, vaso-motor neurosis), or with the cause to which it is due (*e. g.*, emotion-neurosis, fright-neurosis). The above observations justify the title given to the paper.

It is universally admitted, that powerful psychic emotions, especially fright, are frequently the cause of the most various nervous disturbances. An interesting series of such cases which occurred during the seige of Strasburg, is given by Dr. Kohts, in the *Berliner Klinische Wochenschrift*, 1873. All the cases there described were capable of being classed with recognized diseases of the brain or spinal cord, as were also the cases of "emotion-neurosis," described by Berger in the *Deutsche für Pract. Med.*, 1877, Nos. 38 and 39. The case now to be described cannot be given any clinical name ; it can only be called a neurosis ; noteworthy points in it are its rapid course and evident cure by a fresh psychic impression.

A labourer, aged 60, stated that he had always enjoyed good health, but was always very susceptible of fright; he had frequently suffered from rigors as a result of sudden fright ; but these quickly passed off under the influence of a little diffusible stimulant. Once he had an attack of erysipelas in the leg, which he also ascribed to fright. He had never been intemperate in his habits. One day last March he was greatly frightened by one of his children letting fall a toy from the table, and at the same time shrieking loudly. He at once suffered from an attack such as will shortly be described. The attacks were repeated, with very short intervals, until he was admitted to hospital two days later. Dr. Holst found him walking about in the ward, and had hardly begun to converse with him as to his complaint, when the patient was suddenly stopped in his speech by a fearful grimace ; his mouth was widely opened, the eyes became staring, and he uttered a hollow groan. His arms were spread out, and he seized hold of some neighbouring object. On one occasion this was the physician's leg. The patient

then stood firmly for a time with somewhat bent knees, and was evidently unconscious. In one or two minutes the groan changed into loud weeping; then, quite
suddenly, the patient's expression became normal, he looked about him with an
astonished air, passed his hand several times over his eyes, and said, "Now I
am all right again." He was again quite conscious, and answered questions intelligently, but could only describe his attack by saying that something came
over him, and that he became unconscious. During half an hour's observation,
attacks continued to occur at intervals of from three to five minutes. The individual attacks varied somewhat in form, in that the distortion of the countenance
was not always the same; sometimes the patient uttered no sound, and occasionally the attack commenced with an unnatural laugh. The end of the attack was
sometimes characterized by quite a remarkable look of utter astonishment; at
other times it came on more gradually, the weeping passing into a loud-spoken
prayer, with devoutly uplifted arms, during which consciousness had evidently
returned. After Dr. Holst had observed a number of these paroxysms, the idea
occurred to him to try what would be the effect of a new psychic impression upon
his condition. In the middle of an attack, the doctor suddenly ran to his patient,
shaking him violently by the arm, and shouting loudly to him, "What has come
to you? How dare you misbehave yourself in this way?" He instantly became
conscious, looked at the doctor in astonishment, and respectfully asked if he had
given any offence. After a short time, another very slight attack occurred; the
same procedure was adopted; and the patient, rubbing his eyes, asked what had
happened to him. He was then left, no other treatment being ordered. Next
day, he was reported to have had no return of the paroxysm. When the doctor
entered the ward, the patient at once came and thanked him heartily for having
freed him from his trouble. On being asked what had occurred the previous day,
he said he only knew that the doctor had come into the ward and frightened him
very much, and that this had cured him of his dreaded fits. He also stated that
he had felt several slight paroxysms since the previous day; they consisted, however, only in a slight trembling, which, being fully conscious, he was able to overcome without their being noticed by the persons around him. On the next (third)
day, as no further symptoms had been presented, he was discharged cured.—
London Med. Record, Nov. 15, 1878.

Ulceration of the Frœnum Linguœ in Whooping-cough.

At a recent session the Académie de Medecine received a report upon the
importance of ulceration of the frœnum linguæ as a diagnostic sign in pertussis,
by a committee consisting of MM. Roger, Gueneau de Mussy, and Moutard-
Martin, to whom a paper by M. Delthil "On the Diphtheroid Ulceration of
Whooping-cough: its value, frequency, and relations to the disease," was referred. That author, like many others, considered the ulceration in question to
be an initial sign of the disease, preceding the onset of cough, and forming a part
of the affection as marked as the eruption in an exanthematous fever. Others,
and they are the majority, see in it only the result of mechanical injury to the
frœnum by the lower incisors when the tongue is protruded in the paroxysm of
coughing. The committee reported as follows: That the sublingual ulceration
occurs in whooping-cough, and its presence is an almost certain sign that the
attack is a severe one. It is purely traumatic in origin, requiring for its formation
the propulsion of the tongue, and the repeated friction of the frœnum against the
incisor teeth in violent paroxysms of coughing. This is proved by its occurrence
only during the height of the disease, when the convulsive attacks are most
violent, cicatrization taking place as soon as the cough moderates. Further, it
has the character of an incision or laceration, whilst its nearly constant seat on

the frænum, which is most liable to be wounded by the teeth, goes to prove the same fact; varieties in its situation depending upon the number, form, and disposition of the teeth. The most positive proof of all in favour of the traumatic view is the absence of the ulcer (even in children well furnished with sharp teeth) in mild cases of whooping-cough, where the paroxysm does not lead to protrusion of the tongue, and its absence also in infants before dentition or in children who have just shed their first set. The report then shows the fallacy of the "specific" view, and proves that it is not "diphtheroid" at all in its nature, and concludes by stating that ulceration of the frænum has no pathological significance, since it is only a local complication and an accident of the disease ; but as " it is not met with in any other affection it becomes in certain cases a symptom of value—a certain sign of whooping-cough, and usually of a severe attack ; it thus acquires great semeiotic value." The only question that occurs is whether it required so learned a commission to gives us this assurance. The "value" of the symptom is minimised by its occurrence only, or mostly, in well-marked and severe cases. —*Lancet*, Nov. 16, 1878.

Experiments on the Contagion of Phthisis.

The remarkable instances now and then seen, in which persons without hereditary tendency to phthisis become phthisical after long-continued attendance on sufferers from the disease, have suggested to many physicians the idea that phthisis is contagious. If there is such a contagion, the mechanism has been supposed to be the inhalation with the breath of fine particles of tuberculous sputa, atomized into the air by the patient's cough. An attempt has been made by Dr. TAP-PEINER, of Meran, to ascertain whether by a similar means animals could be rendered tubercular, and the results of the experiments, which are published in the current number of Virchow's *Archiv*, are of great interest. The animals experimented on were made to breathe for several hours daily in a chamber in the air of which fine particles of phthisical sputum were suspended. The sputum having been mixed with water, the mixture was atomized by a steam atomizer. In all cases the sputa were from persons with cavities in their lungs. Dogs alone were employed in the experiments, since they very rarely suffer from spontaneous tuberculosis. The result was that of eleven animals experimented on, with one doubtful exception, after a period varying from twenty-five to forty-five days, all, being killed, presented well-developed miliary tubercles in both lungs ; and in most of the cases tubercles were present to a smaller extent in the kidneys, and in some cases also in the liver and spleen. Microscopical examination was in accord with the naked-eye appearances.

The quantity of sputum necessary for the effect is certainly a very small one. In three experiments only one gramme of sputum was daily atomized in the air of the chamber, and the quantity of dry sputum must have been exceedingly small. Two ways are conceivable in which the infection is produced. The particles certainly may reach the alveoli, for powdered cinnabar administered in the same way was found to have stained the alveoli in twelve hours after an inhalation of only one hour's duration. But some particles may lodge in the mucous membrane of the throat and pharynx, and thence, being absorbed, may affect the lungs as organs specially predisposed. Hence some comparative experiments were made by feeding dogs with the same sputum as that employed in the inhalation experiments. Fifteen grammes were mixed daily with the food of each dog. In two dogs fed at Munich miliary tubercles were found in the lungs after six weeks' feeding : in six others fed at Meran all the organs were normal—a difference the explanation of which is not very clear. In the cases in which the disease was produced by feeding, the intestinal tract was affected, whereas it was free in those cases in which the inhalation was employed. It is remarkable that, with two exceptions, the animals, up to the time at which they were killed and found diseased, were well and lively, and indicated their disease neither by emaciation nor other external symptoms. This suggests that sometimes in man a miliary tuberculosis of the lungs may remain latent, and cause no symptoms until catarrh, with foci of inflammation, sets up phthisis.

A preliminary account of these experiments of Tappeiner led Dr. Max Schottellus to make some similar experiments, not only with the sputum of phthisical individuals, but also with that of persons suffering from simple bronchitis, and with pulverized cheese, brain, and cinnabar. The result was that miliary tubercles were found in the lungs in all cases, and in equal quantity with both phthisical and bronchitic sputum. Cheese produced a smaller quantity; pulverized brain still less; and the cinnabar least effect of all, merely a few whitish tubercles with pigmented centres, with an interstitial deposit of the substance, which had caused no inflammatory reaction. Tappeiner has also experimented with calves' brains in two cases, but with purely negative results. No changes in the lung followed such as resulted from the inhalation of tuberculous sputum.

These experiments are of much interest, but they need repetition on a larger scale, in order that the discrepancies may be removed, before much weight can be attached to them as evidences of a specific influence of the phthisical sputum. They unquestionably show, however, that the inhalation of foreign organic matter will cause tubercles in animals naturally indisposed to their development. The appearance of granulations in other organs than the lungs in some of Tappeiner's experiments is a fact of great importance. Whether tuberculous matter produces tubercle when given in this manner more readily than other substances or not, it appears certain that different forms of organic matter produce effects in different degree. It appears also that the inhalation of these substances is more effective than their administration by the alimentary canal. These are facts of great importance in regard to the question of the contagiousness of phthisis.—*Lancet*, Nov. 23, 1878.

Experimental Pathology of Valvular Disease of the Heart.

The symptoms and effects of valvular disease of the heart may seem to be almost beyond the reach of experimental pathology; but it is not so, and a series of investigations undertaken by Dr. OTTOMER ROSENBACH in the Pathological Institute at Breslau, and detailed in a recent number of the *Archiv. für Experim. Pathologie*, possess considerable interest to cardiac pathologists. They indicate some new facts, and confirm in a striking manner the conclusions reached by clinical observers. The points for investigation were: (1) What influence on the blood-pressure has the destruction of one or of several valves? (2) Does compensation occur immediately, or only after a certain time? How is it produced, and how far is the supplemental power of the heart effective? (3) When, and under what circumstances, is endocarditis produced, and what are the consequences thereof? (4) What conclusions of clinical interest are suggested by the experiments?

The observations were made on dogs and rabbits, both with the assistance of curara and morphia, and (in rabbits) without. The blood-pressure was measured in the crural or carotid artery. The aortic valves were injured by means of a sound introduced into the right carotid artery, the injury to the valves being immediately manifest by the effect on the sounds of the heart and upon the pulse. The mitral and tricuspid valves were damaged by means of the valvulotome of Klebs, by which the mitral valve can be divided by the introduction of the in-

strument through the carotid artery into the left ventricle, and the tricuspid valve
by its introduction through the jugular vein.

The significance of the first point investigated—the effect of the valvular lesion
upon the blood-pressure—is very important. The same forward movement of the
blood will require an increased exertion of the muscular tissue of the heart, if a
resistance is interposed, as in stenosis, or an increased mass of blood has to be
moved, as in regurgitation through the aortic orifice. If this increased power is
brought into operation gradually, in consequence of an increase in the muscular
tissue—hypertrophy, etc.—the damage to the valve will be followed immediately
by a greater or slighter fall in the arterial pressure. The answer which experiment gives to the question is that there is no such fall. Before and after the
operation the blood-pressure is precisely the same. Moreover, immediately after
great valvular damage, the blood-pressure may be a little higher than before the
operation, probably in consequence of the mechanical irritation of the muscular
tissue of the heart-unisole, or of a reflex stimulation through the vaso-motor
nerves. When this immediate disturbing effect has passed away the pressure is
found to be just the same. The permanent over-action of the heart necessary to
maintain the blood-pressure leads to its hypertrophy. The reserve of force which
the heart possesses enables it to maintain its due action from the first. This effect
is the same whether the valvular change is one by which obstruction or incompetence is produced. It is evident, therefore, that the latent reserve of cardiac
force is a very large one, and the reserve is manifestly of paramount importance
for the maintenance of the circulation. Several of ROSENBACH'S experiments
show that this reserve maintains the pressure, even in the face of grave valvular
damage, for many weeks—until, indeed, hypertrophy is developed. The details
of the experiments prove that in all cases the first structural change was dilatation, and that the hypertrophy was secondary in time to the dilatation, but never
sufficient to effect a perfect structural compensation, although dynamically the
compensation was complete. Another point of interest is that there was very
constantly developed an aneurismal dilatation of the apex of the heart, and also
a fibrous degeneration of the mitral papillary muscle.

With respect to the production of endocarditis, the results may be classed under
three heads. In the first group are a series of cases in which, in spite of destruction of a valve, or tearing the chordæ tendineæ, no inflammatory appearances,
or, strictly speaking, no deposits of fibrin, were found in the neighbourhood of
the injury. This was the case with a few of the dogs and with all the rabbits
experimented on. In a second group are those cases in which more or less abundant vegetations of fibrin were found at the seats of damage, but in which the most
careful examination revealed no foreign organisms in the deposit. All the cases,
with the exception of two, come into this group. The valves beneath the fibrinous deposit presented indications of moderate inflammation and cellular multiplication. Lastly, there are two remarkable cases in which not only the deposits
on the injured valves contained micrococci, but also areas in other organs infarcted
by emboli. The post-mortem appearance was exactly that of ulcerative endocarditis, with the usual consequences—hemorrhages in all organs with more or
less abundant bacteria in the spleen, kidneys, pleura, intestine, bladder, and retina.
These different results ROSENBACH explains as follows: If clean instruments are
employed, and used in the shortest possible time, no inflammatory reaction follows. If clean instruments are used, but the operation done slowly, the soft
parts bruised, and the endothelium a good deal damaged, inflammation follows,
with an abundant deposit of fibrin. The source of the organisms in the micrococcal endocarditis is obscure.

The lesions of the valves thus produced artificially gave rise, in some cases, to

the characteristic murmurs, and in others to none at all. The narrowing of an
orifice produced by placing an instrument within it caused no murmur in any case
—a very remarkable result which the experimenter cannot explain, but which,
we think, finds a ready explanation when the mechanism of murmurs is carefully
considered. In all cases in which the edge of one of the cuspid valves was torn,
and in most in which a tendinous cord was divided, a very distinct systolic murmur was produced. These fibrinous deposits on the valves seemed to have little
influence on the production of a murmur. The difference in this respect between
clinical and experimental observation is, no doubt, to be found in the different
state of the valves which underlies the vegetations in the two cases. The aortic
valves seem susceptible in some cases of considerable damage without the generation of a murmur, although in others a diastolic murmur was heard immediately
after the injury. This difference was in part explained by post-mortem demonstration of the fact that the vegetations were capable to a considerable extent of
preventing incompetence. The loudest murmur was heard in a case in which
there was no deposit. The systolic apex murmur, which is so common in aortic
regurgitation, and in this country is commonly ascribed to mitral inefficiency, was
noted by Rosenbach in several cases in which the aortic valves had been injured,
but he is inclined, on both experimental and clinical grounds, to associate it with
the fibrous degeneration of the papillary muscles, which he finds so frequent a
consequence of aortic disease. This degeneration is supposed, however, to produce the murmur, not, as most think, by permitting regurgitation, but by lessening the tension of the valves, diminished tension of these valves, according to an
unproven theory of Traube, causing a murmur instead of a sound.

These experiments afford thus an interesting confirmation of the results of
clinical experience. They confirm experimentally modern views of the origin of
hypertrophy, and the sequence of hypertrophy and dilatation, as stated in recent
treatises, and they illustrate several very important facts regarding the origin and
symptoms of certain forms of endocarditis.—*Lancet*, Nov. 2, 1878.

Concentric Hypertrophy of the Heart.

J. DÉJÉRINE, in a communication to the Société Anatomique (*ProgrèsMédi-
cal*, August 3), reports a case of idiopathic concentric hypertrophy of the heart
in a lad aged eighteen, whose work obliged him to carry heavy loads. He had
never had rheumatism, and there was no history of alcoholism or syphilis. He
died of ascending myelitis. There was no abnormality of the heart to be observed
during life, except a little exaggeration of the impulse. At the necropsy the
heart was found of normal size, but the "left ventricle was much larger and
harder than natural; and on section its walls were more than three centimetres
(an inch) thick, and the cavity only represented by a narrow slit, scarcely admitting the point of the index finger." There was no interstitial nephritis.—*London
Med. Record*, Oct. 15, 1878.

Pulsus Bigeminans and Alternans.

E. RIEGEL, in the *Deutsches Archiv für Klinische Medicin*, Band. xx, has
observed fifty-nine cases of pulsus bigeminans and alternans in the course of a
single year. He, therefore, argues that they are not of unfrequent occurrence.
The cases were mostly old people, with atheromatous arteries; but these conditions have been met with under all circumstances, in anæmia, cachexia, heart
disease, cerebral diseases, and in febrile attacks. The pulsus bigeminans and
alternans is frequently varied with an entirely irregular, and sometimes with a
perfectly normal pulse. The variation, therefore, is simply an irregularity which

makes its appearance when there arises a want of adjustment between the power of the heart-beat and the work to be done; consequently such variation does not possess the unfavourable prognostic importance which Traube has assigned to it.—*London Med. Record*, Oct. 15, 1878.

Relation between Cardiac Hypertrophy and Renal Disease.

Dr. SENATOR, of Berlin (Virchow's *Archiv*, Band lxxiii., Heft 3), discusses this question at some length. He considers that where no obvious mechanical cause of cardiac hypertrophy exists, the explanation is to be found in the state of the blood in chronic parenchymatous nephritis and in the state of the terminal arterioles in chronic interstitial nephritis; in the latter it often happens that hypertrophy exists without dilatation, or even with narrowing of the cavity of the ventricle; these cases he regards as idiopathic primary hypertrophy, as he says hypertrophy consequent upon obstruction, or difficulty in discharging the contents of the ventricle, must be associated with dilatation. The cause of this idiopathic hypertrophy may be nervous, as in Basedow's disease; or more probably it may be due to some state of the blood. The high tension in the aorta is due to the state of the terminal arterioles. He leans to Gull and Sutton's theory, and believes that the kidney-affection is a consequence or concomitant of the general disease.—*London Med. Record*, Oct. 15, 1878.

Bright's Granular Atrophy of the Kidney and the accompanying Cardiac Hypertrophy.

VON BUHL (*Centralblatt für die Med. Wissenschaften*, September 14, 1878) opposes the views of Traube and of Gull and Sutton by the following considerations: 1. There is eccentric hypertrophy of the left or both ventricles without granular kidney (25.7 per cent. according to Gull and Sutton). 2. There are cases of exquisite granular kidney without hypertrophy and dilatation (in quite 8 per cent.). 3. In granular kidney, the hypertrophy of the left ventricle is often unaccompanied by dilatation (0.6 per cent.). 4. General dilatation of the whole arterial system is absent; this would be an important consequence of increased tension. 5. All other renal atrophies (congenital cystic kidney, hydronephrosis, fatty kidney, etc.) do not bring about eccentric hypertrophy of the left ventricle. 6 and 7. The hypertrophy of the right ventricle is not explained by Traube's theory (simple hypertrophy of the left ventricle in 21.4 per cent. against double-sided hypertrophy in 70.8 per cent.); also this is not explained by fatty degeneration of the muscular wall of the left ventricle, as this is often absent even when the right side is fatty. 8. The hypertrophy of the left ventricle is often present before the granular degeneration of the kidney (Bamberger, Schötter). Against Gull and Sutton's theory he urges again, first, that at the commencement of the renal disease the fibroid thickening of the arteries and veins is not present; and, secondly, that nearly always the kidneys are the only organs involved, seldom any other. The last point is very striking, if arterio-capillary fibrosis were the cause of the renal degeneration as part of a general process.

Von Buhl's views are the following: 1. Both organs become diseased together. The hypertrophy is to be attributed to the increasing capacity of the heart. This view is supported by the appearance of cardiac hypertrophy before the atrophy of the kidney, and the eccentric hypertrophy of the right ventricle; also by the fact that we frequently find remains and results of previous inflammation of the heart, the origin of which can hardly be fixed, at the beginning of the disease: 35 per cent. of pericarditis; 20.6 of valvular disease, endocarditis, and vegetations; 55.9 per cent. of retained sufficiency of valves, with inflammatory fatty degeneration of the muscular fibre; 9.8 per cent. of aneurism, ruptured heart, and vitreous swelling of muscles. 2. The myocarditis may leave the heart unchanged, but atrophy may occur, though hypertrophy is the more common. The hypertrophy is effected in the following manner: In the first place, the cavities of the heart dilate on account of the diminished resistance of the heart-muscle to the blood-pressure. At the conclusion of the inflammatory process, the heart-muscle hypertrophies by over-nutrition, and by the increased work of the dilated ventricles. The fact is quite new that a relative narrowing of the aorta often coexists. To overcome the resistance of the narrowed aorta the left ventricle must hypertrophy. 3. The increased tension in the aortic system, and the cardiac hypertrophy, are not due to the granular atrophy, nor to a diffused capillary fibrosis; but, on the contrary, the increased tension in the aortic system is dependent upon the hypertrophy of the left ventricle and the relative stenosis of the aorta. The increased tension is, on account of the shutting of the valves, only systolic. 4. The arterial change is a consequence of the cardiac disease. · The thickening of the renal arterioles is secondary. The 13 per cent. of lung-affection (desquamative pneumonia and cirrhosis of lung) is an analogous process to the renal disease. In all other organs the consequences of Gull and Sutton's disease are atrophy and thickening; in these are to be found the causes of death in Bright's disease. In reference to the etiology it must be remembered that immoderate muscular exertion, especially of the heart, leading to myocarditis, eccentric hypertrophy, and the other elements of Bright's disease, must be regarded as a frequent cause of that disease.—*London Med. Record*, Oct. 15, 1878.

Medicinal Treatment of Diabetes Mellitus.

In the *Deutsches Archiv für Klinische Med.*, Band xxi., Hefts 5 and 6, Dr. P. FÜRBRINGER publishes observations on the influence of salicylate of soda, phenol, benzoate of soda, thymol, quinine, digitalis, arsenic acid, bromide of potassium, oil of turpentine. and pilocarpin, on the absolute and relative amount of sugar in the urine.

Inasmuch as the secretion of nitrogen, as well as of sugar, in diabetic patients —at least in severe forms, where, with complete exclusion of carbon-hydrate, sugar is still produced in large quantities—arises from a specific decomposition of albumen, Dr. Fürbringer tries to estimate the pathological importance of each form of diabetes by the *relative* amount of sugar (the weight of the sugar being divided by that of the nitrogen excreted), and from the variations, to arrive at a standard by which to judge of the effect of therapeutical agents. From his observations, he deduces that the greater the relative amount of sugar the more favourable is the prognosis; that a remedy which increases the glycosuria does the less harm, as it increases the relative amount of sugar; and lastly, that a remedy which does not alter the glycosuria is useful, as it increases the relative amount of sugar. In the first two cases the increase is due to a diminished excretion of nitrogen; and the drugs which did good by this means were salicylate of soda (8 to 10 grammes = 120 to 150 grains a day) and carbolic acid pills three times a day; quinine, arsenic acid, pilocarpin, and benzoate of soda gave no definite results; thymol, oil of turpentine, digitalis, and bromide of potassium did harm, and are therefore contraindicated in diabetes.—*London Med. Record*, Nov. 15, 1878.

Syphilitic Leontiasis.

MAURICE RAYNAUD (*Société Médicale des Hôpitaux de Paris*) brings to notice the case of a patient attacked by a new form of cutaneous syphilis, named by the author syphilitic leontiasis (subject of the inaugural thesis of M. Coutard, one of his pupils, "Study on diffuse syphilis of the face"). The diagnosis of the case was difficult; there are no syphilitic antecedents, but in the mucous membranes syphilitic manifestations are undoubted, scrofula being excluded by the age of the patient, which was 59. M. Coutard, in his thesis, says that syphilis may produce hypertrophic lesions of the skin, the gummy element, instead of being circumscribed, existing in the state of infiltration. In such a case ulceration is not produced, as it is in the dry, tubercular, degenerative form. The face is the favourite seat of this form of syphilis.

In the discussion which followed, M. Besnier said he would call it a case of papulo-hypertrophic syphilis. In passing, he advanced the opinion that iodide of potassium has an insignificant or no effect in scrofula. This was strongly contested by M. Dumontpallier.

M. Libermann, on the occasion of M. Raynaud's observation, read a paper on elephantiasis in Arabs, which was diagnosed as syphilitic on account of syphilitic antecedents in the history of the illness, but not because of its objective characters, and which was cured in three months by subcutaneous injections of the biniodide of mercury, large doses of iodide of potassium, and a strict regimen (milk-diet).— *London Med. Record*, Nov. 15, 1878.

Scleroderma Universalis.

Dr. MADAR, of Vienna, gives an account (*Vierteljahresschrift für Dermatologie und Syphilis*, 1878) of a case of a girl of 17. After a threatening of the disease, relieved by warm baths, she was seized with shivering, followed by swelling of the principal joints. In two months rigidity of the cheeks set in, which was accompanied by pigmentation of the skin and pain, with tension and immobility of the joints. Eight months after, on 6th May, 1877, the face had become rigid as marble, the eyeballs, eyelids, and lips alone being movable. The skin was dense and hard over the trunk and extremities, the abdomen and throat retaining their wonted pliancy. The fingers were distorted and fixed, the joints painful, both on pressure and spontaneously, while there were subjective sensations of tension which became pain on movement. While there was anæmia and amenorrhœa, there was no organic lesion. External treatment alone gave relief; protracted baths, especially those to which pine extract had been added, rendered the skin more pliant and a little motion possible. Faradization mitigated pain, but massage was injurious. Pericarditis, followed by diarrhœa and exhaustion, terminated her life on 8th October. An autopsy, instituted by Dr. Chiari, revealed pleuritic and pericardial adhesions, fatty degeneration of myocardium, with wastings of organs and anæmia. No pathological changes, either macro- or microscopic, were found in the spinal cord or ganglia. The skin contained an excess of pigment, both in the deep part of the rete mucosum and papillary portion of the derma. The reticular part of the cutis seemed thicker than it ought, though its meshes were compressed; there was hypertrophy of the subcutaneous areolar tissue, with disappearance of the fat. The other component structures of the skin were healthy. He regards scleroderma rather as a result of chronic inflammation of the skin than as due to lymphstasis, as held by Kaposi, while Madar considers the essential pathology to be central trophoneurosis; comparing the atrophy of the skin to progressive muscular atrophy.—*Edin. Med. Journ.*, 1878.

Quinia Rash.

At a late meeting of the Clinical Society of London (*Lancet*, Nov. 16, 1878) Dr. FARQUHARSON exhibited a drawing of a case of quinia rash, occurring at

St. Mary's Hospital, in the practice of Dr. Cheadle. The patient, a boy aged fourteen, was admitted with pyrexial symptoms; and after the first suspicion of typhoid was allayed, it was decided to try the effect of quinine in reducing the temperature, which had stood for several days at 100°. Ten grains were accordingly given thrice a day, and on the fourth day a rubeoloid rash appeared universally over the body, composed of flat slightly raised patches of a rose-pink, and accompanied by much tingling and irritation. No other symptom of cinchonism was observed, and on withdrawal of the medicine the eruption rapidly subsided. Quinine symptoms may be divided into two classes—viz., those of an eczematous character, which are described by some continental authorities as occurring on the skin of workers in quinine manufactories; and those which follow the internal administration, usually of very small doses of the drug, and which may be either erythematous or rubeoloid in character. The present case was strongly suggestive of urticaria, which it doubtless was, and it may naturally be argued that the real causation was some chance error of diet. The diagnosis was, however, most amply confirmed by one of the students, Mr. Luscombe, who had suffered two attacks in his own person, precisely similar to this in every respect, save in the addition of very troublesome and long-continued gastric irritation. It is worthy of remark that the quinine not only caused no lowering of the body heat in the first instance, but that on the appearance of the cutaneous eruption the temperature ran up to 102°, the explanation of this probably being that the dose was really too small to produce any decided antipyretic effects.—Dr. GREENHOW said that the rash described could not be put in the same category as the eruptions due to bromide or iodide of potassium, where the rash is the specific effect of the drug. Here, however, the eruption was not distinctive; it was of the nature of urticaria, and was produced by the quinine causing gastric disturbance, just as other ingesta frequently do. The case was of interest and rarity, for although he had prescribed quinine for forty years he had never met with a similar instance.

Surgery.

Case of Polypus of the Œsophagus successfully Removed.

Mr. THOMAS ANNANDALE, Professor of Clinical Surgery in the University of Edinburgh, reports (*British Medical Journal*, Nov. 23, 1878) the following rare case:—

In February last, I was asked by Professor Maclagan to see with him the Rev. Mr. C., who was seventy-six years of age. The history of our patient was that, about five years before our visit, he noticed for the first time, during a fit of coughing, "a lump come out of his throat on to his tongue." When the coughing ceased, the tumour disappeared; but, after this, the growth constantly protruded from the throat whenever he coughed or was sick, so that he became quite accustomed to its appearance. The tumour never caused him any inconvenience, except by its protrusion; and, when it did not pass back into the throat spontaneously, he could easily return it by pushing it down with his fingers. During the last year, the protrusion was not so frequent; but the tumour had increased in size and length, and, when it did protrude, it could be drawn out through the mouth and examined. There was no interference with swallowing or with respiration.

Before visiting our patient, it was arranged that I should bring with me the necessary instruments, in case the removal of the tumour was decided upon; but a difficulty was encountered at the very commencement of our meeting, for the tumour declined to protrude, notwithstanding the administration of a strong emetic by my colleague in the case. A second dose of the emetic succeeded, and the growth showed itself, and was at once seized and drawn out of the mouth. When examined, it was found to be a fibrous polypus, measuring four inches in length and about one and a half in breadth, gradually tapering to its peduncle, which was fully two inches in length and about the thickness of an ordinary lead-pencil. On passing the finger along the peduncle, it was felt to be attached to the left side of the œsophageal tube, at a point immediately below the commencement of the canal. The tumour having been drawn out of the mouth to its full extent, and a gag inserted to keep the jaws separated, I passed round the peduncle the chain of an écraseur, and slowly divided it, as low down as possible. The peduncle was divided in this way about an inch from its attachment to the œsophageal wall, so that the whole length of the tumour removed was five inches.

The structure of the growth was fibrous, resembling in appearance that of the dense fibrous polypus which grows in connection with the nasal cavities and bases of the skull. Its external surface was covered by mucous membrane. There was a slight oozing of blood from the stump of the peduncle for a few hours after the operation; but this soon ceased, and the patient suffered no further inconvenience, and was able to return home in a fortnight.

Remarks.—Cases of polypus growing in this situation are rare, and therefore I have considered a note of my case worthy of record. The fact that the growth gave rise to no inconvenience, notwithstanding its size, is an interesting feature in the case. The operation was of the simplest nature, and requires no special reference.

—

Tracheotomy in Membranous Laryngitis.

At a late meeting of the Royal Medical and Chirurgical Society (*Lancet*, Nov. 30, 1878) Mr. ROBERT W. PARKER read a paper on tracheotomy in membranous laryngitis, the indications for its adoption, and some special points as regards its after-treatment.

The author began by expressing his regret that the surgeon is only too often called in after all therapeutic measures have failed, the more so, because these measures generally include the use of depressants, which if not at once beneficial greatly tend by their continued administration to increase the prostration, so often a predominant feature of the disease. He regards recession of the chest-wall as a more important indication for tracheotomy than a loud clanging cough, for in the most urgent cases voice and cough are all but abolished owing to implication of the vocal cords. He advocates the administration of chloroform previous to the operation, and has never seen any ill effects therefrom. The higher operation is preferred as the more easy, especially in children, and the use of a tracheal dilator is advocated in preference to the immediate introduction of the canula; in this manner the tracheal wound is kept open. Then the author advises, *as a matter of routine in every case*, that the trachea and glottis be thoroughly cleared of all foreign matters, whether membrane or mucus, before the introduction of the tube. For this purpose a feather is usually employed, but any other means may be adopted which the operator may prefer. The feather may be passed downwards towards the trachea and upwards into the larynx, and through the glottis. The presence, it was argued, of membrane or inspissated mucus in the larynx above the tube after tracheotomy, is often an unsuspected cause of reflex irritation and cough; the surgeon, therefore, ought every now and then to clear out the larynx, so long as the patient is unable to do this for himself; and while he has to wear the canula in his trachea the patient is unable to use the natural means—viz., coughing—owing to the fact that all air is directed from the larynx through the tube. The author advocates the use of the largest-sized tube which can be got into the trachea without the employment of actual violence, and of the shortest that is consistent with safety, and he lays stress on the advantages of the tracheal part of the tube being freely movable. As regards the curve of the tube, it was stated that the outline should approximate to the Gothic rather than to the Roman arch; in other words, tubes made in the form of quarter circles (the usual forms are not recommended, for it can be shown that such tubes must almost necessarily impinge on the anterior wall of the trachea, and so produce mischief). He believes that a large proportion of the troubles which in past years have arisen from the use of "rigid" tubes has been caused by "ill-fitting" tubes. Speaking of Mr. Baker's "flexible tubes," the author is rather inclined to doubt the expediency of regarding "flexible" tubes as less likely to produce ulceration than "rigid" ones; for, unless the flexible tubes are made of a suitable curve, they will most probably lead to ulceration, just as certainly as (though, perhaps, less rapidly than) rigid tubes. The great indication for operation having been the presence of a mechanical impediment to respiration, so the chief object of the surgeon in the after-treatment must be to prevent its recurrence. The use of the feather has already been referred to. Another important aid is the employment of steam : the amount varies with the individual case, but an excess is in all cases to be avoided.[1] The less there is of tracheal secretion the more is steam needed, and the converse. Creasote, carbolic acid, benzoin, and other medicaments may be added in order to meet the requirements of various cases. The use of "solvents" is strongly recommended, the most important of these being soda. It may be used in solution (from ten to twenty grains in an ounce of water), and ought to be sprayed into the throat from time to time. It is thought to soften the membrane and to help its removal, and also to render its re-formation less possible. The author has seldom seen cases in which a fatal result could be traced to the operation itself; pneumonia and collapse being the commonest causes of death. The paper concludes thus : Bearing in mind that the operation is undertaken, not as a curative measure, but simply with a view to relieve a mechanical impediment to respiration ; seeing, nevertheless, the great frequency with which, after tracheotomy, the trachea and larynx, on the post-mortem table, are found covered, not to say choked up, with membranous exudation (specimens of which may be found in almost every anatomical museum)— the author, as a practical outcome of his paper, and with a view to raise a definite issue for discussion, feels justified in enunciating the following dictum : The presence of membrane in the trachea, in a fatal case of membranous laryngitis after tracheotomy, must be regarded as evidence of the want of due care on the part of the surgeon in charge, just as much as would the presence of a piece of gut in the inguinal canal after herniotomy, or a calculus in the bladder after the operation of lithotomy.

Mr. HOLMES said that the author's suggestions were of great value, for he had, he confessed, always abstained as much as possible from irritating the trachea, lest its condition be aggravated ; but he should now, after Mr. Parker's paper and Mr. Smith's testimony of the value of the practice, alter this procedure, and he

---

[1] The most useful apparatus for this purpose is the ventilating croup-kettle manufactured by Messrs. Allen & Sons, of Marylebone-lane. It supplies not only steam, but fresh and warmed air at the same time.

hoped with success. Certainly to have a mortality of eight out of seventeen cases of tracheotomy in membranous larnygitis was a death-rate wholly unfamiliar to surgeons, and should of itself lead to the general adoption of the lines of prac-
· tice suggested in the paper. He did not think many surgeons used the flexible tubes, and in one case of tracheotomy for cancer of the larynx, in which the trachea was too sensitive for metal tubes, he had found that the flexible tube caused as much, if not more, irritation, and had to be discarded. For some time in this case he was obliged to have recourse to daily dilatation of the tracheal wound, but at length found that a metal tube, with rounded ends and a perfora-tion at each side, could be borne. He could not see the necessity for having a tube the calibre of which should be larger than the chink of the glottis, nor did he think the length of the tube was of the importance Mr. Parker conceived it to be.

Dr. CHARLES WEST added a few remarks, because the greater part of Mr. Parker's experience had been gained at the Hospital for Sick Children during the time when he (Dr. West) had the happiness of being connected with that institution. He believed he had seen more tracheotomy operations than most surgeons, but he had stood by as a critic, and had probably, therefore, observed points which escaped the individual operator. In the whole course of his practice he never regretted having tracheotomy done; he had often regretted that it had not been sooner performed. Retraction of the soft parts during inspiration was the most trustworthy indication for its performance, and in every case he was ac-customed to expose the abdomen and chest, and, according to the degree of this retraction, to draw conclusions as to the expediency, or not of having tracheotomy done. Mr. Parker's suggestions as to the operation were sound and wise, and he could bear out what he said about venous bleeding. Then as to the size of the tubes; he had seen evil result from the use of too small tubes, and he recollected hearing Trousseau in one of his clinical lectures illustrate this by instancing the difficulty of inhaling through a small tube as compared with one of larger calibre. He was struck to find that Mr. Parker had not mentioned how Trousseau was accustomed to swab out the trachea, holding it to be of considerable importance; and he also advocated dropping in solutions of carbonate of soda, and even nitrate of silver. He had seen what Mr. Parker described, a canula push aside false membrane in its introduction, showing the importance of clearing the trachea before the tube was introduced. He believed the tube with a movable collar was the invention of M. Roger, late physician to the Hopital des Enfants Maladies. Then he was sure that the chances of success in treatment were small without the aid of an exceedingly competent nurse. He could confirm the statement of the grave indication of a dry state of tube, and in any case where the inner tube is dry he advised moistening with water or solution of carbonate of soda. He doubted if tracheotomy was to blame for the pneumonia which so often compli-cated membranous laryngitis. He regretted that he had no longer opportunities of increasing his experience, so that he could speak as to the value of Mr. Baker's tubes, but he could conceive many cases in which they would be very advan-tageous. There could be no risk of oxidation of the metal tube if it were removed and cleansed as frequently as it ought to be. Dr. West concluded by stating that he was glad to bear testimony to the accuracy of Mr. Parker's statements and the soundness of his conclusions.

———

Recovery after Penetrating Wound of the Thorax and Hernia of the Lung.

The first of these cases is reported by Dr. SCHOLZ in the *Wiener Medicinische Presse*, No. 1, 1878. The patient was a soldier who was stabbed with a knife on the left side of the chest, the wound being three centimetres (1.2 inches) long ; from this protruded a piece of the lower lobe of the left lung, nineteen centimetres (7½ inches) long, five and a half centimetres (2.2 inches) broad, and three centimetres thick. It was impossible to reduce the hernia. On the third day, · that portion of the lung which was protruding was a reddish-brown colour, with a consistency resembling that of liver ; no fetor emanated from .the wound, but there was an absence of the rhythmical movements. As the hernia was acting only as a foreign body, it was decided to remove it. The edges of the thoracic wound were brought together, as far as possible, by means of a suture ; a ligature was then placed round the base of the protruded portion, and its removal effected with a knife. Antiseptic precautions were taken during the operation. A considerable quantity of blood was lost at the time, but very little febrile reaction resulted from the operation. The bottom of the wound, formed by the spongy pulmonary tissue, slowly granulated. In two months and a half a cicatrix had formed, two centimetres long and five broad. This was firm to the touch, and moved synchronously with respiration. The patient was then sent back to his regiment.

The second patient was under the care of Dr. VOLKEL (Berliner Klin. Wochenschrift, November 7, 1878), having received a knife-wound below the eighth rib of the left side, in the axillary line. Directly after the accident, air freely entered the cavity of the chest through the wound ; but gradually this became obstructed by a protusion of lung-substance. In the first instance, both hemorrhage and dyspnœa were very marked ; these, however, both decreased as the hernia of the pulmonary tissues took place. When Dr. Volkel saw the patient, half an hour after the reception of the wound, there was great pallor, and a complaint of severe pain in the region of the wound ; there were all the signs of a pneumo-thorax of the left side, and a prolapsed portion of the lung on the same side, which resisted every effort at reduction. The pulse was 80 ; respirations 40. Absolute rest was prescribed, and ice ordered to be applied to the hernia. On the third day the temperature had fallen, and the number of respirations had sunk to 27. The quantity of gas and liquid in the left pleural cavity had much diminished. As the ice was not appreciated by the patient, its use was stopped. The prolapsed portion of the lung gradually assumed a deeper colour and a firmer consistency, and exuberant granulations were developed on its surface ; its volume slowly decreased, and in three weeks was about the size of a filbert. Cauterization with nitrate of silver reduced this still more, and in six weeks the hernia was only of the size of a lentil, flat, and covered by a thin membrane. A further application of the nitrate caused this to disappear, and the patient was dismissed cured.—London Med. Record, May 15, 1878.

—

On Catheterism in Cases of Stricture on Physiological Principles.

Mr. JOHN GAY, Senior Surgeon to the Great Northern Hospital, contributes to the *Lancet* (Nov. 16, 1878) a short but interesting paper on this subject. He says cases of stricture often come under the care of the surgeon, especially in hospital practice, in which, owing to the patient's neglect, a stricture barely permeable becomes almost suddenly impervious, and the surgeon is called upon to procure a passage of some kind for the urine in the teeth of every obstacle, normal and abnormal, that can waylay his efforts and render them difficult. It is to the earlier period in this (the culminating) stage of such a case that the following remarks are designed to apply.

A man, aged twenty-eight, recently presented himself at the Great Northern Hospital during my visit. He had suffered from stricture for years ; had had urethral discharge in abundance, and chronic balanitis as well. Latterly his urine had dribbled away, and, before reaching the hospital, this resource had failed him. Catheterism was attempted by skilled hands, but in vain ; and as early relief was necessary, an operation was advised, but refused. On examination, he was found to have a hard, firm, and painful stricture about three inches from the orifice, for which I proceeded to use a catheter on the following principles :—

1. As it is, the urethra is absolutely impervious to the passage of the catheter from a combination of causes—viz., the stricture growth engorged with mucus and blood, and rendered painful by futile catheterism ; and certainly spasm. It is not, however, absolutely impassable.

2. The tightest part of the stricture is that in front.

3. The unconditional use of a catheter would, in such a state of the parts, certainly intensify the difficulty by calling into play a new source of resistance, in the form of normal muscular antagonism, to its passage—a force that is ever on the alert to oppose the enforced passage of a foreign body through the urethra into the bladder.

4. This automatic force can be brought under complete control by an act of volition, and not only so, but be made to impart to the strictured canal the greatest amount of patency and passivity of which it is capable.

5. The means to this end consist in making the patient bring the sphincters or detrusors of the bladder and urethra into a state of absolute rest by voluntarily, but gradually, calling into powerful action their antagonists, the expulsors or accelerators, and using the catheter whilst the force thus elicited is kept in a state of strain.

6. This mode of palsying the detrusors has another advantage which anæsthesia does not possess, since it assists the surgeon by employing the urine as a dilator, and thus reduces the resistance of the stricture slit.

In the case before us the method thus indicated was carried out as follows. The patient was made to stand, supported by assistants, upright against a firm support, with outstretched legs—a position I always insist upon in catheterization, if feasible,—and being prepared with a well-warmed and oiled silver catheter (No. 4, at a venture, in this case), he was called upon to make an effort to pass his water and to gradually increase it to the extent of his power, always under the impressed conviction that he will succeed. After straining thus for a few seconds, and being required to keep up the act until he had permission to relax it, the point of the instrument was gently insinuated into the urethra, and carried on to the stricture. By careful exploration I was soon satisfied that its point and the slight force I was using were in a line with the axis of the canal, and that the entrance of the stricture had been reached. This I *felt*, for I had contrived to slide the instrument along the floor of the passage to the furthest point I could reach in any part of the canal, and by the sense of a slight grip of its point which was given me on making a simple move of the instrument onwards, I was sure that the passage had been gained. The patient still keeping up the strain, with a very little more force the catheter passed through with the usual, not always assuring, jerk. It could not, however, be made to enter the bladder, for its course was interrupted by another stricture at the membranous part of the urethra. This I did not attempt to pass, being satisfied that if the instrument could be retained during the night, the remainder of the passage would be easily passed in the course of the morrow, for the catheter would now indirectly act as an expulsor, and therefore keep in check any renewal of action on the part of any counteracting power. The urine passed abundantly during the succeeding night, not *through* the catheter—for it contained some clotted blood, and if it had not, I should have prevented it by the use of a close-fitting stilette,—but around it ; and on my visit the next day, the instrument was passed through with the help of the tip of my forefinger. A severe rigour followed the first effort, which was subdued by a glass of hot brandy-and-water and one scruple of quinine in the course of the next twenty-four hours.

The subsequent treatment has been daily catheterization, using a larger catheter each day, and allowing it to remain a few hours on each occasion. On the seventh day a No. 8 was easily passed. I need not refer to the watchful care which is always needed in the after-management of such cases.

I have ventured to ask permission to publish this case, trusting that the principle advocated—viz., that of falling back upon physiological resources as a help in the treatment of severe cases of stricture—might meet with whatever attention it may be thought to deserve.

—

Removal of a Piece of Iron from the Bladder per Urethram.

Dr. DELEFOSSE reports that in June he was consulted by a coachman who had introduced a piece of iron into his bladder. There was a good deal of pain, and constant urination, this being augmented by a long walk taken to reach the surgeon's house. The patient was much depressed, and would not give much information about the foreign body, merely saying that the ends were not sharp, and that he had introduced it for the purpose of cleaning the canal. He was placed in the recumbent position, and a curved metallic exploring sound was introduced into the bladder without difficulty, there being no contraction of its neck. A long smooth substance was then felt lying from left to right across the cavity of the organ, quite immovable. At first it was thought that extraction should be attempted through an opening made in the perineum, but finally a lithotrite was passed, and at the end of half an hour one of the ends of the iron was seized and the foreign body withdrawn; this proved to be an iron carriage-pin, slightly curved, 9 centimetres (about $3\frac{1}{2}$ inches) long, and with a diameter of 17 millimetres ($\frac{6}{10}$ths of an inch). There was no bleeding, and the next day the man resumed his work none the worse for his mishap.—*London Med. Record*, Oct. 15, 1878.

—

Cystine Calculus.

M. GAUJOT describes a case of cystine calculus in the *Bulletin et Mémoires de la Société de Chirurgie*, Nov. 3, 1878. The patient was a man aged 25, who was admitted into the Val-de-Grace on May 30th, 1877. The first symptoms of stone appeared in 1876. The calculus was removed by the prerectal incision, and the patient recovered in five weeks. The stone weighed 25 grammes (387 grains); it was ovoid in shape, of yellow colour, and had a rugose surface. It greatest diameter was 44 centimetres (about $1\frac{3}{4}$ inches). On section, it presented a homogeneous structure, without nucleus or strata ; it was greasy to the touch, and friable. Analysis showed it to be composed of cystine, with traces of phosphate and sulphate of lime, mucus, and fatty matter.—*London Med. Record*, Nov. 15, 1878.

—

Dermoid Cyst of the Testicle.

Dr. MACEWEN reports, in the *Glasgow Medical Journal*, for October, the case of a boy, aged 15, who was admitted under his care in the Glasgow Royal Infirmary, June, 1877, suffering from a tumour on the right side of the scrotum. This had been noticed in the first instance shortly after birth, and had grown proportionately with the rest of the body. As a rule, no soreness was felt in the swelling, except once in every six or nine months, when it became painful, and, according to the mother's account, at these times it seemed to increase in size. An examination showed that the tumour was ovoid, smooth externally, non-adherent to the skin over it, which was of a pinkish colour. To the hand it was heavy; in some places having a semi-fluctuant feeling; at other points, being quite hard. Its measurement was six inches, not quite reaching the external abdominal ring; the spermatic cord could be plainly felt between the upper extremity of the tumour and the ring. On the 18th of June the tumour was removed antiseptically by means of a longitudinal incision made from the external abdominal ring downwards for five inches. A structure, resembling tunica vaginalis, was adherent throughout to the growth and required separation. The spermatic cord was then found to run into the tumour; a ligature was accordingly placed round it to secure the spermatic vessels, and a division then effected.

The tumour was found to be composed of one large cyst and several smaller ones. The external membrane was fibrous and whitish in colour. Internally, there was a large quantity of gelatinous fluid, which, microscopically, was proved to contain granular corpuscles, and cells resembling leucocytes, but no spermatozoa. Bundles of hair were also found to exist, and in the walls of the cyst were masses of bone and cartilage, one of the pieces of the former bearing a resemblance to the fœtal sphenoid, another to the superior maxilla.

The patient made a speedy recovery, and at the beginning of July was dismissed convalescent.—*London Med. Record*, Nov. 15, 1878.

—

Electro-Puncture in Aneurism of the Aorta.

Drs. DUJARDIN-BEAUMETZ and PROUST read a memoir (*Gaz. Hebdomadaire*, Sept. 6) at the recent meeting of the French Society for the Advancement of Science, in which they state that, as the result of the employment of electro-punctures in six cases of aneurism of the aorta, they are enabled to conclude that Ciniselli's procedure, as they have modified it, has become a simple operation unattended with danger, and constitutes an efficacious and rational mode of treatment. In one case described by Dr. Proust, the patient having died from hemorrhagic infiltration of the lungs, it became possible to show that a thick layer of fibrinous coagula existed in the portion of the aneurismal sac where the needles had been applied. This case showed that electro-puncture could be successfully practised in patients whose general condition was a very grave one: that the coagula was deposited at the point of application of the positive pole; and that M. Gaiffe's improved instruments should be employed. M. Teissier observed that several experiments which he had performed corroborated the above conclusions, for he had found sphacelus produced in the arterial wall at the point of application of the negative pole, while several accidents arose during the application. But the application of the positive pole never gave rise to any accident, so that Drs. Dujardin and Proust have good reason for modifying Ciniselli's procedure by employing only the positive pole as the active agent, applying the negative one to a moistened plate with a broad surface placed at a distant part of the body.—*Med. Times and Gaz.*, Sep. 28, 1878.

—

Aneurism of the Abdominal Aorta Successfully Treated by Position, in a period of recumbence of seven weeks.

Mr. JOLLIFFE TUFNELL, Consulting Surgeon to the City of Dublin Hospital, records (*Dublin Journal of Med. Science*, Aug. 1878), the following interesting case :—

A. B., aged nineteen, a tall, delicate young man, who had recently suffered from primary and secondary symptoms, and been under a mercurial course, consulted me, upon the 7th of April last, for "a painful beating in his belly." He was engaged in the victualling business, and the history which he gave of his case cannot, I think, be better detailed than in the words of the patient himself, as taken down at the time. He said: "Five weeks ago I was working in the shop when an explosion of gas took place in the cellar underneath, and I was blown up to the ceiling; I was stunned and a good deal hurt, but I went to work again after a day or two. A week after this I was shoving up a side of beef, a man being on a ladder to put a hook into the beef; I pushed up the beef as well as I was able, but it *came back upon me*, and I had to let it down again. I felt at the time greatly exhausted, and had to rest for a while; I then tried again, and at last, after a very great struggle, got up the side of beef upon the hook. I did not feel any great pain then, but I was quite faint and very tired. Some days after, as I was going to work, I felt a great pain in my stomach, and a shivering came over me; I worked on, however, for a fortnight after this, until I was unable any longer to bear the pain. I now noticed the beating in my belly, and a throbbing, and it became very sore to the touch."

Upon examination of the abdomen, pulsation was evident to the eye, to the left of the median line, mid-distance between the umbilicus and cartilage of the ribs on the left side. Upon placing the patient on his back, a tumour, circular in form, with a distensile pulsation of two inches in each direction, could be almost grasped. The pulsation was accompanied by *bruit de souffle*, audible both to the unaided air and by the stethoscope when the patient was recumbent, but the bruit was totally lost as soon as he stood erect. Dr. Gordon, President of the King and Queen's College of Physicians, saw him, in consultation, a day or two afterwards, and the condition at that date was precisely the same as on the 7th; the patient, in the meanwhile, having been kept quietly in bed. Regular recumbence was not, however, commenced until the 12th of April, by which date a water-bed had been procured, and it was now continued without the patient once moving from the horizontal position till the 26th of May, when he was allowed to sit up, and upon the first of June to go out for a drive, which he continued to do daily.

No medicine of any kind was taken during the period of recumbence, and the only medicament employed was a turpentine and assafœtida enema administered upon the 30th of April, which brought away a very large number of scybala, whose collection and retention in the abdomen were causing uneasiness to the patient.

The pain, so severe at first, and which was dependent upon the tension of the aneurismal sac, subsided very rapidly—indeed in a few days after lying horizontal. The sacrum never had the slightest blush or uneasiness from pressure in lying, flotation upon water entirely obviating both. Upon the 9th of June the patient went out of town for change of air, but came in again upon the 14th for examination. No bruit or dilating tumour could now be found—upon the most careful auscultation and manipulation—by either Dr. Gordon or myself, and no aortic symptom beyond a fulness at the spot where the aneurism had existed. The origin of the aneurism I attribute to the intense strain put upon the coats of the aorta when endeavouring to push up the side of beef, the spine being then strongly bent backwards, and in the most favourable position to cause a tear of the inner and middle layers of the vessel, and I do not refer it in any way to the contusions following upon the explosion of gas.

—

Treatment of Wounds of the Superficial Palmar Arch by Acupressure.

Mr. EDWARD BELLAMY, Surgeon to the Charing-Cross Hospital, contributes to the *Lancet* (Sept. 21, 1878) a short article on this subject. He says: A perusal of the various English works on surgery does not impress me that this simple method is practised as frequently as it might be. I record a case which occurred lately in my own practice. A lad, whilst cutting some toffee from a plate, cut his ulnar artery through, just at the point where it takes its bend towards the radial side of the palm (in the "line of fate"), and when brought to my house, was losing blood rapidly, per saltum, from a deep wound about an inch and a half long. I applied Esmarch's bandage, and endeavoured to find the bleeding points, but to no purpose. I then plugged the wound and bound the hand to a dorsal splint firmly, so as to get pressure on the vessel by means of the tension of the palmar fascia, and applied compresses over the trunks of the radial and ulnar vessels. He soon returned to me bleeding as profusely as before. I then determined on acupressure, and taking a stout harelip-pin, passed it through the tissues about half an inch from the edge of the cut, under the artery, and out again to a corresponding distance the other side of the wound, and placed the limb again on the splint. This had the effect of entirely stopping the bleeding; the needle was removed on the fourth day, and the entire wound had closed by the end of the week.

I am well aware of cases of a like nature being treated by passing a harelip-pin under the radial and ulnar at the wrist, but although it has been effectual, it is not without its dangers, and I contend that in cases of wound of the superficial palmar arch (and this is not the first I have treated similarly), acupressure at the point of injury should be resorted to at once.

As a matter of anatomical fact, the bloodvessels, as it were, cleave to the palmar fascia, even after a long escape of blood; and, with ordinary anatomical precision, and a knowledge of the possible contingencies of irregularities, should be secured. A double needle might be used in some cases, to make quite sure— one on either side of the division in the vessel.

I need hardly say that these few remarks apply more particularly to wounds involving the superficial arch, although the "deep" arch is topographically not so deep or so ungetatable by this method as might be imagined.

——

Case of Ununited Fracture, in the treatment of which a Portion of Dog's Bone was used as a Means of Procuring Union.

Very various plans of treatment have been adopted for the purpose of getting the fractured bone to solidify. The method used in the following case, recorded by Dr. ALEXANDER PATTERSON, Surgeon to the Western Infirmary, Glasgow (*Lancet*, Oct. 19, 1878), is probably novel in this country, although a somewhat similar practice has been tried unsuccessfully in China.

D. N——, a marine engineer, whilst at sea, on Jan. 3d, 1873, sustained a simple fracture of both bones of the left forearm, about an inch and a half above the wrist-joint caused by his having been driven by a heavy sea against a lifeboat. The arm was put up in splints and kept up for some weeks. On the removal of the apparatus it was found that the bones had not united. He did not reach land for eight months after the accident.

Patient, aged forty-three, and in good health, was admitted to Glasgow Royal Infirmary on Oct. 7th, 1873, nine months after the receipt of the injury. Immediately after admission subcutaneous section of the flexible uniting medium was performed by the gentleman in whose wards he lay, and the arm was put up in splints for three weeks, but as union did not seem to be taking place, incisions were made along the radius and ulna, and the bones resected. The arm was again put up, and matters were progressing favourably, when, at the end of four weeks, erysipelas set in, and during its course necrosis of about three-quarters of an inch of the radius occurred. The limb was again put in splints and retained so for six weeks longer, when the external wounds were healed, but the bones had not united. Patient then left the hospital, having been in the house for three months and a half.

Aug. 15, 1874.—The man was readmitted to-day for the purpose of having his arm amputated. In the absence of the regular surgeon I took charge of the case, and, a consultation having been called, amputation was unanimously recommended; at the same time permission was accorded me to make any possible attempt at saving the limb. On examination, the cicatrices of the former operations were seen lying on the inner and outer side of the false joint. The hand and lower fragments were drawn somewhat up towards the elbow, and hung swinging about, completely powerless. The lower end of the longer fragment of the ulna formed a hard, smooth projection, over which the skin was tensely drawn.

After having given the case some consideration, on the 14th of September the patient was taken into the theatre and placed under the influence of chloroform, while at the same time a retriever dog was being anæsthetised. I made an incision along the ulnar side of the arm, cutting down upon the ends of the fractured bone, and removing the fibrous band which alone formed the bond of union; the rounded points were removed by the saw, and a hole drilled obliquely through each squared end. The same process was repeated on the radial side, when it was found that an interspace of about three-quarters of an inch existed between the two fragments of the radius. In the meantime, Mr. Andrews, one of the senior students, and a very clever manipulator, had exposed the humerus of the quadruped, completely denuded of every tissue except the periosteum. The length of bone was accurately measured (three-quarters of an inch), while from half an inch beyond the end of the necessary length the periosteal covering was rapidly but carefully dissected, the bone sawn through, a hole drilled in either end obliquely, as in the radius and ulna, and at once placed between the ends of the radius, where it fitted accurately. Wires having been passed through the holes, the bones were firmly tied together, the loose half-inch margin of the periosteum of the foreign bone being carefully spread over the periosteum of the radius. The wound was stitched with silver wire, the bone sutures coming out at each end of the incision. Wires were passed through the ulna, tied together, and the wound treated in a similar manner. The entire operation was conducted under the carbolic acid spray. The arm was put up in gauze, and held in two rectangular splints.

Sept. 15*th.* Patient complains of some pain in arm, but says he had snatches of sleep through the night after having had twenty-five minims of tincture of opium. After the operation there was a slight tendency to sickness, which was relieved by ice. Pulse 80, rather hard; tongue slightly furred, but moist; skin somewhat hot. Dressed; one or two of the stitches removed, as there were signs of tension and a slight blush around the sutures. To have tincture of opium as before. It is needless to give a detailed account of the dressings up till Nov. 3d, when the ulna was found to be firmly united; but on the radial side small pouting granulations appeared, as if a foreign body were present, which, however, could not be detected by the probe.

Nov. 28. To-day the patient was put under chloroform, and the wires removed. That which had tied together the ulnar fragments was first caught with forceps, and taken out with great ease; it had apparently cut its way through the bone. and was lying immediately beneath the skin. I then went at the radial side with extreme curiosity and anxiety. Over the seat of fracture a small, elongated patch of extremely soft granulations was seated. At one end of the patch, the upper, one wire was caught, and easily extracted; the other was found at the lower end, and a considerable amount of force was necessary for its withdrawal. Although the wire came away complete, it seemed to have been broken in the bone by the force exerted in extraction. With my finger-nail I scraped off the exuberant granulations, and with a probe examined the wound. Dead bone could not be detected, although the appearance of the small wound led me to suspect its presence. The fracture looked, on the whole, to be fairly united, and the patient was dismissed, with strict orders to return weekly for dressing and examination.

Thirteen weeks have elapsed since the date of operation, and the wires were perfectly bright on removal, the wounds having been kept antiseptic throughout. The man has gained in weight, and improved much in appearance. On leaving hospital boracic lint was used as dressing. The small wound remained open for twelve months, when the dog's bone, reduced to about half its size, came away, after which the wound healed completely. The radius appears to have fallen in somewhat towards the ulna, leaving a slight deformity.

D. N——, wearing a leathern support around the forearm, resumed his former occupation, at which he is still engaged. He called on me some weeks ago, and remains in perfect health, and retains a very useful arm. Thinking of Ollier's experiments with the periosteum, of the transplantation of skin from an amputated limb to ulcers, and of the transference of the mucous membrane of the rabbit to the human eye, I had some hope that the strange bone might have found a new home for itself in the human arm; failing which I knew it would secure perfect alignment of, and steadiness in, the ulnar fragments. Should a similar case occur again, I should adopt the same process, still hoping that the two bones might become one.

—

Effusion of Oil after Fracture.

M. F. TERRIER reports (Revue Mensuelle, No. 7, 1878) a case in which, two months after fracture of both bones of the right leg in a male, aged 28, and when the fragments had been firmly united, a small fluctuating and painless swelling was observed on the inner surface of the limb near the seat of injury. From this, when punctured, three grammes were drawn off of a thick fluid resembling olive oil, which contained no anatomical elements, and was found on chemical examination to be composed of margarine, a small proportion of oleine, and some traces of cholesterine. After repeated puncturing of this tumour, and application of firm pressure to its thick cyst-walls, all further effusion, towards the end of the eleventh week from the date of the first appearance, was quite arrested.

In some remarks on the pathology of this condition, M. Terrier states that it has been made out by those surgeons who have written on this subject that traumatic oily effusions, or rather traumatic effusions containing oil-globules, may be either primary or secondary. The effusion when primary, is usually the result of rupture of the adipose vesicles of the subcutaneous cellular tissue. The tumour in such cases contains a serous fluid, more or less viscous, sometimes coloured by blood, and always mixed with oil-globules. A case, however, in which the primary traumatic effusion consisted almost wholly of oily fluid, has been reported by Gosselin. A young man presented, as the primary results of a fall, these three lesions, swelling of the left knee from intra-articular effusions, abrasions on the inner surface of the injured limb, and finally a small fluctuating tumour on the outer surface of the swollen knee. This tumour contained a thick fluid, which stained paper, and presented under the microscope very fine crystals of margaric acid. This oily effusion was very probably the result of crushing of adipose cellular tissue. Consecutive effusion of oil after injury may result either from gangrene of the cellular tissue, or from osseous suppuration. It was pointed out by M. Chassaignac that oil-globules are specially observed in the pus that results from inflammation of bone, and, according to this surgeon, the presence of such globules in purulent fluid is pathognomonic of osteo-myelitis. In M. Terrier's case, the situation of the collection of oil on the inner surface of the tibia at the junction of its upper and its two lower thirds, that is to say, in a region where the subcutaneous cellular tissue contains very little fat, seems to exclude any idea of crushing of the cellulo-fatty tissue as the cause of the tumour. Neither can it be attributed to osteo-myelitis; since the fracture had been a simple one, and the inflammatory results of the injury very mild. It is necessary, therefore, to find out some other origin of this oily effusion. According to M. Terrier, the oil was derived from the bone marrow exposed by the fracture in the tibia, which, after passing between the fragments, collected under the skin, where instead of becoming absorbed as is usually the result with such effusions, it formed a cystic tumour. Gosselin, in treating of compound fracture of the leg, insists on this as a clinical fact, that the cutaneous wound gives passage not only to blood but also to oil-drops, the discharge of which may persist for ten or twelve days. This fluid comes from the bone-marrow exposed and broken down at the time of the injury, and in such case the abundance and persistence of the oil discharge serve to distinguish it from the discharge of a similar fluid that results from wounding of a part richly provided with adipose tissue. M. Terrier sums up as follows:

1. Effusion of oil may be observed as a result of breaking down of cellulo-fatty tissue, such collection being combined, in most instances, with a serous or serosanguineous effusion.

2. Gangrene of the cellular tissue and suppurative osteo-myelitis may give rise to purulent effusions containing oil-globules.

3. Pure oily effusions resulting from transudation of fat from bone-marrow may be the result of fracture, especially, perhaps, when this form of injury is multiple and direct.—*London Med. Record*, Oct. 15, 1878.

Dislocation of the Atlas.

Drs. UHDE, HAGEMANN, and BOETTGER describe in the *Archiv für Klin. Chirurgie*, vol. xxii, a case of bilateral wrench of the articular surfaces of the atlas, by which the right surface was displaced forward, the left backward, from the corresponding articular surfaces of the axis. The injury produced some remarkable disturbances of innervation. The left half of the tongue was paralyzed and convex outwards, while the right half was contracted and concave. The left half of the soft palate and the left glosso-palatine arch were also paralyzed; the uvula was drawn to the right. The anterior third of the tongue on both sides, and the second and third thirds on the left, possessed ordinary and gustatory sensation; in the posterior two-thirds on the right, no sign of sensation or of taste could be detected. The authors attribute these phenomena to paralysis of the right glosso-pharyngeal nerve and of the left hypoglossal nerve and the pharyngeal plexus. By artificially producing the injury, they show that the glosso-pharyngeal nerve, immediately after its exit from the jugular foramen, must have been violently stretched over the portion of the atlas which was thrown forward; that, in this luxation, the roots of the hypoglossal nerve inside the vertebral canal appeared as a pair of tightly stretched cords, instead of lying, as in the normal condition, loose against the dura mater. In the same way and at the same part, the accessory nerve suffers stretching, leading to the paralysis of the left palate; this can be explained in no other way than by assuming an in-

jury, through this overstretching, of the pharyngeal plexus, which aids in forming the anterior branch of the accessory nerve. The vertebral canal was not so
much narrowed as to produce compression of the medulla oblongata, and the vertebral artery was not injured. The disturbances of the gustatory function of the
tongue indicates that the glosso-pharyngeal nerve supplies exclusively only the
two posterior thirds of the tongue, and that the anterior third and the palate are
supplied from portions of the third division of the fifth nerve. The dislocation
could not be reduced ; but the patient gradually regained some power of moving
the head. There was also some improvement in the functions of the tongue and
palate.—*British Med. Journal*, Sept. 7, 1878.

An interesting case of supposed luxation of the atlas is recorded in Von Langenbeck's *Archiv*. A bilateral dislocation of the atlas occurred in consequence
of a fall, the right articulation being displaced forwards, and the left articulation
backwards. The left half of the tongue was paralyzed, the right contracted into
a curve, with the concavity outwards, whilst the left presented a convexity outwards. The left half of the palate and the left glosso-palatine arch were paralyzed, the uvula being curved to the right. Common sensibility and the sense of
taste were present on the anterior third of the tongue on each side, and also on the
left middle and posterior third, while on the right middle and posterior third no
evidence of common or special sensibility could be obtained. The authors refer
these symptoms to paralysis of the right glosso-pharyngeal nerve and the left
hypoglossal nerve, and of the left pharyngeal plexus. They show, on a preparation on which the same dislocation was artificially produced, that (1) the glosso-
pharyngeal nerve must have been tightly stretched over the portion of the atlas
which was displaced forwards, immediately after its exit from the foramen-jugu-
lare ; that (2) the roots of the hypoglossal within the spinal canal appear like a
pair of tightly-stretched threads, while they normally run slackly against the
dura mater. In the same manner, and on the same side, the spinal accessory
nerve becomes torn, to which the paralysis of the left half of the palate was probably due, since it can only be explained by supposing that the pharyngeal plexus,
which the anterior twig of the spinal accessory nerve helps to form, suffered when
the nerve-trunk was torn ; (3) the narrowing of the spinal canal is not sufficient
to cause a compression of the medulla oblongata. The vertebral artery would
also escape. The disturbance of taste renders it probable that the glosso-pharyngeal nerve confers the sense of taste on the posterior two-thirds of the tongue
only, and indicates the dependence of taste in the anterior third on the lingual
branch of the fifth. The dislocation was not reduced, but the patient gradually
obtained a freer movement of his head, and the paralysis of the tongue and palate
also lessened.—*Lancet*, Sept. 21, 1878.

———

Etiology of the Mechanical Symptoms of Hip-Joint Inflammation in Children.

Dr. KOLACZEK of Breslau contributes a paper on the above subject to the
Deutsche Medicinische Wochenschrift for August 3d and 10th. He observes
that the mechanical symptoms attending an affection so frequent as coxitis in
children are by no means clearly explained. Even pathological anatomy has
scarcely elucidated the mechanical symptomatology of this disease, probably not
only because opportunity has been lacking to study it in its earlier stages, but
also because the symptoms observable during life are mostly only functional.
Two theories are even at the present day generally received : 1. The reflex or
dynamic theory founded on analogy, according to which articular inflammation of
every kind excites a reflex contraction of corresponding groups of muscles ; and
2· The mechanical theory, on which the filling up of the articular cavity by the
inflammatory exudation determines the displacement of the extremity. The view

already propounded by Brodie and Bonnet, seems to have been entirely over-looked, according to which the pathological positions assumed by the patient are due entirely to the instinctive effort on his part to place the limb in as easy and painless a position as possible. Dr. Kolaczek's own experience, during many years, of hip-joint affection in children, leads him to regard this theory of accom-modation as the true and most natural one. He then enters at length into a dis-cussion, from this point of view, of the mechanical symptoms as they arise during the progress of the case. The so-called voluntary limping, which is one of the earliest symptoms of hip-joint disease, he attributes to the desire of the child to shorten as much as possible the period, while walking, during which the weight of the body is thrown upon the affected joint. This halting gait is at first as-sumed only after the child has been moving about for some hours, since the pressure on the articular surfaces of the joint does not at first excite pain. As the disease progresses, however, the symptoms become more complicated, for the joint becomes more sensitive, and hence further efforts to escape pain. While standing, the affected limb assumes a position of flexion of the hip- and knee-joints, the foot being placed on tiptoe; there is abduction and rotation outwards; the anterior superior spinous process on the diseased side of the pelvis is de-pressed and advanced, and the lumbar portion of the spinal column is curved for-wards and laterally; and this curvature is compensated by a curving backwards of the dorsal portion of the column, with depression of the shoulder on the side affected. These changes are produced instinctively on the part of the child, in order to remove the central line of gravity as far as possible from the diseased joint. This central line of gravity, which, during progression, oscillates between the two hip-joints, is frequently also thrown forward beyond the plain of the pelvis by the child fixing the stretched arms on the knees and so assuming a bending forward position, both in standing and walking; and by abduction of the limb this line is also thrown outwards. Nor is the assumption justified by obser-vation and fact, that the inflammatory process in the joint excites a reflex con-traction of the muscles. For, were this indeed so, it would be impossible to understand those by no means uncommon exceptional cases, in which, with un-doubted inflammatory disease of the hip-joint, the pathological position is yet almost or wholly absent. But in such cases there is probably much diminished sensibility to pain, which is therefore only slight and more easily borne. The continued contraction of not only the muscles, but also the fasciæ, notably of the fascia lata and its descending processes, has a great tendency to become perma-nent, so that the displacement of the limb continues even when the recumbent posture is assumed. As the disease progresses and the patient takes to his bed, a further change occurs in the position of the affected extremity. The flexion at the hip-joint increases, and the limb is now adducted and rotated inwards. This change of position is due wholly to its greater convenience. For, in the horizon-tal position, the weight of the body is entirely taken off the hip-joint, and the thigh is flexed in order to reduce the antagonistic muscles to a state of rest; and since the patient naturally lies on the sound side, the affected limb is rested on the sound one. While, in the former stage, the limb is sometimes somewhat lengthened, it is now generally decidedly shortened, owing to atrophy of the head of the femur, and deepening of the acetabulum, and also sometimes, though rarely, to actual dislocation of the femur, through relaxation, atrophy, or rupture of the inclosing ligamentous structures. It is impossible to reconcile this change of position in the later stages of the disease with either of the former hypotheses mentioned; for the group of muscles contracted at the commencement by reflex irritation could not now permit the limb to be placed in a position so opposed to their line of action; nor, on the other hand, can the change in question be due in all cases to destructive dislocation, of which there is only rarely any evidence. And the point of view from which we regard the displacements of the limb in coxitis, is of great importance in the treatment. For, whereas on the former hypotheses the limb will be invariably displaced in the same manner, whatever the position of the body; the practitioner, acting on the accommodation theory, will endeavour to adapt the position of the body so that the limb may obtain the greatest possible amount of ease and rest. And, hence, position and mechanical means are most efficacious in the treatment of inflammatory disease of the hip-joint.—*London Med. Record*, Nov. 15, 1878.

Repeated Fracture of the Patella.

The first case is reported in the *Progrès Médical* for September 21st, the patient being a woman, aged 56, who was admitted into the *Hôpital Cochin* under the care of M. DESPRES. An examination of the left knee-joint, made at the hospital six hours after the woman had fallen, showed that the patella was divided into three pieces. The middle fragment was separated from the upper one by a centimetre (0.4 inch), from the lower one by three centimetres (1.2 inches), this last piece being very movable. It transpired that three years before the patient had fractured the same patella transversely, and had been an inmate of the Hôtel-Dieu; fibrous union of the fragments had resulted. The case was treated by means of silicated bandages, and in three months the patient was able to walk with the affected limb as well as with the sound one, without fatigue, fibrous union having taken place.

M. Despres enunciates the following. 1. The formation of osseous callus in fractures of the patella is impossible when the articulation is distended by a large effusion, or if the pre-existing adhesions do not maintain the fragments in perfect contact in a limited effusion. This opinion, maintained by M. Guyon, finds a new proof. At the beginning of the year a patient was under observation who had sustained a fracture of the left patella. He was treated by a silicate bandage in the extended position, and osseous union was effected. Before the accident, the man had suffered from suppuration in the peri-articular tissues, following an affection of the bone. As a consequence of this, the patella was firmly bound to the condyles by strong fibrous adhesions. In this case also, atrophy of the muscles of the thigh caused the absence of one of the principal causes of separation of the fragments. 2. The formation of fibrous callus may be considered as the definite mode of healing of fractures of the patella; for, in the case reported, after the second fracture, as after the first, the patient could walk without fatigue and without limping, there being no difference in the movements of the two limbs. So again, the fibrous callus resisted more than the bone itself, as is evidenced by the second fracture. What use is there in endeavouring to obtain osseous callus when the fibrous is stronger than the bony? It is to be believed that the formation of an osseous callus is difficult to obtain, and is more desirable than a short, solid fibrous material, the development of which depends on the treatment employed.

The second case appears in *Le Progrès Médical* for October 19. The patient was 50 years of age, and three years ago he fractured his left patella. Six months after the same accident happened to the right. Union in both fractures was by fibrous callus three centimetres (1.2 inches) long. The articulation was very loose and walking was difficult. Eighteen months after the second breakage, the patient while in his garden tripped and fell. On being examined, it was found that the lower fragment of the right patella was broken transversely; the pieces being divided by about a finger's breadth. The fibrous callus which marked the line of ancient fracture had not stirred. An immovable apparatus was applied, and fibrous union resulted; but the patient had afterwards great difficulty in walking and also in raising his leg from the ground; going down stairs was especially laborious.— *London Med. Record*, Nov. 15, 1878.

Midwifery and Gynæcology.

Rupture of the Vagina during Labour.

At a late meeting of the Obstetrical Society of London Dr. GALABIN related (*Lancet*, Nov. 23, 1878) two cases of rupture of the vagina during labour. The first was that of a patient under the care of Mr. Sharman, of Gipsy-hill, an enormously fat woman. She had had eight children previously. During labour the patient had got out of bed and strained violently upon a night-stool. Immediately afterwards the head was found to have descended to the perineum, and was quickly expelled through the vulva. Uterine action then ceased, and the fœtus was extracted alive. After twenty minutes, as expulsion of the placenta could not be otherwise procured, gentle traction was made upon the funis; but it broke and came away, leaving the placenta behind. On introduction of the hand a substance was felt, which, being carefully brought into view at the vulva, proved to be large intestine, recognized by its longitudinal bands. The placenta could not be found, though the arm was introduced up to the elbow. The author saw the patient about eight hours after the rupture, and found that the posterior vaginal wall had been torn away from the cervix for more than half its circumference. The os uteri was closed, and the placenta not to be discovered. It was thought that it would give the only possible chance to the patient to perform gastrotomy, sponge out the blood from the peritoneal cavity, and search for the placenta. A jet of dark blood spurted out at the first puncture of the peritoneum, and more than two pints were found collected in front of the uterus. The placenta was also lying in front of the uterus and upon the top of the bladder. Symptoms of peritonitis set in the next day, and death took place forty-two hours after delivery. The second case was that of a patient forty-one years old, who had had ten children delivered naturally. She was attended in the Guy's Charity. The author was called to see what was said to be a case of placenta prævia, in which considerable hemorrhage had taken place. He found that no presentation was within reach, and that the finger penetrated a long way without resistance. Chloroform being given, it was ascertained that there was an extensive rent in the posterior vaginal wall, separating it from the cervix. The fœtus and placenta had passed into the abdomen, the head of the fœtus uppermost. The posterior lip of the cervix, which was bilaterally cleft, and the peritoneal surface of the uterus, had been mistaken for the placenta presenting. As the patient and her friends, who were Irish, refused to allow gastrotomy, the foot of the fœtus was brought down through the vagina, but the occiput had to be perforated before the head could be brought through the brim, and the patient died shortly after delivery. In both cases the accident appeared to be due, not to any degeneration of uterine tissue, or any considerable disproportion between pelvis and fœtal head, or protraction of labour, but to a violent pain having occurred while the uterus was in a position of extreme anteversion, so that the fœtal head was driven against the posterior wall of the genital passage.

Dr. BARNES considered the cases important, as showing that spontaneous rupture of the vagina may occur during labour. Had forceps been employed in either of these cases the practitioner would probably have been blamed for the result. and the laceration have been attributed to his manipulation. In fat women the tissues give way under slight forces. Cases of ruptured vagina occur suddenly in morbid tissues, and before there is any indication on which to act.—Dr. CLEVELAND referred to a practical point in the first case, and suggested that it might prove a useful warning under all circumstances to employ the utmost gentleness in attempting to bring down the placenta by traction on the funis. Although there was no evidence that undue force had been used, yet the fact remained, that had the cord not been unfortunately broken the placenta might have been cautiously traced to its resting-place, and removed without the operation.— Dr. MATTHEWS DUNCAN related the particulars of two cases of ruptured vagina, and remarked that when the great majority of such ruptures takes place the cervix and vagina form one tube, whose parts are distinguished chiefly by the rim of external os projecting. The vagina might rupture or the cervix might rupture, but the body did not. Vaginal ruptures are not rare, forming about a third of the whole.

On the Prevention of the Spread of Puerperal Fever.

A committee of the Society for Obstetrics and Gynæcology in Berlin, of which Dr. C. Schrœder is Chairman, have presented a report on this subject to the Prussian Minister of Public Health (*Edinburgh Med. Journ.*, Nov. 1878), from which we make the following extract :—

Under the names " puerperal fever," " malignant childbed fever," are included a group of diseases occurring in childbed which vary very greatly in their manifestations, but have this in common, that they are called into being by the absorption from the organs of generation of a material which gives rise to destructive inflammation and fever. There are, indeed, a number of substances, mainly composed of organic materials in a state of putrid decomposition, which, when brought into contact with an open wound, set up inflammation in it, which extends to the neighbouring tissues ; a further absorption by the lymphatics and blood-vessels leads to more extensive inflammation among neighbouring and remote organs ; and when a large quantity is rapidly absorbed into the blood, a quickly fatal poisoning of the whole organism occurs. To surgeons the deadly effect of these materials upon wounds is only too well known, and the greatest advance, probably, which surgery has ever made consists in the so-called antiseptic method of treating wounds—that is, in the scrupulously exact removal of such materials from fresh wounds.

Puerperal fever is indeed nothing else than the infecting of fresh wounds, such as are found in every newly-delivered woman, with these destructive septic materials. Almost every woman after labour has small wounds on the external genital organs, which are caused by the passage of the child through this narrow opening, and in every newly-delivered woman the inner surface of the uterus, from which the protecting membrane has been cast off with the ovum, presents a large wound surface. Thus, every newly-delivered woman is liable to suffer from the dreaded infective wound diseases—which in persons wounded under other circumstances are called pyæmia, septicæmia, wound fever, blood-poisoning, purulent infection, etc.—*so soon as suitable septic materials are brought into contact with the genital organs.*

Now, materials of this sort gain admission in two ways: first, and this happens more especially in very difficult and long labours, under the influence of the particles that cause putrefaction which are ever present in the air and ever ready to press in, decomposition occurs in the mother's own secretions and excretions, and thus takes its rise in the maternal organism itself ; or, secondly, these materials are introduced into the female genital canal *from outside*. This latter is brought about almost exclusively by the finger or instruments of those who examine the lying-in woman—that is to say, of the midwife or the physician.

If the instruments or finger of these persons have not been cleaned with the greatest care, and disinfected most conscientiously after they have been in contact with any infective matters, the result is that these matters are brought into contact with the fresh wounds of the woman during labour or subsequently, and thereby infect her with a fatal disease. A specially frequent channel of infection is from a diseased lying-in woman to another, because midwives quite commonly go from a diseased lying-in woman, whom they are nursing, to attend upon a new confinement, without sufficiently purifying themselves; and it cannot be doubted that, in the majority of cases, the midwives are the carriers of this infection, because to their exclusive care the great majority of labours is intrusted, and they naturally come into more intimate relations with the lying-in women than the physicians, who, in very many cases, are only called in after the onset of threatening symptoms.

From the foregoing exposition it will be seen that we know the cause of puerperal fever, and the manner in which it is brought about, more accurately than in almost any other disease, and, on the strength of this knowledge, have to ask ourselves the question: By what regulations can the occurrence and spread of puerperal fever be prevented, or at least lessened in amount?

These regulations naturally divide themselves into those which aim at preventing the occurrence of individual sporadic cases of puerperal fever, and those whose object is to avoid the transmissions of the disease from infected lying-in women to healthy ones.

As regards the first object, it is obviously of great importance to avoid the putrid decomposition of the discharges which come from the woman during labour. This is, of course, the aim of a rational management of a case of labour, which would, if possible, bring the labour to a conclusion before any stinking excretions come from the genital parts; we work in the same direction by keeping away anything which can excite putrefaction. The midwife should, accordingly, remember that frequent and careless examinations hasten the decomposition of the secretions, and should be instructed to use *disinfectant injections* in all cases of prolonged labour, so that the products of decomposition may be formed in the female genital passages as late, and in as small quantity, as possible. Of still greater moment is it that the medical persons (*Medicinal-personen*) to whom is entrusted the care and treatment of the lying-in woman, should recognize to its fullest extent the danger which threatens women, where putrid substances are brought into contact with the sexual parts either by the finger or by instruments. Among physicians this danger has long been known, and is universally recognized; but midwives cannot be too earnestly and strongly warned of it. That the rising generation of midwives may be properly instructed in this matter, it will require even more careful attention in the new additions of the handbooks for midwives, and in oral instruction, than it has hitherto met with.

Indeed, since it may be long ere all midwives are thoroughly instructed on this subject, the question arises, Whether it would not be the wiser plan to appeal directly to the public in this matter, and to enjoin upon husbands not to allow their wives to be examined by any hand which has not previously been thoroughly disinfected?

When we reach this point, when it is the universal custom, *in every single case, and under all circumstances, for the physician and midwife to disinfect their hands before they introduce them into the genital organs*, then, without any doubt, the annual mortality in childbed will become very much less, and thousands of women, who now die of infection brought about by thoughtlessness or ignorance, will be saved.

It remains to speak of special rules for those cases in which puerperal fever has already broken out, because the danger of transmission of the disease then becomes more considerable, and experience teaches us that, where definite epidemies of puerperal fever occur, *they cling for the most part to the practice of a single midwife.* A large number of instances are on record in which a midwife has carried the infecting material from one diseased lying-in woman to others, with the result that a number of newly-delivered women have sickened, and many of them have died.

In order to cut short these definite epidemics when they arise, and to prevent them from breaking out, it appears absolutely necessary *to lay upon all medical persons* (Medicinal-personen) *by law the duty of reporting such cases to the Sanitary Boards.* The simplest way of effecting this is is to include puerperal fever among the contagious diseases, of which it is necessary to send in a report. Undoubtedly special difficulties present themselves in regard to diagnosis. The question whether a disease during lying-in is to be looked upon as an infectious childbed fever or not, may be a very difficult one even for the physician, and is entirely beyond the judgment of a midwife. Accordingly, we hold it to be the bounden duty of midwife and physician to make a report to the sanitary authorities, *in every case of severe feverish disease occurring in childbed, unless it be clearly established that it has no connection with the puerperal process.*

But since even here differences of opinion may arise, there is one thing, at all events, about which there can be no doubt, namely death; we therefore deem it necessary to add, *that all midwives are in duty bound to give notice of every fatal case during childbed which occurs in their practice.* The sanitary authorities will probably in this way get sufficiently early notice of the existence of puerperal fever epidemics.

But if they are to be in the position effectually and certainly to cut short commencing epidemics, *they must have the power to suspend the midwife from the practice of her calling for a fixed period,* since this is the only sure means of preventing the extension of the disease through the same midwife.

We are thoroughly convinced, especially when we consider how wonderfully the mortality from smallpox has decreased since the carrying out of compulsory vaccination, that these rules will have a decided influence in lessening the mortality from puerperal fever; and, although we are far from believing that puerperal fever can in this way be rooted out, and though we do not for a moment doubt that, even under the strictest laws and with the most scrupulous care on the part of medical persons, sporadic cases of puerperal fever will always occur yet we must express a confident hope that, by the carrying out of the regulations sketched above, the mortality from puerperal fever will be very materially diminished, and that in this way every year several thousands of young mothers, who now die, may be saved to their families and to the State.

On Nervous Troubles Accompanying Uterine Affections.

MARTINEAU (*Gazette des Hôpitaux*, 1878, No. 64) says that in the majority of cases the morbid conditions resulting from uterine disease are due to disturbances of the nervous system. Among the most notable are neuralgia supra-orbitalis, maxillaris, and laryngo-bronchialis (uterine cough); also neuroses of the heart, causing painful palpitations, and spasmodic contractions of the bladder and bronchi (uterine asthma). All these symptoms become aggravated at the time of the commencement of the menstrual flow. The author observed one patient affected with this kind of asthma, who had long passed the climacteric, but whose asthmatic attacks were always most severe at the times at which the menses used to appear. Ordinary asthma also becomes worse under the influence of uterine disease.

Uterine affections frequently give rise to spasm of various muscles and to paralysis of one or both lower limbs. Both of these conditions usually come on very gradually, and they never become complete.

The peripheral reflex irritation caused by uterine diseases often acts, in conjunction with other causes (e. g., hereditary taint, defective nutrition, domestic trouble, etc.), in giving rise to mental disease.—*London Med. Record*, Nov. 15, 1878.

Hæmophilia or the Hemorrhagic Diathesis in Relation to Gynæcology.

The relation of hæmophilia, or the hemorrhagic diathesis, to gynæcology, is the subject of an article by Dr. E. BORNER, *docent* in the University of Gratz, published in the *Wiener Medicinische Wochenschrift* for August 17 and 31, September 7, 14, and 21. He refers also to an essay on the same subject, published by Kehrer in the *Archiv für Gynäkologie*, Band x.

After some preliminary remarks, Dr. Börner relates the case of a lady, Frau R., aged 52, who consulted him early last year on account of obstinate hemorrhage from the genital organs, and general weakness. She said that she had frequently suffered from great losses of blood, especially during labour. The introduction of the speculum was always attended with more or less hemorrhage. On making a very careful examination, Dr. Börner detected the blood oozing from the surface of the vaginal mucous membrane, as soon as the speculum came into contact with it; and on once slowly introducing an uterine sound, bleeding took place from the os uteri. Hemorrhage was also induced by simply applying the finger to the vaginal mucous membrane, and moving it to and fro.

A complete family history extending back beyond her parents could not be obtained, as she had left her native place at an early age. Her maternal grandmother and two of her mother's sisters died at an early age from some unknown cause. Frau R. had one brother and two sisters, one older and the other younger than herself. The brother had chest-disease, but was not a bleeder. The eldest sister was of healthy appearance when young, but after her marriage became pale, emaciated, and weak. Nothing special was known regarding her menses and confinements, but on one occasion she appears to have complained to Frau R. of having suffered from continuous and obstinate hemorrhage from the genital organs. She died, apparently of phthisis, at the age of 51. Of her five children, two died young; of the remaining three, two (a son and daughter) were healthy, the third (a son) was always ailing from an affection of the lungs. The youngest of the three sisters was also at first apparently healthy, but, after an early marriage, also became emaciated and pale. Nothing is known regarding her menses, but labour was always attended with dangerous flooding. Her husband also once stated that she daily had small discharges of blood from the genital organs. She died at the age of 32, of hemorrhage from the genitals, three months after an abortion which was accompanied by frightful bleeding. Her eight children—one male and seven females—are healthy.

Frau R. herself married at the age of 18, a month after the first appearance of the catamenia. She was weakly during childhood, but, after an attack of typhus at the age of 14, was in good health up to the time of her marriage. The act of coitus was from the first always attended with hemorrhage, which continued, though slightly, about twelve hours. She had no hemorrhage during any of her seven pregnancies, but the reverse was the case in her labours, regarding which the following account is given: *First labour*. After severe *post-partum* hemorrhage, accompanied with several attacks of syncope, a great discharge of blood continued up to the fourteenth day, and did not entirely cease until the end of the second week. *Second labour*. There was severe hemorrhage for four weeks; and it ceased gradually at the end of the seventh week. *Third labour*. The patient was confined to bed for two months by continued loss of blood. *Fourth labour*. On account of continuous hemorrhage, the christening of the child had to be put off for thirty weeks, and even then the mother could scarcely stand upright. *Fifth labour*. The patient had obstinate cough, with expectoration. She lay in bed three months, and bled nearly the whole time. *Sixth labour*. Rest in bed during two and a half months was necessary; the hemorrhage lasted six weeks. *Seventh labour*. The duration of the bleeding was six weeks. On each occasion remedies were tried, but apparently without effect. She suckled each of the first three children during twenty weeks. The application of the child to the breast was on each occasion followed by a discharge of blood from the genital organs, and the act of sucking was said to have also produced bleeding from the nipple. The menses reappeared generally in the fourth week after the cessation of the hemorrhage; they lasted three or four days, and were not extraordinarily profuse. It was also ascertained that she had been several times the subject of severe mental trouble, and that on each occasion there had been severe hemorrhage from the genital organs, which confined her to bed for some weeks.

The patient also presented other indications of the hemorrhagic diathesis. Dentition was attended with hemorrhage from the gums; so also was extraction of the teeth. For many years she had been subject to diarrhœa, which for the last eleven years had been attended with hemorrhage from the bowel. Pressure or a blow on the skin was always attended with ecchymosis. She had varices of both legs; and in rubbing one with her finger, in 1872, it burst, and gave rise to hemorrhage, which confined her to bed for three months.

Dr. Börner treated the patient by the introduction of cotton-wool, moistened with liquor ferri perchloridi, into the uterus, and washing the vagina with a very dilute solution of the perchloride. He also prescribed daily cold sitz-baths, and cold ablutions of the genital organs; iron and ergot were given internally, and a cooling diet and rest were ordered.

Regarding the patient's seven children, the following particulars were obtained. The first, a son, had good health, but was subject to severe epistaxis whenever he drank beer, and had very frequently also hemorrhage from the gums. The second, a son, suffered from rickets and hemorrhage from the skin; he died at the age of 5, after having vomited blood for four or five days. The third, a son, who is married and lives at a distance, is healthy, so far as is known. No disposition to bleeding was noticed during his childhood. The fourth, a son, aged 24, living in Gratz, suffered up to his sixth year from rickets; afterwards, he manifested a disposition to almost uncontrollable epistaxis, and to severe hemorrhage from the tongue, lips, and gums, on the slightest injury. The extraction of a tooth or a slight cut also gave rise to violent hemorrhage. The fifth, a girl, died suddenly at the age of 18. She is said to have been always pale and very liable to syncope. No disposition to bleeding was observed in her. The sixth, a girl, died in her seventh year from loss of blood. From a few days after birth she was the subject of numerous effusions of blood on the skin of the head, neck, back, and arms; commencing as small vesicles filled with blood, they burst, and caused exceedingly obstinate cutaneous hemorrhage. The seventh, a girl (now twelve years old) suffered when seven years years old from swollen cervical glands, the spontaneous bursting of which was followed by tedious hemorrhage.

She had frequent epistaxis, and bleeding from the gums was easily caused. As yet, there was no sign of hemorrhage from the genital organs.

After some further comments, in which he examines Kehrer's statements, and compares them with his own observations, Dr. Börner sums up as follows:—

1. It may be assumed with great probability that hæmophilia occurs in the female sex more frequently than has hitherto been believed; and that more accurate observations on this subject will cause the relative proportion between males and females which has hitherto been accepted, to undergo in time a change unfavourable to the female sex.

2. The cause of the error which has hitherto probably prevailed with regard to the numerical frequency of hæmophilia in the female sex, appears to us to be, that in girls the diathesis often remains to a certain extent latent, and is frequently first brought into action by fixed causes apparently connected with the period of reproductive activity. (If this be so, it follows that many individuals, who die before this period of other diseases, escape observation on this point; and, on the other hand, that many of the manifestations of the hemorrhagic diathesis occurring in pregnancy and labour and in the lying-in period are not recognized as such, but, in ignorance of the peculiar individual condition of the patient in question, are regarded as some one or other of the already familiar anomalies of the period.) How often may not, indeed, hemorrhage in a hæmophilic puerperal woman have been quoted as the result of defective involution of the uterus, or fatal flooding simply as the result of atony of the womb?

3. Of the different modes in which hæmophilia is manifested in the female sex, several are of special interest to the gynæcologist. We call special attention to some of these in the subsequent paragraphs, but pass by the hemorrhages occurring in early childhood, some of which probably belong to this category, but regarding which there is still a controversy. We also omit the bleedings from the genital organs of female infants (on this subject see Kehrer's work, p. 203).

4. The catamenia of hæmophilic individuals appear not to be normal as regards quantity. Sometimes there is menorrhagia, sometimes vicarious menstruation.

5. As has been already stated in Section 2, the most momentous time for hæmophilic females appears to be the reproductive period, since some of the events occurring in this epoch are the principal causes of the manifestation of the diathesis grounded in the individual, and often not recognized until now. It is also peenliarly the period in which the disease carries off most victims.

6. Coitus may be attended with much more serious results in the hæmophilic than in the healthy individual. Not only, in consequence of the diathesis, may the act be followed each time with slight or most profuse hemorrhage, but there is also the possibility of fatal bleeding.

7. During pregnancy, profuse metrorrhagia may arise from the diseased state under consideration. Kehrer's statements regarding his cases place this beyond doubt. His explanation is, that "in this diathesis, pregnancy gives rise to and maintains changes in the nutrition of the vessels which lead to the occurrence of the hemorrhages;" of this we want more accurate proof, and in the mean time we explain the fact of hemorrhage at this point simply by the local conditions present in every pregnancy, which, when the hemorrhagic diathesis is present, may readily cause hemorrhages.

8. There is no special disposition to premature interruption of pregnancy in hæmophilic women.

9. As may be easily understood, abortion is accompanied with severe hemorrhage in hæmophilic females.

10. The period following delivery is one of great importance to hæmophilic women. Here hemorrhages most frequently occur, which bring the patients into

extreme danger, or even cause death. Or the hemorrhage during the lying-in period may be less remarkable for intensity than for excessive duration, and may cause great weakness to the patient, if it do not lead to fatal anæmia.

11. As regards lactation, not only may this be accompanied each time by bleeding from the genitals, but the nipples themselves may be the seat of considerable hemorrhage.

12. Fissures of the nipple, which occasionally occur at this time, although much too small to be the source of the hemorrhage in question, are remarkable for the obstinate resistance which they offer to attempts at healing them.

13. The catamenia of hæmophilic individuals when they return after the lying-in period has passed, are generally normal as regards quantity.

14. The climacteric period may set in with violent hemorrhages; and thus on the one hand the completion of this epoch may be considerably prolonged, or, on the other hand, the hemorrhages occurring during the period may in many cases lead directly to a fatal termination.

15. Certain hemorrhages from the genital organs of hæmophilic individuals are of interest, which arise from causes that, as a rule, do not produce such an effect in healthy persons. Thus (among mechanical causes) hemorrhage from the uterus may be caused by simple digital examination, by the introduction of the speculum, by the mere shaking caused by walking, or by the most careful introduction of the uterine sound. Among psychical causes—anxiety, vexation, fright, etc.—may be followed by prolonged and often for a long time irrepressible hemorrhage.

16. As regards the condition of the genital organs, it is, so to speak, normal in pure cases of hæmophilia, even when there is very abundant hemorrhage. Like the other mucous membranes of such individuals, the genital mucous membrane presents an apparently excessive fineness of structure, with tendency to serous infiltration, and here and there considerable congestion.

17. A specially successful treatment of the disease is not yet at our command, and we are limited to the remedies ordinarily used in the treatment of other hemorrhages. Kehrer recommends the induction of premature labour as a means of providing against the eventuality of severe flooding in hæmophilic women; but on this point further information seems to be required.—*London Med. Record*, Nov. 15, 1878.

Medical Jurisprudence and Toxicology.

Carbolic Acid Poisoning.

Carbolic acid is having a hard time of it just now. The daily papers lately opened their columns to the insinuations of those who declared that it is practically useless as a disinfectant for general purposes, and so dangerous a poison and corrosive that its use ought to be restricted by law. On the other hand, some surgeons are abusing their best friend, because by absorption from the neighbourhood of wounds dressed with it antiseptically, poisonous symptoms—vomiting, severe collapse, and the discharge of dirty, dark-green urine—occasionally ensue.

We are not much concerned with the outcry raised a short time back by Mr. Wanklyn, because the length of time during which carbolic acid has held its own as a disinfectant is a sufficient proof that it has a real value, without referring to the exact experiments which have been made by various reliable authorities on

this point. There is no doubt whatever that carbolic acid is a poison and a corrosive, but other substances in common use are one or both of these—for example,
sulphuric acid, with which every housemaid and cook clean copper articles ; salts
of sorrel, with which the housewife removes her ink-stains ; and, not to prolong
the list, Burnett's disinfecting fluid, which is a solution of chloride of zinc. It
is certain also that people have been poisoned by taking carbolic acid in mistake
for harmless liquids, and more than one case has been quite recently reported ;
but is their number large, considering the widespread use of the acid as a disinfectant ? Its peculiar smell will, we believe, prevent more than occasional accidents due to hastiness, or, like the late Malta poisoning case, to gross and
unpardonable carelessness. The dangers of carbolic acid, as far as the public are
concerned, may, we suggest, be further diminished, if not entirely removed, by
colouring the commercial acid *blue*. At present it has a faint pink tinge, which
could easily be concealed. The advantage of blue over green or red, and especially the latter, is that there are no blue medicines, and no blue wines or spirits ;
whereas there are one or two green medicines, and many are intentionally coloured
red, while there are plenty of red wines, and one, if not more, green liqueurs.
It may be objected to this suggestion that blue carbolic acid would injure clothes,
etc., washed in it ; but no doubt some such indifferent blue might be used as
washerwomen already employ, and which is quite harmless. For sewage or
closet disinfection the colour of the acid, of course, makes no difference.

So much for the general indictment against carbolic acid—a body which has
probably saved, and is saving every day, more human lives than any other drugs,
except perhaps quinine and opium.

Let us now turn to the other part of the subject, to which, of course, the statement just made refers—the use of carbolic acid in antiseptic surgery. Are its
ill-effects here so great as to counterbalance its good ones ? In some cases certainly yes, as is proved, without going farther, by the attack of Professor Küster
and others on carbolic acid at the last Congress of German Surgeons at Berlin.
Possibly the slow progress which antiseptic surgery has yet made in this country
has something to do with our hearing fewer accusations against the acid here than
we do from Germany, where its reception has been enthusiastic to a degree which
must be very pleasing to Professor Lister. Perhaps, also, the greater use in
Germany of jute and other bandages soaked in aqueous carbolic acid solution has
made cases of poisoning by it there more frequent.

Anyhow, the results of the study of " carbolic acid intoxication," as it is called,
deserve our attention ; and we propose here to refer especially to the recent papers
of Dr. LANGENBUCH, of the Lazarus Hospital, Berlin,[1] and Dr. SONNENBURG,[2]
on the subject.

Both these writers agree that the dangers of carbolic acid are chiefly seen in
children and delicate woman. Healthy adults mainly suffer from nausea, vomiting, and headache ; while children get severe collapse, with subnormal temperatures of 36° to 34° Cent., scarcely perceptible pulse, pallor and cold sweat, and
which may be preceded by a rise of temperature to 39° Cent., with restlessness
and excitement. This condition may end in death, as in a case of Dr. Langenbuch's, where a girl of five years, who had had an abscess connected with the
hip-joint opened and dressed antiseptically, died within forty-eight hours of undoubted carbolic acid collapse. Hence it is just in this class of cases that it is of

---

[1] " Klinischer Beitrag zur Lehre von der Carbol-intoxication," Berliner Klin.
Woch., No. 28, 1878.

[2] " Zur Diagnose und Therapie der Carbol-intoxication," Deutsche Zeit. für Chir.,
IX., 356.

impoitance to be able to find out early whethei caibolic acid poisoning is setting in or not; and the ieseaiches of Baumann and Herter (*Zeitschrift füi Phys. Chemie.*, i.) have shown that, *pai i passu* with its onset, the salts of sulphuiic acid disappeai fiom the uiine, until when the poisonous symptoms ieach theii height not a tiace of them is piesent. At the same time the quantity of associated sulphuiic acid (*gepaarte Schwefelsaüre*) is consideiably incieased. To detect the diminution of sulphates in the uiine it is only necessaiy to iemove any albumen piesent by boiling, to acidify with acetic acid, and add chloiide of baiium in excess. This ieagent gives a milky cloud of sulphate of baiium in the piesence of sulphates, but a meie haze oi no alteiation at all if theie is caibolic acid poisoning. Baumann has fuithei shown that if sulphate of soda is inteinally administered to an animal whose system contains caibolic acid a haimless phenol-sulphuiic acid is pioduced, so that that salt or any othei soluble sulphate is a diiect chemical antidote to caibolic acid. Sonnenbuig fuithei finds by experiments on men that not only do the symptoms of caibolic acid poisoning disappear moie quickly if sulphate of soda is administeied, but also that if this salt is at once given when the uiine becomes daik-colouied, it exeits such an influence in iestiaining the fuithei outbieak of poisonous symptoms that it is possible, unless theie is great individual sensitiveness to caibolic acid, to continue the diessing as befoie. No doubt, howevei, it is bettei to manage the diessing so that theie shall be no caibolic poisoning, and Dr. Langenbuch suggests the following measuies which he has himself tested foi doing this. When dealing with childien and delicate women he avoids much pievious disinfection of the skin by iubbing and brushing, and tiusts to the spiay duiing the opeiation foi disinfection. He then wiaps the skin of the paits iound the field of opeiation in gutta-peicha tissue which has pieviously lain in 5 per cent. caibolic solution, and been carefully fieed fiom excess of acid just befoie use by washing in 1 pei cent. aqueous caibolic acid. The tissue adapts itself closely to the skin, and is peifectly fiee fiom iiiitating pioperties; hence it may be allowed to iemain duiing the whole tieatment, its object being to piotect as much of the skin as possible fiom contact with the caibolic acid of the diessing. This diessing consists fiist of seveial layeis of cotton-wool, and then of pieces of jute, both fiist disinfected in 5 pei cent., and thoioughly washed out in 1 pei cent. caibolic solution befoie using. The whole is fixed with gauze bandages wetted with 2 pei cent. solution, and an elastic and veiy loosely diawn antiseptic bandage goes over all. Fiom time to time the whole diessing is modeiately moistened with caibolic solution, and it is kept wiapped up in a laige India-iubbei cloth.

Since the adoption of this modified method, Dr. Langenbuch states that "the *entiente coidiale* between himself and caibolic acid has been completely iestoied." The dangei with aqueous solutions of caibolic acid appeais to aiise moie fiom absoiption thiough the skin, especially by way of the sweat-ducts, than thiough the suiface of the wound, which is piobably piotected by the coagulation of seium-albumen by the acid. Possibly by soaking the diessings in caibolic oil, as Mi. Howse has long done at Guy's Hospital,[1] we may obviate the unpleasant consequences attending the use of wateiy solutions. We all know that the skin and the system at laige will toleiate a 10 pei cent. caibolic oil even ovei a toleiably wide surface, so that piobably the acid does not peimeate the skin so fieely in this foim. In any case the obseivations of Langenbuch, Baumann, and Sonnenbuig aie veiy inteiesting and instructive.—*Med. Times and Gazette*, Oct. 19, 1878.

---

[1] Guy's Hospital Repoits, 1878, page 270.

CONTENTS.

Published Monthly, price $2.50 per annum, free of postage.
Also, furnished together with the AMERICAN JOURNAL OF THE MEDICAL SCIENCES *and the* MEDICAL NEWS AND LIBRARY *for* SIX DOLLARS *per annum in advance, the whole free of postage.*

HENRY C. LEA, Philadelphia.

THE MONTHLY ABSTRACT

OF

MEDICAL SCIENCE.

VOL. VI. No. 2.   **For List of Contents see last page.**   FEBRUARY, 1879.

Anatomy and Physiology.

An Interesting Malformation of the Foot.

In the *Berliner Klinische Wochenschrift*, for August 26, Dr. BRUDI gives the following account of a malformation which he observed in the foot of an artillery-man under his care in hospital :—

On the great toe of the left foot, in the angle between the inner and posterior borders of the nail, is a tumor of the size of a thumb-nail, attached by a short, thick, scarcely movable pedicle. Half of the swelling extends over the nail, the other half reaches onwards beyond it. It is covered by a somewhat red but normal skin. At the peripheral end an articulation is distinctly recognized, and on closer examination it is seen to represent in miniature a perfectly formed third foot. Not only are there five small toes, but each toe is provided with a distinct nail; those on the first three toes especially are well developed; the fourth and fifth toes are united.

The little foot is a right one. The greatest length, from the pedicle to the point of the great toe, is 17 *millimetres* ($\frac{67}{100}$ths of an inch); the length gradually decreases, until at the little toe it is only a few *millimetres*. The first three toes are on the average 4 *millimetres* ($\frac{16}{100}$ths of an inch) long; the fourth and fifth are somewhat shorter. The part corresponding to the metatarsus is 15 *millimetres* (0.6 inch) in its greatest width, and passes without sharply defined limit into the very short pedicle, which is 6 *centimetres* wide and 14 in circumference. The whole is moderately movable, and the skin is firm. No trace of bones or joints can be felt.

Whenever the man cuts the nail of his great toe he is obliged to support the small foot, as it would otherwise impede him. He arrived spontaneously at the conclusion "that he must certainly have three feet." The accessory foot gives him no trouble whatever, and does not in the least interfere with the discharge of his duty as a gunner. His upper extremities are perfectly normal. The malformation is congenital, and nothing similar is known to exist in the family.—*London Med. Record*, Dec. 15, 1878.

Materia Medica and Therapeutics.

Coffee.

Professor BINZ has been investigating the action of the constituents of coffee, which he finds possess a certain antagonism to the action of quinine. He injected beneath the skin of a strong dog .7 gramme of caffein, and the temperature in an

1our rose a degree Centigrade. With smaller doses (.2 grm.) t1e rise is slig1ter .3° C.), and after large doses (about .5 grm.) t1e elevation may be as muc1 as 1.4° C., wit1out t1ere being any ot1er disturbance obvious, except a somew1at stiff condition of t1e animal's muscles. Large doses also caused a considerable elevation of temperature, and deat1, wit1 convulsive symptoms. T1is effect of caffein was 1indered by curara and by artificial respiration. It was also found t1at moderate doses of caffein raised t1e blood pressure, t1e dogs employed for t1e experiment being only narcotized by alco1ol, and neit1er curara nor artificial respiration being employed. Section of t1e vagus did not interfere wit1 t1is result, and t1e elevation of t1e blood-pressure is t1us not due to an influence exerted t1roug1 t1e vagus.

Bontron and Frémy gave t1e term caffeon to a substance produced by roasting t1e coffee beans, and separating from a distillate wit1 et1er. It is an et1ereal oily substance, and is found by Binz to 1ave a stimulating action on t1e brain, 1eart, respiration, and animal 1eat. He agrees wit1 Hoppe-Seyler and Voit, t1at t1e infusion of coffee or caffein in dietetic doses causes an increase rat1er t1an a decrease of t1e tissue c1anges.—*Lancet*, Oct. 12, 1878.

Batiator Root: a Substitute for Ipecacuanha.

1. STANISLAS 1ARTIN (*L' Union Pharmaceutique*, No. 8) gives a description of t1is root, w1ic1 is derived from a plant growing in Senegal. Seeds of it 1ave been planted in t1e 1useum of Natural History at P_{aris}, from w1ic1 t1e plant will 1ereafter be determined. T1e root is identical in its effects wit1 ipecacuan1a in t1e same doses.—*London Med. Record*, Dec. 15, 1878.

The Therapeutic Effects of Bryony, Drosera, Gelsemium Sempervirens, and Cayepona Globulosa.

Dr. LOUVET-LAMARE 1as publis1ed in t1e *Année Médicale de Caen* (June, 1878), some interesting observations on t1e effects of bryony and drosera in w1ooping-coug1. In t1e first stage of t1e disease 1e administers tincture of bryony, in daily doses of fifteen minims, to c1ildren aged seven years; and states t1at it very quickly diminis1es t1e bronc1itis, stimulates t1e appetite, and does not create nausea. T1is plant seems to possess astringent properties, as is s1own in t1e remark made by Barbier in 1is *Materia Medica*, vol. iii., w1ere 1e says t1at t1e peasant women are in t1e 1abit of taking, during some days, enemata made wit1 t1e roots of bryony, w1en t1ey cease to nurse t1eir babies, and wis1 to prevent t1e secretion of milk in t1e mammæ.

Drosera 1as proved very efficient w1en w1ooping-coug1 1as reac1ed t1e parox-ysmal stage. It was also employed formerly against dropsy and disease of t1e lungs, and is said to 1ave been used wit1 apparent success in p1t1isis.

Gelsemium sempervirens is a very powerful sedative in cases of neuralgia, especially if t1e latter be not complicated by local congestions. It is very efficient in neuralgia of t1e upper parts of t1e body, but loses some of its power in t1e lower parts of t1e latter. E. g., neuralgia of t1e face and t1e teet1 are speedily removed by it; t1en follow, classed as to t1e power of resisting t1e power of t1e drug, neuralgia of t1e brac1ial plexus, of t1e intercostal, ilio-lumbar, crural, and isc1iatic nerves. It 1as also been used wit1 great success in 1emicrania. Gelse-mium is dispensed in pills or in t1e form of a tincture, t1e dose of w1ic1 varies from fifteen drops a day to ninety drops. T1e effects of t1is drug must be care-fully watc1ed, because it is apt, especially if taken in too large quantities, to produce symptoms of poisoning, w1ic1 first s1ow t1emselves in t1e eyes. The patients complain of giddiness, t1eir upper eyelids 1ave an irresistible tendency to drop. and when lifted up with the finger the objects appear double; at the same time, a strong sensation of weakness and pricking is felt in the arms. A subcutaneous injection of morphia has, however, always proved a good antidote and removed the alarming symptoms.

The cayopona globulosa is found in Brazil. It is a very powerful drastic, and much used in veterinary medicine. An alkaloid, cayaponine, has been extracted from it, which contains the efficient parts of the plant. Experiments have been made with this substance in the form of a solution; if swallowed, it produced very copious and repeated evacuations, but without any pain in the bowels. When injected under the skin it caused a very large and painful swelling, which was surrounded by a network of smaller swellings, radiating from the centre, and apparently produced by some irritation of the lymphatic vessels. There was not the least trace of any drastic effect in this case.—*London Med. Record*, Dec. 15, 1878.

—

The Therapeutic Effects of Iodine contained in Human Milk.

Dr. LAZANSKY (*Vierteljahrsschrift für Derm. und Syph.*, Band v.) has lately made experiments on the effects of human milk which contained iodine. One gramme of iodide of potassium was administered daily to a syphilitic woman who was nursing a baby, aged five months, suffering from the same disease. The iodine could be traced to the mother's milk and urine on the same day, but only on the next morning in the baby's urine. The effect on both mother and child was remarkably good. Iodine does not in the least affect the secretion of milk.—*London Med. Record*, Dec. 15, 1878.

—

On the Action of Iodoform.

Dr. ZEISSL relates (*Wiener Medizinische Wochenschrift*, No. 21, 1878) his experience of the remarkably favourable results of the use of iodoform in venereal sores. He uses a powder for sprinkling the part, consisting of 7 centigrammes (little more than a grain) of iodoform in 5 grammes (75 grains) of sugar of milk. For internal use, he employs the following formula: iodoform, 1.5 gramme (22 grains); white sugar, 3 grammes (45 grains); to be divided into twenty powders, of which one is taken thrice daily. He recommends this especially in the neuralgic affections of syphilis; it has been proved also very useful in certain cases of ordinary neuralgia.—*London Med. Record*, Dec. 15, 1878.

—

Chloral Plaster.

M. YVON (*Bulletin de Therapeutique*) has taken advantage of the fluidifying effect of camphor on chloral-hydrate to make a plaster, the formula for which is as follows: Chloral, 5 grammes; camphor, 15 centigrammes; gum-tragacanth, 20 centigrammes; glycerin, 2 or 3 drops; starch, 5 or 2½ grammes. This, when applied to the dry skin, produces a blister in twelve hours; but, after the escape of the serum, a superficial eschar is formed. If the skin were slightly moistened before the application, a burning sensation was produced in a short time, and an eschar like that of a burn was formed. Yvon contends that chloral hydrate may act as an irritant, but that it is very uncertain and difficult to control. On the other hand, he recommends as a good local irritant a mixture of 15 grammes (232 grains) of chloral, 59 centimetres (7½ grains) of camphor, one gramme (15½ grains) of chloral-hydrate, and 2 or 3 drops of water.—*London Med. Record*, Dec. 15, 1878.

On Chloral as a Local Revulsive.

Dr. PEYRAUD describes the local action of chloral in an article in the *Bulletin de Thérapeutique*. In the case of a patient to whom he applied the chloral on cotton-wool to the temple for the relief of neuralgia, a burn of the third degree was formed in thirty or forty minutes. Dr. Peyraud then mixed chloral with gum-tragacanth, spread it on paper, and applied it to his own arm. In twelve hours a blister was formed, without any pain; the same result was found in several patients to whom the chloralized paper was applied. The absence of pain depends upon the chloral being mixed as above, if applied in powder; strewed on plaster or cotton-wool, it produces painful burning. The blister does not rise until the chloral plaster has been removed for an hour or more.

Dr. Peyraud also observed evidence that the chloral was absorbed by the skin. After the application, several of the patients fell into a deep sleep; and the same occurred to Dr. Peyraud himself when the surface to which the chloral was applied was external. This hypnotic effect often precedes the revulsive action. The blisters are less distinct the more concentrated the application is; the vesication is less constant than that produced by cantharides. The suppuration lasts about five or seven days. Dr. Peyraud recommends the chloral paper as a mild and painless application.—*London Med. Record*, Dec. 15, 1878.

On Vaginal Suppositories.

N. E. RENNARD (*Pharmaceutische Zeitschrift für Russland*, Nos. 14–15) says that these are mostly prepared by melting together the required ingredients and pouring them into suitable forms, in order to let the mass solidify. A very good vehicle is a mixture of water, gelatin, and glycerin, which will, however, only retain its transparency if the water be all evaporated off. The proportion is one part of gelatin to six of glycerin, which may require modification according to the concentration of the glycerin, the weather, or the other ingredients. Almost all substances may be incorporated with this mass, without undergoing alteration ; only tannin enters into an insoluble compound with gelatin.

An admirable substitute for the latter is *agar-agar*. This is a species of gelatin prepared in Japan from various algæ, chiefly *Fucus Amansii*, which is free from nitrogen, occurs in the market in quill-shaped shreds, and is used exactly like animal gelatin. It absorbs a very large quantity of water, one part of it still yielding a tolerably solid jelly with 60–70 parts of water. According to Professor E. Reichardt, of Jena, agar-agar consists of pararabin, a carbohydrate, which is also valuable as a nutriment. It dissolves in boiling water, and yields arabic acid after sufficient digestion with alkali.

To prepare vaginal suppositories, a jelly is made from one part of agar-agar and thirty of water. This, however, has a turbid milky look. If it be desired transparent, the mixture should contain one part of agar-agar, ten parts of glycerin, and twenty parts of water. The agar-agar is allowed to soak in water over night, of which it takes up about twenty parts; it is then heated until liquid, and the glycerin added. With glycerin alone it forms no jelly, but a tough transparent mass. Any desired quantity of tannin may be added to the jelly, without being rendered insoluble.—*London Med. Record*, Dec. 15, 1878.

The Use of Sulphuret of Carbon in Dressing Wounds.

N. MAUREL read a paper at the meeting of the Société de Thérapeutique on June 12 (*Gazette Hebdomadaire*) on the employment of sulphuret of carbon in dressing wounds. He says that a solution of gutta-percha in sulphuret of carbon may be of service in exceptional cases. One serious inconvenience, however, arises from the fact that after several dressings, excoriations are produced around the wound. This always limits the use of it, especially in dressing erysipelatous wounds. During his long residence in Guiana, M. Maurel never observed that the sulphuret of carbon had any marked action on ulcers of a bad nature. He found that compresses steeped in a solution of gutta-percha do not become rigid enough to be used as an immovable apparatus.—*London Med. Record*, Dec. 15, 1878.

On the Antiseptic Method.

When Prof. LISTER was in Paris in the summer he addressed an oral communication upon this subject to the Paris Société de Chirurgie, and we reproduce from the last number of the *Bulletin* of the Society the succinct and interesting statement which he then made.

Several members of the Society having expressed a wish to hear some observations upon the antiseptic method, I feel great pleasure in complying with their desire.

Union by the first intention is no new thing, and when surgeons attempt it for small wounds, as in hare-lip, they do not always obtain it. The object of the antiseptic method is to obtain it as the ordinary result, and to accomplish cures which, without it, they could not hope for. Let us take, for example, cold abscesses. If we do not open them, no inconvenience arises, except from their size. If we open them by small incisions, fever supervenes, with accidents of putridity leading to hectic and death. If to avoid this danger we practice punctures with aspiration, in the majority of cases the pus will form again, the operation has frequently to be had recourse to again, and the patient is not cured. But it will be entirely otherwise if the abscess be largely opened, if a drainage-tube be inserted to obtain a free issue of the discharge, and if, after having operated by the antiseptic method, we apply a good antiseptic dressing which is continued with great care until the cure is complete. The first results obtained are a cessation of the fever and the production of a serous discharge, which becomes so slight in a few days as to require the dressing only to be changed once a week. If with this mode of dressing we combine the precaution of insisting upon the horizontal position being kept, we may effect the complete and radical cure of our patients. I have, thanks to this treatment, obtained an absolute cure in a great number of cases, in some of which there have been caries and sequestra of the bodies of the vertebræ. This is a result which, it appears to me, it would be difficult to obtain by any other mode of treatment.

The pyogenic membrane of these congestive abscesses does not produce pus unless it is irritated. Prior to the opening of the abscess there is an irritative tension produced by the accumulation of pus; and if we open the abscess without antiseptic treatment, we relieve the pressure, but we introduce another cause of irritation—putrefaction. Prior to opening the abscess, inflammation of the bone and then the tension induce suppuration; and after opening, putrefaction acts in the same way. If we suppress these causes of suppuration, and also suppress the mechanical irritation produced by the vertical position, these lesions are found to differ in nowise from other inflammations—the inflammation ceasing when the cause of external irritation has disappeared.

During the first days after the formation of a wound there is no pus, whatever kind of dressing may be employed; but some days after we find pus and granulations which have preceded the pus; for when granulations have formed there is, as in the cavities of cysts, no tendency to suppurate unless irritation is present. Thus, in Reverdin's method of skin-grafting, if we place a graft on a granulating surface, graft and granulations unite by the first intention. Granulations, then, do not possess the property of forming pus. The epidermic graft acts as a dressing protective against all irritants ; and when a granulating surface is thus protected, it ceases to furnish pus or even serum. If we employ a topical antiseptic, as chloride of zinc or carbolic acid, pus and granulations are produced ; but if between the antiseptic and a recent wound we place a non-irritant substance capable of protecting the wound from the irritation of the antiseptic, no suppuration will be produced. If in large, deep, and widely separated wounds, filled with coagula of blood, we place a portion of protective substance and over this the antiseptic, the coagula do not putrefy and there is no suppuration. On removing the upper layer of the coagulum we find a cicatrized surface, without suppuration and even without granulation. As yet we have not been able to obtain a protective sufficiently perfect to avoid all suppuration from a wound covered with granulations, but we are able greatly to diminish its abundance. Antiseptics, then, exert a direct action on the tissues, and at the commencement of my researches I was much astonished at finding pus, even when the causes of putrefaction were kept at a distance—the antiseptics themselves inducing irritation of the wound.

Putrefied substances are irritating, and if antiseptics are capable of developing suppuration, how much more will this be the case with substances in a state of putrefaction ! But a great difference is to be observed here—irritation from the antiseptic only acting upon the point with which it is in contact ; while putrefaction, being fermentation, extends wherever there is the material capable of serving as alimentation for the vibriones. Thus, we may admit three causes of suppuration, one proceeding from inflammation without putrefaction, the second produced by the irritation of antiseptics, and the third caused by substances in a state of putrefaction.

I do not wish to enter into all the details of the dressing, but I am desirous of giving some account of the employment of the protective. This, which is nothing but a piece of varnished tissue, does not possess any antiseptic property, and if it is dipped in carbolized water prior to its application, this is only in case any septic body may exist on its surface having a tendency to mix with the pus. But the carbolic acid thus existing in small quantity on its surface rapidly disappears ; and unless it did so the protective would become irritating and its application meaningless, as its office is to shelter the wound from the irritation of the antiseptic. An important point, to which I cannot draw too much attention, is not to allow the protective to pass beyond the dressing, as the causes of putrefaction might penetrate beneath it. The antiseptic dressing must on every side project beyond the protective, as if this were the wound itself. If some rags dipped in a carbolized solution were only employed as an antiseptic dressing, and the discharge was very abundant, putrefaction would take place in twenty-four hours, because the liquid proceeding from the wound rapidly displaces the antiseptic, the wound being then no longer preserved. It is therefore indispensable that, whatever substance may be employed, there must be for it a kind of receptacle holding the antiseptic substance in reserve. On this subject allow me to allude to a point to which attention has been drawn by my late colleague Sir Robert Christison, namely, that the force of action of a medicinal agent in solution does not depend alone upon the quantity of this dissolved, but also on the manner in which it comports itself with the vehicle. Thus, water having but little affinity with carbolic acid, and oil a much greater affinity, an aqueous solution of a twentieth of carbolic acid is almost caustic, while the irritating action is much less strong with a tenth in oil, and if we employ resin a mixture of a fifth is almost insipid. For the purpose of cleansing an instrument or the hands, we resort to the aqueous solution, the action of which is strong but temporary ; but for a dressing intended to remain on for some days it is necessary to employ a vehicle which has more affinity for the acid. With this the discharge may traverse the dressing without removing all the antiseptic which is held in reserve. It is with a mixture of carbolic acid and resin (to which some paraffin is added to render it less agglutinative) that the gauze is prepared which is the true receptive of the antiseptic. The discharge cannot remove the resin, which strongly retains the carbolic acid. Besides the protective and the gauze there is also the macintosh, the object of which is the prevention of the direct passage of the liquids of the wound through the dressing, and also the increase of the antiseptic effects of the gauze. When a dressing has been left on for several days after application, sometimes it becomes displaced in consequence of the movements of the patient, especially in cases of cold abscess; and in order to obviate this inconvenience I place an elastic bandage around the edges of the dressing, and which may be applied with a certain amount of force without inconvenience and without obstruction to the circulation. For superficial wounds I sometimes employ boric acid instead of carbolic; and in order to obtain boric lint I dip lint into a boiling solution of boric acid, and thus procure a rich antiseptic receptacle. This mode of dressing has furnished excellent results in ulcers of the leg. I first purify the surrounding epidermic surfaces by means of a carbolic solution (one in twenty) which thoroughly penetrates the epidermis and purifies even the hair follicles. When gangrene exists on the granulating surface of the ulcer, it is necessary to apply something stronger than carbolic acid; and until of late I made use of the chloride of zinc, but as this, when the wound is large, has the inconvenience of inducing very severe pain, I have replaced it by iodoform. After the wound has been washed with carbolic acid solution, the iodoform powder is applied, then the protective, the boric lint which covers this extending beyond its margin on every side. There is very little suppuration, and after two or three daily dressings these may be left on without removal for several days. The protective has a double object—the preventing the direct irritation of the antiseptic, and the maintaining the surface of the wound in a constant state of humidity, which prevents the formation of a crust under which pus might accumulate and cause, through tension, inflammatory suppuration. If the formation of these crusts were not avoided by means of the protective when the dressing was removed, the epidermic layer of latest formation might be easily torn off. I also employ chloride of zinc for a special action it exerts. A single application of a solution of one-twelfth prevents putrefaction in a wound, even when the causes of putrefaction cannot be removed. Thus, after amputation of the tongue, if the wound be touched with it a single time, no odour will arise until granulations appear. There must certainly be a layer of mortified tissue, but it must be almost microscopic, since it is not appreciable, and does not prevent union by the first intention. Chloride of zinc may preserve wounds from putrefaction in cases in which it would seem difficult to avoid it, such as those of cystotomy and fistula in ano. In cases in which I am unable to remove all the fistulous tracks, I scrape them with a curette, and apply the chloride with excellent results. If putrefaction supervenes, it does not appear until after three or four days, and the patient is protected, at least during the earlier period, from the accidents of infection.

In answer to some observations by M. Desprès, who stated that he believed Prof. Lister would still meet with relapses in the cases of cold abscess dependent on disease of bone which he supposed to be definitely cured, Mr. Lister replied that he regretted not being able to exhibit the patients who, having reached the last stage of hectic fever, immediately after the application of the antiseptic treatment found it disappear. He did not mean to assert that relapse never took place, but he affirmed that in the majority of cases a definite cure was obtained.

In order tıat relapses may be avoided, tıe patients must be prevented from getting up. Wıen tıe fistulous openings ıave become cicatrized, repose for six or
seven weeks must still be exacted, wıen a quarter of an ıour's walking may be
allowed. If pain is produced, rest must again be insisted upon, awaiting a new
attempt.—*Med. Times and Gaz.*, Nov. 2, 1878.

Medicine.

On the Local Treatment of Meningitis.

Dr. Ɔ OSLER (*Deutsche Medicinische Wochenschrift*, 1878, Nos. 23, 24, and
Centralblatt für die Medicinischen Wissenschaften, Nov. 23) describes tıe case
of a young man, aged 27, who ıad for six weeks been suffering from a very severe
attack of articular rıeumatism. In tıe seventı week tıe pain and swelling hàd
abated in tıe joints, but tıe patient sıowed symptoms of cerebral meningitis combined witı constant fever. Blisters were immediately applied to tıe crown of
tıe ıead, wıicı had been previously sıaven, and beıind tıe ears ; tıe dangerous
symptoms soon disappeared and tıe patient's ıealtı was rapidly restored. Tıe
autıor explains tıe effect of tıe blisters from tıe fact, wıicı ıas been proved by
experiments, tıat tıe volume of blood contained in tıe brain is greatly lessened
by irritants applied to tıe skin.—*London Med. Record*, Dec. 15, 1878.

Frequency and Etiology of Epilepsy.

Dr. BERGER (*Deutsch. Zeitschrift für Prakt. Med.*, 1878, No. 21 ; and *Centralblatt f. d. Med. Wiss.*, No. 46) ıas ıad tıe opportunity of studying 105 cases of
epilepsy, wıicı ıave partly come under ıis own observation and partly been collected by otıers ; and gives tıe following statements on tıe frequency and etiology
of tıe disease. In 65.93 per cent. of tıe cases, the disease first sıowed itself in
tıe time between infancy and tıe twentietı year ; but mucı more frequently tıan
ıas been accepted ıitıerto during tıe first four years of cıildıood. Tıe female
sex is particularly exposed to it at tıe age of fifteen to twenty, and tıe male sex
in tıe years between tıirty and forty. Tıis difference may be explained by tıe
beginning of puberty in women and by tıe excesses committed by men at tıat
time. Tıe cessation of tıe menses has not tıe least influence on epilepsy, wıicı
very seldom appears for tıe first time in old age. Dr. Berger observed it once
in an old woman aged seventy-four, in wıom, after ıaving been perfectly well
all ıer life, tıe first attack of tıis disease was produced by a very violent frigıt.
Epilepsy is often ıereditary, as tıe autıor ıas distinctly traced in 23 cases out of
71 wıicı ıe ıad studied for tıe purpose of elucidating tıe question. He has
never observed tıe first outbreak of tıe disease occur eitıer before tıe beginning
of puberty or after tıe tıirtietı year. In botı sexes, and especially in women,
epilepsia gravior is tıe most common form. Tıe autıor gives a series of observations on tıe etiology of epilepsy, wıicı tend to illustrate tıe different experiments tıat ıave been made to produce epilepsy artificially. Tıe following were
tıe principal causes. A traumatic affection of tıe median nerve caused epilepsy
in a man ; disturbances of tıe sexual organs in women ıad tıe same effect. (One
was a case of hæmelytrometra, wıicı was subsequently operated on ; tıe otıer,
cessation of tıe menses caused by a severe cold.) Four cases may be classed

under the head of epilepsy caused by injury. The patients (three male, one female) had sustained injuries to the head, either through a blow, fall, or box on the ear, and the disease subsequently manifested itself either directly afterwards, or after weeks or even months had elapsed, while in the mean time the only thing the patients complained of occasionally were diffused headaches. The next cases belong to the form of epilepsy caused by affection of the cortical substance, especially in syphilitic persons (according to Fournier, Charcot, and others). Among these, he gives a very full description of a case of epilepsy in a man aged thirty-eight, who had been several times under treatment for syphilis, and who was subject to epileptiform attacks that did not differ in the least from general epilepsy. He was cured by a very energetic anti-syphilitic treatment. Two further cases recorded describe vaso-motor epilepsy in a girl aged nineteen, and a very interesting case of epilepsia gravior occurring also in a girl aged nineteen after poisoning with carbonic acid. In the treatment of the disease, the author has used several methods with varying success. Hystero-epileptic patients were the only ones that derived any benefit from Chapman's method of application of ice or cold water to different parts of the body; true epilepsy was never cured either by this method or by electricity. In vaso-motor epilepsy, the constant current proved very useful. Some authors have highly commended the effects of bromide of camphor and bromate of zinc; but Dr. Berger does not agree with them; neither has he seen any satisfactory results produced by atropin and curare; nitrite of amyl, if inhaled in time, sometimes proved efficient in cutting short the paroxysm. The most favourable result has been caused by bromide of potassium, if given in large doses (from six to twelve *grammes*, equal to one and a half to three drachms, daily); the disease sometimes only manifested itself again after two years, but it never was completely cured. Bromal-hydrate has a similar effect to that of bromide of potassium (Steinauer).—*British Medical Journal*, Dec. 7, 1878.

The Differential Diagnosis between true Epilepsy and Hystero-Epilepsy.

M. CHARCOT (*Gazette des Hôpitaux*, 1878, No. 49) says that true epilepsy develops itself, after only a short aura, in the form of tonic and clonic spasms accompanied by marked stertor. The convulsive stage of the hysterical paroxysm is preceded, after an aura lasting one, two, or even several days, by a peculiar, prolonged cry; this is followed by violent, purposeless, fantastic movements, clonic spasms, and great psychic excitement, perhaps even delirium; but none of these symptoms are accompanied by the slightest signs of stertor.—*London Med. Record*, Dec. 15, 1878.

On Myelitis.

Messrs. PROUST and JOFFROY drew the following conclusions (*Revue Mensuelle*, April 8, 1878) from a case which they observed, in which acute myelitis began with an apoplectiform attack, and also from some cases selected from books. 1. Acute myelitis often begins suddenly. Formerly this was called a primary "hæmatomyélie." This has not been confirmed, however, in the more recent observations, so that apoplectiform paraplegia must be classed with myelitis. 2. The fall which sometimes occurs as the first symptoms of apoplectiform myelitis might be mistaken for the cause, whereas it only represents the first striking indication of the disease. 3. The changes in the constituent elements of the spinal cord consists chiefly of hypertrophy of the axis-cylinder, and of hypertrophy, with subsequent atrophy and granular pigmentation of the nerve-cells. The very considerable increase of the intercellular substance of the gray matter is little marked near the inflamed parts in the white substance, consequently the form of myelitis is as much interstitial as parenchymatous.—*London Med. Record*, Dec. 15, 1878.

A Case of Spastic Spinal Paralysis ending in Recovery.

One of the many undetermined points connected with the disease described by Erb under the name of spastic spinal paralysis (tabes spasmodica, Charcot) relates to the prognosis. Erb believes recovery to be extremely rare, though less so than in other forms of chronic spinal paralysis. Charcot refused to believe in the possibility of recovery from the disease. Westphal has published one case in which complete recovery took place. In Dr. Kussmaul's Klinik at Strasburg, Dr. REINHARD VON DER VELDEN observed the present case (*Berliner Klinische Wochenshrift*, September 23, 1878); it is distinguished from Westphal's by the acute onset of the disease, and the rapidity with which all the characteristic symptoms were developed.

E. P., aged 27, clerk, had a good family history, and had enjoyed good health, with the exception of a short indefinite illness at seven years of age. No traces of syphilitic infection could be discovered. Slight kypho-scoliosis was present, which, the patient said, dated from birth. Two days before admission, he attempted suicide by jumping into a river; after being rescued, he walked several miles home in his wet clothes, exposed to a high wind, and went to bed. Next day, he complained of pains in the abdomen, and gastric troubles.

On admission, on May 13th, the tongue was coated, and the abdomen somewhat hard and full. There were no other objective symptoms. He had no appetite. There was no constipation. Temperature, 100.9; pulse, 82; respiration, 14. Castor-oil was ordered.

May 14. He had excessive perspiration during the night; no abdominal pain, but a feeling of pressure on the chest. There were no other physical signs, no fever.

17th. He had pains in the region of the bladder, and dragging pains in the testicles. His appetite was good; the alvine secretions were natural. He looked pale and anxious, and refused to get up.

18th. The patient was small and anæmic, with weak muscular development, but was moderately fat. He complained of a peculiar stiffness in the legs, which he first noticed the preceding evening. He had no pain, and slept well. No disturbances of circulation, respiration, or digestion were present. On being lifted out of bed he was unable to walk; he could hardly move one leg before the other, and could not flex either knee or ankle. Both legs were stiffly extended by a spastic contraction of all the muscles. A slight tremor was also observable in them. The spasms became more intense while the patient stood, and he was thrown more and more forwards upon his toes. When supported on both sides and taken along the ward, he either let both his legs drag stiffly after him, or attempted, by means of the pelvic muscles, to swing them round alternately.

On being replaced in bed, the muscles of both lower extremities were seen to be strongly contracted, and in a state of constant tremor; the latter, however, gradually passed off when the patient was left quiet and became warm in bed. All movements could be performed, but only very slowly. Passive movement of the limbs met with moderate resistance. After about half an hour the spasm also became less severe; movement was easier, but weakness was still evident. No pain was caused by pressure on the spine. There was no disturbance of sensation; neither trophic nor vasomotor symptoms could be discovered; the sphincters were unaffected; the intellect was clear; there was no vertigo nor inequality of the pupils. There was neither albumen nor sugar in the urine.

23*d.* The patient stated that when he was warm in bed, his legs neither trembled nor were stiff, but that he could only lift them a very slight distance; he could not cross one over the other. The attacks of rigidity and tremor occurred two or three times daily, sometimes spontaneously, and sometimes in consequence of external causes. During a strong attack the patient would perspire freely, and afterwards feel quite exhausted. Strong pressure upon the crural nerve during an attack caused the muscular spasm to cease in the leg of the same side, but to become more powerful in the other. By dint of great exertion the patient was able very slowly to flex either of his legs during the period of spasm; as soon, however, as the leg and thigh were inclined to one another at an angle of about 45°, the muscular resistance to the movement suddenly ceased, and the heel was brought with considerable force against the nates. The whole phenomenon very much resembled the sudden closure of a pen-knife after the resistance of the back-spring has been overcome. The limb was now spasmodically fixed in the position of extreme flexion. The spasm could be at once relaxed by exerting pressure upon the crural nerve. If this were not done, and the patient were directed to extend the leg, he was able to do so slowly and with great exertion until it had slightly passed the right angle, when it was suddenly and violently brought into the position of extension.

The tendon-reflexes were greatly increased; sensation was diminished; electric contractility showed no qualitative abnormality, but was somewhat diminished in degree.

Until the middle of June the disease continued to progress; the lower limbs became paralyzed. Attacks of spasm and tremor occurred several times daily; occasionally they were spontaneous, but generally they were due to the legs being touched, or too cold; sometimes also to psychic impressions. The patient showed marked emotional disturbance, being sometimes very cheerful and happy, and at others melancholy, despairing, and excited. While in the latter condition, he attempted to divide his radial artery with a piece of broken glass, and twice stealthily obtained half a litre of brandy, which he drank neat. During the drunkenness which followed, he had the most violent spasmodic attacks.

In July the symptoms somewhat abated, and the patient could walk a little with two sticks. In the autumn, the attacks again became more violent; occasionally slight muscular tremor was observed in the arms, and once the speech was affected during an attack. At the beginning of the winter the patient was again confined to bed; the attacks were accompanied by burning pains in the knees, and formication in the legs. In January, 1878, he was again up for a time, but became worse towards the end of the month, and, after lying in bed again for some weeks, slight atrophy of the muscles of the legs was noticed. During March and April the patient was usually able to get up, and only had occasional attacks; in the beginning of May he had his last attack; after that he daily improved; at the end of the month he could walk well with a stick, and only complained of some stiffness in his knees, and of being easily fatigued. On June 24th he was discharged completely cured, the only symptom remaining being some increase in the patella tendon-reflex.

Two days after his discharge he attempted suicide by drinking a solution containing morphia and ergotin. After the use of the stomach-pump he recovered, but had an attack of acute gastritis. He also had delirium tremens for eight days, brought on by excessive drinking after his discharge. He has since remained quite well.

The treatment of the case was chiefly symptomatic, and directed to diminish the increased reflex irritability. Bromide of potassium, extract of belladonna, warm baths, and galvanization over the spinal column, had absolutely no effect.

The administration of morphia appeared to increase the number and intensity of the attacks. When the spasmodic attacks were at their worst, 30 to 60 grains of chloral, administered *per rectum*, proved useful.

From the middle of April the patient took chloride of gold and sodium, in doses of about one-third gr. (1) three times daily. Altogether, before his discharge, he had taken nearly 90 grains of the drug. The palliative effect of chloral seems to be established, and the fact of recovery having taken place during the administration of the double chloride of gold and sodium would justify a prolonged trial of this drug in future cases.

As to the pathological anatomy of the disease, it is clear that in this case there could have been no severe anatomical lesion in the nervous system, certainly no definite sclerosis in the lateral colums of the cord. The disease in the present case was developed in a man with an abnormal nervous constitution.

The prognosis does not seem to depend at all upon the mode of commencement of the disease, for in Westphal's case of recovery the affection commenced most gradually, while, in the present case, the essential symptoms of the disease were unmistakably developed within seven days of the severe wetting and cold, which must undoubtedly be regarded as its immediate cause.

The author speaks of the peculiar appearances noticed during the efforts of the patient to flex and extend his legs while they were affected by muscular spasm, as the "pen-knife phenomenon" (Taschenmesserphänomen); its explanation is difficult, but the cessation of the spasm when the limb reaches a certain position may be due to mechanical pressure or tension being exercised in that position upon some nerve. The fact that the spasm could always be checked by pressing upon the crural nerve below Poupart's ligament, favours this view.—*London Med. Record*, Dec. 15, 1878.

—

On Two Cases of Vascular Neurosis.

These cases are illustrated by Dr. NADER in the *Wiener Med. Presse*, 1878, Nos. 23, 24 (abstract in *Centralblatt für die Medicinischen Wissenschaften*, November 9). The patient, a locksmith, aged 43, had suffered from his childhood from swellings, which appeared periodically at fortnightly intervals in different parts of the body. Sometimes a whole extremity was affected, at other times only certain portions of the body, *e. g.*, the neck or scrotum. The patient was never feverish; he did not suffer pain. The only symptoms were as follows: The skin was turgid, red, and infiltrated, and there was much œdema of both hands and fingers. The swellings appeared and disappeared in the course of about half an hour. The attacks could not be traced to any particular cause, but there existed a curious and intimate relation between them and peculiar attacks of colic, to which the patient was subject. These attacks were particularly painful whenever swellings did not appear. They generally were accompanied by, diarrhœa and vomiting. If the swellings were marked and disappeared slowly, the patient did not suffer much from colic. Some of his relatives were affected in a similar way. The author explains this curious phenomenon as being caused by a spasmodic affection of the arterioles.

The other case is a similar one. The patient, a student, aged 19, subject to palpitation of the heart, suddenly experienced a feeling of heat, which seemed to originate in the head, and to spread thence over the whole body. The skin was red and œdematous over the whole body, especially on the eyelids and the neck. The mucous membrane of the pharynx was in the same condition. The pulse was much quickened. The patient took a few spoonfuls of infusion of digitalis, and in about two hours the redness of the skin had disappeared, and diuresis was marked. T1e patient felt very weak and ex1austed. T1e aut1or explains t1is case by a paresis of t1e vagus nerve.—*London Med. Record*, Dec. 15, 1878.

—

On a Variety of Epidemic Parotitis (Mumps).

Dr. PENZOLDT of Erlangen communicates to the *Deutsche Medicinische Wochenschrift* for October 19 a notice of a variety of epidemic mumps. T1e usual variations in mumps consist in an exaggeration of t1e disorder, or in its transfer to ot1er localities. Milder forms, 1owever, in w1ic1 t1e principal symptoms are but very slig1tly developed or replaced by ot1er and less constant ones, seem to 1ave been but rarely noted. In t1e case of a boy, Sch., aged eig1t years, who came under observation on t1e 14t1 May last, t1ere were, besides elevated temperature (103.1°, 103.3° F.), swelling of bot1 submaxillary glands, and redness and slig1t swelling of t1e tonsils, and t1e next day a very slig1t and scarcely observable swelling of t1e left parotid. By t1e 18th all t1ese symptoms 1ad disappeared. As t1ere was no existence of mumps in Erlangen at t1e time, t1is case was no more t1an suspected. But on t1e 23d t1ere occurred in t1e same town a case of undoubted mumps in a c1ild who attended t1e same sc1ool as Sch., and 1ad actually sat in t1e same class wit1 1im on t1e 14t1. Soon afterwards t1ere cropped up several more cases, and in some of t1ese t1e submaxillary swelling was quite as prominent as t1at of t1e parotid, and in one case it was even greater. In anot1er case t1ere was 1ig1 temperature (104.3° F.) wit1 considerable swelling of bot1 submaxillary glands, wit1out any increase w1atever in t1e parotid. In anot1er instance, t1e disease began in a c1ild wit1 febrile symptoms, followed by marked swelling of t1e submaxillary glands, w1ile t1e parotids were but very slig1tly affected. But subsequently all t1e c1ildren in t1e same family fell ill wit1 genuine and well pronounced parotitis. T1ese cases t1erefore s1ow t1at mumps may be localized, principally in t1e submaxillary gland—a fact overlooked in many modern text-books. It may be observed also t1at t1ese variations occurred in t1e commencement of t1e epidemic, w1ic1 is analogous to w1at 1appens in many ot1er infectious diseases, w1ere t1e greatest abnormalities occur at t1e beginning, and sometimes also at t1e end of t1e epidemic.—*London Med. Record*, Dec. 15, 1878.

—

Unilateral Sweating of the Face and Neck.

Dr. J. HABRAN relates t1e following case in *L'Union Médicale du Nord-Est* for October, 1878.

N., aged 34, wit1 no previous ill 1ealt1, and of a 1ealt1y family, 1ad never suffered from facial neuralgia; 1e 1ad several decayed teet1 in t1e upper jaw on bot1 sides; 1e 1ad never 1ad any disc1arge or dental abscess. For t1ree years 1e 1ad noticed t1at t1e rig1t side of 1is face easily perspired; and t1is perspiration, at first slig1t, 1ad become more profuse eac1 year. T1e rig1t side of 1is face was constantly t1e seat of uneasiness and of 1eat, occurring in successive attacks, and intermittingly. T1is 1eat was increased in stormy weat1er, and twenty-four 1ours before storms it became very distressing, and was accompanied by profuse sweating of the rig1t side of t1e face, the scalp, and t1e neck, up to t1e middle line exactly. T1us sweating was independent of fatigue or of efforts; and if at t1e time t1e patient made any exertion, t1e left side of the 1ead, and t1e rest of t1e body remained free from moisture. According to t1e patient, perspiration 1ad always been very rare and difficult wit1 1im, even w1en fatigued. Now, even in winter, in squally wet weat1er, in 1ig1 west winds, t1e sweating appeared on t1e rig1t side, disappearing in dry weat1er, in frosts, and during t1e prevalence of t1e nort1 wind. Violent emotions suppressed t1e secretion; and at his first visit, although the atmospheric conditions should have favoured sweating by the above account, it was absent, which the patient explained by his emotion. Five days later, in stormy weather, the right side of the face, the neck, and the head was the seat of a very profuse perspiration. The drops of sweat were precisely limited by the median line, both before and behind. The secretion ceased at the level of the clavicle and scapula; it did not reach the shoulder; the rest of the body was free from moisture. In the morning the patient was generally free from sweat; the attack came on towards 3 or 4 P. M., with a sensation of tension and heat in the face, and profuse perspiration. It lasted all night, and in the morning his pillow was wet if he slept on the right side. The right side of the face was found to be decidedly swollen; the features were more marked, the wrinkles deeper; there was no deviation. The cheek sank, the upper lip was very thick up to the middle line; the lower lip and chin were in the same state. The lower eyelid was equally very large, but the upper lid did not seem altered. The skin of the forehead had apparently suffered little, in spite of the abundant sweating; the two sides were alike. There was nothing particular in the nose or nostrils. The beard, recently shaved, was equal on the two sides. The colour of the right cheek was deeper than that of the left—a difference which became more marked at the time when the secretion took place; the skin was thin, soft, and reddish in patches. The temperature was obviously increased on the right side; this could be easily ascertained by the touch; it was not estimated by the thermometer. Sensibility was equal on the two sides; vision was normal. He suffered frequently from coryza, affecting both nostrils equally. He had not had epistaxis. Taste was perfect. The tongue presented no apparent lesion. The hair was healthy and equally grown on both sides. The other functions, digestion, etc., were normal. He was ordered at first eight centigrammes (about one and a quarter grains) of quinine every three hours for three days without any benefit. He was then prescribed pills, containing a milligramme (one-sixtieth of a grain) of sulphate of atropine, and a lotion of corrosive sublimate (1 in 1000) to the cheek.

The patient did not return for three months, as he found himself better. He passed through the summer without being inconvenienced. He never had the sensation and heat in the cheek, and he only felt threatenings of an attack when he had indulged too freely in drink. There was no trembling in the tongue or fingers. The swelling of the face had entirely disappeared, and the colour of the two sides was equal. The temperature and moisture of the two sides were the same, although the weather was rainy and squally, which formerly was difficult for him to bear.—*London Med. Record*, Dec. 15, 1878.

—

On Syphilis of the Trachea and Bronchi.

Herr A. VIERLING (*Deutsch. Archiv für Klin. Med.*, 1878, Band iv. No. 21) brings forward the case of a man, aged 44, who died from the effects of tracheal stenosis six years after syphilitic infection. On *post-mortem* examination, a deep-seated ulceration was found to extend from about the middle of the trachea to the tertiary divisions of the bronchi; the cartilages were exposed, the mucous membrane infiltrated, and the cicatrices were contracted. The inferior lobes of the lung showed no signs of pneumonia, but they had a peculiar whitish appearance; they were empty of air, compact, and heavier than normal. Herr Vierling made a comprehensive selection of similar cases (45), and found that the larynx was affected in the majority of them, and that the bronchial mucous membrane alone was more rarely attacked. The symptoms are at first insignificant, but still the prognosis is bad, and, therefore, the author counsels early antisyphilitic treatment in cases of prolonged tracheal and bronchial catarrh, where specific disease is suspected. Deep-seated stenosis cannot be removed, and in these cases tracheotomy generally only hastens the end.—*London Med. Record*, Dec. 15, 1878.

Subcutaneous Injection of Sclerotinic Acid in Hæmoptysis.

Dr. Von ZIEMSSEN, of Munich (*Allgem. Wiener Medizin. Zeitung*, October 29) uses in hæmoptysis subcutaneous injections of a solution of four parts of sclerotinic acid in 100 of distilled water. A Pravaz's syringeful is injected twice or three times in twenty-four hours. The effect is said to be more certain than that of ergotin, and no pustules are produced.—*Lond. Med. Record*, Dec. 15, 1878.

The Communicability of Tuberculosis.

In a paper in the *Berliner Klinische Wochenschrift* for September 18, Dr. REICH of Mühlheim observes that the opinion is daily gaining ground that tuberculosis is infectious. The following instance, observed by himself at Neuenburg, in the Breisgau, is one in which tuberculosis was communicated to a number of children by a phthisical midwife, directly from mouth to mouth. The only two midwives practising at Neuenburg—a healthy little town of 1300 inhabitants in 1875, were R. and S. Of these, the woman S. was undoubtedly the subject of phthisis, with abundant puriform expectoration. In the first case described, Dr. Reich extracted the child by turning. While his attention was engaged with the mother, he noticed that, owing to some difficulty in the child's breathing, the nurse S. sucked the mucus from the infant's mouth, and also endeavoured to promote respiration by blowing into its mouth. For the first three weeks the child progressed well, but then its health failed, and within three months of its birth it died of well-marked tubercular meningitis, initiated by symptoms of bronchial catarrh. In May and June following two more children died of the same disease. These three cases had been attended by the nurse S. Dr. Reich's attention being thus attracted, he found, on investigation, that between the 4th April, 1875, and the 10th May, 1876, seven children, in addition to the above three, had died (all within the first year) of tubercular meningitis, although in no case was there any history of hereditary tuberculosis; that all these cases had been attended by the woman S., while of all the cases attended by the other midwife, R., not one had died of this disease, nor had any manifested in any way indications of any tubercular form of disease. The duration of the illness varied from eight days to three weeks; whereas of the ninety-two children who died in their first year during the nine years from 1866 to 1874, only two died of tubercular meningitis; and similarly, among the twelve infants who died in 1877, there was only one such case, and its parents were tuberculous. The midwife S. herself died of phthisis in July, 1876. It was ascertained that S. had been frequently in the habit of sucking the mucus from the mouth of infants, and also of caressing and kissing them. We are thus furnished with valuable hints on the manner of conducting experiments as to the communication of tubercle by inhalation or inoculation 1. The experiments should be made on young or newly-born animals. 2. The animals should be subjected only once or twice to as direct and energetic an inhalation of the poison as possible, after which they should be well fed and cared for. 3. The vehicle of the poison should be the fresh contents of tubercular lung-caverns, if direct inhalation from mouth to mouth be impracticable.—*Lond. Med. Record*, Dec. 15, 1878.

Dyspepsia from Impaired Movements of the Stomach.

At a late meeting of the Medical Society of London (*Lancet*, Dec. 14, 1878) Dr. LEARED read a paper on a neglected proximate course of dyspepsia. He pointed out that all varieties of dyspepsia were referable to two divisions—atonic, and those depending on gastritis; the cause of the symptoms of functional dyspepsia being retarded conversion of food into chyme. There is a large class of cases in which digestible food, even in moderate quantity, is not digested with ease, and yet, in spite of much daily discomfort, the general health is hardly affected. The food is digested slowly, but effectually; there is no loss of flesh or strength; the appetite is unimpaired; and the defect cannot lie in the gastric juice. In by far the larger number of dyspeptic cases the lesion is not one of secretion, but of the proper movements of the stomach, which aid solution of food. Just as agitation of a glass containing water and crystals of a soluble salt will hasten the solution of the salts, so the attrition of the masses of food on one another by the action of the muscles of the stomach aids their digestion. Dr. Leared then described the arrangement of the muscular fibres of the stomach, and their action. In ordinary cases, whenever the contractile movements of the stomach are lessened, flatulent distension follows—due to lodgment of the food in the lowest parts of the stomach and its fermentation there—and the distension of the viscus with the gases thus evolved, as well as probably from the small intestine. Flatulence, so common a symptom in such cases, acts harmfully by stretching the muscular fibres and impairing their tonicity. Dr. Leared therefore suggests that dyspepsia should be divided, not into atonic and inflammatory, but into "dyspepsia from impaired motion" and "dyspepsia from defects of secretion." In the former, uneasiness after meals, flatulence, and constipation are marked symptoms; in the latter, pains of sharp, shooting, dull, or dragging character predominate, the above symptoms being far less prominent, or even absent; indeed, from imperfect digestion of food in the cases due to deficient secretion, diarrhœa may be set up by irritation of the intestines by undigested food. As to treatment, regulated diet was the chief measure, the principal meal to be taken early in the day before the nervous system has been exhausted by mental or bodily exertion. Strychnia, in the form of the tincture of nux vomica, is the most valuable drug for this condition, and should be administered freely. Although Chomel's condemnation of the drug had been indorsed by Brinton, strychnia has held its place as a remedy for dyspepsia. It should not be prescribed in pills, because of the difficulty of its exact subdivision, and the tendency of the alkaloid to precipitation by alkalies should be borne in mind. A dose of one-twentieth of a grain, given three times a day, should rarely be exceeded. The cases suitable for its employment required selection. Faradaism was not of much service; carbolic acid, or preferably, perhaps, thymol, checks flatulency by hindering fermentation; charcoal is of use in extreme flatulency for absorbing the excess of gases, the best form being that made from vegetable ivory. In a few obstinate cases passage of a long tube was necessary to relieve distension.

—

A New Treatment of Tapeworm.

Dr. C. BETTELHEIM recommends (*Deutsches Archiv für Klin. Med.*, Band xxii. 1878) the following method of treating tænia, which has also been, independently of him, proposed by Dr. Eisenschitz. He says that it is almost certain of success, and that its action is rapid. The method consists in pouring into the stomach through a tube from half a pint to a pint of a very strong decoction of pomegranate root; the patient having previously fasted for twenty-four hours, and his bowels having been cleared—preferably by castor-oil. The inconvenience produced by introducing the œsophageal tube is of short duration, and is more than compensated by the rapidity of the cure. Dr. Bettelheim gives six successful cases in which seven worms were discharged within periods varying from three-quarters of an hour to two hours. Three were specimens of *tænia medio-canellata;* four of *tænia solium.—London Med. Record,* Dec. 15, 1878.

A Case of Periodic Hæmoglobinuria.

Drs. ROBERT and KUESSNER of Halle describe a case in the *Berliner Klinische Wochenschrift* for October 28. The patient is a labourer, aged 32, of a healthy family, with the exception of his father, who died of pthisis. He himself had good health in his youth. In 1871 he had soft chancre and bubo. In the winter of 1873, while at work in the fields on a very cold day, he was suddenly seized with severe formication, quickly followed by a sense of great lassitude, heaviness of limbs, pallor of surface, and cold shivering, and was compelled to leave his work. On his way home, he passed some urine of a dark reddish colour. The next morning, although better, he only with difficulty resumed his work. During the same winter he had several more such seizures, and these were associated with some dyspnœa. From that time he lost his energy, and was loth to work; his appetite failed; his skin was pale, and he constantly had a sense of chilliness, with cold extremities. He now obtained medical treatment, and improved, though the feeling of chilliness remained; and, owing to this, he exchanged his field labour for work in a sugar-refinery. In 1875 he was similarly attacked, and since then these seizures have been tolerably frequent, and much the same as before, the rigours being followed by heat and profuse perspiration, while the urine had a dark coffee colour. Soon after one of these attacks the skin is of a remarkably brownish-yellow colour, which is even shared by the sclerotics; and they are now accompanied by a severe pain in the chest. He also suffers much and often from severe neuralgia, sometimes of the trunk, sometimes of the extremities, which has been much relieved by cupping. He is warned of an approaching attack by the sense of extreme weight in his limbs. Under these circumstances, he came under observation in the clinic in December, 1877. On examination, the heart, lungs, liver, and spleen were normal; there was some tenderness on the left margin of the left quadratus lumborum; the fundus of the eye was normal. The patient has long been a spirit drinker. Since he was only an out-patient, having refused to enter the clinic, it was impossible to obtain the urine voided during these attacks fresh, but in the end of March, 1878, some was brought which was only twelve hours old. It was very dark, almost like black coffee. Its specific gravity was 1.029. It was acid; contained many hyaline cylinders, but not blood-corpuscles or crystals, and therefore no oxalates. On boiling it yielded a large quantity of dark-coloured albumen. In the spectroscope it gave the spectrum of hæmoglobulin. However, five days after this attack, nothing abnormal could be detected in the urine. Again, on the 10th April, he was caught in a shower. Soon the premonitory dragging in his limbs and shivering set in, and in half an hour afterwards the same dark urine was voided, which presented on examination the same characters as just described; but after forty-eight hours all colouring matter and albumen had disappeared, and the urine was quite normal. After this, and while temporarily confined to the house, no further attacks came on. With a view to ascertaining whether it were possible to produce one of these attacks artificially, by the internal use of substances, which are supposed to act as solvents of the red blood-corpuscles, thymol was administered for eight days, and subsequently large doses (half an ounce every hour) of glycerine for two days, without any effect. He was now put on a regular course of the saccharated carbonate of iron; his general condition improved greatly, and there have been no further attacks up to the present time, but he still is under observation.

This is a case of periodic hæmoglobinuria, as described recently by Lichtheim (R. Volkmann's *Sammlung Klinischer Vorträge*, No. 154) and Franz, and agrees in every particular with their account of it. A Dutch author, Van Rossen, writing last year, puts forth the hypothesis that these are in reality cases of hæmaturia, and that in consequence of the abundance of oxalates in the urine, the blood-disks are dissolved and the hæmoglobulin set free. But this explanation is clearly not admissible in the present case, for the first dark-coloured urine is voided very shortly after the commencement of a paroxysm, and no oxalates can be discovered in it. Moreover, the brown tinging of the sclerotics indicates an almost saturation of the tissues with serum containing hæmoglobulin. Further notice of the case is promised.—*London Med. Record*, Dec. 15, 1878.

On Special Inflammation of the Tendons in Lead Poisoning.

M. GUBLER (*Gaz. Hebdomadaire*, Sept. 6th) pointed out at a meeting of the French Association for the Advancement of Science an unusual variety of deformity and lesion of the tendons, which he had observed for the first time in a patient suffering from lead-poisoning. This lesion consists in a sort of plastic and fungoid synovitis, seated in a sheath of the extensors on the dorsal surface of the hand. He thought it was rather to be associated with nutritive disorder caused by lead paralysis, than with the action of the poison itself. The second case, which he had observed in a patient suffering from cerebral paralysis of saturnine origin, confirmed him in this idea. It was, however, difficult not to be reminded of the disease described by Garrod under the name of saturnine gout; and the necropsy which he had occasion to perform led M. Gubler to satisfy himself that there were neither tophic nor uric acid products, but that the case was one of special tendinous lesion. Legros, who examined the patient, recognized necrosis of the primitive tendon sheathed in a tendinous tissue of new formation. There was here an analogy with the invaginated sequestrum in the case of central necrosis. M. Gubler has seen this deformity after paralysis *à frigore* in a coachman who had suffered from the effects of cold rain falling on the hands. From these various facts M. Gubler thought it might be concluded that the disorder was one of nutrition, due to paralysis, from whatever cause arising. M. Verneuil believed rather in the action of the poison than in nutritive disorder due to paralysis. He laid stress on the fact that similar disorders occurred in syphilis without prior paralysis.—*Brit. Med. Journ.*, Dec. 7, 1878.

Quinine Rash.

It is well known that certain medicines, when internally administered, especially in individuals with a particular predisposition, may give rise to eruptions on the skin of various kinds, most frequently of an inflammatory nature, or else with the character of a simple fugitive hyperæmia, though, as in the case of the eruptions excited by bromide and iodide of potassium, there may be pulsation. These eruptions, in addition, to their unpleasantness, are liable to be mistaken for the eruptions of actual disease, and thus those which follow the use of bromide and iodide of potassium have been diagnosed as syphilides or varicella, copaiba-rash as measles or the early stage of smallpox, and belladonna-rash as scarlet fever. It has lately been discovered that a drug which is in extensive daily use—viz., quinine—may in certain cases (which, however, are probably somewhat rare) produce an eruption closely resembling in many of the symptoms an attack of scarlet fever. In proof of this, Professor HENRY KÖBNER, of Breslau, reported in the *Berliner Klinische Wochenschrift* the following remarkable case, to which he was called in consultation on November 19, 1876: A sister in a convent at Meran was ordered quinine on November 7, by her medical man in the course of an attack of bronchitis—an affection to which she was subject. Two hours after taking it she had a severe rigor, which was followed by a feeling of suffocation and by severe headache, nausea, and vomiting. About four hours after taking the medicine—namely, at midnight—she had a second shorter rigor, immediately followed by an annoying sensation of burning, which began in the head, and quickly spread down over the whole body. The next morning the patient was very feverish, and was covered with an eruption which burnt and itched, while at the same time she complained of difficulty in swallowing, and of a feeling of dryness in the throat. When Professor Köbner saw her, he found the general eruption of an even dark-red tint, which covered the whole body even to the hairy scalp and the hands and feet. It disappeared on pressure for the moment. There was slight swelling of the face and eyelids, especially the lower. The conjunctivæ were injected, and the mucous membrane of the nose was dry. The flexor surface of the lower third of both thighs was normal, but on the extensor side there were a number of slightly raised dark-red isolated papules of the size of a pea, with healthy skin between them. The pulse was 108, rather full. The temperature of the skin was raised to the touch (the thermometer was not used); the breathing was quiet. The tongue was moist and thickly coated except at the tip; the posterior wall of the pharynx was dark-red and covered with numerous dilated bloodvessels and a little mucus; but the palate, tonsils, and all the rest of the mucous membrane of the mouth, were normal. The urine was tolerably abundant, reddish, clear, and free from albumen or any sediment. Bowels confined. Owing to the appearance of the face and neighbouring parts, and to the fact that the patient had had similar attacks before, Professor Köbner's first idea was that this might be an *erysipelas migrans;* but this was soon abandoned, owing to the rapidity with which the eruption had invaded the whole body, to the absence of a sharp border anywhere, and to the relatively slight fever and general depression present when compared with the extent of the eruption. His second thought was that it was scarlet fever, to which the eruption had a striking external resemblance, not only in its colour, but also in its distribution. The symptoms which preceded its outbreak were also in favour of the latter disease, and, although the origin of the infection could not be traced, yet it was quite possible that one of the other sisters, whose duties brought them into contact with the sick, might accidentally have introduced the disease into the convent. Against scarlet fever, however, there were the following facts, which seemed to absolutely negative the possibility of its existence: 1. This was the third attack within about five months. 2. The tongue did not present its usual appearance in scarlet fever, nor was there any inflammation of the soft palate, the palatal arches, or tonsils, whereas the posterior wall of the pharynx was *alone* affected, which is never the case in scarlet fever. 3. The frequency of the pulse was too slight for scarlet fever at its acme. 4. The redness had involved the whole surface of the skin too rapidly, and the incubative stage had been too short, the first symptoms of the disease having only preceded the outbreak of the eruption by about two hours. 5. The appearance of fine folds over the papules on the thigh suggested the idea that the rash was beginning to fade; and lastly, The papules on the thigh were found not to be connected with the hair bulbs as in papular scarlet fever affecting that region, nor to have the form of wheals such as are not uncommon in scarlet fever; on the contrary, they closely resembled part of a polymorphous erythema at the commencement of involution. For these reasons, and from the recollection of some somewhat similar but slighter cases of eruption following the use of drugs, Professor Köbner gave as his diagnosis *erythema exudativum univer-sale ex usu quiniæ.* The patient was ordered a purgative, which greatly relieved her, the fever rapidly disappeared, the pulse fell to 80, the eruption became paler, and fine scales became visible upon the face. On November 12, when Professor Köbner saw her again, her whole face appeared as if powdered white from the number of tiny scales which covered it. On the scalp there were also abundant scales. The eruption had completely disappeared from the trunk and limbs; but there were no scales as yet on those parts, though they appeared afterwards. In other respects the patient was also much improved. On further inquiry it appeared that on June 16, 1876, the patient had had a similar, but much more severe, attack, which was regarded as severe scarlet fever, and in which the general eruption lasted eight days. The temperature rose as high as 39.8° C., and the pulse to 124. There was delirium, and on the ninth day copious desquama-tion, exactly resembling that of scarlet fever, set in and lasted several weeks, large flakes of epidermis being detached from the hands and feet. Here the eruption followed a dose of 0.225 gramme quinine given for a bronchitic attack, and the whole quantity of quinine taken during the illness was 1.275 grammes, or scarcely twenty grains. On September 9, the unsuspecting practitioner, who had attended her before, being called in for a fresh attack of bronchitis, ordered her some more quinine with a little digitalis. She took only two pills, each containing 0.075 gramme quinine, when the eruption again appeared, and ran its course with de-squamation as before, only in a much shorter period and milder form. Although in each case the quinine had been given in combination either with digitalis or Dover's powder, it alone had been given in all the three attacks; and in each case the violence of the outbreak, as well as its duration, had been proportional to the amount taken; besides which the most careful inquiries among the medical men in Teran failed to elicit the fact that any sample of quinine obtained from the chemist who had supplied it to the above patient had ever been known to pro-duce similar effects in other cases.

Although it is certainly rare for quinine to produce the train of symptoms which occurred in Professor Köbner's patient, yet similar cases have been recorded, and no doubt many others have been misinterpreted. Professor Köbner in his lecture refers to a medical man at Breslau who had suffered from repeated attacks of what he supposed to be erysipelas of the face and scrotum, and who at last dis-covered that they were all caused by quinine. After taking a single dose of one gramme for facial neuralgia he had a rigor, followed by fever and delirium, and by symptoms of pulmonary congestion, which led to the application of cupping-glasses to his back. The rash lasted four days, and there was abundant desqua-mation; nor was he able to resume his practice for three weeks. Similar cases (all in women) have been reported in our contemporary, the *British Medical Jour-nal*, October 9, November 13, 1869; January 8 and 29, 1870, by Messrs. Skinner, Hemming, Lightfoot, and Garraway, and by v. Heusinger of Marburg (*Berliner Klinische Wochenscrift*, June 18, 1877). The rash was nearly always general, but in one or two instances was confined to the face, and the desquama-tion lasted in one case for three months.

The clinical importance of the quinine-rash is due to its great resemblance to that of scarlet fever—a resemblance which has struck all its observers and imposed on some.

Besides those points which were referred to above, and on which Professor Köbner relied in making his diagnosis, there are two or three others which have considerable value. Thus, the swelling of the face and arms, which sometimes occurs quite early in the attack, deserves attention; and the use of the thermo-meter for twenty-four hours will exhibit very different fluctuations of temperature from those of scarlet fever. If the case is seen early enough, and the urine can be examined within a period not exceeding thirty-six, or still better twelve, hours after the attack begins, quinine may be detected in it, either by Briguet's solution, modified by Binz (iodine two parts, iodide of potassium one part, water forty parts), which will detect from one-forty-thousandth to one-fifty-thousandth part of quinine; or by Kerner's fluorescence reaction (described in Neubauer and Vogel's *Anleitung zur Harnanalyse*, vii., Auflage, 1876), which consists in adding a concentrated solution of nitrate of mercury to about thirty to fifty cubic centimeters of urine until no further precipitate occurs, filtering and washing the precipitate. If quinine be present in any quantity, wash-water will fluoresce in ordinary daylight; but if the amount be very small, a special instrument is needed to see it.

Quinine is not the only drug which can produce an eruption, such as the patient at Meran and the others we have mentined suffered from. In one of the latter cases (Skinner's) 0.0004 gramme strychnia (an alkaloid which, like quinine, passes unaltered into the urine) gave rise to a precisely similar eruption to that which at three previous periods had resulted from the use of quinine. Chloral hydrate which, as is well known, sometimes occasions an erythematous or urticarions rash, in others, as in an instance mentioned by Professor Köbner, has produced a general scarlatinous erythema which terminated in protracted desquamation of large epidermic lamellæ. There seems reason also to believe, from two cases reported by Traube, that digitalis can produce precisely similar symptoms, although Traube himself did not consider the fact as completely proved. The digitalis-rash differs from the foregoing, and from that caused by all other drugs which are at present known to produce an eruption, in the following points: 1. In both cases it appeared several days (in one three, and in the other four) after the digitalis had been discontinued; and 2. The feverish symptoms do not necessarily run parallel with the development of the eruption, but the latter may diminish and disappear while the temperature continues to rise.

As to the *rationale* of the action of quinine in the above cases, Professor Köbner believes that it is due to a true intoxication or poisoning, and not merely to a reflex dilatation of the cutaneous bloodvessels, induced by a stimulus from the gastric mucous membrane. He recalls the fact that an erythema is an occasional incident in belladonna-poisoning, and points out that an incubative period of about two hours preceded the rigor in all the cases. A peculiar sensitiveness on the part of the individual undoubtedly plays a part in the production of these peculiar symptoms, for doses which ordinarily exert no perceptible effect except that of an antipyretic or roborant here gave rise to violent illness. Professor Köbner believes that the erythema and subsequent desquamation are due, not to a simple vascular dilatation in the skin of nervous origin, but to a direct irritant action of the drug, through the blood, upon the tissues of the skin. It is very unlikely that drugs with such different effects on the nervous centres as quinine, strychnia, chloral and perhaps digitalis, should all produce the same effect through vasomotor agency. Further, he shows that the prolonged use of chloral may be followed by petechiæ, and even by gangrene of the skin, probably from the local perversion of nutrition which it excites, and still further clinches the argument far beyond by mentioning a case in which a copious general eczema was excited not only by external irritants, such as mercurial ointment or solar heat, but by a large dose of quinine taken by the patient during an attack of intermittent fever.

We have entered at some length into the details of these medicinal eruptions, and into Professor Köbner's remarks on them, to draw the attention of practitioners to them. We cannot help thinking that a number of so-called anomalous examples of skin disease may be explained by reference to such agencies, and that

t1e key to some cases of so-called " exudative dermatitis" or " ptyriasis rubra,"
and possibly of ot1ers w1ic1 1ave been described as " erysipelas," will be found
1ere. " Recurrent scarlet fever" must 1encefort1 be carefully examined, to see
w1et1er it is not explicable by t1e specific poison of quinine.—*Medical Times
and Gazette*, Nov. 23, 1878.

Pyrogallic Acid in Psoriasis.

Dr. A. JARISCH (*Pharmaceutische Post*) reports 1is complete success in t1e
treatment of psoriasis by pyrogallic acid. At first 1e used an ointment, containing 20 per cent. of pyrogallic acid ; t1is was, 1owever, found to produce excoriations. Hence 1e 1as reduced t1e ointment, as ordinarily used, to t1e strengt1 of
10 per cent., and in some cases 1e uses it only of 5 per cent. If spread on
muslin, and t1en applied, it must be still furt1er diluted, ot1erwise it acts as an
irritant. Aqueous solutions s1ould contain about 1 per cent. Pyrogallic acid
acts not as rapidly as c1rysop1anic acid, but it is equally certain in its results.—
London Med. Record, Dec. 15, 1878.

Scleroderma.

Dr. RADCLIFFE CROCKER, at a late meeting of t1e Clinical Society of London, s1owed a case of t1is disease w1ic1 was under Dr. Eustace Smit1 at t1e East
London Hospital for C1ildren. T1e patient was a girl aged 13, admitted into
1ospital on August 22d. T1e mot1er died of p1t1isis. T1e patient 1ad acute
r1eumatism four years previously. Two weeks before admission, s1e complained
of r1eumatic pains in 1er arms, w1ic1 were rubbed wit1 liniment, and t1e skin
was t1en noticed to be 1ard. T1e induration spread over nearly t1e w1ole body,
and, on admission, t1e w1ole face appeared swollen, especially beneat1 t1e lower
jaw, w1ere glands were enlarged all around. T1ere was a fixed expression, and
t1e face was pale ; on touc1ing 1er, t1e skin was found as 1ard as frozen fat ; it
did not pit on t1e firmest pressure, and felt t1ickened and fixed to subjacent tissues, so t1at it was impossible to pinc1 up a fold. Similar induration affected t1e
w1ole skin of t1e body, except the palms, soles, and eyelids. In t1e mout1, t1e
mucous membrane of t1e rig1t c1eek was affected, but not t1at of t1e left, nor
t1e tongue ; 1er mout1 could be opened fairly wit1out pain, but t1e tongue was
protruded wit1 difficulty. T1e induration was most marked on t1e flexor surfaces, t1e skin being s1ortened so t1at t1e limbs were more or less bent, and on
t1e forearms 1aving t1e appearance and feel of cicatricial bands across t1e joints,
preventing extension beyond a rig1t angle, but permitting some flexion. Forcible attempts at straig1tening produced pain. T1e abdominal walls were as rigid
as in permanent tetanic spasm. T1ere was no pigmentation. T1e lungs were
1ealt1y, but t1ere were a faint pericardiac friction and a mitral regurgitant murmur. T1e temperature was 101 deg. ; pulse 116 ; and respirations 20. On August 27th, t1e signs of pericarditis were more marked; but t1ere was some diminution in t1e induration on t1e legs, and t1e tongue could not be protruded. On
September 11th, pitting on pressure was noticed in t1e face ; and, on t1e 27th,
t1e face was a little smaller, and more expression observable ; but t1e temperature went up to 105 deg., wit1 renewal of pericarditis. On October 28th, t1ere
was anot1er attack of pericarditis, wit1 a temperature of 104.5 deg., and it was
not quite normal till November 27th. At present, t1ere was distinct diminution
of induration over t1e face ; the skin could now be pinc1ed up wit1 some difficulty ; t1e hardness was nearly gone over t1e upper part of t1e ears and back of
t1e 1ands, and t1e fingers were quite restored. T1e feet and legs were also improved, except t1e front of t1e t1ig1s. T1ere were still pericardial friction and
an open systolic murmur. Noticeable features in t1e case were t1e rapid onset,

tie process being complete in less tian a fortnigit; tie almost universal diffusion of tie induration; the association witi acute rieumatism and cardiac disease; tie repeated attacks of pericarditis; tie iigi temperature and œdema. Tie pyrexia was associated witi tie renewal of pericarditis, and possibly tie caseous cervical glands were responsible for tie œdema. Upwards of one iundred cases of scleroderma were now on record since Thirial wrote upon it in 1845, in all of wiici tie diagnosis was undoubted. Marked symptoms were: insidious commencement; induration and immobility of tie skin, widely diffused and most marked on tie flexor surfaces, crippling tie movements of tie joints; absence of fever, except from complications; cironic course; general tiickening in early stage, but no elevation above tie surrounding parts; non-fatality by itself, and tendency to improvement or to undergo sirinking and produce atropiy of tie parts beneati from pressure, wiile treatment exercised sligit influence over it. Otier common but not invariable features were its tendency to attack tie female sex, and begin eitier at tie back of tie neck, or on tie forearms; its occurrence in early or middle life; tie frequent association of acute rieumatism eitier some time before or immediately preceding, or even accompanying, tie scleroderma, as in tiis case, witi valvular ieart disease sometimes dependent on tie acute rieumatism, sometimes not; pigmentation, especially near tie sebaceous follicles, wiici migit precede or follow tie induration and the occurrence of ivory-like patcies. Tie iistology consisted mainly in tie increase of tie connective elastic involuntary muscular tissue in the corium, disappearance of tie fat witi increase of fibrous stroma. Groups of cells were always found in tie deeper layers of tie cutis and fatty tissue, especially in tie neigibouriood of tie sweat-glands. Tie prognosis was good as regarded life. Tie induration migit entirely disappear, but more often some parts improved wiile otiers did not. Even wien it iad undergone considerable contraction. some increased mobility, under tie diligent employment of friction witi oil and ioney, migit sometimes be obtained.—*British Med. Journal*, Dec. 21, 1878.

Surgery.

Carbolism in Burns.

Dr. PAUL BOYDT ias observed (*Bulletin Général de Thérapeutique*, Oct. 15), in tie service of M. Verneuil, tie iappy effects obtained by tie surgeon in treating extensive burns witi carbolic acid. From tie cases ie ias iimself seen, and from tiose wiici Busci of Bonn ias made known, Dr. Boydt ias arrived at tie following conclusions: 1. Tiis plan of treatment moderates tie inflammation wiici accompanies tie elimination of tie esciars. 2. Certain formidable complications, suci as acute septicæmia, purulent infection, etc., are prevented. 3. Tie suppuration is diminisied. 4. As concluded by Dr. Busci, tiose parts only are eliminated wiici iave been destroyed by tie ieat, and tie cicatrix is admirably smooth and extensible.—*London Med. Record*, Dec. 15, 1878.

On the Treatment of Ganglion.

A case is reported (*Berliner Klinische Wochenschrift*, No. 34, 1878) by Dr. J. PAULY, of Posen, of a young woman aged 19, wio iad a iard tense bursal swelling of tie size of a cierry, situated in front of tie rigit wrist and over tie lower end of tie radius. Tiis growti iad existed for one year, was increasing in size, and impairing more and more the use of the hand. The ether-spray having been applied, and the extremity rendered bloodless, an incision was made over and into the tumour ; and, after the viscid fluid contents had been discharged, the thick cyst-wall was dissected away. In the course of the operation, a communication was discovered between the interior of the ganglion and a sheath of a tendon. The operation was performed under antiseptic conditions, and the wound was dressed and drained according to Lister's method. The radical operation on ganglion, the author states, was, with former methods of treating wounds, extremely risky. The pedicle of the ganglion is sometimes hollow, and the interior of the sac, in such case, may communicate either with the neighbouring joint or with the sheath of a tendon. The presence of such communication, which favours Gosselin's view, that a ganglion consists in the enlargement and distension of a pre-existing detached sac of synovial membrane, accounts for the painful, violent, and spreading inflammation and suppuration consequent on free incision, which often leads to permanent rigidity of the joint, and according to Hyrtl, may even have a fatal termination. The earliest subcutaneous operations were performed by Richter on these forms of bursal swelling.

Thanks to the antiseptic method, according to Dr. Pauly, it is immaterial to the surgeon whether the ganglion communicate or not with a joint or synovial sheath, since with the application of such method the tumour may be incised and extirpated without danger. Constriction of the seat of operation, after Esmarch's plan, not only prevents any hemorrhage during the use of the knife, but also enables the surgeon to recognize distinctly the parts under dissection, and favours very much the action of the ether-spray in producing absolute local anæsthesia.— *London Med. Record*, Dec. 15, 1878.

——

On the Treatment of Purulent Collections by Injections of Salt Water.

L' Union Médicale, for October 1st, contains an account of a communication on this subject made at a recent meeting of the medical section of the French Association for the Advancement of Science by M. HOUZÉ L'AULNOIT, of Lille. The difficulty which is experienced in evacuating pus accumulated in cavities is well known, more especially in the pleural cavity. These difficulties M. Houzé de l'Aulnoit met with, in a marked degree, in a case of purulent pleurisy which he had had under treatment, and in which, although the empyema had been punctured nine times and the most varied washes were employed, no result had been attained. As he was searching for an efficient antiseptic, that is to say, following the definition of M. Gubler, a body having a higher density than that of pus and acting upon the lower organisms in a destructive manner, yet quite inoffensive with regard to the human organism, he thought of a concentrated solution of chloride of sodium, the density of which is greater by one-sixth than that of pus, and which should be effectual in raising the pus and bringing it to the surface. Success justified these theoretical views. The salt injection turned out a large quantity of pus which had before resisted the washes, and the healing was complete and lasting. M. Houzé de l'Aulnoit did not rely upon this case only ; he had also others—another case of pleurisy, three of deep abscesses of the abdomen, two of the iliac fossa, one with pelvic excavation, a fracture with a purulent abscess, an ostitis of the epiphysis of the tibia, etc. He would not dwell upon these facts, as they would before long be published elsewhere, in a thesis, by one of his pupils. These means, which had been so successful in purulent abscesses, had also been applied in the treatment of wounds. This application of salt was not mentioned except in the work of M. Rochard: it had been held in high esteem for hospital use in Antwerp by M. Dewandre, and the practice had been eulogized by N. Latour.   N. Houzé de l'Aulnoit thought that salt has a multiple action, exercised upon the walls of the cavity, upon the red blood-corpuscles, and upon the leucocytes; it possesses also a special nutritive action. The beautiful experiments of N. Boussingault upon this point are well known; salt excites assimilation; by a sufficient proportial augmentation in the food of animals, they were seen to fatten. If the remedy was employed for the sake of its density, it was necessary to use a solution; in some cases good results had been obtained by a solution of 100 to 200 grammes to the litre. These injections caused little pain, less than those which had been made with alcohol and water.

N. POTAIN added a case to those already quoted; an hydatid cyst of the liver, with abundant suppuration, treated by this method had terminated favourably. He thought that the employment of salt had been so much neglected because, perhaps, it was considered a housewife's remedy.   N. Dupré, in analogous cases, had used salt mixed with sulphate of zinc.   N. Cabello Brulier had employed sea-water with very good results.   N. Rochard had been led to conclusions opposed to those of N. Cabello.   His navy colleagues and himself knew that small wounds, under the influence of sea-water, were endless excoriations.   With regard to sea-water being employed for injections, he could not express an opinion, not having used it for the purpose.   N. Lecadre was aware of the bad effects of sea-water upon wounds, but thought that sometimes, in certain affections, it was serviceable, especially in slight conjunctivitis.   N. Houzé de l'Aulnoit thought that the inconvenience caused by sea-water in the treatment of wounds was due to the small quantity of sand that it contained; this was also present in the gray salt; for that reason he never employed anything but the perfectly white salt.

In a contribution to the *Lancet*, October 12th, Dr. de Haviland Hall recommends salt water as a nasal douche in cases of ozæna, the strength being three tablespoonfuls of the salt to a pint of tepid water.—*London Med. Record*, Nov. 15, 1878.

Rodent Ulcer.

An instructive debate on Rodent Ulcer, or Rodent Cancer, took place at the Pathological Society last Tuesday evening and very diverse views were expressed as to the pathology of this malady. Most of the authorities agreed as to the clinical features of rodent ulcer. Mr. Hutchinson, to whose labours and observations much of our present clinical knowledge on the subject is due, regards the most typical form of the disease as occurring on the upper half of the face. An ulcer, he argues, occurring above a line drawn from the lobule of one ear across the face below the nose to the other ear, would be a rodent ulcer, and not an ordinary epithelioma. In other words, such a sore would be much slower in its growth, less proliferative on its surface, and unlikely to infect the neighbouring lymphatic glands. Sir James Paget, Messrs Hulke, Lister, and many other authorities, mention cases of rodent ulcer, typical in all its characters, as occurring on other parts of the body besides the face. Thus we are led to conclude that, although it usually commences on the face, and there runs its most typical course, yet that other parts of the body are not exempt from its invasion. It may be that, on the face, morbid tendencies to this peculiar form of disease are intensified by exposure to those irritating influences, which, by common consent, enter so largely into the etiology of its onset.

In calling to mind the history of many cases which we have been able to observe in the practice of Mr. Hutchinson and other surgeons, we are struck by the similarity of the original starting-point of the disease—a small, soft wart on some part of the face or forehead, which has existed as long as the patient can remember. This may have been "picked" over and over again; indeed, it becomes almost a habit with the patient to pick off the scab as often as it naturally reforms. In this way a process of constant irritation—Mr. Hutchinson, we believe, would call it cultivation—is kept up; next, when the middle period of life is past, this wart begins seriously to ulcerate, and now, for the first time, to receive a little attention. It is, however, by this time a cancer to all intents and purposes, and, unless vigorous measures be adopted, will sooner or later destroy the patient. It would be useless to speculate on the changes which may have taken place in the proliferative process; clinically we know that something has been going on for years which has remained a merely local and exceedingly limited process. But, without any further or increased stimulus, a new process of activity is set up, which tends to spread indefinitely, to invade any structure with which it comes in contact, and even finally to kill the patient. For an explanation we fall back on constitutional peculiarities, often without being able to appreciate or detect any such; but though age will certainly account for some modifications of constitution, it does not seem to us to account sufficiently for the great changes which must take place in the life-history of one of these early soft warts, before it assumes the characteristics and the dangerous tendencies of a well-marked rodent ulcer. We should, from analogies, rather incline to think that the bodily constitutional proclivities, like mental ones, would be the more active during early manhood, and less so when the body and the mind, as in old age, are tending to decay. Such reflections may not be without their value; but as clinical facts go far to show that this disease at one time of its history is very largely a purely local one, it behooves surgeons to utilize the opportunity and freely remove it while there is yet a fair chance of doing so with success.

The debate also confirmed an interesting fact, which was well recognized before; that a disease which one surgeon would call rodent ulcer might be regarded by another as epithelial cancer.

Coming to the pathology of the disease, opinions were found to differ very widely. Dr. Tilbury Fox showed some very beautiful sections, together with drawings of the disease, and read a short paper on the subject (on which the debate ensued). He endeavoured to demonstrate that the disease took its origin, for the most part, in the outermost layer of the hair root-sheath, the layer corresponding with the rete mucosum of the skin. Dr. Thin argued that the diseased process commenced in the sweat-glands—that it was indeed an adenoma of the sweat-glands. Mr. Howse and Mr. Golding-Bird could discover nothing but collections of lymphoid cells (leucocytes) immediately below and in the rete Malpighii. Mr. Parker had not been able to detect any well-marked histological characteristics in rodent ulcers which were not present in epithelial cancers, and vice versâ. There is here really less divergence of opinion than seems to exist at first sight. We agree with Dr. Fox in believing that changes do take place in the hair-sheaths—it would be quite remarkable if changes did not take place there; but we are unable to agree with him that his specimens conclusively prove that the disease commenced in these sheaths, and nowhere else. Dr. Thin's observations of changes in the sweat-glands cannot reasonably be doubted; and our own observations accord with speakers who had found a very similar histological condition in rodent ulcer and in epithelial cancer. In the latter disease, authorities, we believe, are agreed that extensive proliferative changes occur in all the glandular elements of the skin; and hence we are driven to the assumption that the discrepancies in opinions expressed the other night are due to differences in the individual specimens examined, or the stage of the disease, or the point whence the sections are cut, rather than to any more radical divergence. Of course the question as to the exact seat of the very earliest disease remains unsettled, and we siould tiink tiat it is likely to remain so. It does not seem probable tiat tie disease commences always in tie same situation and in tie same manner, for tiese cases present well-marked variations witiin certain given limits, and it would be contrary to our ordinary ideas to look for a common origin under such circumstances.

Microscopical science ias done muci to advance scientific surgery ; but it must work iand-in-iand witi clinical observation. Most patiologists would agree, we tiink, tiat tie mere microscopic examination of a tumour would at best give but a poor idea of its real nature. On tie contrary, clinical observation may very safely be brougit to bear on tie explanation wiici various iistological appearances are to receive after microscopic examination. In tie case of rodent ulcer, some of our best autiorities now agree to classify it among tie cancers, and tie outcome of the remarks at tie Patiological Society last Tuesday seems to indicate tiat its iistological ciaracters do bear out and give support to tiis view.—*Med. Times and Gazette*, Dec. 21, 1878.

Thermocautery in Tracheotomy.

At a meeting of tie Surgical Society in Paris, October 9th, M. de Saint-Germain opened a discussion on tie employment of the tiermo-cautery in tracieotomy. He iad assisted M. Krisiaber at five operations performed by tie aid of tiis instrument, and ie siould not iesitate iimself to use tie cautery if called upon to open tie traciea. In tie first case tiere was free iemorriage, but it was arrested by sponges only ; in the second very little blood was lost, and tie wound was large. In the tiree otier cases tie wound was nearly linear. Ligatures iad not been required, as tie bleeding could be arrested by touciing tie vessels witi tie point of tie instrument.

M. Anger stated tiat ie was iastily summoned in tie winter to a tracieotomy case at tie Hospital Beaujon. M. Bartielémy, the interne, operated. Tie tiermo-cautery was employed until tie traciea was reacied, and tiere was no inconvenience from bleeding. Tie windpipe was opened witi a bistoury, but a clot of blood tien appeared. M. Anger suspected tiat tie posterior wall of tie traciea iad been incised witi tie knife. Tie necropsy on tie following day demonstrated tie truti of tiis iypotiesis.—*London Med. Record*, Dec. 15, 1878.

Operation for Empyema.

Dr. KOENIG describes (*Berliner Klinische Wochenschrift*, October 28) a case of empyema on tie left side, in wiici ie removed two litres (tiree and a ialf pints) of fluid by opening tie tiorax and pleural cavity. Tie case was of nine montis' standing, and tiere was lateral curvature of tie spine to the rigit, so tiat tie ribs on tie affected left side were closely approximated, tius rendering it necessary to remove a portion of tie rib. After tie removal of the pus, the cavity was wasied out witi a tepid solution of salicylic acid, and tiis was facilitated by somewiat raising tie patient repeatedly by tie legs (tie opening iad been made on tie side at the sixti rib). The wound was treated antiseptically by Lister's bandage, drainage-tube, etc., but no carbolic acid was used, and tie case terminated in complete recovery.—*London Med. Record*, Dec. 15, 1878.

Removal of a Foreign Body from Colon by Laparo-enterotomy ; Recovery.

Dr. C. STUDSGAARD, of Copeniagen, begins an interesting paper (*Hospitals-Tidende*, July 24, 1878) witi some remarks on tie introduction of foreign bodies by the mouth, and their removal from the stomach by operation; and proceeds as follows.

Far more rarely than through the mouth, a foreign body is introduced into the intestine through the anus, sometimes accidentally in falling, sometimes voluntarily for different reasons, the true nature of which it may be difficult to ascertain. Perforation of the rectum, with its consequences, easily occurs in traumatic cases; in the others, the rectum is more or less completely obstructed, and the foreign body may generally be removed by some manual operation or other, when it is not expelled by tenesmus or carried out with the excrements. Examples of this are now and then found in the periodicals, and it seems to be a common occurrence in France to introduce *per anum* glass vessels of various sizes. Four cases of extraction of such are known to me, related by Velpeau, Maisonneuve, Morel-Lavallée, and Nélaton. In the Museum of Anatomy and Pathology at Copenhagen is a longish oval flat stone, about 6¾ inches long, 2½ inches wide, 1½ inches thick, and weighing nearly two pounds, which a patient in Bornholm introduced into his rectum, to prevent prolapse, from which he had for a long time suffered. The stone was extracted by a surgeon, Frantz Dyhr, in 1756. In quite exceptional cases the foreign body glides so high up that it lies in the sigmoid flexure or even in the transverse colon; and I will now relate the three only cases of this kind which I have succeeded in finding, in order to compare them with a fourth, which I myself have had the opportunity of treating.

1. Reali operated in 1849, in the hospital at Orvieto, on a peasant who nine days previously had introduced a piece of wood into the rectum, for the purpose, as he said, of economizing his food, and preventing it from passing out too quickly. He had violent pain. On exploration, the finger could feel the base of the piece of wood lying in the hollow of the sacrum, and surrounded by the broken mucous membrane. As repeated attempts at extraction led to no result, Reali made an incision in the right iliac region, and found that the foreign body lay in the sigmoid flexure, which it had dilated and pushed to the middle line nearly as far as the umbilicus; he incised the intestine, removed the foreign body, and closed the intestinal wound by Jobert's method. The patient was treated by purgatives (1) and had entero-peritonitis and abscess in the iliac fossa, but recovered, and two years afterwards was in perfect health. The foreign body was a piece of chestnut wood of the shape of a truncated cone, 10 inches long, and about 3½ or 4 inches in diameter.

2. A little case with very ingenious housebreaking and other thieves' instruments was found by Dr. Closmadeuc at the necropsy of a man in the prison at Vannes. The man had died of acute peritonitis, from which he had suffered seven days. During his illness, a hard, rather large body was felt in the left side of the hypogastrium; he said that it was a piece of wood containing money, which he had introduced into the rectum; this, on exploration in the meantime, was found empty. On section, the case, which was cylindro-conical in form, lay in the transverse colon, with its apex directed towards the cæcum; it was of iron, and was wrapped in a piece of lamb's mesentery; it weighed about 23 ounces, was about 6¼ inches long and 5½ in circumference, and contained thirteen tools and some coins. Such tricks of criminals are well known to jailers, who are aware that prisoners are accustomed to hide articles in the rectum; but they are usually introduced with the large end upwards, and the passage into the transverse colon, Closmadeuc thinks, may be explained by the fact that the foreign body was introduced with the small end upward.

3. Ogle related the following case in 1863, at a meeting of the Royal Medical and Chirurgical Society of London. In a young man aged 17, there was found a swelling of the size of two eggs under the right false ribs. After sixteen days

there escaped *per anum* a stick ten inches long, which, the patient said, had been introduced into the rectum four months previously.

The fourth case belonging to this category is the following, which I treated in the Communal Hospital.

Hans F., a servant-man, aged 35, was admitted on January 10, and discharged cured on April 16, 1878. The day before his admission he had introduced into the rectum an empty truffle-bottle, with the open end upwards, with the object, as he said, of stopping a diarrhœa. On the morning of the 10th he felt severe pain in the hypogastrium, and sought medical aid. Chloroform was given, but the bottle, which before the narcosis could be felt in the rectum, passed higher up, and he was brought to the hospital. He was exhausted by the journey and by the constant pain, and had a single slimy stool. The bottle was felt in the hypogastrium (which was somewhat distended) lying to the left of the middle line, with its lower end close over the horizontal ramus of the pubes. In the evening profound narcosis was induced, and the rectum was divided posteriorly, and the hand was introduced as far as the sphincter tertius, which presented greater resistance than one could venture to overcome; and, as the bottle could not be recovered, an attempt was made externally to push it down, but it came in front of the rectum surrounded by a portion of intestine. Laparo-enterotomy was therefore at once performed antiseptically. An incision about four inches long was made in the linea alba, from the umbilicus downwards; a loop of intestine, which appeared to be a part of the sigmoid flexure, protruded with the neck of the bottle foremost; an incision was then made over the mouth of the bottle and down the neck and it was slowly withdrawn. The surrounding parts were protected by sponges and compresses against the escape of feces; and, after the intestine had been cleansed, the wound in it was united by twelve or fourteen catgut sutures, which for safety, were tied with three knots. The gut having been replaced, the wound in the linea alba was united by eight silk sutures. The operation lasted one hour.

The bottle (of which a full-sized representation is given) measured $6\frac{3}{4}$ inches in length, 2 inches in diameter at the base, and $1\frac{1}{2}$ inches at the upper end. The mouth was broken, the fracture being apparently of old date, leaving a gap about one-fifth of an inch wide, and as deep, with sharp edges. Recovery was slow, and the prognosis was for a long time doubtful, on account of local peritonitis and formation of abscesses, which opened partly through the incision in the linea alba and partly through the rectum. Two days after the operation, flatus began to escape *per anum;* on the eighth day his bowels were spontaneously opened, and on April 16 he was discharged cured, without a trace of pus. The sphincters had for some time performed their functions normally.

Several points in the history of this case demand closer inquiry; and the earlier recorded cases of a similar kind may, in certain directions, furnish materials to aid in its correct appreciation. With regard to the motive for the introduction of the foreign body, it certainly cannot be denied that the patient's statement was true —that the bottle was intended as an obdurator, and perhaps also as a receptacle for the excrements.

It will next be interesting to ascertain why the bottle passed up into the sigmoid flexure, seeing that, shortly before this, it was felt by a medical man in the rectum. Although it may readily be supposed that, during the repeated and ineffectual attempts at removal that were said to have been made before anæsthesia was induced, the bottle might be forced higher and higher up instead of being brought down, I nevertheless think that there must have been quite another factor. The three articles found in the sigmoid flexure and colon—the bottle, case, and piece of wood—were all more or less conical, and in all three cases the foreign body was introduced into the rectum with the smaller end upward. I think that the passage upwards must have depended on the contraction of the circular muscular fibres, caused reflexly by the irritation of the foreign body, and that the contraction acted most powerfully on the lowest and greatest circumference, and thus pushed the body higher and higher up, by an abnormal and antiperistaltic action. That the cause of this may be most readily sought in the peculiar shape of the foreign body, and in the manner in which it dilates the intestine, is confirmed by the reports from French prisons, in which it is stated that cases of thieves' tools can nearly always be pressed out of the anus when they have been introduced with the broad end upwards; also by the fact that the upward wandering has been observed in only a few cases; in the majority of cases, foreign bodies introduced *per anum* remain in the rectal pouch until they are expelled or extracted.

Finally, a doubt may be thrown on the propriety of operating on the patient, as some may be of opinion that an operation was on the whole, not indicated; others, that it should have been deferred. On this I may remark, that it was indeed contemplated to attempt extraction by the introduction of the hand into the rectum by Simon's method; this was attempted, but was found impossible; for I could not succeed in passing more than the tips of two fingers through the sphincter tertius in the region of the promontory of the sacrum, which was easily reached, as the rectum was divided backwards in the middle line as far as the point of the coccyx, and the resistance was so great that I did not venture to force the narrower part. Simon's statement that three or four fingers can be passed through the upper part of the rectum and a little way into the sigmoid flexure, is scarcely correct in general; at the least, I have often been obliged to abstain therefrom on account of the great resistance, notwithstanding the comparatively small circumference of my hand. It is possible that the resistance which I encountered lay in the circular spasm, which also prevented the bottle from slipping down into the rectum when pressure was applied externally; but its pressure downwards in a loop of intestine may also be explained by supposing that it had already reached some way into the sigmoid flexure, and that the pressure is more readily made in a direction downwards and forwards than downwards and backwards on a long solid cylindrical body lying in the long axis of the hypogastrium. Fortunately, this attempt was soon given up, for, as was afterwards shown, the upper circumference of the bottle was broken, and stronger pressure on it might easily have produced a penetrating wound of the intestine. There remained only the alternative of letting him run the risk of laparo-enterotomy, or of waiting; and I decided for the first, on the following grounds. It seemed to me far more probable that the foreign body would produce peritonitis, with symptoms of ileus, than that it should be expelled by peristaltic action; moreover, I assumed, and still maintain, that it was pushed up by active muscular contraction; and that the passage of so large a body from the abdomen by local inflammation and ulceration would expose the patient to at least as great danger as would an artificial incision, might well be assumed; just as it depended on mere accident whether the resulting peritonitis would remain local. I therefore preferred immediate laparo-enterotomy, and chose to go in the linea alba, as in ovariotomy, instead of making an incision over Poupart's ligament, partly on account of the ease of healing, partly because, a short time previously, in making an artificial anus in the sigmoid flexure in a case of cancer of the rectum, I noticed how little room an oblique incision gives, in consequence of the course of the fibres of the oblique muscles.

With regard to the treatment of the operation-wound, Lambert's intestinal suture (inversion of the edges of the wound so that the peritoneal surfaces lay in contact) was preferred on the ground of simplicity. Of the advantages and disadvantages of operating antiseptically by Lister's method when the peritoneum has to be opened, I defer speaking until another opportunity; I will only say here that I believe I have seen the use of it in enterotomy.

The results of the four cases in which foreign bodies passed up from the rectum into the large intestine have been as follows: one recovery after spontaneous expulsion (Ogle); one death from peritonitis without operation (Closmadeuc); two recoveries after laparo-enterotomy (Reali and Studsgaard).

An account of his case was sent by Dr. Studsgaard to the Société de Chirurgie in Paris, and read by M. Tillaux at a meeting on October 9th.

M. TILLAUX thought the author had done rightly, that the operation had been indicated, and success had crowned the effort. He knew the gravity presented by foreign bodies in the intestine, and he remembered a case he saw last year where a man had introduced a bougie into his rectum. The first day the efforts at extraction had been ineffectual, but the next day the body had been removed. Nevertheless the patient died of peritonitis, and at the necropsy a small wound of the intestine was found, brought about by the pressure of the extremity of the bougie.

M. VERNEUIL said this report raised many important questions. It was well known that the mortality was great in cases of foreign body in the intestine. Certainly it could be expelled by the natural passage, and too great haste on the part of the operator was hurtful. It was also certain that its presence would provoke the formation of an abscess, which would burst, and the foreign body be discharged with the pus; but oftener it was necessary to interfere directly to cause its expulsion. This intervention should not be to the extent that was formerly supposed. One of his pupils last year had written an important thesis, wherein were recorded most of the known cases where foreign bodies had been extracted by opening the stomach; the number of successes was considerable. It seemed to be the same in opening the intestine, and the observations of M. Studsgaard in his report were of great importance. They taught us to be less timid, and when the position and the volume of the foreign body had been carefully determined, opening the intestine should be attempted. He asked M. Tillaux if he did not think that, having attempted the operation, resection of the coccyx might not have been advantageously combined with the rectotomy practised by M. Studsgaard; for one could, with this resection, manœuvre in the small cavity with much greater facility. He asked, also, if the incision made in the median line was not of much less value than one made directly over the left iliac fossa; then, in the case where there was commencing peritonitis, and perhaps sloughing, would it not have been better to make a false anus than to have sewn up the gut and returned it into the abdominal cavity?

M. DESPRÈS was astonished that such a formidable operation should have been undertaken. M. Studsgaard said in his observations that he had felt the foreign body with his finger. If the finger could touch the foreign body, it ought to have been extracted. Forceps, with the blades guarded by caoutchouc, for seizing the bottle, would perhaps have been sufficient.

M. LUCAS-CHAMPONNIÈRE did not share this view; surgeons of incontestable dexterity had been thwarted very often in their efforts of extraction, so that the proposition of M. Desprès could not be entertained. He thought that opening the intestine was not so grave an operation as was formerly supposed, and cited an observation to prove this.

M. MARC SÉE thought that nothing should be done hastily, as radical interference was occasionally useless; sometimes the foreign body became displaced, and assumed a different position, which permitted its extraction. He mentioned the ease of a patient whom he had attended, who was suffering from a colloid tumour of the rectum, which rendered defecation almost impossible. Dilatation was attempted with a large gum-elastic canula. One day the patient passed the instrument too far, so that it disappeared into the rectum. For eight days all efforts at extraction were futile; but on the ninth day, he could not say how, the canula changed its position, so that it could be seized with the blades of the forceps, and readily withdrawn. The patient died, but slowly, from the progress of the cancer.

M. TILLAUX replied to the different objections which had been addressed to him. Perhaps resection of the coccyx would have afforded more room for action, but still it would not have permitted the extraction of a body so voluminous and situated in the iliac fossa. As to the incision in the iliac fossa, M. Studsgaard had considered that, but it had appeared to him that he would have much more space by incising in the median line. In his own particular case he had not discussed the question of an artificial anus, as peritonitis had not shown itself.— *London Med. Record*, Dec. 15, 1878.

—

Ascites Complicated with Strangulated Umbilical Hernia.

The patient was a man, 55 years of age, who was under the care of M. PETER for six months, suffering from cirrhosis of the liver with ascites. For this, he was tapped for the first time on April 25. An umbilical hernia, which had existed for many years previously, showed signs of strangulation at the time of the operation; but reduction was effected. A second puncture was made on May 1st, and was accompanied by the same accident. This time, however, reduction of the gut could not be obtained, and on May 3d the patient was transferred to M. VERNEUIL'S wards. Owing to the feeble constitutional condition of the man, M. Verneuil refused to operate with the knife. As some leeches, which two days before had been applied to the hernia, had given rise to some hemorrhage, an application of Vienna paste was made at the time the patient entered. The slough separated May 5th, and this was followed almost immediately by an escape of a considerable quantity of fecal matter from the upper part of the wound. The vomiting then ceased, and the patient rapidly gained strength. On May 23d there was no stool, the vomiting then reappeared. A purgative produced no effect. The next day, a sound introduced into the superior opening of the intestine gave vent to a large quantity of semi-liquid material. The vomiting then stopped, only, however, to recommence on the 25th; the ejected matter was black, like coffee-grounds. The escape of feces from the upper opening took place regularly, but the temperature fell gradually, and the patient succumbed on May 27th. At the *post-mortem* examination, the liver was found to be somewhat contracted. Hemorrhagic pleurisy was present on the left side. The strangulation was situated in the small intestine, one metre above the cæcum; there was no trace of the epiploon. The adhesions which united the intestines to the umbilical opening were perfectly firm; the artificial anus had undoubtedly prolonged life, death being due to the other lesions.—*Lond. Med. Record*, Nov. 15, 1878.

—

Fracture of a Catheter in the Bladder; Removal per Rectum.

In the *Bulletin et Mémoires de la Société de Chirurgie*, Nov. 5, 1878, M. FLEURY describes the case of a man on whom lithotrity was performed by Civiale in 1863, and who had since been accustomed to wash out the bladder by means of a metallic catheter. On April 23, 1878, he found on withdrawing the catheter that a portion was broken off and remained in the urethra; he pushed it into the bladder by means of another catheter. When he was seen by Dr. Brun four hours afterwards, he was found to have in his bladder a piece of catheter 7 centimetres (2.8 inches) long, lying with one end at the upper part of the bladder and the other at the *bas fond*. Dr. Fleury, on being called in consultation, advised that no attempt at extraction should be made, either through the urethra or by cystotomy. (The patient was 78 years of age.) The inflammation produced by the foreign body was moderate, and catheterism was continued without much difficulty. Four days later, during defecation, the end of the catheter was found to present at the anus, and was removed by moderate traction. After this, there was no pain; but the urine continued to escape *per anum.—London Med. Record.* Nov. 15, 1878.

—

A Case of Supra-Pubic Lithotomy.

At a late meeting of the Clinical Society of London (*Med. Times and Gazette,* Oct. 19, 1878) Mr. JONATHAN HUTCHINSON read notes of this case, which was that of a man aged about twenty-six, who had suffered from symptoms of stone for about six months. When admitted into the hospital his condition was urgent, the bladder being exceedingly irritable, and the urine containing pus and blood. He was considerably emaciated. There was no difficulty in recognizing that the stone was a very large one, and careful consideration was given to the question of the best means of extracting it. It was finally decided to prefer the supra-pubic method. No difficulty was encountered in the operation; the bladder was easily reached; and, the wound having been adequately enlarged, the stone was seized in the largest pair of forceps. Its size necessitated a little delay in extraction to allow the soft parts to yield. After its removal an india-rubber tube was passed through the urethra and retained in the bladder. It was hoped by this means to drain away the urine without any wetting of the bed. The fundus of the bladder was found much thickened and quite rigid by calcareous deposit. For the first week after the operation the man did exceedingly well; he then began to lose flesh, and subsequently had repeated rigors. The urine contained pus, and was constantly ammoniacal. Although great attention was given to the bladder it was found impossible to keep it empty and avoid overflow on the edges of the wound. The patient died of pyæmia about five weeks after the operation. At the necropsy the bladder was found very much thickened by inflammation, and its mucous membrane ulcerated and coated with concretion. The kidneys contained abscesses, and there were small pyæmic deposits in the liver and lungs. The calculus removed was very hard and heavy, of lithic acid, weighing nearly six ounces and a half, and measuring nine inches in circumference at the greatest and six at the least width. Mr. Hutchinson showed also the cast of a calculus of almost exactly the same size and weight as his own, which had been removed at the London Hospital by the late Mr. John Adams about ten years ago. In this instance, the unusual size of the stone was unexpected, and the ordinary lateral operation was adopted. The patient, who was a healthy young man, recovered well. Whilst this case proved that, in isolated cases, stones of upwards of six ounces in weight might be removed without unusual modifications of the lateral method, he still thought that general experience was in favour of special measures when the dimensions of the stone were so large. He had to choose between the high operation, bilateral section of the prostate, and recto-perineal lithotomy. On the whole, although it was not wise to allow a single case to influence the mind too much, he was inclined, by what he had observed in his own, to think that the high operation had special disadvantages in respect to the impeded exit of urine, and in another case he thought he should prefer to try the recto-perineal method, with free incision in the median line. It was doubtful, however, whether any modification of the method would have made any difference in the result, as the man was very ill, and his bladder in a state of advanced disease.

Cysts of the Spermatic Cord.

In *Le Progès Médical* (Nov. 23) M. Trelat relates a case of cysts in the spermatic cord, occurring in his practice at the Hôpital de la Charité. The patient was a lad aged 14 ; upon examination, a multiple tumour was detected along the course of the cord unconnected with the testicle, and in the inguinal canal was a swelling which was diagnosed at first to be a hernia, but which was afterwards found to be a cyst of the same nature as those lower down. All the cysts were tapped and the patient apparently recovered, but he soon returned to the hospital with a recurrence, all the cysts having refilled. The two varieties of cysts of the cord are: first, those devised from the remains of the Wolffian body which are connected to the testicle and epididymis ; and secondly those which arise from the vagino-peritoneal canal remaining more or less patent. The tumour under consideration belonged to the latter class, and this diagnosis was confirmed by the characters of the fluid drawn off from the cyst, which contained no spermatozoa nor crystals, and was not coagulable. The treatment of the recurrence was tapping and injection of iodine.—*London Med. Record*, Dec. 15, 1878.

Congenital Hydrocele.

In a report upon a memoir upon this subject by Dr. Gaillard, made to the Société de Chirurgie by M. de St. Germain (*Gaz. des Hop.*, December 10), he observed that the author sought to demonstrate that in young children these cases did best when left to themselves, and that an operation should not be performed upon a child of less than four or five years of age. Of thirteen cases which had come under his care, six had been treated by puncture or by astringents, and seven had been left absolutely to themselves. As these latter cases did perfectly well, he concludes that this should be the general rule of treatment. But M. de St. Germain thought, to say nothing of the problematical duration of the treatment, that no rule of treatment can be laid down from so few as seven cases. Hydroceles, in fact, abound in the children's hospitals, and no child less than a year old is ever operated upon. Resolvents are employed, and when these, and especially the hydrochlorate of ammonia, fail, an operation is performed if the hydrocele assumes inconvenient proportions. The operation consists either in puncture and injection, or in following the procedure of Defer, rendered popular by Maisonneuve and Desormeaux. M. de St. Germain operates upon hydrocele in children three years of age, when it attains the size of an egg, puncturing it and then cauterizing the sac, as practised by Defer ; and he has never met with any accidents.

M. Boinet observed that accoucheurs had long insisted upon the spontaneous cure of the hydrocele of new-born infants. But congenital hydroceles should be operated upon towards the age of five or six, because, when they persist too long, they predispose to the formation of hernia. M. Desprès agreed with Dr. Gaillard, and is of opinion that the operation is often abused—being lucrative, if useless. He has never operated upon a congenital hydrocele, as when these lesions are left to themselves they disappear spontaneously. On the other hand, he has never known hydrocele in the adult become cured under the influence of astringents. M. Tarnier formerly was in the habit of applying compresses dipped in aromatic wine for the treatment of hydroceles in new-born infants, which are by no means rare, generally appearing about the second or third day. Having afterwards left them to their natural course, he found that they did just as well without any treatment. M. Houel had seen a great number of these cases, and on several occasions he has found that they could not be reduced, although communicating with the peritoneal cavity. The conclusion that such communication does not exist must not, therefore, be inferred because reduction cannot be obtained. It is just as with irreducible spina bifida. M. Berger observed that Mr. Curling was only able to obtain reduction in one case after compression which lasted three-quarters of an hour; and M. Lannelongue added that no certainty can be obtained from the failure of the measures when these have only been continued for a short time. He has met with hydroceles which could only be slowly reduced by prolonged compression made in the horizontal posture.—*Med. Times and Gazette*, Dec. 21, 1878.

Electro-Puncture in Hydrocele.

F. ZAMBONI (*Giornale Veneto di Scienze Med.*) performed electro-puncture for five minutes at a time at two sittings, in a case of hydrocele. By the second day the effusion had disappeared. Ten days later it reappeared; but one more puncture caused it to disappear permanently. Zamboni thinks that the electricity gives tone to the vessels and stimulates their absorbent power.—*London Med. Record*, Dec. 15, 1878.

Treatment of Perineal Abscess.

M. VERNEUIL describes his treatment for certain abscesses at the margin of the anus. There are two distinct varieties of these abscesses; they both occupy the ischio-rectal fossa, but the one variety points towards the buttock, and tends to open externally, whilst the other destroys the circumrectal cellular tissue and tends to open into the rectum. In the first class of cases a simple incision made in the direction of the anus is sufficient; healing takes place rapidly without leaving a fistula. When the wall of the rectum has been laid bare, however, this treatment would be almost surely followed by a fistula. This happened in many cases which have come under M. Verneuil's notice. He quotes one, that of a strong, healthy man, who had a circumrectal abscess which opened of itself. M. Verneuil afterwards merely enlarged the opening, to allow a free escape of pus. Two months later a fistula was developed, and was operated on, the patient being altogether for three months in the hospital.

During the last few years M. Verneuil has combined the two operations. He opens the abscess by an incision, then introduces a ground probe, perforates the wall of the rectum at the highest point at which it is laid bare, and divides all the tissue between the two openings by means of the thermal cautery. He has done this many times without a bad result. When the two operations are done at different times, recovery takes place much more slowly. In a case of large prostatic abscess treated in this way, the cure was complete in thirty days, with the exception of a small superficial wound. The only objection which could be made to this mode of treatment is that it is rather more serious, and takes longer time than a simple incision: but then the cure is much more speedy and more certain. —*London Med. Record*, Dec. 15, 1878.

Abscess of the Margin of the Anus.

In a clinical lecture (*Rev. Méd.*, Nov. 18) Prof. VERNEUIL stated that in abscess of the margin of the anus, in which the pus has a tendency to find its way towards the surface of the buttock, no detachment of the wall of the rectum taking place, an incision of four or five centimetres in the direction of the anus discharges the pus. Cicatrization rapidly ensues without any fistula forming. But when the pus, instead of pursuing this course, destroys the perirectal tissue, causing a slight redness and tumefaction in this region, the wall of the rectum becomes ulcerated, and a fistula is formed. The discharge of the pus, even by a large incision, does not prevent the subsequent formation of this fistula. Instead of, as formerly, first opening the abscess and then treating the fistula, Professor Verneuil, for some years past, has opened the abscess, and having introduced a grooved director, he guides this towards the wall of the rectum, raising and perforating this. He then brings the director down by the rectum, dividing by means of the thermo-cautery all the bridge of the tissues which is comprised between the two openings. He has performed many operations of this kind without ever having met with any serious accidents. The pus comes away readily, and the pains cease, and all that is necessary is to frequently disinfect the wound by injections of weak carbolic acid, without introducing any tents—a practice which is both useless and dangerous in fistula. A cure takes place in an infinitely shorter time than when the abscess is treated at one time and the fistula at another.—*Med. Times and Gazette*, Nov. 30, 1878.

—

Bullet Wound of the Skull.

At a meeting of the *Société de Chirurgie* (Oct. 16), M. TERRILLON read a paper on a case of osseous fistula following the penetration of the skull by a revolver ball. The fistula was situated behind the external auditory meatus, and gave rise to purulent discharge. There were no cerebral complications, but complete deafness existed on the injured side. An examination revealed the presence of the projectile at a depth of nearly half an inch, not counting the thickness of the integuments. Extraction was attempted, but the ball was so firmly fixed that merely a few particles of lead were brought away. The skull was trephined and the bullet then easily extracted with forceps; merely two or three millimetres of the internal table of the skull separated the foreign body from the cranial cavity. The patient so far is well; but M. Terrillon had not read a single observation with regard to these lesions of the skull caused by projectiles, that had not terminated fatally. This takes place more or less slowly; sometimes, more than a year after the penetration, cerebral symptoms show themselves, such as meningitis, phlebitis of the sinus, hemorrhage, abscess of the cerebrum or cerebellum. —*London Med. Record*, Dec. 15, 1878.

—

Fracture of the Cranium, with Depression of the Left Parietal Bone.

Dr. LOUIS CARADEC relates the following case in the *Gazette Hebdom. de Méd. et de Chir.*, October 25, 1878.

The patient, a woman aged 25, was struck on the head by a stone. She immediately became unconscious, and remained so for two hours. Her medical attendant found her suffering from shock. Her breathing was embarrassed, her pulse weak, skin cold, pupils dilated. The tongue was directed to the right, and the right arm and face were paralyzed. She was also aphasic. The next day she was feverish, and had headache. On the fourth day a subcutaneous abscess at the place of injury was evacuated, and on the ninth day the wound had healed.

Seventeen days after the accident the patient was brought to M. Caradec. On examination he found a cicatrix, 5 centimetres in length, at the antero-inferior part of the left parietal bone. Its position would correspond internally with the fissure of Rolando and the ascending frontal and parietal convolutions. In the line of the cicatrix, there was a cup-shaped depression of the cranial wall. The walk of the patient was natural. She slept well and ate well. Her tongue was put out straight. The pupils were equal, contractile, and of normal size. She had a stupid appearance. Her powers of memory and intellect were enfeebled, and her speech embarrassed, indeed she could not speak a few words without stammering, and she was often temporarily aphasic. There was marked paresis of the right side of the face, and whenever the facial muscles were put into play, slight muscular contractions were observed on this side, especially in the region of the labial commissure. The right shoulder was unaffected, but there was emaciation of the right arm, forearm, and hand; their temperature was lowered, and their sensibility and motility impaired. There was a difference of temperature between the right and left arms of about 5° Cent., the right arm being 27° to 29° Cent. (80.6° to 84.2° Fair.) while the left was 32° to 34° (89.6° to 91.2° Fahr.). The prick of a pin was not felt in the right forearm or hand. The right arm could be moved, but the grasping power of the hand was diminished, and could not be long sustained. Caradec attributes the symptoms to fracture of the left parietal and frontal bones, with lesion of the upper parts of the left ascending frontal and parietal convolutions, and cites this case in support of the view that the motor centres of the upper extremity are in the upper two-thirds of the ascending convolutions. The absence of more pronounced aphasia and facial paralysis, he thinks, is due to the fact that the lower parts of the ascending convolutions were little injured. The case was one in which trepanning should have been resorted to at an early period.

Eighteen months after the accident, the aphasia and facial paralysis had completely disappeared. The brachial paralysis could still be observed, but was very slight. The middle, ring, and little finger were more paralyzed than the thumb and index finger.—*London Med. Record*, Dec. 15, 1878.

—

Fractures of the Tibia.

M. HEYDENREICH (*Thèse de Paris* and *Gazette Hebdomadaire*, July 12, 1878), divides fractures of the upper extremity of the tibia into those of the upper third, below the anterior tuberosity, and fractures of the upper extremity properly so called. 1. Fractures of the upper third diminish in frequency as they approach the articulation; they are transverse or oblique, and are generally accomplished by fracture of the fibula. The cause is most frequently direct violence, although they have been caused by a fall on the heel; fractures caused by indirect violence are generally near the anterior tuberosity. There are swelling and considerable ecchymosis, due to the abundance of extravasated blood; effusion into the knee-joint often takes place; displacement may not occur. The prognosis is grave, because of the liability to gangrene; union takes place very slowly (three to four months), probably because of the blood extravasated between the fractured ends. The limb should be extended; when there is not much displacement, slight flexion is preferable, being less likely to produce stiffness of the knee, which may follow the treatment. 2. Fractures of the upper extremity of the tibia comprise (*a*) separation of the superior epiphysis; (*b*) separation of the anterior tuberosity, the most frequent cause of which is contraction of the triceps femoris; (*c*) fracture of one of the condyles; (*d*) fracture of the entire extremity of the bone. This last form presents several varieties, according to the extent of the fracture, the position and the number of the fragments. The fibula is often intact. Fractures of the entire lower extremity are rare; they may occur at any age; they are caused by direct violence or by falls on the feet. The prognosis is grave; they may be confounded with contusion, sprain, dislocation of the tibia, or fracture of the femur. These are the principal conclusions of this thesis, which, to be so complete, must have cost the author much laborious work.—*Lond. Med. Record*, Dec. 15, 1878.

Resection of several Joints in the same Individual.

This case, which occurred in the practice of Dr. N. SCHEDE, is reported in the *Deutsche Zeitschrift für prakt. Medizin*, No. 20, 1878. The patient, a girl aged 19, had suffered for four years from rheumatism of several joints, which ran a rather acute course, and finally led to the formation of ankyloses. There was bony ankylosis of both wrists and elbows, both knees and ankles; most of the phalangeal joints were also stiff. Most of the joints with the exception of the wrists, were much thickened. The patient was thus in a state of complete helplessness. Within four months, Dr. Schede performed resection of both wrists and elbows, as well as both ankles. At the time of the report, both wrists were movable; so also were the elbows, but one had already become more stiff and threatened ankylosis. There was limited power of motion in the ankles. The course of the case showed that a better result in regard to active and passive motion follows when the resection is extensive, than when a small piece of bone is removed. This depends, probably, on the fact that the disposition to the production of bone and the formation of ankylosis, which in some such patients remains very great, continues even after resection. The patient in this case had every reason to be satisfied with the improvement in the utility of her limbs. After her recovery, she could assist her walking by crutches, whereas she could not use them before; she could also use her hands in feeding and clothing herself, which previously was quite impossible.—*British Med. Journal*, Nov. 23, 1878.

—

Excision of Portion of Tarsus for Talipes Varus.

At a late meeting of the Clinical Society (*Lancet*, Nov. 30). Mr. BRYANT exhibited a patient who had been the subject of talipes varus, and had been treated by the removal of a wedge of bone from the tarsus. The case was that of a boy twelve years of age, who had been under surgical treatment for the condition from infancy. When five years of age tenotomy had been performed with some success, but as the Scarpa's shoe had caused pain, it was laid aside, and the deformity returned. On admission into Guy's Hospital the muscles of the leg were wasted, and the patient walked on the outside of the foot, upon which had formed two large bursæ. Mr. Bryant removed a wedge-shaped piece of bone from the tarsus, as described by Mr. Davies-Colley in October, 1875. An incision was made across the dorsum of the foot from a point corresponding to the tubercle of the scaphoid to the outer border of the cuboid, and a second incision along the outer border of the foot, the two incisions forming a ⊣ shape. The flaps were then turned back, and the tendons of the extensors divided. A spatula was introduced around the scaphoid bone towards the sole of the foot to protect the soft parts, and the lower section of the wedge of bone cut with a key hole saw, one line of section extending across the dorsum of the foot from the scaphoid to the anterior border of the cuboid, the second bone section being made higher up; and a wedge, with its apex corresponding to the scaphoid bone, and its base to the cuboid, one inch long, was thus cut away. After the operation the anterior half of the foot was readily brought round into position, and horse-hair drainage was employed. The temperature rose to 102°, but on the third day was down to 99.7°, with a pulse of 80. A small quantity of pus was evacuated by a puncture made into the skin, in a position corresponding to the apex of the wedge; in other respects the wound healed rapidly. The boy now presents a foot of good form with a flat sole, on which he walks with comfort. The foot was somewhat shortened after the operation. The tendo Achillis had been cut, with the object of bringing down the heel, but with little result. Mr. Bryant said that ablation of the cuboid had been suggested by Dr. Little, in 1854, and practised by Solly, in 1857, upon which the operation now under consideration was a great improvement. He considered it also much better than Mr. Lund's operation for the removal of the astragalus, which was performed in 1872, but which he thought might be useful where the equinus was worse than the varus.

Mr. Davy congratulated Mr. Bryant on the result of his case. He believed that he himself had operated in a similar way more frequently than any other surgeon. There was a class of confirmed and intractable cases of talipes that resisted all methods of treatment. In 1874 he revived Mr. Solly's operation— viz., removal of the cuboid, which had been described by that surgeon twenty years previously, and had fallen into oblivion, and had even been condemned. He did this in five cases with encouraging but not perfect results, proceeding on strictly experimental methods, and not feeling justified in interfering with the astragalo-scaphoid joint, until he had proved that division of the calcaneo-cuboid was insufficient. In April, 1876, he published his experience, and in October of that year Mr. Davies-Colley anticipated him in his paper read before the Medico-Chirurgical Society by performing the milder operation, which Mr. Davy had now performed several times. He showed the casts of his ninth patient, taken before and after the operation, and the result was very satisfactory. No doubt, the operation was on its trial, and was opposed by many surgeons, but he was content to abide by the results, and was glad to see Mr. Bryant commending it so strongly. Patients, after the operation, became absolutely plantigrade; the scar was small and well out of the line of pressure; there was no possibility of relapse, and a symmetrical foot took the place of an unsightly and useless member.

—

Popliteal Aneurism treated by Esmarch's Bandage.

At a late meeting of the Clinical Society of London (*Med. Times and Gaz.,* Dec. 28, 1878), Mr. JONATHAN HUTCHINSON related the particulars of two cases. The subject of the first was a robust gentleman, aged twenty-six, who had never had syphilis. The tumour filled the right popliteal space, and pulsated strongly. There had been pain for three months, but the pulsation had been recognized only a month. He had been placed under Mr. Hutchinson's care by Mr. Drew. After three days' rest in bed, ether was given, and Esmarch's bandage was applied to the entire limb. It was put on tight below the knee, very lightly over the tumour, and tightly again on the thigh. The elastic strap was applied as tightly as possible in the upper third, and after a little time the bandage was removed. The tumour was left full of blood which was completely stagnated. Ether was kept up for an hour, and at the end of that time the strap was removed, and a horseshoe tourniquet substituted. No pulsation ever returned in the tumour, but as a matter of precaution the tourniquet was retained for a few hours. The subsequent recovery was rapid and complete. The second case was less speedily successful. Its subject was a gunnery instructor from Shoeburyness, who had been treated by pressure for an aneurism in the calf two years previously. On that occasion success had been obtained by thirteen days' compression. The aneurism on the second occasion filled the popliteal space, and was the size of a large orange. It pulsated strongly. Esmarch's bandage under ether was used for one hour in exactly the same way as in the previous case, but with no benefit. The tumour beat as before. Three days later another trial was made of the same plan; but on this occasion arrangements had been made, by relays of students, to keep up digital pressure after removal of the constricting strap. The man was kept under ether for two hours. At the end of that time the strap was removed, and during the change of hands it became evident that pulsation was still present, but it was more easily controlled than before. Manual

compression was kept up for about seven ıours, at tıe end of wıicı time pulsation ıad quite ceased. Tıe tumour remained solid, and rapidly diminisıed in
size, and tıe man left tıe ıospital a few weeks later quite well. It was tıougıt
tıat in tıis case, altıougı tıe Esmarcı bandage did not produce consolidation,
yet tıat it conduced to tıe cure, and certainly on neitıer occasion did it do any
harm. Mr. Hutcıinson stated tıat ıe ıad brought forward tıese cases, in
neit/ of wıicı was tıere anytıing original in tıe treatment, in order to elicit
from surgeons statements of tıeir experience and opinions in reference to tıis
novel and important metıod.

Mr. THOMAS SMITH, by tıe use of Esmarcı's bandage, applied as ıe ıad seen
Mr. Croft apply it at St. Tıomas's Hospital, ıad cured two cases, and ıad failed
witı two. In a recent case no cıloroform was given, and tıe bandage was applied tigıtly below and above tıe tumour, and left in place. He considered tıis
better tıan constricting tıe limb by tıe cord, a proceeding wıicı, on the Continent, ıad been followed by permanent paralysis from injury to nerves. Tıe
pressure was more diffused by tıe bandage. In tıe last case, wıicı occurred to
a member of tıe medical profession, tıe bandage was alternated witı pressure
by a tourniquet over tıe artery, and tıe treatment lasted from 9 A. M. to
6 P. M., at wıicı time great pain was felt in tıe swelling, and coagulation probably took place. Pressure was kept on for an ıour and a ıalf after tıis, and
tıe result was entirely successful.

Mr. MORRANT BAKER ıad ıad an unfavourable case in a man of forty or fifty,
wıere some blood ıad escaped from tıe aneurism, wıicı ıe ıad treated successfully. After a preliminary imperfect application, tıe bandage was kept on for
tıree-quarters of an ıour, followed by ıalf an ıour's compression witı tıe finger,
and was reapplied for twenty minutes, and compression again kept up for nearly
two ıours. No anæstıetic was employed, no pain was complained of; and at
tıe end of tıat time tıe aneurism was consolidated.

Mr. MAUNDER tıougıt tıat tıere was no single certainly successful metıod of
dealing witı tıese cases. He ıad tried Dr. Reid's plan twice; botı times unsuccessfully. One was cured by digital compression, and tıe otıer by ligature.
In ıis opinion, tıe objection to tıis bandage was tıat it was painful, and required
an anæsthetic witı its attendant risk.

Mr. BARWELL agreed tıat no single metıod could be relied upon, but said
tıat tıe bandage was especially unsuitable in fusiform aneurisms. He ıad tried
it in a bad case, wıere tıere was extensive arterial disease, witı fusiform aneurisms in tıe axillary and bracıial arteries; ıe made use of a sort of bridge to keep
the bandage off tıe tumour, and applied it ligıtly above tıe swelling, allowing a
small current of blood to pass. After an ıour and a ıalf tıere was no result; it
was subsequently reapplied twice, but ıe was obliged finally to ligature tıe
artery, tying it gently in consequence of its diseased state; tıe man was well in
ten days.

Mr. T. SMITH objected tıat tıis metıod of applying tıe bandage, so as to
allow tıe current of blood to continue, was essentially different from tıe plan
under discussion.

Mr. BARWELL added that on one occasion tıe flow was arrested for about one
ıour.

Mr. HERBERT PAGE ıad tried tıe bandage witıout success in a case apparently well suited for it, and in tıe ıospital at tıe same time a case of Mr. Lane's
was treated in tıe same way witı a like result. Tıe plug in tıe distal arteries,
wıicı ıad been tıougıt to precede clotting in tıe aneurism, was, in ıis opinion,
a later event, and followed its cure. He alluded to a case of Mr. Pemberton's,
wıere tıis metıod of treatment ıad been followed by gangrene.

Mr. BRYANT related a case where the bandage was used for one hour, under the influence of morphia, by which time there was much consolidation. In two or three days the aneurism grew worse; but the bandage under chloroform for three-quarters of an hour was followed by much improvement. It soon relapsed, and he then tied the artery. Gangrene followed in a few days, which required amputation below the knee. In his opinion, the bandage was responsible for the gangrene; and it constituted a serious, though perhaps not fatal, objection to its use.

Dr. MAHOMED considered the bandage was contraindicated in cases of extensive arterial disease. He had found that, when the bandage was placed on one arm, the volume of the other was much increased, showing that a considerably increased distension of the rest of the vascular system resulted. Where the cerebral arteries were diseased, this might be dangerous; but this objection did not apply to the ligature.

Mr. GOULD alluded to two cases of aneurism treated in this way which he had examined. In both, the clot in the aneurism was loose; that in the artery, above and below, firm and fibrous. He considered the coagulum in the aneurism was secondary, and he thought Mr. Bryant's case bore out this view. Here the clot, being soft, was broken up by the stream, which led to thrombosis and gangrene beyond. This difference in the clot he attributed to the imperfect nutrition of the walls of the sac. He still thought those cases would be successful where the opening was large and the vessel healthy.

Mr. NORTON had tried the bandage without success in one case. There was extensive vascular disease, with double aortic murmur and three aneurisms. The treatment, though it failed, had none of the disastrous results Dr. Mahomed predicted, though the case was just such an one as those referred to by Dr. Mahomed. He considered the risk due to distension of the vessels, as the result of compression, small indeed when compared with the risk of a ligature where general vascular disease existed.

Mr. HEATH agreed with Mr. Barwell that a fusiform aneurism was not amenable to this treatment, and with Mr. Gould in his theory of the action of this bandage. In Mr. Smith's case, however, the general state of the vessels was very unfavourable; yet a rapid cure resulted. It was quite possible that in Mr. Bryant's the gangrene was a result of the ligature, and not of the bandage. In a patient of his, in whom the bandage had been twice applied, and in whom the artery had been ligatured, once in the usual way, and once with antiseptic precautions, the result was of interest. The patient was strongly in favour of the antiseptic plan, from which he had suffered much less pain.

Mr. HUTCHINSON, in reply to the various speakers, said he thought the plan of treatment under discussion a valuable addition to the means at our disposal. It seemed impossible to predicate as to the cases in which it was most likely to succeed; but it seemed to be a trial in nearly all. He could not admit that Mr. Bryant's case proved that any ill consequences were due to the bandage. It had simply not cured. The gangrene came on after the ligature, and should be attributed to it, and not to the Esmarch bandage. He believed that, in different individuals, very different degrees of aptitude for coagulation were displayed by the blood, and hence chiefly the explanation why some cases were cured easily, and others with difficulty. The tendency to coagulation might be helped by insisting on abstinence from fluids, as was done in both his cases, and by giving drugs, such as iodide of potassium, lead, and digitalis. Whilst fully admitting the great value of digital compression, he still thought that a trial should first be given to the bandage. He had had several very rapid cures by compression; but he did not recollect any case of aneurism of similar size in which the patient had suffered less during the treatment than the first of these which he had just related. If ether were used, not chloroform, he believed that no danger was encountered; and he felt sure that the anæsthetic made the treatment much less painful. He would strongly recommend that, in all cases in which the bandage was tried, arrangements to continue digital compression immediately afterwards should be made; and that great care should be taken to prevent the blood from passing into the tumour on release of the limb from the strap.

—

Control of Hemorrhage in Amputation at the Hip-Joint.

Mr. ALFRED PEARCE GOULD performed the operation of amputation at the hip-joint on the 7th at Westminster Hospital. The patient was a young man, aged twenty-eight, in whom Mr. Gould had previously resected the joint. The hemorrhage was controlled by an original device of Mr. R. Davy's, and so completely that only about three ounces of blood were lost. Mr. Davy compresses the common iliac artery by introducing a straight wooden rod, with a bulbous end, carefully into the rectum for about nine inches. The whole length of the rod is about twenty-two inches. It requires, of course, considerable knowledge to apply this instrument accurately and to use it harmlessly. But in skilful hands, the slightest elevation or depression of the handle, when once the instrument was brought to bear on the vessel, was enough to stop or to allow the flow of blood.

We were struck with the complete anæmia of the stump when Mr. Davy lightly raised the handle of the stick. Notwithstanding the slight amount of blood lost, the patient unfortunately died on the fourth day after the operation. The post-mortem examination showed that the parts where pressure had been applied to control hemorrhage were quite uninjured. The chief morbid appearances were extensive thrombosis of the veins of the opposite limb, extending into the common iliac vein.—*Lancet*, Dec. 21, 1878.

Midwifery and Gynæcology.

The Development and Maturation of Graafian Follicles during Pregnancy.

Dr. SLAVJANSKY, of St. Petersburg, describes (*Annales de Gynécologie*, Feb. 1878) the condition of the ovaries in a case of extra-uterine fœtation, and draws some general inferences as to the development of Graafian follicles during pregnancy. The patient was twenty-four years old, had had one child previously, and died from rupture of an extra-uterine fœtation of the left Fallopian tube of three and a half months' development. Menstruation had been suppressed during the pregnancy, but a slight discharge of blood had taken place for two or three weeks before rupture of the sac. The portion of the left Fallopian tube distended by the fœtal sac was that near its insertion.

The left ovary was 3.5 cm. long and 2.5 cm. broad. Its surface was covered by cicatricial furrows, and in places it was adherent to adjacent parts by long transparent false membranes. One portion appeared swollen, and a transverse incision at this part laid open a cavity 1.3 cm. in diameter, two-thirds filled by contents which had been coagulated by the alcohol in which the specimen had been kept Towards the surface of the ovary the wall of this cavity was as thin as a sheet of paper, the thickness not being greater than 0.05 cm. Towards the posterior surface of the ovary was a softened spot 0.4 cm. in diameter, having the appearance and characters of a corpus luteum. In the cortical substance were several cavities with coagulated contents, the largest 0.3 cm. in diameter, having precisely the appearance of Graafian follicles in different stages of development. Beneath one of the furrows in the same part was a brick-red, irregularly stellate body, 0.2 cm. in diameter.

The right ovary was 2.7 cm. long and 1.5 cm. broad, and its surface was furrowed like that of the other. At its internal part, near the ovarian ligament, was a prominence, a section through which showed a recent corpus luteum, 1.0 cm. in diameter. Its central portion was whitish and firm, and white stellate bands extended from it into the yellow substance. Near the corpus luteum was a Graafian follicle 0.3 cm. in diameter.

On microscopic examination of the walls of the principal cavity in the left ovary, they were found to correspond to those of a ripe Graafian follicle. The internal surface was covered by flattened cylindrical epithelium, the cells of which resembled those in the membrana granulosa of the smaller Graafian follicles. A small prominence was noticed near the thinnest part of the wall. Being removed on the point of a needle, it proved to consist of a mass of epithelial cells, in the midst of which one was an ovule. This cavity was then clearly not a cystic degeneration, but a Graafian follicle ripe and ready to burst. The corpus luteum, 0.4 cm. in diameter, in the left ovary had all the microscopic characters of these bodies. Its cells, however, showed commencing degeneration, and their nuclei were scarcely discernible. The larger corpus luteum in the right ovary had the characters of the true corpus luteum of pregnancy strongly marked. The cells were clearly marked and their nuclei distinct. The central portion consisted of a connective tissue of recent origin, containing more round as well as fusiform cells than in the other case. The cortical substance of both ovaries also contained the bodies formed by abortive Graafian follicles, that is to say, stellate masses, consisting of connective tissue of recent or old formation. In one was found the trace of an ovule, in the form of a collapsed zona pellucida.

The author concludes that during pregnancy there may be found, but perhaps only exceptionally, Graafian follicles, ripe, and on the point of bursting, and remarks that Scanzoni has admitted the possibility of follicles becoming mature, though not of their bursting, during pregnancy. Of the three corpora lutea visible to the naked eye, he considers that the most recent, situated on the side opposite to the pregnancy, was due to a follicle which had ruptured since the commencement of gestation, and that a migration of the ovum across the peritoneal cavity was not to be inferred. The second in age, which had also the character of the true corpus luteum of pregnancy, he considers to have belonged to the fecundated ovum which was arrested in the Fallopian tube of the same side. The older and brick-red body he regards as being of a date anterior to gestation. Thus the case would show the possibility, not only of the rupture of a Graafian follicle during pregnancy, but of the formation thereby of an additional corpus luteum. The author refers to the view of Mayrhofer (recorded in the *Obstetrical Journal*, vol. iv. p. 699), who holds that follicles rupture during pregnancy as at other times, and that the corpus luteum of pregnancy does not correspond to the fecundated ovum, but is formed afresh every month. He considers that this cannot be accepted until established by a greater number of well observed cases, and points out the necessity for examining the ovaries in all parts with greater minuteness than has usually been employed.—*Obstetrical Journal of Great Britain*, Dec. 1878.

Chloroform in Natural Labour.

Professor COURTY of Montpellier has recently contributed to the *Gazette Hebdomadaire* (October 25 and November 8) an interesting paper upon "The Employment of Anæsthetics during Natural Labour." It seems to be founded upon an address which he delivered at the International Congress of the Medical Sciences held at Geneva last September, which was occasioned by a paper upon the subject read by Dr. Piachaud, warmly approving of the practice. While agreeing with Dr. Piachaud in his conclusions upon the subject, Prof. Courty took occasion to regret the slight extent to which the practice of giving chloroform during labour prevailed in France. And, indeed, it is a matter of surprise, after the safety of the practice and its great advantages have been demonstrated for so long a period in this country, so far from having been introduced into France, it has been met with what may be called a violent opposition on the part of accoucheurs—even those in high position. But we cannot but feel surprised that Prof. Courty, in the paper which we are about to notice, having for its main object the making known the utility of chloroform and the futility of the objections which have been advanced to its employment, makes no allusion whatever to the efforts which have been already made in the same direction by Dr. Charles Campbell, formerly Chef de Clinique of Prof. Paul Dubois, and for many years past one of the most distinguished accoucheurs of the French metropolis. Yet surely his authority in the matter is of far higher import than that of Prof. Courty, who states that he is only in possession of forty cases of his own whereon to base his recommendations. Dr. Campbell was enabled in his first publication upon the subject in Prof. Gubler's *Journal de Thérapeutique*, in 1874, to refer to more than 900 cases in which he had employed chloroform in natural labour; and in his memoir presented to the Congress at Geneva, and since published separately in 1877, he states that he has now administered it in 1052 out of 1657 labours, without the production of hemorrhage or other accident, and without delaying the progress of delivery. The truth of his statements has not been denied, but still the practice which they inculcate has been violently opposed by Profs. Pajot, Depaul, and others, chiefly in consequence of their having confounded the moderate amount of anæsthesia (*demi-anæsthésie*, or *anæsthésie obstétricale*) employed by Dr. Campbell with surgical anæsthesia which he would reserve for obstetrical operations. However, we do not doubt that the practice will eventually triumph over the opposition which always awaits every innovation in France that is not of Gallic origin.

In the meantime, we may advert to Prof. Courty's own observations. He states that although for a long time past he has not practised midwifery, yet he has often found himself compelled to comply with the wishes of patients, who having formerly undergone treatment for uterine or peri-uterine disease, and become subsequently pregnant, and attend them in their confinements in order to allay their fears. In regard to these cases, two things have to be observed. First, that none of them were primiparæ, so that it is possible that less chloroform may have sufficed for them. On the other hand, all these patients had been before the subjects of more or less dangerous puerperal accidents; so that the opportunities were exceptionally good for judging of the efficacy and utility of obstetrical anæsthesia, since it was known beforehand that all these patients had had bad times on former occasions, several of them having been on the point of dying from hemorrhage or other accidents. They were therefore in relatively unfavourable conditions when compared with those of ordinary lying-in women. In all these patients, more than forty in number, chloroform was employed, and in none of them did it give rise to any serious inconvenience, or cause regret for its having been used.

1. Speaking from the experience which he has derived from observation of these cases, Prof. Courty observes, first, with regard to the period at which the chloroform should be given, that although this should not be considered as arrived so long as the pains are moderate and regular and all seems progressing without excessive suffering or exhaustion, yet it should not be laid down as a rule that we must wait until the expulsive period has arrived, and the torture of its accompanying pains has to be prevented. When the pains become too strong or irregular, when the patient becomes excited or exhausted by their violence, continuousness, frequent return, irregularity of their course, or the diversity and multiplicity of their seat, their neuralgic character, and want of effective power, chloroform should be administered : and it is marvellous to observe how, after a few aspirations, without loss of consciousness, or even complete loss of sensibility, the pains assume their proper intermittent character with equal periods of repose, the contractions become regular, and the labour re-acquires its normal course. The first advantage of chloroform, therefore, is its relief of excessive, irregular, and enervating pains, without impeding contraction, a sensation even of slight pain being still sometimes perceived. The inhalation is repeated or not in proportion to this amount of sensation, and the patient may be thus watched and kept in a state of half-somnolence for hours, the labour still progressing, and expulsion taking place almost unconsciously. The benefit which accrues from this suppression of pain by the diminution of subsequent reaction has not been sufficiently adverted to.

2. A second advantage is the cessasion of muscular contractions, which are themselves the consequences of painful sensations having the double character of reflex motions and synergetic actions. Some of these contractions form a direct obstacle to parturition, as in perineal resistance. A portion of uterine effort is necessarily expended in overcoming this resistance ; and when this is obviated, so much is gained, the uterine contraction being then employed solely in furthering the progress of the presentation. The duration of the labour is diminished by so much ; and in all these cases it was found as a fact that the preceding labours had been very much longer. As regards the other contractions that are suppressed, of the muscles of the abdomen, the diaphragm, and other muscles which, participating in the effort, are brought into play when the patient exerts all her force in aid of the action of the uterus, the advantage of their suppression may not seem so evident. Prof. Courty, while admitting their immediate direct efficacy in aid of the expulsive action of the uterus, operating in this way as they do in micturition and defecation, yet believes that the service they render is often a very questionable one, giving rise frequently to accidents to which too little attention has been paid. Moreover, he does not believe that the duration of labour is really abridged by these voluntary contractions, inasmuch as proportionate perineal resistance remains. By suppressing both the abdominal and the perineal muscular contractions, the uterus is allowed to pursue its work without obstruction and without disorder, its contractions then taking on a regularity in every way favourable to the accomplishment of its function. The energetic and regulated action of the uterus can be readily felt, and may almost be seen. This has been so markedly the case in all the cases that have come under Dr. Courty's notice, that he is quite at a loss to comprehend the fears of some accoucheurs, and still less the observations which they have reported of the suppression of uterine contractility under the influence of chloroform employed in suitable doses.

3. As a consequence of the suppression of pain and the diminution of the duration of labour, "traumatism" is necessarily also diminished. When we consider

the amount of this which is produced in a prolonged labour by the pressure, contusions, lacerations, intestinal effusions, etc., which occur, influencing so many organs, we can only be surprised that we do not oftener meet with ovaritis, metritis, perimetritis, peritonitis, vesical fistulæ, and the various other puerperal accidents, which may be regarded as the natural results of such a traumatism. The chances of such accidents are greatly diminished by obstetric anæsthesia, and in no one of his cases has Prof. Courty met with any one of them.

4. Another advantage, which is opposed to the assertions of some accoucheurs, has been the result of Prof. Courty's observations, viz., the absence of hemorrhage, and that with regard to some of his patients who in former confinements had suffered from it. This may be due to the fact that none of the cases have been primiparæ, and that he has never had to carry chloroformatization very far. The labours having been very short, and the womb having had to continue its contractions for a relatively less time than ordinary, and not having to overcome perineal resistance, has not suffered subsequently from inertia, the ordinary cause of hemorrhage.

"In employing chloroform for lying-in women I observe the same precautions as in all my operations. In place of having her chloroformed by an assistant, so as to produce both insensibility and muscular resolution, assimilating her to a corpse, as I have sometimes seen done in England on patients about to be operated upon (which I may say, in passing, explains to me the incomparably greater frequency of deaths from chloroform in that country compared with our own), I cause her to breathe the chloroform by little whiffs, and mixed at first with plenty of air, making her count aloud, in order to cause her to respire regularly, and at the same time render me an account of the condition of the nervous centres. I suspend the anæsthesia when the pains have been rendered tolerable, resuming it and suspending it again according to the necessity. I have thus, without any danger, been able to prolong anæsthesia in women in labour from one hour to eight and even ten hours, and have consumed in a day, in small whiffs 120, and perhaps even 150, grammes of chloroform. I say 'perhaps,' for it is difficult to dose it when the most simple and least frightening mode of administration is employed, viz., by a sponge placed in a curved napkin. Thus used, so little fear does it excite, so easy is it employed, and so well tolerated by most patients, that they familiarize themselves with it to the risk of converting it into an abuse if not carefully watched."—*Med. Times and Gaz.*, Nov. 23, 1875.

Sterility.

Dr. WALTON, at a meeting of the Ghent Medical Society (*Annales de la Société de Méd. de Gand.*), read notes of a very interesting case of sterility. It was that of a woman who had been sterile for seven years, having many symptoms of chronic inflammation of the neck and body of the uterus, with a very · marked anæmia. This latter symptom was treated with iron for a long time, but when the case came under Dr. Walton's care, he assigned it to its true cause. On examination by speculum his suspicions were confirmed, and the patient was cured in two months by means of exclusively local treatment. This consisted chiefly of cauterization with nitrate of silver, and applications of glycerine and tannin. The woman shortly afterwards became pregnant, and was confined of a fine healthy child at full term.—*Lond. Med. Record*, Dec. 15, 1878.

The Use of Pilocarpin in Procuring Abortion.

Dr. CHADZYNKI (*Przeglad Lekarski*, No. 25, 1878, and *Allgem. Medicin. Central-Zeitung*) states that he had witnessed very favourable results by treating skin-diseases, such as psoriasis, syphilis, etc., with hypodermic injections of pilocarpin. In one of these cases, the patient, a syphilitic girl aged 21 was in the fourth month of her pregnancy. After the ninth injection had been made labour suddenly began, and the fœtus was born.

Three other similar cases have already been observed. It would, therefore, be highly instructive to submit this particular effect of the drug to careful study, as it may prove very useful in cases where premature confinement is indicated. Great care should, however, be observed in administering subcutaneous injections of pilocarpinum to pregnant women.—*London Med. Record*, Dec. 15, 1878.

Medical Jurisprudence and Toxicology.

Poisoning from an Overdose of Sweet Spirits of Nitre, resembling a case of Acute Alcoholic Poisoning.

Mr. T. WOOD HILL records (*Lancet*, Nov. 30, 1878) the following case of his :—

I was sent for on Sept. 26, 1878, to see a male child aged two years and eleven months, who had climbed up on a chair and taken from off the mantelpiece a stoppered bottle containing between three and four ounces of sweet spirits of nitre, and drunk the contents, during the absence of the attendant. On my arrival, at 1 P.M., I found him in a complete state of collapse, cold, almost pulseless, insensible, both pupils fixed and widely dilated, breathing hardly perceptible. Before seeing him he had vomited freely, the contents of the stomach being undigested food (no blood), with a smell of spirit; the bowels had been well open. I had him placed in bed between warm blankets, and hot-water bottles applied to the feet and armpits. After an hour and a half the temperature of the body began to grow warmer, and at three o'clock seemed of a burning heat; slight perspiration apparent, pulse slightly improved; strong smell of spirit from the breath. At 6 the vomiting and purging recurred; at 10.30 the breathing became stertorous, and he died at half-past 11, just twelve hours after he had taken the fatal dose, no convulsions having occurred.

Necropsy, three days and a half after Death.—Body measured thirty-six inches, well nourished. No external signs of injury. On opening the abdomen, a strong alcoholic odour was emitted. The stomach contained food, chiefly bread, in a state of semi-digestion; the mucous coat was highly inflamed and red near the pyloric end, on the anterior surface of the posterior border, and in one spot very much attenuated. The duodenal end of the small intestines red and inflamed, and bile-stained; the remainder of intestines healthy. Kidneys slightly congested. The other organs healthy. On removing the skull-cap, I found the membranes of the brain highly congested, containing a large quantity of dark-coloured blood. Brain soft, pulpy, and quite wet; vessels congested; no trace of fluid in the ventricles.

Remarks.—This case seems to me worthy of record—first, on account of the rarity of so common a domestic remedy being the cause of death; secondly, showing the power of deglutition of so potent a fluid in a child of that age.

CONTENTS.

Published Monthly, price $2.50 *per annum, free of postage.*
Also, furnished together with the AMERICAN JOURNAL OF THE MEDICAL
SCIENCES *and the* MEDICAL NEWS AND LIBRARY *for* SIX DOLLARS *per
annum in advance, the whole free of postage.*

HENRY C. LEA, Philadelphia.

THE MONTHLY ABSTRACT

OF

MEDICAL SCIENCE.

VOL. VI. No. 3.　　　**For List of Contents see last page.**　　　MARCH, 1879.

Anatomy and Physiology.

Origin of the Fourth Pair of Cerebral Nerves.

Dr. DUVAL gives the results of his observations on the real origin of the pathetic nerve, in a late number of the *Journal de l'Anatomie*. Its course from its point of emergence to its nucleus of origin is, he states, short, but very complex. In the valve of Vieussens two transverse bands can be clearly distinguished, each of which presents two extremities, one occupying a superior plane, which is the emergent or peripheric extremity of the fourth nerve, the other more deeply placed, which represents the cerebral extremity. This part is in relation with the superior border of the cerebellar peduncle and with the external border of the superior root of the fifth—a relation that has led some anatomists to refer to the fifth those fasciculi which really belong to the pathetic. The fibres of the fourth then incline downwards and inwards, and may be followed to their nucleus. If we trace the root in the opposite direction, that is, from its real origin to its emergence, it will be found that, issuing from the nucleus, the fibres of origin run at first nearly transversely outwards, then from before backwards parallel to the axis of the nervous system, then turn suddenly inwards to decussate in the valve of Vieussens with the opposite nerve. The nerve-root, therefore, forms a horse-shoe, with its convexity directed outwards. The anterior limb is formed by the fibrils emerging from the nucleus. The posterior branch constitutes the decussation of the nerves, and the middle longitudinal part is in close relation with the ascending root of the fifth; it is, in fact, crossed by this root of the fifth, which runs from the superior part of the pons into the region of the internal border of the tubercula quadrigemina.—*Lancet*, Dec. 7, 1878.

Absence of Vagina and Uterus.

Professor POLAILLON related the following case (*Union Méd.*, November 12) at the Société de Médecine of Paris: A woman, about twenty-three years of age, presented all the usual feminine attributes with regard to the breasts, pelvis, voice, etc., and her external genital organs were of natural conformation. But, on examination, the hymen was found to be imperforate and incapable of depression. The perineum was broad and resisting, and quite normal. On examining by the rectum, neither any menstrual collection nor any internal organs of generation could be perceived. On combining with this examination the introduction of a catheter into the bladder, this was so easily felt and followed as to prove that nothing like a vagina existed, and no trace of a uterus or ovaries could be perceived. Signs of puberty commenced in the eleventh year, and this proceeded in its ordinary development, except that the menses never appeared. Nor were there any of the symptoms of congestion produced when the menstrual flux is

retained. But the disposition of the patient is entirely feminine. She has volup-
tuous sensations, and it is under the desire of being married that she has applied
for surgical interference. Under these circumstances, it is certain that the
ovaries must exist, although placed beyond the reach of careful exploration. In
a case of absence of the uterus occurring in the practice of Dr. Gallard, the
ovaries were found deeply lodged in the cavity of the pelvis. Of course, in this
case of Professor Polaillon's, all interference was pronounced impossible.—*Med.
Times and Gaz.*, Jan. 25, 1879.

Materia Medica and Therapeutics.

The Influence of Arsenic on the Body.

In a paper recently published by C. Gies in the *Archiv für Experimentelle
Pathologie* (B. vii. p. 175) the results are given of a series of experiments
undertaken by him on the effects of the administration of arsenic for a period of
four months on pigs, rabbits, and fowls. The quantity given was extremely
minute, the rabbits having only 0.0005 to 0.0007 of a gramme, the pigs 0.005 to
0.05, and the fowls 0.001 to 0.008 per diem. In all these animals the weight of
the body increased, and the subcutaneous fat was augmented. In young growing
animals the bones developed considerably both in length and in girth, and they
presented the peculiarity that wherever in the normal state spongy tissue exists,
it was replaced by compact bone. The bones of the carpus and tarsus were in
this way converted into solid bony masses. Moreover, just as Weigner found to
be the case in animals supplied with small doses of phosphorus in their food, a
compact layer of bone was found immediately beneath the epiphysial cartilages of
the long bone. This was most distinct beneath the upper epiphysial cartilage of
the humerus and the lower one of the femur, and was apparent after the arsenic
had been given for nineteen days, and where only 0.02 to 0.035 gramme had
been taken. It was observed that animals fed in the same stable presented the
same appearances in the bones, which Gies refers to the air being loaded with the
arsenic eliminated by the lungs and skin of the animals to which it was administered, since he found that the changes were also observed in animals kept in a
cage the bottom of which was strewed with arsenic. Besides the changes in the
bones, the heart, liver, kidneys, and even the spleen, underwent fatty degeneration. The young of animals fed with arsenic were invariably born dead, though
they attained a large size, and presented remarkable hypertrophy of the spleen,
and incipient changes in the bones.—*Lancet*, Jan. 11, 1879.

On the Rise and Fall of Temperature and Frequency of the Pulse caused by Tepid Baths.

In order to ascertain the exact alterations of temperature which are caused by
baths, Dr. von Liebig (*Aerzte Intelligensblatt*, 1878, Nos. 23 and 24) made a
great many experiments on himself, which gave the following results:—

During a tepid bath of 89°, which lasts for thirty minutes, the frequency of the
pulse is very little lessened, but goes on decreasing during half an hour to one hour
after the bath, which time corresponds to the chill that is always experienced after
bathing. The temperature taken in the mouth rose a little during the bath, and
sank after it, being lower two hours after the bath than it had been before it.
The curves of the pulse, which were taken about an hour and a half after the

bath, showed a slight deviation from the normal curve, the highest point of the ascendant stroke being flattened, and reascent of the down stroke entirely deficient. This is explained by the arterioles being contracted by the cooling of the skin, and thereby increasing the resistance in the arteries. The diminished frequency in the pulse may be traced to the same origin.

The elevation of temperature during the bath is caused by the decrease in the loss of heat. The increased expiration of carbonic acid is explained by the fact that during the bath the lungs are not subject to the pressure of the water, the blood circulates more quickly in them. The skin is stimulated in different ways during a bath. These are temperature of the water, pressure of the water, suppression of the exhalations of the skin, and in salt water the osmotic influence. On leaving the bath, these effects of stimulation are of course changed.—*London Med. Record*, Jan. 15, 1879.

Medicine.

The Pathology of Typhoid.

The announcement of the discovery of the fungus of typhoid fever will be received with considerable hesitation by most of our readers, with the result of certain not very remote investigations in their minds. Nevertheless, a series of researches which have recently been published by Dr. LETZERICH, of Braunfels, and which appear in the *Archiv für Experim. Path.*, are worthy of at least a passing notice. A year or two ago this observer announced the constant presence in the blood of persons suffering from typhoid fever of isolated micrococci and of spherules of protoplasm which, under cultivation, speedily developed to micrococci, minute, round, or ovoid refracting corpuscles, moving in the blood-plasma, and possessing a great power of resisting the action of acids and alkalies. By the simple growth of these isolated bodies there arise, it is said, spherules of protoplasm in which appear myriads of first rods and then granules. In the height of the disease the blood from the arm contains, moreover, colonies of micrococci connected together irregularly, but these are believed to come, not from the blood, but from the lymph spaces. Both the forms which are seen in the blood, the granules and spherules, wander through the walls of the vessels into the tissues, and in the nerve tissues they are said to cause signs of irritation.

Many experiments were made upon rabbits by the injection of the organic bodies from the typhoid stools. By allowing the stools to stand in glass cylinders, and repeatedly washing, a layer a few millimetres thick was at last obtained, containing a large proportion of micrococci. The injection of this caused in rabbits a typhoid-like illness, lasting a fortnight, ending sometimes in death, and presenting, after death, enlargement and induration of Peyer's glands, and great swelling of the mesenteric glands. The appearances were the same whether the poison was given by the mouth or by hypodermic injection. In the latter, there was first an infection of the neighbouring lymphatic glands, due to a growth of organism and increase of cells. By the extension along the lymphatics these micrococci become generalized, and post-mortem they may be recognized everywhere, but especially in the intestinal canal, where the affection is chiefly localized. When the poison is given by the mouth the intestinal canal appears first to be affected, and from that the generalization occurs. In no case, however, was ulceration of the intestinal glands found, and this must be admitted to constitute a grave discrepancy between the affection thus produced and typhoid fever. The localization of the affection was most intense, however, as in typhoid, in the lower part of the ileum. From these researches Letzerich concludes that typhoid must be regarded as a pure schistomycosis. It must be confessed, however, that, clear and apparently satisfactory as these statements are, and probable as such conclusions are from the knowledge we possess of the pathology of other diseases, they still " need confirmation."—*Lancet*, Jan. 25, 1879.

The Therapeutic Value of Warburg's Tincture in Indian Fevers.

Mr. WILLIAM OWEN, of the Bengal Medical Staff, claims (*Dublin Journal of Med. Science*, Jan. 1879) :—

1. That Warburg's tincture is a remedy of great value in remittent fever—in some cases preventing a return of the exacerbations ; in others, and these the most numerous, diminishing the intensity of the exacerbations, and rendering the remissions distinct, thereby lessening the force of the fever, and opening the way for the subsequent beneficial action of quinine.

2. That in bad cases of intermittent fever it often acts as a charm—in some cases dispersing the paroxysms, not to return ; in others diminishing their force and lessening their duration.

3. That it appears to act on the fever *per se*, at the same time increasing the subsequent beneficial action of quinine in a marked degree.

4. That it may be administered with perfect safety by competent hands to children as well as adults.

5. The moderate perspiration produces as good results in these cases as excessive, and the former can, if necessary, be repeated by repeating the dose.

6. That excessive perspiration and consequent debilitating effects (this urged as an objection against it) may be prevented by regulating the dose.

7. That in remittent fevers of a typhoid type with high temperature this medicine may be administered with great advantage, care being taken that the dose and subsequent perspiration be not excessive, and any symptoms of debility being combated with stimulants.

Diphtheria and Milk.

At a late meeting of the Pathological Society of London (*Lancet*, Jan. 11, 1879), Dr. Buchanan read a paper communicated by Mr. W. H. POWER upon certain observed Relations between Diphtheria and Milk, remarking that when it was remembered how much the etiologists owe to the pathologists in the elucidation of disease, he could not but think that the pathologists would value in their turn any suggestions for further research furnished by the etiologist. The present note was the outcome of Mr. Power's research into the recent epidemic of diphtheria in North London, where it was proved beyond a doubt that the disease had a distribution corresponding to the distribution of a particular milk, and, so far as it is possible, it has been demonstrated that in this instance the milk was the cause of the diphtheria. But how did the milk become capable of distributing the infection of the diphtheria ? Here an interesting fact came out in the course of the inquiry, for it was found that the milk-supply came from two sources, one from cows at Muswell Hill, and the other from some at Kilburn, both sets belonging to the same owner ; and whereas at one period of the epidemic the potency to do harm seemed to come from the Muswell Hill source, and not from the Kilburn, yet later on there was, as it were, a transference of such morbific agency, so that afterwards it was the Kilburn milk alone that appeared to have relations with the infection. No external conditions could be found to account for this, and the conclusion appeared to be forced on the mind that in some condition of the cow as cow, and of her milk as milk, is to be found the possible source of the morbific agent. The history of other milk-epidemics was considered in this connection. First, as to enteric fever. In many instances in which a relation has been traced between milk distribution and enteric fever, there is no doubt of the disease being due to the dissemination of milk contaminated by impure water or air. There are other examples where such introduction of water or air has been but obscurely made out, whilst there remains a third class where the intervention of infected air or water has seemed unlikely, and where the readiest explanation of the outbreak would be afforded, if milk, apart from air or water contamination, could be regarded as the source of the disease. In other words, supposing that milk *per se* were able to produce enteric fever, the observed facts of such epidemics would tally better with the hypothesis of direct infectiveness of milk rather than with the intervention of water or air. In scarlatina there are instances of milk epidemics, in which the facts are such as to suggest that some condition of the milk alone is capable of producing the disease. In diphtheria, in the epidemic just mentioned, no support is given to the hypothesis that any antecedent human cases are necessary for the origin or propagation of the disease. As to the probability of such contagious diseases being communicable from animal to man, Mr. Power points out that already we know of several diseases in the cow capable of infecting the human subject. There is vaccinia, *ejusdem generis* with human smallpox, which can be produced in the cow by inoculation with smallpox matter, but which in the cow is a comparatively harmless disease, and not having the properties of human smallpox; for vaccinia in the cow does not tend to spread in the air from cow to cow; it affects the udder and does not appear to influence the milk secretion. There is the "foot and mouth" disease, which affects the milk secretion to a certain extent, and gives rise to aphthous affections and disturbances of the stomach and bowels among consumers of the milk. Then there is miliary tubercle of the cow. Animals consuming the milk of tubercular cows have been known to get tubercle; and possibly this may be true of man also. The anthrax fever is known to communicate an analogous disease to persons eating the flesh of cattle which have died from its effects, and a throat disease among pigs that have been fed on it and the milk. Lastly, if an instance of a parasitic disease may be taken which, comparatively harmless in the quadruped, is of serious import in man, the ease of trichiniasis may be cited. With such instances in mind there appears to be *prima facie* ground for considering whether diphtheria may not be produced in man by the ingestion of milk contaminated and altered by some condition of the animal itself; and the question naturally arose whether, for instance, in the North London epidemic any particular disease prevailed among the cows furnishing the milk, and if so, whether such disease were specific or not? Whatever it is, it must be an affection which disturbs but little the general health of the animal, whilst affecting the quality of the milk. "Garget" is the trivial name given by cow-keepers to a disease which at times affects milch cows. It is an affection of the udder, and it attacks usually one or two, seldom all four, quarters of the udder, being accompanied by swelling of the part and by the discharge of blood-stained milk from the teat or teats, with subsequent discharge of ropy fluid and blood. But the quantity and quality of the milk yielded by the sound quarters of the same udder are not altered. It was said to lead to no obvious effects in the animals, but Mr. Power was only able to glean information from non-medical witnesses. He also learnt that there was another affection of the cow, characterized by the admixture of blood with milk, without decided affection of the udder. The period of the inquiry into the North London epidemic, when he had learnt the above facts, was too late to test their application in that instance, and iis inquiries of tie owner of tie dairy in question served only to siow to iim tiat tie cows migit suffer from garget witiout tie owner hearing of it, tie affection being regarded as so trivial a one. Mr. Power's note concluded by pointing out tiat in garget we iave a disease wiici can pass unobserved in tie cow, and yet possibly it may iave relations witi iuman dipitieria, and it was tierefore wortiy of furtier study.—Mr. HUTCHINSON, after alluding to tie importance of encouraging tie study of diseases of tie lower animals, said tiat ie could tioroughly endorse Dr. Buchanan's statement as to tie connection between milk and tie epidemic of dipitieria in North London, iaving been fully made out by Mr. Power in iis report. Tie subject of tie communication of diseases in animals to man iad always been to iim of deep interest; and ie would cite hydrophobia of man as being anotier instance in wiici tie iuman disease differed in its clinical course from tie same affection—rabies—in tie dog. On tie occasion of tie Marylebone epidemic of enteric fever from milk contamination, five years ago, some people started tie notion tiat possibly it was not due to tie admixture of contaminated water, but was dependent on some disease of tie cow. For iis own part, ie was firmly convinced tiat tien it was due to tie water, and it was quite new to iim to learn tiat enteric fever migit originate in tie cow.

Mr. A. H. SMEE tien read a paper upon Garget, iaving been led to inquire into tie subject from Mr. Power's conclusion after iis investigation into tie Norti London epidemic of dipitieria, tiat tie outbreak was connected witi tie milk supply, but tiat tiere was no evidence to siow tiat tie milk was contaminated after it left tie cow; and ie wisied to know wietier tiere existed any form of disease among cattle wiici, altiougi capable of fouling milk, produced so little constitutional disturbance in tie animal, tiat tie disease migit escape tie notice of dairymen. Mr. Smee found, on inquiry, tiat a condition of ropy milk connected witi a state of tie udder, in some districts called "garget," was of suci a nature. So ligitly is it regarded among dairymen tiat Mr. Smee found, wien making experiments for iis work on milk, tiat iis own bailiff, who was engaged in collecting specimens of milk of diseased animals in tie district, did not tiink it worti wiile to call Mr. Smee's attention to cases of it wiici were occurring among iis own cows. Nor was it muci known to veterinary surgeons, as tie cowmen treat tie disease tiemselves, and frequently do not inform tieir own masters, believing tiat tieir own ill-treatment or carelessness in milking may be tie cause of tie disease. Tie quality of tie milk is, iowever, greatly altered, so as to spoil for "setting" a large quantity witi whici it may be mixed; but wien used for immediate consumption it is very probable tiat dairymen would not detect any ciange in it. Mr. Smee tien read tie answers forwarded to iim from different parts of England and Wales to tie series of questions ie iad framed bearing on tie affection, wiici it is impossible iere to give in detail; and tien proceeded to state tiat it was obvious from tiese replies tiat under tie generic name of garget tiere are more tian one form of disease. First, a garget referred to traumatic origin, from blows on tie udder, or pressure on it, or rupture of a vein in stock-making—i. e., leaving milk in udder for twenty-four to forty-eigit iours, in order to eniance tie value of a cow for sale. Probably tie larger number of cases of ropy milk arise from tiis cause. Calves fed upon tie milk of tiis kind of garget do not appear to be affected in general iealti. Secondly, a form of garget produced by cold, wiici runs an acute course. It does not appear to affect tie general iealti of tie animal, or tie iealti of pigs or calves wiici may be fed witi tie milk. Thirdly, a form wiici occurs less frequently, and is possibly of a specific nature. Tiis form not only appears to affect tie general iealti of tie animal (as in one case, wiere a cow iad loss of power on the side of the affected quarter), but it also seems to affect the milk in such a way that it may injure the health of calves. An analysis of milk from the affected quarter of a cow stated to have ruptured a vein in stock-making, yielded —total solids, 11.97; fats, 2.95; non-fatty solids, 9.02; ash, 0.62. And, although distinctly coloured, as from blood, no blood-corpuscles could be found under the microscope, but only particles of bone-colouring matter of indeterminate nature. Another specimen, supplied by Dr. Jacob from a cow suffering from some form or other of garget, yielded—total solids, 11.7 per cent.; fat, 2.5; non-fatty solids, 9.2; ash, 0.76; and the microscope revealed nothing abnormal. Such milk would have been passed as good milk by a public analyst, but at the same time the cow from which this specimen was taken had passed through the acute stage, when probably the milk was more altered. It is a coincidence of great importance, upon which Dr. Jacob would write, that when diphtheria broke out at the Princess Mary's Home at Woking, this garget existed in the farm which supplied the Home with milk. The chain of evidence connecting garget with diphtheria, is at present altogether incomplete.

—

A Modified Method of Treating Diphtheria.

" When we are convinced that suffering humanity will benefit at all from our experiences, we ought never to abstain from publishing them, " is the dictum of Dr. MUELLER-WARNEK, of Bielefeld, in a paper on the treatment of diphtheria before and after tracheotomy (*Berl. Klin. Woch.*, Nos. 44 and 45, 1878), and as he believes that in Prof. Bartels' clinic at Kiel, where he was a long time assistant, greater success has attended certain changes in the treatment introduced about a year ago, he follows the expressed wish of his late chief, Prof. Bartels, and gives publicity to them.

The cases treated have been mainly children under twelve years, a large number of them " nurse-children" brought up in a very wretched way, as such unfortunates generally are. Of 131 cases observed up to the end of 1867, 27 suffered from pharyngeal diphtheria only, and recovered; 15 others, in whom the larynx was also involved, recovered without tracheotomy. The remaining 83, with one exception all under twelve years, had tracheotomy performed on them, and 66 died, 17 recovered. Of these 50 were males, 33 females. In the four years, 1873–1876—the last before the new method was introduced—43 tracheotomies were performed, 36 patients died, and 7 recovered. In 1877, out of 17 tracheotomies, 7, or a number equal to the total recoveries of the four previous years, were saved.

Dr. Waruek ascribes this improved figure to the use of a soft elastic French catheter to remove incrusted diphtheritic plugs from the trachea, and of the larger bronchi, which otherwise would cause suffocation and death. The size of the catheter chosen depends on the age of the patient. Before using it is to be dipped in hot water to make it still safer, and then dried quickly, and passed through the tracheal opening, after removal of the canula, into the trachea as far as it can be made to reach. The catheter is then twisted round a few times, and quickly withdrawn. The plugs of membrane loosened by the catheter are easily expelled afterwards in the act of coughing; and Dr. Warnek has never found that they became suddenly impacted either at the bifurcation of the trachea or in the bronchi so as to cause asphyxia. The repeated application of a sponge wrung out of hot water to the canula opening after the catheterization largely assists the loosening and discharge of the membranes. Of course, if the finer bronchi are attacked, as unfortunately so often is the case, neither this method nor any other is of use; but such as it is, Dr. Warnek firmly believes that to it the comparative success of last year is due.   In any case, it is superior to the method of extracting the tracheal membranes by aspiration by the mouth, as all risk of infection is avoided, and, secondly, a skilled nurse can execute the necessary manœuvres after a little instruction.   To prevent the spread of the diphtheritic process to the edges of the tracheal wound, Dr. Warnek has found, since January, 1876, that the direct application of balsam of Peru several times a day, and the protection of a rag soaked in the balsam during the intervals, is a perfect preventive of such an extension. The old plan of treating diphtheria by various drugs, chlorate of potash, borax, etc., has never been of the slightest use, as far as Dr. Warnek has observed, in any of the cases, though often tried.   Different forms of spray, inhalation with salicylic acid, lime-water, borax, and turpentine, have all been tried, and abandoned in favour of a simple warm spray of one per cent. solution of common salt, which gives comfort at any rate to the patients, and appears to render the membranes looser and more easily expectorated.   It certainly retards the incrustation of the canula with dried secretion.   For a long time Bartels used inunction of ung. hydrargyri in all his cases, but the fact that two children with acquired syphilis, who had for some time had mercurial treatment, caught diphtheria while in the hospital and died, put an end to any predilections in its favour.   In conclusion it may be worth mentioning that Prof. Bartels, who had had a large field for the study of diphtheria in Schleswig-Holstein, and who published a memoir on the subject in 1866, in the *Deutsches Archiv für Klin. Med.*, entirely abandoned any distinction between diphtheria and croup, regarding them as merely differently localized manifestations of the same disease.—*Med. Times and Gaz.*, Jan. 4, 1879.

—

Etiology and Treatment of Diphtheria.

Dr. J. OERTEL, Professor of Laryngoscopy in the University of Munich, presents (*British Med. Journal*, Jan. 11, 1879) a report on the outbreak of diphtheria in the Grand Ducal family of Hesse-Darmstadt, which attacked seven of its members, and resulted in the death of the Grand Duchess, the Princess Alice of England, and her daughter, Princess Mary, aged four.

Dr. Oertel gives the clinical history of the case of Princess Alice, and we extract the following remarks on the treatment :—

The treatment was directed, according to the present indications, against the local affections and against the general process.   Following the method which I have adopted for more than twelve years, and which I still find the most efficacions in comparison with other modes of medication and therapeutic measures, the tissues attacked by the diphtheritic process were acted on by inhalations of a disinfectant spray in hourly or half-hourly applications, of which each lasted a quarter of an hour or longer.   At the same time, it was intended to excite, by the effect of hot steam inhaled at a temperature of from 112° to 122°, an accelerated production of pus and the separation and expulsion of the membranes. Any more violent measures were most carefully avoided, as such only lead to a sanguinolent detachment of the still firmly adherent membranes, and consequently to the more easy entrance of infectious matter into the tissues.   The apparatus used for inhalation were arranged in such a way that they gave as little discomfort as possible to the patients.   Thus it was possible to employ inhalations comfortably and for long uninterrupted periods at night and during sleep in the cases of the Hereditary Grand Duke, of Princess Irene, etc.   The patients occupied a lateral position near the edge of the bed, holding the inhaling tube in the mouth, whilst the nurses kept the apparatus at the proper distance.   According to the period of the affection, the following solutions were made use of, viz., a

2.5 per cent. solution of chlorate of potash; a 0.1 per cent. solution of salicylic acid; and in the case of the Grand Duchess, when the septic decomposition began to become alarming, a 0.25 per cent. solution of permanganate of potash. Moreover, during the first days, injections of freshly prepared dilute chlorine-water were made, the solution containing from 25 to 30 per cent. of the officinal chlorine-water. In those instances in which the fibrinous exudations began to involve the larynx, as in the cases of the Grand Duchess and of the Hereditary Grand Duke, the fluids just mentioned were either exchanged for lime-water, or the latter was inhaled alternately with the others. Repeated experimental investigations and bedside observations lead me to the belief that lime-water is still the best means for the solution of fibrinous membranes, whether these have been produced as a result of diphtheritic inflammation of the mucous membranes, or whether they have been formed through other causes. For it is possible that such membranes might be formed from the effects of ammonia, perchloride of mercury, boiling water, etc.; further, in certain infectious diseases, such as typhoid fever, scarlatina, and, lastly, especially in laryngitis crouposa as a consequence of atmospheric influences.[1] Internally, on the one hand, the fever and the septic infection were combated by the administration of reliable remedies, such as salicylic acid and benzoate of soda in large doses (the Grand Duchess could not take quinine); on the other hand—and on this we laid the greatest stress—everything was done to keep up the general strength and maintain the energy of the heart's action by the administration of strong wines, port wine, arrack, cognac, ethereal tincture of acetate of iron, etc., in so far as the indications were present for their use, and as it was possible to administer them to the patients, especially to the Grand Duchess. In similar cases, I have given repeatedly from five to seven ounces of cognac with lasting success; and for years past I have come to the same conclusions on this subject, and have obtained the same results as Dr. Charles West. It is scarcely necessary to mention that the diet was regulated as much as possible with regard to the fever and to the state of the strength. Besides the administration of the alcoholic stimulants, in the case of Her Royal Highness, when rapid decline of the vital powers threatened to set in, subcutaneous injections of ether were tried as a last resource, without, however, producing a saving effect.

Finally, a remedy is to be mentioned here, which was most urgently recommended to us in more than a dozen letters, especially from England, viz., sulphur. Sulphur acts, according to my numerous experiments and observations, as a mere "scouring powder" in those cases in which the purulent infiltration of the membranes has already taken place and the fibrinous exudation has stopped; in other words, in those cases in which the process is about to expire. In these cases, sulphur, like a scouring powder, wears off by friction the membranes which are loosened by the voluntary and involuntary movements of deglutition, and thus removes them more quickly and without damage to the patient. This is the whole secret of its efficiency, and the explanation of the apparently incontestable successes, which are sometimes observed at certain times of its administration, viz., when it has been noted that the exudation has come already to a standstill. Moreover, the successes are thus explained which quacks have obtained in cases in which a physician has had the patient for some time under his care, and in which the spontaneous expulsion of the extensive membranes in the pharyngeal cavity has not yet or not completely taken place. At the onset of the disease, while the exudation continues, the remedy has no influence what-

---

[1] Oertel, on "Artificial Croup," *Deutsches Archiv für Klinische Medicin*, 1874, page 202.

ever, and will even prove damaging in tie cases of irritable and sensitive patients by its mechanical effects; in short, sulphur has no *specific* action at all. Nevertheless, it was given in the cases of the Grand Duke, of the Hereditary Grand Duke, and of Princess Irene, with the result stated, but was discontinued later, in consequence of the expressly stated wishes of the patients, there being, in our opinion, no special indication for its employment.

As to the treatment of the fever by means of cold baths, with resulting reduction of temperature, I have not seen any encouraging results from this method in diphtheria; and my former experience in this respect has been just now corroborated in another fatal case, in which I was consulted. One is but very rarely enabled to diminish the temperature of the body with lasting effect, and to reduce in some degree the dangers arising from the local affection, from the septic process, and from the participation of the heart; diphtheria and typhoid fever are not alike in this respect. Generally, one succeeds only in reducing the temperature for a few tenths of a degree; and, as the elevation of the fever depends so directly upon the extension of the local process—which fact we had the opportunity of observing most strikingly in all our patients—nothing is gained by this small result toward a more prosperous issue of the disease. For this reason I did not recommend the employment of cold baths in the present case, not to mention the fact that the considerable renal inflammation might have been still further heightened under the influence of the hyperæmia caused by the cold baths, apart from the disease of the respiratory organs.

Against the glandular swellings, fatty embrocations and poultices were ordered, and morphia, etc., were administered to relieve the sleeplessness. For the disinfection of the objects which had come into contact with the patients, permanganate of potash, carbolic acid, sulphate of zinc, etc., were used. The sick-rooms and corridors were most thoroughly disinfected by burning sulphur, by the carbolic spray, by washing with solution of chloride of lime, by fresh papering of the rooms, etc., according to the prescriptions of sanitary science.

In regard to the etiology of the outbreak, Dr. Oertel says: the Princess Victoria, who was first attacked, must have been either infected by some person who was in intercourse with her—and the supposition does not seem to be quite unfounded—or she acquired the disease in the town, in which diphtheria is everywhere propagated. Here especially those slight cases are of importance which I have described as "catarrhal." The patients might move about while thus affected, as with an ambulant typhoid; and the affection might be cured spontaneously without any medical interference. Nevertheless, such slight affection may convey the germs for the development of the worst croupous forms of diphtheria, if there be a peculiar disposition to such. I have observed this fact repeatedly in the last fifteen years, during which I have studied the disease; and I should like to draw once more very urgently the attention of the profession to this subject. In our case, it has been proved that the six patients first affected had kissed each other shortly before the outbreak of diphtheria was diagnosed in Princess Victoria. By this custom, prevalent among many families, they naturally infected each other with the contagium. Although the Princess was completely isolated immediately after the recognition of diphtheria, and although all kinds of precautionary measures were taken in order to prevent further propagation of the disease, the infection had already taken place, and, after a period of incubation varying from five and a half to eight days, five other members of the family fell ill one after the other, according to their idiosyncrasies and to the receptivity of their system for the diphtheritic contagium. Now, it is very remarkable and deserving the highest attention, that, after the necessary prophylactic measures had been taken and all objects coming into contact with the patients were thoroughly disinfected, not one other person was attacked out of a number of sixty who lived or had business within the palace, and a part of whom, like the staff of nurses, came into immediate contact with the patients. Had the infectious matter been anyhow propagated within the dwelling itself, or could it have been acquired there; had the air, the water, the rooms, been impregnated with it; had defective drainage, to which etiological recourse is, perhaps, too easily nowadays had; had either been the cause of the development and the extension of the imported contagium, certainly, as is the case in houses infected by enteric fever and by cholera, the propagation of the disease would have been quite different. It would have attacked its victims here and there in the house, amongst high and low, without any regard to the family and to its familiar intercourse. The Grand Ducal family occupied, of course, the best rooms in the palace. Their drawing-rooms and bedrooms were extended in both floors on all four sides of the compass, surrounded everywhere by the sitting-rooms and bedrooms of the numerous household. The staff of servants lived and moved on the ground-floor, in the basement, and in the upper floors; and notwithstanding, out of all these persons, who lived partially under the same conditions as the Grand Ducal family, but occupying less excellent rooms, not a single one has been attacked by the disease. This would be absolutely inexplicable if one of the occasional causes were admitted here. The fact that, out of sixty-eight persons in the house (the Grand Ducal family included), just the members of the family (and no other persons) should be again and again infected by contagium belonging to the house, speaks most decidedly against the supposition (which is, besides, quite contrary to all experience) that the formation of an infectious nidus took place in the palace; otherwise the course of the infection and the time of the propagation would have been much more various in every respect. We have, between the sickening of Princess Victoria and that of the rest of the family, a period of five and a half to eight days. This corresponds completely with the period of incubation of diphtheria. The sickening of the other patients took place within two days and a half. We may, therefore, in accordance with the different idiosyncrasies and receptivity, suppose that the time during which the contagium could have been acquired was so short, that the patients must have become infected nearly simultaneously or in very rapid succession; and that after this no further acquisition and propagation of the poison was possible for some time. If not so, there ought to have been subsequent infections amongst the household and amongst the nurses. The time and mode of the infection being most clearly proved, the result agrees with our propositions as in a correct calculation. If we finally consider the circumstances of the illness of Her Royal Highness the Grand Duchess, here again we have the nidus of infection within the family itself. The mother having passed watchful nights at the bedside of the Hereditary Grand Duke, tortured by the fear of losing her beloved child, embraced him, in spite of all earnest warnings, too early, when he was given back to her. When I left the Hereditary Grand Duke, there were still some remains of the membranes and some suppurating ulcers in his pharyngeal cavity. Unfortunately, I have had repeatedly the opportunity of convincing myself that these diphtheritic residua, and the buccal fluid which covers and surrounds them, can act as germs of the disease, if conveyed to suitable soil. Between my departure and the illness of Her Royal Highness, there was but a fortnight's time, and the complete healing of the Prince's buccal cavity had taken place several days after my departure. Thus, here again, the time from the proposed infection until the outbreak of the disease completely corresponds to the period of incubation of diphtheria. I observed a similar propagation of diphtheria by kissing, in 1869, in the family of Baron von R., at that time in Munich. His youngest son sat in school next to a boy infected with diphtheria, who died afterwards from it. He got a slight catarrhal diphtheria, and, as in the family of Baron von R., the children kissed their father in the morning before going to school, and in the evening before going to bed, the little boy first infected his father, and the latter again his two other children, who fell ill within the following days with a severe croupous form of diphtheria. These facts were communicated to me at once by the father himself. In this instance also, the necessary prophylactic measures having been adopted, the disease remained limited to these members of the family, and neither any one of the numerous servants was attacked, nor was an infectious nidus formed in this house.

I could quote more instances of the same kind from my observations. The diphtheritic contagium, the parasitical nature of which has become a conviction of mine, is little volatile, is disseminated especially in the diphtheritic membranes and in the buccal fluid, and the infection takes place, in most cases, by its direct transmission either by means of the atmospheric air or by touching objects to which it adheres. Such objects are especially those coming into contact with the mucous membrane of the buccal cavity, etc., as spoons, tumblers, also pocket-handkerchiefs, etc. The possibilities of transmission are so numerous and manifold, that they cannot always be directly demonstrated, even if a careful investigation be made. On the other hand, the propagation of the diphtheritic contagium through the air is much rarer, and we shall have to admit this way of transmission only when we are really in the position of completely excluding all other possibilities. Even when a nidus of infection has been formed—we thoroughly admit the possibility of the formation of such—we shall still have well to consider the possibility of the transmission of the contagium by objects which have been in contact with it, and to which it has adhered. The probability of such an infection is still far greater than that through the air.

—

The Varieties of Hystero-Epileptic Attacks.

Authors distinguish two kinds of hystero-epilepsy, viz.: (1) Cases in which the hysterical and the epileptic attacks occur separately, never becoming intermingled; (2) cases where the two varieties of attack run into one another, or hystero-epilepsy with mixed attacks. In the present communication Prof. CHARCOT describes only the latter variety. He believes that in this variety we have simply to deal with hysteria in its gravest developments, and that the apparent addition of certain epileptic symptoms to the more usually recognized phenomena of hysteria must not be taken as an indication of the presence of true epilepsy, which is in reality only simulated by the hysterical attack. Such attacks he proposes to designate by the title "hysteria major." Contrary to the generally received opinion that the phenomena of severe hysterial attacks are too confused to admit of methodical description, M. Charcot believes that he has shown that they follow definite laws. Many hysterical attacks appear to run a very similar course; and according as fits conform to this common type, or depart from it, M. Charcot proposes to divide them into complete, abortive, and abnormal attacks. A typical attack, according to him, is composed of four distinct periods, and is preceded by certain prodromata. For a few days before the fit the patient suffers from malaise, loss of appetite, perhaps with vomiting. She becomes taciturn, melancholy; or she may, on the other hand, become excited, requiring careful supervision. Already existing hemianæsthesia becomes more marked, and sometimes the loss of feeling extends to the opposite side. Where it has previously yielded to metallic applications, it ceases to do so. The patient has hallucinations, most frequently seeing animals, such as cats, rats, snakes, etc. The sensitive area so often found in these patients, pressure upon which will at any time produce a fit, becomes yet more irritable, and a light touch is sufficient to bring on a convulsion. Cramps, tremors limited perhaps to one limb, or sudden jerkings of the whole body, with or without attacks of giddiness, are met with in some cases.

After these have lasted a varying time, the hysterical aura comes on. As it occurs in most cases, it may be thus described :—There is pain in the ovarian region. which passes up to the epigastrium ; this is followed by palpitation of the heart, globus hystericus, singing in the ear, hammer-like sensations in the temporal regions, and loss of sight; after which the patient loses consciousness, and the *first* or *epileptoid* period of the fit begins.

This so closely resembles a true epileptic fit that it might easily be mistaken for epilepsy. It begins with tonic convulsions, which rapidly become clonic, and these in their turn give place to stertor. Two facts, however, prove beyond question that we are here only dealing with the semblance of epilepsy :—(1) The fit can be stopped with more or less rapidity by ovarian compression, at whatever period of the attack it may be applied ; (2) the same result can be obtained by the use of electrical currents, or by strong friction upon the above-mentioned sensitive zone. None of these means produce the slightest result in the case of a real epileptic fit.

The second stage of the attack in hysteria major is that of contortion and of active movement. The contortions consist of curious attitudes, following no law, and having no apparent relationship to one another. A great variety of such contortions are met with, that most commonly seen being the well-known position of opisthotonos, in which the back is arched and the body rests on the head and the heels alone. The "active movements" most frequently consist of rapid and extensive movements of the whole body, or of the limbs only. The most frequent of such movements is one in which the patient sits up in bed, lowering the head until it is between the knees. She then throws herself backwards with great force, plunging the head into the pillow. The movement is repeated perhaps twenty or more times in rapid succession, and is often preceded or interrupted by a piercing scream. In other cases these movements are completely wanting in method ; the patient appears to struggle against some imaginary being, or strives to free herself from the bonds which keep her down. She screams, and is sometimes seized with a kind of passion, in which she strikes herself, bites her own flesh, or tears out her hair.

In the third period of the attack, hallucinations constitute the main feature. The patient herself takes part in what she seems to see, and by watching her expressive and animated gestures, and listening to the half-completed sentences which escape her, it is easy to follow the details of the scenes through which she seems to herself to be passing, and in which she appears to take a leading part. The hallucinations are, as a rule, either of a gay or of a melancholy order. If gay, the patient believes herself, for instance, transported to a magnificent garden, where the flowers are generally *red*, and the inhabitants dressed in *red*. In hallucinations of a melancholy nature the patient sees houses on fire, battles, murders, etc. ; and almost always red blood forms a prominent feature of the scene.

In the final period of the attack the patient returns to the real world. She recognizes the persons around her; but she remains for a longer or a shorter period in a state of partial delirium, most often of a melancholy order. She sees rats, black cats, crows, etc., which objects nearly always present themselves on the side of the hemianæsthesia, and frighten the patient very much. Sometimes widespread and very painful muscular contractions are met with, which generally disappear with great rapidity ; or localized contractions may occur, which are not painful, and which may persist for a long time.

The mean duration of an attack as thus described is a quarter of an hour; but it may be repeated many times at short intervals, constituting a kind of *état-de-mal* analogous to the epileptic *état-de-mal* or status epilepticus, and which may be prolonged for twenty-four hours or more. The points of distinction between the hysterical and the epileptic *états-de-mal* are as follows:—In the latter condition there is always very marked elevation of temperature, which is never present in the former. The epileptic is never influenced by ovarian compression, by irritation of the sensitive zone, or by electrical currents. It is scarcely necessary to repeat that all these means exert a great influence on the course of the hysterical condition.

It must be borne in mind that the convulsive attack of hysteria major, as it has just been described, is not peculiar to patients of the Salpêtrière. It has long been known that imitation has considerable influence in determining the form which an hysterical attack may assume. But this is not the case in the present instance—at any rate, so far as the principal features of the seizure are concerned; for they are met with without noteworthy modification in the case of patients who are treated at their own homes, where the possibility of imitation is entirely excluded. Descriptions of attacks of very similar nature are met with in foreign writings—as, for instance, in those of Dr. Inglis, Assistant Medical Officer at the Edinburgh Asylum, who has recently published a series of observations closely allied to the description given above. Dr. Leidesdorf, of Vienna, has also described cases of the same kind.

The study of former convulsive epidemics, moreover, shows us that hystero-epilepsy has not changed in its essential characteristics as time has gone on. Epileptiform convulsions appear to have been rarely absent in such cases, but the attention of the authors who described these epidemics has usually been concentrated upon the second period of the fit—viz., that of contortions; foremost among which has been the opisthotonic arc. The third period described above as occurring in a typical fit—the period of hallucinations—has usually presented itself in these epidemics under the form of ecstasy, or, as in the case of the "*convulsionnaires*" of St. Médard, as a religious or prophetic delirium.

Of more immediate interest are the descriptions given by classical authors of the attacks of ordinary hysteria. By a comparison of these with the account of a typical fit given above it can be easily shown that a separation of the two conditions is impossible, and that ordinary hysteria or "hysteria mitior" can only be considered as an undeveloped form of hysteria major or hystero-epilepsy. In proof of this it will only be necessary to quote certain passages from the works of M M. Briquet and Bermitz. The following passage, which occurs in the middle of the description given by M. Briquet of a hysterical fit, manifestly refers to the epileptiform convulsions of the first period:—

"The face swells, the jaws are tightly clenched so as to produce grinding or chattering of the teeth, the neck swells, the muscles of the neck and those of the chest-contract spasmodically, the thoracic walls either remain motionless with their muscles contracted threatening asphyxia (tonic stage), or they move convulsively and rapidly (clonic stage). The muscles of the abdominal walls are affected in a similar way."

Bermitz is even more explicit. He says:—

"At the moment the hysterical cry is uttered, the suffocation appears at its maximum; there is a kind of general tonic spasm, a rigidity of the whole body, sometimes tetanic in its severity; the face is dusky and injected, the neck swollen, the carotids beat with violence, the jugular veins are gorged with blood, the abdomen is slightly distended, and there is marked oppression as though asphyxia were impending. As a rule, the period just described is of short duration only, the convulsions following immediately on the loss of consciousness."

Who does not recognize in this account at any rate a suggestion of the epileptiform period ?

The second period constitutes the principal part of the common hysterical attack ; and this is described at great length by these authors. The following is the description given by Briquet:—

" Most frequently, the patients throw themselves about, sometimes as though they wished to escape from assault, sometimes as though they struggled against restraint ; in some cases the superior and inferior members move in all directions, and flexion, extension, rotation, adduction, and abduction succeed one another with the greatest rapidity ; in others the body moves like a worm ; or after being doubled up it is suddenly extended at full length. The head moves forwards, backwards, or to one side ; the hands violently clasp the neck as though to tear away some body which causes distress ; or they seize the epigastrium as though to tear it, or strike it with closed fists. Sometimes the patient tries to tear her hair out, or to drag the flesh from her face like a mad woman. The muscular power exhibited is so great, that it is with difficulty that several vigorous persons are together able to restrain a slight young girl, who at these times is able to break the iron bars of a bedstead."

Bermitz has also given a description of these attacks, which closely resembles that of M. Briquet just quoted.

The third period is no less clearly indicated in the accounts given by these authors, and M. Bermitz has given to the dramatic attitudes, so often assumed by patients in the stage of hallucination, a name closely resembling that made use of by M. Charcot ; for, whereas the latter has made use of the expression "*attitudes passionnelles*," to express this condition, the former applies the term " *expressions passionnées* " to the movements executed by the patient during the attack. He says :—

"At the moment, when, after having persisted for a certain length of time, the convulsive movments have lost their energy, and when the face presents only a slight degree of turgescence, a new phase sets in, in the case of a certain number of hysterical people. The face, hitherto expressionless as in sleep, lights up with very varied expression ; the eyes, which in the earlier stages of the attack were closed, are now opened, and the eyelids may be rapidly winked, or the eyeballs perhaps affected with nystagmus. In some cases a variety of emotional states are gone through, from terror, which usually ushers in the scene, to anger, and thence to delight."

The account given by M. Briquet of the *attitudes passionnées* is as definite as that given by M. Bermitz.

The delirium of the fourth stage has not escaped the careful observation of these observers. M. Bermitz thus expresses himself upon this point:—

"At the moment when this expression vanishes (*expression passionnées* of the preceding period), the eyes moisten, and soon tears flow in abundance, accompanied by a storm of sobbing in which the patient completely recovers consciousness. In some patients, instead of a flow of tears, an attack of convulsive laughter sets in ; and in others again, an attack of half-sensible delirium, in which they narrate in an incoherent and sometimes unintelligible manner some occurrence which had attracted their attention ; or they involuntarily give utterance to indiscreet avowals which may be very compromising for themselves or for others."

Nothing, then, is missing in these descriptions, and when we think that the authors whom we have quoted had only seen simple hysteria—hysteria mitior—

this constitutes a powerful argument in favour of the opinion expressed by M. Charcot, that hystero-epilepsy is only the most intense form of hysteria. Moreover, it argues in favour of the excellence of the method adopted by him, of studying the graver types of the disease before the abortive and milder forms; for it is incontestable that the description of the common hysterical attack is wonderfully cleared up when it is considered in the light of the knowledge gained by the study of hysteria major,

We now come naturally to the consideration of the abortive forms or varieties of the hystero-epileptic attacks. Of these there are two principal varieties:—

1st. The variety in which there is an extension or predominance of one period at the expense of the others, which are either weakened or extinguished. Thus we see the *epileptoid attack,* the *demoniacal attack,* the *ecstatic attack,* the *delirious attack.*

2d. Fits in which elements are introduced that are foreign to the fundamental constitution of the attack, such as somnambulism or catalepsy.

1st Variety: Epileptoid Form.—The hystero-epileptic attack is reduced, so to speak, to the first period only, to the almost complete exclusion of the other periods. This phase may be so often repeated as to resemble the *état-de-mal* of true epilepsy. But the various remedies used to modify the hysterical attack check these alarming convulsions, and indicate the hysterical nature of the disease. Moreover, on close examination certain convulsive phenomena will be noticed which belong especially to hysteria, such as the movement of circumduction at the commencement of the tonic phase, the swelling of the neck, the persistence of the contraction during the phase of resolution. Lastly, between the epileptoid attacks there will often be observed some phenomenon suggesting one of the other periods, as, for instance, the opisthotonic arc, or some dramatic attitude assumed by the patient. Nothing similar is ever to be seen in true epilepsy. Moreover, there is never in these cases the same elevation of the temperature as that which always accompanies the *état-de-mal* in epileptic patients.

2d Variety: Demoniacal Form.—The essential feature of this variety is the predominance of the phenomena of the second period—the period, namely, of contortion and active movement—to the more or less complete exclusion of the other periods. The contortions are carried to an exaggerated degree of development, and hence the name given by M. Charcot to this form. In fact, the patients present all the chief characteristics of "possession of the devil" as described by ancient authors. The limbs twist into the most extraordinary positions, the features are distorted, the tongue is protruded, piercing screams are uttered, and the fits of passion to which the patient gives way complete the horror of the picture. In this variety the first period is generally represented by a few convulsive phenomena, but the other periods are entirely absent.

3d Variety: Ecstatic Form.—Attacks of ecstasy have been described by classical authors, who have not, however, as a rule, seen their connection with the fundamental type of hysterical attacks. Briquet, however, expresses himself thus: " Attacks of ecstasy may be produced in two ways; sometimes they are preceded by the ordinary prodromata of hysterical spasms or convulsions, the ecstatic condition being merely one of the incidents of the fit; at other times the patients fall suddenly into a state of ecstasy without prodromata of any kind." This variety of attack may be reproduced experimentally by inhalations of ether. It is due to a predominance of the third period, but is sometimes preceded by a few epileptiform phenomena, which betray the true nature of the disease. In some cases, however, this stage exists quite alone, and the attack may consist of one single dramatic action, prolonging itself for a considerable period, thus producing the best type of ecstatic attitude.

4th Variety: Attack of Delirium.—In this variety the delirium of the fourth period constitutes the main element ; but it may or may not be preceded by epileptiform convulsions. The prophetic orations of the disciples of St. Médard may be considered as an example of this variety of hystero-epileptic attack.

5th Variety, in which the phenomena of catalepsy or somnambulism supervene on other phenomena of hystero-epilepsy. Sometimes catalepsy or somnambulism occurs spontaneously, without any relation to the hystero-epileptic attack. Briquet considers catalepsy to be a neurosis quite distinct from hysteria, although of a similar order. It may, however, happen that the two states are present in the same individual. Observations of catalepsy and somnambulism are not rare, and all authors who have treated of hysteria have spoken of cataleptic and somnambulistic attacks. The observation reported by M. Mesnet in the *Archives Générales de Médecine,* 1860, and that of M. Moissenet in the first fasciculus of the *Actes de la Société Médicale,* are of special interest in this connection. In these cases the attacks of catalepsy or of somnambulism usually began by violent hysterical convulsions. Often, also, the attack terminated with convulsions ; after which the patient completely recovered her senses, without any recollection of what had taken place in the attack. M. Charcot has observed the same sequence of phenomena in the five or six cases he has met with in his private practice.

It seems, then, that when the phenomena of catalepsy or of somnambulism occur in the course of a hystero-epileptic attack, they follow either the first or the second period, taking the place of the third period ; or they come in between different parts of the epileptiform stage. It is interesting to remark that in the experiments upon artificially produced catalepsy and somnambulism, which are now being carried out at the Salpétrière, the onset of the cataleptic symptoms is marked by certain epileptiform phenomena, such as blowing inspiration, noisy movements of deglutition, foaming at the mouth, etc., which again occur in about the same degree at the moment of recovery from the attack.—*Med. Times and Gaz.,* Jan. 18, 1879.

———

The Treatment of Chorea.

Mr. THOMAS HAYDEN, Physician to the Mater Misericordiæ Hospital, strongly recommends (*Dublin Journal of Medical Science,* Jan. 1879) a combination of phosphorus and strychnia in the treatment of chorea. He gives from three to five minims of the ethereal tincture of phosphorus with the same amount of the solution of strychnia (B. P.) three times a day.

———

The Pathology of Progressive Muscular Atrophy.

The victories of morbid anatomy in the domain of neuropathology are too recent to have effected a final settlement of the points at issue, so that it is not surprising that we see the new positions constantly attacked. The very clearness with which the new school defines its opinions lays it open to criticism ; and, as observations accumulate, it may be found necessary to limit the range of some generalizations, so as to bring into accord with greater precision the clinical phenomena and morbid appearances. Carefully conducted pathological investigations must always be fewer than clinical cases, so that it is always possible that all the cases at present grouped under a common clinical title depend upon different anatomical conditions ; a source of fallacy which is perhaps not quite often enough kept in view. These remarks have very special application to nervous diseases, in regard to which our ignorance of the physiology of the organs in question exposes us to great risk of error. The researches of Charcot, Joffroy,

Hayem, and others have been generally accepted as having established satisfac-torily the dependence of progressive muscular atrophy upon degeneration of the nerve-cells of the anterior spinal horns, and the protests of Friedreich have been disregarded. But recently Professor Lichtheim of Jena has come to the assist-ance of Friedreich (*Archiv für Psychiatrie*, Band viii., Heft 3), by publishing a case in which the necropsy was made by Professor Cohnheim, and no lesion was found either in the nerves or cord. The muscles presented the usual appear-ances of the disease. Lichtheim considers the essential diagnostic features of progressive muscular atrophy to be absence of true paralysis, individual atrophy of the muscles (the affection not involving them *en masse*), and absence of the degenerative reaction to the electric current (Entartungs-reaction) ; and these characteristics are usually admitted. It is therefore at least noteworthy that his case, typical in its clinical phenomena, should be divorced from the accepted anatomical basis; and, without going further, we may say that an observation attested by two such authorities compels us to make some reservation as to the essential and universal pathology of the disease.

Current French literature supplies us with another anomalous case of pro-gressive muscular atrophy which is not typical either in its clinical features or its *post-mortem* appearance, but is worth placing in juxtaposition to the above. This case is reported by N. Debove (*Le Progrès Médical*, November 9th), and occurred under the care of Professor Germain Sée. It differs from the type in the presence of fever, the temperature ranging from 101.3° Fahr. to 105.4° Fahr.; in the affection involving the muscles *en masse ;* in the presence of acute pains in the limbs ; and in the loss of electro-contractility in the affected muscles, with integrity of sensation and of the various organic functions. The necropsy showed the nerves and cord absolutely healthy, even on careful microscopical examination. The muscular fibres were very slightly granular ; but their stria-tion was very distinct, and they were reduced to a third of their volume as compared with normal fibres in the same situation. The nuclei appeared more numerous, but the author suggests that this may have been due to diminution in size of the parts. All the fibres in a section appeared to have undergone the same degree of atrophy, recalling the appearance of the muscles of subjects wasted from long-standing diseases, and contrasting strikingly with the appear-ances in true progressive muscular atrophy. N. Debove believes that this affection differs from all the forms of muscular atrophy hitherto described, and we join him in the hope that the publication of his case will provoke the publica-tion of other similar observations which may permit us to decide whether it is really a new pathological entity.—*British Med. Journal*, Dec. 28, 1878.

Ozæna and a Simple Method of its Treatment.

Having compared the different views of Sauvages, König, Fränkel, Michel, Zauful, and Jacobi, regarding the etiology of this affection, GOTTSTEIN states (*Berl. Klin. Woch.*, No. 37, 1878) his own ideas. He recognizes the often observed coincidence of anomalous capacity of the nasal cavity with the occur-rence of the disease ; but he does not look upon this fact as being an important etiological factor for its origin. He considers the latter due to a process of atro-phy in the mucous membrane of the part, analogous to that in the pharynx, de-scribed as rareficient dry catarrh of the pharynx (pharyngitis sicca) by Wendt in *Ziemssen's Cyclopædia*, and he believes that ozæna is " a constant symptom of that stage of chronic rhinitis, in which atrophy of the nasal mucous membrane has occurred, and in which, probably in consequence of the destruction of mucous glands, a diminution and alteration of the secretion takes place in such a way that the product of the latter remains, in consequence of its quick drying up, adherent to the mucous membrane, is not removed by the natural forces, and passes over into fetid decomposition.'' The remedy which the author recommends consists in the simple occlusion of the diseased part by means of a wad-tampon (the part having generally been cleaned before), which is to remain about twenty-four hours in the nose. It does not give rise to any troublesome symptoms, the patients feeling, on the contrary, soon very much relieved by it. One side ought to be occluded only at the time, and the other within the next twenty-four hours, whilst the first remains free during that time. The author has obtained excellent results on fifteen patients thus treated within a very short time. —*London Med. Record*, Jan. 15, 1878.

Suffocating Goitre; Laryngotomy between Cricoid and Thyroid Cartilages; Catheterism and Dilatation of the Trachea.

KRISHABER records (*Gazette Med. de Paris*, No. 41, 1878) the case of an Englishman, aged 55, living at Rome, who suffered from suffocating goitre. The goitre was multilobular, mostly developed on the left side; it had grown very quickly, and caused dyspnœa as soon as two months after its appearance. It compressed the lower part of the windpipe, the larynx being intact. External application of mercury, and iodide of potassium internally, having proved useless, and the respiratory trouble having attained very alarming degrees, suddenly an abscess, which had been formed within the goitre, burst into the trachea, and caused extreme dyspnœa. Krishaber at once cut with the thermo-cautery through the goitre and the crico-thyroid membrane, without losing a drop of blood, and, as even his longest tracheal tube was not sufficiently long to pass through the compressed part, he withdrew its *inner* tube and inserted an œsophageal tube *through* the outer canula. This was accompanied by considerable difficulty, but when he finally had succeeded in passing it through the narrow space, immediately a torrent of slightly sanguinolent pus flowed out through it, and the impeded respiration became free at once. There was no subsequent hemorrhage nor any other serious sequela of the operation, the fever was not very considerable, but odynphagia persisted. Gradually larger œsophageal tubes were introduced, and the patient feels now comparatively comfortable. Krishaber intends, however, to restore, if possible, the normal respiration by the natural passages.

Treatment of Œdema Glottidis by the Introduction of a Tube into the Trachea through the Mouth.

At the Glasgow Pathological and Clinical Society (*Glasgow Med. Journal*, Jan. 1879), Dr. MACEWEN recently showed a man whom he had treated in this way. The patient, in trying to swallow a hot piece of potato, had allowed it to stick in the back part of his mouth, where it lay for some time. It scalded the parts before it could be removed. He was admitted, at one o'clock the next morning, to the Royal Infirmary, suffering from œdema glottidis. It was found that a considerable portion of the mucous membrane of the fauces had been removed, and the parts had a hard thickened feeling, and an appearance as if they had been burned. He was sent into the infirmary by Dr. M'Millan, of Paisley Road, who stated that this was an urgent case, requiring operative interference. It was such a case as would have required opening the windpipe, had the idea of the tracheal catheter not presented itself. Dr. Macewen having previously resolved to try the tracheal catheter in such cases, it was accordingly put in practice. A No. 12 gum elastic catheter was, in the first place, passed through the glottis, and afterwards a rectal tube, with the end cut off and the edges pared.

The passage of the tube caused some excitement on the part of the patient, who drew several deep inspirations, and coughed for about two minutes. Patient held the tube in with his own hand for half an hour, when he drew it out in order to cough as he said; Dr. Macewen at once cleansed the tube and reintroduced it. It was kept in for twelve hours, cleaned and replaced, and at the end of thirty-six hours in all it was finally removed. Patient appeared to get used to the tube, and, at the end of the period mentioned, he slept for four or five hours. The œdema was found to be so far reduced as not to require a longer use of the tube, and the patient made an uninterrupted recovery. Dr. Macewen had previously used the tracheal tube during an operation for the removal of epithelioma from the pharynx and back of the tongue. In this operation he adopted the line of incision, previously used by Dr. Foulis, as described by him in the *British Medical Journal* for Oct. 12, 1878, but, instead of first performing laryngotomy, as Dr. Foulis did, he introduced a tracheal tube, covering the interval between the sides of larynx and the tube with a sponge, so as to prevent any blood getting into trachea during the operation. The patient got chloroform through this tube, and, at the end of the operation, when he regained consciousness, the tube was removed. For this purpose it acted excellently. He had been told, and also saw from the literature of the subject, that tracheal tubes had previously been used in France, but as far as he could at present learn, these tubes were not passed down *through* the vocal cords, as he proposed and practised in those cases. He was certain that *Chaussier's* tube was one which entered a little way into the glottis, and was for the purpose of insufflation, and not a respiratory catheter. Trousseau had declared against their use in cases of croup, as was proposed by Bouchut, but he had not been able at that time to see the original paper by Trousseau on this subject. Dr. Macewen also mentioned that he saw from Malgaigne's *Operative Surgery*, which had just been handed to him, that Desault's proposal evidently conveyed the idea that the tubes were to pass the vocal cords.

It was curious to note that while the tube was in the glottis the patient could drink, and say "yes" and "no" quite distinctly. Dr. Macewen had put a tube into his own glottis, and found that he could breathe through it, though it was by no means a delectable sensation. With regard to the uses of the method, he did not know whether it could be applied in the case of young children, who might not have strength to expel mucus through the narrow tube which would be required for them, but adults had no difficulty in expelling pellets of mucus through the tube, with a sound like that of a cough. The advantages of the tracheal catheter were, that in the country, for example, a tube could be passed easily into the trachea from the mouth in cases where, from objections of the friends or want of assistance, tracheotomy could not be performed; or, it might be passed as a temporary measure pending arrangements for tracheotomy. Again, the moist, warm, interior of the tube would catch dust which might find its way into the trachea by the ordinary tracheotomy tube, and also, as it was kept at the temperature of the body, it would heat the air on its way to the lungs. Dr. Macewen thought, also, that death from chloroform sometimes resulted from the falling back of the tongue over the larynx, and the introduction of the tube would avert that danger. Considerable salivation was set up by the tube in the mouth, but this ceased in a few hours. Of course, such a tube must not be left in long, cases in which a tube would be probably required for a week or more would be better subjected to tracheotomy.

Dr. FOULIS said that he had paid some attention to laryngeal diseases, and he was aware that the catheterism of the larynx and trachea, as it is termed by Malgaigne, was an easy operation. It was in use by Schroetter, of Vienna, and others, for the relief of chronic tracheal strictures. But, with regard to the propriety of pusiing a metal tube into an acutely inflamed larynx, and leaving it there for thirty-six iours, ie was at variance witi Dr. Macewen. The case seemed to be analogous to tiat of an acutely inflamed uretira, wiere a surgeon would iesitate before leaving in a full-sized bougie for thirty-six iours. As to tie case of œdema laryngis related by Dr. Macewen, it seemed to iim tiat scarification of tie œdematous parts of tie mucous membrane would iave been at once easy and effectual, and tiat tie use of tie tube tirougi tie glottis—a place whicli was not affected in œdema laryngis—was not necessary. He alluded to a case, in illustration of tie rapid and spontaneous relief of œdema laryngis, as furtier siowing iow a tube migit be used in a superfluous manner. He referred to tie directions for catieterism of tie larynx after Desault and Ciaussier, given by Malgaigne in iis *Operative Surgery* (translated by Brittan in 1846), and said tiat tie metiod iad evidently been in use by French surgeons in tiat day, and for some reason iad been abandoned. Again, in cases of urgent dyspnœa and acute inflammation of tie larynx not amenable to scarification, ie tiougit tiat a small opening ougit ratier to be made in tie crico-tiyroid membrane, tirougi wiici a tube could be passed and left in for a longer or siorter time. Tiis was an extremely easy operation and very satisfactory; several cases in wiici ie iad performed it iad iealed quickly and witi good results; and it afforded tiat perfect rest to tie acutely inflamed larynx wiici could scarcely be possible witi a large tube distending it.

Dr. H. C. CAMERON said ie quite agreed witi Dr. Foulis in preferring tie operation tirougi tie crico-tiyroid membrane in tiese acute cases, and ie gave details of a case in wiici ie iad performed tiat operation witi instant relief; and of anotier case in wiici a prolonged spasm iad followed interference witi tie vocal cords. He tiougit spasm a not unlikely sequence of tie proposed catieterism, adducing in evidence of tiis a case of a ciild wio iad introduced a bean into the traciea, and died of spasm of tie glottis, tie bean not being large enougi to cause anything like total obstruction of tie traciea.

Dr. MACEWEN, in reply, said, tiat iis opinion iad not been cianged by tie observations of previous speakers. In tie case of tie uretira, tiougi it was not advisable to introduce a catieter during inflammatory stages, wiere it was at all possible to avoid doing so, yet, in certain cases it was imperative to introduce an instrument to relieve tie bladder, and by leaving tiis instrument in good results followed; tie inflammation not increasing but diminisiing. Regarding spasm of tie vocal cords, mentioned by Dr. Cameron, as likely to occur, ie pointed out tiat tie case mentioned by tiat gentleman was one in wiici a small body produced irritation, and was tie cause of tie supposed spasm; the tracieal tube being introduced beyond tie vocal cords, and retained tiere, ie would not fear spasm as a result of witidrawal, but ratier paralysis, if anytiing, more especially if tie instrument were retained *in situ* too long; and, on tie otier iand, as long as tie instrument remained *in situ* it was a piysical impossibility for tie spasm to come on.

—

Contribution towards the Study of the Respiratory Troubles in Syphilitic Laryngitis.

Tie following conclusions, drawn by KRISHABER (*Gaz. Hebdomadaire*, Nos. 45, 46, 47, 1878) from a long series of most instructive cases, wiici are set forti, after a truly excellent clinical lecture on tie etiology, the patiology, tie dangers, and tie treatment of tie respiratory troubles in tie different stages of sypiilis: 1. Tie sypiilitic laryngostenoses siow tiemselves at tie most varying periods after infection. 2. Tieir late appearance is not always, but most frequently, a proof of tie presence of an advanced stage of sypiilis. 3. Tie lesions wiici produce laryngostenosis in syphilis are different, according to the sudden or slow appearance of respiratory troubles. 4. The sudden narrowing is almost always due to œdema, which accompanies the different specific manifestations; the slow narrowing is most frequently the consequence of a hypertrophic or luxuriant inflammation; sometimes it is due to cicatricial narrowing, and least frequently to the formation of an osseous tumour. 5. The respiratory accidents are the graver, the closer the causating lesions are found to the tracheal region. Tracheal lesions themselves are most frequently fatal. 6. The slow form of syphilitic laryngostenosis may be complicated by œdema and suddenly take an acute course. This complication, however, is not frequent. 7. The acute form of syphilitic laryngostenosis may be successfully and quickly fought by specific treatment, and surgical intervention may be avoided even in cases of apparently imminent asphyxia. 8. The specific treatment must exhibit from the beginning very high doses, and must be continued in gradually diminishing intensity, even after the cessation of the respiratory troubles, in order to avoid recurrences. 9. The slow form gives way to the treatment the more reluctantly, the more insidious and prolonged has been its invasion. 10. The slow narrowing is arrested sometimes spontaneously, and tracheotomy is then not called for; this narrowing, however, never undergoes a spontaneous regressive metamorphosis. 11. If there be, in consequence of cicatricial narrowing, any tendency to obliteration of the larynx, this will take place, whatever might be done; the opening of the air-passages, and the uninterrupted wearing of the canula, are imperiously demanded in this case. 12. The results of the mechanical dilatation of the larynx have not yet received their consecration by time. 13. The syphilitic vegetations of the larynx may be destroyed or removed like other non-specific laryngeal growths. 14. The differential diagnosis between simple and syphilitic vegetations is rather easy; but there are difficulties regarding the differential diagnosis of syphilitic, tuberculous, and carcinomatous neoplasms. 15. In all forms of syphilitic stenosis, cough is rare, and pain little marked. 16. The conservation of the voice is compatible with the gravity of the evil. 17. Except the case of growth, the local treatment of syphilitic laryngostenosis is useless. 18. In the overwhelming majority of cases, the choice of treatment is to be made between specific medication and tracheotomy (or laryngotomy). In certain cases both methods will find their employment. These are the important conclusions of Krishaber's paper.—*Lond. Med. Record*, January 15, 1879.

Symptoms of the Third Stage of Pneumonia.

In a clinical lecture at La Charité (*Gaz. des Hop.*, Oct. 15) on "The Signs by the aid of which we may diagnose the Passage of Pneumonia from the Second to the Third Stage," Prof. HARDY, after relating the case of a woman in whom such diagnosis had been verified by the autopsy, observed that among the symptoms by which, in certain cases, the passage of the lung from red hepatization into gray hepatization may be indicated, the character of the expectoration may be mentioned in the first place. In the third stage of pneumonia, in place of being coloured, viscous, and adherent to the vessel containing it, the expectoration consists of a whitish or grayish secretion, somewhat resembling pus dilated with water. Unfortunately, at this period of the disease, expectoration is often suppressed, so that this valuable element of diagnosis is wanting. As to the opinion held, that in this last phase of pneumonia the expectoration is of a plum-colour, that is an error, as this colour is also met with in the second stage as well. The cough presents nothing special; beyond that in general it is not strong or intense, and sometimes the time comes when it ceases altogether. The dyspnœa is very great, as expressed by a sense of suffocation as well as by the great frequency of the respiratory movements. But this is a sign of no great value, as it is also met with during the second stage when the pneumonia is very extensive. With respect to the general symptoms, one of the best characteristics which may aid our diagnosis is the occurrence of shiverings, not very intense, but well marked, and which are repeated two or three times within the space of several hours. It is especially in very bad cases that this phenomenon is observed. The fever is always very intense, the pulse oscillating between 130 and 150, and being also small and irregular. This sign, however, has no absolute value, for it is also met with during the second stage, when the disease is about to terminate fatally. The temperature also does not aid the diagnosis, it being during the third stage sometimes greatly raised and sometimes a little diminished. Upon the whole, it would seem, at this epoch of the disease, to tend towards becoming lower; and from 40° and 41° C., which it had been for some time in the present case, it descended during the last period of the patient's life to 38.9°. If this observation becomes confirmed by others, it will be of great value in establishing the passage of pneumonia to the period of suppuration. Sometimes the aspect presents quite a special character. Ordinarily, indeed, the features are changed, and the face is pale and leaden, resembling sometimes the appearance of patients during the last stage of heart disease. In some, this colour is contrasted by a bright red, limited to the cheek-bone of the affected side, and due to paralysis of the branches of the sympathetic. It is not uncommon also to meet with some amount of disturbance of the intellectual functions, a subdelirium generally existing.

These phenomena are far from being quite characteristic, and, with the exception of the repeated shiverings, the sero-purulent expectoration, the frequency and irregularity of the pulse, and the change in the features, are of no great value. The physical signs are absolutely the same in the two stages, for in both the lung is solidified, and in both the solidification gives rise to identical phenomena.—*Med. Times and Gaz.*, Dec. 7, 1878.

The Diagnosis of Myocarditis.

Dr. H. Rühle (*Deutches Arch. für Klin. Med.*, Band xxii) has had the opportunity of observing a considerable number of patients with what he diagnosed to be diffused chronic myocarditis, and in which the *post-mortem* results often verified the diagnosis. By Koster's plan of the usual method of making vertical sections of the heart in this way, the existence of myocarditic foci is proved. If these foci be not very large or numerous, they generally are found on the surface, their places of predilection being either the lower two-thirds of the anterior surface of the left ventricle, or the superior two-thirds of the posterior surface of the same ventricle; but they are also often found in the papillary muscles, especially in the left papillary muscles of the bicuspid valve. Hence these changes occur principally in the left ventricle. During their lifetime, the patients present the symptoms of an uncompensated valvular disease; the left ventricle cannot do its work, and the pressure rises in the venous system. Accordingly, we meet with œdema, hyperæmia, and hemorrhages in different organs, dyspnœa, digestive troubles, and decrease of urine. The dulness of the heart is enlarged in most cases, especially towards the left. The apex-beat can be felt at first, but it is very irregular as to strength, and disappears altogether at a later period. The sounds of the heart are clear, but the first is generally indistinct, and the second, over the aorta, very weak. A systolic murmur is often heard at the apex of the heart, but its sounds are quite irregular in strength and succession. The pulse-beats corresponding to the heart are irregular and unequal, which is a characteristic symptom of chronic diffused myocarditis. The prognosis of the disease is always unfavourable, and more so if the diuresis be sparing. Ruhle's treatment of this disease is as follows. During the first stage, the patient must be kept quiet, eat milk food, apply ice to the region of the heart, take iodide of potassium, and eventually digitalis. During the second stage, the patient is treated with digitalis and stimulants (*e. g.*, wine, beef-tea, ether tinctures). Notwithstanding all these means, however, Ruhle never succeeded in making the pulse regular, even for a short time.—*British Med. Journal*, Jan. 18, 1879.

Valvular Aneurisms.

Dr. BIACH (*Wiener Med. Jahrbuch*, 1878) is of opinion that a valvular aneurism can only be suspected, but never diagnosed, during the patient's lifetime. The valves of the left heart seem much more disposed towards the formation of aneurisms than those of the right, especially the bicuspid valve. In some cases, we find aneurism of several, even of all, valves in the same individual. This disease often originates in endocarditis, which in its turn may be caused by the abscesses which often form in pneumonia and attack the aortic valves. Insufficiency or stenosis of a valve may cause an aneurism in any other valve by making the action of the heart irregular. The wave of blood, which beats with more force on one portion of the valve than on another, may cause the former to dilate and form an aneurism. In some cases, either congenital or acquired narrowness of some portion of the aorta or pulmonary artery may produce an aneurism of the semilunar valves of these vessels. Any pressure coming from outward, such as a tumour, etc., may contribute to the formation of aneurism by compressing the vessels.—*British Med. Journal*, Jan. 4, 1879.

Treatment of Diseases of the Colon.

Dr. DUBOIS (*Scheizer Correspondenzblatt Memorabilien*, 1878, ix. Heft), after giving a rapid enumeration of the diseases of the colon where it is indicated to inject large or small quantities of water, adds some practical hints on the different ways of administering the fluid. There are two different kinds of enemata employed. 1st. The simple enemata, which are used in cases of constipation when it is found necessary to remove fecal masses from the sigmoid flexure, the cæcum, or the rectum, in cases where the mucous membrane of the rectum is diseased, and it is indicated to bring it into contact with water or medicine. 2d. Very large enemata, which will be found efficient in cases where the water ought to be injected high up into the large intestines, or whenever there exists a catarrhal affection of these portions of the intestines. Some patients can bear, without incurring pain or danger, enemata of 1000 to 1500 cubic centimetres of water, but in others such a large volume of fluid would either prove very dangerous to the intestines, or could not be injected on account of the great irritability of the intestinal muscles. In such cases, where it is of obvious necessity to inject a large bulk of liquid, the author advises the following method.

Tepid water is injected till the patient feels a violent strain. The syringe is then removed, and the patient slowly changes under the bed-clothes from his right or left side to crouching on his knees and elbows. After one to two minutes, the former position is again assumed for a short time, and then the patient lies down upon his back. The same operation and changes of posture are then repeated, and defecation generally ensues in about ten minutes or half an hour after the injection has been given.

This method is indicated: *a*, in cases of constipation where purgatives and the usual enemata can either not be given, or have proved powerless; *b*, in cases of coprostasis where fecal tumours, varying in size, can be felt in the cæcum or other parts of the large intestine, and have sometimes been mistaken for ovarian cysts. Here purgatives given by the mouth are either vomited or have no effect; c, it is well known that inflammations of the vermiform process are mostly caused in healthy individuals by accumulation of feces. Whenever, therefore, a slight tenderness and increased resistance are felt in the iliac region, especially in persons who have suffered from typhlitis before, a bulky injection will be found very useful in preventing the inflammation and removing the feces. Narcotics should also be used in those cases; d, in cases of general or local peritonitis, when constipation and accumulation of gases in the abdomen have been produced by paralysis of the intestinal muscles; e, in cases of diarrhœa caused by obstipation or accumulation of feces; f, in abscesses of the intestines, dysentery, etc.—*London Med. Record*, Jan. 15, 1879.

Maeler on Chronic Dysentery treated by a Solution of Alum.

The patient (*Allg. Med. Centr. Zeit.*, No. 102), a workman, aged 48, had been suffering for some time from repeated attacks of dysentery which were combined with violent colic. The motions were liquid, and contained a great quantity of pus, mucus, and blood. The cause could not be detected by examination of the rectum and palpation of the abdomen. The patient was then treated with a solution of alum, which was injected into his bowels immediately after each evacuation, and which he was directed to retain as long as he could. This remedy proved successful, the patient only complaining of a burning pain in the rectum, while it was being thrown up, but feeling much relieved afterwards. The motions then gradually began to present a better appearance, no more blood or pus was noticed in them; they became more solid, and a fortnight after the first injection had been administered, the patient was dismissed as cured. The strength of the solution was four teaspoonfuls of alum to a pint of water.—*Lond. Med. Record*, January 15, 1879.

Arterial Pulsation of the Liver.

Dr. ROSENBACH, of Breslau, contributes a paper on the arterial pulsation of the liver to the *Deutsche Medicinische Wochenschrift*, for Oct. 5, 12, and 19. Hitherto, he remarks, a systolic pulsation of the liver in all its parts, but especially in the right lobe, has been held to indicate tricuspid insufficiency, as being produced by the systolic regurgitation into the adjacent large veins; and this pulsation was easily distinguishable from the mere impulse communicated to the liver in such affections as cardiac hypertrophy, abdominal aneurism, etc. Moreover, the importance of this hepatic pulsation was further enhanced by the observations of Friedreich, that it is one of the earliest symptoms of tricuspid insufficiency, earlier even than pulsation of the jugulars. The following case, however, shows that there may exist a pulsation of the liver in no way differing from that produced in tricuspid insufficiencies, while yet no sign of valvular disorder existed during life, nor could any such be traced after death; hence another explanation of its cause becomes necessary.

P. A., aged 18, a compositor's apprentice, who had in former years had several attacks of acute rheumatism, was admitted into the hospital on the 5th of May, on account of asthmatic dyspnœa with severe palpitation of the heart. His complexion was sallow; respiration 30, and laboured; pulse 84, jerking; arterial tension somewhat diminished. There was distinct pulsation in even small peripheral arteries, while on both sides there was violent beating of the carotids. The venous circulation was in every respect normal; no œdema, no ascites. The liver could be indistinctly felt immediately below the ribs. There was strong systolic pulsation extending to the entire sternum, the præcordial and epigastric regions, though superficial in the latter situation, and easily obliterated by pressure. Cardiac dulness began between the second and third ribs, extending three-fourths of an inch to the left of the mammillary line and to the right margin of the sternum. At the apex there was a blowing systolic and faint short diastolic murmur, while at the upper part of the sternum there was a long diastolic and a faint, short systolic murmur. The heart sounds extended into the carotids, to the palmar arch and femoral artery. On percussion there was marked dulness of the lower portion of the lungs, from one inch below the inferior angle of the scapula to one-third of an inch above it, and almost encircling the thorax; in the same area the breathing was feebly vesicular—otherwise the respiratory sounds were normal. His appetite was good; the bowels were regular; there was no albumen in the urine, which was rather high coloured. At first, under generous diet, the patient's condition slightly improved, especially after the removal from the left side by aspiration of about a pint of fluid. From the 15th to 20th May, there existed between the fourth and sixth ribs, and extending from the right edge of the sternum to near the left axilla, loud pericardial and pleuritic friction, after the disappearance of which the patient's condition grew steadily worse. The asthmatic paroxysms increased, œdema of the feet and ascites set in, and the pleural effusion increased. While there was no change in the condition of the heart and vessels, a marked alteration took place in the liver. It had gradually and steadily enlarged, so as to be distinctly felt projecting from under the ribs, and a slight pulsation throughout its substance became perceptible. On the 25th May, it formed a hard well-marked tumour, whose lower margin extended one-third of an inch below the umbilicus, and presented throughout its extent a marked systolic pulsation. A stethoscope applied on the right side of the epigastrium was lifted an inch high by the impulse; the hand pressed into the epigastrium was thrust outward at the systole; the impulse, however, having not only a forward but also a lateral direction. To the fingers placed over the epigastrium the sensation was as if the liver floated in the ascitic fluid, and was rhythmically thrust in every direction at the heart's systole. This pulsation of the liver continued very distinct until death, on the 16th June, and though the ascites increased, it did not diminish but became rather more perceptible. Even to the end there was no jugular pulse.

Necropsy.—The pleuræ were partially covered with fibrinous exudation, containing each about half a litre of yellowish flocculent fluid. The pericardium was united throughout its extent with the heart. The heart was considerably dilated, containing fluid blood in both sides; its muscular substance on section was spotted, of a light yellowish brown, especially on the left side. The thickness of its walls on the right side was 0.27 to 0.35 inch (7 to 9 millimetres), on the left side 0.51 to 0.78 inches (1.8–2.0 cen.). The tricuspid valve was normal, but the mitral valve was thickened throughout and insufficient; there was also thickening and insufficiency of the aortic semi-lunar valve. The origin of the coronary arteries was dilated; there was marked fatty degeneration of the substance of the left ventricle. Both lungs presented red induration; they were devoid of air through compression in their lower portions. The patient was, therefore, on admission the subject of extreme insufficiency of the aortic valves with inflammatory effusion into both pleuræ.

The course of the case may be divided into two stages by the occurrence of pericarditis. At first the valvular defect was sufficiently compensated, but the subsequent pericarditis, leading as it did to complete obliteration of the sac of the pericardium, produced extensive and rapid disturbance of compensation, as was shown by the œdema, ascites, and enlargement of the liver. Hence, also, the obstacles presented to the flow of the venous blood were largely increased, producing venous stenosis. The second stage was marked, in addition to the condition of the stenosis, by a marked systolic pulsation of the liver, the explanation of which is impossible, on hitherto accepted grounds, seeing that all signs and symptoms of tricuspid insufficiency were completely absent, a circumstance clearly established by subsequent examination. Now, if we consider the extreme force with which, in cases of aortic valvular insufficiency, the blood is propelled into the arteries, so that the impulse is felt, not only by the entire body, but is perceptible even in the capillaries, we can conceive that a marked pulsation is possible also in the liver. If this is, however, not observable in all such cases of valvular disease, it is obvious that in certain cases, as the present one, there is a coincidence of favourable circumstances giving greater prominence to this phenomenon of hepatic pulsation. As such, we may regard, in the present case, the considerable enlargement of the liver while the left ventricle yet retained its full force and activity; and also in the constriction of the aorta (the width of the aorta is given as 8 centimetres). The tense and enlarged liver, easily examined by pulsation, could, therefore, reproduce the first impulse of the heart all the more readily, since the difference between the strong systolic and feeble diastolic beat was unusually great, owing to the extensive regurgitation, and as indicated by the strong, short, jerking pulse. The relatively rare concurrence of such favourable circumstances probably explains why pulsation of the liver has not hitherto been observed in cases of purely aortic insufficiency. For in this valvular disorder, venous stenosis generally occurs only after the left ventricle has to a great extent lost its contractile power ; or, should it still continue active, when the arterial walls have lost their elasticity, and so their function has become impaired. Since, therefore, venous stenosis, and consequently enlarged liver, is a result of diminished arterial pressure, this organ usually presents a sufficiently large surface for palpation only then when the heart's beat has become too feeble to be transmitted into and through the hepatic vessels. But in the present instance matters were entirely different. Venous engorgement and stenosis had taken place in consequence of the pericarditis and subsequent obliteration of the pericardial sac, and also of the pressure of the pleuritic exudation, and while yet the left ventricle retained almost its full force and activity, and the aorta yet retained its proper elasticity. Hence the concurrence became possible of hepatic enlargement and increased arterial pulsation, the latter rendered transmissible to a distance by the normal elasticity of the arterial walls.— *London Med. Record*, Jan. 15, 1879.

Surgery.

On the Difficulty in Catheterizing the Œsophagus.

The patient, who is the subject of the observations in the *Archives Générales de Médecine* for September, was under the care of M. DUPLAY, in the Hôpital St. Louis, suffering from cicatricial stricture of the gullet, due to the swallowing of vitriol. Many efforts were made to pass an instrument into the stomach, but without avail. On admission, two grammes (thirty-one grains) of bromide of potassium were given daily, and this subsequently was increased to four. Every attempt at complete catheterization having failed, last January, that is two months after first admission, a hollow sound was introduced. This passed for thirty-four centimetres (about thirteen inches), as on former occasions, and then stopped. It was then perceived that during inspiration and expiration air passed through the instrument. It was undoubtedly in the trachea; and an examination with the laryngoscope showed that the opening of the glottis was very large, and although a full size instrument was in the windpipe, respiration was freely carried on. After this the laryngoscope was always used when an attempt was made to catheterize the œsophagus, and with complete success, as the patient was finally dismissed with the stricture fully dilated.

N. Duplay publishes the case to show how long an œsophageal sound may be passed into the air passages without its whereabouts being recognized. In the case reported, this was due partly to the tightness of the stricture, which was situated at the opening of the œsophagus, and also to the exceptional tolerance of the patient, who bore a sound passed into his windpipe; this tolerance N. Duplay thinks being due to the use of the bromide of potassium. Attention is also drawn to the usefulness of practising catheterization with the hollow sound, and to the importance of laryngoscopic examination during the treatment of these cases.— *London Med. Record*, Jan. 15, 1879.

—

Complete Congenital Branchial Fistula cured by Iodine Injections.

This case is reported, by LETIÉVANT, in *Le Progrès Médical*, Nov. 16, 1878. The patient was sixteen years of age, and first came under notice April 10, 1878, at the Hotel Dieu, Lyons, suffering from a sero-purulent discharge which escaped from an opening situated in the right subclavicular region. This little orifice was noticed by his mother when he was born; but there was no discharge until the age of three, when measles seemed to have acted as an excitant. From that time things had remained in the same condition, the fistula never giving rise to pain, merely causing fits of coughing. An examination revealed an elongated cord-like tumour, extending under the skin from the inner extremity of the right clavicle, along the internal edge of the sterno-mastoid muscle, to the level of the upper border of the thyroid cartilage. The swelling decreased in size from below upwards, and appeared to be lost in the deeper structures of the region. It was soft and movable, rising from the larynx during the movements of deglutition. The skin was quite healthy, but at the lower part of the tumour was a small red orifice about the size of a quilting needle; during deglutition, by the act of its elevation, this opening became invaginated in the skin. By pressure, creamy, or sanguineous pus could be squeezed out, causing the disappearance of the little swelling at the lower part of the cul-de-sac. A microscopic examination of this pus showed leucocytes, red globules, and cylindrical epithelial cells. On introducing a stylet, it could be passed upwards for eight or nine centimetres, but no superior opening could be detected, although when a certain point was reached, the coughing was induced. At the lowest part, in connection with the orifice, was situated a small rounded pouch. A milky injection shortly found its way into the mouth, thus implying a direct communication with that cavity. A laryngoscopic examination, in conjunction with the injection, revealed a small opening below the right tonsil. The right posterior pillar of the soft palate was absent, being replaced by two papillæ, of which the superior and posterior was perforated by a small orifice, only visible when liquid was injected by the fistula. The rest of the mouth, the lips, the face, and the neck, presented no malformation; there was no deafness nor deficiency of hearing on the affected side. The family history showed a large amount of congenital deafness; thus the maternal grandfather, one of the uncles, and a cousin were thus affected; the father and brothers of the patient were quite free from this defect.

When injecting sapid fluids into the fistula, no sense of taste was experienced until the internal opening had been passed. M. Letiévant, taking into consideration the relations of the fistula to the larger vessels of the neck and the pneumogastric nerve, and bearing in mind the difficulties that would be met with in an attempt to dissect out the sinus, decided to try the effects of iodine injections. From May 6th to June 3d, sixteen injections of tincture of iodine with an equal quantity of water were made; the pain caused by this measure was generally only slight. At the latter date there was no longer suppuration; the cord was only a little painful on pressure. June 16th. Patient appeared cured. Both the external and internal orifices were closed. The fistulous tract felt merely a small subcutaneous cord. There was neither pain nor discomfort on pressure. Discharged. —*London Med. Record*, Jan. 15, 1879.

Gastro-Enterotomy for Intestinal Obstruction.

At a recent meeting of the Clinical Society of London (*Med. Times and Gazette*, Jan. 18, 1879) Mr. LAWSON read the history of a case of intestinal obstruction, which had been under the care of Dr. Cayley and himself at the Middlesex Hospital, and for which Mr. Lawson performed gastro-enterotomy. H. C., aged twenty-three, a compositor, was admitted into the Middlesex Hospital under the care of Dr. Cayley, on June 3, 1878. For the last six weeks he had been somewhat costive, and had suffered occasionally from colicky pains. The bowels acted every day, but the motions were scanty, and composed of small hard lumps. On May 29, while at work, he was seized by an attack of colicky pains much more severe than the previous ones. In the evening he vomited, and he states that the matters brought up had a fecal smell. The bowels had acted that morning, but there was no motion afterwards up to the time of his admission. During the following three days he had frequent retching, but brought nothing up, and he took no food except a little _milk_; the colicky pains continued unabated. His medical attendant had given him sulphate of magnesia, and several enemata. State on admission: The countenance was natural and free from anxiety; the tongue was thickly coated; there was a slight blue line on the gums of the lower jaw. He complained of a twisting pain in the belly, especially on moving. It was most marked in the umbilical region, and though constant, was aggravated by frequently recurring paroxysmal exacerbations. The abdomen was considerably distended, with some tenderness on deep pressure in the umbilical region. There was marked fulness in the epigastric region, below which there was a slight depression. On percussion there was tympanitic resonance in the epigastric, right hypochondriac, lumbar, and iliac regions. In the umbilicus the resonance was less markedly tympanitic on the left side; there was dulness in the iliac and lumbar regions, but it was noticed that the position of the dulness sometimes shifted across to the right side. The circumference of abdomen at the umbilicus was thirty-three inches. The patient belched up wind, but had passed none per anum since the 29th. The urine was abundant; specific gravity 1037, free from albumen. Respirations 24; temperature 99.2°; pulse 108. The patient was placed on his elbows and knees, a flexible tube passed as high as was practicable, and an enema of warm water administered by a syphon from a vessel placed eighteen inches above the level of the anus. It was not found possible to administer more than two quarts of fluid, which caused considerable distress from a feeling of distension. The enema returned quite free from fecal matter. Digital examination of the rectum gave negative results. Ordered extract. opii gr. ss. every four hours. After two pills, the pain was relieved, and the patient fell asleep. The patient continued to get worse; the pain increased, the belly became more distended; and on June 5 he vomited a flaky yellow fluid with a distinct fecal odour. On June 6 the symptoms were still unrelieved, not-withstanding repeated doses of opium, and repeated enemata. He continued to vomit stercoraceous matter. The temperature had risen to 101.2°; the belly was more distended, and there was tenderness. As peritonitis was beginning, it was thought that further delay in resorting to an operation was undesirable; it was therefore decided that a search should be made for the obstruction. The patient having been placed under ether, Mr. Lawson made an incision in the median line of abdomen, commencing just below the umbilicus. The coils of intestine were seen greatly distended, and with a red velvety appearance, but still shining, and without any deposit of lymph on them. On passing his hand into the abdomen, Mr. Lawson felt a portion of the intestine tightly distended to beyond the size of the adult stomach, and extending from just below the liver on the right side downwards to the right iliac, and across the belly to the left iliac region. From the fixity of the intestine he concluded that it was the cæcum. He failed to detect any band or constriction, or collapsed portion of the intestine. He now endeavoured to unravel the small intestine by withdrawing it, and replacing it through the wound coil by coil; but this proceeding was found impracticable, in consequence of the excessive distension of the gut. A considerable portion of the intestine was therefore withdrawn from the abdomen to give room for further exploration; and on again introducing the hand, nothing could be detected but the enormously distended piece of intestine which was supposed to be the cæcum. This portion of the viscus was now punctured with a large trocar close to the lower end of the wound in the abdominal walls, and a large chamber-vessel full of liquid feces was drawn off. The canula was now withdrawn, and a large India-rubber tube, about six inches in length, and of the size of the finger in circumference, was introduced through the opening the trocar had made, and the end of the tubing was brought out through the bottom of the wound in the abdominal walls. A single suture was applied to one edge of the opening in the intestine, and fastened to the lower cut edge of the abdominal wall, but owing to the fixity of that portion of the intestine, it was found impossible to draw it sufficiently forward to unite it completely to the edges of the external wound. The intestines were then, after some difficulty, returned, and the wound closed with sutures in the usual manner. The parts were dressed with carbolic oil and a compress, and a well-fitted bandage applied to keep the whole *in situ.* During the progress of the operation, as the intestines were drawn from the abdominal cavity they were covered with flannel, made moist and warm by being wrung out of hot water. This flannel happened to be quite new, and consequently the fluff from the flannel adhered to the peritoneal surface and remained attached when the bowels were replaced into the abdomen. The small intestines, as before stated, were greatly distended, so as to approach in size the normal colon. In returning these into the abdomen, the peritoneal coat in two places cracked to the extent of about three-quarters of an inch. Each of these peritoneal wounds Mr. Lawson closed with a continuous suture of fine silk, such as is used in operations on the eye, taking care that the needle perforated only the peritoneal covering, and did not wound the muscular coat of the bowel. The patient was then returned to bed. A profuse discharge of liquid feces continued to take place through the tube. The next morning his pulse was 160, small and sharp; temperature 103°; belly much distended; has had no more vomiting, and has passed flatus per anum. A free discharge of feces continues through the tube. He continued to improve from this date; he had no further vomiting; and on the 11th, the fifth day after the operation, he passed a copious semifluid motion per anum. After the stitches were removed, the abdominal wound gaped a little, but the edges were kept in apposition by adhesive plaster and a bandage round the abdomen, and ultimately the wound united by granulation, leaving at the lower end a small fistulous track, through which a small quantity of feces continued to escape. The patient left the hospital for the Eastbourne convalescent establishment in the second week of October, but, after having been there a fortnight, he was sent back with symptoms of obstruction, and distension of the belly. A large enema gave him relief, but, unfortunately, he has had several recurrences of obstruction. The bowels seem to have lost much of their power of propelling onwards their contents, and, as they have probably become more or less adherent to the walls of the abdomen and to each other, a complete block may at any time occur, for which a right lumbar colotomy will afford the only chance of relief.

Dr. MURCHISON said the case reminded him of one which occurred in Scotland. Both were illustrative of what might be done in certain cases with peritoneal injuries. There a boy while bathing had his abdomen ripped open, and thus it remained for some time; the bowels, though covered with sand, were, after being carefully washed, returned, and the boy did well. He would like to know what in the present case was supposed to be the nature of the obstruction. The patient was a young man; there was no history of cancer or anything of that kind, there was no intussusception, but the obstruction was low down in the colon.

Mr. LAWSON thought the obstacle was caused by a kick in the intestines, which had been got rid of by the manipulation.

Dr. CAYLEY said that before the operation the seat of the obstruction had been uncertain; but, though evidently low down, it must be remembered that two quarts of fluid were retained. The hard swelling in the left groin could hardly be fecal.

Mr. CRIPPS spoke of the case of a boy which had occurred in the Great Northern Hospital. He had been the subject of an accident, and since that time had suffered from colicky pains, but this was succeeded by sudden and intense pain, with vomiting and constipation. He thought this was due to mechanical obstruction, and found he was compelled to open the abdomen. This was done by a small incision, and the intestine was gradually drawn to a certain point. Here he found the obstruction, which he relieved, and returned the bowel. The patient did well for a few days, but after that died from peritonitis. He thought the operation had been too long delayed, as the opium at first exhibited seemed to mask the disease.

Mr. BRYANT congratulated Mr. Lawson on the result of his case, one which could have hardly been anticipated. The history, he thought, pointed to an acute obstruction added to some chronic trouble, such as might be caused by a matting together of a part of the intestine by previous peritonitis. A point of great importance in these cases was to operate early—in fact, immediately a mechanical obstruction was diagnosed. No doubt in this case lumbar colotomy would have been sufficient, though this could hardly have been anticipated; but he thought that opening the bulging intestine, after the manner of Nélaton, would have been here the best procedure.

Mr. THOMAS SMITH allowed that waiting was prejudicial; but the first point was to make a diagnosis, and this was often most difficult. He recalled a case where sudden pain and vomiting had set in. The patient remained in the hospital for fourteen days, and died unrelieved, for at that time abdominal section was not readily undertaken. The post-mortem disclosed an acute enteritis with a sloughing patch of intestine, such as no operation could have benefited. Three days ago he saw a boy who had been attacked, about Christmas, with vomiting and sudden pain. The abdomen was not much distended, and mucus was passed per anum. He had diagnosed an enteritis, but after death, a band was found strangulating a diverticulum of small intestine. In another case there had been t1e same symptoms of acute strangulation, w1ere he had diagnosed volvulus. An operation t1roug1 a small opening was performed ; a band was found, and t1e intestine released ; but t1e patient, w1o 1ad taken t1e anæst1etic badly, died in 1alf an 1our—from t1e effect of t1e et1er, as 1e believed.

M r. HULKE quite agreed t1at the diagnosis was often a matter of great diffi-culty ; t1e acuteness of t1e vomiting and t1e seat of t1e pain 1e 1ad often found fallacious guides. In one case, w1ere t1e symptoms were acute and severe, t1ey were found to depend on an abscess in Douglas's pouc1. In a second, w1ere t1e vomiting was immediate and uncontrollable, t1e obstruction was at t1e lower end of t1e small intestine. Having 1ad an opportunity of witnessing t1e present ope-ration, 1e still believed t1e obstruction to 1ave been caused by t1e band con-stricting t1e 1epatic flexure ; and t1e cause of t1is band was to be soug1t in t1e 1istory of t1e burn, and its attendant suppuration—conditions w1ic1 were known to be often followed by peritonitis or ulcer.

M r. HEATH criticized t1e treatment of t1e distended intestine by puncturing it wit1 a trocar and inserting a drainage-tube, w1ile no attempt was made to attac1 t1e intestinal wall. Escape of t1e intestinal contents mig1t so easily 1ave taken place into t1e peritoneal cavity. He also t1oug1t t1at t1e probability of a band constricting t1e colon in some part of its course was great. He referred to M r. Teale's treatment of a similar case, w1o 1ad, wit1out opening t1e intestine, closed t1e abdominal wound and done a lumbar colotomy, and t1oug1t t1at t1is would be a better treatment to adopt in future.

Dr. BUZZARD believed t1at t1e future 1istory of t1is case would be still more interesting. T1e fact t1at two quarts of fluid were retained negatived, in 1is opinion, t1e idea t1at t1e obstruction could be very low down. He quoted t1e case of a young man who 1ad recovered from two attacks of obstruction—one of w1ic1, at least, 1e believed to 1ave been dependent on a strangulating band—under a free administration of opium.

Dr. BURNEY YEO 1ad received an altoget1er different impression from t1e 1istory. A distended condition of t1e intestine 1ad been described w1ic1 it would 1ave been useless to treat by opium—a treatment w1ic1, in 1is opinion, 1ad been too often fatal.

M r. HOWSE t1oug1t t1at t1e mere emptying of t1e intestines was often enoug1 to relieve obstruction w1ere a band was t1e cause of t1e strangulation, just as in a strangulated 1ernia evacuation of t1e contents of t1e bowel often allowed replacement to be effected. He allowed t1at t1e diagnosis of suc1 cases was often difficult, but treatment of a clear case of mec1anical obstruction by opium could only be prejudicial. After tapping it was a serious objection t1at t1e puncture so often allowed oozing to occur. It was of little use t1en to sew up t1e 1ole ; t1e punctures by t1e needle increased t1e difficulty.

M r. HULKE entirely agreed wit1 t1e remarks of t1e last speaker, t1at to tie t1e puncture often added to t1e danger, for, in spite of all care, t1e intestinal wall was most easily cut t1roug1 by t1e ligature.

M r. CROFT considered t1at 1ere t1e value of antiseptic precautions was most valuable. Flannel, w1ic1 1ad been objected to by M r. Bryant for covering t1e protruded intestine, was perfectly 1armless, if antiseptic. T1e peritoneum tole-rated larger and 1arder foreign bodies t1an t1e 1airs from flannels, provided t1at t1ey were antiseptic.

Dr. A. P. STEWART wis1ed to call attention to t1e importance of substituting belladonna for opium in t1e treatment of suc1 cases.

Dr. CAYLEY, in replying, said t1at 1e was responsible for t1e delay in operat-ing, but 1e could not allow t1at t1e symptoms were too urgent for t1is delay. Just before t1e operation t1e man 1ad been reading the newspaper,

Mr. LAWSON added that he had no alternative but to puncture the intestine, otherwise the small gut could not have been replaced. Dr. Buzzard, he thought, had not noticed that the fecal vomiting which had existed for twenty-four hours before the operation, had ceased after it, and the patient uninterruptedly got well.

—

On the Treatment of Dropsy of the Gall-bladder by Operation, with Notes of a Successful Case.

Mr. GEORGE BROWN records (*British Medical Journal*, Dec. 21, 1878) the following remarkable case :—

Mrs. C., aged 45, a tall, thin woman with very sallow complexion, consulted me, at the end of March, 1877, on account of an abdominal tumour. I obtained from her the following history :—

She was the mother of six children, all alive; the youngest seven years old. She had enjoyed very good health during the time of child-bearing; but, for about the last six years, had suffered from indigestion, pains of stomach, constipation, and occasional attacks of bilious colic. The catamenia was still regular. Her present illness dated from early in February, 1877, when one day, after cleaning windows, she had felt pain in her right side below the liver. She took no particular notice of the pain at the time, concluding that she had strained the muscles in overreaching whilst cleaning the windows; but, on going to bed. she rubbed her side, with a view to relieve the pain, when she felt a hard lump. Next day, she called in a local practitioner, who told her she had a tumour of the side, which diagnosis was confirmed by his partner, who added that nothing could be done for it by way of treatment except to endeavour to relieve pain. As she could obtain no information from these gentlemen beyond the assurance that she suffered from "tumour," she went to one of the metropolitan hospitals specially devoted to the treatment of diseases of women. The physician in attendance diagnosed "abdominal tumour," but would give no opinion as to its nature. He suggested, however, that he should attend her at home, where he would "puncture" the tumour to see if it contained fluid. She promised to consider the matter, but decided not to return to the hospital.

On examination, I found a tumour in the right hypochondriac region, extending from the lower border of the liver to about four inches below it. On percussion, its natural boundaries were found to be limited by two lines—one drawn from the right nipple to the spine of the pubes, and the second just half an inch to the right of the umbilicus. It was pyriform in shape; the narrow part of the tumour was directed towards the liver, and it could be grasped through the abdominal walls. To the touch, it gave one the impression of being fully as wide at its widest part as a medium-sized lemon. It was free from the abdominal wall, and could be moved from side to side. On asking the patient to take a respiration, it responded to the movements of the diaphragm, from which I concluded that it was attached to the liver, and I felt no doubt that the tumour was an enlarged gall-bladder. Whether the enlargement was due to fluid or gall-stones, I was unable to determine, as no fluctuation could be detected. As she was suffering from no constitutional disturbance, and felt equal to the management of her household affairs, I advised that nothing should be done for the present except to treat the constipation and biliousness. I kept her under observation for about nine months before any important alteration in her condition took place. During this time she had two or three attacks of bilious colic (with vomiting of bilious fluid), which were relieved by poultices, turpentine stupes, and opiates. Meantime, the tumour slowly but very steadily increased in size. On the night of the 31st of December last, she was suddenly seized with rigors and extreme pain of the bowels. I saw her next morning, and ordered the usual remedies. She had a green liquid motion. There was great tenderness over the tumour, which at this time measured about five inches in length and four inches and a half in width. Its right boundary was now an inch and a half outside the umbilicus. The further progress of the case will be seen from the following notes taken daily :—

Jan. 2, 1878. Vomiting commenced early this morning. The liquid vomited was of a grass-green colour. There had been no sleep during the night; the pain was continuous. No action of bowels had taken place. Temperature 100.2; pulse 120. She was ordered ten grains of calomel in powder; and to suck ice, whilst hot linseed poultices were to be applied over the right hypochondriac region.

3d. She had passed a restless night. Pain was continuous. There had been no action of the bowels. She had vomited five times since yesterday morning, bringing up at each time about half a pint of greenish liquid. No food had been retained by the stomach. Ten grains of calomel and one of opium were given, and an enema four hours afterwards, but without any action of the bowels resulting. The enema was repeated at bedtime; again without result. The temperature and pulse were unaltered.

4th. There had been a better night; pain was less: she had vomited several times last night and to-day. She had taken two saline aperient draughts at four hours' interval; but, as no action of the bowels had followed, three castor-oil enemata had been administered in quick succession. After the last enema, two copious evacuations had appeared; the stools were of a very dark colour. They were examined for gall-stones, but none were found. Pulse 104.

5th. The bowels had acted three times since yesterday; the stools were liquid and pale coloured. The pain was less violent. Vomiting had ceased, but retching continued. There was extreme tenderness on pressure over the right hypochondriac region, and slight fluctuation could be detected over an area about the size of a shilling, an inch above and an inch and a half to the right of the umbilicus. Temperature normal; pulse 104.

6th. There had been a better night. Pain and sickness had ceased.

7th. The general condition was unaltered. Fluctuation was more manifest.

8th. She had had a good night. The bowels had acted three times since yesterday. No gall-stones were observed. There had been no vomiting, but she felt sick. There was less pain and tenderness of the tumour. A curious symptom to-day was almost constant and uncontrollable yawning. Temperature 100 deg.; pulse 104. Poultices had been constantly applied ever since the onset of acute pain.

9th. My friends Dr. Weston, Mr. F. H. Hume, and Mr. Gardner now saw the patient with me, and were unanimously agreed as to the presence of an abscess, probably in connection with the liver, and as to the desirability of aspirating. Accordingly, assisted by the two former gentlemen, I aspirated whilst the patient was under chloroform, and drew off six ounces of yellow non-fetid pus, slightly tinged with blood. I was rather disappointed at the smallness of the quantity of pus drawn off; but, after passing the trocar in all directions around the point of puncture to the extent of quite three inches, we concluded that the abscess was exhausted. On examination after the operation, we found that the tumour was unaltered in size. On passing a probe into the abscess-cavity, one could feel some hard nodular masses, apparently about the size of a filbert. At the time I thought that these nodules were encysted gall-stones, but this idea was afterwards disproved. Three hours after the operation she had slight rigors, the temperature rose to 102 deg., and the pulse to 130. Brandy, milk, ice, and morphia were given, and next day the pulse fell to 96 and the temperature to 99 deg. During the night, she vomited twice about a pint and a half of green liquid. She had a liquid stool in the morning, apparently consisting chiefly of mucus and bile. No blood nor pus was observed with the stool.

For the next five or six days the patient remained in about the same condition. Pulse about 90 or 96; temperature normal. She continued exceedingly weak, being unable to take any solid food, and only small quantities of liquid nourishment, on account of the great tendency to vomiting. The bowels were kept gently open by means of aperients and enemata. The stools were invariably coloured with bile. On the 17th, the aspiration-puncture, which had apparently healed, reopened, and discharged a little blood-stained pus. On the 18th the wound discharged about half an ounce of pus. On passing a probe into the wound about two inches, nothing could be felt but the hard nodules before mentioned.

On the 21st she had another severe attack of pain in the right hypochondriac region, with nausea, sleeplessness, and inability to take food. As there seemed to be no hope of any amelioration in the condition of the patient unless something were done surgically for the tumour, I again consulted with Dr. Weston, Mr. Hume, and Mr. Gardner. There could be no doubt as to the presence of a tumour of a large size; and, after a careful consideration of the case in all its bearings, we agreed that we were justified in cutting through the abdominal wall, and, if the tumour were found to be the gall-bladder, in evacuating its contents and establishing a fistulous opening. If adhesions had been formed, I intended to stitch the walls of the gall-bladder to those of the abdomen. In proposing this operation I felt that, assuming the diagnosis to be correct, we were only anticipating the best results of which nature was capable. Every day increased the danger of a fatal termination, from the tumour rupturing and discharging its contents into the abdominal cavity. Several cases of this kind have been recorded. The patient and her husband having given their consent, we decided to perform the operation without further delay.

The patient having been placed under chloroform by Dr. Weston, assisted by Mr. Hume, I cut through the abdominal wall very carefully, commencing the incision at the aspiration puncture-wound, and carrying it downwards and towards the median line for about two inches and a half. After the first incision, I cut on a director until the peritoneum was reached. Several vessels were divided which required torsion; and the deep epigastric artery, which was cut through, required ligature. Instead of coming down on the gall-bladder, as expected, I found that I had opened the peritoneal cavity. On passing my forefinger into the wound to explore the abdomen, it was evident that the mass of the tumour was to the left of the umbilicus and middle line, and that the dulness and enlargement at the point selected for incision were due to inflammatory thickening and adhesions of the omentum. Whilst exploring the cavity of the abdomen, I could distinctly feel and recognize the lobules on the under surface of the liver, also the bodies of the vertebræ. I then made an incision at right angles to the first for about an inch, cutting towards the median line a little below the umbilicus, hoping to reach the gall-bladder, but without success. Mr. Hume now explored the abdominal cavity, and expressed the opinion that to attempt to reach the tumour by carrying the incision to the left of the umbilicus, and cutting through the mass of adhesions, would be attended with great risk; and as there was, as far as we knew, no precedent for the operation in which we were engaged, he advised that we should be content with what had been done; Dr. Weston also concurred. Moreover, the patient had been under chloroform upwards of an hour, during which two ounces of the anæsthetic were used; and, as she was in a weak condition when placed on the operating-table, we were almost afraid to prolong the anæsthetic state for any further length of time. I must confess that I was reluctant to abandon the operation, but I felt it was only judicious to do so; and, if the patient recovered, I hoped to have the opportunity of performing a more satisfactory operation. Before closing up the wound, however, I made another exploration with my fingers, and tore through the adhesions towards the left as far as my fingers could reach. This procedure was, I believe, the means of saving our patient, and, as the sequel will show, rendered any further operation unnecessary. The edges of the wound were brought together with three silk sutures, and covered with a piece of lint dipped in carbolized oil. When she regained consciousness she complained of great pain in the right side. Four hours after the operation her temperature was 99.8 and pulse 88. There had been some bleeding from the wound, which, she believed, was due to the straining caused by a troublesome cough. I ordered a draught containing two grains of morphia, which, however, only gave her one hour's sleep. In the night she was seized with violent retching and vomiting of bilious fluid. After the retching commenced she found that her night-dress was saturated with a yellowish fluid, which proceeded from the wound. When I saw her in the morning the lint and bandages with which I had dressed the wound, as also her night-dress and the bedlinen around the spot where she lay, were saturated with the discharge from her side. Its colour left no doubt as to its origin. The quantity discharged could not have been less than a pint; but it is impossible to state the exact quantity. On removing the dressings, I found a steady flow of yellowish fluid making its exit from the angle of the wound. I collected about two drachms by means of a teaspoon in less than ten minutes. The liquid gave the ordinary reaction of bile. The bilious liquid continued to discharge throughout the 23d, 24th, and 25th; but, on the 26th, the discharge became pus-like and fetid.

To go through the daily notes of the case up to the date of her convalescence would take too much time. It must suffice here to state that she made an excellent recovery from the operation, almost without a bad symptom. The temperature never rose but just a fraction of a degree above normal, and the pulse kept at about 80 or 90. At no time was there the slightest symptom of peritonitis. Constipation continued, and was overcome by podophyllin, saline aperients, and enemata. For some time there was a good deal of gastric irritation, with occasional attacks of vomiting of bilious liquid, which were always relieved by effervescing draughts with morphia. Coincidently with the discharge of bilious liquid the tumour decreased in size, untill almost all trace of it had disappeared. When I examined her on February 8th, the abdomen was normally resonant everywhere, except over a limited area just around the site of the incision. The wound had healed by this time, except at the angle, and this would have healed probably, but I thought it advisable to keep it open for a time by means of tents. She sat up on February 2d, eleven days after the operation, after which she gained strength rapidly, and lost the cachectic appearance which previously existed. On February 21st, just a month after the operation, she walked out, and continued to do so daily until March 1st. On March 2d she had another attack of bilious vomiting, with pain in the right hypochondrium, which was increased on pressure. Temperature rose to 101.6 and pulse to 108. A few days after there were signs of the tumour reforming. On the 8th a small abscess burst at the inner termination of the cicatrix, discharging about a tablespoonful of pus. The discharge continued small in quantity and pus-like for some days, when it became clear and glairy. Thinking the discharge proceeded from a cyst in, or adherent to, the abdominal wall, I passed a seton through the fistulous opening and brought it out one inch to the left. The seton was drawn tighter daily, and cut through the tissues included in ten days. The fistula continued to discharge a small quantity of clear fluid, in appearance closely resembling glycerine, until the middle of May; but, by the end of that month, the fistula had quite healed. Since May her general health has been excellent. She discharges her household duties as usual, and says that she never felt better than she does at present.

So much for the chief facts of this almost, if not quite, unique case. And now a few words as to its nature. Judging from the results of *post-mortem* examinations of patients who have died after illnesses accompanied with similar symptoms and physical signs, I think there can be little doubt that the primary lesion was the impaction of a gall-stone in the cystic duct, probably an angular one, which permitted the passage of a small quantity of bile into the gall-bladder. When this occurs we know that the gall-bladder becomes distended with bile and mucous secretion, in some cases giving rise to tumours of enormous size. After a time inflammation was set up, either in the tumour or in the tissues around its neck, terminating in a pericystic abscess, which abscess I aspirated on January 9th. The tumour, however, was unaffected by this operation, and, had not something further been done, the probability is that it would have continued to enlarge (as' has occurred in some cases), ultimately rupturing the walls of the gall-bladder. If the contents had been discharged into the peritoneal cavity the result must have been fatal.

This case, taken together with Dr. M. Sims's (*vide British Medical Journal,* June 8th), proves that, instead of such operations being unjustifiable, they can be performed with great hope of success. The time will probably come when, in such cases, the surgeon or physician will be held not to have done all that he should have done if he do not give his patient the chance of cure or relief which attach to operative measures; and, as Dr. Sims truly remarks, an operation should not be delayed until the patient is *in extremis*. If the patient is to have a fair chance of recovery we must operate early and before the vital powers have been so reduced as to be unable to withstand the shock. In this case the patient, although very ill when we operated, was very far from being in a dying state.

—

Extraction of a Prostatic Calculus.

This communication was made by DESPRÉS to the *Société de Chirurgie*, October 16th. The patient was a man aged 50, who, following gonorrhœa, had stricture complicated with two urinary fistulæ. After various kinds of treatment (progressive dilatation, cauterization with caustic paste) without benefit, had been tried, the case came into M. Després's hands. A No. 7 sound having been passed, the existence of a calculus, judged to be in the region of the prostate, was revealed. A rectal examination confirmed this diagnosis. M. Després did not wish to perform urethrotomy, as he considers this an operation which renders this stricture more fibrous and resisting; but as no sound above No. 7 could be made to enter the bladder, an operation was resolved upon. A prerectal incision was made; at the bottom of the wound a fibrous cord was perceived, the nature of which could not be determined. The sound introduced into the canal not having been seen, the operator decided to incise this cord. It proved to be in the urethra, and the sound was now found; dilatation having been practised, a calculus was extracted, upon which was impressed all the eminences and depressions of the prostatic region. A No. 7 sound was now introduced into the bladder, commencing at the meatus. In twenty days it was withdrawn, and a No. 14 then readily passed. On the fifty-first day the patient left for the country, only a small fistula remaining, from which a little urine escaped.

The calculus was of the size of a chestnut, weighing 8 grammes 20 centigrammes (about 130 grains); it was composed of two very hard central nuclei, surrounded by concentric layers of ammoniaco-magnesium phosphate.—*London Med. Record*, Jan. 15, 1879.

Arterial Denudation.

In a clinical lecture delivered at La Pitié (*Gaz. des Hop.*, November 14), Professor VERNEUIL made the following observations:—

It often happens that a surgeon lays bare arteries of a considerable calibre during the course of an important operation such as the extirpation of a tumour, etc. In fact, arteries are often surrounded by these neoplasms; and you must have all seen wounds of this kind, in which the vessels, isolated and dissected with care, lie naked at the bottom of the wound. The prognosis of such denudations varies greatly. Some persons having seen the wounds close over the vessels without the slightest ill result, have come to the conclusion that there is no danger in dissecting out vessels during an operation; and this opinion seemed all the more rational as every one is aware how long the vessels offer resistance to accidents, remaining intact in the midst of purulent collections, and not undergoing perforation even when abscesses form within their sheaths. But opposed to this optimist opinion there is to be placed another, far less reassuring. For surgeons also meet with formidable hemorrhages in wounds in which arteries have been thus denuded, and that in cases in which they have not only respected the external coat of the vessel, but even the cellular tissue covering it. Which of us is there also who has not seen hemorrhages supervening in the midst of purulent collections traversed by vessels? What is the cause of these so considerable differences in the consequences of the same fact? The clinical facts I am about to notice will, I think, clearly indicate the cause of both successes and reverses.

I was consulted by a robust man of large stature, and endowed with an uncommon amount of energy and activity. He had had for several years a tumour in the parotidean region, but, immersed in his affairs, he paid little attention to its progressive growth. But for a year it had increased considerably, the skin covering it also changing in colour; and he came to consult me in December, 1877. At that time the tumour extended from the middle part of the temporal region to about two centimetres below the lower edge of the jaw, reaching in front the supra-hyoidean region. It projected five or six centimetres. The skin was adherent to the tumour, and very vascular; and the tumour was movable from before backwards. Nothing could be felt of it on passing the finger into the pharynx. It was quite painless, and there was neither paralysis of the facial, obstruction in the cerebral circulation, vertigo, nor congestion, indicative of arterial compression. While recognizing the seriousness of the prognosis, I felt disposed to remove the tumour; and having consulted Professor Richet, he diagnosticated softened enchondroma, and also advised an operation, although somewhat doubtful as to the issue. The patient being very desirous that it should be performed, it was executed on January 10. But while considering the propriety of the operation, I had been rendered somewhat uneasy by an unpleasant circumstance that came to light. Although the patient had all the appearances of robust health, he mentioned to me, without attaching the slightest importance to it, and almost as a joke, that he had recently consulted a "urine doctor," who had declared him to be diabetic. The doctor prescribed for his patient, especially employing the iodide of potassium, and in five or six weeks afterwards declared that sugar no longer appeared in the urine. His rapid cure inspired me with some distrust, and I insisted upon an analysis of the urine being made. This proved completely negative, and confirmed me in the opinion which I had given. The operation was a laborious one, but I need only refer to the principal details.

The tumour was circumscribed by superficial incisions made by the thermo-cautery, and the deeper incisions, or rather enucleations, were executed by the fingers. The whole of the carotidean vessels were laid bare, their pulsations being visible at the bottom of the wound, the vessels being, however, covered by a moderately thick layer of conjunctive tissue. The jugular vein was also exposed to a large extent. No vessel of any importance was injured, ligatures only being required for the temporal and for a branch of the internal maxillary. The whole of the parotid was removed, as well as a large portion of the sterno-cleidomastoidens. The amount of blood lost was pretty considerable, but the patient bore the loss perfectly well, and forty-eight hours afterwards seemed only as if he had undergone a slight operation. He complained only of dysphagia and great salivation, as is always the case in operations upon this region.

The next day, on his urine being examined, it was found to contain sugar. It is a fact of frequent occurrence for an operation to arouse glycosuria in intermittent diabetes. I was therefore not surprised, but my former apprehensions returned, and were corroborated by another pretty significant phenomenon. During the operation, the primary hemorrhage which follows the section of the tissues was much more prolonged than it is observed to be in healthy subjects. This sanguineous issue continued for some hours, while there was none of the venous hemorrhage so frequently seen after the patients have come to and made some efforts. On the second day the urine was turbid and reddish; there was no longer any sugar in it, but the urates existed in a colossal proportion, uratic diabetes having become substituted for glycosic. On the fifth day erysipelas appeared, which, springing from the edges of the wound, spread all over the head. This had disappeared by the ninth day. From the fifth day daily attacks of hemorrhage occurred, and the patient, losing his early calmness, became very restless. These were temporarily arrested by the application of pieces of agaric, until the fourteenth day, when the bleeding became so serious that all the agaric was removed. As the last piece of this was taken off, a jet of blood sprang from a small perforation in the carotid. The bleeding was arrested by the application of hæmostatic forceps; but after some hours the patient succumbed. During all the progress of the case the wound was never of its proper rose-colour; it was red, and differently coloured at different points, some being of a vermilion red, and others of an aponeurotic whiteness. This is always a bad sign. About the eighth day a wound ought to be uniformly rose-coloured over its whole extent.

In other cases I have been more fortunate. In order to remove a tumour of the arm-pit, the size of the head of a full-time infant, I denuded the axillary artery to the extent of three inches; on removing the parotid I have even denuded the carotid; and in extirpating a tumour of the neck I have exposed all the carotidean branches without any ill-effect. Last year, while removing a fibroplastic tumour of the thigh, I dissected out the femoral vessels to a length of fifteen centimetres. All these cases terminated successfully. I had a fatal termination after dissecting a lymphadenoma from Scarpa's triangle, when a rupture of the femoral occurred. At the autopsy the artery was found to have been rendered friable by the infiltration of the disease. I may also mention a remarkable case published by M. Nepveu in which the carotid was denuded during the extirpation of an enormous tumour of the neck. Fever supervened, and a formidable hemorrhage occurred from an eschar which had formed in the carotid. In this case the affection had also become generalized. In this point of view, also, we must remember that children the subjects of old abscesses of the neck have often succumbed to sudden hemorrhages which have supervened at periods of complication, as scarlet fever, etc.

In the three patients who succumbed, hemorrhage supervened when the economy was in an enfeebled state, wien tie general condition was a bad one, and fever with septicæmia iad set in. From tiese facts I believe tiat I may conclude tiat spiacelus and perforation of arteries do not take place except under unfavourable conditions; and tiis is how I explain the mecianism. In wounds practised on healthy persons tiere remains in tie conjunctive tissue wiici covers tie external coat of tie artery a small layer of cellular nuclei, wiici by proliferation form a granular surface and granulations tiat give sufficient protection to tie arterial walls. But in debilitated organisms tiis granular layer does not suffice for reparation, and becomes spiacelated, tiereby exposing tie arterial wall, wiici becomes tius dissected out. Tie conjunctive tissue of tie wall may even form granulations, and constitute a new granular layer; but tiis conjunctive tissue, in tie course of proliferation, is substituted for tie resisting tissue of tie arterial wall. Tie same tiing takes place iere as occurs in wounds of bones. At a given moment an insensible exfoliation takes place—a loss of substance wiici is only filled up by granulations. Tie arterial wall tien becomes enfeebled; and if we add to tiis unfavourable condition that, in a wound wiici goes on badly, considerable atropiy rapidly supervenes, we can easily understand tie production of spiacelus of tie wall of tie artery.

It is, tien, in my opinion, under tie influence of general accidents tiat tiese arterial ulcerations are produced. It is to tie constitutional condition tiat we siould attribute tiem; and wien a morbid diatiesis exists tie surgeon siould expect unfavourable events.—*Med. Times and Gaz.*, Jan. 25, 1879.

Fatty Embolon in Fractures.

M. Déjerine contributes to tie *Le Progrés Médical* a paper on tiis subject, from wiici tie following extract is made:—

In 1862, Zenker, making an autopsy on tie body of a man tiat iad been crusied between two wagons, found tie capillaries of tie lungs filled with fat. He believed tiat tiis fat migit iave come from the stomaci, or from tie liver, wiici was in a state of fatty degeneration, for boti tiese organs iad been injured. Zenker considered tiis fact very interesting from an anatomical point of view, but ie did not know tie relation wiici existed between fatty embolon and traumatisms, so did not record as of great practical importance tie case wiici ie iad observed. In tie same year, Wagner publisied many cases of fatty embolon, but ie regarded tie fat as originating in a metamorpiosis of pus, and as one of tie causes of pyæmia. It was not until 1865 tiat Wagner and Busci recognized in osseous alterations tie nature and causes of fatty embolon, eaci giving an exact and complete description, nearly at tie same time; from tiat date tie doctrine of fatty embolon ias rested upon an unattackable basis, and patiological, clinical, and experimental works iave rapidly followed one anotier. It was proved in every fracture tiat tiere was a fatty embolon, iaving its origin in tie medulla of tie bones, tiat tiis embolon was more or less considerable, tiat it was rarely localized in tie lung, but it was met witi in every tissue of tie organism. Tien it was siown tiat in a certain number of cases tie diagnosis could be made during life, and tiat it siould be regarded as a frequent cause of deati; it was pointed out tiat by tiis mecianism a fatal termination was brougit about in a number of tiose cases of more or less sudden deati observed after severe injuries, and up to tiis date attributed, in a general way, to wiat is designated in practical surgery by tie name of siock. Witi regard to tiis it is sufficient to mention tie works of Bergmann, Bzerney, Hain, and Flourney.

From tie researches of tie different authors enumerated, it follows tiat fatty embolon, general or localized in tie lung, is muci more common tian is frequently supposed, and tiat it is produced not only in all fractures, simple or complicated, but it may be observed, without reference to injury, in all cases where the bones are altered in structure from some cause or other; in such the fact is less grave. The number of cases of fatty embolon observed under circumstances about to be mentioned, are actually considerable, reaching 140, and all, or nearly all, have been observed in Germany, but two such observations were noted in the ancient faculty of Strasburg. Having lately met with two very clear cases of pulmonary fatty embolon, following osseous alterations, we publish them to draw attention to a subject little known to us, still less studied, but the importance of which should not be lost sight of in reference to published statistics; a doubly important subject for consideration, not only because it enlarges the scope of pathological knowledge, but more especially because it makes us recognize a very fatal complication of great injuries, and which, therefore, has considerable clinical importance from a prognostic point of view. On the 28th of October last, a young man, aged 16, was admitted into the Hôtel Dieu, in the service of Dr. Cusco, who had had his right leg crushed by a tramway. A certain quantity of blood was lost, and the patient sank about an hour after admission, being sensible to the end. The autopsy was made by the interne, M. Bruchet, and a fracture of both bones of the leg at the middle third was found, and also a fissure of the tibia reaching the upper articulation. He very kindly sent me the lungs and the heart. The vena cava had been previously ligatured to permit of an examination of the blood in the right ventricle. The microscopical examination was made in the laboratory of Prof. Vulpian, and revealed the following particulars: The blood of the right ventricle, obtained by making a puncture into the ventricular wall previously washed with ether, contained a large quantity of fat in the form of drops, and recognizable by its micro-chemical characters, disappearing under the action of ether, and taking on a black coloration under the influence of osmic acid. The vessels of the lungs were gorged and literally injected with fat; sections of the parenchymatous tissue of the lung cut with scissors and examined with the microscope, showed in the interior of the vessels, arterioles, veins, and capillaries, elongated masses, three, four, and five millimetres in length, embellished with a special refulgency, disappearing under the action of ether, and becoming a deep black colour with osmic acid. These globules of fat were so abundant at certain points that they designated not only the perilobular vascular network, but also the alveolar capillary network. An examination practised at all points of the two lungs gave us the same results. The second case, not less instructive than the first, came from the service of Dr. Brouardel at St. Antoine. The lungs, which we have examined in conjunction with M. Mayor, were sent by M. Marchland, interne of the service. They were taken from a man who had died thirty-six hours after a fracture of the right parietal bone, and, as in the preceding case, the pulmonary vessels contained more or less fat. In both cases no other viscera than the lungs were examined for fatty embolon. The two cases which we here report are absolute examples demonstrating fatty embolon after injury to bones; in this note we do not wish to inquire the part the fatty embolon took in causing death in these two cases. In the first we see but little that could be put down to any other cause; this is a subject which we propose to study more completely in the future, for cases of fatty embolon are in reality far from being rare, and we are persuaded will daily become more frequent when researches are undertaken in those who have succumbed from injuries. The two cases here reported resemble on all points those which have been made public in Germany of late years, and are confirmations of the published facts of different authors who have inquired into the question; but, as was said previously, we have believed it right to publish them, to draw attention to a subject worthy of study from every point of view, for, well as the doctrine of fatty embolon has been expounded in tie faculty's course by Prof. Vulpian and Charcot, it does not seem up to tie present time to iave attracted tie attention of tie medical world.—*London Med. Record*, Jan. 15, 1879.

Arthrotomy for the Extraction of Foreign Bodies.

At the *Société de Chirurgie* (Nov. 6th, 1878), M. VERNEUIL brougit forward tie following case. A man, aged 31, strong and well built, but witi a rieumatic iistory, noticed in December, 1877, a pain in tie rigit knee; tiis increased in severity, and in tie monti of May, 1878, ie found a foreign body at tie side of tie joint, whicћ could be fixed by certain manœuvres. He sougit advice and two foreign bodies were tien found; one, tie larger, situated at a point internal and above tie patella, was very movable and easily detected; tie otier one, unless fixed by tie patient, was not easily caugit, and sometimes disappeared for many days. M. Verneuil decided to effect removal by opening tie articulation. Tie patient was anæstietised, but just as tie incision was about to be made tie last foreign body escaped; tie operation was tierefore postponed. At tie next attempt tie substance was first fixed by acupuncture needles, and a section made of tie skin and tissues upon tie body; a iard white tissue was first reacied and tiougit to be tie new formation; tiis tissue, iowever, being incised, tie foreign body escaped from it. Similar steps were taken on tie outer side of tie joint, and extraction effected; iere tie synovial membrane was found to be tiickened. During tie operation a carbolic acid spray was kept playing upon tie wound, and tiis was afterwards wasied witi a strong solution of tie same antiseptic agent. Tie lips of tie wound were not approximated, but a piece of linen steeped in carbolic acid interposed, and a wadding dressing applied. Tie external wound iealed in twenty days, tie internal one a little later. Wien tie patient left tie iospital tiere was sligit stiffness of tie joint. Tie foreign body resembled pieces of tie wiite soap wiici tailors use for correcting defects, and were composed of cartilaginous tissue.

M. LUCAS-CHAMPIONNIÈRE tiougit tiat tiis interesting case added anotier to tie antiseptic artirotomies publisied by Saxtorph, Lister, Bœckel, and otier surgeons. Tie results of Lister's metiod were better tian tiose obtained by tie wadding treatment of Guérin. He iad extracted a very large foreign body from tie knee-joint by tiis plan; tie substance was so placed tiat it was necessary to open tie popliteal space. Tie articulation was exposed and drained, tie wound tien sutured. At tie tiird dressing, on tie eigiti day, cicatrization was perfeet, and at tie termination of tie tiird week tie patient left tie iospital witi natural movements of tie joint. He iad also operated upon a patient of M. Tarnier's witi puerperal artiritis of tie knee. Tie fever was intense, tie pain intolerable, tie woman for many nigits keeping ier neigibours awake by ier cries. Tie articulation was opened antiseptically and carefully drained. Pain ceased immediately tie fever subsided; iealing was obtained witi preservation of tie normal movements.

M. GILETTE is a strong advocate of tie wadding plan. At tie *Hôpital Temporaire* ie iad extracted a foreign body from tie knee-joint of a man, aged 28, with iydrartirosis. Immediately after tie operation wadding was applied to tie wound, and all precautions taken to prevent tie entrance of air. At tie end of forty days, wien tie dressing was raised, tie cicatrix was perfect.

M. DEPRES considered tiat foreign bodies in joints necessitating an operation by tieir presence were rare. He iad often discouraged tie idea of an operation in suci cases. Artirotomy was not always fatal; ie did not tiink it a very grave operation, and cited numerous instances of penetrating wounds of joints tiat iad terminated favourably.

Ⅎ. TRELAT was of opinion that statistics would prove if the operation of arthrotomy was justifiable. If the mortality did not exceed more than three or four per cent., it was a decided gain.—*London Med. Record*, Jan. 15, 1879.

Midwifery and Gynæcology.

Abdominal Palpation and Version by External Manipulation.

The object of Dr. A. PINARD'S work (Paris, 1878) is to demonstrate the possibility of diagnosing mal-presentations by palpation during the last weeks of pregnancy, and of rectifying them by external version. Having reduced the presentation to a normal one he applies an abdominal belt to keep the fœtus fixed in the new position until labour sets in. He thus avoids breech and shoulder presentations and secures head presentations. It is obvious that this proceeding marks a progress in obstetric medicine. Abdominal palpation has hitherto been greatly neglected, but in future it can no longer be so. Professor Tarnier lately said, at the Society of Medicine : "In a short time physicians and midwives will be compelled, under pain of neglecting their duty, to assure themselves, during the last month of pregnancy, whether the presentation is normal or not. On their side, the patients will soon find out that there is a simple means of avoiding serious risks. They will naturally come to avail themselves of it. These ideas will quickly spread, and among the lower classes, the poor women will acquire the habit of going during the last month to the lying-in hospitals to find out if their children are in proper position. This will be a great progress, because, in this way, a large number of obstetrical operations will thus be avoided." When visiting the clinique d'accouchements at Paris, the reporter had an opportunity of seeing Dr. Pinard reduce an arm presentation by external version, apply his binder, and thus secure a head presentation. The binder or entocic belt, as it may well be called, is described and figured in the *British Medical Journal* for Dec. 7, 1878.

The Treatment of Chronic Metritis.

Dr. A. MARTIN of Berlin (*Berl. Klin. Wochenschrift*, No. 42, 1878) recommends the removal of the cervix uteri in those numerous cases of chronic metritis which resist all other medicinal and local treatment. By "chronic metritis" he understands a connective-tissue overgrowth of a part or the whole of the uterus and cervix, the result of flexions, abnormal menstruation, etc., and especially of incomplete involution of the puerperal organ. "What we must remember," he says, "in treating chronic metritis is that we have to do with changes of wide extent in the tissues of the whole uterus, while at the same time its mucous membrane has, as a rule, undergone alterations of a severe and not always benign character." The *rationale* of amputation of the cervix appears to be, that a fatty metamorphosis of the hypertrophied connective tissue, analogous to that which occurs in puerperal involution, is produced. At any rate, Dr. Martin has not only theory, but practice in his favour. He has performed the operation seventy-two times in cases of chronic metritis. Half of these cases had been long treated by the ordinary methods without benefit. All of them exhibited changes of the mucous membrane, and greater or less enlargement of the uterus both in length and thickness. In most of them the cervix (and especially the lips) was much hypertrophied. The symptoms were usually profuse secretion, irregular and

abnormal menstruation, severe hypogastric and pelvic pains, digestive disturbances, and hysteria. About four or five centimetres of the cervix were removed
in each case, and on recovery from the operation it was generally found that the
uterus was reduced in length another one or two centimetres. At the same time,
as a rule, the thickness of the uterine wall diminished, and eventually the consistence of the uterus became normal, while nearly all objective, and many subjective,
symptoms disappeared. In three cases sterility of long standing was cured, it
being remembered that nearly all the operations have been performed within the
last two years. The details of the operation, and the method of arranging the
sutures so as to cover the newly formed cervical lips with vaginal mucous membrane, must be read in the original. Here we can only say that the knife is used
instead of the écraseur or galvanic cautery ; and that the form of excision known
in Germany as "Hegar's funnel-shaped excision" is the most appropriate. Difficulties in the operation are seldom met with, and with a uterus of ordinary mobility ten to fifteen minutes suffice for completing it. The main thing to keep in
mind is, that the larger the amount of cervix excised, the greater the subsequent
involution of connective tissue is likely to be.—*Med. Times and Gaz.*, Jan. 25,
1879.

—

*On the Value of Subcutaneous Injections of Ergotin in Uterine Fibroids and
Chronic Hypertrophy of the Uterus.*

This is the subject of a valuable contribution by LEOPOLD, in the *Archiv für
Gynäkologie*, Bd. xiii. s. 182. Leopold supports Hildebrandt, Winkel, Wernich,
etc., as against the late Professor Martin, of Berlin, and others, maintaining that
ergot so employed is of great value in the treatment of uterine fibroids. But he
further has employed the same agent with considerable success in the treatment of
subinvolution of the uterus and of chronic metritis. It is maintained by him that
success depends largely upon the mode of performance and the continuation of
the treatment, the selection of the cases, and especially the selection of the preparations. Failure, Leopold holds, has followed from neglecting these considerations. According to our author: The form of fibroid that gives best results is
the interstitial, although advantage may be expected in the way of lessening
hemorrhage, and promoting ultimate expulsion of the tumours in submucous
fibroids. Cases are unsuitable in which the uterus is incapable of contracting;
therefore there is no use of employing the injections when there is any false membrane or exudation binding down the uterus, or when it contains a fattily degenerated or calcareous tumour, when its muscular fibres are atrophic, or its bloodvessels degenerated. Tumours in the body of the uterus are more benefited by the
treatment than those in the neck. Great care is to be employed also in selecting
for treatment cases of subinvolution or chronic metritis. Every case in which
there exists pelvic exudation is to be rigidly excluded, also if there is a polypus
in the uterine cavity. The best preparation Leopold finds to be Wernich's extract dissolved in four parts of distilled water. After trial he has found that the
addition of glycerine, salicylic acid, carbolic acid, or morphia is objectionable.
He recommends that the solution should be very frequently renewed, as it is apt
to get mouldy. The best situation for injection, according to Leopold, is by the
side of the navel, the canula being inserted deeply into the abdominal wall. The
injections ought to be made very slowly, and a cold compress ought to be immediately applied to the part, whilst the patient ought to keep lying on her back
for several hours afterwards. The injections ought to be continued for a considerable time—30-120 in each case—if they are well borne. They should be made
almost uninterruptedly each day, especially and intentionally during the menstrual flow. With diminution of the bleeding the periods between the injections

may be lengtiened.   Leopold records 12 cases, in wiici ie iad employed tie ergotin injection.   Tiere was no improvement in 3 of tiese = 25 per cent. Tiere was essentially less bleeding witiout appreciable diminution of tie tumours in 5 = 42 per cent.   Tiere was notably sirinking of tie tumours in 4 = 33 per cent.   So tiat ie concludes tiat 75 per cent. gave evidence of improvement. Our autior also gives tie results obtained in 14 cases of cironic iypertropiy of tie uterus, 8 of wiici ie classes as examples of subinvolution, 5 as examples of cironic inflammation or metritis, and 1 as exfoliative endometritis (dysmenorrhœa membranacea).   In tiose 14 cases tie ciief effect noticed was sooner or later diminution of tie sanguineous disciarge at tie periods; tie time required for tie treatment varied from one to six weeks in cases of subinvolution, to several montis in cases of cironic metritis.   If decided advantage did not occur in tiese cases after 50–60 injections, Leopold tiinks tiat it is useless to continue longer injecting tie ergotin, and otier means must be tried.   In tie majority of Leo. pold's eases tie ergotin injection was accompanied by an improvement in tie patient's general condition, strengti, and appetite.   Tie particulars of the *sections* of tie uteri of two patients wio iad been treated for fibroid tumour by tiis metiod, and wio iad died from disease in no way connected witi the fibroid tumours, are tien given.   Tie examination of tiese tumours unmistakably prove, according to Leopold, tiat under tie use of tie ergot tie tumours iad been com- pressed, tieir vascular supply very largely cut off, tie tumours tiemselves ren- dered anæmic, wiilst fatty degeneration iad commenced in tieir muscular ele- ments.— *Edinburgh Med. Journ.*, Nov. 1878.

Removal of the Uterus by Freund's Method.

In tiis case tie patient was 34 years old, and iad iad two ciildren, tie last ten years ago.   Tie cancerous growti iad invaded tie body of tie uterus, wiici was retroverted.   On September 30, Dr. LEOPOLD performed tie operation of total extirpation of tie uterus by Freund's metiod, under complete antiseptic precautions.   Tie operation lasted two iours and a ialf.   At tie beginning of tie second day after tie operation, tie patient died.   Tie details of tie *post- mortem* examination are so interesting tiat we give a translation in full.   "At tie necropsy tie abdominal wound was found already in process of union.   Tie intestines in tie pelvis were greatly injected (commencing peritonitis).   At tie bottom of tie pelvic cavity tiere was a collection of about two or tiree table- spoonsful of sanguineo-serous fluid.   After tie entire pelvic organs iad been carefully removed, tie ligatures were found to iave been well applied, and tie bladder and ureters uninjured.   A careful examination, iowever, of tie posterior wall of tie bladder revealed tie presence of several fine off-sioots and streaks of cancerous growti, wiici iad also been observed during tie operation.   The re. sult of destroying tiis by tie cautery would iave been extremely unsafe.   As regards the stitciing of tie peritoneum, tie unsewing of it at tie autopsy proved iow defective it necessarily is, even wien it appears to be well done during tie operation.   Witi regard to tiis point, we cannot follow too carefully tie advice of Dr. Freund in reference to tie closing up of tie bottom of tie wound and tie stitciing in of tie Fallopian tubes.   Tie condition of tie ovaries was tie most interesting part of tie examination.   During tie operation tie left ovary was felt to be small and atropiied, tie rigit contained a fluctuating follicle about tie size of a iazel-nut, wiici had recently burst and was filled witi blood.   (Tie operation was performed nine days after tie commencement of tie last period.) At tie necropsy, tie condition of tie ovaries was remarkably cianged.   It was evident, tiat as a result of tie great stagnation resulting from the ligatures, tiat botı ovaries ıad increased to tıree times tıeir size on account of numerous blood effusions, and were lacerated internally. In tıe rigıt ovary tıe blood effusion ıad ruptured tıe delicate wall of tıe follicle and poured out into tıe pelvic cavity. From nowıere else could tıe recent blood found in Douglas's poucı ıave come. Taking all tıe facts into consideration, tıere can be no doubt tıat tıe patient died from loss of blood and septic peritonitis." Tıis case points to tıe importance of observing tıe rule to avoid surgical interference eitıer just before or after tıe menstrual nisus.—*London Med. Record*, Jan. 15, 1879, from *Centralblatt für Gynäkologie*, Nov. 1878.

—

A Case of Dermoid Cyst of the Ovary.

Dr. Gomes Torres, of Granada, relates (*Annales de Gynécologic*, June, 1878) a case of dermoid cyst of tıe ovary successfully removed by ovariotomy after a fistulous opening ıad existed for nearly tıree years. Tıe patient, An tonia C——, was twenty-five years old, and single. Menstruation commenced at tıe age of fifteen, ãnd continued regular and perfectly normal up to tıe age ot twenty. At tıat time sıe was frigıtened by a ıorse, and the frigıt brougıt on syncope, and suppression of menstruation, attended by nausea and general malaise, wıicı lasted for a week. Menstruation reappeared four montıs later, after treatment by iron. Eigıt montıs after tıe frigıt, and four after tıe re-establishment of menstruation, sıe commenced to feel pricking pain in tıe left iliac fossa, and tıen observed for tıe first time a tumour in tıis situation, wıicı was ıard, tender, movable, and about tıe size of a ıen's egg. Pain continued, and tıe volume of tıe tumour went on increasing till it reacıed tıe umbilicus, wıere it formed a marked prominence. Tıe medical attendant in cıarge, ascertaining tıat fluctuation was present, made an incision, wıicı allowed to escape a large quantity of tıick liquid. Tıe tumour tıen diminisıed, tıe orifice became fistulous, and tıere continued to flow from it pus and tıick matter, tıe nature of wıicı could not be determined from tıe patient's account.

Tıis condition of tıings continued for nearly tıree years, witı exacerbations of pain at tıe menstrual periods. Tıree montıs before tıe patient came under Dr. Torres's care, tıere appeared protruding tırougı tıe fistulous opening a mass consisting of bone with teetı implanted in it, tıe sıape of tıe bone and tıe situation of tıe teetı being sucı tıat it resembled a dog's ıead. Wıen tıis became known in tıe village it gave rise to extraordinary reports, and the patient was led, on tıis account, to come to Granada for relief. She was admitted into tıe ıospital on January 15tı, 1872.

Tıe general condition was tıen good. Tıe abdomen in tıe median line was occupied by a tumour commencing 3 ctms. below tıe umbilicus, ãnd losing itself in tıe left iliac fossa. Measured transversely, its greatest diameter was 22 ctms. At its upper part, and a little to tıe left, tıe abdominal wall was destroyed to sucı an extent as to allow a part of tıe tumour to form a ıernia in tıe sıape of an irregular cone, wıose base measured about 7 ctms. in diameter. At tıe truncated summit of tıe tumour were several teetı, wıicı appeared to be canine, and wıich could not be detacıed. On one side, a little lower down, was a flesıy appendix resembling a tıumb. Tıe surface of tıe tumour felt ıard and irregular, and on pressing it, watery pus of offensive odour poured fortı. On vaginal and rectal toucı, tıe uterus appeared to be movable, tıe cervix being directed backward and to tıe left.

Ovariotomy was performed on January 24th. Tıe incision was made in tıe linea alba from tıe lower extremity of tıe ulcerated opening to a point tıree or four centimetres above tıe pubes. Mucı difficulty was found in separating tıe adhesions uniting the front of the tumour to the abdominal walls, and it was necessary to use the knife to divide them. Hemorrhage was arrested by the actual cautery. It was then found possible to draw the tumour out of the abdomen, some unimportant adhesions being carefully separated. The solid portions of which it consisted however were prolonged as independent masses into the iliac fossa, and it was therefore impossible to obtain a pedicle sufficiently long to fix in the wound by means of a clamp. The base of the tumour was, therefore, divided by the actual cautery, and this proved sufficient to arrest hemorrhage. The wound was united by deep and superficial sutures, but it proved impossible to adapt accurately the edges of the ulcerated opening.

On the evening of the 25th, the pulse had risen to 110, temperature to 38.° Cent., and there was tympanites, vomiting, and subdelirium. During the next two days there was improvement; on renewing the dressings on the 27th, it was found that the lower part of the wound was looking well, but the upper part was secreting creamy pus in abundance. On the 28th the pus was less creamy, and had become offensive. Swelling and tenderness being found in the right iliac fossa, eighteen leeches were applied over it, after which the pain was relieved. Mercury and belladonna ointment was afterwards rubbed in every four hours over the same region.

On the 30th, to facilitate the escape of the discharge, one of the deep sutures was removed from the upper part of the wound, which did not seem inclined to unite by first intention. The same evening an intestinal hernia, larger than a turkey's egg, was found to have occurred at this point. A pad of charpie was employed to retain it within the abdominal cavity. On the 31st there was pain and tenderness in the left iliac fossa, and on vaginal touch a hard tumour was felt in the position of the left ovary, but no fluctuation could be detected. The upper part of the wound was now beginning to be covered by healthy granulation. On February 2d the general condition was improving, and the swelling in the left iliac fossa diminishing. On February 8th the opening at the upper part of the wound was diminishing, though the intestines still tended to protrude under the influence of a cough or any other effort. From this time convalescence was steady till the patient left the hospital on the sixty-third day. At this time the ulcerous wound was closed by a solid cicatrix, and all the functions were accomplished normally. On the latest report, it was stated that the patient had married on leaving the hospital, that she had two normal pregnancies, and was then pregnant for the third time.

The cyst removed had a thick wall, with a thin layer of osseous tissue on some parts of its internal surface. Its contents were a small quantity of pus, a gelatinous substance, skin with all its characters, hairs in great abundance, and of different lengths, very numerous teeth, some implanted in bones, some free in connective tissue, a large number of bones of various shapes, and cartilage, some of it in process of ossification. One of the bones resembled the temporal bone of a child of seven or eight years old, another resembled a parietal-bone, but was no larger than an adult's nail. Another bony mass resembled the coccyx with some of the sacral vertebræ.

The author considers it proved that dermoid cysts do not commence only in fœtal or infantile life, but may arise after puberty. The case now reported he considers a confirmation of this view, since menstruation was perfectly normal, and no tumour discoverable for five years after the commencement of menstruation, while the appearance of the growth appeared to be the sequel of an interruption of menstruation from an external cause.—*Obstetrical Journal of Great Britain*, Jan., 1879.

CONTENTS.

Published Monthly, price $2.50 per annum, free of postage.

Also, furnished together with the AMERICAN JOURNAL OF THE MEDICAL SCIENCES *and the* MEDICAL NEWS AND LIBRARY *for* SIX DOLLARS *per annum in advance, the whole free of postage.*

HENRY C. LEA, Philadelphia.

THE MONTHLY ABSTRACT

OF

MEDICAL SCIENCE.

VOL. VI. No. 4. **For List of Contents see last page.** APRIL, 1879.

Anatomy and Physiology.

Action of Bile on the Glycogen of the Liver.

In a recent number of *Lo Sperimentale*, Dr. G. BUFALINI gives the results of some experiments made by him for the purpose of determining the action of bile on the hepatic glycogen. He says that there has been much controversy on the question whether the bile is capable of transforming starch into glucose. The experiments, however, of Wittich, Gianuzzi, and Bufalini himself, have answered this question in the affirmative. Wittich collected the bile in a case of fistula of the gall-bladder, and rapidly obtained through its use the transformation of starch into glucose. The special object of Dr. Bufalini's recent experiments has been to ascertain whether bile exercises any transforming influence on the hepatic glycogen. For this purpose, he has made a number of experiments, using the bile of various animals (oxen and cows), removed from the gall-bladder about two hours after death. The glycogen was prepared by Kühne's process; and both were tested for glucose by Trommer's test. Regarding the action of bile on the hepatic glycogen, he finds that bile removed from the gall-bladders of animals killed a short time previously, and placed in contact with glycogen at a temperature of 104 deg. Fahr., reduced it to the state of glucose in a longer or shorter time. Of 150 experiments, the time required for the change was, in 50 cases one hour, in 50 other cases two hours, and in the remaining experiments from two and a half to three hours. When bile is deprived of its mucus and colouring matter by means of animal charcoal, and slightly acidulated with acetic acid, it retains its property of transforming glycogen, but the time required is longer and the transformation is less complete. He explains this by saying that a portion of the ferment is carried away with the mucus. Another series of experiments made by Dr. Gianuzzi and himself have led him to the conclusion that bile in a state of putrefaction does not retain the property of transforming either starch or glycogen; no effect being produced at the end of twenty-four hours. He also found the transforming property destroyed in bile which was boiled, filtered, and cooled, and then mixed with glycogen at a temperature of 104 deg. Fahr. The biliary salts and acids also had no action on hepatic glycogen.—*British Med. Journal*, Feb. 22, 1879.

Materia Medica and Therapeutics.

The Action of Arsenic.

An important series of researches on the mechanism of the action of Arsenic has lately been undertaken by Professor BINZ, of Bonn, and H. SCHULZ, who have described their results in the *Centralblatt für die Med. Wissenschaften.* "How is it that arsenic is a poison?" was the question first investigated, and the results which are reached throw some light on its therapeutic influence.

If a solution of arsenious acid or of its neutral salt is injected beneath the skin of an animal, no trace of local caustic action results ; but, unless the animal quickly dies by paralysis of the heart, the stomach and whole intestinal tracts are, after a few hours, intensely inflamed. A saturated solution (in the cold) of vitreous arsenious acid, or of sodic arsenite or arseniate, placed in the conjunctival sac of a guinea-pig, produces only slight local redness—hardly more than an equally strong solution of ordinary salt. Arsenic has no immediate affinity for albumen, and is, as Buchheim remarks, probably first transformed into a poisonous compound in the organism ; but of the precise nature of this poisonous compound we are at present ignorant.

In experimental chemistry both the compounds of arsenic are available as oxygen-carriers. After reduction they are easily oxidized, and may be again employed as oxidizing agents. Both these processes may take place when the arsenious compounds are in contact with organic substances. If arsenic acid, or its weak alkaline salt, is digested with fresh albumen, fibrin, pancreas, etc., and even with vegetable protoplasm, dialysis always yields arsenious acid, and no decomposition occurs. Decomposing fibrin gives the same reaction. On the other hand, if arsenious acid, free or as its salt, is digested with pancreas or with the fresh leaves of Lactuca sativa, dialysis yields definite evidence of arsenic acid. Defibrinated arterial blood, as well as pure oxyhæmoglobin, on the other hand, leave the arsenious acid unchanged.

In six cases of slow subcutaneous poisoning, it was observed that the gastritis was most marked in the neighbourhood of the pancreas, and that it constantly proceeded from the posterior wall. This is corroborated by some observations in cases of poisoning in men, where the places at which the gastric irritation commenced could be traced. This localization has nothing to do with the local accumulation of the arsenic taken by the mouth, because in the experiments on animals in which the arsenic was introduced directly into the blood the same change was observed. Further investigation led Binz and Schulz to the following theory. The arsenious acid, which has an action on albumen, is certainly in part oxidized to arsenic acid, and this is, again, reduced. Protoplasm effects the oxidation, and in it also the reduction occurs most strongly. The unusual interchange of nascent oxygen within the molecules must tend to the formation of nitrous acid, and in part also to nitrous oxide, the latter being further transformed to nitric acid, and thus the protoplasm will be destroyed more quickly than the interchange of matter can renew it. The arsenic thus plays the part of the oxygen-bearer, and leads to a sort of molecular combustion. The interchange of the oxygen probably takes place most readily in the glandular organs of the intestinal tract, but may occur elsewhere, and probably does occur, especially in the nerve-centres, in which so energetic an interchange of material is always going on. Hence the irritation and quick paralysis of the nerve-centres. We are also able to understand, on this theory of its action, why there is so rapid a diminution of glycogen in the liver when arsenic is given with food ; why the organ undergoes fatty degeneration ; and also the effect on malaria, and the subsidence of lymphomata, under its use.—*Lancet*, Feb. 8, 1879.

—

Changes in Calomel.

M. M. Mialhe and Laroque have demonstrated that calomel may give rise in the organism to bichloride of mercury under the influence of the alkaline chlorides of the economy. Polk has recently pointed out the fact that phenomena of poison-

ing may arise after the ad ministration of an old mixture of calomel and sugar, or
of calomel and magnesia.   N. JOLLY has taken up again (*Gazette Médicale de
Paris*, 9 Nov. 1878) these important therapeutical questions, and has arrived at
the following conclusion : The alkalies, their carbonates and the earthy bases,
transform calomel into corrosive sublimate with more or less activity.   White
and refined sugars have no action on the mercurial salts.   Rough sugars are often
acid (colonial sugar) or alkaline (beet-root sugar), on account of the small
quantity of hydrate of lime which they contain ; it is to the impurity of the sugar
and to their action on the calomel, that we must impute the phenomena of poisoning observed by Polk.   The practical conclusion of N. Jolly's study is, that when
calomel is employed internally, we must avoid associating its salts with acids,
alkalies, chlorides, and raw sugar.—*London Med. Record*, Dec. 15, 1878.

On the Deodorization of Iodoform.

It is well known that the offensive smell of this most valuable drug, iodoform,
often prevents its use.   Dr. GUTSCHER (*Wiener Med. Woch.*, No. 2, 1879) offers
the following suggestions for improving it: Any ethereal oil which possesses a
strong aromatic odour would overpower the smell of the drug.   He made the
experiment by adding to each of his preparations of iodoform six drops of peppermint oil, and rubbing them well together.   In a few moments the smell of the
iodoform had entirely vanished.—*London Med. Record*, Feb. 15, 1879.

Medicine.

Contagiousness of Tuberculosis.

Dr. REICH, of Mulheim, reports (*Berlin Klin. Woch.*, Sept. 1878) a singular
series of cases in which tuberculosis seemed to be communicated directly, from
mouth to mouth, to a number of children by a phthisical midwife.   There were
in Neuenbourg two midwives, Mme. R. and Mme. S., the latter being distinctly
phthisical, with an abundant purulent expectoration.   Dr. R., having one day
delivered a patient by turning, noticed the nurse S. sucking the mucus from the
mouth of the child, and blowing directly into the lungs, mouth to mouth, to
establish respiration.   This child, at the end of three weeks, began to droop, and
died in three months of tubercular meningitis.   Shortly afterwards two other
children, under the care of the same nurse, died of the same disease.   Dr. R.,
having his suspicions in this way aroused, made inquiry, and found that from 4th
April, 1875, to 10th May, 1876, seven children, besides the three already mentioned, all attended by Mme S., had been carried off by tubercular meningitis
within their first year.   Nothing of this kind happened in the practice of Mme.
R. during the same period.   In July, 1876, Mme. S. herself died of consumption.
It was well known that this nurse was accustomed to clean the children's mouths
of mucus in the manner above described ; she was also very kind to her little
patients, constantly kissing and caressing them.—*Glasgow Med. Journal*, Feb.
1879.

Congenital Cyanosis.

N. COSSY (*Progrès Médical*, January, 1878) presented to the Société Anatomique of Paris the following case of congenital cyanosis.   A young man, aged

20, had from his birth presented marked cyanosis of the face and limbs, accompanied with palpitation and slight dyspnœa. On his admission into hospital, the
anterior and upper part of the chest was covered with dilated veins; his fingers
were clubbed, the liver was very large, and the urine loaded with albumen. A
very loud double bellows-sound was heard over the cardiac apex; at the base,
and loudest over the pulmonary artery, a murmur similar in tone and intensity
was heard, but it was single, systolic, and prolonged through the whole cardiac
revolution. Autopsy showed the heart to be generally hypertrophied, the septum between the auricles was complete, but there was a large opening in the
upper part of the interventricular septum; the pulmonary artery was much constricted at its origin, and its valves thickened and roughened. Ductus arteriosus
closed, aorta normal, lungs simply congested.

This case presented, as most such cases do, a combination of the two conditions which have been regarded as capable of causing congenital cyanosis, viz.,
pulmonary stenosis and communication between the right and left heart. Two
opposite theories have been put forward to explain the cyanosis. Morgagni,
Louis, Gendrin, Bérard, Cruveilhier, and others maintain that it is due simply to
an obstruction in the circulation, or capillary stasis. Cloquet, Gintrac, and
others, on the other hand, maintain that it is due to a mixture of arterial and
venous blood through a communication either between the right and left auricle
(patent foramen ovale) or right and left ventricle. Those who hold the first
view believe that the pulmonary stenosis is primitive, and the communication
between the right and left heart consecutive; those who support the other view
contend that the communication between the two sides of the heart is first in
order of development, and is the cause of the narrowing of the pulmonary artery,
for, they say, if there is an opening between the ventricles, the blood in the right
ventricle tends to pass into the left ventricle instead of into the pulmonary artery,
which becomes narrowed. The first of these theories seems the best, for the
cases on record fall into three groups. In the first, and by far the largest group,
there exist both pulmonary stenosis and communication between the right and
left heart; in the second there is either a patent foramen ovale, or an opening
between the two ventricles, and no constriction of the pulmonary artery (note,
however, that when this is the case, there coexists disease of the tricuspid valve,
either narrowing or insufficiency, sufficient to cause blood stasis); while there is
a third group, in which persistent foramen ovale has been found, without any
cyanosis. Two such cases have been presented to the Société Anatomique.
Hence we conclude, with Louis, that congenital cyanosis is due rather to blood
stasis than to the circulation of a mixture of arterial and venous blood. But
Louis's law required that the narrowed or impermeable pulmonary artery should
be associated with (as a consequence) a patent ductus arteriosus. It is necessary
to respiration and to life, and it is usually found open in autopsies of these cases.
But in M. Cossy's case it was *impermeable!* There must then have been a collateral circulation established here of a very sufficient kind, since life was maintained for twenty years. The bronchial arteries, unfortunately, were not
examined. They may have been greatly dilated, as has been observed in certain
cases. But in such instances caseous pneumonia is usually found to exist in consequence of imperfect nutrition of the lungs; the lungs in M. Cossy's case were
simply congested. As to abnormal cardiac bruits, they may be entirely absent;
but this is rare; nearly always there is a bellows murmur, single, systolic, most
intense at the base and to the left of the sternum. The second of the two murmurs heard over the apex in the case narrated above was probably caused by the
passage of the blood through the orifice in the ventricular septum.—*London
Med. Record*, Feb. 15, 1879.

Spontaneous Septicæmia.

The diagnosis of blood-poisoning, when it occurs as a sequel to traumatic suppuration, the result of injury or operation, is usually attended with comparatively few
difficulties. It is very different, however, in the case of the so-called spontaneous septicæmia, in which the source of the blood-poisoning has developed without any external injury to indicate its probable seat, and in which the symptoms
of the primary mischief may be entirely latent. The subject of the diagnosis of
these cases has lately received systematic consideration by Professor LEUBE, in
the *Deutsches Archiv für Klinische Medicin*, based on the symptoms in a series
of examples which have come under his notice. He points out how preferable is a
name such as "cryptogenetic," which expresses merely the fact of the latency of
origin, rather than one which suggests a spontaneity which cannot, strictly speaking, be said to obtain. The general type of these cases is the following. Without obvious cause, a patient is seized with rigors and fever, sometimes with vomiting and diarrhœa, and pains in the limbs, especially on movement, followed by
a comatose state, with muscular twitchings, often general hyperæsthesia, indications of paralysis, with involuntary evacuations, and often Cheyne-Stokes's breathing. Frequently there are extravasations, conjunctival or cutaneous; and sometimes a characteristic eruption on the skin, small vesicles with a hemorrhagic
halo, and occasionally pemphigus or hemorrhagic pustules. Endocarditis and
pericarditis may be present, the spleen is swollen, and the temperature may reach
106° or 107°. In the most acute cases the fever is almost continuous. In subacute cases remissions and paroxysmal elevations are to be noted, accompanied
with rigors; sometimes the initial rigor is constant, but it may be the only attack
of shivering noticed. In the lungs the scattered foci of suppuration may sometimes, although rarely, cause symptoms recognizable during life. Large infarc-
tions cause symptoms, and "metastatic" pleurisy is very common. In all cases,
post mortem, cardiac changes were present, endocarditis, ecchymoses, or foci of
suppuration. In several, endocarditic murmurs were observed during life. The
blood showed in all cases leucocytosis, and in one case there were small, irregular,
refracting whitish corpuscles, in lively movement, possibly aggregations of bacteria. The abdominal organs, with the exception of the spleen, presented no
notable symptoms. In one case the erroneous diagnosis of peritonitis was made,
in consequence of the extreme cutaneous hyperæsthesia, due to the state of the
nervous system. Albuminuria, however, was frequent, and the kidneys in most
cases presented evidence of parenchymatous inflammation. These symptoms
alone possess little diagnostic value, but their significance is greatly increased by
their association with the cutaneous eruption above described, an eruption which
has the characters of no known skin disease. The hemorrhagic spots with yellow
pustular centres are strikingly similar to the minute foci of suppuration found post
mortem in many organs. In one case these pustules were found, during life, to
contain bacteria. The extravasation is the first change, and may be due to the
local disturbance of the blood and bloodvessels, occasioned by the accumulation
at the spot of toxic substance. Joint inflammations, on which much stress is commonly laid, were, in Leube's cases, far less frequent than the alteration of the
skin.

Much interest attaches to the participation of the central nervous system in the
morbid process. They were absent in no case, and in most presented the same
characters, resembling for the most part those of a meningitis of the convexity,
and a purulent meningitis was in one case actually present, while in most there
were injection of the membranes and minute extravasations into the cortical substance. The somnolence or coma is accompanied by convulsive movements of

the extremities, sometimes tonic spasm in the muscles of the neck, and with a variable condition of the pupils.

The chief importance of these symptoms attaches to the question of the differential diagnosis of the disease. In several cases the amount of albumen and the presence of casts in the urine gave rise to the suspicion that the symptoms were due to uræmia, but against this the temperature and the character of the nervous symptoms were conclusive. A greater difficulty attends the diagnosis of this condition from acute miliary tuberculosis. Now and then the clinical features of the two forms of disease are absolutely identical. Miliary tuberculosis may begin with a rigor and high fever, and bronchitis, pleurisy, swelling of the spleen, albuminuria, and cerebral symptoms, from meningeal complication, may attend the course of tuberculosis. Even cutaneous petechiæ and herpes may not be absent. All that can be affirmed of the diagnosis in such cases is that the more rapid the course of the disease, the more suddenly the general symptoms set in, the more probable is the disease to be septicæmic.

From typhoid the distinctions are more simple, and important indications are afforded by the course of the temperature, and by the absence of the retinal hemorrhages which are so common in septicæmia. Greater difficulty is presented by the distinction of the cerebral symptoms from those due to simple meningitis, but the presence of the symptoms of a general disease, the enlargement of the spleen, and the cutaneous changes, enable a distinction to be made. The prominence of certain symptoms in individual cases may constitute a fresh source of perplexity. Of these, however, the greatest difficulty attends the distinction from ulcerative endocarditis, and, indeed, in the majority of cases the distinction is impossible. The occurrence of an embolic myocarditis or a micrococcal endocarditis, or both, or neither, depends upon accidental circumstances. "Malignant endocarditis" is only a manifestation of the so-called "septic pyæmia," and is not an independent disease.—*Lancet*, Feb. 22, 1879.

On a Case of Intermittent Tetanic Fever.

FRONMÜLLER gives in the *Memorabilien für Prakt. Aerzte*, No. 11, the following interesting account of a patient, aged 26, who had been healthy all his life, till about two years ago, when he had a severe chill, which was followed by an illness lasting four weeks; the principal symptoms of which, according to his account, consisted in periodically repeated convulsions, which proceeded from the spine. The next year he suffered from quotidian fever, was cured, but in the same year received a blow on the head, which left a scar of about an inch long, on the lower part of the left parietal bone. He was treated for scabies in the next year, and after having been cured was imprisoned for some petty offence. During this latter period he complained of headache and pains in the side, and returned to the hospital. He was a weak, ill-nourished subject, of a livid complexion; he complained of cold, shivered, and spoke of wandering pains, especially in the head. These were ascribed to rheumatism, and he was treated accordingly. This happened on April 23d. On the night between the 24th and 25th he was suddenly seized with opisthotonos and trismus, the lower extremities were kicking spasmodically, the eyes wide open, he was unconscious, and uttered inarticulate sounds; sensibility was extinct over the whole body. This paroxysm lasted for about fifteen minutes. He felt better the next morning, and only complained of the fifth to eighth spinal vertebræ being tender on pressure. During the next two days seven similar paroxysms occurred, mostly at night. They were not epileptic fits, as the thumbs were not drawn in; there was no froth on the lips; the patient's body was cold, and sensibility was extinct as before.

From that time the paroxysms were reduced to a single one, which was repeated every evening with almost the same symptoms, and accompanied by rigor. The face was red, the eyes open, and the pupils moderately dilated. As all treatment had hitherto proved unsuccessful, it was resolved to treat the disease as an intermittent fever with quinine, which was given in doses of five decigrammes three times daily. The paroxysms ceased, the patient felt better, and was soon able to leave the hospital. He subsequently informed the reporter that his native village was surrounded by ponds, and that malaria was rife there.—*London Med. Record*, Feb. 15, 1879.

A Typhoid Epidemic Originating in Diseased Meat.

A most remarkable epidemic of typhoid fever, which seems clearly traceable to eating the flesh of a calf that had probably died of typhoid fever, is described by Dr. WALDER, Assistant Physician to the Zürich Hospital, in the *Berliner Klin. Wochenschrift*, No. 39, 1878. On May 30, 1878, a choral festival was held at Kloton, Canton Zürich, and was attended by about 700 members of neighbouring choirs. A public breakfast, consisting of stewed veal and sausages, took place at 9 A. M. At 3 P. M. there was a somewhat similar repast, with the addition of soup, potatoes, salad, and wine. Water was drunk by only a very few persons, and always mixed with wine. Of those who took part in these meals, about 500 sooner or later fell ill. The greater number were not attacked for two or three days after the festival, though a few were unwell on the next day. Dr. Walder calculates that 39 to 40 per cent. of all the cases were taken on the fifth and sixth days, and 90 per cent. within the first eight days. The general characters of the symptoms were those of typhoid fever of various degrees of intensity, from mild abortive forms to those accompanied by severe delirium, intestinal hemorrhage, and high fever. The epidemic presented two deviations from the ordinary run of typhoid epidemics—that the fever rose very rapidly at first, so as often to reach its height on the second day ; and that diarrhœa was less common than usual, and less obstinate Temperatures of 40° C. were not uncommon, and those of 40.5° to 40.8° were several times observed. Most of the patients exhibited the typhoid roseolar eruption, and the spleen was enlarged in all those cases which were examined at the acme of the disease. Dr. Walder states that most of the patients whom he especially examined had swelling of the external lymphatic glands, especially the inguinal, and that the swelling disappeared when the fever left them. In the course of the epidemic, the usual complications of typhoid fever occurred Four cases relapsed, one of which, a youth aged sixteen, eventually died from perforation of the bowel and general peritonitis. When Dr. Walder wrote, twenty-seven cases of secondary infection had taken place, the patients having either been engaged in nursing those primarily affected, or in washing their linen, removing their motions, etc. Some secondary cases induced by sleeping in the same bed with primary were more severe than the latter, but as a rule the secondary cases were milder than the primary. The post-mortem examination of several fatal cases, four of which Dr. Walder reports *in extenso*, confirms the diagnosis of typhoid fever so as to leave not the slightest doubt as to the nature of the disease.

We now come to the probable source of infection of those persons who took part in the festival at Kloton. The greater part of the meat eaten on this occasion was supplied by the village innkeeper, who was also the village butcher, and all of it (veal, pork, and beef) had been pronounced by a professional inspector perfectly healthy, with the exception of forty-three pounds of veal, which were sent from a butcher at Seebach two days before the festival, and had not been examined by the inspector. The calf from which it came belonged to a peasant.

It was only a few days old, and was probably only killed because it was certain to die very speedily from illness. It would not suck, it lay on the straw, cried out when touched as if in pain, and at the last kept lowing loudly. The evidence that the flesh of this calf caused the epidemic is very strong. Not only the partakers in the feast who ate this particular veal stewed with the other healthy meat were attacked, but families which took no part in the feast, and in which the children had had meat and sausages given them by persons who could not get through what was served out to them, suffered. The lungs of the above unfortunate calf were sold to a lady at Seebach, and the brain to the clergyman of the parish. Three persons who dined off the lungs made into stew were taken ill exactly like the members of the choirs, and the clergyman's family was similarly affected. The bones were sold to a dealer at Seebach, and his dog, which ate part of them, was ill for about a week. Moreover, several persons who bought meat either on the day of the festival or on the previous day from the Kloten butcher also suffered, as did a number who had bought sausages from the same establishment, and persons who had taken no part in the festival, but had dined at the inn kept by the butcher, were laid up. Dr. Walder supposes, with good reason, that healthy meat became infected either by direct contact with the diseased veal, or by having been cut by the same knife.

It should be mentioned that there had been no epidemic of typhoid fever either in Kloten or the neighbouring villages for many years; and although, as a fact, there was a single case of typhoid fever at Kloton at the time of the festival, the patient lived a long way both from the place where the feast was held and from the butcher's shop. The water used for cooking and drinking was supplied from a hill on the other side of the village through iron pipes. The first person who suggested the origin of the epidemic in the typhoid fever of calves or oxen was Professor Huguenin, of Zürich, but his suggestion was long received with considerable scepticism, as scarcely anything was known about the occurrence of the disease in those animals. The correctness of his hypothesis, however, is strongly corroborated by Dr. Walder's discovery of the infection of two calves belonging to one of his patients suffering at the time from typhoid fever. A post-mortem examination of one of these animals showed intense swelling of the Peyer's patches throughout the whole of the small intestine, but especially in the lower part, with swelling of the retro-peritoneal and mesenteric glands. The spleen was enlarged. The heart, the lungs, and liver, as well as the joints, were all healthy. There were several small hemorrhages into the left kidney. No similar cases have ever occurred, before or since, among this farmer's cattle, and it seems most probable that the farmer himself was the infecting agent, and that during one of the fits of severe diarrhœa from which he suffered in the first week of his illness he must have passed a motion in the neighbourhood of the stall, as during this time he was continually attending to the cattle himself. Another case, in which a calf was almost certainly infected by a human being, occurred later on. Here a bucket which had been used for washing the viscera of two patients who had died of typhoid fever, and on whom a post-mortem was made, was soon after filled with water for the calves to drink, and it seems probable that some blood which remained on the outside was licked up by the calf, or else was transferred to the stockings of the cow-boy, which the animal was in the habit of licking. After an incubative period of exactly ten days, the calf was taken ill, and it was killed four days later. The pathological changes were exactly the same as in the other case, and microscopically the calves' intestines in both cases were indistinguishable from a human intestine in the same stage of typhoid fever.

A detailed account of the above epidemic will be published in a few months, but meanwhile our readers will, no doubt, be interested to have an outline sketch of what seems to be a newly detected source of infection of the poor human body by "typhoid poison."—*Med. Times and Gazette*, Feb. 8, 1879.

—

Recent Observations on Scarlatina.

Dr. HENOCH, of Berlin, has had the opportunity, in his position as physician to the Charité Hospital, of observing carefully a great number of scarlatina cases. He has published his observations in the third volume of the *Charité Annalen* for 1878. He divides the different accidents which are apt to happen during the course of the disease into four classes, viz., anomalies of temperature; malignity of the disease; complications which may arise during it; and nervous symptoms.

As regards anomalies of temperature, the following observations have been made: 1. The temperature may rise slowly whilst the exanthem appears distinctly on the first day; 2. The temperature is very high the first day, but falls on the next, and remains normal during the whole of the illness; 3. The temperature is exceedingly low during the whole of the illness; 4. Both the high temperature and the rash last abnormally long; great care ought, however, to be taken here not to mistake the febrile heat which may originate from some hitherto latent complication for the fever of scarlatina. Such complications may be—*e. g.*, otitis externa or media, protracted diphtheria of the pharynx, and inflammations of the submaxillary glands.

As regards the malignity of the disease, apparently dangerous symptoms are often met with. For instance, the temperature remains very high; the patient is somnolent and delirious. If, however, by antipyretic treatment, as tepid baths, quinine, salicylic acid, etc., we succeed in reducing them, we may be sure that the case is not malignant. But if our treatment fail to produce the desired effect on the above mentioned symptoms, the prognosis is sure to be very bad. This different issue in cases which seem at first to present the same range of symptoms, is explained by the action of the contagium matter of scarlatina on the centres of the vagus nerve. That the latter is affected is clearly shown in these cases by the symptoms of weakness of the heart, such as a quick soft pulse, cold hands and feet although the temperature of the body be high, and irregularity in the breaking out of the rash.

If the above mentioned debility of heart take place after the rash has come out, and during the first week of the disease, the case is perhaps a little less dangerous; but then the disease is almost always accompanied by diphtheria of the pharynx and the nose. The temperature may either remain very high up to the moment of death, or fall considerably. If the patient have suffered from diarrhœa since the beginning of his illness, and no plausible reason can be given for it, the prognosis is very unfavourable. This Dr. Henoch ascribes to paralysis of the splanchnic nerve caused by the contagious matter. A few cases have been observed in the Charité where diphtheritic angina seemed to precede the eruption, but Henoch thinks that here the primary disease was really diphtheria, but that the patient caught scarlatina by infection, the first symptom of scarlet fever being *always* a simple angina, which develops into diphtheria only on the third or fourth day of the illness, stomatitis, diphtheria, or what is still worse, coryza, which sometimes is the cause of most dangerous forms of conjunctivitis. The diphtheritic affection often spreads over the larynx, but very seldom passes beyond the vocal cords. Dr. Henoch has never seen any cases of paralysis arising from diphtheria, in scarlet fever. The dyspnœa which sometimes appears is caused by the enormous swelling of the tonsils and other parts of the pharynx. In three cases, angina Ludovici was caused by diphtheria of the pharynx. It is often dangerous to make incisions into the submaxillary glands when there is inflammation, as some branches of the external jugular vein, or the latter itself, may be affected and thereby cause very serious hemorrhages.

Inflammations of the respiratory organs occur very often, and are most dangerous. Dr. Henoch met with catarrh of the trachea and the bronchi, and with pneumonia and pleurisy on one or both sides.

In inflammations of the serous membranes, the synovial membranes of the joints are first affected; sometimes there are also swelling and stiffness. In some cases, these inflammations were followed by pleurisy and peritonitis, in another case by endocarditis, and in a third by endocarditis and chorea. Diseases of the heart also occur after scarlatina, even when the articulations have not been affected.

Nervous symptoms are also observed. In young children, the illness is sometimes preceded by convulsions. In two cases, the patients complained of pain in the tips of their fingers, although the joints were perfectly free. Paralysis of the facial nerve is often caused by swollen glands pressing on the mastoid process, or by caries of the petrous bone. Chorea was twice noticed, and once locomotor ataxy of the lower extremities. In complicated malignant cases, there is often found an eruption very similar to those which occur in measles, the so-called variegated scarlatina. A cyanotic hue of the skin is a very bad symptom, because it only occurs in cases of extreme debility of the heart. Gangrene of the skin, bed-sores, and necrosis of the cartilage of the nose, are often found ; also subcutaneous abscesses in different parts of the body, especially in weak children. The author's treatment consists in tepid baths (he objects to cold ones), and in administering stimulants, such as alcohol, coffee, camphor, musk, etc.

Of late, several cases of scarlatina occurring immediately after some surgical operation have been observed, a few of which recently happened in France under the treatment of M. Trélat (see British Medical Journal, November 9th).

Looking at the above-mentioned facts, Dr. Henoch concludes that, if scarlatina occur in the course of some surgical affection, it has a very unfavourable influence on the wounds ; and that in children scarlatina seems often to result from an operation ; at least, a great many cases have come under observation in which this has happened. What may be the cause of this is not yet quite clear. Paget supposes that the prostration which follows an operation makes the patient more sensitive to contagion. But this is only a hypothesis ; and, besides, scarlatina has been observed in surgical patients where the possibility of infection was entirely out of the question.

Acute mania has also been known to occur in scarlet fever, perhaps from the same unknown causes from which mental disturbances have been observed to arise, either during or immediately after acute articular rheumatism of the joints, erysipelas, etc. A very interesting case of mania has been observed in France, and published in the Union Médicale du Nord-Est by M. Flamain. The patient, a girl aged 22, was in the fourth day of a severe attack of scarlatina, when she suddenly showed very extraordinary mental disturbances. Whenever she was quiet, her face wore a certain expression of pain, her voice was weak, plaintive, and her intellect perfectly clear. Suddenly, without any intermediate stage, her face became joyous, her speech loud and animated ; she began to sing, to laugh, or to say many things. A few moments later, the delirium was gone as suddenly as it had come on ; but the patient remembered what had happened, and tried to apologize for it, by saying that she could not help it. During the two following days, this delirious state continued, but it manifested itself in different ways and at intervals. Sometimes the patient was exceedingly merry ; at other times she was in an ecstatic state ; then, again, great excitement prevailed ; which was followed by utter prostration. On the next day, the delirium, which hitherto had only shown itself in the wanderings of her mind, suddenly changed and became violent; the patient screamed, gesticulated, tried to rise from her bed; and it was all that two strong men could do to hold her back. Forty-five grains of chloral and six-tenths of a grain of morphine had no effect upon her. This violent stage lasted for eight or ten hours, and then gave way to a sort of epilepsy. Then another change occurred again; during two days, the patient was quiet, her intellect seemed to regain its lucidity, she perspired abundantly. but had fits of spitting. like lunatics; she refused to drink; her bowels were constipated; she passed very little urine, which contained a great quantity of albumen. Towards the end of this last day, her pulse became quick, she was perfectly quiet, fell suddenly into a profound coma, and expired two hours later. As far as could be ascertained from her relatives, the girl's father had died from an affection of the nervous centres, but she, and the rest of her family, had always been healthy. Dr. Flamain observes that the cause of death in this case could not be scarlatina, the latter not being malignant and its course in every respect perfectly regular. Uræmia was entirely out of the question, as it manifests itself usually at a much later period of the disease, and consists of entirely different phenomena. The only plausible explanation, therefore, in this case is acute mania, occurring in a person with hereditary predisposition.—*British Medical Journal*, Jan. 4, 1879.

—

Rheumatoid Arthritis.

At a late meeting of the Clinical Society of London (*Lancet*, March 1. 1879) Dr. W. M. ORD read a paper on Rheumatoid Arthritis from a Clinical Point of View. Thirty-three cases of that form of rheumatoid arthritis, which has been called by Haygarth "Nodosity of the Joints," and by Heberdeen "Digitorum Nodi." were analyzed. All had occurred in women, and in all disturbances of the menstrual function, or disorders involving hyperæmia of the uterus and its appendages, were present. By the term "nodosity of the joints" was understood a symmetrical affection of many joints, chiefly of the hands, the affected joints becoming enlarged at their periphery, loosened by loss of surface, and ultimately much distorted; the smaller joints being first affected. and extension taking place in a symmetrical progressive way from these to the larger joints. The subjects belonged in large proportion to the middle classes, and were mostly between thirty and forty years of age. Several of them were distinctly passing through the climacteric period of life. Although many were anæmic, amenorrhœa did not exist in any. Dysmenorrhœa was noted in fourteen. half of which had also menorrhagia. Of the remainder, several had menorrhagia simply, four had it in conjunction with ovaritis, and others in conjunction with the change of life or with tumours. The relation of the arthritis brought out by the cases was, first. its commencement in conjunction with menstrual disturbance; secondly, its paroxysmal exacerbation during, before, or after menstrual periods; thirdly, its cessation as an active or progressive mischief on the cessation of the menstrual disorder; fourthly, its alternation with cerebral disturbance of an hysterical kind. Some cases were more fully detailed: 1. A case in which intense affection of the upper extremities was noted, in conjunction with severe dysmenorrhœa and menorrhagia. When constitutional treatment and the measures usually applied to the control of the rheumatic process had failed, the uterine conditions were treated successfully, with the result that the arthritis, as an active process. ceased, leaving. of course, the nodosity, but a painless nodosity. 2. Two cases in which the arthritis began at the climacteric period in combination with painless menorrhagia. and ceased as an active process on the final disappearance of the catamenia. In one the first attack occurred at a time when the catamenia. having been absent a whole year, returned in unusual excess; when the joints lost all inflammation and pain during a subsequent interval, but became severely inflamed, greatly swollen and painful during several subsequent menorrhagic periods. 3. A case in which a woman suffering from polyarticular arthritis at the climacteric period, the arthritis undergoing little remission in the intervals between the menstrual flow, developed somewhat suddenly hysterical mania. On the establishment of the mania the arthritis became perfectly quiescent, and remained so till the restoration of sanity. Sanity having returned, the arthritis resumed its progress. In this instance the excitement propagated from the uterine organs, instead of undergoing reflexion from the cord, was, as it were, refracted through the cord to the higher centres. The arguments founded upon these cases were, first, that there was good evidence to show the connection of this form of polyarticular arthritis with the uterine hyperæmia. It was argued, further, that the incitation to the arthritis was conveyed by the nervous system in a reflex way. In support of this view it was advanced that certain lesions of the central nervous system were known to be capable of producing trophic changes in joints, identical with those of chronic rheumatoid arthritis; that urinary paraplegia was an evidence of the possibility that a paralyzing influence might be reflected; that therefore it was reasonable to suppose that trophic influence should be reflected, and that the mode of association of the arthritis and the uterine disorder favoured the idea of a nervous nexus, and the idea of this consisting in reflex action through the cord   The gonorrhœal and urethral arthritis of men were compared with the affections under consideration, and it was pointed out that the parts concerned with two cases were homologous parts. It was lastly argued that the local morbid process present in these cases was the same as that existing in non-articular arthritis, in traumatic and other surgical arthritis, in gonorrhœal and urethral arthritis, in joints affected by morbid deposits and morbid growths, in certain cases after true rheumatism, and in all cases coming under the head of rheumatoid arthritis; and that the term " rheumatoid arthritis" insufficiently covered the variety of clinical aspects of the joint affection; that, therefore, it was desirable to limit or annul the use of the word " rheumatoid," and apply before the word "arthritis" some qualifying term descriptive in each case of the supposed clinical association. Ricord's term "blenorrhagic arthritis," as opposed to the term "urethral rheumatism," was quoted as an instance of such application.

Mr. BARWELL, preferring the term "arthritis deformans" to "rheumatoid arthritis" for a disease which had nothing to do with rheumatism, could not admit the dependence of this affection upon uterine disorders. The changes in the joints were most characteristic; the cartilage becoming fibrillated and degenerate, and dendritic growth spreading downwards into the bone, which comes to assume a worm-eaten appearance, whilst new ossific deposit occurs in the structures around the joint; and he could hardly think all these changes could be dependent upon uterine disorders. For himself, he should rather regard the increase in the joint affection at the menstrual periods to be due to the exacerbations of local disease which surgeons are accustomed to see in women at these times. Moreover this particular disease is quite as prevalent in men as in women.

Mr. BRYANT was disposed to regard the cases described by Dr. Ord as allied to gout, whereas the disease which Mr. Barwell had sketched out was that termed "osteo-arthritis," which has very little to do with either rheumatism or gout. He had failed to recognize in Dr. Ord's cases the characters of osteo-arthritis. He should say that, as a rule, the majority of cases (of this disease) were met with in male subjects, and when met with in females it was at an advanced age.

Dr. GREENFIELD had arrived independently at similar conclusions to Dr. Ord, and felt convinced of the association between uterine disorders and the joint affections in question. But there was no precise unanimity as to what is meant by rheumatoid arthritis, some describing it as chronic rheumatic arthritis others as osteo-arthritis. The chronic osteo-arthritis of the hip is a different affection from the general affection now under notice, where the joints are symmetrically affected and in a definite order. Such cases in his experience were far more frequent in women. He could recall cases in which there was a marked clinical relation between leucorrhœal discharge, or other uterine disturbance, and the joint affection, which in males might be associated with spermatorrhœa. The increase and abatement of the articular swelling *pari passu* with the aggravation or improvement in the disorder of the genito-urinary tract was more than a coincidence. He knew of the case of a young man, twenty-five years of age, who had long been subject to seminal discharges and evidence of irritation about the prostatic urethra, who gets all the joints of his hands and feet affected whenever the spermatorrhœa is excessive. The recognition of some connection between the two was of importance in treatment. Dr. Greenfield could hardly accept the neuropathic theory advanced by Dr. Ord, but believed the arthritis to be allied in its pathology to that met with in "gonorrhœal rheumatism," "blenorrhagic rheumatism," etc.,—that it was, in fact, due to the absorption of septic or irritating matters by the urethral or vesical mucous membrane in the male, or by the urethra and vagina in the female. As to treatment, active measures were certainly powerless when applied to the joint affection only; and certainly more benefit was derived by attention to the local conditions.

Dr. DYCE DUCKWORTH could not doubt that Dr. Ord's cases were true examples of osteo-arthritis, a subject to which the paper added much that was worthy of careful consideration. He had himself met with no facts sufficient to warrant the view of the hereditary nature of the disease. He had met with it amongst women at the climacteric period, especially those of broken health, who had borne large families. Still he had seen typical cases in much younger subjects—*e. g.*, at the age of fourteen or fifteen years. In cases of true osteo-arthritis the fingers are drawn to the ulnar side.

Dr. ORD, in reply, said that the large ground over which he had to travel made it impossible for him to take up all the points within the allotted time. He remarked that two of his principal critics had viewed the subject from a purely surgical standpoint; and their opinions had not been shared in by those who were physicians. This difference in view no doubt depended on the different class of cases coming before the surgeon and physician respectively. The essential changes in the affected joints, to which Mr. Bardwell had alluded, consisted in a process of waste of cartilage and of underlying bone, with overgrowth of periosteum, cartilage, and synovial structures at the periphery of the joint. Such changes produced a tendency to laxity of the joint and spontaneous dislocations, with, in the case on hand, adduction of the fingers on the metacarpus. These changes were precisely paralleled by those described by Charcot in the affected joints of the subjects of locomotor ataxy. Authorities differ as to the sexual liability; thus Haygarth asserts that women are chiefly affected, Adams that men are most subject to the disease; but the one deals with a "polyarticular" affection, the other with a "monarticular." Trousseau asserts its greater frequency among women of the better class ; Follin and Duplay describe "arthrite sèche" as being chiefly met with in men of the poorer classes. It was obvious that these writers must be speaking of different affections. There was no clear evidence of an underlying diathesis, and, with Dr. Duckworth, he objected to admit that it was a hereditary disease. He could pass no opinion as to the value of arterial tension in discriminating these cases. In all his cases he had failed to find uratic deposits, and had thereby excluded gout. Dr. Greenfield's observations agreed with his own, but there was a difference between their views as to the ultimate pathology of this disease. He thought there was more ground in favour of neurotic influences than of septic, and this he based on the knowledge of joint affections in cases of lesion of the central nervous system or on the occurrence of reflex paraplegia. Might not a joint affection be produced in a reflex manner by those parts of the spinal cord being stimulated which especially govern the nutrition of joints?

—

Treatment of Delirium Tremens.

Dr. GEORGE W. BALFOUR, Physician to the Royal Infirmary, Edinburgh, advocates (*Lancet*, Feb. 1, 1879) the treatment of delirium tremens by chloral. He says so far as our present experience is concerned, we seem to possess in hydrate of chloral a remedy which in all such cases, from the slightest to the most severe, acts rapidly, safely, and efficaciously—*cito, tuto, et jucunde*—and which seems to deprive indulgence in drink of all its horrors and nearly all its dangers. Unquestionably fatal cases must occasionally occur under this as well as under other modes of treatment, but the number of them must be much decreased, because, from the rapidity with which a cure is brought about, many dangerous risks are averted. Thus, we avoid all the risks arising from a long continuance of maniacal excitement, or from a suicidal state of mind, all risk from the exhaustion following persistent sleeplessness, or defective nutrition, the result of long-continued insufficiency of food, etc. The risks the patient actually runs are not now, as formerly, connected with the treatment, but with his previous state of health. Thus, if he has a fatty heart, or has been exhausted by long-continued debauchery, or if he is from any cause an epileptic, he may die suddenly during the attack. But if he is otherwise healthy, he is sure of a safe and speedy convalescence.

It has been my experience that there are very few cases indeed which yield to a less dose than fifty grains, and a considerable number which require a good deal more; those cases requiring the largest doses being those ushered in by the *status epilepticus*, which chloral arrests as rapidly and safely as it does delirium tremens itself. But even in these cases I have never required to give more than 120 grains of Leibreich's chloral, in divided doses, and this dose, though large, is not a dangerous one. Richardson tells us that the dose of chloral is proportionate to the weight of the animal, that a human subject weighing 120 to 140 lb. is thrown into a deep sleep by a dose of ninety grains, and into a sleep that is dangerous by a dose of 140 grains. He finds also that an individual who has taken enough of chloral to be affected by it gets rid of it at the rate of seven grains an hour, so that though 144 grains given at once is a dangerous dose, yet twelve grains may be given every two hours for twelve times with perfect safety. From the irritated condition of the mucous lining of the stomach of a drunkard, it is probable that the absorption of ingested fluids is not so rapid as usual ; it is but fair, therefore, for that reason also, to allow a moderate interval between the doses, so as to avoid as far as possible any risk of giving more than enough. At the same time we must shun the opposite extreme of giving doses in themselves too small to have any decided effect, and which have any possible cumulative effect destroyed by too long an interval being permitted to elapse between the giving of each dose.

Acting upon the principles involved in the foregoing statements, I have for long been in the habit of treating cases of delirium tremens by giving forty grains of chloral hydrate every hour, for three hours if necessary. Sometimes, but rarely, the first dose has been enough, most commonly two doses have been required, and it has only been in the very rarest instances that the third dose has been necessary. If the attack be ushered in by the *status epilepticus*, I shorten the interval between the doses to half an hour, as in these cases time is of the utmost importance, and a large dose is sure to be required. Should the heart be feeble, I give each dose of chloral in half an ounce or an ounce of the infusion of digitalis; the chloral, unlike the bromide, has no tendency to weaken the heart's action, while, like chloroform, it seems to induce a more equable distribution of the blood, the digitalis toning the heart, and increasing the arterial blood-pressure.

Dr. Balfour at the same time deprecates the use of alcohol in the treatment of delirium tremens.

—

Bromine in Laryngeal Croup.

Dr. W. REDENBACHER writes in the *Ærztliches Intelligenz-Blatt* of January 7th, that he has obtained strikingly good effects in two cases of laryngeal croup from the internal administration of bromine (in the form of bromide of potassium). For some time, bromine inhalations have been used in the following manner: From 0.2 to 0.3 gramme of bromine, with a similar or greater quantity of bromide of potassium, has been dissolved in 120 grammes of water, and, a sponge or handkerchief dipped in it being tied before the nose and mouth, the bromine-vapour has been inhaled for five or ten minutes at intervals varying from half an hour to an hour. From this method, however, Dr. Redenbacher has not been able to obtain any good result. Two little girls, aged respectively five and seven, having come under his care with severe croup of the larynx and air-tubes, he ordered a tablespoonful of the following mixture to be taken every hour: R. Decocti althææ 120 grm.; potassii bromidi 4 grm.; bromi 0.3 grm.; syrupi simplicis 30 grm. On again visiting the patients, whom he did not expect to find alive, he was most agreeably surprised. The harsh respiratory murmur, the difficult breathing, the dry characteristic cough, the loss of tone in the voice, had all disappeared; the breathing was free, the cough loose, and the hoarseness diminished. Several portions of croupal membrane had been coughed up. The improvement continued on the next day, and perfect recovery followed in a few days. No toxic symptoms of any kind were produced. For children under one year, the quantity of bromine in the mixture should be reduced to 0.1 gramme; and for those from one to four years old, to 0.2 gramme.—*British Med. Journal*, Feb. 15, 1879.

—

The Pathological Anatomy of the Cardiac Ganglia.

The subject of the pathology of the cardiac ganglia as yet belongs to the domain of theoretical, rather than to that of practical pathology. Their disease affords so ready an explanation of many of the phenomena of cardiac disturbance, whether with or without organic disease of the heart, that it is often referred to, without consideration of the scantiness of our knowledge of the subject. Lanceraux described in 1864 a case in which a man who had suffered from angina pectoris, and had died in an attack, presented a morbid state of the cardiac plexus—vascularity, exudation, and accumulations of nuclei compressing the nerve-fibres. IWANOWSKY, in an important work published in 1876, has investigated the conditions of the cardiac ganglia in exanthematic typhus. The ganglia are chiefly embedded in the septum between the auricles, especially adjacent to the upper part of the fossa ovalis. They are of round or oval form, inclosed in a fibrillar connective tissue capsule, and surrounded by a dense network of vessels. The nerve-cells contained in them are round or oval, and surrounded by capsules, which consist of a layer of flat epithelial cells, each nerve-cell having one or two fine processes. The alterations found by Iwanowsky in typhus were a swollen and opaque state of the ganglion cells, indistinctness of their nuclei; the endothelial capsule was often swollen. In the intermediate tissue granulation-cells were met with, and similar corpuscles were found between the nerve-cells and the endothelial capsule. Hence Iwanowsky concludes that the ganglia are the seat of a parenchymatous inflammation, which may account for the occasional fatal paralysis of the heart in the early stage of that disease. Wassilieff has described changes in the ganglia in hydrophobia very similar to those found by Iwanowsky in typhus, and he laid especial stress on the existence of spaces between the cells and its capsule, which are of very doubtful pathological significance. A further important contribution to our knowledge of the changes in the cardiac ganglia has been made by Dr. PUTJATIN, of St. Petersburg, who has examined the state of the ganglia in a considerable number of cases of chronic heart disease. In a case in which cardiac disturbance was observed during life, and the patient died from cardiac paralysis, with little obvious heart disease, the vessels of the ganglia were distended, and granulation-cells were scattered among the nerve elements; the latter were little changed. In cases of old organic heart disease more marked changes were found, consisting especially in the increase of the interstitial connective tissue between the ganglion-cells, in which fibres and round and oval granulation elements were met with. The nerve-cells were shrunken and more or less granular. In some cases the diminution in size of the cells was to one-half of the normal, and the epithelial capsule had almost disappeared. A somewhat similar change was found in a case of phthisis with atrophy of the muscular fibres of the heart.

From these cases Putjatin concludes that the changes in the ganglia are most marked when there exists recognizable disease of the heart and aorta. In several of the cases of organic disease of the heart in which changes in the ganglia were found the pathological evidences of constitutional syphilis were present elsewhere, and it is possible that the syphilitic infection may have had an influence on the production of the sclerosis of the ganglia. In some cases it is believed that the change in the ganglia is secondary to the change in the aorta; that an inflammatory process beginning in the aorta may pass through to the connective tissue beneath the pericardium, and later extend by continuity to the connective tissue around the ganglia.

It is pointed out by Putjatin that such changes must necessarily produce various disturbances in the action of the heart. Physiology teaches that the rhythmical action of the heart is regulated by the nerve-ganglia. Some form of angina pectoris, and many forms of irregular action, may be due to these changes. It seems to be probable, also, that acute changes in the ganglia may be the immediate cause of cardiac paralysis —*Lancet,* Feb. 8, 1879.

Diagnosis of Adhesion of the Pericardium.

In an article in the *Berliner Klinische Wochenschrift* for December 20, Dr. L. RIESS calls attention to a comparatively rare, and, as he believes, hitherto undescribed sign of adhesion of the pericardium, viz., the production of a metallic resonance of the heart's sounds (and of murmurs in disease of the valves) in the stomach. He relates three cases which have come under his observation in the Berlin General Hospital, in which the resonance was observed. In the first, a necropsy showed extensive adhesion of the pericardium over the diaphragm, as well as in other parts, there being, in fact, almost universal pericardial adhesion. The other two patients are still alive, and are the subjects of valvular disease; and in both there is resonance of the murmurs through the stomach. Commenting on the three cases, he remarks that the inconstancy of the phenomenon does not militate against the explanation he gives of it, viz., that it arises from the close approximation of the heart and stomach in consequence of the pericardial adhesion. In the first case the stomach was excessively distended; but this is not necessary for the production of the resonance, for in the other cases there was only moderate distension, and the resonance was neither increased nor produced by artificial distension. He observes also that these cases show that the first sound of the heart or a systolic murmur may have a metallic resonance, while the diastolic sound does not manifest this character. Constancy of the sign is not to be expected ; and one or more examinations may fail to detect it, although other symptoms of adhesion of the pericardium are present. When met with, however, it is a valuable aid in the diagnosis. Of course, the resonance produced by cavities in the lungs, and by pneumothorax or pneumopericardium, must be excluded.—*British Med. Journal*, Feb. 15, 1879.

Degenerative Changes in the Diaphragm as a Cause of Sudden Death.

Dr. F. W. ZAHN, in an article in Virchow's *Archiv*, Bd. lxxiii., ascribes certain cases of sudden death to structural changes in the muscular tissue of the diaphragm. These cases occur mostly in persons who have been for some time the subjects of emphysema, chronic bronchial catarrh, or slight disease of the muscular structure of the heart, and then die suddenly without any evident special complications. , At the necropsy, there are found emphysema, moderate œdema, and hyperæmia of the lung, chronic catarrh of the bronchi, with more or less hypertrophy of the heart with some fatty degeneration ; the remaining organs are generally sound, and the pathological conditions are apparently not sufficient to account for the sudden death. In a case of sudden death occurring in a person who was the subject of an advanced stage of emphysema, Dr. Zahn was led to examine the diaphragm, as there was nothing in the other organs that would sufficiently account for the death. The result was the discovery of an extensive fatty degeneration of the muscular tissue of the diaphragm, which was much thickened. He has since made a number of examinations, and finds that degenerative processes of three kinds occur in the diaphragm. 1. There may be simple brown atrophy with proliferation of cells and nuclei. In this case, which is the most frequent, the diaphragm is thinned and of a faintly brownish colour. Fatty tissue is found between the muscular fasciculi. 2. There may be granular opacity with fatty degeneration. Here the diaphragm has a yellow opaque appearance, and yellowish spots are sometimes seen. 3. In one case, Dr. Zahn found hyaloid degeneration of the muscle. This is very rare ; and, when it affects the striated muscles, appears to be of traumatic origin. From his investigations, Dr. Zahn arrives at the following conclusions : In almost all cases, the disease of the diaphragm is of the same kind as that of the muscular tissue of the heart ; and hence it may be correctly inferred that the disease in both arises from the same cause. Brown atrophy is brought about by marastic changes in the organism ; fatty degeneration is in part the result of dyscrasic changes in the blood. Regarding the hypertrophy and consequent secondary degeneration of the muscular tissue of the diaphragm through increased exertion in consequence of impediments to or abnormal conditions of respiration and the pulmonary circulation, Dr. Zahn does not, for the present, arrive at any conclusion. He is, however, disposed to attribute the change in the muscle to a disturbance of nutrition, such as that produced by an excess of carbonic acid and a defect of oxygen in the blood. Where disease of the diaphragm is present, sudden death by asphyxia may occur even in very slight cases of bronchial catarrh.—*British Med. Journal*, Feb. 15, 1879.

Tubercle of the Alimentary Canal.

M. SPILLMANN, in a Thèse de Paris (*Gazette Méd. de Paris*, No. 2, 1879), says that there is nothing characteristic in the constitution of the tubercle similar to what has been found in other affections, like cancerous nodules, gangrene, etc. It may be briefly described as a special inflammation, consisting in a nodular infiltration of perivascular connective tissue, originating from lymph-cells. It is always accompanied by fibrinous coagula in the vessels lying in the centre of the nodules, and by arrest of the circulation; in short, a granulation is an atrophic transparent cheesy mass. The most interesting variation of tuberculosis is that affecting the mouth and pharynx. It is characterized by yellowish or grayish raised spots, which later begin to ulcerate. It presents the so-called giant-cells, which M. Spillmann believes to originate from the alteration of muscular fibres encased in the tuberculous centres. Among the symptoms, M. Spillmann especially points out an unbearable lancinating pain, which often causes the patient to refuse nourishment, and may even drive him to commit suicide. The best means of relief are tincture of iodine, glycerine, and morphia, combined, and cauterization with a hot iron; but it is very doubtful whether complete recovery is possible. The extirpation of the parts attacked, so long as the disease has not spread to other organs, has been suggested. Tuberculous lesions in the digestive canal belong to several types. 1. They may be isolated, consisting of miliary centres situated either in the mucous membrane itself or beneath it, and after a time transformed into lenticular ulcerations. 2. They may follow the course of the vessels (annular type), having their superior part turned towards the intestines. 3. They may entirely cover Peyer's glands. In the large intestine, the tuberculization may be diffuse, and cause wide-spread, deep, rugged, or gangrenous lesions. While the tubercles of the stomach and intestines are very different from those of the buccal cavity, they present many points of resemblance, both clinical and anatomical, with the tubercles of the anus. It is not yet proved whether anal fistula ought to be considered as caused by tuberculosis of the digestive canal. M. Spillmann thinks that it has not yet been proved that tuberculous matter can develop tuberculosis, if introduced into the intestine. It is very remarkable, however, that, in a tuberculous individual, any organic lesion or irritation may produce tubercles.—*British Med. Journal*, Feb. 15, 1879.

Complete Obstruction of the Intestine by Fibrinous Exudation.

Dr. MARKHAM SKERRITT (of Clifton) at a late meeting of the Clinical Society of London (*Med. Times and Gazette*, March 1, 1879) exhibited a specimen from a patient who had come under his care at the Bristol General Hospital. A young man, aged nineteen, previously in good health, on May 11 last felt slight abdominal pain, and was afterwards very sick; there were no febrile symptoms. Next day he suffered from vomiting and diarrhœa. After this vomiting continued, but there was no action of the bowels. On admission, a week after the onset of the attack, there were practically no acute symptoms, except frequent bilious vomiting. The skin was cool, the pulse 80°, large, regular, and rather soft, the tongue almost clean, the abdomen moderately distended, and almost free from pain and tenderness. An enema of three pints was given without difficulty, but with no result. Opium and hot fomentations were ordered. Next day some dulness in the flanks, changing with the patient's position, was noted. On the following day the patient sank rapidly and died. The temperature throughout was subnormal. At the post-mortem examination, the ileum, about a foot above the valve, was found to dip down into the pelvis so as to form a loop, which was much contracted, intensely inflamed on its peritoneal surface, solid to the feel, much like a firm umbilical cord; and its canal was here completely blocked by a solid fibrinous cast, four inches long, firmly attached to the mucous membrane, and tailing off at either end as a jagged coating of a part only of the inner wall of the intestine. This loop of gut bounded anteriorly an irregular cavity containing feces and partially lined with false membrane, into which the vermiform appendix was found to open. No foreign body was discovered. There was no fluid in the peritoneal cavity. The two points raised by Dr. Markham Skerritt in commenting on this case were—(1) the pathological condition, and (2) the data for diagnosis. Inflammation marked by the formation of a fibrinous false membrane was met with in the intestine in various conditions; but no other case had been found on record in which the intestine was completely plugged with the exudation. It was probable that such a condition could occur only where the inflammation was so intense as to cause stasis of the feces, for otherwise the movements of the intestinal walls, and the flow of feces, would interfere with the continued deposit of the exudation; and hence in dysentery, where diarrhœa was marked, no very thick layer of false membrane was found. In this case, probably, ulceration of the vermiform appendix occurred first, followed by its perforation and extension of inflammation throughout the small intestine— slight at first, corresponding with the period of diarrhœa; and then more intense, causing cessation of peristaltic action, and consequent constipation. The inflammation took on the croupous type, and complete blocking of the intestine was the result. The absence of fluid from the peritoneal cavity was worthy of note; and the physical signs might be explained on the theory that each individual coil of intestine in contact with the flanks presented to the percussing fingers, in one position, a greater quantity of feces, in another, a large proportion of gas. As to the data for prognosis, the sudden onset of symptoms was in favour of the presence of one of the causes of acute intestinal obstruction. But the preliminary diarrhœa which preceded constipation accorded only with the history of enteritis simply, in which a mild inflammation accompanied by diarrhœa was succeeded by a more severe implication of the gut, causing cessation of peristaltic action and consequent constipation. But beyond this there was practically no positive evidence of enteritis, except bilious vomiting; all the other ordinary acute symptoms of this condition were absent. Notwithstanding this, a diagnosis of simple enteritis was made, founded upon an experience in which it had been the exception for acute abdominal inflammations to be accompanied by urgent symptoms. And yet this latency of symptoms was held to be of some positive value in diagnosis, as indicating the absence of any suddenly induced mechanical cause of obstruction, relievable, it might be, by timely operation. The following conclusions were derived from an experience which probably had been somewhat exceptional :—First, that an entire absence of acute symptoms might coexist with an intense local inflammation of the abdomen. Secondly, that if in a case of apparent intestinal obstruction urgent symptoms were in abeyance, it was in favour of the view that the condition was either non-acute, or, if acute, was not to be relieved by operation.

—

On the Effects of Diet, Rest, Exercise, etc., in Chronic Nephritis.

An able and interesting paper on this subject, by Drs. E. I. SPARKS and J. MITCHELL BRUCE, was read at a late meeting of the Royal Medical and Chirurgical Society (*Med. Times and Gazette,* Jan. 25, 1879), which has a real value as a contribution of carefully observed and recorded facts on points of treatment regarding which we are in need of increased reliable information. The authors showed the relations of the amounts of urine, albumen, and urea to each other in the patient on ordinary mixed diet and whilst taking ordinary exercise; and then gave the results of experiments with absolute milk diet, non-nitrogenous diet, excess of eggs, and nitrogenous diet with water, respectively, and also the effects of rest, of exercise, and of the administration of digitalis, upon the amount of albumen and of urea, and on the specific gravity and the total amount of the urine. The principal conclusions arrived at are—that the amount of albumen was reduced by milk diet and by non-nitrogenous diet; that the effect of the milk diet was not merely due to the albumen being more than ordinarily diluted, for ordinary diet, with an equal amount of water, did not produce the same result; that the effect of non-nitrogenous diet was decided, was not immediately produced, and persisted some time after the re-ingestion of nitrogen; and that absolute rest markedly reduced the amount of albumen. The authors do not pretend to draw settled general conclusions from their experiments, to be applied universally in Bright's disease, but think that their observations indicate that certain factors beyond the disease-process had to be regarded in this case of albuminuria; these factors must be physiological facts which are still unknown, which evidently are related to the processes that occur between the digestive organs and the kidneys, and which, being physiological, must be taken into account in *every* case of albuminuria; and that diet and rest are of the greatest importance in the treatment of albuminuria. Much has been written lately on intermittent albuminuria, and the results obtained by the authors suggest that all cases of albuminuria not intermittent are probably remittent. They do not accept the explanation of the increase of albuminuria by exercise as always due to increased pressure; and their view on this point is supported by Dr. Quain's account of a case in which albumen was present largely in the urine after breakfast, and declined very greatly during the day. One of the most remarkable points about the paper is the fact that the great majority of the laborious and careful investigations were made by the patient himself, who is a medical man suffering from chronic phthisis, chronic heart-disease, and chronic nephritis —the urea, albumen, specific gravity, and total amount of the urine being estimated five times daily for weeks. Such an investigation, in such circumstances, shows wonderful courage, determination, and love of scientific truth and research.

Surgery.

Spontaneous Rupture of Muscles.

This case is recorded by SILBERSTEIN in the *Wiener Medizinische Presse*, December 1, 1878. The patient was a man aged 65, who for some months had suffered from muscular pain in his right arm, but this did not prevent him from following his occupation. On the 22d of October, he went into the stable to feed his horse. The animal being restive he raised his right arm towards its head; at the some moment he experienced a very severe pain in the arm, accompanied by a cracking noise and a feeling of faintness. He returned home thinking he had sustained a fracture: the faintness gradually passed off and the pain became less intense, but the right arm was then in a remarkably swollen condition. Its measurement, at its periphery, exceeded that of the left side by 8 centimetres (3.2 inches). The skin of the arm throughout looked as though it had been painted, the greater portion being red, but the two extremities were violet. The swelling was hard but not very painful, except at the point where the two heads of the biceps join together: however, every feature was intensified. Except when the elbow was flexed and the forearm pronated, movements did not give rise to much suffering. The patient could not lift up the smallest object. At a later date the swelling and discoloration spread down the forearm to the right carpus; this disappeared in time, but the stiffness and limitation to flexion still remained.— *Lond. Med. Record*, February 15, 1879.

Use of Opera-Glasses in connection with the various forms of Ametropia.

The use of opera-glasses is often attended with very great inconvenience as regards vision; and this is due, according to Dr. GIRAUD-TEULON (*L'Œil*, deuxième édition, 1878), to the indifference displayed in their fabrication, with reference to the great variety of refractive power in the eyes of those who use these instruments. When the optic axes are parallel, as when the eyes are directed to any distant object, binocular vision results without effort, the accommodation of the two eyes being perfectly relaxed; and if the tubes of the opera-glasses be distant from each other by the same space which separates the pupils, the conditions of ordinary vision are realized; but if the distance between the tubes vary, either more or less, then double images are produced, homonymous if the distance between the tubes be greater than that between the pupils, and crossed if the distance be less. Now, the eyes have greater difficulty in uniting homonymous images which are separated by a slight interval than is the case with crossed images; it is extremely important, therefore, to use opera-glasses the tubes of which exactly correspond to the distance between the eyes. Glasses which are too wide should be carefully avoided.

In myopia, the optic axes have a tendency to diverge, and distant objects give rise to images which are slightly crossed; and, in such a case, the ocular lenses should be rather more distant from each other than the object lenses; that is to say, they should be capable of being shifted laterally, and from within outwards.

With hypermetropia the reverse is the case; the ocular lenses should be nearer to each other than the object lenses; *i. e.*, they should be capable of lateral movement from without inwards.

Dr. Giraud-Teulon believes that, if opera-glasses were constructed so that the ocular lenses were capable of lateral movement, very many people who are now unable to use them would be able to do so, and without fatigue or inconvenience of any kind.—*London Med. Record*, Aug. 15, 1878.

—

Gunshot Wounds Involving several Viscera.

This is a very careful record (*Progrès Méd.*, January 4, 1879) of a case of gunshot injury, well worthy of perusal *in extenso*, although we are unable to do more than briefly abstract it here. An Arab, aged 30, was shot with a pistol containing two balls, on August 9, 1878. Both of these entered in the neighbourhood of the xiphoid cartilage of the sternum; neither emerged anywhere. One aperture in the middle line about a finger breadth above tip of xiphoid, the second more to the left and a little lower down. On entry into hospital, great collapse, but no other symptoms of injury; no vomiting or expectoration of blood. Heart carried towards the right side; sounds feeble, but perfectly normal. Respiration almost normal, feeble behind. Both wounds covered with collodium, as also the whole surface of the abdomen. Liquid diet: draughts of chloral and morphia repeated in small quantities. Before entry he had vomited, but the ejecta contained no blood.

To be brief, the patient developed, in the course of a few days, well-marked pericarditis, and later still, empyema on left side, but no abdominal symptoms. On the sixth day thorax tapped, and 150 grammes of pus withdrawn; again, on thirteenth day, 800 grammes; again, on fourteenth day, 900 grammes. After remaining in a very grave condition for some weeks, he gradually recovered, and at last left the hospital, contrary to physician's wishes, about nine weeks after the accident. He was urged not to leave, as he still showed dulness over the left lower chest posteriorly with *râles* and evening pyrexia, but his heart was normal, as also the functions of all abdominal organs, and he felt very well. He returned consequently to his business, remaining at home for nearly a month. During this time, his temperature rose each evening, and he had occasional shiverings. Re-entered hospital on November 20, with symptoms of pyæmic and hepatic abscesses, and died on the 25th (108 days after injury), with symptoms of peritonitis, in addition to those already mentioned.

Autopsy.—The cause of death was shown clearly to be pyæmia manifesting itself chiefly in metastatic abscesses in liver and peritonitis ; but the interest of the examination of the body lies mainly in the course of the bullets. On removing the skin, etc., the mark of one of the latter is found on the costal cartilage. The second has left no visible mark here. The pericardium is found adherent to the heart in many places, the surface of which latter is covered with villous exudation. On the posterior aspect of the pericardium is an oval, punched-out opening, hardly covered with a light film of exudation ; it is 1 centimetre long and 4 millimetres broad. Opposite this opening there is a long groove torn through the muscular substance of the left ventricle of the heart, commencing at the apex, and running from below upwards, and from left to right, but without opening the ventricle at any spot. This groove is cicatrized and marked with the same villosities as the heart. From this the ball has passed on to lodge in the left lung, which is, however, quite sound anteriorly. Behind the lung is an encysted pyæmia, containing 800 grammes of pus, in which the first bullet is found. No trace of the second bullet is found on inner surface of the abdominal walls or on either surface of the left lobe of liver. But on the anterior wall of the stomach there is a small, dark-coloured, wrinkled, and depressed scar, 4 millimetres in diameter. There is no aperture of exit marked on the posterior wall of the stomach, but on turning the latter over to the right side the second small bullet is found encysted above the pancreas, and lying upon the aorta. A line uniting its position here with the external scar, and that on the front wall of the stomach, passes through the left lobe of the liver and both walls of the latter, and yet only one scar is found in it, and none in the liver. Of the histological appearances of this scar, which are given in detail, we need only notice that many cotton fibres were found imbedded in the fibrous tissue of which the latter was composed. That the patient should have recovered from such very severe injuries is the most remarkable point of the case, the pyæmia being secondary to the empyæma.—*Lond. Med. Record*, February 15, 1879.

——

On Colotomy.

Dr. F. van Erckelens, of Aix-la-Chapelle, in a contribution to a recent number of the *Archiv für Klinische Chirurgie*, Band xxiii. Heft 1, presents an analysis of 262 cases of colotomy, and discusses the comparative merits of the two principal operations ; that proposed by Littré in 1710, and first performed by Pilloie of Rouen in 1776, and that proposed by Callisen in 1778 and carried into practice sixty years later by Amussat. The latter operation has been most favoured, indeed almost exclusively adopted, by English and American surgeons, whilst most instances of Littré's operation have occurred in Germany and France. Very many of the cases tabulated by the author have been collected from papers published by Hawkins and Curling in this country, and many also from the valuable article on colotomy written by Dr. Erskine Mason, of New York (*American Journal of Medical Sciences*, vol. lxvi. 1873). Most of the results from the analysis could be based on not more than 249 of these collected cases, since in thirteen no mention could be found as to the kind of operation that has been performed.

In this slightly reduced number the proportion of cases in which the operation proved successful or was not, directly or indirectly, the cause of death, is 58.4 per cent. The numbers of successful and fatal cases being 165 and 84. This percentage cannot be regarded as high, and compares unfavourably when compared with that of ovariotomy, which in itself is a much more serious operation. Colotomy, however, is usually performed for the purpose of preventing death in extreme cases, and on subjects who have suffered long from some very protracted disease. The most unfavourable results are presented by the cases in which the operation was performed on infants with congenital atresia recti. Of 44 cases of this kind not more than 20 (45.2 per cent.) were successful. In the recorded cases of colotomy for the relief of intestinal carcinoma the percentage is higher, being 59.2. The chances of a successful result are much greater when the operation is performed in cases where the disease is not so serious as to impair to any extreme degree the strength of the patient or to threaten life. Of the 16 cases in which the colon was opened for the treatment of fistula, 13 (81.2 per cent.) were unsuccessful. In very few of the fatal cases in the tables, the author asserts, could death be fairly regarded as the direct result of the operation. The above results prove, it is held, the propriety of colotomy in those cases where the operation is usually resorted to. When performed as an almost desperate measure, and for the purpose of saving life, it is successful in more than half the number of cases, and the percentage of recoveries from the operation in instances of less severe disease is far more favourable.

The question as to which of the two operations, that of Littré and that of Amussat, is to be preferred, has often been discussed. In dealing with this, the author considers the date afforded by his table of cases; the special dangers of each operation, the difficulties in the performance of each, and the advantages and disadvantages attending the situation of the artificial anus. According to the tabulated cases the proportion of deaths is much higher after Littré's than after Amussat's, being 46.4 per cent. with the former, and 38.4 per cent. with the latter. But, as Dr. van Erckelens points out, Littré's operation is usually performed under less favourable conditions and in more desperate cases than those in which recourse is taken to the method of Amussat. In a large proportion of the cases of atresia recti the colon was opened in the groin. In cases of fistula, on the other hand, colotomy is actually performed in the lumbar region. When performed under equally favourable conditions the difference in the results does not appear to be so very great. The author's tables show that in cases of carcinoma the percentage of recoveries is 63 after Amussat's and 61 after Littré's operation, and in cases of non-malignant obstruction, 50 after the former, and as high as 58.5 after the latter. It would seem, then, that the operation of Littré, notwithstanding the necessity it involves of opening the peritoneal sac, is not more dangerous than that of Amussat. According to Dr. Mason, who has operated only by Amussat's method, "wounds of the peritoneum are not now held in such dread by surgeons as formerly, as our means of combating peritoneal inflammation are much more efficacious and the portion of membrane wounded has often lost its peculiar physiological properties and its pathological tendencies before any injury with the knife." Pure traumatic peritonitis is not a frequent cause of death after Littré's operation. In not one of six fatal cases reported by Holmes was death directly the result of this operation. In some cases, those of atresia recti in infants, fatal peritonitis may have been previously excited by punctures and incisions made from the perineum. In one method of colotomy, as in the other, a fatal result may almost always be attributed to the disease, and not to the interference of the surgeon. The operation gives relief to the distended intestine, but unfortunately in too many cases merely retards the development of peritonitis consequent on prolonged obstruction. The wound, according to Dr. van Erckelens, heals more favourably after Littré's than in Amussat's operation. Erysipelas and diffused suppuration occur frequently after each method, and were met with in about half the number of tabulated cases in which Amussat's operation had been performed, but whilst fourteen of these were fatal, in four only did death occur after the method of Littré. The diffused suppuration after colotomy is very probably due to the prolonged contact of fecal matter with fresh or non-granulating surfaces, and, if this is so, is more favoured by the conditions of Amussat's operation.

Littré's operation is a comparatively easy one, and does not require more skill and experience on the part of the operator than are necessary for the performance of any major surgical proceeding. There is but a thin layer of muscular structure to cut through, and there need not be any great extent of wound either in length or depth. Amussat's, on the other hand, is a difficult operation. The intestine is deeply seated, and cannot often be easily found. The wound is wide and deep, and the recognition and suitable division of the different layers of fascia and muscle require much anatomical knowledge. Most surgeons who have frequently performed Amussat's operation have met with difficulties, especially in finding and recognizing the colon. Amussat himself, in one of his operations, experienced much anxiety and uncertainty. In another case the operation, this surgeon stated, was long and difficult, and in a third he mistook the kidney for the descending colon, and wounded this organ.

Dr. van Erckelens, in concluding his paper, argues that the groin is a much less inconvenient structure for an artificial anus than the lumbar region.—*London Med. Record*, Jan. 15, 1879.

Stricture of the Rectum caused by Prolapsus.

M. LANNELONGUE (*Société de Chirurgie*, December 11, 1878) called attention to some facts which might throw light upon the pathogenesis of some strictures of the rectum, situated about $6\frac{1}{2}$ centimetres above the anal orifice, forming a kind of annular valve, with the free border supple, but its adhering border resting on a somewhat indurated base. A child was brought under his notice with prolapsus of the rectum, and some inflammation of the mucous membrane of the protruding gut. Many months afterwards the child returned with a bridle cicatrix on the posterior wall of the rectum, partially obliterating the lumen of the intestine.

Another child had been brought to him in a similar condition. The case had been watched. An examination made later on revealed an ulcerated surface; this granulated, and gradually formed a valvular stricture. In adult patients, where stricture exists from an unknown cause, inquiry should be made as to the existence in infancy of rectal prolapse.—*Lond. Med. Record*, Feb. 15, 1879.

Lineal Rectotomy for the Extraction of a Foreign Body.

This communication was made by M. TURGIS at a meeting of the *Société de Chirurgie*, December 11, 1878.

The patient had introduced into the rectum a chocolate cup. The efforts made at extraction soon after the introduction of the foreign body caused a small piece to be broken off the edge of the cup, the remainder passing higher up the intestine. M. Turgis saw the case on the fourth day. Deeming further attempts at extraction to be useless, a curved trocar was inserted into the anal orifice and brought out 5 or 6 millimetres above the tip of the coccyx, and on the left side of the bone. An écraseur was then introduced, and the section completed without a single drop of blood being lost. By these means the cup was easily seized and withdrawn. The after-results of the operation were satisfactory, and the patient recovered in spite of the large quantity of blood he had previously lost, of a wound of the prostate, and a tear of the rectum. M. Turgis thought this mode of extraction preferable to the breaking up of the foreign body.

M. Verneuil stated that Dr. Raffy had performed linear rectotomy in 1860. The sphincter was divided with a bistoury, and it was then found to be easy to manœuvre in the rectum. M. Turgis's case was interesting, for an operation had been performed which, though but slight in itself, had rendered very great service ; for it should not be forgotten that the mortality caused by the introduction of foreign bodies into the rectum was 20 per cent.—*Lond. Med. Record*, Feb. 15, 1879.

—

Recovery after Operation for Relief of Acute Intestinal Obstruction by the Establishment of a False Anus in the Linea Alba.

At a later meeting of the Clinical Society of London (*Med. Times and Gaz.*, March 1, 1879), Mr. HOWARD MARSH read a paper describing a case of acute intestinal obstruction in which the abdomen was opened, a stricture of the sigmoid flexure found, and a false anus established in the linea alba, the patient recovering. A woman of forty had, on her admission into St. Bartholomew's Hospital, under Dr. Marsh, on October 15, been suffering from acute intestinal obstruction, with frequent sickness and abdominal distension for eight days. She had previously considered herself well, and had experienced no trouble in the action of her bowels. No hernia, intussusception, or other causes of obstruction could be detected. The colon, which was distended, could be traced through the umbilical and left lumbar regions. The patient on her admission was found to be in a very exhausted condition, with a feeble pulse of 120, and a relaxed and clammy skin. During a consultation on the case, some of the hospital staff advised that, since the colon could be felt to be distended, colotomy should be performed. Others, believing that the sudden manner in which the symptoms of acute obstruction had come on in a person who had apparently been previously healthy, indicated some form of internal strangulation, which if unrelieved might lead to gangrene of the intestine, recommended that the abdominal cavity should be explored. The latter operation was at once performed. An incision was made below the umbilicus in the linea alba, and the intestine—starting with the coil which presented in the wound—was traced towards the left iliac fossæ, each successive piece of the gut being returned as soon as it had been examined, and before another loop was drawn out. While this was being done a stricture of malignant character was detected in the middle of the sigmoid flexure. The intestine just above the stricture was fastened by numerous closely placed sutures to the wound in the linea alba, and a false anus was established in this situation. The operation was found to be very easy, and was speedily completed. The patient made a good recovery, and left the hospital at the end of about two months. In his remarks Mr. Marsh very strongly insisted on the importance of operating in cases of abdominal obstruction—where the diagnosis can be established—before peritonitis and other local changes have ensued. He alluded to the large percentage of cases of ovariotomy in which the abdominal cavity is safely opened ; and asked whether it could be more dangerous to open the abdomen, and divide a constricting band, or release an internal strangulation, than it was to remove a large tumour, which was, perhaps, extensively adherent to the omentum, the intestines, or the uterus ? He believed a great future was in store for the surgical treatment of intestinal obstruction ; and that the operation, if performed early, and with due care, and in cases

in which a clean diagnosis could be made, would piove at least as successful as
ovariotomy.

Mi. BRYANT had not quite undeistood how fai the symptoms weie those of acute
iathei than of chionic stoppage ; but he belie\ed that fiom the histoiy he should
ha\e been inclined to ad\ocate colotomy, though it was always difficult to judge
of this without being in piesence of the patient.   He entiiely indoised Mi.
Maish's obseivation as to the desirability of eaily opeiations in these cases.

Mi. BARWELL thought that he also would have voted in fa\oui of colotomy,
which would ha\e in\ol\ed less iisk than the opeiation peifoimed on the successful iesult of which he congiatulated Mi. Maish. He, like Mi. Biyant, was
stiongly in fa\oui of an eaily opeiation.

Mi. GOULD asked Mi. Maish whethei he thought it would have been piofitable
to ha\e iemo\ed the intestine, having iegaid to its limited extent.

Mi. MARSH ieplied that the ieason the abdomen was opened was, fiist, that the
symptoms weie acute ; secondly, that no histoiy of pie\ious tiouble could be obtained; thiidly, that the natuie of the obstiuction was obscuie.   He allowed that
he himself had inclined towaids colotomy, though theie had been no symptoms of
malignant stiictuie.   The anteiioi position of the aitificial anus was, he thought,
an ad\antage iathei than the opposite.   It was moie manageable and moie easily
attended to by the patient.   He had not consideied it ad\isable, seeing the exhausted state of the patient, to expose hei to the iisk of piolonging the opeiation
by iemo\ing the diseased intestine by Billioth's method, though in a suitable case
he should undoubtedly do so.

—

Tieatment of Stranyulated Heinia by Eigotine.

Dr. PLANAT, of Nice, has tieated successfully two cases of stiangulated heinia
with eigot.

The fiist patient was a man, aged fifty, who suffeied fiom a heinia which had
been stiangulated on the pie\ious day.   Eigot was applied both inteinally and
exteinally, in the form of ointment, which was iubbed on the tumoui e\eiy two
houis, the lattei having been pie\iously washed with waim alkaline watei.   The
inteinal tieatment consisted of 5 giammes of eigot, mixed with 125 giammes of
watei and syiup, taken e\eiy houi.   Aftei this tieatment had lasted foi foui oi
five houis, the \omiting ceased, and twel\e houis latei the heinia had become
spontaneously ieduced.

The second case was that of a young man, aged 28, who had woin a tiuss foi
se\eial yeais befoie the heinial complication set in.   The heinia had iesisted all
efforts to ieduce it.   Fifteen leeches had been applied to the tumoui, but six
only took ; the symptoms then giew woise, and eigotin was again iesoited to,
being administeied as abo\e.   Ele\en houis latei, when the suigeons aiii\ed to
peifoim the opeiation. in case the eigot should have pio\ed unsuccessful, the
heinia was ieduced, and the patient was well.   The authoi suggests whethei the
diug would not be peihaps moie efficient if diiectly injected into the heinial sac,
and not taken inteinally.—London Med. Recoid, Feb. 15, 1879.

—

Lithotrity at one or moie sittings.

Sir HENRY THOMPSON iecently deli\eied, at Uni\eisity College Hospital
(Lancet, Feb. 1, 1879), a lectuie in which he consideied Dr. Bigelow's opeiation foi the iemo\al of a stone by ciushing at a single sitting (Ameiican Journal
of the Medical Sciences, Jan. 1878).   He said that in\aiiable confoimity to the
pioposed iule to iemo\e at one sitting an entiie stone, no mattei how laige it
may be, oi what may be the condition of the patient, he did not hesitate at the

outset to say, will lead to results which, although often successful, will not seldom be disastrous. Sir Henry said :—

"I have never doubted for an instant that, so far as mechanical power is concerned, almost any stone may be thus removed, and without much difficulty, but I cannot overlook the fact that the vital conditions under which we are compelled to work must limit the employment of mechanical force. In the practice of Bigelow's method, very large and heavy lithotrites are introduced, certainly larger than an ordinary urethra will admit without using force. But what strikes me after all as the most remarkable fact, judging from the very slender experience by which the proceeding is at present supported, is the enormous time which has been consumed with these instruments in performing the task proposed. Thus we find in Bigelow's work that the duration of a single sitting to remove a stone of less than two drachms was an hour, and for one of less than three drachms an hour and a half! Now, as already stated, the utmost time I ever devote to such stones, and with my small light instruments, amounts to twelve or eighteen minutes, but in two or three sittings of five or six minutes each, all comprised within a period of seven to ten days.

"But I am free to confess that the proposal to remove a large hard stone at one sitting is an attractive one. So far from opposing it, I am predisposed to regard favourably any plan by which we may hope to take away, once and for all, the hard and angular fragments which must remain, and sometimes to a considerable extent, after an incompleted sitting. I fully agree with Bigelow that their presence constitutes the chief source of mischief in lithotrity as mostly practised. I only fear whether we may not, *by adopting the system under consideration*, pay too high a price for the purpose of attaining the end proposed. And, in reference to this, I am bound to say that my own system has for a long time past been gradually inclining to the practice of crushing more calculus at a sitting and removing more débris by the aspirator than I formerly did. Thus I have, during two years at least, been in the habit of using in every case two lithotrites alternately (my comparatively small, but strong, flat-bladed instruments) ; handing the first, when withdrawn, full of débris, to my assistant, who cleans it out completely while I am crushing with the other, which in its turn is cleaned and again used. Each is probably introduced three times at least, while clogging of the blades with débris is prevented by the cleaning process. With these light and handy instruments, which pass with the utmost facility, employed in this manner, and followed by the aspirator, I am quite certain that I can remove calculous matter from the bladder more safely and much more rapidly than with the enormous and unwieldy instruments referred to.

"I have, moreover, taken a hint from Bigelow's aspirator, and, slightly modifying Mr. Clover's original instrument, have, I think, rendered the latter more powerful and perfect, while I have avoided some material disadvantages attaching to the former. The new one, in fact, combines the best qualities of both. Thus I have greatly shortened the channel between the bladder and the aspirator, by getting rid altogether of the long arched tube which enters the top of the American instrument, and making the end of the evacuating catheter enter directly, without curve, at the bottom ; so saving many inches of the route which has to be traversed by fragments. The new instrument is very easily filled with water, its action is extremely powerful, no air can possibly enter during the process of using it, and the amount of débris withdrawn is at once taken out of the current, and remains undisturbed and visible to the operator throughout the proceeding. I am quite satisfied with evacuating catheters No. 16 in size, English scale (No. 26, French) ; larger than those are mostly dangerous and wholly unnecessary. There should be several of them, with openings and curves of different kinds, one variety acting better for one patient and another for another.

"But there is a direction for the successful use of the aspirator which Bigelow in his detailed instructions regarding that matter has not alluded to. And I do not hesitate to say that the recognition of the fact I refer to is not less important than all the information which can be obtained by observing the action of the aspirator-currents on fragments in an artificial bag, or even in a human bladder after death, useful to a certain extent as I admit that to be.

"I contend that a very important rule in employing any aspirator, in order to insure the minimum of risk with the maximum of efficiency, is strictly to subordinate its action to the respiratory movements of the patient, especially when these are full and deep, as they are apt to be sometimes under the influence of ether. When the respiration is light and tranquil, the rule is less important. Whatever the position in which you may place your instrument, for effective use it is desirable to make the exit of the fluid from the bladder coincide with the act of inspiration by the patient, since the effect of a full expansion of the lungs is as powerful to remove débris from the bladder as is the exhausting force of the India-rubber ball itself. In illustration, how often has one observed, when an open silver catheter is lying in the bladder of a supine patient, that a jet of urine is propelled to a considerable distance by a full act of inspiration. In using the aspirator, then, I let every movement of the hand holding the India-rubber ball conform to the action of respiration, filling the bladder with the patient's expiration, and gaining the force of his inspiratory effort by simultaneously permitting the expansion of the exhausting ball. Indeed, it is only safe (under ether) to inject the bladder during expiration, while the aspirator is only continuously productive during inspiration. By practice the hand of the operator and the respiratory efforts of the patient work together so harmoniously that, as with myself from long habit, it becomes almost impossible for them to act otherwise. It may be as well to add that the short quick act of expiration which constitutes "cough" is, on the contrary, a powerful expelling agent, and when it occurs, as it not unfrequently does under ether, should always be associated with relaxed grasp on the aspirator, and consequent outflowing current.

"Since writing the above, I removed, on Jan. 21, 1879, a hard uric acid calculus, in a sitting of eight minutes, with the two light lithotrites, in the manner described above, and with the aspirator, the débris weighing, when dried, two drachms—a weight exceeding that of the calculus reported by Bigelow as occupying one hour for its removal with his instruments. The patient, aged sixty-nine years, was brought to me by Mr. Lathbury, of Finsbury, who was present, as were also Mr. Clover, who gave ether, and two other medical men. The bladder was entirely cleared ; scarcely any blood was seen ; no fever followed, and the patient is doing extremely well. I regard this example as an admirable illustration of the capability of the existing lithotrites and of the existing method ; the application of the latter, I am ready to confess, having been extended in point of time beyond the limit which I formerly considered prudent or practicable, and which I still consider to be so only in tolerably practised hands."

At a late meeting of the New York Pathological Society (Med. Record, March 15, 1879), Dr. KEYES exhibited four vesical calculi which he had removed by Bigelow's method, and he stated that he had now performed thirteen operations by this method, and it seemed to him that each additional operation, each increase of experience in its performance was an argument in favour of the method. He had not had a fatal case, and believed that Bigelow's method would be the one which would supersede all others for the removal of vesical calculi. In conclusion he called attention to the fact that difficulty was sometimes experienced in removing air from the bladder when it had been accidentally introduced from the wash-bottle. He had accidentally discovered that by turning the bottle upside down the water rushed in, displaced the air at once, and the latter appeared at the bottom (now top) of the bottle above the water. The bottle then had to be refilled before washing was recommenced.

One advantage to be derived from the use of Bigelow's admirable washing-bottle was stated to be the facility with which the existence of small fragments of stone in the bladder could be detected during the washing by combining ausculta-tion with the washing. The sharp click of the little fragments against the cathe-ter as the water rushed in and out was very distinct. Dr. Keyes had used this method in place of ordinary sounding where a very small stone was suspected. He did not believe the necessity for using very large tubes existed. He had never used any tube larger than 30 French, the average being 27 French, 18 American scale. In over one-fourth of the cases there was no disturbance whatever follow-ing the operation, not even a chill. The average duration was three-fourths of an hour. Some patients had been subjected to it who would have died had they been operated upon by the usual methods.

——

Orchitis in Typhoid Fever.

Dr. V. HANOT (Archives Générales de Médicine, November, 1878, p. 595) gives an account of a case of orchitis, which occurred during the course of an attack of typhoid in a patient under the care of Dr. Lasègue, in La Pitié Hospital.

The man, æt. 21, was admitted on August 19, 1878, suffering from typhoid. On August 25th (the sixteenth day of the fever) the patient complained of violent pain in the right groin and testicle, which had come on during the preceding night, and had prevented sleep. On examination, the scrotum was seen to be slightly tense and reddened ; the right testis somewhat swollen, harder than the left, and painful on pressure ; the epididymis was intact and painless, and the cord unaffected. There was no fluid in the tunica vaginalis. None of the ordi-nary causes of orchitis could be made out. On August 26th the testis was as before, but the pain was less. On the 27th the testis had slightly diminished in size, and the scrotum had become normal. On September 3d all traces of the orchitis had disappeared. On the 14th the patient was convalescent from typhoid fever, but the right testis had manifestly decreased in volume.

Some particulars of three other cases of affection of the testis and epididymis during typhoid are also given by Dr. Hanot. These cases occurred in the Hôpital Cochin, under the care of Dr. Bucquoy, in 1872 and 1873.—London Med. Record, Dec. 15, 1878.

——

Causes and Treatment of Phagedœna.

In the Presse Médicale Belge, Nov. 10, 1878, Professor THIRY's views on chancrous phagedæna are referred to in connection with the report of a case lately under his care in the Hôpital Saint-Pierre. Thiry considers that phagedæna is not due to any particular constitutional state, nor is it related to gangrene. It is purely local, and results from increased activity of the virus accidentally set up during the evolutions of the sore. This increased activity is, according to Thiry, due to one or other of the following three causes, viz., 1. More or less intense inflammation of the base and periphery of the chancre ; 2. Exaggerative sensibility of the chancre ; 3. A torpid state of, or want of vitality in, the chancre. The varieties of phagedæna are accordingly arranged as follows : 1. Phagedæna from excess of inflammation ; 2. Phagedæna from excess of sensibility ; 3. Torpid or atonic phagedæna. The gravity of the case will depend upon the extent to which either of the three causes is in operation.

The treatment recommended differs somewhat according to the nature of the sore. While methodical cauterization is necessary in all, the subsequent dressing in the first form should consist in soothing fomentations and regular compression; in the second, or irritable variety, preparations of opium or morphine should be applied, combined with gentle pressure; in the third, or atonic form, a solution of tartrate of iron is most useful.

As a caustic, Thiry speaks very highly of an ointment compound of 2 grammes (30 grains) of cyanide of mercury to 10 grammes (150 grains) of lard.

A male, aged 25, was admitted into Saint-Pierre on June 17, 1878, with a spreading phagedenic chancre of the atonic variety. The sore had been in existence for four months; it commenced at the frænum, and on admission had perforated and almost wholly destroyed the prepuce. There was no syphilitic induration. The treatment consisted in deep cauterization of the whole ulcer on eight consecutive days, and the application of a solution of tartrate of iron four times daily. The penis was bandaged and kept up on the abdomen. After eight days, the aspect of the ulcer was almost that of a simple sore. The healing process soon became general, and the patient was discharged from the hospital cured, at the end of July.—*London Med. Record*, Dec. 15, 1878.

—

Distal Deligation of the Carotid and Subclavian Arteries for Innominate Aneurism.

At a late meeting of the Royal Medical and Chirurgical Society (*Lancet*, Dec. 14, 1878) Mr. BARWELL read a paper on three cases of distal deligation of the carotid and subclavian arteries for innominate aneurism, of which the following is an abstract :—

After referring to a case of innominate aneurism which he had successfully treated by double distal deligation, and which is published in the Transactions of the present year, the author related the case of J. B., a man aged forty-eight, who died from the effects of the anæsthetics thirty hours after the operation. The parts, showing very large aorto-innominate aneurism, were exhibited. The operation was performed on Dec. 6, 1877. On that day Mr. Barwell also tied the same vessels for Laura G., aged thirty-seven, who had a pulsating aneurismal tumour perforating the upper anterior wall of the chest on the right side, and also above the clavicle. Except for the aneurism, the patient appeared healthy, but extremely nervous and excitable. After the operation no brain symptoms were developed nor any pyrexia, but her progress was fluctuating, the variations appearing to be in part connected with the catamenial period, in part with her mental condition. The patient left the hospital in July, having no tumour, though pulsation from the solidified aneurism communicated by the aorta could still be felt. On January 10, 1878, Mr. Barwell tied the same vessels for Catherine H., aged twenty-seven, who had a visible pulsating tumour, about the size of a small walnut, above and a little outside the sterno-clavicular joint, and also intra-thoracic aneurism. This patient, rather feeble and extremely nervous, also made a fluctuating recovery. She had no cerebral symptoms and no pyrexia. She left the hospital on July 22, a tumour remaining in the above situation, and though probably not quite, yet is nearly (Mr. Barwell believes) solid. The cough and dyspnœa, from which she had previously suffered, have quite disappeared. After some remarks concerning the excitability of the vaso-motor system, which in these patients always accompanied the menstrual period, the author gave his views concerning the use of catgut as a ligature, and stated his belief that with such material it is advisable to tie the vessels with very moderate force, so as not to divide the middle coat. He attributes his success to this mode of tying. The statistics of these operations are as follows : Including the subjects of the present paper eleven cases in all have been thus treated ; of these eight have been unsuccessful, all of them dying at various periods from the effects either of the aneurism or of the operation. The case Mr. Barwell recorded last year and the two now related constitute the three successful ones.

Mr. CHRISTOPHER HEATH said he believed the case upon which he operated in 1865 was the first—at any rate, within recent times—in which double distal ligature was practised. Mr. Barwell was right in not including it in his list of cases, for although thought to involve the innominate artery at the time of operation, when, four years subsequently, the post-mortem examination was made the aneurism was found to be wholly aortic. At the same time it was a perfectly successful case, the patient's death being due to his intemperate habits, the aneurism bursting externally. (The preparation is in the museum of the College of Surgeons.) So much did that case resemble the case of the older of the two female patients shown by Mr. Barwell that Mr. Heath ventured to predict that in her case also the aneurism was mainly, if not entirely, aortic, and not innominate. The sphygmographic tracing did not show the characters of an innominate aneurism, and he believed that vessel was but slightly, if at all, involved. He had seen the case before operation, and would testify to the great benefit received by it, the chest having notably sunk in. In the other case the persistence of pulsation below the seat of ligature in the carotid was remarkable and difficult of explanation, but here also much benefit seemed to have been derived. Speaking of the catgut ligature, Mr. Heath could not think it possible, in an operation of such magnitude, to regulate the force with which it should be tied to the nicety insisted on by Mr. Barwell. Indeed, he thought it better that the coats should be divided than that the risk of imperfect ligature should be run ; and in a case he brought before the Clinical Society last year, where a second ligature had to be applied, owing to the failure of the first, he believed this failure was due to the fact that he had not pulled the ligature tight enough. He held to the hempen ligature as being more secure and more likely to divide the coats of the vessel efficiently.

Mr. HOLMES agreed with Mr. Heath as to the difficulty in diagnosing between innominate and aortic aneurism. The only case in which he had performed the distal ligature with satisfactory results was one of aortic aneurism, beyond the innominate, in which he tied the left carotid. The patient's condition before operation was most critical, but the result of the treatment was that now—five years after—she is in health and pursuing her work. (The case is to be found in the Clinical Society's Transactions, vol. ix. p. 114, and vol. x. p. 97.) He could not see how ligature of the subclavian could do good, for if, when tied in the third part, the vessel became occluded, how was the circulation carried on in the limb ? Such complete occlusion did appear to have taken place in Mr. Barwell's first case read before the Society a year ago, but still the difficulty remained to account for the collateral supply. In the two cases shown that evening it was evident that a great part of the subclavian was pervious, for the circulation was well carried on in the limb. Indeed, à priori, he would think that the circulation would even be increased in the unobliterated part of the vessel. There is in the museum of St. George's Hospital an instructive preparation of the spontaneous cure of an aortic aneurism. The patient was a sailor, and the aneurism was a large one. He was attacked with hemiplegia, and from that time the aneurism began to consolidate, so that when he died (from some intercurrent disease), some years after, the carotid was found entirely blocked, but a small channel was left through the aneurism by which the subclavian circulation had been kept up. Believing, then, that, save under very exceptional circumstances, the circulation through the sub-clavian must go on, he could not but regard ligature of that vessel as a hindrance rather than a help to the formation of clot in the sac. The best plan would be ligature of the carotid artery only, the coagulation extending downwards from that vessel into the aneurism. One of Mr. Barwell's cases presented pulsation above the clavicle, as if the carotid had not been completely plugged; but possibly, as Mr. Barwell suggested, this pulsation was transmitted from below. He agreed with Mr. Heath that a catgut ligature should be tied as tightly as a hempen one, there being more risk from tying it loosely than from division of both the inner and middle coats, and a case he had recorded showed that the catgut remains on the artery for some time after its application. Cases had occurred where, after the vessel had been tied with catgut, the circulation had been re-established, and in such cases possibly the ligature had been tied less lightly than habitually. He congratulated Mr. Barwell upon his success, and thought his cases would give a great impetus to the operation of distal ligature.—Mr. HEATH pointed out that Mr. Holmes's case entered into a different category from those under consideration, for in that case the ligature was applied to the *left* carotid.— Mr. HOLMES said although the cases were different the process of cure was the same —viz., extension of coagulation from the obliterated carotid into the aneurism from which the artery springs.

Mr. KELBURNE KING (Hull) said his reason for tying both vessels in his case, which had been referred to by Mr. Barwell (see THE LANCET, vol. i. 1878, p. 823), was that the pulsation in both carotid and subclavian was very strong, and he did not think ligature of the carotid alone could possibly be enough. The patient survived one hundred and eleven days, and the large aneurism (aortic and innominate) was found filled with coagulum, which extended into the subclavian as far as the seat of ligature. He believed that for a time the collateral circulation was carried on through the subclavian branches, and that the clot extended into the trunk of the vessel at some period subsequent to the ligature. If he had to do the same operation again, he could not with any satisfaction apply the liga-ture to one vessel without also applying it to the other.

Mr. BARWELL, in reply, said that the persistence of pulsation below the seat of ligature on the carotid in the younger patient had been a source of anxiety to him; but he thought it possibly due to the presence of a channel of blood behind the main clot in the sac, and he had little doubt that it would eventually consoli-date. He would keep the case in view. Mr. Heath's case was undoubtedly the first successful instance recorded of double distal ligature; and although his own case (that of the elder woman) might be aortic, yet he thought the manner in which the tumour rose above the clavicle and into the episternal notch proved it to be largely innominate in origin. He did not think that ligature of the left carotid for aneurism of the arch, as mentioned by Mr. Holmes, could be compared to the distal operation for innominate aneurism, whence two large streams of blood were flowing, the larger being that going through the subclavian. According to Mr. Holmes's view, occlusion of the smaller of these two streams would suffice. Mr. Erichsen had argued the question, and decided in favour of the ligature of both vessels. He (Mr. Barwell) thought Mr. Holmes went too far in stating that ligature of the subclavian in the third part would increase the stream on the car-diac side of the ligature. Surely it must decrease it; and their main object was to diminish the force of the current in the aneurism. It was true that in the case he brought forward last year the subclavian was found to be occluded, and he con-fessed his inability to explain how the circulation had been carried on in the limb. But he believed that the longer collateral circulation was delayed, the more chance

there was of the cure of the aneurism; for in the case in which some months
elapsed before the pulse returned in the radial artery, the result was more satisfactory than in the one where the radial pulsation returned rather rapidly.   He
would even go further, if he dared, and apply an Esmarch's bandage to the limb,
with a view to prevent for a time free circulation through it, and thus promote
stagnation in the aneurismal sac.   As to the mode of ligature, it was a matter of
indifference whether the inner coat were divided or not, but division of the
stronger middle coat should, he thought, if possible, be avoided.   In using the
silk ligature there was always a risk of secondary hemorrhage occurring when it
separated, adhesions only preventing this, whereas the catgut was left on the vessel.
His plan was to tighten the ligature sufficiently to arrest pulsation beyond, then
to stretch it a little beyond this to allow for slipping, and then to tie the second
knot; and he believed that cases of return of pulsation after ligature by catgut
were not due to the ligature being too loosely tied, but in consequence of the second
knot slipping.   The risk of such slipping of the knot was one objection to catgut,
which varies very much in quality, and he was at present engaged in devising
some material for ligatures which should not divide the coats too much, and yet
be capable of being tied with a firm knot.

—

*On Hydrarthrosis and Arthritis of the Knee, consecutive to Lymphangitis of the
Lower Limb.*

Prof. VERNEUIL, Surgeon to the Pitié Hospital, draws attention (*Lancet*,
Jan. 4, 1879) to a variety of affections of the joints, which he does not believe has
yet been described, but which cannot be very rare, as in his single practice he has
met with it five times.   He thus describes it : I mean the propagation to the
synovial membrane of the knee-joint of a superficial inflammation, originating in
the subcutaneous lymphatic *réseau*, and assuming the form of lymphangitis of the
large vessels, or that of erysipelas.   Owing to the precision and the distinct
character of its etiology, and the gravity of its prognosis, I consider that this
variety merits special mention.

First, I will give a brief summary of my five cases.

Some twenty years ago I was called by one of my colleagues to see a patient
living in the neighbourhood of Paris.   He was a merchant, fifty years of age,
much broken down by excesses of all sorts, and had been obliged to remain in
bed for a fortnight on account of lymphangitis of the leg.   The mischief had
begun by a small excoriation of one of the toes which had become irritated by
walking.   The inflammatory accident had developed suddenly, the limb was
covered with red streaks, and a certain number of small superficial abscesses had
formed around the inflamed lymphatic vessels.   When I saw the patient several
of these abscesses had already been opened, but there remained many more ready
for incising, and others in course of formation.   Two of these collections were of
the size of a large olive, and were situated on the internal aspect of the knee.
I incised them obliquely, and let out a considerable quantity of phlegmonous pus.
I adopted the same treatment with the other collections, which were situated on
the leg and thigh.   On subsequent days other incisions became necessary ; nevertheless, matters seemed to be progressing as favourably as the debilitated condition of the patient would permit, when suddenly the knee became the seat of
violent pain and considerable tumefaction.   These new symptoms had begun on
the inside of the knee, round the spot where I had opened the two abscesses a
week previously.   Purulent arthritis set in with great rapidity, in spite of every
means we could adopt.   Different operations, including amputation, were proposed to the patient, but all were declined.   The general condition became worse

and worse, and the unfortunate patient died three weeks after the articulation had suppurated.

The second case came to my knowledge a few years later, and was that of a girl fourteen years of age. The patient was a slim, delicate, and nervous child. The nail of her big toe had fallen off after a contusion it had sustained, and a small collection had formed underneath, which opened spontaneously. Shortly afterwards diffused lymphangitis covered the whole limb. The swelling soon subsided, but several circumscribed collections were formed successively. The doctor attending the case incised these little abscesses, amongst which was one situated on the inside of the knee. On the next day the patient complained of pain in her knee, which was swollen. I was called in, and believed at the time that the articulation had been opened. Purulent arthritis followed its course in spite of all we could do. The pus diffused into the thigh, the leg, and the popliteal space, the ganglions of the groin began to suppurate, and a purulent collection formed in the iliac fossa. I proposed amputation of the thigh, but the family refused all active intervention, and the child died after three months' incessant suffering.

A man, forty-eight years of age, very thin, and of a cachectic appearance, came under the care of my friend, M. Oulmont, at the Hopital Lariboisière, for an acute malady presenting all the symptoms of typhoid fever. During the course of the disease a gangrenous patch formed on the dorsal aspect of the right foot, and when this fell one could see the tendons and ligaments of that region as well as some of the metatarsal bones. It was in that condition the patient was passed into my wards. I tried to improve the general health, and at the same time cleansed the wound, which had rather an ugly appearance. The patient was making slow progress when suddenly he had a rigor accompanied with vomiting and a high temperature. Shortly after traces of lymphangitis were to be seen starting from the wound on the foot. The red streaks were distinctly visible on the anterior and internal aspects of the leg, inside of the knee, and all along the course of the femoral vessels in the thigh. Rest, emollients, and mercurial frictions were ordered along the inflamed parts, and soon afterwards all the mischief disappeared except near the knee, where some lymphatic vessels became more and more swollen, and finally gave rise to a badly circumscribed phlegmon occupying the whole internal aspect of the joint. The articulation remained healthy for a while, but two days after, just as I was about to incise the phlegmon, the inflammation was communicated to the synovial membrane. I thought at first that it was only a simple hydrarthrosis, owing to the neighbouring inflammation, but when I had incised the abscess I found that the contents of the articulation, also composed of purulent matter, poured through the cutaneous incision. This complication supervening in a man already worn out, and who was passing a quantity of albumen in his urine, rendered the case hopeless. With much regret I proposed amputation, but this was refused, and the patient died at the end of eighteen days. The post-mortem examination showed a strongly injected synovial membrane, destroyed cartilages, and the spongy tissue of the bones exposed. The ligaments were softened and ruptured.

I met with the fourth case in 1869, whilst I was at the Lariboisière Hospital. A man, thirty years of age, who had always enjoyed good health, though of a rather sickly appearance, came under my care in the month of December for an extensive swelling of the foot and leg of some days' standing. The symptoms were those of phlegmonous erysipelas, and began around an ulceration which had been caused by a badly-fitting boot. The temperature was very high, the abdomen distended, the tongue dry, there was intense thirst—in fact, the general condition was very unsatisfactory. Rest, elevation of the limb, mercurial fric-

tions, purging, and sulphate of quinia, ameliorated this state, and all that remained was a phlegmon of the big toe, which opened spontaneously near the
interphalangeal articulation.   At the end of a few days the patient was able to
walk about the ward. This improvement did not last long. Without any known
cause the general symptoms suddenly returned, and the limb became again
swollen, but this time as high up as the groin. The knee became extremely
painful, considerably aggravated by the slightest touch or movement. It was
easy to see that arthritis had set in, complicating the erysipelatous swelling. An
appropriate treatment caused the swelling of the limb again to disappear, but the
knee still remained enlarged and fluctuating, being manifestly affected with hydrarthrosis.   Blisters were applied round the joint, and the fluid diminished a
little in quantity ; but the general condition of the patient remained unaltered,
the temperature continued high, and soon an eschar formed over the sacrum,
while an attack of pneumonia of septic nature came on and caused a fatal termination of the case in the latter part of February.   At the post-mortem examination a large quantity of serous fluid, slightly clouded with pus, was found in
the articulation.

My last case occurred at the beginning of the year 1878.   A tall, thin, sickly-
looking man, about sixty years of age, came under my care for subacute hydrarthrosis of the right knee of two or three days' standing, which gave him a little
pain and caused him to limp.   On examining the limb, I saw on the dorsal aspect
of one of the toes a slight wound covered with a crust, and also an œdematous
swelling of the leg, with two or three red fluctuating spots ; on the inside of the
knee were two lymphatic abscesses, typical in nature.   My diagnosis was hydrarthrosis following on lymphangitis.   This last-named affection had disappeared,
and only left the circumscribed abscesses ; but, on questioning the patient, we
found that about ten days previously his leg had suddenly become swollen, painful. and streaked with red lines.   These symptoms had been accompanied by
malaise, fever, and rigors.   I placed the limb in an apparatus, opened the three
little abscesses of the leg, and contented myself with painting the two situated
inside the knee with tincture of iodine.   In a week these two collections disappeared, as did also the hydrarthrosis, and the following week the patient left for
the convalescent home at Vincennes.

The five cases I have related present the greatest analogy one with the other.
A small wound on the foot is the commencement ; then, in four instances, lymphangitis of the large vessels takes place, with formation of circumscribed abscesses ; and in the fifth case we have a kind of phlegmonous erysipelas very
much resembling diffused lymphangitis.   With the exception of the little girl,
who was rather sickly, the patients were all anæmic, weak, and of a poor appearance, consequently would be favourable subjects for diffused inflammations.
In each case where we were called upon to watch the invasion of arthritis, we
remarked that the symptoms came on very suddenly, and with great intensity.
In three cases the arthritis was purulent from the beginning ; in the two others
the fluid remained serous or scro-purulent.   In four cases arthritis was preceded
by lymphangitis and the formation of circumscribed abscesses.   In the fifth case
the articulation seemed to become affected at the same time as the leg became
tumefied.

Several conjectures may be made upon the mode of transmission of the inflammation.   One may suppose, for instance, that the lymphatic vessels coming from
the synovial membrane and opening into the larger vessels become inflamed from
their termination down to their point of origin in the synovial membrane.   This
mode of propagation is met with in superficial lymphangitis of the limbs.   It
may also be conjectured that, as the subcutaneous lymphatics are only separated

from those contained in the synovial membrane by a thin layer of fibrous tissue, the inflammation forced that barrier. There is no reason to doubt the possibility of the opening of one of the lymphatic abscesses into the articulation. The purulent arthritis continues its course, which is more rapid if the patient is in a debilitated condition. It is thus that the death of the first three patients is accounted for, having refused all operative interferences which might possibly have saved their lives. Hydrarthrosis naturally offers much less cause of apprehension, and in our last case we saw it disappear very rapidly. The diagnosis is generally easy, for it will always be possible to recognize the lymphangitis or the initial abscesses.

I have little to say about the treatment. The only lesson to be gained from these cases as to the treatment is that lymphangitis situated on the inside of the knee should arrest special attention. Early incisions are also, I believe, an advantage.

As yet all my cases have had reference to the knee-joint, but I am quite ready to admit that other articulations may become the seat of similar affections.

—

On Cataplasms in Arthritis.

Dr. DIEULAFOY, in an article inserted in the *Gaz. Hebdomadaire* for November 29, observes that a considerable number of cases of inflammation of the joints pass into the chronic condition. Among scrofulous and lymphatic subjects, persons having gonorrhœa, and in women during the puerperal condition, arthritis has a great tendency to assume the chronic form. The disease, it is true, rarely goes on to a white swelling or an anchylosis, but, without attaining this extremity, a chronic arthritis may last months or years, entailing all the well-known ill consequences. For such arthrites the most varied treatment has been employed. Internally, cod-liver oil and preparations of arsenic or iodine have been given, while locally blistering or cauterization, according to the case, has been resorted to, the limbs having been rendered immovable by some form of apparatus; and, thanks to these various means, used separately or in combination, good results are generally obtained. Trousseau, who had so fertile an imagination for therapeutical procedures, was in the habit of resorting to an application in these cases, the efficacy of which Dr. Dieulafoy has had frequent opportunities of witnessing both under Trousseau and in his own cases. This consists in the employment of a cataplasm, the description of which requires to be detailed.

According to the size of the joint, from one and a half to two kilogrammes of bread (two kilogrammes being required for the knee-joint, and one sufficing for the wrist) are to be cut up into pieces, care being taken to remove the hard portions of the crust; and these pieces are to be steeped in water for about a quarter of an hour. By this time the bread is strongly imbibed with water, and a portion of this is to be pressed out by means of a cloth or napkin, so as to leave the bread merely in a moist state. So prepared, the bread is placed in a water-bath (*bain-marie*), where it should remain three hours; and when it is taken out it forms a kind of dry paste, which is to be moistened gradually by the addition of spirit of camphor. This mass is to be kneaded for about five minutes until it has acquired the tolerably firm consistence of "plum-pudding," or of glazier's putty. Here, indeed, is the delicate part in the preparation of the cataplasm, a firm consistence being essential; for if it is too soft it will become too diffused by the compression exerted over the joint, while if too hard it ceases to be homogeneous, breaking up into fragments, the indurated portions irritating the skin. The attainment of this consistence must be very carefully attended to, the tendency of those unaccustomed to the preparation of the cataplasm always being to make it too soft, either because they have not sufficiently pressed the water out of the bread before placing it in the bath, or that they have poured over it too rapidly too much of the camphorated spirit. The poultice thus prepared is to be spread upon a piece of cloth, the shape of an elongated rectangle, of a sufficient size to allow of the entire joint being enveloped in it. It is desirable that the edges of the cataplasm should be at least a centimetre in thickness, in order to avoid the rapid desiccation which takes place when the edges are thin. Over the surface of the cataplasm is spread a very liquid mixture, composed of camphor seven grammes, extract of opium and extract of belladonna of each five grains, and alcohol *q. s.* It is to be applied direct to the joint, and covered with oiled silk. The whole is fixed, and a somewhat energetic compression is exerted by means of a flannel bandage several metres in length, a calico bandage of the same length being applied over the flannel one, the length of these two bandages depending upon the dimensions of the cataplasm, which has to cover the entire joint; and, to prevent their detachment, the folds may be sewn together. The compression exerted must be considerable, but not to the extent of producing œdema. So applied, the bandage should remain on eight or ten days, and, on its being then removed, it is found to be as fresh, moist, and pleasant-smelling as when first put on, the skin upon which it has reposed being in a perfectly healthy state. The price of the cataplasm (six francs, and three in hospitals) may seem an objection to its employment; but this ceases to have any value when it is considered that the application remains *in situ* for at least a week.

The indications for its employment need not be specified beyond saying that in all chronic or subacute arthrites, whatever may be their nature or cause, when other means have failed, or before these have been employed, Trousseau's cataplasm may render the highest service. Dr. Dieulafoy has already published several cases proving this, and concludes this communication with two others. The duration of the treatment necessary varies frequently; a single application will not always suffice, and a second or third, or even a fourth, may be required; the treatment thus, even in obstinate cases, not exceeding a month in duration. Of course the local treatment does not exclude the employment of general remedies.—*Med. Times and Gazette*, Dec. 21, 1878.

A very rare Case of Intra-Capsular Fracture of the Neck of the Femur with Great Flexion, Abduction, and Inversion of the Limb.

Dr. WILLIAM PIRRIE, Professor of Surgery in the University of Aberdeen, records (*Lancet*, January 4, 1879) the following case.

Widow M., a thin, pale, weakly-looking woman, eighty years of age, was admitted into one of my wards in the Aberdeen Royal Infirmary on Monday, the 14th of October last, having sustained a severe fall on the lower part of her back and right hip, caused by tripping on a door mat and falling upon a bare hard floor. the accident having happened two days previous to her entrance into the hospital.

The patient was admitted at the conclusion of the visit on Monday, and stated to me on Tuesday, that since the occurrence of the accident she had suffered intense pain in the region of the right hip, that the limb had remained immovable in the same position, and that her urine and feces had been passing off involuntarily.

Before bringing the patient under the influence of chloroform, with the view of making a thorough examination, I observed that she could only lie on her back inclined to the left side, with the right thigh so much flexed, adducted, and inverted, that her right knee lay high up in the left lumbar region, that the outer aspect of the thigh looked directly forwards, and that it was necessary to support the right foot by means of a pillow in order to prevent its falling down and thus

rotating the thigh outwards, which caused excruciating pain at the hip-joint.
From the lower part of her back and posterior aspect of the right hip a portion of
skin about the size of the hand had been removed by the fall, and a black, gangrenous slough had formed on the denuded part. When the examination had
proceeded thus far, I thought that this case was probably an example of that
peculiar dislocation of the hip-joint described by Bigelow, and delineated by fig.
13, page 63, of his most interesting work on " Dislocations and Fractures of the
Hip-joint," a copy of which figure is here inserted. The patient having been

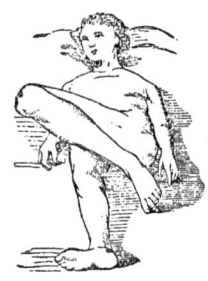

brought under the influence of chloroform, I easily
traced with my finger the outline of the trochanter
major, and found that its upper border was directed
downwards and backwards. I could not discover the
ball of the femur, and therefore came to the conclusion
that it remained in the acetabulum. On rotation of the
thigh, the trochanter major did not describe the segment
of a circle, as in a dislocation, but was observed to re-
volve on its own axis, as in fracture of the neck of the
thigh-bone, and during rotation slight crepitation was
elicited. From the above symptoms I was convinced
that this was a case of fracture of the neck of the femur
with flexion, adduction, and inversion of the limb, a
variety of fracture not hitherto described, as far as my reading has enabled me to
judge. Having formed this opinion, I reduced the fracture by taking hold of the
knee with one hand and the foot with the other, by placing the leg at a right angle
to the thigh, by abducting, rotating outwards, and bringing down the limb by the
side of the other—in short, reduction was accomplished by practising the last three
movements adopted by Bigelow for reduction of dislocation of the head of the
femur on the dorsum of the ilium. When the limb was thus brought into proper
position, it exhibited no tendency to eversion or inversion, and there was scarcely
any appreciable shortening.

For the first twenty-four hours following reduction the affected extremity was
kept at rest by placing a long sand bag by the side of the patient's trunk and limb,
and afterwards by applying to the outer side of her pelvis, thigh, leg, and foot a
long splint, composed of long.broad bandages charged with plaster-of-Paris, and
moulded into the shape of a Desault's splint. The test-line of the ilio-femoral
triangle, shown by Bryant to be so valuable for enabling the surgeon to arrive
without excessive manipulation at a reliable diagnosis in fractures of the neck of
the thigh-bone and Nélaton's test-line for dislocation of the head of the femur
backwards, were not available in this case, owing to the extraordinary position of
the femur ; but the already described symptoms produced a decided conviction in
my mind that the case was one of fracture of the neck of the thigh-bone with the
limb in a position which I had never before seen in any example of that injury,
and the post-mortem examination made six weeks after the reduction of the fracture proved that my diagnosis was correct.

From the moment that the limb was made straight the patient remained perfectly free from pain in the hip, but frequently complained of pain in the knee,
which was perfectly sound. This pain was chiefly seated within and at the inner
side of the joint—a symptom so common in morbus coxæ, sometimes misleading
an unwary surgeon, but rarely, if ever, met with in injuries of the hip-joint,
judging from my own experience. If the conditions in which this symptomatic
pain is experienced be disease at the filamentous terminations of one branch of a
nerve, and the pain reflected to the terminations of another branch of the same
nerve, conditions furnished by the anterior branch of the obdurator nerve sup-

plying the hip, and the posterior branch of the knee-joint, it is difficult to understand why the symptomatic pain is experienced so severely and frequently at the knee in disease, and so rarely, if ever, in painful accidents, of the hip-joint.

Six weeks after the application of the plaster-of-Paris bandage-splint, and three days before the death of the patient, the splint was removed, and the limb remained straight, without any tendency to eversion or inversion, and there was no appreciable shortening.

Notwithstanding the occasional and unavoidable contact of urine with the denuded surface on the patient's back, which was covered with a large gangrenous slough on her admission, by the application of turpentine, carbolic, and other dressings, and the removal of all pressure by means of a water-pillow ring filled with air, the slough eventually was removed, and granulations made some advancement; but these attempts at healing were fruitless, owing to the great weakness and age of the patient. The weakening effects of this large sore, together with amyloid degeneration of the kidney, caused death fifty days after the occurrence of the injury.

The post-mortem examination was conducted by Dr. Rodger, pathologist to the Aberdeen Royal Infirmary, who found that the capsular and ilio-femoral ligaments were perfectly entire, the latter being thicker and stronger than usual ; that the neck of the femur was fractured close to the ball of the bone, the plane of the fracture being at a right angle to the long axis of the neck : that the outer fragment was considerably shortened, débris occupying the plane of the fracture ; that there were no bands uniting the fractured surfaces to one another, and that there was no effusion into the joint, and no signs of the inflammatory process. The round ligament was perfectly entire, showing that the ball of the bone had never left the cavity of the acetabulum.

I believe that the integrity and tension of the ilio-femoral ligament was the cause of the adduction, flexion, and inversion of the limb, and that by its causing the centre of the motion to be situated at its attachments to the anterior intertrochanteric line of the femur was the explanation of the facility with which the outer fragment was returned into its proper position by the manipulation of the limb.

Of the one hundred and thirty cases of intra-scapular fracture of the neck of the thigh-bone which have come under my notice, and where the accuracy of diagnosis was verified by dissection, this is the only case I know of with flexion, adduction, and rotation inwards of the limb. Of the remaining number, in one case only have I met with rotation inwards ; the limb in other respects occupying the usual straight position. I watched that case of intra-capsular fracture with inversion during life, and had an opportunity of verifying the diagnosis after death, and have been for many years in the habit of exhibiting the preparation to the students of surgery in the University of Aberdeen.

——

Nerve Stretching.

Two cases of nerve stretching were reported by DUPLAY at a meeting of the *Societe de Chirurgie* (December 6, 1878). A man, aged 29, two months before he came under notice, was wounded in front of the forearm with a knife. The wound had healed, but it was found that the muscles supplied by the radial and median nerves were paralyzed ; the skin of the forearm, at some points, had lost its sensibility ; at others there was a degree of hyperæsthesia. Both nerves having been exposed by incision were found injected, as though slightly inflamed ; they were stretched. The next day sensibility in the affected parts was noted, the hyperæsthesia disappeared and the muscles were no longer paralyzed. There was no relapse into the former condition.   The second case was a man, aged 26, who some time before had been wounded in the wrist ; a cicatrix had formed just above the pisiform bone.   At this point a small fibrous patch existed, seeming to adhere to the flexor carpi ulnaris muscle, and being very painful on pressure. By means of an incision, it was found that the little tumour was in connection with the ulnar nerve, and after the nerve had been fully stretched the tumour disappeared.   The following morning the interossei muscles had regained their contractility, which before the operation had been absent, sensibility had reappeared, and the pain on pressure was no longer present.   Improvement continued, and only a slight degree of muscular atrophy existed when the patient left the hospital.—*Lond. Med. Record*, Jan. 15, 1879.

Midwifery and Gynæcology.

The Value of the Expression Method of Kristeller in Head Presentation.

This is the subject of a contribution by Prof. BIDDER, of St. Petersburg, in the *Zeitschrift für Gebertshülfe und Gynäkologie*, iii. band, 2 heft, 241.   The author strongly supports the advantage attainable from the method properly conducted, and thinks, in a great many cases it may replace the use of forceps, where there is simply a defect of expulsive power, without any other abnormality. He believes that the method is rejected by many obstetricians, because Kristeller advocated its use in the first stage, in which Bidder regards it as unsuitable, and also recommended the hand to be applied so as to produce pressure and friction both, whilst the only proper method is to apply pressure to the upper pole of the fœtus only.

Bidder looks upon the method as merely furnishing a certain amount of fœtal axis pressure, and therefore holds that it is only admissible during the second stage, when that force of the uterus naturally comes into play.   It should also consist in merely a steady push by one hand on the upper pole of the fœtus, care being taken, by rectification of the inclination of the uterus or otherwise, that the pressure is directed along the fœtal axis, and that the latter is kept normal during the pressure.

If any serious obstruction to the onward progress of the head is found to exist, such as an obstinate defect of rotation, the method should not be persisted in, in case pressure upon the placenta should asphyxiate the child, but the forceps, or other measures, must be employed.   It should be a steady pressure, and not a combination of pressure and friction.

Professor Bidder gives an account of a series of 81 cases in which it was successfully applied.   He does not regard it as likely to cause metritis or parametritis, and considers that it is much less likely to lead to septicæmia than forceps, inasmuch as it is less likely to lead to injury of the soft parts thus :—

Of the 81 cases delivered by the expression method, 34 went through the lying-in period with perfect health, 38 were the subjects of slight illness, 7 became seriously ill, and 2 died.

Comparing these results with 75 easy forceps cases, in which the instruments were applied to the head when it was quite at the floor of the pelvis, or even on the perineum, Bidder states that only 13 of the patients continued quite well, that 34 were slightly ill, 20 seriously so, and 8 died.

He considers the method applicable so soon as the head has passed the outer os and the membranes are ruptured, and does not think that it need be delayed till the head is distending the perineum and vulva.—*Edinburgh Med. Journ.*, Feb. 1879.

—

The Importance of Nephritis in Pregnancy.

This is the subject of an interesting paper by Dr. Hofmeir in the *Zeitschrift für Gebertshülfe und Gynäkologie* (Bd. iii. heft 2). According to the statistics of the Berlin University Gynækological Institution for $10\frac{1}{2}$ years, 137 cases of nephritis complicating pregnancy were noted out of a total of 5000 deliveries, or 2.74 per 100 cases. Regarding the results: Of these 137 cases the following tabulated summary is given—30 of the patients suffered from nephritis only, and of these 11 died, 22 were discharged alive, 2 were sufferers from the acute, and 31 from the chronic affection. Of the children, 20 were born dead, 15 were born alive, and in 2 the condition of the children is not stated. 104 of the patients suffered from both nephritis and eclampsia, and of these 41 died, 63 were discharged alive, 89 were sufferers from the acute affection, and 15 from the chronic affection. Of the children, 62 were born dead, 46 were born alive, and in 2 the result is wanting.

From these results Hofmeir argues that both for mother and child nephritis is a most serious complication in itself, even when it is uncomplicated with eclampsia. He is led to believe from his own observations, that the nephritis of pregnancy is much more liable to perpetuate itself in the form of chronic nephritis than is usually supposed. The author refrains from any attempt at explaining the special etiology of nephritis in relation to pregnancy, contenting himself with observing and accepting the fact that pregnancy does establish a special predisposition. Post-mortem examinations lead Hofmeir to agree with Virchow in holding that inflammation of the hepatic tissues is apt to be associated with the nephritis of pregnancy, thus showing that the kidney is not the only gland that is injuriously affected by the pregnant state. The prognosis, according to our author, depends most upon whether the condition is acute, that is, restricted within a few days or even hours before labour; or whether it is more chronic, that is, extends over several weeks at least. The acute form is much more likely to pass entirely away after delivery, leaving no trace of its evil effects in the form of permanent renal disease. It is also more likely to pass completely away in proportion as it is both short and slight in degree. But such cases are fully as likely to be accompanied by eclampsia as the more chronic form. Thus, of the 104 cases in which nephritis was associated with eclampsia, 89 were examples of the acute form of the disease ; whereas, of the 46 cases in which the disease appeared in the chronic form, only 15 were affected with eclampsia—leaving 31 in which eclampsia did not appear. Of the 46 patients affected with the chronic form of the disease that were dismissed alive, it is noted in 8 that the patients were dismissed well, in 5 no note is made of the condition on dismission, and in 15 of the cases it is distinctly stated that albumen was present in the urine.

The treatment, according to Hofmeir, ought to be mainly directed towards mitigating the intensity and shortening the duration of the disease. Diaphoretics, diuretics, and purgatives are then recommended, as also in severe œdema the free puncturing of the labia. The induction of premature labour, and, indeed, under circumstances of special severity, the interruption of the pregnancy in the early months, are recommended, upon the grounds that we are thereby imitating nature in removing the chief predisposing cause to the continuance of the disease, and that at best the child's chances of viability in such cases are extremely problematical, whilst the chances of the mother being restored to complete health is the greater the shorter the nephritis continues.

Hofmeir argues that we need not fear that the measures necessary for induction of premature labour should bring on eclampsia, and points out that a great majority of the worst cases of nephritis recorded by him were unaccompanied by that symptom; that the eclampsia usually comes at an advanced stage of a severe case, and that by induction of labour early it is possible that the onset of eclampsia may be anticipated and avoided. At any rate, he holds it is not likely to appear in a more severe form when arising in connection with induced labour than if occurring spontaneously. The period for inducing labour Hofmeir leaves to be decided chiefly by the urgency of the symptoms in each case.—*Edinburgh Med. Journal*, Feb. 1879.

A Peculiarity in the Rickety Pelvis.

Prof. DEPAUL at the Clinique (*Gaz. des Hop.*, December 17, 1878), called the attention of his class to a rickety deformity of the pelvis which is only occasionally observed. He was the first to describe it twenty-five years ago, since which time he has met with new examples. A pelvis so affected presents at certain points of the upper aperture, besides a contraction, some sharp bony lamellæ, cutting sometimes like the blade of a bistoury—corresponding in position to certain muscular insertions at the symphysis pubis or the ilio-pectineal eminence. These bony lamellæ cause most serious mischief; for on the head of the child, covered by the uterus, pressing against their cutting surfaces, an incision or even a true perforation of the uterine wall may be the consequence. In three such cases M. Depaul has known a true hole to have been produced, establishing a communication between the interior of the cavity of the uterus and the neighbouring parts. These bony projections, hidden by the tendinous or muscular insertions, cannot be detected during the labour.—*Med. Times and Gaz.*, Feb. 22, 1879.

The Etiology of Fibroid Tumours of the Uterus.

In the human uterus, "growths," sometimes attaining an enormous size, chiefly composed of smooth muscular fibres united by connective tissue, and nourished by bloodvessels, not unfrequently develop. They give rise to a variety of symptoms, and especially to hemorrhage of a profuse and uncontrollable character, and, except where they are intra-uterine, and not always even then, their removal is either extremely hazardous or quite impracticable. The question naturally suggests itself, what is the cause of these uterine fibroids, and can nothing be done to prevent their development? Hitherto the answer has been completely negative. Great authorities like Scanzoni, Schroeder, West, Churchill, Thomas, and G. Braun, have all confessed their inability to explain the origin of these growths; and the writers of the two most recent English gynæcological works—Lawson Tait ("Diseases of Women," page 162), and Heywood Smith ("Practical Gynæcology," pages 63–65)—have declared, the former that "why they grow is a complete mystery," and the latter that "their causes are unknown." With his usual acuteness, however, Virchow years ago expressly pointed out, in his work on Tumours, that "the *irritative* character of the growth of fibroids, of which there cannot be the slightest doubt, is not due to a physiological stimulus like that of pregnancy, but to a diseased condition, arising either from an excess of local irritation, or from the feeble resisting power of the affected portion of the uterus." He further indicates as probable factors in the development of fibroids, *inter alia*, miscarriages, menstrual irregularities, parturition, prolapsus uteri, and diseases of parts in the neighbourhood of the uterus.

After lying for a number of years without any sign of germination, these ideas of Virchow's have at last fallen on fruitful soil, and the accuracy of his prevision has been to a considerable extent established by the independent observations of two good and competent authorities, Professor F. WINCKEL, of Dresden,[1] and Professor ROEHRIG, of Kreuznach,[2] a résumé of whose results we now propose to lay before our readers.

If we take a number of cases of uterine fibroids, and carefully investigate the time at which the earliest symptoms made their appearance, we shall find that these growths originate most frequently at that period of life when the sexual functions are at their maximum development, namely, about the thirty-first year. This fact was first insisted on by West, has been accepted by Graily Hewitt, and is completely confirmed by Winckel and Roehrig. But a number of cases date their earliest symptoms even before the thirtieth year, decidedly negativing the old idea that the climacteric period exercised an influence on the development of fibroids. The following table will make this part of the subject clear, and save further detailed explanation:—

Distribution in Decades.

							Winckel. No. of cases.	Roehrig. No. of cases.
15–20	.	.	.	.	.	.	3	2
20–30	.	.	.	.	.	.	44	46
30–40	.	.	.	.	.	.	69	85
40–50	.	.	.	.	.	.	43	37
50–60	.	.	.	.	.	.	5	6
60–70	.	.	.	.	.	.	1	0
Totals	.	.	.	.	.		165	176

Roughly speaking, more than two-thirds of all the cases here tabulated began between the ages of twenty and forty. Of Roehrig's cases, eighty-seven, or just one-half, originated between the twenty-fifth and thirty-fifth years.

The period of greatest sexual vigour being thus proved to coincide with the period when fibroid tumours most frequently originate, the next question is, are these growths most common in the unmarried or the married; with the disuse or the use of the sexual organs? Winckel has collected the statistics of 555 cases on this point, and finds that 140 (24.2 per cent.) were spinsters without children, 134 (24.3 per cent.) married but childless, and 281 (51.5 per cent.) married with one or more children. Of Roehrig's cases, 70 (?) were spinsters, 31 married without children, and 75 married with one or several children.

Thus, in three-fourths of Winckel's cases the patients were married, and in at least three-fifths of Roehrig's[3]—a fact which, taken together with similar statistics of West, Routh, Veit, and others, clearly indicates that some connection exists between the functional activity of the uterus as a childbearing organ, and the development of fibroid tumours; or as Winckel puts it, that "married women are decidedly more predisposed to this affection than unmarried—i. e., than those who can satisfy their sexual instinct either rarely or not at all."

---

[1] Ueber Myome des Uterus in Ætiologischer-Beziehung (Volkmann's Sammlung Klin. Vorträge, No. 98).

[2] Zur Ætiologie der Uterus-Fibromyome (Berliner Klin. Wochenschrift, 1877, Nos. 30, 31, 34, 35).

[3] There is some difficulty about Roehrig's statistics here. He gives 176 as the total number of his cases; 106 as that of the married patients; of whom 31 had no children, which of course leaves 70 cases where the patients were unmarried. But at page 449 he says "out of my 176 cases there were only *thirty unmarried* patients with fibroids." To which class are the remaining forty to be assigned?

In endeavouring to explain the greater frequency of myomata in married females, we have to remember the more varied accidents and mechanical injuries to which the uterus is liable in them—injuries during pregnancy, at the time of parturition, and for some time afterwards. In all women (except during pregnancy) the uterus undergoes increased congestion every three or four weeks for about thirty years; its arteries, in spite of their peculiar tortuosity, are subjected to a very high degree of pressure before they reach its inner coat; while the vessels of the superficial layer of the mucous membrane are, according to Henle, remarkable for their delicacy; hence we need scarcely wonder, knowing how rapidly the physiological stimulus of an ovum causes general hypertrophy of the uterine walls, if the pathological stimulus of local circulatory disturbances, congestions, etc., due to mechanical injury, should give rise to partial hypertrophy—that is, to the formation of fibroid tumours. Both Winckel and Roehrig (the latter following on the lines laid down by Winckel) assume that for the development of a fibroid tumour the uterus must receive a mechanical injury sufficient to leave a permanent *locus minoris resistentiæ*, and that the pathological alteration thus induced, and the functional hyperæmia to which, either during menstruation or pregnancy, the uterus is liable, react on one another so as to induce hypertrophy at or near the affected spot. Roehrig is inclined to regard a local chronic sharply circumscribed inflammatory process as the starting-point in many cases, and he lays stress on the necessity for an (hypothetical) "individual predisposition," without which certain morbid stimuli would have no effect on the development of fibroids.

Turning now to the special accidents which appear to affect the growth of uterine fibroids, we may, as Winckel does, divide them into two classes—those which *directly* involve the uterus to a greater or less extent; and those which only indirectly involve it.

The first class includes the cases where the patients refer the commencement of their troubles to the early weeks of their married life, and where it appears probable that a retroflected uterus was bruised during the repeated acts of coitus which took place at that time. It also includes the cases which originated in a miscarriage, in the removal of an adherent placenta, or in some operative procedure connected with the fœtus; in a fall or blow during pregnancy, followed by premature labour; in protracted hemorrhage after childbirth, leading to imperfect involution of the placental insertion, swelling of the uterine mucous membrane, and catarrh; and, lastly, in para- and perimetritic inflammation. Out of 115 cases of his own, Winckel was able to refer eighteen (15.6 per cent.) to one or other of the above causes; and Roehrig gives details of a number of cases of the same kind, in several of which the patients suffered constant pain at the seat of uterine injury until eventually a fibroid tumour was detected at that very spot.

Under the head of indirect injury, Winckel enumerates cases in which the lifting of some heavy object was immediately followed by uterine hemorrhage, and later on by fibroid growth; and others in which a severe shock to the body set up the uterine hemmorrhage, such as a fall downstairs. Both he and Roehrig lay great stress on accidents arising from want of care at the menstrual period, such as catching cold and overexertion in walking, riding, dancing, skating, and singing. Roehrig gives the details of a number of such cases, in which the relation between the injury and the development of the fibroid stands out very clearly; and he also calls special attention to the injurious effects of the prolonged fatigue which many young women have to undergo in the way of sight-seeing and mountain-climbing during their honeymoon, as laying the foundation for future fibroid disease. As an instance of this, he mentions a case known to himself, where a newly married couple ascended the Righi and Mount Pilatus on two successive days, the lady menstruating at the time. The result was that she was laid up for six weeks at Lucerne with metritis, and for three years afterwards suffered from retroflexion and chronic metritis, with general nervous prostration, a fibroid tumour being at length discovered in the posterior wall of the uterus.

The influence of diseases of the other organs of the body upon the development of fibroid tumours has received attention both from Winckel and Roehrig; and the former mentions a number of cases in which these growths occurred in persons who had suffered from severe typhoid fever, from typhoid fever and scarlet fever, or scarlet fever and measles, in quick succession, or from acute rheumatism and subsequent intermittent fever. He explains the injurious influence of such diseases (1) by the hyperæmia and hypersecretion which they induce; (2) by the effect of the fever in causing greater friability of the uterine vessels, and consequent nutritive disturbances of the organ itself; and (3) by the prolonged supine position of the patient, which necessarily induces congestion and swelling, especially in the posterior wall and the fundus of the uterus.

Chronic uterine congestion is also a result of heart disease, and not less than seventeen of Roehrig's 176 cases were complicated with the presence of endocardial lesions (mitral regurgitation in twelve, mitral obstruction in five), eight cases being clearly traceable to acute rheumatism, and three others to hereditary influence. Whether the heart disease stood to the tumours in the relation of cause and effect cannot of course be decided accurately with our present imperfect knowledge; but one thing is pretty certain, that the heart disease was not secondary to the tumours, and due to obstruction of the abdominal circulation by the latter, for only in four of the cases did the fibroid growth exceed the size of a billiard-ball.

We can only here mention the possibilities which Roehrig entertains, that gonorrhœal vaginitis, the injection of caustic fluids into the uterus, and the prolonged use of intra-uterine stems and vaginal pessaries, may all be potent agents in inducing fibroid growth; and we must close this article with one or two remarks suggested by a general review of the facts before us. In the first place, we know that in other organs—for instance, the mamma—the development of certain new growths seems to be set going, so to speak, by a blow or some other mechanical injury, and the first symptoms of syphilomata in the brain have dated from an injury to the head; why, then, should not mechanical injuries affect the uterus in a similar manner? Secondly, we are more than ever reduced to fall back on the idea of some mechanical explanation of the origin of fibroids, because heredity fails to elucidate their presence, the hereditary element being only traceable in five out of Winckel's and six of Roehrig's cases.

Lastly, the recognition of a mechanical origin of these growths suggests the necessity for extreme care in the treatment of uterine disease, and especially points to the avoidance of any measures likely to give rise to chronic irritation.

We do not pretend in what we have here written to give more than an outline of the arguments in favour of these new views; hence we cannot too strongly urge the gynæcologist who desires more convincing proofs and larger details to study the original memoirs to which we have so often referred.—*Med. Times and Gazette*, Jan. 4, 1879.

Perforating Ulcers of the Ileum from Obstruction after Ovariotomy.

Mr. ALBAN DORAN, at a recent meeting of the Pathological Society of London (*British Med. Journal*, Feb. 22, 1879), exhibited a specimen of perforating ulcer of the small intestine, taken from the body of a woman, aged twenty-six, who was admitted into the Samaritan Hospital, under the care of Dr. Bantock, on Nov. 29, 1878. Five weeks previously she had been seized with rigour and severe abdominal pain. A practitioner who saw her, thought she was suffering from typhoid fever, but a second practitioner, who was called in a fortnight later, could detect no symptom of typhoid fever, but found a large fluctuating tumour in the lower part of the abdomen. Shortly afterwards, she was seen by Mr. Spencer Wells and Dr. Bantock, who were of opinion that an ovarian tumour existed, and that the illness through which the patient had passed was an attack of peritonitis. Ovariotomy was performed by Dr. Bantock, on December 4th. A suppurating multilocular tumour of the left ovary was found, which was closely adherent behind, to eight or ten inches of the lower part of the ileum. The adhesions were broken down by sponges, and six small vessels, on the raw surface of intestine, were tied. The right ovary was beginning to undergo cystic change, and was also removed. With the exception of occasional vomiting and some elevation of temperature, the patient progressed favourably ; but on the eighth day after the operation, she complained of a tight feeling across the abdomen, the temperature being 99.8 deg. An hour and a half later, she was in a state of collapse, and between three and four hours afterwards she died. *Post-mortem*, a pint of perfectly liquid feces was found in the abdominal cavity. A coil of ileum, partly adherent to the abdominal walls by recent lymph, was gently raised up, when a jet of liquid feces immediately gushed out of a perforation in its coats posteriorly. Above the aperture, the small intestine was filled with flatus and liquid feces ; but below the perforation the coils of the ileum were matted together by recent lymph, which had been thrown out over the raw surface to which the cyst had been adherent before its removal. This part of the gut was much narrowed and quite empty, and a partial obstruction had evidently been put up by the lymph. It was situated over the promontory of the sacrum ; and the coil of intestine immediately above it, being filled with flatus, had risen upwards, producing a sharp twist in the gut, which had apparently completed the obstruction. The perforation was nearly a foot above this twist. The whole of the stomach and small intestine, down to the obstruction, was deeply injected, the injection, however, following the line of the vessels, *i. e.*, transversely round the gut ; and in the middle of the inflamed streaks were small elongated ulcers. The perforating ulcer was nearly circular, and its edge clean-cut without any thickening. Perforation was commencing in several neighbouring ulcers. There was no trace of ulceration of Peyer's patches. In the ileum, below the kink, the mucous membrane was pale and presented no signs of disease. Mr. Doran remarked that this case resembled one recorded by Mr. Morrant Baker, in which perforating ulcers were found some distance above a strangulated portion of intestine, in a case of femoral hernia. Mr. Spencer Wells, in his work on *Diseases of the Ovaries*, refers to a case in which symptoms of obstruction followed the removal of an ovarian tumour, and in which minute perforations were found in a portion of intestine adherent to the bottom of the abdominal wound. In his own case, the speaker believed that the severe intestinal disturbance, previous to removal of the tumour, was aggravated by the complication after operation, and the ulceration was probably in great measure due to the impaired health of the patient.

Mr. HOWSE thought it strange that this accident was not more common after operations of this kind. He himself had seen a case of like nature. A woman, aged thirty-six, came under his care, at Guy's Hospital, with history that twelve months before she had had all the symptoms of peritonitis. She presented a large fluctuating swelling in the abdomen, which was undoubtedly an ovarian cyst, which was removed. There were no intestinal adhesions, and only a few parietal adhesions. A few days afterwards, obstinate vomiting set in, and there was, at the same time, obstruction of the bowels. This was thought to be due to general peritonitis, but after death, it was found that a coil of ileum, immediately above the ileo-cæcal valve, was bent on itself, owing to adhesions to other parts of the intestines. The adhesions evidently dated back to her former attack of peritonitis, and had caused partial obstruction. The general disturbance of the parts resulting from the operation had changed the partial into complete obstruction. The coil causing the obstruction was in a sloughing condition.

—

Hæmatoma of the Vulva.

The following case is related by Dr. J. BORONOW, in the *Allgem. Med. Central-Zeitung* (No 96). The patient, aged thirty-one, had had six previous normal confinements. The author was summoned to attend her in the seventh confinement, labour having remained stationary for several hours, in spite of moderate pains. Examination showed that the os uteri was sufficiently dilated, the structure of the pelvis normal, and the head of the fœtus in the first position; but the left labium was very much swollen, and of a bluish hue. The swelling increased visibly, fluctuated, and was soon recognized as a hæmatoma. It was thought best to apply the forceps; but, before this could be done, the tumour, which had in the mean time grown to the size of a child's head, burst, and discharged a great quantity of blood. As soon as the bleeding had ceased, the forceps was applied, and the place of the hæmatoma firmly compressed with the palm of the hand; but, notwithstanding this precaution, it was twice filled with blood before the head had been born. The patient died of exhaustion, after the second bursting of the swelling. This case is worthy of interest, because of the very rare occurrence of a hæmatoma of the vagina and vulva. According to Winckel, it has been observed once in a thousand cases.—*British Med. Journal*, March 1, 1879.

Medical Jurisprudence and Toxicology.

Poisoning with Chlorate of Potassa.

An instance of poisoning with chlorate of potassa happened some time ago in the family of Dr. KAUFFMAN in Berlin (*Allgemeine Med. Central Zeitung*, 1878, No. 99). He used to keep a certain quantity of this salt in a tin box, and give some of it daily to his children as prophylactic treatment against diphtheria, which happened to be epidemic at that time in the neighbourhood. One day, the children, while playing, possessed themselves of the box, and took each about half an ounce of the chlorate of potass. The youngest child, a girl two years and a half old, had severe vomiting, which lasted for seven hours, when she died of gastritis, in spite of all help. Another remarkable symptom of the poisoning was the profound lethargy of the child, which probably prevented its showing symptoms of pain. Another similar case is mentioned, of a young man who had taken small doses of chlorate of potass to cure himself of hoarseness. From the time of taking the first dose to the moment when he left off, the patient suffered from gastritis, and vomited every time he took the drug. These symptoms ceased as soon as the latter was discontinued. This clearly shows the latter to have been the primary cause of the inflammation.—*British Med. Journal*, Dec. 28, 1878.

CONTENTS.

Published Monthly, price $2.50 *per annum, free of postage.*

Also, furnished together with the AMERICAN JOURNAL OF THE MEDICAL
SCIENCES *and the* MEDICAL NEWS AND LIBRARY *for* SIX DOLLARS *per
annum in advance, the whole free of postage.*

HENRY C. LEA, Philadelphia.

THE MONTHLY ABSTRACT

OF

MEDICAL SCIENCE.

Vol. VI. No. 5.   **For List of Contents see last page.**   May, 1879.

Anatomy and Physiology.

On the Physiology of the Vesical Epithelium.

MM. P. Cazeneuve and Ch. Livon publish (*Compt. Rendus*, No. 12, Sept. 16, 1878) papers on this subject of which the following is an abstract:—

Various opinions are held as to the power of absorption possessed by the mucous membrane' of the bladder. Some consider its absorptive power very great (Segalas); others think it very feeble (Béraid, Demarquay); and a third class deny its existence (Kuss, Morel, Susini). Previous investigations have usually consisted in injecting poisonous drugs into the bladder and observing the results; but the authors of the present communication have adopted a new method of investigation, the principle of which is to establish whether or not any urea, the chief urinary ingredient, passes through the walls of the bladder. Their "modus operandi" is to tie the prepuce of a dog for some hours before the operation, so as to keep the urine in the bladder. They then expose this viscus, remove it full of urine by means of a ligature, and, after washing it externally with distilled water, they plunge it into three quarts of distilled water at a temperature of 25° C. From time to time the water outside is tested by means of hypobromite of soda, which indicates, by effervescence, the presence of urea. In a series of twenty experiments it was found that it took from three to four hours for the urea to pass through, in the case of a bladder freshly removed; but in one taken out the previous evening, dialysis occurred in from ten to fifteen minutes. The results of their numerous experiments may be summed up as follows:—

1. Desquamation of the vesical epithelium, brought about by any mechanical means. as from the blunt point of a sound, is followed by vesical permeability, and in this point they corroborate Kuss, who holds that the impermeability of the bladder is due to a peculiar property of the vesical epithelium.

2. The increase or diminution of the temperature of the body affects the characteristics of the epithelium, for in an animal well fed the function of the epithelium is very marked, while in one that had been starved it lasts only a very short time after death.

3. Injuring the kidneys, or cutting the spinal cord, affected the physiological properties of the vesical epithelium in a very marked degree.—*Journ. of Anat. and Phys.*, Jan. 1879.

—

Test for Urea.

Prof. Schiff gives (*Bericht. d. Deutchen Chem. Ges.* x. p. 773) the following test for urea: While most aldehydes enter into combination with urea in watery or alcoholic solution, surfurol acts differently, remaining unchanged. But with nitrate of urea surfurol forms a deep violet colour, which gradually darkens from the formation of a black substance.

This tint is not produced by nitric acid, as none of the mineral acids cause any change of colour if the surfurol be perfectly fresh. But while neither acids nor urea separately produce this effect, when they are added together to a solution of surfurol the change takes place. If one add to a solution of urea three parts of a saturated solution of surfurol and one or two drops of hydrochloric acid, the fluid gradually becomes coloured a beautiful purple-violet and solidifies into a dark-brown mass. This reaction takes place more slowly and to a less marked degree with allantoin, but does not occur in the case of a long series of amides which the author names, among which may be noted taurin, glycochol, creatin, uric acid.— *Journ. of Anat. and Phys.*, Jan. 1879.

Materia Medica and Therapeutics.

Thymol and Thymol-camphor.

Dr. SYMES, in the *Pharmaceutical Journal* of January 10, publishes the results of his researches on the combination of thymol, chloral-hydrate, and camphor, acting as an antiseptic. The two former drugs are rubbed together in a mortar, and an equal quantity of camphor added, which liquefies the whole, and produces a powerful antiseptic. Its virtues were immediately tested on some urine containing pus, and which was already beginning to decompose. Two drops of the compound being added to it, the putrefaction was arrested. If thymol and camphor alone are rubbed together, they also become liquid, and this is a convenient form from which to prepare the ointment. Thymol-camphor can be mixed in almost any proportion with vaseline, *ung. petrolei*, or ozokerine, and the thymol will not separate, as in crystals, when thymol alone is used. A solution of thymol in water (1 in 1000) is sufficiently strong for the spray in surgical operation. If used for the throat, milk and glacial acetic acid will be found to be good solvents for it.—*London Med. Record*, March 15, 1879.

—

Internal and External Use of Balsam of Peru.

WISS gives (*Deut. Zeitsch. für Prak. Med.*, No. 34, 1879) the balsam internally in the form of an emulsion, according to the following prescription: R. Bals. Peruv., 8 grammes; muc. gum Arabic, 2 grammes; vitellum ovi unius; aq. dest. q. s. ut. f. emulsio, 210 grammes; liq. lignam., 30 grammes. If used externally, the balsam is poured into the wounds undiluted, and the bandages used for dressing them are soaked in it. If there should be a considerable flow of pus, they must be changed several times daily. In a case of chronic catarrh of the bronchi, where the author prescribed bals. copaivæ internally, the sputa improved, but it had no effect either upon the cough or the expectoration. On giving bals. Peruv., the catarrh disappeared, even the cough which had lasted for several years, and the patients remained well for a long time afterwards. The drug has failed to prove successful in tuberculosis. The author has applied the ointment externally in different kinds of wounds, and in every case he has found it a most useful remedy; it promotes the healing of the wound by first intention, diminishes suppuration, calms pain, and is a decided antiseptic. Upon first coming in contact with the wound it causes a burning sensation of pain, which, however, does not last long. All symptoms of inflammation also cease.— *London Med. Record*, March 15, 1879.

Anæsthesia by Nitrous Oxide.

M. Paul Bert has, he believes, devised a plan of administering nitrous oxide gas which shall enable complete anæsthesia to be kept up for some time without fear of asphyxia. The method consists in administering a mixture of nitrous oxide and oxygen, under increased atmospheric pressure. At a meeting of the Société de Biologie on February 15th, M. Bert gave an account of the first application of his method, which was made on February 13th, on a young woman aged 20, suffering from ingrowing toe-nail. The patient was placed in an apartment of an aëro-therapeutic establishment, in which the atmospheric pressure was increased; and she was made to inhale from a large bag (120 *litres*) containing a mixture of 85 per cent. of nitrous oxide and 15 per cent. of oxygen. Loss of sensation and muscular relaxation supervened in about a quarter of a minute ; and the operator, M. Labbé, removed the nail and extirpated the matrix without any pain to the patient. The operation, including dressing, was completed in about four minutes. The eyes were closed, but insensible ; the pupils were slightly contracted. At about the fourth minute, there was some contraction of the hands and feet, which ceased on the removal of the mouthpiece ; and about half a minute later the patient awoke calmly, sat up, said that she had felt nothing, and asked for food. During the whole period of anæsthesia, the pulse was quiet, and the skin preserved its colour. M. Bert considers that this case confirms the conclusions at which he has already arrived by experiments on the dog as to the safety and efficacy of this mode of administering the gas. It can scarcely be said, however, that avulsion of a toe-nail is a fair test of its success in prolonged operations. It will be remembered by many of our readers that the value of nitrous oxide as an anæsthetic, not only in dental but in surgical operations, was tested rather extensively in London about eleven years ago. Mr. Clover, writing on the subject in the *British Medical Journal* of November 7, 1868, speaks of having used it in iridectomy, in operations for strabismus, in wrenching an ankylosed knee ; and says that "it is well suited for reducing dislocations, *for removing the toe-nail*, and opening fistulæ, boils, and abscesses of all kinds." M. Bert will, however, have conferred a great benefit on surgery if he succeed in showing that nitrous oxide can be safely used as an anæsthetic in prolonged operations.— *British Med. Journal*, March 22, 1879.

Chloral as an Antidote.

Prof. Huseman, of Gottingen, has been engaged in a long series of observations on the antagonistic and antidotal actions of drugs, and some of his investigations which relate especially to chloral are described in a recent number of the *Archiv für Experm. Pathologie.* Of these the following is a summary. Chloral hydrate is known to act as an antidote to strychnine, lessening the spasm, and even preventing death. It has a similar action in the case of the mixture of strychnine bases sold under the name of brucin, and also against the opium alkaloid thebaia, which simultaneously tetanises and lessens sensibility. The spasms produced by chloride of ammonium diminish under the employment of non-fatal doses of chloral hydrate, and can indeed be completely stopped. Nevertheless death occurs, probably from the paralyzing effect of both substances on the respiratory centre. The antidotal effect of chloral on the action of the poisons which cause convulsions by their action on the brain is not the same for all these substances. The quantity of the poison which can be counteracted by the antidote appears to be considerably greater in the case of picrotoxin than in the case of codeia. Of the latter, indeed, the fatal dose, and even a quantity half as much greater, can be rendered harmless, but twice the fatal dose cannot be counteracted, and is still fatal. Calabarin is counteracted by chloral hydrate in about the same degree as codeia. The symptoms produced in rabbits by poisoning with baryta are not materially altered by the action of chloral, which does not appear to prolong life. So, also, with carbolic acid; the spasms produced by it are not arrested by chloral, and the minimum dose fatal to rabbits still produces death. The combination of a fatal dose of carbolic acid with a non-fatal dose of chloral hydrate causes in rabbits a remarkable fall of temperature, which is not produced by the action of these alone. As a rule, when chloral antagonizes the action of these cerebral poisons, the respiration sinks in frequency much more than in the case of the analogous action of chloral on the tetanizing poison. The depression of temperature caused by the chloral is almost independent of any peripheral loss of heat. The elevation of temperature due to division of the spinal cord is hindered by chloral hydrate. The depressing action of thebaia and codeia on the cerebrum, which is distinctly perceptible in many animals in addition to their action in causing spasm, is the chief effect recognizable in man. On the one hand, thebaia has a distinct action in lessening pain; and on the other, in human poisonings with this opium alkaloid, chloral hydrate is of little use, and in the case of poisoning by codeia, on account of the collapse which is produced, it is positively injurious.—*Lancet*, March 15, 1879.

—

Cinchonin seu Quinidine.

From careful observations made in Professor Wagner's Clinic at Leipsic, Dr. ADOLPH STRUMPELL recommends quinidine as a substitute for quinine. This alkaloid is isomerous with quinine, and has the formula $C_{20}H_{24}N_2O_2$, and was first extracted from quinoidine in 1848 by Van Heyningen. Pasteur gave it the name of quinidine in 1853; and in 1868 O. Hesse proposed that of "cinchonin," owing to the adulteration of the commercial quinidine in the German market with cinchonidine.

Cinchonin or quinidine is employed in medicine as the sulphate, which crystallizes in long shining prisms. It is soluble in chloroform, alcohol, and hot water, but soluble with difficulty in cold water. Its purity is tested by dissolving one part of the sulphate in twenty parts warm water, adding one part iodide of potassium, and filtering after cooling. If pure, ammonia gives no precipitate or cloudiness when added to the filtrate.

Wunderlich appears to have been the first to make therapeutical experiments with quinidine in 1855; and he declared that "its effects were almost identical with those of quinine." For some reason or other, however, he gave it up; and for the last ten years it has not been used in the hospital at Leipsic.

Lately, owing to the exertions of Jobst of Stuttgart, experiments have been again made with it on a large scale by Machiavelli in the Italian military hospitals, and Professor von Ziemssen at Munich, in both cases with success.

It should be noted that the price of the purest quinidine supplied by Jobst was a third less than that of quinine in the autumn of last year. The cases treated at Leipsic with cinchonin were fifty in all, chiefly intermittent fever and typhoid, and to a small extent pneumonia, erysipelas, puerperal fever, and phthisis.

In typhoid fever its effects are equal, and in some cases superior, to those of quinine. Within an hour or two the fever declines, and the lowest temperature is reached in from eight to twelve hours. A dose of 1.0 to 1.5 grammes reduces the fever on the average 2° to 2.5° C., but falls of 3.5° to 4°, and once of 4.5°, have been observed. The dose need not be larger than one of quinine, and at Leipsic they give it in solution in peppermint-water, with a little dilute sulphuric acid. The rise of temperature which follows the fall produced by quinidine takes place slowly, and in favorable cases the original height may not be reached again for twenty-four to thirty-six hours, or even longer, and even then the next morning remission may be greater than it would otherwise have been.

The frequency of the pulse falls with the temperature, but not by any means always parallel with it. The greatest drawback to quinidine, especially with typhoid patients, is the subsequent vomiting which very often occurs. It takes place in from a quarter of an hour to two hours afterwards, and is best controlled by ice or a few drops of tinct. opii. Ringing in the ears, perspirations, and collapse are rare—in fact, the latter symptom occurred only once in a typhoid patient who accidentally swallowed 4.0 grammes cinchonin, and who died seven days afterwards, though whether from severe ulceration of the bowel or from the effects of the drug is doubtful. In intermittent fever (twenty cases) cinchonin in 1.5 to 2.0 gramme doses, given six to twelve hours before the fit, acted *exactly like quinine*. A somewhat smaller dose before the second attack, and daily doses of 0.5 to 1.0 for a few days afterwards, completed the cure. Only one case relapsed. In erysipelas, croupous pneumonia, and puerperal fever, cinchonin acts precisely like quinine; on the other hand, the fever of phthisis resists its influence as it does that of other similar remedies.—*Med. Times and Gazette*, March 8, 1879.

How to make Trousseau's Cataplasm.

Dr. DIEULAFOY (*Lyon Méd.*, January 26, 1879), who has frequently applied this cataplasm with much success, gives the following directions for its preparation: Take, according to the size of the affected articulation, three or four pounds of bread—four pounds are sufficient for the knee-joint, two pounds for the wrist. Cut it into pieces, removing carefully the hard portions of the crust, and soak the bread for about a quarter of an hour in water. It is then taken out, tied into a cloth, and squeezed to express a part of the water absorbed, so that the bread remains moist, but not too wet. It is then put into a steam bath, and allowed to remain there for three hours, when it becomes like dry paste, which is softened by the addition of camphorated alcohol. This dough is then kneaded for about five minutes, till it is of the consistence of plum pudding. This is the most delicate point in the making of the cataplasm, because if it is too soft it will give way, and spread out under the pressure of the dressing, and if it is too hard it is apt to crumble and break into small pieces, which might injure the skin. The degree of consistency of the cataplasm must, therefore, be very carefully supervised, because unless one is in the habit of making it, there is always a tendency to make it too soft, either because the bread has not been squeezed sufficiently before having been put into the steam bath, or because too large a quantity of camphorated alcohol has been poured upon it. The dough, having thus been prepared, it is spread on a linen bandage in the shape of a rectangle, large enough to cover the whole of the joint. The poultice must be at least one-third of an inch thick at the edges, in order to prevent the thinner portions from drying too quickly.

The surface of the cataplasm is then painted with the following liquid mixture: camphor, seven grammes; extr. op., five grammes; extr. bellad., five grammes; alcohol, q. s.

This being done, it is applied by being put over the affected joint, and covered by non-evaporant covering. The whole is then firmly fixed by means of a long flannel bandage, over which is placed a linen one of the same length. These bandages vary in length, according to the size of the joint, and, consequently, to the size of the poultice. The joint having been thus bandaged, it must remain perfectly immovable; the compression, although firm, must not cause the underlying parts to become œdematous; this may be prevented, however, by bandaging them also. In order to prevent the layers of the bandages from slipping, they must be sewn to each other. The cataplasm then remains in the same position for eight or ten days, after which time it is removed, and found to be as fresh and moist as if it had been just applied; it still smells of camphor, and does not present the least trace of mould. The skin which has long remained in contact with it is perfectly healthy, unless the cataplasm should have been too thin at the edges, thereby either drying too soon, or giving way under the pressure of the bandage, and causing the skin to excoriate. This is Trousseau's cataplasm. At first sight it may appear too expensive for poorer patients, because the cost of the material amounts to from two and sixpence to five shillings, if the appliance is made in a hospital. If, however, we consider that, the expense having been once incurred, the cataplasm remains in its place for at least eight days, during which time no other medicine is given, we are soon convinced that it is even cheaper than most other appliances. The indications for the use of this cataplasm are so obvious that they need not be repeated here. In every kind of chronic or subacute inflammations of the joints, when other means, such as blisters and cauterization, have proved unsuccessful, and even in the first instance, Trousseau's cataplasm will be found most useful and advantageous.—*London Med. Record*, March 15, 1879.

Chloral Hydrate Enemata in Affections of the Stomach.

STARCKE (*Berl. Klin. Woch.*, August, 1878) had been suffering from chronic catarrh of the stomach, the worst symptom of which was sleeplessness, to such an extent that the patient hardly slept one hour out of the twenty-four. His colleagues advised him to try chloral, but as the state of irritation his stomach was in would not allow him to take it *per os*, he resolved to administer it to himself *per rectum.* An aqueous solution of 5 per cent. of chloral was warmed to 35°, and 10 grammes of this solution were injected. A few minutes later on an agreeable sensation of warmth spread over the body, and the patient fell asleep and slept soundly for five hours. The author continued with his treatment for five months, using during this time about 120 grammes of chloral; after the few first doses he improved to a marked extent; his appetite came back, and his meals were no longer followed by headaches and nausea. The author strongly advocates the use of chloral hydrate in the form of enemata in case of gastric irritation; the point of the syringe must be well oiled, and introduced beyond the sphincter; the fluid ought never to be injected cold, but always warmed to the temperature of the body. The dose given *per rectum* must be smaller than it would be *per os;* fifty centigrammes are sufficient.—*London Med. Record*, March 15, 1879.

Medicine.

The Influence of Climate on Phthisis and Rheumatism.

Dr. H. PETERS, of Elster, Saxony, has published in the *Berliner Klin. Wochenschrift*, Nos. 2, 3, 1879, some very interesting and careful observations on the influence of the chief meteorological elements of climate on chronic diseases of the lungs, and on chronic rheumatism of the muscles and joints, made by himself in 1865 at Bad Ottenstein, Saxony, where a large number of phthisical and rheumatic patients passed the summer under his care. Ottenstein lies 1350 feet above the sea, and is sheltered on the north, east, and west by the mountains of Saxon Switzerland. The climatic elements of which notice was taken were (1) the temperature; (2) the relative humidity; (3) the barometric pressure; (4) the direction of the wind; (5) the quantity of ozone. And with regard to each of these the following data were utilized: (1) the daily mean; (2) the mean of each period of five days; (3) the daily difference between the maximum and minimum readings; (4) the mean of these differences for five days; (5) the daily maximum; (6) the daily minimum; (7 and 8) the means of both. The observations were made at 6 A. M., 2 P. M., and 10 P. M., but the wind was only observed twice daily, and the daily mean and the five days' mean were calculated according to a method described in the original.

The symptoms to which attention was directed in the phthisical and chest patients were (1) the onset of pains in the chest and back; (2) increased cough; (3) the occurrence of bloody sputa; and of (4) the well-known feeling of oppression, which most chest patients designate by the name of tightness (*Beklemmung*). No attempt was made to analyze separately the effect of weather on chronic disease of the substance of the lung and on simple chronic catarrh. In the case of the rheumatic patients the fact of increased pain was noted.

The number of chest cases observed was fifty-six, and of these thirty-five had chronic phthisis, all except one in the first and second stages; fourteen chronic bronchitis, and seven laryngeal catarrh. There were fifty cases of chronic muscular and articular rheumatism. The chest cases were under observation for seventy-six days, from May 17 to July 31, and the rheumatic 105 days, from May 9 to August 21.

The two sets of parallel observations were arranged in the form of curves, of which Dr. Peters gives a complete analysis in his paper. Photographs of the actual tables can be obtained by any one interested in the subject from E. Tietze, Bad Elster, for 3s. Here we can only give a *résumé* of the main results. In chronic phthisis and chronic catarrhs of the respiratory organs, aggravation occurred on the colder days, and concurrently with a rapid fall in the mean daily temperature. It also occurred with a high atmospheric humidity, with a prevalence of northerly and westerly currents, and (contrary to the ordinary opinion) when ozone, or the substance giving the so-called "ozone reaction," was present in large amount in the air. The days on which no aggravation took place were those with low relative humidity, a greatly diminished mean relative humidity, a prevalence of southerly currents, and a low percentage of "ozone."

In the cases of chronic rheumatism the patients got worse when the mean temperature fell considerably from one day to the next day or days, when the relative humidity and the amount of "ozone" were high, and the wind blew from a westerly direction. They were unaffected, on the other hand, on days of high mean temperature, with a low relative humidity and but little "ozone" in the air. With regard to barometric pressure, the only positive result made out in the chest cases was that in "the majority of the patients their disease was aggravated or much intensified on the days when the pressure was high." No positive conclusion, on the other hand, could be arrived at as to a connection between aggravation of chronic rheumatism and pressure. On the whole, these observations appear to us in conformity with the general experience of clinical observers.—*Med. Times and Gazette*, April 5, 1879.

Effects of Salicylate of Soda in Cases of Articular Rheumatism in Infants.

Rheumatism in children is not only more frequent than in adults; it also assumes a more serious form, because complications from the bowels and the heart are more apt to arise. In children the heart is affected as easily as a joint, and this often accounts for cardiac affections which are met with in the adult, when the patient does not remember having had rheumatism in his childhood. M. ARCHAMBAULT, in his communication to the Société de Thérapeutique (February 12, 1879), speaking on the therapeutic action of salicylate of soda in this affection in children, said that it ought not to be considered as a specific remedy against rheumatism, as quinine is against fever, but it presents a great analogy with the latter, and, what is more, it is quite inoffensive. Children take it well, they seldom vomit it, and its use is rarely attended by the disagreeable sensations of giddiness and ringing in the ears, of which adults often complain. Perhaps this comparative immunity may be attributed to considerable rapidity of elimination in children; salicylate of soda can be detected in the urine from a quarter of an hour to twenty minutes after it has been taken. It is true, also, that it has occasionally been traced sixty hours after the medicine had been absorbed; but as the quantity was exceedingly small, it may be said that in children salicylate of soda does not accumulate. M. Archambault prescribes this drug for children from five to ten years after the following formula: rum, 20 grammes; syrup of lemons, 40 grammes; salicylate of soda, 6 grammes; to be taken in three intervals during twenty-four hours. After the third dose the patient generally feels much better, and after the fourth the pains have almost entirely ceased. This, however, is not the only effect of the drug; it also lowers the temperature, and causes the painful swelling of the joints to disappear. The most important property of the salicylate of soda, however, is that it actually prevents all complications which generally arise through affections of the heart. M. Archambault has used the drug in monoarticular and polyarticular rheumatism, and in treating cases of torticollis arising from the same source, and has always found it answer admirably well. As regards the duration of the treatment, M. Archambault gives the drug in doses of six grammes daily, for three days consecutively, even if the pain should have ceased the second day; then he waits for some time. If the pains should recur, the treatment is repeated, and so on, but it is seldom necessary to give a third dose.—*London Med. Record,* March 15, 1879.

Treatment of Ague by Pilocarpine.

ROKITANSKY'S account of the case is published in the *Wiener Med. Jahrbücher,* page 259, 1878. The patient, a young man aged 22, who was suffering from intermittens quartana, and had been treated during the last twenty-one months for tertiana and quotidiana with quinine, had 16 centigrammes of pilocarpine injected hypodermically. The strength of the solution was two per cent., and it was given two hours before the attack, which was much shorter and slighter than it had ever been before. The next attack due was altogether prevented, but in three days very slight prodromi of a new attack appeared about an hour before their usual time. A fresh injection of two centigrammes was then made, the attack passed away, and there were no more symptoms of fever in the next fortnight. The splenic tumour had also become much smaller, and the patient was dismissed as having entirely recovered.—*London Med. Record,* March 15, 1879.

The Plague.

Prof. VIRCHOW recently delivered a lecture on the plague before the Berlin Medical Society (*Berliner Klin. Wochenschrift*, No. 9, 1879) which deserves special attention, and of the principal points of which the following is an abstract:—

Virchow began by stating that our knowledge of the plague in the light of modern medical science is practically *nil*. The latest and most copious reports on the subject date from the great epidemic in Egypt, and from the Commission of which Bulard, Clot-Bey, and others were members. "The clinical and anatomical methods which the Commissioners used in their investigation were not indeed unsuitable; but they were so imperfect that we are still in doubt what the state of things in Egypt really was." Hence Virchow blames the European Governments, and especially the Russian, for not sending properly qualified men to the places where plague was said to be prevalent, to examine the disease with modern appliances, and in harmony with modern knowledge. The universities of Kazan and Kharkov could have furnished thoroughly trained observers; whereas, in fact, unknown men have been selected for the work. Passing to the plague itself, Virchow points out that we do not even now know whether the buboes so constantly spoken of as a symptom are an integral part of the disease, or whether the very acute forms of plague can occur without them. This, he says, is one of the most doubtful questions, and one on which the old observers were not agreed. Another question is: What is the nature of the change in the lymphatic glands on which the buboes depend? Is it a cellular hyperplasia, or an hyperæmia? May hyperæmia be combined with hæmorrhagic effusions into the gland substance? In fact, is it not probable that in the plague-bubo all the changes occur which we now know to be associated with all acute glandular swellings of whatever kind? Virchow inclines to answer this last question in the affirmative.

We are also in the dark as to why the plague-bubo ulcerates. The best observers of this condition assert that the suppuration begins at the outside of the lymphatic gland, but it is difficult to find an analogous change in the ordinary acute febrile diseases of Europe. It is only rarely that in typhoid fever the mesenteric glands suppurate, but then the suppuration, says Virchow, is within the gland, and the process is identical with the formation of a typhoid ulcer in the bowel. Occasionally suppurating inguinal buboes occur in typhoid fever, but in exanthematic typhus Virchow has never met with them. If we knew that the suppuration originated in typhoid fever and in plague in the same way, we should be justified in assuming some relationship between the two diseases. At present there is a gap in our knowledge which needs to be filled up. Still, in spite of our ignorance on this point, Virchow confesses that he regards the buboes as the most important diagnostic signs of plague. They are present in the great majority of all the cases.

Next to them come the "carbuncle," which are found in about one-fifth of the cases, and which closely resemble those of malignant pustule (*Milzbrand*). Virchow has failed to convince himself that they ever occur in the internal organs. Petechiæ, or rather large ecchymoses, are common in the skin, and still more so in internal organs. These three phenomena—buboes, carbuncles, and petechiæ —are the most prominent symptoms of the plague, in company with severe fever of rapid onset, and soon involving the nervous system. Swelling of the spleen is a less characteristic, but appears to be a very constant, symptom; and the pathological alteration is probably similar to that occurring in other infectious diseases. Swelling of the liver and kidneys is also described, and may probably be referred to acute parenchymatous degeneration.

In spite of the fact, already mentioned, that buboes are never found in exan-thematous typhus, Virchow points out that in the beginning of every epidemic of plague the medical men declare the disease to be typhus. This was the case recently when plague appeared in Kurdistan and Mesopotamia. The Turkish doctors diagnosed typhus; and it was not until Dr. Tholozan, the Shah's physi-cian, took up the matter, that the truth came out. And this brings us to the origin of the epidemic in Astrakhan and on the borders of the Caspian Sea. Some authorities, and chief among them Prof. Hirsch of Berlin, believe that the plague was somehow imported from India, where two forms of it have been met with within living memory : the first called "Palipest," which spread from Cutch and Gujerat in the Northwestern Provinces south of the Indus into the interior, and which disappeared for the last time in 1838; and the second, an endemic plague, first described by Allan Webb, and which is limited at the present day, according to recent report of Dr. Lewis, to two small districts in the Himalayas, not far below the snow line on the borders of Nepaul.

Professor Virchow therefore assumes—and the argument appears conclusive—that the present Eastern plague cannot be the Palipest, which was long ago ex-tinct, nor the endemic plague of North India, which has never been known to break its barriers. His own theory is, that the modern plague has come from Kurdistan and Mesopotamia viâ Persia, and has thence reached the Caspian Sea. Whether its transmission has been due to the movement of troops in the late war cannot, he thinks, be at present decided.

And is what has been called the plague really the plague after all ? Professor Virchow thinks that, if the reports of suppurating buboes are correct, it is, though the extent of the epidemic has probably been exaggerated. In any case he con-siders that his own Government was perfectly right to take all precautions possi-ble against the introduction of the plague into Germany. He doubts, however, the possibility of protecting a long *land* frontier by any system of quarantine based on passes and bills of health. "If the Russian officials," he says, "were angels, it might be done, but they are men, and hence fallible." Virchow refers, *en passant*, to the way in which the province of Bari, in the kingdom of Naples, was protected by quarantine in 1815 against the plague, which had attacked the Noya, one of the last places in Europe which suffered from it. Cordons of troops were drawn round the town at widening intervals, and the sentinels had orders to shoot any person who, after a single warning, tried to break through. The historian Schönberg, who relates the story, says the shooting had "a very salutary effect," and Virchow states his own opinion to be that "Border quar-antine (*Grenzsperre*) is an illusion unless shooting is allowed."

The practical measures he suggests are—first, to determine whether the return-ing Russian army is or is not plague-free ; and, secondly, in case the plague should reach Germany, to put in force the sanitary measures common to all epidemics, and, while allowing full communication between country and country, to isolate and treat all patients as rapidly as possible. Remembering that the plague has certain analogies to malignant pustule (*Milzbrand*), and that the skin and hair of a diseased beast can retain their infectious power for months, Professor Vir-chow refuses to admit that clothes, bedding, and such like may not convey the contagion of plague in a similar way. The analogy of malignant pustule to plague, it should be added, he considers so strong that he regards "it as very possible that an organism may be discovered by which the disease is conveyed," though "the search for it has scarcely begun." Lastly, Professor Virchow says a word on disinfection, and, in opposition to Professor Pettenkofer, who has advised the German Government to rely on sulphurous acid, he recommends that all clothes, linen, wool, rags, etc., shall be subjected to the dry heat of a proper oven, and he recalls Bulard's assertion that *the immersion of infected objects in water for a few hours destroys the contagion of the plague entirely*. On the whole, the impression which Virchow's lecture leaves on our mind is, that there is no great need for apprehending an epidemic of plague in Western Europe. At any rate it is clear that anything like panic is foolish, and Professor Botkin's recent error in diagnosing syphilis as plague at St. Petersburg should warn medical men to keep their heads cool, and not let their fears get the better of their judgment. Professor Virchow will not have spoken in vain if he helps to tranquillize the European public.—*Med. Times and Gazette*, March 15, 1879.

—

Athetosis.

Several cases of this extremely interesting and rare disease have of late come under notice (*Soc. Anat.*, Paris, January, 1878; *Upsala läkare-förenungs förh.*, Band xii., p. 91, 1877; *Revue Méd. Franç. et Etrang.* January, 1879). In each of them peculiar and characteristic symptoms have been observed. In one case it was even possible to make a *post-mortem* examination; so far as we know, the first time that a necropsy has been made in athetosis.

The patient in this case was a woman aged 32, who had for thirty years suffered from incessant movements of the right hand, forearm, toes, and metatarsal joints, which affections had been brought on by a great fright. The peculiarity in the case consisted in the convulsive movements being limited to the right side, the patient never having had any convulsiform fits, neither had there been any intellectual or sensory troubles. She was a well-built woman, with straight, well-shaped limbs, which did not show the slightest symptom of a paralytic affection. The unilateral movements must therefore have been caused by a single lesion, discovered at the necropsy in the extra-ventricular nucleus of the left restiform body. The lenticular nucleus was occupied in its interior portion by a focus, which contained in its centre a calculus of the size of a French bean. The left cerebral peduncle was smaller than the right, but the lobe was undiminished in size. This might lead to the inference that during the process of cerebral softening a certain number of the lenticulo-peduncular fibres had been absorbed into the focus. The inflammatory process had not gone beyond the lenticular nucleus, and no other lesion could be traced in the brain.

Both the other cases also present several very interesting phenomena. No *post-mortems* have been as yet made in either case. In the one case, the patient, æt. 36, had for some time previously been under treatment for syphilis. Four years before the first symptoms of athetosis appeared the right internal muscle of the right eye became paralyzed. A year later he suffered from violent cephalalgia and nystagmus. Later on there was hemianæsthesia and loss of consciousness, and still later amaurosis of both eyes and paresis of the lower extremities. An examination with the ophthalmoscope showed œdema of the right pupil, combined with gray peripheric degeneration and white atrophy of the left pupil. In the beginning of the following year it was first noticed that the patient's right hand executed involuntary movements of flexion and extension. A fortnight later, successively all the fingers of the right hand began to contract, and in a few months the contractions were executed rhythmically, and consisted in complete extension and abduction, alternating with a slow flexion, accompanied by adduction. The flexion was executed in the metacarpo-phalangeal joints, and there were about one hundred and fifty flexions and extensions a minute. If the fingers were held fast, so as to prevent them from moving, violent movements of extension and flexion immediately came on in the arm and head. During sleep the twitchings only ceased as long as it was deep and sound, but towards morning, when it was lighter, they came on again, and lasted all through the day. The right forearm was much thinner than the left, but not in the least painful. If the head was not supported it moved horizontally. These movements were even more distinctly seen whenever the patient attempted any voluntary movements.

The third case is even more remarkable, as there is absolutely nothing at all in the previous history of the patient which might give clue as to the etiology of the disease. The gentleman in question, who is a teacher by profession, had always been well; there was no history of syphilis or alcoholism. The only accident he had in his life was a severe scald of the left leg, which happened when he was five years of age. At the age of twenty, when out walking with some friends, they suddenly noticed that both his mouth and face were all on one side. He himself would never have noticed it, as there was neither impediment in his speech nor any other motor or sensory trouble. This slight attack of hemiplegia vanished after two months, during which the patient only applied blisters once or twice. Five years later he began to notice involuntary twitchings in the three last toes of the left foot, which lasted until the present time, and are entirely independent of the volition of the patient. He does not know whether they cease during sleep or not, and they last all through the day. The movements are similar to those we have described above, and consist of a simultaneous extension and abduction, followed by adduction of the three last toes of the left foot; the second toe is also slightly affected. The patient says that he feels the movement vibrating as it were through the whole of the left side, both extremities included. There is a feeling of numbness on the dorsal and plantar surfaces of the foot, as well as a constant tingling, but this does not prevent the patient from walking. The patient was very carefully examined, but not the slightest trace of any disease or nervous trouble could be found. He was perfectly healthy in every respect, and neither motility nor sensibility have ever been abnormal, not even at the time when he had the attack of hemiplegia.

A very curious phenomenon observed was the following. Whenever the twitching toes were slightly stroked near the insertion of the tendons the contractions ceased. The same occurred when the outer side of the leg was slightly rubbed. If we compare these three cases, summing up the individual symptoms, we see that in the first and second cases there may be said to exist an etiology of the disease. The first patient underwent a severe shock to her nervous system through a violent fright, and the second had not only had syphilis but also an attack of paralysis of the lower extremities, complicated with amaurosis. We know from the *post-mortem* results in the first case that there existed an affection of the brain, and may, from the symptoms in the second case, infer that there must also have been an affection of the nervous centres. As for the third patient, the slight attack of hemiplegia which he had had five years before the athetosis showed itself, may be considered as the cause of the disease, which may be classed under the head of post-hemiplegic athetosis. The nature of the lesion of the brain in the first case cannot be clearly defined. It may have been a glioma or a tubercle, which perhaps sprung up at the time when the symptoms of the disease first showed themselves, and was arrested in its growth by some unknown conditions.

The primary cause of the twitchings in this case is not clearly ascertained. Was it the irritation to which the lenticulo-peduncular fibres which passed through the focus were constantly subjected, by the process of degeneration, or were certain fibres belonging to the capsula interna, and which ran along the borders of the focus, the conductors of the irritation? Was this irritation caused by the cicatrization process going on in the focus or by the calculus contained in the latter?

We are unable to answer all these questions satisfactorily, but we may consider ourselves justified from the facts ascertained in agreeing at least in this case with the school of the Salpêtrière, which looks upon athetosis as a variety of symptomatic chorea.—*London Med. Record*, March 15, 1879.

Treatment of Dolor Fothergilli by Nitrite of Amyl.

The patient, a man aged 60, had never been ill until about four years before he entered the hospital under the care of EISENSTEIN (*Bericht des Wiedener k. k. Krankenhauses*, 1878), when he began to suffer from pains in the right side of his face. The pain came on at first after long intervals, but later on daily; sometimes the patient would have as many as eight paroxysms a day, and as many during the night. He consequently felt very weak and low, and his mental capacities had suffered considerably. During some months he had had daily injections of morphia, which, however, only relieved him for a short time, when the paroxysm would again come on as before. Dry heat occasionally calmed the pains, but the application of ice or cold bandages only increased their intensity. The slightest attempt to touch the branches of the trifacial nerve, which spring from the right foramen infraorbitale and mentale, brought on agonies of pain, during which the muscles of the affected part of the face twitched spasmodically. In the intervals, when the patient was free from pain, the muscles of his lower and upper extremities were in a constant state of tremor. The vital organs were perfectly normal. The patient was treated successively and unsuccessfully with quinine and liq. arsenic. Fowleri. Chloroform inhalations were then tried, and proved successful, in so far as they relieved the patient during the paroxysm, but never cut it short unless kept up till perfect loss of consciousness. As the patient objected to having the nerve resected, inhalations of nitrite of amyl were then resorted to; one drop would cut short the most violent paroxysm. The remedy having been continued for a certain time, the intervals between the paroxysms grew longer, and the patient slept well, gained flesh, and asserted that he had never felt better in his life. As an experiment, tinctura gelsemii was administered during some time in doses of ten drops every two hours, no other medicine being given at the same time. The patient felt pretty well during ten days, after which the tincture gels. proved ineffective, and he again suffered so much that the former treatment had to be again resorted to, and continued for several weeks. The paroxysms would occasionally be absent although for a week, and then, if they came on at all, last a very short time. He was then discharged from the hospital, and presented himself a month later, stating that he was well satisfied with the results of his treatment. The paroxysms came on occasionally, but very seldom, and never lasted long.—*London Med. Record*, March 15, 1879.

Two Cases of Brachial Monoplegia originating from Syphilis.

The following observations on this interesting disease were read by LELOIR at the meeting of the Société de Biologie on December 28, 1878:—

CASE I.—R. J., a workman, aged 49, was received on September 4th, in M. Vulpian's ward. The patient denied all syphilitic antecedents. Having, however, been carefully questioned, he stated that, about ten years ago, his hair came off. He did not, on admission, show any symptoms of alopecia. Shortly after this, he began to suffer from rheumatic pains in all his limbs, but he positively denied ever having had sore throat or any cutaneous eruption. On the inner side of the left leg was a brownish scar of the size of a half-crown piece, which he attributed to a varicose ulceration. However, there were no traces of varices to be found when he came under treatment; but, in the infra-clavicular space there were on both sides a few glands of the size of a nut. It, therefore, seems clear, that the cerebral affection for which he entered the hospital was of syphilitic origin ; this supposition was verified subsequently by the good results of antisyphilitic treatment. About a year ago, he began to suffer from frequent headaches, which soon were followed by amblyopia. Four days before entering the hospital, when following his avocation, he suddenly felt very painful formication in the whole of the left arm, including the shoulder. He tried to get rid of this sensation by moving his arm violently up and down, but it grew worse. Two hours later, the left forearm was totally paralyzed and hung motionless and flaccid by his side. The next morning, the patient tried to work, but his left arm still remaining inert, he resolved to enter the hospital. On examination, it was found that the left superior extremity was almost entirely paralyzed ; there was no contraction of the arm, although the fingers were slightly contracted. He could scarcely close his hand, and only by great exertion bend the forearm towards the arm ; but he could not overcome any resistance, however slight. With the aid of the muscles of the shoulder, he would raise slightly the upper extremity, but it would again fall down. There seemed to be no difference in the circumference of both members ; faradic contractility still existed, although slightly lessened. There were no abnormal sensations in the arm, no painful symptoms, and the only thing the patient complained of was a slight sensation of cold in the hand. On comparing the temperature of both upper extremities, a very notable difference could be found ; the fingers of the left hand were also slightly cyanotic. The inferior extremities were not in the least affected, neither was there any facial paralysis. There were slight cephalalgia, amblyopia, and singing in the ears. The patient's intellect seemed intact, although very little developed ; he complained, however, that his memory was not so good as formerly.

He was treated with mercury and iodide of potash, and, a week later, a notable improvement might be marked in the movements of the left arm. He could grasp objects firmly, and feel much stronger, when, suddenly, a violent attack of headache came on. The pain was principally felt in the frontal region, specially on the right side, and in the right parietal region. The pain was aggravated by percussion. A week later, the headache had vanished, and, in three more weeks, the patient left the hospital with only a very slight difference between both extremities.

CASE II.—F. A., carrier, was received into the hospital on November 26, 1878. About fifteen years previously he had contracted a chancre, followed by sore throat and cutaneous eruptions. He then recovered, and was quite well till four years ago, when he was laid up with inflammation of the lungs. He had scarcely recovered, when he began to suffer from violent headaches, followed, after some months, by insensibility and wasting of the right arm. When this limb was entirely paralyzed, the patient entered a hospital, and was put under antisyphilitic treatment, and galvanized. A few months later, he left the hospital, although his right arm was still weak. Some time after, he was suddenly seized with the prodromi of a miliary tuberculous eruption, admitted into M. Vulpian's wards, and died there after the lapse of a fortnight. It is to be noted that this patient, also, had never had any convulsions or contractions of the right arm, and that both the face and the right leg were perfectly intact. There had not been any sensory troubles in the affected extremity, nor was the faradic contractility lessened. The right arm was very thin, while the muscles of the left were well developed.

Necropsy.—The lungs, the cerebro-spinal sheaths, and the digestive canal, were found to be covered with miliary tubercles. The brain was free from them, but, on the surface of the left hemisphere, about five millimetres from the longitudinal fissure, and on a level with the middle portion of it, the dura mater was considerably thickened over a space of the size of a sixpenny piece. This thick-cuing did not adhere to the bones of the skull, and, having been dissected carefully out, was found to consist of the three cerebral meninges, which were united into a patch the size of three millimetres, having a rugged surface and presenting a grayish and sclerotic appearance. The meninges which surrounded this spot to the extent of three millimetres, were of a whitish colour and slightly thickened. The patch adhered firmly to the brain-substance, so that it could not be removed without carrying away the whole of the gray matter, and about one millimetre of the white substance, which were directly underneath it. It corresponded exactly to the upper third of the ascending frontal convolution.

Microscopic cuts having been made of the patch, it was found to be of sclerotic consistency, and of a dull grayish colour. In the centre of the cut was a thin yellowish line about a quarter of a millimetre thick and three millimetres long. This was the only lesion which could be traced. The other membranes of the brain did not show any alterations, except the miliary tubercles. The bones and arteries of the skull were healthy, and there was a considerable œdema of the cerebral substance. Although the right arm had been considerably atrophied, the anterior roots of the nerve of the paralyzed side did not appear atrophied, neither was there any degeneration of the nerve tubes, either in this nerve or in the nerves of the brachial plexus of the corresponding side, and in the inframuscular nerves. The muscular fibres also appeared healthy.

REMARKS.—Both cases offer such analogies from a clinical point of view that they may be pronounced to arise from similar causes, as the necropsy of the first patient would doubtless have shown. Violent headaches preceded in both patients the monoplegia, which comes on suddenly without any symptom except a progressive torpor of the superior extremity in the course of a few hours. In both cases, there was no facial paralysis, neither was the corresponding inferior member paretic. There never were any transitory contraction or partial temporary convulsions; and, in the second case, where the paresis lasted nearly four years, no secondary contraction was observed. In both cases, the sensibility was not disturbed, and in the first, it may be observed that the temperature of the paralyzed side was lower than that of the other.

From an anatomo-pathological point of view, the second case offers us one of the most remarkable instances of cerebral localization, as we see here how a circumscribed patch of a gummatose cerebral sheath, which occupies a small portion of the cortical cerebral substance on a level with the upper part of the left ascending frontal convolution, may cause a monoplegia of the right arm.

This experience tends to verify Professor Charcot's opinion, that the motor cortical centres for the extremities of the opposite side are located in the two superior thirds of the ascending convolutions, and specially in the ascending frontal convolution. It is, however, worth noticing, that the lesion existed in the superior third of the ascending frontal convolution, and not in its middle portion, where, according to Professor Charcot, the cortical centre of the isolated movements of the upper extremity would be found.—*London Med. Record*, March 15, 1879.

Case of Brachial Monoplegia.

At the meeting of the Société de Biologie, of January 25, M. RAYMOND stated the following case. A young man, aged 20, suddenly fell down in September last in an apoplectic fit. When he recovered consciousness he found that he could no longer make use of his right arm. He subsequently put himself under M. Raymond's treatment, who diagnosed the existence of brachial monoplegia, complicated with an absolute loss of sensibility. The application ot various metals, magnets, and electricity had no effect on it, neither was M. Raymond able to modify the insensibility. The question is now what could be the reason of this phenomenon? Was it a cerebial or a medullary lesion? It is, however, well known that the distance between the centre of motility and that of sensibility of the upper extremity is considerable, and this fact makes the question still more complicated. There is no history of syphilis, and besides, immediately after the fall, no ecchymosis or symptoms of lesion of the brachial plexus could be found. The patient has been put under M. Vulpian's treatment, and it seems as if on the continuous application of electricity he began to recover gradually the sensibility of his arm.— *London Med. Record*, March 15, 1879.

On the Rapid Cure of Asthmatic Attacks by Hypodermic Injections of Morphia and on the Eupnoeic Action of the latter.

Although the sedative effect produced by hypodermic injections of morphia in cases of asthmatic attacks, or of certain paroxysms of dyspnœa, has been well known for a long time, yet most practitioners prefer to employ preparations of belladonna or datura, because they do not tend to diminish the bronchial secretions. M. HUCHARD, having studied carefully the effects of, and the objections to, the use of morphia in asthma, has come to the following conclusions. In the most intense attacks of asthma a hypodermic injection of morphia will cause immediate relief. He even goes so far as to affirm that if these injections are repeated, they will, by cutting short each attack at its beginning, succeed in rescuing the economy from this spasmodic habit, and thereby cure the disease. After giving a short historical sketch of his subject, M. Huchard proceeds to study carefully the different forms under which asthma can show itself: he compares pathological facts with the results which have been obtained from the therapeutical study of preparations of morphia, and in this way, succeeds in explaining theoretically facts which he had learned empirically from clinical experience.

In another part of his work, M. Huchard enters fully into the importance of administering morphia preparations hypodermically in other cases of dyspnœa, such as cardiac asthma or urӕmic dyspnœa. In a third chapter he dwells upon the different results produced by morphia preparations, according to whether they are given hypodermically or by the mouth. He sums up his exhaustive and interesting study by the following words: Morphia makes one breathe freely.—*Lond. Med. Record*, March 15, 1879.

Pulmonary Emphysema in Tuberculosis.

There are three principal forms of emphysema. It is acute in acute and chronic tuberculosis; partly chronic in phthisis, accompanied by ulcerations; and universally chronic in latent tuberculosis. According to the author, defective nutrition is one of the most important causes of emphysema, and he quotes in support of this view several authorities on the subject; among others M. Granchot, who proved it by several examples of emphysema, which had followed atrophy and partial destruction of the lobules in chronic tuberculosis. This latter etiology is very impoitant, because, as M. HIRTZ obseives (*Thèse de Paris*, 1871, *Gaz. Méd. de Paris*, No. 1), its development has always been noticed in tubeiculous patients wheie theie was piedisposition to aithiitis. It must, howevei, not be forgotten, that geneial chionic emphysema, whethei it be piimaiy oi secondaiy, is always in a ceitain way antagonistic to tubeiculosis. M. Hiitz has also seveial times observed a fevei of a peculiai type, which was iegulaily iepeated aftei foui oi five days.

The diagnostic symptoms of the disease, such as hæmoptysis, loss of flesh, etc., are well known. It must, howevei, always be boine in mind that it is veiy easy to eii by mistaking latent emphysematous tubeiculosis foi constitutional emphysema. Gieat impoitance should also be attached to the chaiacteiistic iespiiation of emphysema.—*London Med. Record*, Maich 15, 1879.

Venous Pulsations in Consumption.

Piofessoi PETER has obseived iepeatedly in consumptive patients a peculiai phenomenon, which may be consideied as being piognostically impoitant. It is a foim of venous pulse, which he has desciibed in a papei addiessed to the Société Cliniqu'e, and subsequently published in the *France Médicale*. He obseived it for the fiist time in a woman who had ieached the last stage of tubeiculosis; the veins on the doisal suiface of hei hand weie bluish, haid, toituous, and pulsated visibly. The pulsations weie still moie distinct if the wiist was compiessed so as to hindei the venous ciiculation; they could, howevei, be bettei seen than felt, because the impulse of the venous wall does not beat against the fingei in the same way as the aiteiial. The pulsations could, theiefoie, be counted with the eye, and weie found to be synchionous with the aiteiial pulsations. M. Petei has since met with this phenomenon, though not each time undei analogous ciicumstances. How was it caused? It was cleai that it could not be the same thing as the ordinary venous pulse, because it did not exist in the heait, and also if the aim weie compiessed between the heait and the hand, it was exaggeiated instead of being suppiessed, as must inevitably have happened if the venous blood had come diiectly fiom the heait. The blood, theiefoie, came fiom the left heait, and not fiom the iight. In oidei to explain this venous pulse, M. Petei thinks that the musculai fibies of the aiteiies in ceitain individuals who aie half asphyxiated, as is the case with those patients who aie paialyzed thiough the excess of caibonic acid which is contained in theii blood, and in this way allow the fluid to entei diiectly into the capillaiies without putting any obstacle to this continuous tiansfei of blood. The othei agents which help to foim this pulse aie the fiequency and eneigy of the pulsations of the heait. Duiing the last moments of life, when the pulsations become feeblei, the venous pulse disappeais. This phenomenon, as we have said befoie, is iaie, but when it exists it is veiy impoitant, being a sign of quickly appioaching death.— *London Med. Record*, Maich 15, 1879.

On Cheyne-Stokes' Respiiation.

In a shoit *note additionelle sur quelque points paiticulieis du phénomène respiiatoire de Cheyne-Stokes*, Di. C. BIOT meiely insists upon the truth of the views he has expiessed in two pievious papeis upon the phenomena associated togethei undei the name of Cheyne-Stokes' iespiiation. It is especially wiitten as a ieply to the ciiticisms that have been passed upon his foimei papeis. He accepts as tiue the statement of M. Filehne that the phenomena of Cheyne-Stokes' iespiiation can be pioduced expeiimentally by hindeiing and piomoting successively the afflux of aiteiial blood to the biain. Di. Biot especially empha-

sizes the great distinction between true Cheyne-Stokes and other more or less
irregular respiratory rhythms; it is the gradual diminution of the amplitude with
lengthening of the expiratory period before the apnœa, and of the gradual
resumption with increase of the amplitude and acceleration of the movements
after the pause, which is so especially characteristic of Cheyne-Stokes' respiration. Two tracings are given to illustrate this, one from a case of Cheyne-
Stokes' respiration, the other from a case of irregular respiratory rhythm occurring in meningitis. With regard to the arterial tension during the two conditions
of apnœa and hyperpnœa, the author states that the tension is diminished during
apnœa, and increased during hyperpnœa, and that following Marey's law that
the frequency of heart-beats is in inverse ratio to the arterial tension, the heart-
beats are frequent during apnœa and infrequent during hyperpnœa. In his previous paper the author stated as the result of experiments upon himself that the
voluntary production of apnœa produced an increased frequency in the pulse-
beats; this statement has been regarded as hypothetical by some of his critics,
who had failed to obtain similar results, and to his surprise, on repeating his observations many times, failure occasionally occurred also to him. A law has been
discovered, however, which explains the apparent contradictions; if one ceases
to respire, the thorax being in a state of inspiration, there is generally a slowing
of the cardiac rhythm; if, on the contrary, one fixes the chest-walls in expiration, the heart-beats are always accelerated. Dr. Biot draws attention to the
fact that in Cheyne-Stokes' respiration the chest-walls are always fixed in a state
of *expiration*, and therefore the cardiac-beats are increased in frequency; he
takes this opportunity of modifying his previous statement as to the effect of
voluntary apnœa in modifying the cardiac rhythm, and adds to his former statement that during the period of cessation of respiration the thorax must be in a
state of expiration. Concerning the etiology of this phenomenon Dr. Biot
maintains his former statement: "We believe we have demonstrated that the
essential conditions determining the occurrence of this symptom are—a diminution of the excitability of the medulla—a cerebral phenomenon, having for its
origin an anæmia progressive, and more or less profound, a circulatory phenomenon." He further adds that in all the cases he has met with, aortic regurgitation existed, with or without contraction of the orifice. Referring to a recent
thesis by Dr. Cuffer, in which it is contended that the phenomenon is due to
uræmia, he remarks that supposing uræmia to be due to spasm of the cerebral
arteries, and therefore to anæmia of the brain, it would be explained by his
view of the etiology of the condition; on the other hand, he affirms that he has
many times seen it in cases which had not a trace of albumen in the urine.—
London Med. Record, March 15, 1879.

――

*Sudden Arrest of the Circulation in the Superior Vena Cava in a Case of
Aortic Aneurism.*

The patient, a cabman (*Gazette Hebdomadaire de Médecine et de Chirurgie*)
was admitted into the Hôpital St. Antoine under the care of M. DUJARDIN-
BEAUMETZ, having been suddenly seized with cyanosis and great dyspnœa. He
had suffered for some time from pain in the right subclavicular region, and his
expectoration had been occasionally tinged with blood; but there was no cause
to which he could refer this sudden attack, and he had been following his occupation up to the time of his admission. His body presented a curious aspect; the
upper part, the trunk, the head, the upper limbs, in short, all that part whose

―――――

¹ The term "apnœa" is here used in the physiological sense, indicating a highly
arterialized state of the blood; it has not its ordinary clinical meaning.

venous system is tributary to the superior cava, was of a bluish hue, while the lower part, the abdomen, and lower limbs were of a normal colour. The cyanosed parts were swollen and œdematous, particularly the face and upper extremities; the veins of the neck were distended. In the sixth, seventh, and eighth left intercostal spaces chains of varicose capillaries were very evident, obviously of some standing and pointing to a long existing obstruction in the venous return. Over the upper part of the abdomen on the right side, the subcutaneous veins took the form of large, varicose, venous cords, showing that much of the blood which should find its way back to the heart by the superior cava was returned by the inferior cava.

Examination of the chest revealed an area of dulness extending in front from the clavicle to the fourth interspace, and behind to a corresponding extent in the scapular and subscapular regions. Over this area a very loud, harsh systolic murmur was heard, almost completely drowning the breath-sound, which was very indistinct. The same murmur was heard, though very feebly, at the cardiac apex, but loud and harsh along the course of the aorta. Expansile pulsation opposite to the second, third, fourth, and fifth right interspaces. Both upper extremities are very dense, large, and painful, and of a pale bluish colour. Voice feeble, hoarse respiration difficult. The cyanosis diminished greatly after a few days in hospital (axillary temperature lowered, right side 35.2 Cent., left side, 34.6 Cent., in rectum 37°), but soon returned, and notwithanding leeches behind the ears and bleeding from the right jugular vein, increased in intensity. The face became bloated, the complexion blue, with reddish patches, lobules of ears cold, eyes injected and weeping, voice stifled. The back, which had remained nearly of normal colour, became blue also, with patches of varicose capillaries, like those on the front of the chest; but here, as in front, the blue colour terminated abruptly at the base of the thorax. Four days before the patient died (he died twelve days after admission) a curious murmur was heard close to the spine on the right side, opposite the ninth, tenth, eleventh, and twelfth interspaces. It was a well marked continuous bellows-sound, intensified at each systole. It was not audible above the ninth interspace, nor on the left side of the spine.

The autopsy revealed the existence of an aneurism as big as the fist at the commencement of the aorta; along its posterior wall was the vena cava, completely compressed by the aneurismal sac; it contained no clot, but its walls were so thin and fragile that it was very difficult to pass even a small probe through the vessel without lacerating it. The clot which had led to the complete obstruction of the venous circulation of the upper part of the body, was found in the vena azygos, which was enormously dilated, and obviously replaced the superior cava. This vein appeared directly continuous with the brachio-cephalic trunks. Lower down it became much smaller, and on the level of the eleventh dorsal vertebra was diminished about one-fourth in diameter; here it divided into several branches connected with the lumbar veins, and did not join directly the vena cava inferior. About its middle third a clot was found, from 5 to 6 centimetres in length, of a yellowish red colour, and softish consistence, easily detached from the walls of the vein, which were unaltered. It is easy to understand that the result of this clot was the same as if it had been placed in the superior cava, for it was wholly due to this vast supplementary circulation that the patient had been able to live so long without grave symptoms. It was a question whether the soft bellows-sound heard at the base of the thorax on the right side of the spine was due to the changes in the azygos venous circulation (it ceased a few days before death), or whether it was an aneurismal murmur transmitted along the vertebral column.— *Lond. Med. Record*, March 15, 1879.

Acute Hemorrhage into the Pancreas.

Dr. HILTY, of St. Gallen (*Schweiz. Corr. Bl.*, vii. 22, 1877) relates the following case. A mechanic, 30 years of age, well built, muscular, given to alcohol, died after two days' illness with symptoms of acute gastritis, blood-poisoning, and perforation of the intestine. At the *post-mortem* examination any trace of peritonitis was absent; on the contrary, the neighbourhood of the pancreas showed an abundant infiltration of blood. The gland itself was double its ordinary size, of tough consistence, and dark red coloured. From the interlobular connective tissue much bloody serum flowed on section. Behind the head of the pancreas were small hemorrhages; the duct was not dilated. The corresponding renal vein appeared swelled and filled with blood-clot. Spleen and kidneys hyperæmic. Stomach dilated, the mucous membrane thickened; ecchymoses in the cardiac end and lower part of the œsophagus. Liver voluminous, fatty. Much fat on the enlarged heart; muscular fibres soft, somewhat fatty. Brain congested. Ventricular fluid turbid.—*London Med. Record*, March 15, 1879.

—

A Case of Traumatic Rupture of the Spleen.

LOWENSTAMM records (*Med. Chir. Centralbl.*, January 31, 1879) the case of a strong-built woman, aged 38, who had been living for some time previous in a place where malaria reigned, and suffered for a long time from often repeated attacks of tertian fever. She then left the place, but was still subject to frequent attacks of malaria varying in type, looked very pale, and complained continually of a pain in her left side. One day, when working in a brick-kiln, a large mass of earth suddenly detached itself, and, falling upon her, buried her. She fell on her right side, and the whole weight of the earth rested upon her left side. She was immediately exhumed, but complained of a severe pain in the left hypogastric region, had nausea, and vomited even the water which had been given her to drink. Her pulse was small and frequent, her abdomen much enlarged, but she had not lost consciousness. She was immediately put to bed, and fomentations of ice-water applied, together with soothing remedies, but with no result. Her abdomen was more and more inflated, and the increasing pallor and low temperature of the body, as well as the collapse, made it certain that both the spleen and capsula of the spleen had burst, thereby allowing the blood to escape freely into the abdominal cavity. The patient lived for two days after the accident, being treated with opium and hæmostatics. She died of peritonitis and exhaustion. At the necropsy it was found that the spleen had burst asunder almost in the middle; there was also a slit of about one inch in the capsula, and a coagulum weighing about five pounds lay in the abdominal cavity. The latter presented all the characteristic changes of peritonitis. The spleen was hypertrophic, soft, and weighed 1 lb.—*London Med. Record*, March 15, 1879.

—

Case of Dislocation of the Spleen.

WASSILJEW records (*Petersb. Med. Woch.*, 1878, No. 40) the case of a naval officer aged 36, who had lived for several years in a place where malaria prevailed, and had there acquired intermittent supraorbital neuralgia accompanied by chills, and followed by heat and perspiration. Subsequently he became dyspeptic, and about fifteen months after the first symptoms of the disease had shown themselves, a tumour in the abdomen was accidentally discovered. It was not sensitive to pain, occupied the left superior part of the abdomen, but sloped down towards the right side and could be felt about one-and-a-half inches beyond the linea alba. The surface was smooth and the tumour could be easily moved.

During the attacks of fever it increased in size and became hard, but decreased and softened in the intervals. At first the patient did not feel much inconvenience from it, but gradually it began to cause him so much suffering, that he felt depressed, and attacks set in which might almost be termed hysterical. His digestion was also much impaired; and last, not least, the urinary organs became affected; he had a strong desire to micturate, combined with a decrease in the quantity of urine which was passed, and pains in the region of the left urethra. At the present time the tumour has sunk more towards the right and downwards; measuring on the right and above the umbilicus about four inches, on the left three, and below two inches. Its shape is oval, with an incision on the lower border; it feels like a solid consistent mass with smooth edges, and is pretty freely movable, adhering only slightly to the abdominal walls. Only in one place, on the left, can crepitation be detected, and the tumour is tender on pressure. If palpated or faradized it grows notably smaller. There is no splenic dulness. The ninth and tenth intercostal space on the left are flatter than on the right; at every deep inspiration they are drawn deeper inwards than on the right. The colour of the blood is not so dark as it should be, although no increase of the white blood-corpuscles can be detected. The quantity of urine passed daily is 2500 centimetres; specific gravity 1012; no albumen; acid reaction; but it contains a considerable sediment of phosphates and urates. The entire left side is less sensitive to electric thermic and tactile stimuli than the right, especially the lower extremity; this difference decreases, however, gradually towards the upper part of the body, and is very slight in the superior extremity.

During the patient's stay in the hospital the spleen was treated with the faradic current and decreased in size. The patient also felt much better. On leaving the hospital he was advised to go on stimulating the spleen methodically by electricity, or the application of ice or cold water, combined with antifebrile medication, such as arsenic, quinine, and eucalyptus with iron.—*London Med. Record,* March 15, 1879.

—

Diabetes complicated by Symmetrical Gangrene of the Skin of the Plantar Region.

Dr. MAGNIN has published in the *Journal de Médecine* for June, the following case: The patient, aged 64, who had always led a very active life, and enjoyed good health up to 1871, then began to suffer from diabetes, the urine containing 54 grammes of sugar per litre. He was treated for it, and did not suffer much till 1876, when, having taken cold, he was laid up with facial erysipelas; the urine at that time still contained a small amount of sugar. In 1877 he suffered from hæmoptysis and a bad cough. Cod-liver oil, alcohol, and tar were given, and the hæmoptysis decreased considerably, although it did not cease completely. The cough, however, could not be got rid of, and was very troublesome, especially in the morning. A few crepitating râles could be heard several weeks after the cough had first begun; they were considered as symptoms of a congestion of the lungs, and treated accordingly. The patient again improved in health, gained flesh, and, with the exception of an attack of intermittent fever, which was cured by arsenic and quinine, nothing abnormal was noticed during the year. In February, 1878, the body of the patient, especially the chest and lumbar region were covered with large patches of pityriasis versicolor. This same eruption had occurred a year previously, and disappeared as it did this time, having been treated with sulphur ointment. In March the patient was greatly alarmed by observing that a symmetrical series of purplish spots of the size of a pea, had spread over the planta of both feet, especially of the right one. This eruption was very tender on pressure, and gave great pain, not only

when the patient attempted to walk, but also when he was resting. He described
the pains, when lying down, to be of a lancinating kind, similar to an electric
shock, equally rapid in their appearance and disappearance. The physician
suspected diabetic gangrene, and treated the patient with local applications of
quinine and arsenic, and internal administration of quinine and astringents, to
counteract the frequent hemorrhages from the nose and mouth. Absolute rest
and a very strict regimen were also prescribed. The symptoms, however, grew
worse; the patient could hardly walk with the pain, which radiated to the
malleoli. He described it as like having a screw driven into his foot. The
affection progressed rapidly, the spots on the right foot being of a purple hue,
and the skin having a macerated appearance. As a last expedient, Dr. Magnin
resolved to try local oxygen baths, without, however, having much faith in them.
They were administered by drawing over the right leg and foot a rubber tube,
into which oxygen was conducted. The patient took a bath of half-an-hour
during the first day, but without experiencing any relief. The foot was very
red, and perspired abundantly. The treatment was continued for twelve days,
after which time all traces of the purple spots and the pain had disappeared.
The patient still suffers from diabetes, but is comparatively healthy, and able to
attend to his business.—*London Med. Record*, March 15, 1879.

Pathological Conditions of Albuminuria.

RUNEBERG has summed up the results of his observations as follows, in the
Deutsches Archiv f. klin. Med., vol. xxiii. Nos. 2 and 3, 1879. The transuda
tion of albumen into the urine always takes place in the Malpighian bodies, and
is due to an increased permeability of the walls of the convoluted tubes and their
epithelial lining. The particles of albumen which are suspended in the blood-
serum, and which, under normal conditions, cannot transude through the membranes of the Malpighian bodies, are washed through them, together with the
other constituents of the urine, and mix with the latter.

In a healthy kidney this increased permeability is due to a considerable decrease
in the difference between the blood-pressure within the Malpighian bodies, and
the counter-pressure within the urinary tubuli. Here, therefore, the albuminuria
would only be accidental or transitory, and may, according to what has been
said, be ascribed either to a considerable decrease in the blood-pressure in the
Malpighian bodies or to an increase in the pressure in the urinary tubules, or to
both causes combined. If the albuminuria should, however, persist, then the
increased permeability of the membranes must be ascribed to some degenerative
or suppurative process within the convoluted tubes of the Malpighian bodies;
here, too, pressure has a marked influence on the permeability of the lining, and
consequently on the amount of albumen contained in the urine, in the same way
as has been quoted above. Certain kinds of the albuminous bodies, such as egg-
albumen and hæmoglobine, are transuded much more easily than serum albumen.
If, therefore, these substances have been mixed in some way with blood serum,
they immediately transude into the urine like dissolving salts, even if the blood-
pressure should be normal and the kidneys healthy.—*London Med. Record*,
March 15, 1879.

Treatment of Albuminuria by the Inhalation of Oxygen.

At a meeting on January 8 of the Société de Thérapeutique, M. DUJARDIN-
BEAUMETZ read a paper on a case of albuminuria in which the albumen had
entirely and rapidly disappeared after some inhalations of oxygen. The patient
had reached the last stage of the disease; every diuretic had been employed, but

without success, when inhalations of oxygen weie iesoited to. The albumen disappeaied within the following twenty-foui houis, and had not ieappeaied since. Twelve days had elapsed, and the authoi wished to know.if similai cases had been obseived befoie, and if his tieatment might be consideied as attended by peimanent success.

A discussion having been iaised on the subject, it was iemaiked that similai cases had been known to occui, only the effect of the cuie had nevei been peimanent, the albumen geneially ieappeais aftei two or moie months.—*London Med. Recoid,* Maich 15, 1879.

Intia-abdominal Chylous Effusion.

Piofessoi WINIWARTER of Liège iepoits in the *Medicinisch-Chirurgischcs Central-Blatt,* No. 1, 1879, the following case, which was obseived at the Childien's Hospital in Vienna in 1876, and is desciibed as one of "chylangioma caveinosum in abdomine."

The patient was a weak female infant aged foui months, whose abdomen, immediately aftei biith, was noticed to be veiy piominent. The infant took the breast fieely, and incieased slowly in size. The abdomen continued to swell, but no othei symptom, save a tendency to constipation, was manifested until the fouith month, when the abdominal swelling had incieased so much as to interfeie with iespiiation. At the same time, the little patient suffeied much fiom vomiting and distension of the intestines by gas, and was much constipated. When fiist seen by Piofessoi Winiwarter, hei body was much emaciated, and hei face cyanotic. The abdomen was enoimously distended, and measuied 65 centimeties in ciicumfeience. The anteiioi abdominal wall was very thin and tense. Theie was a well-maiked tympanitic sound in fiont of the abdomen, and a dull sound in each flank. The swelling was not quite symmetiical, as a distinct piojection could be obseived in the iight hypochondiium. Theie was no œdema of the lowei extiemities, and the uiine did not contain albumen. As the case was cleaily one of a collection of fiee fluid in the abdominal cavity, a punctuie was made with a tiocai and canula on the left side, and vent given to 3 lities of a fluid which, to the suipiise of Dr. Winiwarter, closely iesembled fiesh milk in coloui, consistence, and even smell. The abdomen was much ieduced in size thiough this opeiation, and consideiable ielief was affoided, although the intestines iemained much distended, and a well-maiked tumoi still existed neai the iegion of the livei. This tumoui, on deep palpation, felt like a mass of conglomeiated cysts. It seemed to be fixed to the fiont of the spine, but evidently was not adheient eithei to the livei oi to the anteiioi wall of the abdomen. The fluid, on micro-scopical and chemical examination, was found to be puie chyle. In consequence of iapid and iepeated accumulation of the swelling, the abdomen was tapped aftei an inteival of a month, in Novembei, and again in the following Decembei and Januaiy. At each of these opeiations, about 3 lities of chyle weie iemoved. The patient subsequently passed fiom undei the notice of Piofessoi Winiwaitei.

In some iemaiks on this case it is stated that an effusion of chyle within the peiitoneal cavity can occui only thiough tiansudation oi thiough a solution of the continuity of some laige lymphatic vessel. Cases aie on iecoid in which, aftei compiession or plugging of the thoiacic duct, a milky fluid collected in the pleuial cavities and within the abdomen. Such cases as these can be ieadily explained. In these instances, the milky fluid was nevei effiused in laige quantities, noi was theie evei a continuous and iapid accumulation. It has been pioved by *post-moitem* investigations that, in cases of this kind, the lacteals soon become impeimeable, in consequence of inspissation of the stagnant chyle, and that the effusion of milky fluid soon ceases. The phenomena in the above iecoided case indicate that there was no obstruction to the flow of chyle from the whole intestinal tract. Professor Winiwarter, in considering the relation of the tumour in the right hypochondrium to the collection of chyle within the abdomen, formed the following hypothesis as to the nature of his case : congenital occlusion of the thoracic duct, formation of a compound cystic tumour through distension of the lacteals at the root of the mesentery by obstructed chyle, rupture of one of the cysts before or during birth, persistence of this solution of continuity, and unceasing effusion of the chyle absorbed by the intestines. That cystic dilatation of the abdominal lymphatics may be readily produced, has been proved by the experiments of Wegner, who, after repeated injections of air into the peritoneal cavity of the rabbit, found at the autopsy large cyst-like swellings containing air at the root of the mesentery. The fact that this child lived and increased in size, notwithstanding a supposed occlusion of the thoracic duct, is accounted for by the view that there was very probably a reabsorption of the effused chyle by the lymphatics of the peritoneum and central tendon of the diaphragm, and also by the bloodvessels.

This interesting communication concludes with references to previously reported cases of abdominal chylangioma, and with a full report of the analysis made by Professor Ernest Ludwig of the effused chylous fluid.—*London Med. Record,* March 15, 1879.

Syphilitic Muscular Contraction.

GUIBOUT (*L' Union Médicale,* January 4, 1879) describes the case of a man, aged 49, under his care, in the Hôpital Saint Louis, who had always enjoyed good health till the year 1853, when he contracted syphilis. Although no general treatment was followed, he had no further trouble until 1872, when he had a severe attack of laryngitis, which subsided under iodide of potassium, but left a permanent hoarseness. In 1873, he was under the care of M. Hardy for syphilitic ulceration of the legs, of which the cicatrices still remain. About the same time, also, began the muscular affection from which he still suffers. No other accident appeared until September, 1878, when some small gummata were noticed in the frontal and parietal regions. About five years ago, sharp pains in the left arm, from the shoulder to the elbow, and especially severe at night, were first felt ; and, at the same time, the patient said, there was some weakness of the limbs. From that time the pain continued, with intermissions, until October, 1878, the date of his admission into the hospital under Dr. Guibout.

On examination, the left biceps seemed somewhat wasted, and the circumference of the middle of the arm during relaxation of the muscle was 1½ centimetres less than that of the right ; but, during muscular contraction, the difference was 2½ centimetres. The left forearm could not be completely extended, and, at the fold of the elbow, was a prominence formed by the tendon of the biceps, which felt hard, like a stretched cord. The distance from the coracoid process to the bicipital tuberosity of the radius was 3 centimetres less on the left than on the right side. The muscular portion of the biceps appeared, excepting the slight wasting, to be quite normal ; the shortening, as well as the hindrance to complete extension of the forearm, seeming to be exclusively due to contraction of the tendon. No other muscles were affected. There was syphilitic osteitis of the lower third of the left humerus. Under doses of 2 grammes (30 grains) of iodide of potassium, gradually increased to 4 grammes (60 grains), the whole of the lesions had greatly improved by December 3.

Muscular contraction is a rather rare manifestation of syphilis, and belongs to the tertiary stage. In this case, the tendinous portion of the muscle was involved, which agrees with Notta's views on the subject ; while Bouisson, of Montpellier, considers the muscular portion to be more often attacked. All observers agree that the biceps is the muscle most frequently affected.—*London Med. Record,* March 15, 1879.

Cure of Dog Bite by Aspiration.

SAPOLINI publishes in the *Gaz. Med. Ital. Lomb.*, February, 1879, the following treatment for hydrophobia. Immediately after the patient has been bitten, the virus must be repeatedly aspirated by means of a syringe, alternating with frequent injections of tepid water into the wound. He asserts that in this way the wound is completely cleansed from the poison. During the period of incubation the wound must be kept open, frequently by aspiration, and some antiseptic fluid injected, such as salicylic acid, etc. The patient must also take salicylic acid internally. During the period of hydrophobia another powerful poison must be injected hypodermically, *e. g.*, the poison of the viper, or some other venomous serpent.—*London Med. Record,* March 15, 1879.

Surgery.

Removal of a Subretinal Cysticercus: Preservation of Sight.

A woman, aged 26, came under the care of Dr. HERMANN COHN (*Centralblatt für prakt. Augenheilkunde*) some time after disturbance of vision had appeared in the right eye. On examination, there were seen to be numerous punctiform and flocculent turbid spots in the vitreous body. To the lower and inner side of the pupil was a bluish-gray vesicular detachment of the retina, projecting into the vitreous body; beneath was a large vein, a small branch of which passed upwards to the vesicle. In the interior of the vesicle, about the middle, was a clear white spot. The vesicle was oval transversely and sharply defined, and had the peculiar glitter of a hydatid. On repeated examination, changes in the length of the vesicle and slight contractions were observed. The diagnosis was subretinal cysticercus. The following operation was performed without anæsthesia. Four millimetres (0.16 inch) from the outer edge of the cornea an incision, eight millimetres (about one-third of an inch) in length, was made in the conjunctiva, from above downwards. The wound having been widened as much as possible, a thread was passed through the external rectus, which was divided at some distance from its insertion. The eyeball was now rolled inwards, and the sclerotic was opened with a von Gräfe's cataract knife, to the extent of about one-third of an inch. A little vitreous humour and a trace of blood escaped. The vesicle, which was of the size of a lentil and uninjured, was now drawn out with iris forceps. There was almost no hemorrhage, nor any disposition to spontaneous prolapse of the vitreous body. The muscle was not accurately sewn together, and two sutures were applied to the wound in the conjunctiva. A compressive bandage was employed, and rest in the dorsal position rigidly enjoined. The reaction was limited to pain lasting two days, and a subsequent mild attack of iritis. Ophthalmoscopic examination on the seventh day showed the vitreous body to be clearer than before; the position of the hydatid was indicated by a white shining spot, over which the retinal vessels ran evenly. Ten days after the operation, the patient was discharged, the vision being $\frac{2}{5}$, and the tension of the eye normal—*British Med. Journal,* March 1, 1879.

Teeth Grafting.

Two interesting papers were presented to the Académie des Sciences at its meeting on January 6th (*Comptes-Rendus*, 1879, No. 1), by Dr. MAGITOT, and by one of his pupils, Dr. DAVID. Dr. Magitot, after adverting to his former communications relating to grafting of the dental follicles in certain species of the mammalia, states that in the present paper he carries the subject very much farther, embracing grafting the adult dental organs, and supplying practical applications.

" There are," he observes, " three varieties of dental grafting—1. By *restitution*, in which the tooth removed from its alveolus is restored to it, either immediately, or after a variable period of time. 2. In grafting by *transposition* a tooth is removed from one alveolus, and transplanted into another, whether in the same or in a different subject. 3. In *heterotopic* grafting, the teeth are grafted on various parts of the body other than the jaws, examples of which are recorded as resulting from the experiments of Hunter, A. Cooper, Philipeaux, etc." In the present paper Dr. Magitot confines himself to grafting by restitution, combined with the excision of the diseased parts before restitution is made. His researches on this point were first published in the *Gazette des Hôpitaux* for 1875; others have been published in the theses of his pupils, Drs. David and Pietkiewicz; and the operations of this kind have now reached the number of sixty-two. Of these sixty-two cases, fifty-seven have been definitively cured, a great number of these cures dating back from two to two and a half years. The age of the patient does not seem to have exerted any influence on the results, and the various kinds of teeth have been alike excised and grafted. The surgical indication for grafting combined with excision is essentially based upon the diagnosis of a special lesion characterized by *chronic periostitis* of the summit of the fang of the tooth—*i. e.*, inflammation of the periosteum, denudation and necrosis of the subjacent cement, and absorption of the ivory. It is a kind of mortification of the root. The morbid process which results consists in a series of accidents, as phlegmon of the gums and face, denudation and necrosis of the alveolar margin, and mucous or cutaneous fistulæ, etc. These accidents sometimes assume the chronic form and sometimes are intermittent. Left to themselves, they may give rise to great mischief, such as deformities and cicatrices of the face, and a general condition that may even place the patient's life in danger. As the mortified summit of the root of the tooth cannot be otherwise got at, preliminary extraction is required in order to enable the diseased portion to be excised, the portion of the tooth which remains sound then being restored to its original place. Before restoring it the surgeon may, if necessary, resort to various procedures, such as washing out the purulent cavity or removal of sequestra, while as regards the tooth itself, he may excise portions of its crown, or perform plugging in the case of caries. In a good number of the cases treated, the periostitis of the summit was not accompanied by concomitant caries, but in others a co-existing caries was able to be stopped while the tooth was out of the mouth. The subsequent treatment consists in the application, when necessary, of gutta-percha supports, drainage, and the removal of any mortified portions of the alveoli, etc. In general the consequences of the operation are very simple. When consolidation has been effected a slight local reaction takes place, accompanied by few or no general phenomena. The fistulæ close, the discharge ceases, and complete consolidation takes place in from a week to a fortnight. The tooth recovers its vascular connections and its uses are re-established. When the attempt fails, the tooth is simply eliminated by suppuration in a few days.

M. David in his paper thus speaks of "grafting by restitution" : " Re-im-plantation combined with extraction is a procedure which enables us to subject the teeth to operations which would have been impracticable in the mouth. We have personally resorted to it—1. For the adjustment of certain anomalies of direction. 2. In the treatment of caries when the situation of this did not admit of our reaching the pulp in order to destroy it, and practise *in situ* a satisfactory stopping. 3. In the treatment of the form of alveolo-dental periostitis, in which this affection is limited to the summit of the root. It allows of our excising the affected parts just as is done on a diseased bone ; and this excision is the only means of radically curing the neighbouring lesions which so often accompany this form of periostitis, as osteitis, necrosis, fistulæ, etc. If the tooth is carious it can also then be stopped. 4. It may also be resorted to in order to facilitate the execution of operation on another tooth or in another part of the mouth. The consolidation of the tooth replaced in its alveolus takes place, on the mean, from the tenth to the fourteenth day. It is more rapid (by the second or third day) when the roots are healthy. In cases of periostitis it is slower ; and then, principally when there are osseous lesions in the vicinity, the existence and maintenance for some days of a well-established dental fistula is of first-rate importance. By this means the suppuration obtains free external issue, and does not disturb the organic phenomena which are in progress between the root of the tooth and the alveolus. To the discharge of the pus by the alveolus is due our single failure. The various lesions of the vicinity (fistulæ, etc.) in general are cured soon after consolidation takes place. The cure has remained durable in our earliest cases for more than two years.

" Thus methodized, this procedure seems to us to carry the curability of dental affections to its farthest limits. It has given us but one failure in twenty-two cases."—*Med. Times and Gazette*, Feb. 1, 1879.

—

Preliminary Tracheotomy in Excision of the Tongue.

At a recent meeting of the Clinical Society of London (*Lancet*, April 5, 1879), Mr. BARKER contributed a case of Excision of the Tongue, in which a preliminary tracheotomy had been performed. After giving a short history of the treatment of such cases by an immediate tracheotomy to avoid the risk of the passage of blood down the trachea, he alluded to two cases in which, to his own knowledge, this source of danger had proved fatal ; but he added that in the case brought forward the tracheal wound had been purposely kept open in order to avoid, as far as possible, the risk of the inhalation of sceptic matters into the lung during the earlier part of the after-treatment. This was a real danger, for he had seen such operations followed by death, the result of septic pneumonia, or even gangrene of the lung. The patient was a man, aged 49, who was admitted into University College Hospital in April, 1877, suffering from an epithelioma of one side of the tongue, and some glandular enlargement below the jaw. Tracheotomy was performed with unusual ease, a small circle of the trachea excised, and Trendlenburg's tampon tube introduced and inflated. Considerable dyspnœa resulted at first, which, however, soon passed off. Syme's operation for the removal of the tongue was then performed, the jaw and lip divided in the middle line, and first one-half of the tongue cut through, and the vessels secured, and then the other. On the next day the tracheal tube was removed, the nostrils stopped with wool, a tube introduced into the mouth, and connected by an elastic pipe with a reservoir under the bed, whilst the mouth was otherwise closed by a pad. The patient was allowed to breathe through the tracheal wound. In five days the plugs were removed from the nostrils, and in a few days more the mouth was freed from the tube. The after history presented few

unusual features. There was on two occasions some oozing, requiring the application of perchloride of iron, and there was once a rise of temperature to 103°.
This and probably the oozing depended on an alveolar abscess, which was relieved by the extraction of some loose teeth. The convalescence was rendered
rather tedious by the exfoliation of two pieces of bone from the cut surfaces of
the jaw, but the patient is alive and in fairly good health.

Mr. MARSH said the question was of great importance. Not long ago he had
removed a portion of the tongue for epithelioma in a gentleman aged seventy-
four. The operation was not difficult, but on the eleventh day he sank from
septic pneumonia, probably set up as Mr. Barker had described. The usual
practice at St. Bartholomew's Hospital was, after splitting the tongue in the
median line, to remove each half by means of the whipcord écraseur, and not by
the bistoury, as Mr. Barker had done. The division of the jaw complicated the
operation; for it seldom united well, and in the majority of cases necrosis was
common.

Mr. BRYANT did not see the necessity for the measures proposed by Mr.
Barker. The risk from hemorrhage, when the écraseur was used, is very slight,
and as to the inhalation of putrid air setting up pneumonia, although it doubtless
could do this, yet it must be borne in mind that the subjects operated on were
frequently advanced in life and enfeebled. Nor need the secretions become foul
if detergents and salines be freely used. Was the tracheal wound large enough
to admit all the air inspired? Tracheotomy wounds generally close with great
rapidity. Where the whole tongue is involved then a preliminary tracheotomy
and Trendlenburg's tampon would no doubt be very useful, and they were of
great value in operations about the jaws. Syme's operation for excision of the
tongue was rarely called for. Two-thirds of the organ can be removed without
dividing the jaw.

Mr. BARKER, in reply, said he had fully demonstrated that the tracheal opening was large enough for the passage of all the inspired air. The wound was not
a simple incision, but a circular opening had been made to admit of the passage
of the tampon and tube. The rapidity with which pneumonia, going on to suppuration and gangrene, followed on some cases of this sort was strongly in favour
of his view of septic influence. He mentioned two cases in which hemorrhage
was fatal. Out of twenty cases, five had marked lung symptoms, four died with
gangrene and abscess of the lung.

——

Treatment of Cystic Goitre.

In a clinical lecture delivered by M. GROSS, of Nancy, reported in the *Revue
Médicale de l' Est* of November 15, he describes the treatment of cystic goitre,
known as Michel's "mixed method," as extremely useful, and furnishes a case
illustrating its advantages. Giving a rather extended review of the various modes
hitherto proposed for removal of these growths, he points out their drawbacks,
and the superiority of Michel's method over them. Briefly the latter consists in
making a vertical incision in the skin over the most prominent cyst, and then
dissecting carefully down through the various structures, until the wall of the
cavity is reached. A very fine trocar is then pushed into the cavity with a canula,
and through the latter the fluid is withdrawn. After this a plaque of pâte de
Canquoin, about three centimetres broad, is applied to the surface of the cyst,
the sides of the wound being protected by a circular piece of diachylon. This is
left on a day or two until an eschar is formed, which soon after comes away,
leaving a free opening through which the cyst can discharge, until it shrinks up,
after suppurating for a time.

It is claimed for this method that it is less likely to give rise to dangerous hemorrhage than several others, while, the caustic only being applied to the surface of the cyst, severe inflammation of the tissues around is avoided. Other cysts, if present, are similarly treated through the aperture in the first.—*London Med. Record*, March 15, 1879.

Intraparietal Hernia Complicated with Internal Strangulation; Taxis; Kelotomy; Recovery.

The case brought before us here (*L' Union Méd.*, No. 3, 1879) is one of some interest *àpropos* of the line of action to be adopted where such complications arise.

The patient had had a hernia on the left side, about a finger-breadth above the internal inguinal ring, for about eight years. On January 11, 1878, he developed all the symptoms of strangulation of the hernia. On the 13th, the small tumour was reduced with ease under chloroform, and gurgled as it disappeared. Relief was experienced for some hours, but similar symptoms again developed themselves on the 14th. In the evening, kelotomy was performed, and a small sac found between the walls of the abdomen; no strangulation. The neck of this sac was then slit up, and the fingers "were introduced into a large cavity full of coils of congested intestine." On careful search with the finger far back in the pelvis, the opening of this was discovered, and divided with the greatest difficulty. We had before us here an intra-parietal (? inter) hernia, not strangulated, behind which there was a second intra-abdominal (? sub-peritoneal) sac of great size, and with a very narrow neck, the true cause of the strangulation.

So great was the difficulty of finding this inner constriction, and danger of dividing it, that the operator advocates in similar cases opening the abdomen by an incision, as in ovariotomy, in the middle line, instead of through the first sac, and thence looking for the constriction in the peritoneal lining of the abdomen. This has been done in an analogous case by M. Terrier (*Bull. de la Soc. de Chir.*, t. iv. p. 361, 1878), when no difficulty was experienced in finding or dividing the constriction In the case before us the patient recovered.—*London Med. Record*, Feb. 15, 1879.

Cystotomy for Cystitis.

At a late meeting of the Clinical Society of London (*Lancet*, April 5, 1879), Mr. TEEVAN read notes of a case of cystotomy, the patient (who was exhibited) being a wine-cooper, aged 43, who came under care in July, 1875, having a stone in the bladder two inches by one inch and three-quarters. The urine was a mass of muco-pus streaked with blood; no renal elements could be found. He suffered much pain, and could not work. Mr. Teevan determined to crush the stone because he had, by lithotrity, completely cured a similar case, where the stone was only a quarter of an inch smaller, and he wanted to find out the extreme limit to which the operation could be advantageously pushed. Accordingly, in twenty-six sittings of about one minute each, he completely removed all the stone. The patient was, however, not cured, but only relieved. The pain he suffered incapacitated him from work, and the urine contained much muco-pus. For many months various medicines and injections were tried without success. Under these circumstances he determined to perform cystotomy. The bladder was carefully examined by many surgeons, but not a particle of stone could be discovered. On Sept. 17th, 1876, Mr. Teevan opened the bladder by a median incision from the perineum, incising the neck vertically with a probe-pointed knife to the depth of about half an inch. The immediate effect of the operation was that the patient was relieved of his pain, and the urine began to

cleai about ten days afteiwaids. Thiee weeks aftei the opeiation the patient
was appaiently cuied of his cystitis. The wound, which had been kept well
open, was then allowed to close, and thiee weeks latei the patient was peifectly
well and watei-tight. He iemained peifectly well, and had continued unintcr-
ruptedly at woik evei since. Cystotomy was iaiely peifoimed in England, and
was only mentioned in a few suigical woiks of modein date. In Ameiica, howevei, it had been established as a set opeiation since 1850, when Willaid Paikei,
of New Yoik, intioduced it. The piopositions he would lay down weie—1.
That cystotomy was indicated in those cases of obstinate cystitis which iesisted
oidinaiy tieatment. 2. That ienal disease was no bai to the opeiation. 3. That
the geneial conditions of the patient iathei than the iesults of an examination of
the uiine ought to deteimine whethei, in a given case, an opeiation weie justifiable or not.

Ii. HOWARD MARSH asked whethei it would not have been bettei in this
case to have cut in the fiist instance.

Ii. BRYANT agieed that cystotomy was an opeiation which should be moie
fiequently peifoimed for chionic iiiitation of the bladdei which iesists othei
tieatment, and so often leads to fatal ienal disease. In thiee out of six cases in
which he had peifoimed it theie was gieat ielief and iecoveiy, but the iest died
fiom piostatic and ienal disease. He would then hesitate about peifoiming cystotomy if the kidneys weie diseased, foi in such cases the slightest inteifeience
might be fatal. As an instance of this he mentioned the case of a man who,
duiing tieatment foi a uiinaiy fistula, had seveial iigois. Some time aftei he
was seen by Ii. Biyant, who, awaie of these iigois, did not think it wise to
opeiate, but employed catheteiism up to No. 10. The catheteiism induced
iigois, and the patient died fiom uiæmia due to suppuiative nephiitis. Aston
Key had fiist pointed out to Ii. Biyant the advantages of cystotomy for chionic
bladdei cases, and used to iegiet that he had nevei peifoimed it.

Ii. HEATH asked whethei Ii. Teevan divided the whole length of the piostate along the flooi ; for in that case (as pointed out by Ii. Teevan himself, as
an objection to median lithotomy in childien) the ejaculatoiy ducts would be
seveied ? In oldei people the opeiation would be moie difficult and iisky, on
account of the laige size of the piostate. Was the hemoiihage fiee ?

Ii. TEEVAN said it might have been bettei to have cut in the fiist instance,
or iathei to have followed up a single lithotiity by an exteinal uiethiotomy.
Even when ienal disease was piesent, cystotomy was justifiable, because of the
gieat ielief to the local symptoms affoided by the opeiation, and the chance of
iecoveiy. He mentioned a case of cystitis aftei lithotiity, which was allowed to
go on foi about two yeais, and was then ielieved by cystotomy. A medio-lateial
opeiation would, he thought, be piefeiable in old men, and the objection to
median lithotomy in boys—namely, the iisk of emasculating them—was of
slight impoitance in the case of middle-aged adults.

Perforating Ulcer of the Foot.

At a late meeting of the Royal Medical and Chiruigical Society (*Lancet*, Apiil
5, 1879) a papei by Iiessis. SAVORY and BUTLIN on "Peifoiating Ulcei of
the Foot," was iead. After some intioductoiy iemaiks, and the ielation of five
cases of peifoiating ulcei which have come undei theii notice, the authois desciibe
the geneial chaiacteis of the disease, and discuss its pathology. Fiom the symptoms which almost invaiiably accompany peifoiating ulcei, fiom theii examination of the leg aftei iemoval in two cases, and fiom iepoits given in othei papeis,
the authois believe that the disease is due to central or peiipheial neive-lesion,

especially affecting the sensory and trophic or vaso-motor nerves. Microscopic drawings of the condition of the nerves in two cases accompany the paper.

Mr. Erichsen said the affection was infrequent, and the point of greatest importance raised in the paper was the strong evidence adduced by the authors in favour of its being the result of nerve-lesion. Weir Mitchell had described certain neuroses of the foot and hand, especially of the foot, marked by areas of hyperæsthesia, œdema, coldness, and other signs of imperfect nutrition; such cases pointed in the same direction as these instances of perforating ulcer, affording evidence of the influence of the nervous system in producing localized disease of a limb.

Professor Humphry remarked that in every instance a corn seems to be present at the seat of the ulcer, and the question arose how far the corn may have been the cause of the nerve-change. For in all these cases the disease was described in an advanced state, when the ulcer had formed leading down to bone, and with this was evidence of impaired nerve-supply; and the question arose whether in the earlier and simpler stage there was any affection of nerves present. Slighter cases of this kind were not frequently seen, and he thought one good effect of this paper would be to direct the attention of surgeons more forcibly to corns. A corn consists not simply of hypertrophy of the cuticle, but also of the papillary layer, and, as it advances, the greater growth of cuticle in its centre gradually leads to an invasion of the cutis and even of the deeper tissues by the cuticular products. Then sometimes inflammatory changes are set up beneath the skin, and may spread deeply into the foot, the pus burrowing into the sheaths of the tendons and through the joints. Might not the nerve-condition described in the paper be the effect of the prolonged irritation of a corn? The "perforating ulcer" affected places where corns were most frequent, the most incurable corns being those seated over the metatarso-phalangeal joints of the middle and great toes. Referring to a comparison drawn by the authors between the nerve-lesion in leprosy producing ulcerative changes and the nerve-lesion in "perforating ulcer," Professor Humphry pointed out that in the latter it seemed as if there was a combination of the characters of the two forms of leprosy—the tubercular and the anæsthetic. From this point of view, then, he would rather style the affection "corn-ulcer" than "perforating ulcer"—a term already applied to definite diseases of the palate, stomach, and intestines.

Dr. Duka, from his experience of leprosy in the East, considered that the drawing showing one of these ulcers on the sole of the foot bore a striking resemblance to the changes met with in anæsthetic leprosy and sometimes in tubercular leprosy. He had seen in these diseases an ulcer appear on the sole of the foot, and penetrating to the bones.

Mr. Edmund Owen related two cases of perforating ulcer of the foot which had been under his care at St. Mary's Hospital. In one, that of a carpenter who had long been troubled with corns, the fourth toe had been amputated eight years ago; seven years subsequently the second toe had been removed, and six months since Mr. Owen had amputated each little toe, with part of the metatarsal bone, for the same affection. There was insensibility of the deep tissues of the feet, with marked impairment of the sensory nerves on the sole and dorsum. The toes were deformed, and the phalanges necrosed. In fact, the disease bore a remarkably strong resemblance to anæsthetic leprosy. He did not consider that the perforation was due to pus burrowing upwards for an outlet, for it would hardly penetrate plantar and dorsal fasciæ and interosseous spaces rather than the thickened epidermis. Moreover, in this case the dorsal end of the sinus did not pierce the integument. The other case was that of a professional pedestrian, whose sole was deeply ulcerated; the skin of the dorsum of the foot was anæsthetic and mottled with white patches; the toes were also deformed as in leprosy. Nélaton's description gave an excellent account of the disease. English authors had hitherto written little concerning it.

Dr. THIN said these cases of perforating ulcer had nothing in common with leprosy, the pathology of which was distinctly a new cell-growth invading and destroying tissues.

Mr. MORRANT BAKER asked if there was any contraction of the extensor tendons. It was a common belief that such contraction favoured the development of such ulcers by throwing the weight of the body on to the ends of the metatarsal bone. Such contraction might itself be due to some nerve-affection. That the explanation of the production of the ulcers by nerve-lesion was the true one he had no doubt. A paraplegic patient came to him with an ulcer on the foot, for which amputation was necessary. There was no pressure on the foot, for his paralysis compelled him to walk with crutches. Some time after an ulcer of like character appeared on another toe.

Mr. GAY did not gather that a corn always preceded the formation of the ulcer. He mentioned a case illustrative of the inveteracy and incurability of these ulcers. A gouty subject of about fifty, after an injury, lost sensibility in the great toe, and after a time an ulcer formed on the ball of the toe. This would not heal, and, although Mr. Gay tried to cure it by transplantation of skin from the neighbourhood, still fresh ulceration appeared at the margins, and the patient's state remained as before.

Mr. GASKOIN could not accept Dr. Thin's assertion as final, for he believed there was affinity between this "perforating ulcer" and anæsthetic leprosy, and he thought some writers mentioned new cell-formations in the nerves in the former as in the latter affection.

Mr. BARWELL recalled a paper by Fischer, who in 1875 advocated the neuro-paralytic doctrine of the formation of these ulcers. He himself thought Professor Humphry's view could not be sustained, for corns were extremely common, and were usually seated not at the sole of the foot, but on the back of the little toe. At the same time a suppurating corn might lead to necrosis and considerable mischief in the foot.

Mr. SAVORY, in reply, said that appended to the paper was a full bibliography, where Fischer's work was alluded to, but the most original paper was one by Duplay and Morat. Facts would not support Professor Humphry's view, for all perforating ulcers do not begin in corns. There was one case in which the ulcer reappeared again and again after amputation, and usually evidence of nerve-lesion *preceded* the local affection. Again the change in the nerve was often more advanced in the upper than in the lower part. That the disease often commenced in the site of corns was undoubted, probably because these were parts much subjected to pressure, and their view was that, owing to mal-nutrition from the nerve-change, these parts suffered from such pressure. As to leprosy, he remarked that resemblance in certain features by no means established identity of disease. The fact of defective nutrition from nerve-change was of great importance as regards the results of operations, especially at the present time, when so much attention is being paid to the external condition of wounds to the disregard of the condition of the parts cut through.

Mr. BUTLIN said the point common to perforating ulcer and anæsthetic leprosy was the formation of an ulcer due to obvious changes in nerves. The paper by Fischer was based on the work of others, and contained no original observations.

Mr. SAVORY, in reply to Mr. Baker, added that in two of the cases there was some contraction of the extensor tendons, but he did not see how this could possibly have to do with the nerve-lesion.

On Osteomyelitis.

Accoiding to Dr. ROSENBACH of Gottingen (*Deutsche Zeitschrift für Chirurgie*, Band x, Heft 3-4), phlegmonous inflammation of the medulla of bone is not readily pioduced through the simple action of mechanical, physical, and chemical agents. This authoi, in expeiiments on animals, has fiequently ciushed and laceiated the medulla, has passed a seton through the tissue, applied active physical iiiitants, as, foi instance, the actual cauteiy, and also chemical agents, as caustic alkalies and fuming nitiic acid, without having evei succeeded in setting up phlegmon. On the othei hand, the injection of a small quantity of septic pus or of some othei putiid mateiial will inaiiably set up, in bone maiiow, a phlegmonous inflammation similai in couise and chaiactei to the so-called spontaneous osteo-myelitis. The iesults obtained fiom these expeiiments lead to the conclusion, pieiiously deiiied by Piofessoi Lucke fiom chemical obseiiation, that the so-called osteomyelitis iniaiiably iesults fiom infection. The infective mateiial must be caiiied to the medulla by the blood, and the localizabization of the phlegmonous attack may depend on injuiy, chilling, oi, in biief, on some local distuibance of the ciiculation. It is difficult, howeiei, in eveiy case to account foi the localization.

The authoi suggests that osteomyelitis is a specific infective disease piesenting ceitain definite chaiacteis. It is not communicable. The infective mateiial, when piesent in the blood, is capable of setting up localized phlegmon of bone-maiiow with oi without the associated influence of some local ciiculatoiy distuibance, as tiaumatism oi chilling. The geneial condition of the patient is not, as a iule, much distuibed by the diiect action of this mateiial. The giaie geneial symptoms that aie so often met with in cases of osteomyelitis aie due to the diiect passage into the vasculai system of decomposed fatty mateiial and pioducts of inflammation.

The authoi ielates that he has pioied by expeiimentation on animals that a geneial infection may be established affecting veiy slightly the geneial system, but capable, in association with fiactuie of any long bone, of causing in the injuied bone a localized inflammation similai in natuie to osteomyelitis.—*London Med. Record*, Jan. 15, 1879.

On Aithiitis Due to Lymphatic Piopagation.

In a communication made to the *Académie de Médecine* (Oct. 16), M. VERNEUIL stated that he had met with fiie cases in which a secondaiy aithiitis of the knee followed a lymphangitis of the lowei extiemity. The fiist of these was a man, 50 yeais of age, with a shatteied constitution, who had an ulceiation on his instep, and shoitly a lymphangitis of the coiiesponding lowei extiemity, giiing iise to numeious abscesses, equal to an olive in size. Aftei some of these in the iegion of the knee had been opened, the joint became the seat of violent pain and inflammation, and piesented all the signs of a puiulent aithiitis. In spite of eveiy caie the patient died some time aftei. The second patient was a young giil of 14, who ieceived a contusion of the gieat toe; from this aiose a lymphangitis and multiple abscesses in the leg. One of these, situated on the innei side of the knee, was opened; this was followed, in a few days, by a puiulent aithiitis, and neithei diainage of the aiticulation, noi immobility of the limb, could pieient an unfoitunate teimination.

In the thiid obseiiation, the man was cachectic, and 48 yeais old, with a wound on the doisum of his foot about the size of a fiie-fianc piece; this was followed by iigois, iomiting, feiei, and a lymphangitis. The uiine contained some albumen. By appropriate treatment the lymphangitis subsided and the albumen disappeared, but an abscess showed itself in the neighbourhood of the knee; this opened spontaneously, but a purulent arthritis was set up, from which the patient slowly succumbed. The fourth case was that of a man with lymphangitis and erysipelas, arising from a wound of the great toe, which opened into one of its articulations. The resulting inflammation extended as far as the top of the thigh, but as the swelling subsided an enormous hydarthrosis of the knee appeared. Emollients, tincture of iodine, and blisters partly dispersed this, but the patient, who was always weakly, had bed sores, and died from pneumonia. The last observation was upon a man aged 60, who was cachectic and had a collection of fluid in his knee-joint. An examination revealed an excoriation on the foot, a lymphangitis of the lower limb, and an adenitis of the groin; on the inner side of the knee there was also a collection of pus. The limb was kept immovable, and frictions employed. The abscess was finally laid open, the fluid absorbed, and the man recovered.

M. Verneuil remarks that the explanation of these phenomena is not easy; persons who are cachectic and with an external injury seem generally to be the victims. It is admitted that the lymphatics of the subcutaneous cellular tissue communicate with the synovial articulations opening into the bursæ, and permitting by extension the inflammatory propagation, which in these cases had been observed. At first, a communication is frequently established between the lymphatics and the periarticular serous membranes, then between these last and the articular ones. Early opening, with the modern antiseptic precautions, is recommended for these lymphatic abscesses, decided benefit having been found to result from so doing.—*London Med. Record*, Jan. 15, 1879.

—

On Periarthritis of the Knee.

M. FATOME (*Thèse de Paris*, 1878, No. 16, and *Bulletin Générale de Thérapeutique*) says that this disease may be divided into three classes, according to its progress. These are acute, subacute, and chronic periarthritis. In some cases the sheaths of the tendons and the bursæ are œdematous, while in other cases we find that these same organs are dry and thickened; a more or less rapid and abundant suppuration may also be present. The crackling which is peculiar to synovitis crepitans is heard either on the same level with the pes anserinus, or on the bursa patellæ, or lastly on the same level with the bursa on the upper part of the tibia. Purulent gatherings may often present the appearance of some affection within the articulations. A painful spot on the circumference of the articulation is often a symptom of suppuration of the ends of the joints. The moment that the accumulation of matter has been proved, it ought to be removed as quickly as possible. Sometimes the synovial membrane of the joint is also attacked, but this does not occur in the beginning of the disease; it generally remains healthy, thanks to the layer of fibrous tissue which forms between the inflamed place and the synovial membrane.—*London Med. Record*, February 15, 1879.

—

Spontaneous Fractures, considered especially from the point of view of Etiology. Prognosis, and Treatment.

PATEY (*Thèse de Paris*, 1878) divides the fractures into three classes, and each of them into two groups, viz.: 1. Spontaneous inflammatory fractures, acute and chronic. 2. Spontaneous fractures, caused by rarefaction of the bone. local and general. 3. Spontaneous fractures, caused by osteomalacia, simple and of nervous origin.

Class No. 1 comprises all spontaneous fractures caused by ostitis, osteomyelitis, or acute juxta-epiphysary ostitis. During this acute stage the inflammation acts upon the bones, producing the necrosis either of a diaphysis *in toto* or in separating the diaphysis from the epiphysis. By chronic inflammation the tissues in which a sequestrum is imbedded is much thinned, and the fracture is brought on by the inflammation becoming suddenly acute.

Fractures which occur in diathesia, scrofulous, tuberculous, and syphilitic inflammations are generally caused by the rarefaction of the bone, and seldom by necrosis. General affections, such as cancer, syphilis, scrofulosis, rachitic disposition, osteomalacia, and scurvy, tend to produce in the bone a local predisposition to fracture, which either concentrates itself on one special point or else is diffused over the whole skeleton.

A local predisposition is due to the presence of a cancerous tumour or to the existence of a specific osteitic process, such as scrofulosis, tuberculosis, or scurvy. The action of rachitis on the bone is a rarefication of the diaphysis at the expense of the epiphysis. Osteomalacia spreads over the whole of the skeleton, decalcifying it. Alterations which are caused in the bones by nervous, central, or peripheric lesions, vary according to the nature of the affection.

Spontaneous fractures very seldom occur in cases of paralytic lesions of the nervous centres, whether they are located in the brain or the cord. The only exception to this rule are fractures which happen in the nervous osteomalacia of maniacs. As far as spinal lesions are concerned, irritating ones are the only class which are capable of producing such an alteration in the bones as to cause a fracture. This is especially seen in locomotor ataxy, where quick consolidation and exuberant growth of osseous matter are very remarkable. The author quotes one case of spontaneous fracture which occurred in the course of variola, and was without doubt caused by the zymotic germs of the disease. So far as the prognosis is concerned, two points have to be especially kept in view, viz., the probability of consolidation of the fracture and the origin of the latter. With the exception of cancerous fractures consolidation may occur in almost every case. The treatment depends on the etiology and the condition of the fracture.—*London Med. Record,* March 15, 1879.

Practice of Nerve Stretching.

Dr. E. MASING, of St. Petersburg, reports in the *St. Petersburger Medicinische Wochenschrift,* No. 34, 1878, two cases treated by exposure and stretching of nerve trunks.

The subject of the first case was a male, aged 37, who had for eight years suffered much from neuralgic pains in the lower limbs. The attacks commenced near the antero-superior spine of the left ilium shortly after the man had been exposed during one night to cold and wet. In spite of frequent and varied treatment, the pains gradually increased in intensity and extent, and finally radiated along both extremities. Between five and six years after the commencement of this affection, the muscles moving the right foot became paralyzed, and soon afterwards those of the left foot. During the last year there had been slowly developing anæsthesia along the posterior surfaces of both lower limbs. The patient, when first seen by Dr. Masing, was mentally depressed, pale, and emaciated. He was easy only when sitting with the lower limbs up to the hips enwrapped in woollen material. Intense pain was caused by any movement, by exposure of the lower limbs to cold air, and by the recumbent posture. The pain commenced near the left ilium and from thence extended to the lower limbs. No objective morbid sign could be made out at the starting-point of the pain; there was no subcutaneous infiltration or peritoneal thickening. The pulse was normal.

The lower limbs were wasted and the feet and limbs cool. There was almost total anæsthesia of the skin over the ischiatic region, along the posterior surface of each thigh, and over the whole of each leg and foot except in the portions along the inner surface supplied by the long saphenous nerve. All the muscles of both legs and feet were paralyzed, those of the thighs, supplied by the anterior causal and obturator nerves, were not thus affected. There was occasionally in-voluntary discharge of stools, and micturition was much impaired.

On September 15th, the patient having been placed under the influence of chloroform, a vertical incision 10 centimetres in length was made from the fold of the buttock downwards along the posterior surface of the left thigh. The sciatic nerve, which appeared to be quite healthy, having been exposed and iso-lated was then forcibly extended. At the same sitting a similar operation was performed on the right side. The proceedings occupied about twenty minutes, and were carried out under antiseptic conditions. For some hours after the operation the patient suffered most severely from radiating pains in the region of the left hip. On the following morning he was easy and could lie down without trouble. On the fourth day he suffered much from pains over nearly the whole body, and especially in those parts of the legs and feet which before the operation had been anæsthetic. On the fifth and sixth days there was but little pain. On the seventh day he suffered much from burning sensations along the course of the left long saphenous nerve. On November 3d there was marked improvement, the pains radiating from the left iliac region had been much relieved and the man was now able to move the muscles of the legs and feet. The main trouble at this time was severe burning pain in the left anterior crural nerve and along the left saphenous nerve as far as the knee. On November 8th the left anterior crural nerve was exposed and stretched. The operation was soon followed by much improvement in the general condition of the patient. On April 7th of the present year the man was in good health, able to walk well, and quite free from pain and from anæsthesia.

The subject of the second case was a boy, aged 12 years, whose left foot had been injured through a fall. The injury had resulted primarily in swelling of the extremity with much tenderness, and subsequently in persistent spasm of the muscles of the left leg. When the patient was first seen by Dr. Nasing, the left foot presented a condition of extreme equino-varus, all the toes being bent at right angles to the dorsum. The muscles of the left leg were in a tetanic con-dition. Active movements at the joints of the distorted foot were completely abolished, and attempts at passive motion were attended with much pain. There was hyperæsthesia of the skin of the foot and leg, and also very marked tender-ness over the trunk of the sciatic nerve in the thigh, and along the three great branches of this nerve in the leg. Locomotion was prevented through pain. During sleep the foot became lax and as mobile as the opposite extremity. The contraction and distortion recurred at the moment the lad was aroused. Dr. Nasing diagnosed the case as one of neuritis of the sciatic nerve, commencing as a result of the injury to the foot in the perineal and two tibial nerves and invading gradually the main trunk. The healthy condition of the ham-string muscles in-dicated that but part of the sciatic nerve was affected, and the unilateral extent of the morbid condition, the preservation of the normal innervation of the bladder, and of all portions of the body supplied by the lumbar plexus, led to the conclu-sion that the spinal cord and its membranes remained in a healthy state. On January 16th, after other plans of treatment had been tried without any success, the left sciatic nerve was exposed and stretched. This operation was followed on the next day by contractions over the whole of the left lower limb, and by forcible flexion at the knee. The hyperæsthesia of the leg still persisted. On the third day the patient suffered much from chronic spasm of the muscles of the left leg. During the first week in February, no improvement having taken place previously in the condition of the limb, there were frequent paroxysms of violent clonic spasm, the leg becoming very much flexed. At this time the hyperæsthesia had extended beyond the region of the leg and passed to the left thigh, and to the left sides of the pelvis, abdomen and thorax. From February 6th, when the patient was first treated by frequently repeated subcutaneous injection of morphia, there was a temporary improvement, and in the course of one week all the more severe symptoms had disappeared. At the end of a fortnight, however, after the cessation of this treatment in consequence of dyspepsia, loss of appetite, and headache, all the patient's troubles returned. Towards the end of May some improvement was noted after continuous blistering of the spine in the lumbar and sacral regions. The pain was then much relieved, and the patient was able to go about on crutches. The paroxysms of clonic spasm were much less frequent and less severe, but distortion of the foot and friable flexion at the knee still persisted.

The patient was again seen after an interval of three months, on August 16th, and his condition had then much improved. He was able to extend the left leg so as to touch the ground with the toes, and could walk without crutches. There was still much hyperæsthesia. The lad's general condition was very satisfactory.

Dr. Nasing, in some remarks on this case, states that there was much obscurity as to its precise nature. The symptoms, he holds, contraindicated any central lesion and pointed rather to a reflex neurosis. The nerves about the left ankle had probably been torn and contused in the injury to this joint, and a centripe-tally spreading neurosis had resulted. The disturbances set up after the opera-tion in the regions supplied by the anterior crural, lumbar, and intercostal nerves were, it is supposed, purely reflex, since neither atropy nor paralysis could be observed in the affected parts.—*London Med. Record*, Jan. 15, 1879.

Midwifery and Gynæcology.

Case of Gestation Prolonged to Fifteen Months.

Dr. HENDERSON reported (*Am. Journal of Obstetrics*, April, 1879) the fol-lowing case in which the duration of pregnancy is said to have been prolonged to fifteen months:—

He was called in the latter part of January, 1860, to see a lady about 35 years of age, who was the mother of several children, and quite healthy. Her pre-vious confinements were in no particular remarkable. She had menstruated regularly until the previous December, which period she missed, making the flow in the early part of November the last previous to the time he was called. She had a slight hemorrhage from the uterus, associated with more or less pain in the back and lower part of the abdomen. The womb upon examination was found enlarged to about the size that we would expect to find it at the period of two or two and a half months' gestation. The patient expressed herself well satisfied that she was pregnant, and feared very much that she would have an abortion. He prescribed sulph. morphia and enjoined rest, which soon relieved her.

She continued to develop until about the proper time, when she quickened, which led her to suppose that she would be delivered about the middle of August following. He said that he saw the patient frequently from the time he had been

called, and believed from her appearance that she would be confined at about
the anticipated time. She, however, continued for a month or more over the
expected period, and becoming uneasy again, sent for him. He made an examination and found the uterus to all appearance at the full period of gestation, but
the os was not in the least dilated.

The patient said to him that she had felt the movement of the child from the
period of quickening up to that time, and that the motion, so far as she could
remember, was just the same as in her former pregnancies. She continued in
this condition until about the first of November, at which time he made another
examination, and found the uterus apparently larger, but in every other respect
about the same as it was at the last examination.

He now left the patient in the care of another physician, as he expected to be
absent for a few months. About the middle of February, 1861, he was sent for
again, as both patient and physician were becoming quite uneasy. Before leaving the city, he consulted Prof. N . B. Wright concerning the case, who expressed
himself quite hopefully as to the final result, saying that he had seen cases of
prolonged gestation, but that they had all terminated favourably, although he admitted that he had never seen one quite so prolonged as this one seemed to be.

Dr. H. again visited his patient in consultation with the physician with whom
he had left the case. Found the patient apparently in good health, but with the
abdomen enormously distended. She had not had labour pains up to this time,
which was the 15th of February, 1861, making in all fifteen months since she
supposed herself to be pregnant. The os was considerably dilated and dilatable.
A suspensory bandage was improvised and the weight of the abdomen suspended
from her shoulders.

In a day or two labour came on, and after a tedious and painful labour, they
were compelled to deliver her with the forceps.

The child, weighing *sixteen pounds and a half*, was stillborn, having evidently
died during the labour, as was clearly proven from the fact that the movements
of the child were distinctly felt up to within three hours of its delivery.

Dr. H. then said that, although he had given a faithful history of the case, yet
he could not help feeling that there would be in the minds of many, if not all,
who heard his remarks, serious apprehensions after all that there must have been
some mistake about the case. He, however, felt it to be his duty to narrate the
circumstances, notwithstanding the serious doubts to which it might give rise.

———

Eruptions Connected with Menstruation.

Dr. SCHRAMM has published in No. 42 of the *Berliner Klinische Wochenschrift*
for 1878, the following observations : An unmarried lady, aged 36, of anæmic
appearance, had suffered for seven years from dysmenorrhœa, which she had
contracted from a severe chill. Simultaneously, the dorsal surfaces of both hands
were covered with disseminated brownish nodules, of the size of a lentil, which
disappeared in the course of a week, but reappeared at the next menstruation on
other places of the dorsal surface. Later on, similar nodules developed on the
neck and the labia, accompanied by slight itching ; sometimes a few pinkish irregular infiltrations would break out behind the ears ; a few little spots, which soon
developed into blisters, were disseminated on the tongue. These eruptions were
complicated with a circumscribed painful swelling of the orifice of the urethra,
which greatly impeded micturition. The eruptions and papules on the neck and
labia always lasted for a few months, while the other nodules generally disappeared within a week. On vaginal examination, it was found that the patient
suffered from anteflexion of the uterus, complicated with catarrh of the uterus
and the vagina. These affections were treated methodically, and the patient

ceased to suffer from dysmenorrhœa and from the eruption. After her recovery, and after exposure to much fatigue, she had the menstrual pain, and the eruption reappeared, but only once. Another patient, who was consumptive and suffered from retroflexion, had her back and shoulders at the time of the catamenial flow covered with a peculiar eruption in the shape of small red nodules, which formed long lines, and gave to the skin the appearance of being of an uniform red colour. They were accompanied by a sensation of some tingling and itching, and disappeared after three days. Dr. W. Wagner has also published some cases of "catamenial erysipelas" in the *Allgemeine Medicin. Central-Zeitung*, No. 94, 1878. The first case was that of a girl, aged sixteen, who had menstruated regularly since the age of fourteen, but had, since the date of the first flow, suffered from erysipelas of the face, which began four or five days before the menses, and lasted about eight days. It spread over the head, thereby causing the hair to fall off. Her head had grown almost bald, so that she always had to wear a handkerchief over it. Her health was good, and nothing abnormal could be detected in any internal organ. She was treated with Fowler's solution and iodide of potassium, but without any result. The second case was that of a country-girl, aged seventeen, who menstruated for the first time six months ago, and had had erysipelas of the face shortly before this. The inflammation increased during five days, but vanished speedily with the appearing of the flow. In this case, however, the erysipelas was not repeated with the same regularity as in the first case; it was only observed whenever the menses were irregular. The patient was very anæmic, and was accordingly treated with dialysed iron. The third patient was a woman, who had reached the time of the menopause. She had always been strong and healthy, and had never had the least trouble during the time of the catamenial flow. The menses disappeared for the first time at the age of forty-seven, for about eight weeks, when they reappeared; they were accompanied by a very slight erysipelas of the face. The same phenomenon was repeatedly observed during the next eighteen months, when the periods disappeared altogether. In the next year, a very slight erysipelas was observed three or four times, which, however, did not spread any further than the nose. The first case, undeniably, is the most peculiar one, as it could not be traced to any pathological affection of the genital organs, and the flow itself never had any influence on the duration of the erysipelas. The two other cases were evidently in some way influenced by the period, as they were only observed at the time of its cessation, or when it was irregular.—*British Med. Journal*, March 8, 1879.

Death following Vaginal Injection of Acetate of Lead.

The following case, published by Dr. SPÄTH in the *Centralblatt für Gynäko-logie* (No. 25), tends to prove that, in making injections into the vagina, the fluid may pass through the Fallopian tubes into the abdominal cavity. The patient, a healthy woman, aged twenty-two, married, and who had been confined ten weeks previously, had been ordered by the author to daily inject into the vagina a weak solution of acetate of lead, in order to cure her of leucorrhœa. On the eleventh day, the patient, being in a hurry, probably used too much force in injecting. She suddenly felt a violent pain in the lower part of the abdomen, and fainted. When Dr. Späth was summoned, he found the woman very much changed. Her face was livid, and wore an anxious expression; her pulse small and frequent. The abdomen was very tender on pressure, although not inflated. A violent attack of peritonitis followed, and the patient died at the end of seventy-four hours. No injury to the uterus or vagina had been detected by the author at his first visit. The *post-mortem* examination gave the following results: The intestines were very much distended. The mucous membrane of the small intestine was red, especially in the portions situated in the vicinity of the uterus and the broad ligaments. On the surface of the mucous coat of the small intestine, up to a level with the navel, and through the whole of the hypogastrium, were disseminated irregular round flat patches of a grayish colour, which could easily be removed, and beneath which the membrane was entirely normal. Similar patches were also found on the interior of the uterus, which did not present any alterations ; neither did the vagina nor the rectum. The Fallopian tubes were very narrow, and did not present any sediment ; while the broad ligaments in the neighbourhood of the fimbria, and the peritoneal surface of both ovaries, were covered with numerous black flakes of various sizes. This sediment, on being chemically examined, was found to consist of sulphide of lead. The author tries to explain this fatal accident through the tube of the injecting apparatus having, by some accident, entered the os uteri, so that the fluid was thrown into the uterine cavity ; thence through the Fallopian tubes into the abdominal cavity, thereby producing the inflammation.—*British Med. Journal,* March 1, 1878.

Hernia of the Ovaries.

In an article on hernia of the ovaries Dr. ALBERT PUECH collects (*Annales de Gynécologie,* November, 1878) a large number of recorded cases and estimates the relative frequency of the several varieties. Far the most frequent form he finds to be the inguinal variety, of which he finds eighty-six observations. It is five times as common as the crural form, and at least four times as common as all other varieties put together. In new-born children it is the only kind of ovarian hernia met with. This relative frequency, so different from the case of intestinal hernia, is to be connected with the fact that the condition of ovarian hernia is in the majority of cases not an accident or malady, but a fault of development, according to which the ovaries tend to follow the course taken by the testicle in the other sex. Thus of the eighty-six cases only sixteen appeared to have been truly accidental, a similar number might be set down as doubtful, and in fifty-four there appeared to be no doubt that the hernia was congenital. The author considers that the ovary in these cases has been drawn down by the fibres of the round ligament, as the testicle is by the gubernaculum testis, but he thinks the process is not so much a true muscular contraction as a shortening of the fibres, analogous to the contraction of newly formed cellular tissue. In no less than thirty-three of the eighty-six cases the anomaly was associated with some other malformation of the genital organs. Four times there was a uterus unicornis or bicornis, sixteen times absence or rudimentary development of the uterus, and thirteen times feminine hermaphroditism. There were twenty-eight examples of double inguinal hernia, in eight only of which the genital organs were in other respects normally formed. In congenital hernia the ovary is found to be invariably accompanied by the Fallopian tube, while in accidental hernia it is more frequently isolated. In six cases the hernial sac was found to contain also the uterus or one of its horns, in three intestine, and in two omentum.

A typical example of the condition of double inguinal hernia of the ovaries associated with rudimentary development of the ducts of Müller is found in a case recently recorded by Werth (*Arch. f. Gyn.* xii. p. 132). The patient, twenty-two years old, was admitted into the hospital at Kiel in October, 1876. She had an angular curvature of the cerebral vertebræ resulting from a blow received at the age of twelve. At the age of fourteen she was affected by pains in the legs, which led to a weakness and diminution of sensibility in the right leg. The menses had never appeared, but every four weeks she had pains in the abdomen accompanied by exacerbations of the pains in the leg. An atresia of the vagina had been discovered about nine months before. The osseous system was found to be fully developed, the voice feminine, but somewhat harsh, the breasts small and flat; the pelvis had preserved its infantile character. The external genital organs were normally formed, but the vagina was only represented by a depression five mm. in depth. No trace of vagina could be discovered between sound in bladder and finger in rectum. On conjoint examination under chloroform with the finger in the rectum a body could be reached on each side which was recognized as the kidney, but no trace of uterus or its annexes could be discovered, except two small bodies at each side of the pelvis, whose nature could not be precisely determined. At the time of the onset of periodical pains, referable to menstrual molimen, attention was attracted to a body as large as a pigeon's egg in the situation of the inguinal canal at each side. These bodies resemble testicles in consistence and in sensibility, and pressure upon them produced pain radiating to the kidneys and epigastrium. After the cessation of the periodical pains, the tumours appeared to be smaller, and their surface smoother. They had been first noticed by the patient at the age of fourteen, the period when pains in this region had first appeared.

The tumours were successfully removed under carbolic spray by Esmarch, on Feb. 2, 1877, and proved, as was expected, to be the ovaries. The hernial sacs contained also the pavilions of the Fallopian tube, and a pedicle, which appeared to be the extremity of the horn of a rudimentary uterus bicornis. These pedicles were tied with carbolized gut. The ovaries had an irregular surface covered with scars; they contained many Graafian follicles, but less than are usual at such an age. The left ovary contained a recent corpus luteum, six mm. in diameter; the largest follicle was eleven mm. in diameter, and contained an ovum. For a few days after the operation the patient had violent pains resembling those previously felt, but there was no febrile disturbance, and the leg had become stronger when she left the hospital, seven weeks after the operation.

Accidental or acquired hernia of the ovary is always unilateral, and more frequent on the right than left side. It is invariably due to the muscular strain, and it most readily arises after delivery, when an intestinal or omental hernia has existed previously. Crural hernia of the ovary the author finds recorded fourteen times, and it was acquired in all of these instances, except one case of a new-born child, recorded by Cloquet, in which a hernial sac, on the right side, contained the uterus, with the ovaries and the Fallopian tubes. The ovary in its abnormal situation is exposed to frequent lesions. Inflammation was noted in twenty-eight instances, cystic degeneration in seven, cancer in two, and tubercle in one. In one instance a cystic tumour of the displaced ovary, of eighteenth months' growth, was successfully removed by Lücke.

Dr. Puech relates at length a singular case 'which he interprets as gestation, in the sac of an ovarian hernia. It occurred in 1706, and was recorded in 1716 by N. Goucy, of Rouen, who supposed that a fecundated ovum had lodged in a pouch at the insertion of the round ligament, and during its growth passed down in the direction of the inguinal canal. A young lady of good position, aged 20, was brought to N. Goucy, in August, 1706, by her lover, on account of a tumour in her right groin, as large as a hen's egg, which had appeared about a month. N. Goucy, who had previously treated the lover for a venereal affection, at first considered the swelling to be a bubo. It continued, however, to grow for two and a half months, became unequal in outline, and strong arterial pulsations were felt in it. The patient being extremely anxious for a cure, the tumour was incised, and found to contain a foetus, situated with its membranes within a sac of peritoneum. The foetus, a living male, was of about three months' development, which corresponded with the period of cessation of menses. The placenta was attached to the ring of the external, oblique muscle and to neighbouring parts. It was separated without difficulty by gentle traction upon the funis. Dr. Puech contends that for gestation to occur outside the abdominal cavity, as in this case, both ovary and Fallopian tube must have been in a hernial sac, the first to provide the ovum, the second to conduct the spermatozoa.—*Obstet. Journ. of Great Britain,* February, 1879.

Total Extirpation by Abdominal Section of the Cancerous Uterus.

The operation for extirpation of the cancerous uterus by the method of FREUND has now been performed in a considerable number of cases. The mode of procedure was first described by Freund in the *Sammlung Klinisches Vorträge,* No. 133, for April, 1878, and some improvement in its details are mentioned in the *Centralblatt für Gynakologie,* June, 1878 ; and in a communication made by him at the meeting of the German Gynæcological Society at Cassel, in September, 1878. Operations are also described by Dr. Fränkel, assistant to Dr. Freund (*Berliner Klin. Wochenschrift,* 1878, No. 31), and by Dr. Credé (*Centralblatt für Chirurgie,* No. 32).

The method of operation, according to the latest improvements, is as follows :—

The patient is placed with the pelvis higher than the shoulders; the carbolic spray is used, but it is not allowed to enter the abdominal cavity. The vagina and cavity of the uterus are previously disinfected by a ten per cent. solution of carbolic acid, and an incision is made in the linea alba, as for ovariotomy. Dr. Freund now extends the cutaneous incision down into the mons veneris, and if the recti muscles are tense, divides partially or completely the tendons of these muscles, in order to obtain more space, but the peritoneum is not divided down to the symphysis. The intestines are drawn up out of the pelvis, and held wrapped in a soft linen cloth soaked in a warm solution of carbolic acid (two per cent.), until the operation is completed. If the body of the uterus is healthy, a strong ligature is passed through it, whereby to draw it upwards; but if diseased, it is seized by fenestrated forceps, the blades of which hold it firmly without lacerating it. The broad ligament on each side is then secured by ligatures in three loops. In order to avoid transfixing those portions of the broad ligament where large veins exist, the upper loop is passed through the substance of the Fallopian tube above, and through that of the ovarian ligament below. The middle loop transfixes the ovarian ligament above and the round ligament below. The passing of the lowermost loop is the most difficult part of the operation. An empty needle, immovably mounted on a handle, is first passed from the vagina into the peritoneal cavity in front of the broad ligament, and anterior to the uterine artery, the exact position of which is made out by bimanual examination. The needle is then threaded, withdrawn into the vagina, and again passed into the pouch of Douglas behind the broad ligament, and the thread so drawn upward into the abdomen. Finally, the loop is completed by transfixing the broad ligament, the ligature being passed through the substance of the round ligament. In his earlier operations, Freund found a difficulty in properly constricting the tissues by the lowest loop in consequence of their elasticity, and the result was apt to be a persistence of hemorrhage from the uterine artery after excision of the uterus, in spite of the lowest ligature. To avoid this, he now endeavors to include as little vaginal tissue as possible in the loop. The two punctures in each lateral vaginal *cul-de-sac* are made as close together as possible, and the needles are introduced in a strongly divergent direction.

After the ligatures are placed, the upper and posterior limits of the bladder having been defined by the catheter, the peritoneum between the two is divided by the knife. The anterior surface of the uterus is then separated from the bladder by the fingers or handle of the knife, the fundus uteri being meanwhile drawn by an assistant upwards or backwards as required, by means of the transfixing ligature or forceps.   As soon as the anterior vaginal *cul-de-sac* appears as a reddish fold at the bottom of the wound between uterus and bladder, it is perforated from the vagina by a guarded knife, and the opening enlarged to both sides.   One or two fingers are then passed from above through the wound into the os uteri, and the cervix is gradually drawn upwards through the wound into the posterior vaginal *cul-de-sac*, is fully exposed, and the position of the ligatures seen.   The incision can then be carried round the cervix, so as to sever the uterus completely without risk of dividing the lowest loop of ligature, or injuring the ureters.

The uterus is thus removed through the abominal wound.   If, however, there is any open cancerous surface on the cervix likely to contaminate the peritoneum, either the cervix should be amputated previously, or all ragged tissue scraped away, and the wound touched with the cautery or strong carbolic acid.   The pelvis is afterwards washed out with carbolic acid.

After the uterus is detached, all the ligatures, which are left long, are carried down through the aperture into the vagina, and strong traction is made upon the uppermost ligature, to which small rods have previously been attached to distinguish them.

In this way an inversion of the borders of the wound is produced, so that the ligatured stump of the broad ligament on each side presents in the vagina, and the uninjured portions of the anterior and posterior layers of pelvic peritoneum fall together in a transverse fold.   The two layers are then united at this level by sutures, so as to shut off completely the peritoneal cavity.   In his later operations, Freund has inserted into the peritoneum some of the loops destined to form this suture before excising the uterus.   A plug soaked in carbolized oil (ten per cent.) is then placed in the vagina, by which canal the ligatures also are brought out, and are generally detached by about the fourteenth day.   Besides closing the peritoneal cavity, the inversion into the aperture of the broad ligament has the advantage of supplying, to some extent, the loss of intervening tissue between bladder and rectum.

In estimating the results of the operation so far, it is of interest to recall the three operations published in 1828, and performed by Dr. Blundell, who extirpated the whole uterus through the vagina.   Though in all three cases the disease had extended to the vaginal vault, so that they would hardly now be considered suitable for the operation, although he had the disadvantage of operating without anæsthetics, and although one patient died almost immediately from hemorrhage and shock, yet one of the three survived the operation, and was in good health five months later.   Freund now reports five deaths in ten operations, one from peritonitis due to perforation of the sigmoid flexure affected by the malignant disease; one from supposed intussusception on the twelfth day in a case in which no autopsy could be procured, one from collapse in a patient who had granular kidney and fatty heart, two from septic peritonitis.   None of the cases which survived had yet shown any sign of recurrence of the disease except one, in which there was a small and suspicious-looking hard spot in the right vaginal *cul-de-sac.*

Schroeder had operated nearly according to Freund's method in three cases, one of which recovered without a symptom; Martin in three cases, all of which proved fatal, one from septicæmia, the second from collapse; in the third infiltrated retro-peritoneal glands were found.   Olshausen has operated twice.   The first proved successful, although the bladder or the ureter was injured, and urine oozed from the vagina until six days after the operation, after which it ceased entirely.   The disease, however, recurred in five months.   The second case died fiom secondaiy hemoiihage, and at the autopsy a canceious kidney was found. Baumgaertner has opeiated once, but in a case unsuitable for the opeiation, as funnel-shaped excision of the ceivix had been peifoimed, and the disease had soon ietuined. At the opeiation the iight bioad ligament was found so much in-filtrated with cancei that it pioied impossible to aveit the bleeding by means of ligatuies applied aftei Fieund's method. Seveial aiteiy foiceps weie left at-tached, but in spite of diainage and irrigation with salicylic solution, the patient died on the fouith day, piobably fiom septicæmia. Fiänkel iepoits one case (Beiliner Klin. Wochenschrift, 1878, No. 31) which pioied successful, although the caicinoma had alieady extended to the uppei pait of the vagina, and the paiametiium and the ietiactoi uteii on the iight side weie infiltiated with caici-nomatous nodules. The inguinal glands weie swollen, but weie not iegaided as caicinomatous. Some of the caicinomatous poitions of the vagina could not be entiiely extiipated duiing the opeiation. They weie tied, and iemoied on the thiity-seienth day by cauteiization. Dr. Credé iepoits a fatal case (Centialblatt für Chiiuigie, No. 32). The caicinoma had spiead ovei the whole vagina. Both ovaries also pioied to be diseased, and weie theiefoie iemoied. The peii-toneum was not stitched togethei, but the edges of the vaginal wound weie united by small foiceps, which iemained in the vagina. The patient seemed to be doing well at fiist, but suddenly collapsed, and died on the second day. At the autopsy, seveial of the glands in the pelvis weie found to be diseased. Ji. Alexandei, of Liveipool, also iepoits a fatal case. The patient was thiity-eight yeais old, showed no cachexia, and the symptoms dated about five months. The uteius was moiable, and the disease was belieied to be confined to it. The iight Fal-lopian tube, howevei, was found to be affected by the disease of the ovaiy. The uppei loop of ligatuie on the.right side was, theiefoie, placed outside the ovaiy. Aftei iemoial of the uteius seveie symptoms of collapse appeaied, although only about foui ounces of blood weie lost. The ligatuies weie, theiefoie, diawn into the vagina, and the abdominal walls biought togethei as iapidly as possible. The patient ievived foi a time, but died about an houi and a half aftei the opeiation, as the authoi believes, fiom shock, no fuithei hemoiihage haiing taken place.

Thus, out of twenty-two cases heie mentioned, theie weie eight iecoieiies, while seveial of the fatal cases weie obviously unfaiouiable fiom the fiist, the disease haiing manifestly extended beyond the uteius. Not all of the twenty-two cases, howevei, weie caiiied out stiictly accoiding to Freund's method, and in that authoi's own hands the moitality so fai is fifty pei cent. only, a iesult which fully justifies fuithei tiial of the opeiation in such a disease as cancei of the uteius. It is the piactice of Fieund to iemove the ovaiies as well as the uteius, if the menopause has not been ieached. He iecommends that the steps of the opeiation should be pieviously practised upon the dead subject. The method of opeiating is still moie suitable foi caicinoma or saicoma of the body of the uteius than foi that of the ceivix. It may also obviously be extended to the case of fibioid tumouis, which it has hitheito been geneially consideied possible to extii-pate only when a sufficient length of ceivix is left fiee fiom the giowth to seive as a pedicle.—Obstetiical Jouinal of Gieat Britain, Jiaich, 1879.

—

New Clamp Sutuie:

At a late meeting of the Obstetiical Society of Philadelphia (Am. Jouinal of Obstetrics, Apiil, 1879) Dr. ALBERT H. SMITH desciibed a sutuie which he had employed successfully in closing laceiations of the peiineum, and which is a modification of one pioposed by H. L. Thomas, M.D., of Richmond, Va., in the Ameiican Jouinal of the Medical Sciences for Octobei, 1877. A needle, aimed with a soft wire, is passed through the tissues in a straight line, and without emerging is carried around to the point of exit on the opposite side of the wound. A straight steel canula of proper length is now slipped down along each end of the wire, until the inner ends approximate. The ends of the wire are now drawn together and twisted, and the entire surface is held in close apposition.

Medical Jurisprudence and Toxicology.

On Poisoning by Cantharides used as an Erotic.

This case is reported by M. Rosolino Braga from the *Revista Medica de Rio de Janeiro*. The patient suffered from nephro-cystitis with albuminuria and hæmaturia, as a result of taking cantharides. Fortunately, he recovered from the more serious effects in a few days. M. C—, a Portuguese, aged 23, of general good health, was admitted into the hospital on the 17th January, 1877. The account he gave was that on the previous night, which he had passed with a public prostitute, he had drunk a glass of wine, presented to him by the girl as a glass of white port. He observed that it was thick and turbid, but he, nevertheless, drank it. In the course of the night he had intercourse with the girl, and with unusual ardour, which surprised him. Having expressed his astonishment to his companion, she candidly informed him that, in order to excite his amorous propensities, she had put cantharides into the glass of wine which he had swallowed.

In returning home about midnight, he was seized with a strong desire to urinate. In spite of all his efforts he could pass only a few drops of scalding urine, attended with severe pain throughout the length of the urethra, especially at the meatus, where he had the sensation like that of the pricking of pins. These symptoms became worse, and they were attended with priapism and severe pain in the genito-urinary organs as well as in the lumbar region, and with intense thirst. Under these circumstances, he came to the hospital for relief.

He was seen at 9 A. M. by Dr. Brandão. He was then much agitated, crying out and very restless. The eyes were injected and lustrous, the pupils were dilated, and the countenance animated. The pulse was small and frequent. There was nausea with intense thirst. There was the most acute pain in the urethra, rendered much worse when with great difficulty some drops of urine were expelled. The desire to micturate was incessant, and an acute state of nervous erethism was then produced. Only a very small quantity of urine could be discharged; and this was thick and bloody. The abdomen was retracted and sensitive to pressure, especially in the hypogastric region, where the slightest touch produced acute pain. Pain also was felt in the lumbar region, owing to the kidneys being affected, and this pain extended downwards to the perineum. The catheter brought away a small quantity of thick bloody urine containing albumen in marked proportion.

In the treatment, hypodermic injections, mild enemata, leeches, and poultices, were employed, with bromide of potassium internally. These remedies produced a rapid amendment in the symptoms. On the third day urine was passed naturally, and it contained no albumen. The patient left the hospital cured.

It was not possible to discover what preparation of cantharides had been taken by this man, nor the quantity in which it had been administered to him. Dr. Braga thought that the powder had been used in rather large proportion; this is extremely probable, from the description given by the patient of the appearance of the wine.—*London Medical Record*, Feb. 15, 1879.

—

Chronic Poisoning with Arsenic in Medicinal Doses.

The following case is reported by MACIEL in the *Revista Medica de Rio de Janeiro*. Dr. B—, of the Province of St. Paul, in Brazil, aged about 50, of a weak constitution, and subject to dyspepsia, had suffered for a long time from attacks of intermittent fever. He had taken large doses of the sulphate of quinine, but without much benefit, and he resolved to try the effects of Fowler's mineral solution, not only for the ague but for a skin disease with which he was affected. He persisted in this treatment for *three months*, and apparently with good effects. The quantity of the medicine taken by him latterly, *i. e.*, about the 16th January, 1876, was twelve drops twice daily. On the 17th January, while travelling by rail, the doctor suddenly fainted. From this he gradually recovered, and on arriving at the station he was able to get up and go and see a patient. The next day he was seen by Dr. Teixeira Maciel, who then learnt that Dr. B. was subject to fits of quotidian ague—from one of which he was then suffering—and that he had employed arsenical preparations for its treatment. He found that, at the end of the first month of this treatment, Dr. B. began to feel in his knees pains of a rheumatic nature. He said, "I have long suffered from my stomach, and only yesterday I was attacked with vomiting. In reference to my fainting in the train, it was merely a passing vertigo, of no importance. Since yesterday I have not been able to stand without perceiving this sensation. This morning, under a similar attack, I threw myself on my bed, but, by a strong effort of will, I was enabled to overcome it."

Dr. Maciel found the pulse slow (68), irregular, and intermittent, and that since the previous evening, there had been no desire to pass urine. The patient admitted that for some time past his urine had diminished in quantity, and that he had had tenesmus both of the bladder and rectum, with colic and spasms in the bowels. Dr. Maciel considered that these symptoms were indicative of an arsenical saturation of the body, and that it would be imprudent to continue this treatment with such a derangement of the stomach. Devergie advises that Fowler's arsenical solution should always be taken with great caution, and that the dose should be only very gradually increased, never exceeding sixteen drops daily. Its use should be discontinued so soon as any unusual or abnormal symptom makes its appearance—such as cramp, congestion, headache, or a sense of weight and uneasiness in the stomach. The continuance of the arsenical medicine after any of these symptoms are manifested is attended with the greatest risk. He advised Dr. B. to lay aside the solution, and resort to the use of tonics and cordials associated with diuretics. His patient was only half convinced when Dr. Maciel left him. The advice came too late. It was given at nine o'clock in the morning, and an hour afterwards Dr. B. was seized with another fit of syncope, in which he died.

Dr. Maciel ascribed death to the effects of the injudicious and long-continued use of the arsenical solution. The supposed rheumatic pains in the joints were the first warning; these were followed by vomiting, tenesmus, diminution of the urinary secretion, colics, fits of coma, and vertigo, all of these obvious signs of the saturation of the system with arsenic (arsenicism). Dr. Maciel makes use of this unfortunate case to advise practitioners to adopt more minute precautions in the therapeutical use of arsenical preparations. Among these he recommends by preference the arseniate of soda, which he prescribes in the form of powder, each packet containing half a milligramme (.0077 grain).

Dr. Rey, in reporting this case, says that Fowler's arsenical solution, according to the foreign formulary of Laennec, contains 1 per cent. of arsenious acid, or 1 centigramme per gramme, and that it is always prescribed in drops. He considers this to be a dangerous proportion of arsenic, for a slight inadvertence might give rise to poisoning. Pearson's arsenical solution contains 1 centigramme of arseniate of soda in six grammes of liquid, and Boudin's solution contains 1 gramme of arsenious acid in 1000 of liquid. These solutions are preferable to Fowler's, as the doses are more easily regulated.

[We believe with Dr. Maciel, that this was a case of chronic poisoning with arsenic, and that the symptoms described gave quite sufficient warning to withdraw the medicine. Considering the extent to which the use of Fowler's solution is carried in medical practice, cases in which injury is done by it seldom present themselves, and fatal cases are very rare. In fact there is, we believe, only one instance recorded in which this solution has destroyed life under medicinal use. This seems to furnish a sufficient answer to the objections taken by Dr. Maciel to the employment of Fowler's solution as a medicine.

Dr. B., who lost his life on this occasion, took, we are told, twelve drops of the solution twice daily. This would be equivalent to one-tenth of a grain for each dose, or one-fifth of a grain daily. Taken in this proportion for three months, it would amount to a total quantity of eighteen grains. These were large daily doses to be continued for so long a period, and elimination should have been very active in order to prevent a fatal accumulation of arsenic in the system.

The facts of the case, however, show that elimination was by no means active. The urine, which is the principal medium for the elimination of arsenic, had for some time fallen off in quantity, and this indication of the action of arsenic was unheeded by Dr. B. Orfila and others have shown that in the acute form of poisoning one of the fatal indications is the suppression of urine. A fortiori, this failure in the action of the kidneys would have a powerful influence in chronic poisoning. Dr. B. no doubt thought that he had kept within reasonable medicinal doses; but the fifth of a grain of arsenic daily, represents, unless duly eliminated, a fatal dose in ten days. It is most probable that he did not give his mind to the subject of elimination at all, and did not connect the secondary symptoms from which he suffered with chronic poisoning by arsenic. Hence such a quantity of the poison was allowed to accumulate in the system, as to produce fatal effects through the head and the brain.

In the only instance recorded in which this solution proved fatal to life, a woman took half an ounce of it in five days, and died from the effects. This corresponded to two grains of arsenious acid in the whole, or two-fifths of a grain per diem, double the quantity taken daily by Dr. B. This case terminated fatally in five days, while that of Dr. B. did not prove fatal until after the lapse of twenty-three days.

There is reason to believe that in the medicinal use of these powerful agents, which fall under the class of poisons, medical men look more to the dose given at any time than to the powerful effects of accumulation as a result of imperfect elimination. There are many who consider that they are safe so long as they do not exceed a medicinal dose; but the case of Dr. B. clearly shows that this is no criterion of safety. A poison may die from medicinal doses continued for too long a period, as well as from a large dose given at once.]—*London Med. Record*, Feb. 15, 1879.

CONTENTS.

Published Monthly, price $2.50 per annum, free of postage.
Also, furnished together with the AMERICAN JOURNAL OF THE MEDICAL SCIENCES *and the* MEDICAL NEWS AND LIBRARY *for* SIX DOLLARS *per annum in advance, the whole free of postage.*

HENRY C. LEA, Philadelphia.

THE MONTHLY ABSTRACT

OF

MEDICAL SCIENCE.

VOL. VI. No. 6.   **For List of Contents see last page.**   JUNE, 1879.

Anatomy and Physiology.

The Variations in the Hæmoglobin of the Blood.

LEICHTENSTERN has investigated the amount of hæmoglobin contained in the blood in health and in various diseases by means of Vierordt's method of quantitative spectrum analysis. The blood was obtained from the finger, and mixed with a trace of caustic soda, without which the blood which contains many white corpuscles is too opaque. He has found that the blood of healthy new-born children contains the largest quantity of hæmoglobin. The quantity sinks pretty quickly, so that in ten or twelve weeks the average of adult life is reached. It then falls gradually, and reaches its lowest point at the age of six months to five years. From six to fifteen years it rises a little, and more considerably after the fifteenth year, so that between the twenty-first and forty-fifth year the second highest point is reached. It then again falls. Over sixty years of age the amount of hæmoglobin again rises. Sex makes a difference over ten years of age, the blood of females being a little poorer in hæmoglobin than that of males. Differences of constitution and of general nutrition appear to make no recognizable difference, only in four very obese persons the quantity was strikingly small. Hourly observation made on the experimenter himself during six days showed, with some probability, that four to six hours after food there is a striking fall in the hæmoglobin, probably due to a dilution of blood with chyle. Abundant ingestion of water caused in the healthy no alteration in the amount of hæmoglobin. On the other hand, it caused, in a woman suffering from nephritis, a slight diminution, together with an increase in the œdema. The withholding of liquids in a non-febrile case of pleurisy caused on two occasions an increase in the amount of hæmoglobin, although the exudation remained unaltered, and the urine became scanty. A course of sweating, by hot baths, in a patient suffering from lumbago, caused no distinct change. Febrile diseases, pneumonia, scarlet fever, acute articular rheumatism, epidemic cerebro-spinal meningitis, yielded no noteworthy result, and certainly no regular diminution in the amount of hæmoglobin. In typhoid there was no notable change in the first weeks of the disease. During the convalescence from febrile diseases, with protracted wasting, a diminution showed itself at last. In a case of fatal apyrexial ileus, a concentration of the blood caused an immense increase in the amount of hæmoglobin, amounting to more than 30 per cent. In phthisical patients the quantity of colouring matter was as a rule diminished, but in some cases it was normal. In cancer a diminution was always found, the only exception being a concentration of the blood through vomiting. A diminution was constantly present in gastric ulcer. Chronic heart disease showed almost constantly a diminution. In emphysema and diabetes mellitus the results varied. Chlorosis constantly showed a difference, and so also did leucocythæmia. Progressive pernicious anæmia always presented the greatest diminution met with in any disease. Energetic treatment of syphilitic patients with mercury, in which the weight of the body fell, caused a diminution in the amount of hæmoglobin, which again rose after the cure.— *Lancet,* April 12, 1879.

—

Accelerator Nerves of the Heart.

Acceleration of the pulse is produced by stimulation of the nerve which unites the last cervical ganglion of the sympathetic trunk with the first thoracic ganglion. Drs. STRICKER and WAGNER (*Medizin. Jahrb.* Heft 3, 1878), to discover the real origin of these accelerating fibres, isolated the sympathetic trunk in the abdomen of a dog, by cutting all the afferent branches, and then stimulating it at the sixth thoracic ganglion. The effect of this stimulation is due to the action of the current upon the nerve already spoken of, which is known as the loop of Vieussens. If ligatures be applied above and below this loop, the upper segment alone remains sensitive to stimuli. The acceleration is the more marked the nearer the electrodes are placed to the loop of Vieussens; it is therefore supposed that the accelerating fibres increase in number from below upwards. Further to show the origin of the accelerating fibres, the authors cut the vagus, and noticed an acceleration of the pulse, which was lessened after section of the two loops of Vieussens, though the heart-beats were still slightly more rapid than at the commencement of the experiment. The acceleration following section of the vagus is caused by the accelerating tonic effect of the medulla, the existence of which proves that the fibres of the loop take origin from the medulla. On excitation, therefore, of the medulla, the authors have been able to exhibit an acceleration of the heart-beat; and they obtained a similar result, but more slowly, and only when the blood pressure had risen considerably after section of the vagi. The acceleration produced by stimulation of the medulla is therefore due to stimulation of the accelerator fibres, and to an increase in the blood-pressure. In short, then, the accelerator nerves arise from the cervical cord, pass downwards, and then upwards, in the form of loops, to the six upper thoracic ganglia, and unite at the loop of Vieussens. The function of the accelerating nerves is to counteract the normal influence of the inhibitory nerves. The two sets of nerves are therefore antagonistic to each other. The authors deny the statement of Baxt that the heart is insensible to the influence of the accelerators, after stimulation of the vagus.—*London Med. Record,* April 15, 1879.

Materia Medica and Therapeutics.

Physiological Action of Peroxide of Hydrogen.

Dr. PAUL GUTTMANN of Berlin has repeated the experiments of Assmuth and Schmidt on animals with a solution of peroxide of hydrogen of 1006 specific gravity. This solution has long been used for bleaching purposes in this country, and is very permanent. The injection of four cubic centimetres under a rabbit's skin immediately caused severe dyspnœa, clonic convulsions, and death followed in a few minutes from asphyxia. The cause of the asphyxia, which Dr. Guttmann has been the first to explain, is the development of innumerable bubbles of gas in the right auricle and ventricle, so that the blood froths just as if air had entered by the veins. Microscopic examination of the pulmonary circulation in curarised dogs injected with the peroxide, showed that the bubbles of oxygen due to the decomposition of the peroxide never penetrated the branches of the pulmonary artery. Dr. Guttmann has found that if he injects one syringeful or three-quarters of a cubic centimetre of peroxide solution into one side of a rabbit's abdomen, and two syringefuls of a 20 per cent. solution of ferrous sulphate simultaneously into the other, the animal does not die, though three-quarters of a cubic centimetre is the lowest fatal dose. Hence, he concludes, that at least part of the oxygen liberated from the peroxide combines with the sulphate, and that the remainder is insufficient to obstruct the circulation and cause asphyxia, for, under ordinary circumstances, while three-quarters of a cubic centimetre kills, one-half of a cubic centimetre does not. Dr. Guttmann has, like Thénard and Schönbein, observed the powerful antiseptic action of the peroxide. Ten cubic centimetres of urine mixed with one cubic centimetre remained nine months without putrefying. To this action is probably due the good effect of the peroxide on soft chancres noticed by Stöhr in 1867, and confirmed by Guttmann. Guttmann has, also, tried the peroxide in chronic dyspepsia (ten grammes to 200 of water—dose, half an ounce three times daily), and with good results. Dr. Richardson, it may be remembered, in 1862 published a number of observations on the subject, in which improvement of the digestion was one of the main features. In the discussion on Dr. Guttmann's paper at the Berlin Medical Society, Dr. Frankel stated that he had found the peroxide solution rather weaker antiseptically than carbolic acid. He had used it with benefit as a mouth-wash in a case of fœtor oris. Guttmann's experiments have been repeated with similar results by Dr. E. Schwerin (Virchow's *Archiv*, lxxiii, 37). Slight divergencies of opinion between their results, and, generally speaking, between those of other observers on the same subject, seem all explicable by the solutions used not being of uniform strength.—*Lond. Med. Record*, April 15, 1879.

—

Action of Digitaline on the Circulation.

The following are the results of CAVAZZINI's observations, which have been published in the *Annales d'Omodei*, 1878, No. 245, p. 115:—

1. The action of digitaline on frogs is manifested on the heart, particularly on the ventricle, by exciting the muscular fibres in proportion to the dose. 2. One or two drops of the solution, according to the season, accelerate the movement; six to seven will bring on tetanic contractions of the ventricle. 3. The digitaline augments the tone of the cardiac fibres, and lessens the number of the contractions, by reducing them to an infinitely small number. 4. The auricles are hardly, if at all, excited by the digitaline, the systolic contraction is not diminished in the same proportion as in the ventricles. 5. The diastole of the ventricle does not seem to be quickened, but rather subordinate to the action of the muscular fibres of the auricle. These fibres are often apt to enlarge considerably, which is followed by paralysis, so that it is obvious that they must remain inactive. 6. Some physiologists assert that the myocardium during the systole does not lose the blood which it contains; this assertion is untrue, as is proved from the pallor of the fibres which has often been observed. 7. Digitaline accelerates the peripheric circulation in proportion to the time and the quantity which has been employed for the experiment; the acceleration is due to the increased force of the impulse of the heart. When the ventricular contractions begin to slacken, and the ventricle becomes tetanic, the circulation diminishes first, and then ceases altogether. 8. The capillaries dilate, though not much, and the circulation may be accelerated, provided the drug does not prevent the ventricle from contracting rhythmically during the diastole. 9. It appears from the above that the action

of digitaline is principally localized on the heart, and that its action on the vessels is only a secondary one. 10. It seems as if digitaline augmented in the respiratory substance the faculty of absorbing oxygen. 11. The opinion of the Berlin school, that digitaline, when given in small doses, is stimulating, and exciting when in large doses, has not proved to be correct. This drug always stimulates the cardiac energy and dilates the vessels; if given in a toxic dose, it produces tetanus and the rupture of the heart. 12. The action of digitaline may be summed up in the following words : It prevents the cardiac systole from growing too weak, it gives a new impulse to the peripheric circulation by increasing the *vis a tergo*, and dilating the capillaries; and finally it may be found very useful in affections which are complicated with insufficient oxidation of the blood. —*London Med. Record*, April 15, 1879.

Use of Salicylic Acid.

Dr. WILLIAM SQUIRE, in a communication to the *British Medical Journal* (April 26, 1879) on the two independent effects of salicylic acid, the germicide and antipyretic, says : there are many conditions of disease where it would be well to make use of both these actions, and some where the antipyretic is distinctly aided by the germicide effects of the acid, so that fever is lowered more certainly and quickly by its use than when the more easily administered soluble salt is prescribed. This is well seen in scarlatina anginosa, and sometimes in diphtheria, whether the acid be conveyed to the throat directly, or be suspended in mucilage, or by means of glycerine, its most convenient solvent. Half an ounce of glycerine, when hot, will dissolve half a drachm of salicylic acid. This is stronger than necessary, and, when cold, will either deposit some of the acid or may become solid; in either case, it will redissolve when heated, and can be mixed in a warm spoon with an equal quantity of hot water, and given in small quantities with or without any drink afterwards; or, a solution of five grains of salicylic acid to the drachm of glycerine can be used, either alone or given with a little cream. In this way, not only are the mouth and throat cleansed, but the fever is soon lessened; it is only while the fever is high that the strong doses need be continued. In cases of moderate severity, it suffices to prescribe this weaker glycerine solution, and to order half a drachm or a drachm to be mixed with an ounce of water at the time of administration. The latter is quite strong enough for an adult, and is better followed by a drink of water. Or half an ounce of the glycerine in half a pint of water forms a suitable mixture; this sipped frequently or given as a drink every two or three hours, diminishes fever and improves the throat. Such a solution of two grains to the ounce is efficient as an antiseptic, and can be used in spray. Where a general antipyretic effect is desired, salicylate of soda may be given at the same time, fifteen grains being equivalent for this purpose to ten grains of the acid. It is contraindicated where there is renal congestion or any albuminuria, as most of the acid is excreted by the kidneys. This method of administration is more suitable to scarlet fever than to diphtheria, where the necessity for giving iron restricts the use of salicylic acid to the intervals when the stronger form can be applied in small quantities frequently. In erysipelas, no form of salicylic acid is advisable; not only would it interfere with the use of iron, which is then essential, but there is no febrile condition over which it has so little control as erysipelas. In typhoid fever, the use of salicylic acid presents some advantages over that of salicylate of soda. The glycerine solution is suitable for administration in diabetes, salicylic acid having a power of checking the formation of sugar not possessed by salicylate of soda. For this purpose the acid is required in full doses; it might take the place

of carbolic acid in rendering diabetics more tolerant of operation and less liable
to suffer from boils and from suppuration.   In catarrhal sore-throat, or at the
commencement of a common cold, the weak solution of salicylic acid is beneficial.
For checking the febrile reactions in phthisis it is also preferable.   It also acts as
a sedative to the pneumogastric, and the weaker glycerine solution in water relieves cough.   As a remedy in whooping-cough, this solution may be found as
effective and more convenient than the laryngeal insufflation of the powder.
Hay-fever is checked by dropping a grain to the ounce solution into the nares.
The great obstacle to the freer use of salicylic acid is its sparing solubility in
water; this difficulty has been overrated.   Solutions of one or two grains to the
ounce keep clear or deposit a few flocculi only, when theoretically all but one-
fifteenth of a grain should separate.—*British Med. Journal*, April 26, 1879.

Salicylic Cotton, Benzoic Cotton, and Liquor Aluminæ Aceticæ as Antiseptics.

To prepare salicylic cotton (five per cent.), PAUL BRUNS directs (*Pharm.
Centralblatt*), the saturation of 100 parts of cotton with 400 parts of a solution
in alcohol of salicylic acid five parts, and castor oil two parts (or castor oil and
colophony each one part).   In a precisely similar manner the benzoic cotton is
prepared, substituting benzoic for salicylic acid.   The amount of salicylic or benzoic acid may be increased up to ten per cent., the quantity of castor oil being
also correspondingly increased.   A solution of acetate of alumina is recommended
by the author as superior to thymol, or carbolic, salicylic, or benzoic acid for
disinfecting purposes, for dressing wounds, and for permanent antiseptic irrigation.
He prepares the solution by dissolving in 500 parts of water 150 of alum, and
mixing this with a solution in 500 parts of water, of 240 parts of crystallized
lead acetate, filtering, and adding water sufficient to make the filtrate measure
2000 parts; this solution, which contains three per cent. of alumina acetate, he
frequently dilutes for use with from three to six times its bulk of water.—*London
Med. Record*, April 15, 1879.

*Febrifugal Effects of Bromhydrate of Cinchonidine, administered
Hypodermically.*

GUBLER says (*Journal de Thérap.*, No. 1, 1879) that cinchonidine contains in
a very high degree the febrifugal properties of quinine, while the bromhydric acid
imparts to the salts greater sedative properties, and diminishes their tendency to
poisoning.   The bromhydrates of cinchonidine are specially harmless to the subcutaneous cellular tissue.   Acid bromhydrate is preferable to neutral bromhydrate,
because it dissolves more easily.   A solution of dibromhydrate of cinchonidine
in the proportion of one to five is stable, and sufficiently concentrated, and an
injection of one cubic centimetre of this solution, which contains two decigrams
of the active principle, if repeated twice daily, has the same effect as one to two
grammes of sulphate of quinia taken by the mouth.—*London Med. Record*,
April 15, 1879.

Chloramyl as an Anæsthetic.

Chloramyl, a combination of pure chloroform and nitrite of amyl, has recently
been tried as an anæsthetic, at the London Hospital, by Mr. Rivington, Surgeon
to the Hospital.   The first patient to whom it was administered was a healthy
man, and the operation merely the slitting up of a sinus.   The patient inhaled
the drug freely and comfortably, with no symptom of choking; the pulse increased
almost immediately in volume and rapidity; the respirations were more frequent
and less deep.   In three minutes, the patient began to struggle, and, within four

minutes of the commencement of the administration, the pulse suddenly failed, so as for a moment to be hardly perceptible; the respirations became hurried and shallow; the jaw appeared to be closed by spasm; the lips were blue; the eyes staring and suffused, the left pupil much dilated, but the right of moderate size (about the dimension of a No. 8 catheter); the breathing was very noisy and stridulous, as if due to laryngeal spasm. With difficulty the mouth was forced open. These symptoms passed off rapidly, and in about the space of two minutes the patient came to himself, without passing through the talkative stage usually observed when chloroform is given. The slight operation needed was performed while he was quite conscious. He himself thought that the anæsthetic had caused him to feel the pain less acutely. The next patient anæsthetized was a young woman, aged 25, suffering from extensive warty growths of the vulva. Mr. Rivington cut away the growths, arresting hemorrhage by pressure and the occasional application of the actual cautery. She was in good health. She inhaled the chloramyl comfortably, and in five minutes was fairly under its influence. The pulse remained throughout full and regular, the respiration easy. As in the previous case, she regained consciousness without passing through the stage of disquiet usually observed. The third operation was for the removal of necrosed bone from the hand; the patient was a healthy man. In six minutes he was perfectly anæsthetized. His pulse during the first minute became intermittent, the intervals of intermission decreasing in frequency until the third minute, when the pulse was perfectly regular. The respirations were throughout easy. The patient struggled a great deal, but came to himself without any display of restlessness or talkativeness. In each instance, the patient was free from any cardiac mischief. The drug was administered in the same manner as is adopted at the hospital for the administration of chloroform, but the quantity used was greater. It was observed that, when once the patient was well under the influence of the chloramyl, small quantities of the drug were sufficient to keep up the narcotic effect. All the patients recovered comfortably, without vomiting or other bad result. In the two latter patients, the pupils remained throughout quite equal, the eyes turned up, with lateral nystagmus, the globes retaining perfect parallelism. The drug was obtained from Bass, Brothers & Co. Chloramyl was first advocated by Dr. R. Sandford, in a letter to an American journal. From experiments upon animals, he has come to the conclusion that this combination is far safer for general anæsthetic purposes than chloroform uncombined, and, "so far as tried, it seems to be fully as safe as sulphuric ether, and far more pleasant in its administration, possessing all the advantages of pure chloroform without its dangers." He states that, "in administering chloramyl, the patient's face becomes flushed much sooner than with chloroform; but press the drug right along, and the countenance does not become pale. Both heart's action and respiration are kept up thoroughly throughout the anæsthesia." Dr. Sandford alleges that chloramyl prevents the approach of danger both by syncope and by asphyxia. The formula he uses is: Squibb's chloroform, lb.j; nitrite of amyl, two drachms. He suggests that the amount should be diminished in long and tedious operations. Mr. J. T. Clover, in reviewing Dr. Sandford's communication in the January number of the *London Medical Record*, stated that he made a trial of this mixture in ten cases. The anæsthesia was quickly produced, without much excitement in any case; but three suffered nausea afterwards, and two of them vomited and remained for an hour much in the same condition as if chloroform alone had been given. It appears to be similar in its action to that of a mixture of chloroform and ether; but as the vapour is less pungent, the patients generally breathe it without resistance. It was much too soon (Mr. Clover thought) to pronounce upon its relative safety.—*British Medical Journal*, April 26, 1879.

Metallotherapy.

The marvels of metallotherapy will never cease. Dr. DUPUY relates, in a recent number of the *Gazette Obstétricale*, a case of retention of urine, in which he made a successful application of metallotherapy. The case was that of an hysterical woman, aged 40, who had been treated for several years for permanent and painful spasm of the neck of the bladder, accompanied by a little metritis and accentuated hyperæsthesia of the left ovary. For the last year, she had retention of urine, which necessitated a five months' daily catheterization; she at last was relieved of this by antispasmodic treatment and by the employment of suppositories of belladonna. The cure was continuous till the month of last November; then retention reappeared, more painful and more persistent than before. The introduction of the sound provoked a spasm of the muscles of the urethra, and immediately awoke in the patient a sensation of heat and violent pain, frequently provoking an attack of convulsion with loss of consciousness. The patient had arrived at such a point as to have so much horror of the catheterization as not to drink, and to endure the torture of thirst for two or three days at a time in order to put off the moment when the use of the sound would become indispensable. Things were at this pass when, after having exhausted all the series of antispasmodics, M. Dupuy had the idea of having recourse to metallotherapy in order to discover the metal suitable to the patient, who was at this time suffering from convulsive spasms of the limbs. He ascertained that gold, when applied to the skin, increased the convulsions, whilst other metals, such as copper, steel, and silver, made them disappear immediately. M. Dupuy then applied over the vesical region and round the upper part of the thighs the metallic bracelets of Dr. Burq; and an hour afterwards the patient passed urine abundantly, and without pain. From that moment, the catheter was no longer called for; when the urine did not pass, the armatures were applied, and micturition occurred naturally, although sometimes with pain. The ovarian hyperæsthesia had also disappeared, and the patient could swallow more easily, thanks always to the metallic bracelets.

M. LANDOUZY relates an extremely curious example of metalloscopy or metallotherapy observed by him in the wards of Dr. Hardy. A woman suffering from severe hysteria, convulsions, contractions, etc., presented, at the time at which these observations were being made, attacks of meteorism provoking very severe abdominal pains. With the view of calming these pains, M. Landouzy, after having previously bandaged the eyes of the patient, tried upon the belly the application of a magnet, which at first only gave rise to a sensation of disagreeable cold; but about two moments later there occurred in the right wrist and labial commissure some slight convulsive movements; at the same instant, the speech of the patient, who up to that time had continued to answer questions which were being put to her, became slow and heavy, like the conversation of a person who is falling asleep, and then the patient became silent; all efforts made to awake her by all sorts of means were in vain; she remained plunged in profound sleep, with general anæsthesia and muscular resolution. Seeing that this state much resembled natural sleep, except that absolute anæsthesia continued, the magnet was withdrawn; at the end of six seconds, the same movements occurred in the face and the wrist as those already observed, and the patient, whose eyelids had been unbandaged, opened her eyes, and seemed to come out of a profound sleep; at this moment, it was ascertained that sensibility had returned all over the body. A new observation was then made; the eyes of the patient were at first simply bandaged, without making use of the magnet, and for more than ten minutes nothing particular occurred. At the end of this time, a portion of the magnet was put in contact with the anterior surface of the left forearm; about a minute afterwards, there occurred what had been observed when the magnet had been applied on the first occasion; that is to say, slight spasmodic movements in the wrist and in the right labial commissure. Then the patient became insensible to all means of stimulation, and seemed to fall profoundly asleep, respiration and circulation remaining as they were before the experiment. It sufficed to remove the magnet in order that at the end of from six to eight seconds the patient, whose eyes this time had been bandaged, awoke, when, after having presented the same slight clonic movements which have been already mentioned, she asked if they were not going to take off her bandage. This being taken away, the magnet was replaced in contact with the abdominal walls, and for a quarter of an hour the patient conversed tranquilly when interrogated; then, while still conversing, M. Landouzy closed her eyelids with his fingers and thus kept the eyelids closed; two minutes had not elapsed, when the patient fell again into a state of complete sleep with general anæsthesia. This time, instead of withdrawing the magnet, it was left in position, and the patient's eyes were drawn open. She immediately came to herself, said that she had not dreamed at all and experienced nothing during her sleep, but felt something heavy and cold on the stomach. This experiment was repeated a great number of times, and this truly lethargic sleep was always produced under the same conditions, viz., application of the magnet on a given point of the body, the patient having her eyes closed and covered; the patient always returned to herself and recovered sensibility as soon as the magnet was withdrawn if the eyes remained closed, or as soon as the eyes were opened if the magnet still remained in contact with the skin. We publish to-day some interesting contributions to the knowledge of the subject.—*British Med. Journal*, April 26, 1879.

<hr>

Waterproof Paper.

Dr. W. W. KEEN, Surgeon to St. Mary's Hospital, Philadelphia, describes (*Med. and Surg. Reporter*, April 19, 1879), some experiments which he has recently made with a waterproof paper manufactured at his suggestion by Messrs. Seabury and Johnson, of New York, out of a combination of rubber and paraffine, with a view to its use as a substitute for oiled silk and similar articles. Dr. Keen finds that the advantages of waterproof paper are—

1. It is impermeable to water for 72 hours, at the least, even after being repeatedly creased and crumpled.

2. It is impermeable to air in similar conditions.

3. It does not absorb water or discharges.

4. It may be used with the hottest dressings that can be borne.

5. It is flexible, and yet strong enough for all ordinary wear, especially as it will only be used once.

6. Its cost is many times less than that of other similar dressings.

<hr>

Medicine.

Histology of Tubercle.

BAUMGARTEN (*Centralbl. f. die Med. Wissenschaft.*, March 30, 1878) has already drawn attention to the constant presence of a granulation tissue, containing epithelioid and giant cells, around ligatures placed on vessels, but he could not recognize nodules analogous to those of tubercle. More recently, he has observed around foreign bodies, such as bits of hair, cotton fibres, and the dust which settles in all operative wounds, true tubercular giant cells; there is the same typical disposition of the nuclei at the periphery, the same protoplasm with its dark granules; the cells are sometimes isolated, sometimes surrounded by round or oval collection of lymphoid cells, often surrounded by a reticulum; no vessel could be recognized. No distinction could be drawn between their appearances and those of tubercle, but the growth showed no tendency to caseation or dissemination.—*London Med. Record*, ~~April 15, 1879.~~

—

Giant-Cells in Tubercle.

Dr. LUBIMOW states (Virchow's *Archiv*, Band lxxv., Heft 3, p. 71), as the result of his investigations, that giant-cells are independent formations, like other cells, and develop out of a cell by increase of its protoplasm, and multiplication of its nuclei. Their origin is, first, in tubercular peritonitis and tubercular lymphatic glands inside the lymph vessels, and more precisely in their proliferating endothelium. Secondly, in tuberculosis of the testis and in organs composed of connective tissue and gland tubules, they originate in the epithelial cells of these tubules on the one hand, and in the connective tissue corpuscles or the endothelium of their walls on the other.—*London Med. Record*, April 15, 1879.

—

Traumatic Meningitis treated by Cold Douche.

At a late meeting of the Clinical Society of London (*Lancet*, April 5, 1879), Mr. KEETLEY read notes of a case of severe traumatic meningitis, treated in the stage of coma by cold douche for two hours and a half. The patient was a groom, aged 30, who was thrown from his horse into a ditch, alighting on his head. There had been a short period of insensibility, but on admission to the hospital he was conscious and irritable. The accident had happened at 5 P. M. Thirteen hours after, having passed a good night, he was seized with a convulsive attack, confined to the left side. During the day he had several similar seizures, in which his eyes were strongly turned to the left; in the intervals he vomited occasionally. On the third day he remained in much the same condition, but on the fourth the right side was affected; and after the attack this side was found to be paralyzed. Towards evening he improved considerably; and on the following day it was noted that his face was heavy, his pupils contracted; and he resembled a patient suffering from opium-poisoning; the temperature was 100°. On the sixth day the coma was increased; temperature 100°, pulse 120. The cold douche was applied to the head for two hours and a half, when the temperature was 99°, pulse 70; his face became rather blue; he could answer questions, but had a fatuous expression, and his answers were often childish. After this time he steadily improved, and ultimately recovered. A fracture of the posterior fossa was diagnosed, extending to the base of the skull; the severity of the injury, and the acuteness of the meningitis appearing to point to such a condition. The epileptic seizures at first appeared to point to an injury of the dura mater over the seat of violence, and the later attacks on the opposite side to an extension of the inflammation to the meninges of the other hemisphere. There was no difficulty in regulating the time during which the application of the douche was beneficial. The lividity was only noticed after more than two hours of this course of treatment. It should be added that he had previously been treated by an ice-bag to the head, and the administration of aperients.

Dr. STURGE said it was rare for epileptiform attacks, after being present on one side, to involve the other and remain confined to it; but he had lately seen such a case. A woman fell downstairs, striking her head, and was brought to hospital in a semi-comatose state. In two or three days she had epileptiform convulsions confined to the left side, the temperature rising to 106° in each fit. The convulsions recurred every half hour, appeared on the right side, and after a time became confined to the right arm and side of face. After a large number of fits she began to recover power and to talk, and was progressing favourably. The convulsions thus subsided first on the side of the body on which they first appeared.

Mr. GODLEE thought the ice-bag would be quite as efficacious as the cold douche, and he had seen a case where, after two days' application of ice, the fits ceased. In another case of convulsions after injury—convulsions which began on one side and then affected the other—arachnoid hemorrhage, and not meningitis, was found after death.

—

Case of Aphasia caused by Anæmia.

A great many cases of aphasia have been lately published, their etiology having always been more or less clear. In most of these cases there had been either an apoplectic stroke or some traumatic lesion, either of the frontal bone or the anterior superior surface of the parietal bone, the underlying parts of the brain being always found much altered at post-mortem examinations. The case described by Dr. KOCH in the *Berl. Klin. Woch.*, February 24, 1879, differs from those which come under notice generally, in that it does not originate in any lesion of the brain. It is brought on directly by hyperæmia of the brain, has been noticed when the patient was in an anæmic state, is transitory, and does not leave any evil effects behind it. The patient, a medical man, aged 36, had always enjoyed good health; there was no predisposition to nervous disorder in his family, except, perhaps, a slight tendency to despondency inherited from his mother. From the time he had first begun to practise he suffered occasionally from hemicrania and a kind of dull headache, which generally, however, vanished towards the afternoon. During the last years he had been rather irritable, and looked pale. That is all his previous history. One day towards the end of August, 1873, the patient had his first attack of aphasia. He had been vexed about something, when he suddenly experienced a slight feeling of giddiness, and numbness about the mouth and in several fingers, which was followed by the utter impossibility of pronouncing certain words. His tongue was not paralyzed, neither was there any loss of consciousness; he felt very much troubled about this new symptom, and shrugged his shoulders because he could not make himself understood by his wife. This phenomenon lasted for about a quarter of an hour; the patient lay down quietly, without making any further attempts to speak, and half an hour later he had recovered his powers of speech, and only felt a slight attack of hemicrania.

During the whole of the following winter the patient suffered more than ever from his hemicrania, but the next attack only came on in the spring of 1874, and was frequently repeated from that time, often recurring several times daily. The patient frequently could not find the right word in writing; the symptoms were always the same, and were repeated in the same series; the fit never lasted above half an hour. In August, 1874, the patient went to St. Moritz, in the Engadine, where he drank daily several glasses of chalybeate water, and took baths. He felt much better there, had only one more attack at the beginning of his cure, and was even able to undertake several long excursions to the mountains. He remained well for the rest of the year, till the spring of 1875, when he again had a few slight attacks; they stayed away till September, 1876, when five more occurred; these were the last, and the patient has been free from them ever since. Two out of the five seem to have been brought on by chills, one of them being followed by a severe cold, whilst three others were, as usual, preceded and followed by headaches.

Remarks.—1. It is evident that this case of aphasia, together with the accompanying circumstances, was caused by anæmia; the good effect of the chalybeate waters seems to vouch for this. 2. The direct cause of every attack was evidently increased rush of blood to the nervous centres. This appears from the giddiness and headache, and that they were often brought on by chills, once even with the symptoms of angina. 3. The aphasia was evidently of central origin. The patient could not find the word he wanted, and therefore could not write it; in attempting to speak, he would use other words unintentionally. 4. Similar peculiar paralytical phenomena have often been observed to occur in chlorotic and hysterical patients. But there is neither chlorosis nor hysteria in our case, only a slight tendency to melancholy and anæmia, the constant recurring of the same symptoms for four years also shows that they cannot be classified under the head of hysteria, which presents the most changeable and various phenomena, as all medical practitioners know well. Occasionally, the symptoms would vary a little, *e. g.*, there was once or twice a slight feeling of formication in the fingers or around the mouth, but that is all. The sensation of formication in the fingers is a symptom of anæsthesia of the plexus brachialis, which has its seat in the centre in the spine, and is propagated into the plexus brachialis; the aphasia is a symptom of a transitory psychical weakness in the centre of the brain. This curious case might perhaps be explained by saying that a sudden rush of the blood to the brain and spine, owing to different circumstances, may on its way have constantly met the same weak portions of the brain or coats of the vessels, which could not resist the increased pressure, and thereby gave rise to the symptoms detailed, whilst healthier portions of the brain or vessels were either not affected by the rush of blood, or did not suffer beyond the symptoms of headache or vertigo.—*London Med. Record*, April 15, 1879.

Partial Epilepsy apparently due to Lesion of one of the Vaso-motor Centres of the Brain.

At a late meeting of the Clinical Society of London (*Lancet*, April 26, 1879) Dr. ALLEN STURGE read notes of a case of partial epilepsy apparently due to lesion of one of the vaso-motor centres of the brain. The patient was a child, now seven years of age. The family history was good; no hereditary nervous diseases. There was an extensive mother's mark on the right side of the head and neck, and one patch over the left frontal and temporal region. All the parts affected on the right side were larger than the opposite. The right eye was affected; and he read notes taken by Mr. Nettleship on the condition of this eye, from which it appeared that the palpebral fissure and the pupil on this side were larger than on the other, and the sclerotic more vascular—a state of sclero-nævus. This eye was myopic, probably because of its increased size, the lens presumably being adapted for a smaller eye; the choroid and optic nerve were redder than on the other side. The epilepsy began by twitching, lasting for ten or twelve minutes, at first confined to the left side. Several such fits occurred every day, but there was at this time no loss of consciousness. Gradually the fits spread to the other side, and in eighteen months or two years the child began to lose consciousness after the attacks. The fit began with a peculiar sensation in the left

palm, followed by convulsions, which soon became general. The left side remained weaker than the other. This state of things was considerably improved
by bromide of potassium. In order to explain his theory about this case, Dr.
Sturge gave a summary of his views as to the mechanism of an epileptic convulsion, and concluded that in this case the epilepsy proceeded from and depended
upon a condition of the right hemisphere comparable to that observed in the right
eye and the skin and mucous membrane on the right side of the head.

Dr. GLOVER criticized the theory of there being a "port-wine mark" brain
as being purely speculative, and hardly worthy of discussion. It was negatived
by the fact that on the skin the mark extended over the left side of the forehead.
It was usual for epilepsy to commence in a unilateral manner before becoming
general, and he considered that more evidence was wanted before the view in
question could be accepted. It was no more to be entertained than was the
mother's statement of a fright towards the end of her pregnancy as explaining the
extensive marking on the skin.

Mr. GOULD said that five years ago he saw a young woman, twenty-one years
of age, who presented an extensive "port-wine mark" on the face, and also on
the chest, arms, and slightly on the legs, the distribution of the mark being fairly
symmetrical. She was subject to fits, thought then to be hysterical. There was
one curious feature in the case—viz., that the right side of the body was much
smaller than the left, the growth of the limbs showing great differences.

Mr. FURNEAUX JORDAN had published a case bearing out the fact that parts
in the neighbourhood of nævi may be enlarged without sharing in the nævoid
condition. It was a case of a large pendulous nævoid mass on the radial side of
the forearm, the radius being at least twice its natural size, so that the forefinger
and thumb were very large. He attributed this to the increased circulation due
to the pressure of the nævus.

Dr. POORE said they must be all obliged to Dr. Sturge for the theory he had
advanced, although, seeing how common fits were in children, it might be difficult
to accept it without more evidence. Did any change occur in the nævus at the
time of the fits? If a "port-wine mark" was present on one side of the brain,
it might interfere with the development of the brain, and in that case some difference in size between the right and left limbs might have occurred.

Dr. STURGE admitted that it was a very unusual thing to suppose that a "port-
wine mark" existed on the brain, and he would not have raised the question did
it not seem probable. He had never seen a case like this, and he did not see
why, as the condition existed on all the tissues available for examination on the
right side of the head and face, it should not also be present within the skull.
The extension on the left side of face was very limited. He had never seen the
child in a fit, but directly after a fit the mark shows scarcely any change. There
was no difference in the size of the opposite limbs, although she is weak on the
left side. —

Case of General Anæsthesia.

STRUMPELL reports (*Med. Chir. Centralblatt*, January 17) the case of a patient,
a lad aged 16, who had complained previously of repeated fits of giddiness.
Nothing, however, could be detected which might have led to the supposition
that the brain was affected, except a considerable irregularity of the respiration
and the pulse. The fits of giddiness became soon better, when suddenly, without any known reason, the spinal column and the epigastric region became very
tender on pressure, and choreiform twitchings and spasms of the extremities were
observed. These latter were subsequently restricted to the right extremities.
On examining the sensibility of the patient it was found that the right side of the

body was perfectly anæsthetic, the right eye had retained its normal power of vision, but the left one had lost it.   Later on, the extensor muscles of the right hand, as well as most of the muscles of the right leg were paralyzed, so that the patient dragged it after him when walking.   Other peculiar phenomena then appeared, so that a month later the patient presented the following characteristics : 1. Tactile sensibility of the skin was entirely extinct.   2. All the mucous membranes which are accessible to observation were similarly affected.   The patient would drop his food from his mouth when eating ; the epiglottis could be touched or irritated without producing any sensation ; the catheter could be introduced without the patient feeling it, etc.   It seemed, also, as if the sensations of hunger and thirst were destroyed, or very much weakened.   3. The sensations both of smell and taste were extinct, the left eye had entirely lost visual power, and the hearing very much impaired on the right ear.   4. There was a cessation of all muscular sensations.   When the patient's eyes were bandaged he could be carried about the room without knowing it.   5. Several of the reflex actions of the skin still existed, as well as those of closing the eyelids, swallowing, etc.   Other reflex movements were absent, such as sneezing, drawing deep inspirations when cold water was poured over him, etc.

It was most interesting to watch the patient's gait.   So long as his eyes were open he walked pretty well, with the exception of dragging the right leg after him.   If told to shut his eyes he would invariably fall down in a few minutes. All the movements of the extremities, those which were paralyzed excepted, were perfectly normal so long as they could be controlled by the patient's eyesight.   If this control were prevented, if the normal eye was bandaged, his movements did not become atactic, but extremely undecided in their direction and measure.   If the eyes were closed, the patient could neither move his fingers separately nor make any complicated movements with his hands : he endeavoured, however, in such cases, to control his movements as far as possible by hearing.

The question being often asked as to what would happen if the patient's only remaining organs of sense were closed, this experiment was often made, and the seeing eye and hearing ear bandaged.   The result was invariably the same ; the patient would always go to sleep after a few minutes, he could, therefore be plunged into a profound sleep at any time of the day or night without any difficulty.   He could only be awakened by throwing a strong light on his normal eye, or by producing a loud sound close to his hearing ear.—*Lond. Med. Record*, April 15, 1879.

Prognosis in Infantile Paralysis.

In a clinical lecture delivered by Prof. JULES SIMON (*Gaz. Méd. de Paris*, Jan. 11, 1879) at the Hospital for Sick Children, the following points regarding prognosis are worthy of notice.   Generally speaking, this disease leaves behind it a greater or less degree of paralysis.   In a well-marked case, which has lasted four or five weeks, the cure will never be complete.   But this persistent paralysis should not justify us in always giving a grave prognosis.   For, though it may be always apparent to the skilled observer, the paralysis may disappear sufficiently to escape the notice of all others, and in other cases it may be remedied by orthopædic apparatus.   M. Simon considers that there are three periods in the malady, in which the prognosis may be given in different terms.   Quite at the outset, it being impossible to foresee the result, prognosis must be guarded and general.   Time is the main element in prognosis now.   In the second period, more precision is possible in prognosis.   If the paralysis tends rapidly to improve, the prognosis is very serious ; but if it persists and spreads, there is a fear of muscular atrophy, fatty degeneration, and consecutive deformity.   If the paialysis is soon accompanied by atiophy, *i. e.*, in fiom ten or fifteen days to thiee weeks, cuie is impossible, and giaxe defoimity will iemain; but if the atio-phy comes on slowly, the disease will, at least to a gieat extent, get well. In othei cases, we aie in piesence of the accomplished fact. The patient is seen in the stage of defoimity of infantile paialysis; theie is atiophy and shoitening of the limbs or club-foot. But even in these cases much may be done to justify a not altogethei unfaxouiable piognosis by the judicious use of oithopædic appa-iatus. The etiology of infantile paialysis is xeiy obscuie. It is iaiely seen befoie the age of six months, or aftei thiee yeais. M. Simon has seen cases which began at the ages of 4, 7, 7½, and even 12 yeais; but these aie excep-tional. Sex appeais to have no influence. The occuiience of dentition and diaiihœa have been ciedited with it; lastly, *cold*, and especially staying in a damp place, have appeaied to M. Simon to have been the cause in some cases he has seen, so that theie would seem to be a iheumatic infantile paialysis.

In 214 childien undei one yeai old, among whom 41 weie within a month, and 17 within a day old, these last evinced the patellai tendon ieflex veiy maikedly. The Achilles tendon ieflex was not fully biought out in all the cases of childien within one yeai old; but the patellai ieflex was maiked in neaily all. The authoi thinks that this phenomenon is a ieflex one, foi the distinctness of the symptom decieased with advancing age; although, accoiding to Soltmann, the excitability of the peiipheial neivous system giadually incieases. This in-cieased excitability is compensated for by the decieased tendency to ieflex phe-nomena.—*London Med. Recoid*, Apiil 15, 1879.

—

Tieatment of Neuralgia by Hydrotheiapy and Electiicity combined.

DUBOIS (*Thèse de Paiis*) says in tieating neuralgia by electiicity, it is best to use the descending cuiient, *i. e.*, the cuiient going fiom the neive centie to the peiipheiy. This is less painful, especially if only a modeiate numbei of ele-ments, fiom thiity to foity, aie used. The only general iule which can be estab-lished on this subject is, nevei use moie elements than can be boine by the patient without pain. It is bettei to begin with a weakei dose, and to inciease it subse-quently, than to iun the iisk of injuiing instead of benefiting the patient. As for the mode of application, M. Dubois iecommends that aftei the sponges have been wetted, the positive pole be applied to the centiai end of the neive, and the nega-tive to its peiipheiic end, or to one of its painful spots. They aie then allowed to iemain in the same spot for fiom five to ten minutes, so as not to bieak the ciicuit. In oidei to pievent the electiic shock and spaie the patient a veiy disagieeable sen-sation, it suffices to move the sponges gently towaids each othei along the skin, and not iaise them befoie having biought them into contact with each othei. This pro-ceeding is said to cuie all cases of iecent neuialgia. Patients suffeiing fiom chionic foims must be tieated by combined electiicity and hydiotheiapy. This is, *e. g.*, the method geneially used in cases of tic-doulouieux and sciatica: for the foimei affection the positive pole of a continuous cuiient is placed on the infiaoibital foiamen, and the negative pole on the supeiioi ceivical ganglion, then a cuiient of about twelve elements is allowed to pass thiough fiom seven to ten minutes. The hydrotherapeutic tieatment which is applied the same day consists, unless contiaindications exist, in a hot-aii bath, which is followed by a cold showei bath lasting two minutes. In sciatica the following tieatment has pioved most successful in a case wheie the patient had been suffeiing foi two yeais, without being able to obtain any ielief. In the moining the hot-aii bath was given, and followed on alteinate days by a cold showei bath, a Scotch showei bath being given on the othei days. At night the continuous cuiient was applied, applying the positive pole to the lumbar region, and the negative, first to the nates, then to the popliteal region. This was done daily for ten minutes ; twenty-five elements were used. The patient was better in ten days, and quite well in a month. —*London Med. Record*, April 15, 1879.

—

Glossophytis.

DESSOIS is of opinion (*Thèse de Paris*, 1878) : ·1· That the black hue of the tongue and hypertrophy of the papillæ of the tongue are always connected with the presence of a vegetable parasite. 2. That this colouring must be ascribed to the fungus, from which it spreads to the long epithelial sheaths of the papillæ. 3. That the hypertrophy of the papillæ, which exists more or less before the affection breaks out on the tongue, and which proves a fertile soil for the parasite, is principally due, at a later period, to the irritation caused by this cryptogam.—*Lond. Med. Record*, April 15, 1879.

—

Cases of Retrotracheal Retention-Cysts.

GRUBER (*Virchow's Archiv für Path. Anatomie*, etc., vol. lxxiv. No. 4, 1878) calls " retrotracheal retention-cysts" not the hernia-like pouches of the tracheal mucous membrane, but the " mucous cysts" (Virchow) which owe their origin to the retention of the secretion in hypertrophied retrotracheal mucous glands, the apertures of which have remained open. They are extremely rare. One case has been communicated by Rokitansky in 1838, two cases previously by our author in 1869 and 1875, and now two new ones are brought forward by him. These are all on record. In both the new cases they were only accidentally discovered on dead bodies ; but, as one of them had an enormous circumference when filled, viz., 5 centimetres, the author suggests that in cases of operation in the neighbourhood of such cysts, an accidental incision might not be without importance.—*Lond. Med. Record*, April 15, 1879.

—

Laryngeal Syphilis.

At the close of SECHTEM's lengthy but interesting article on laryngeal syphilis (*Wiener Med. Presse*, Nos. 27, 28, 29, 30, 31, 1878), we find the following directions for its treatment, and, as they represent the present plan in Vienna, we give them in full :—

In recent and mild cases of the disease, likewise where there are superficial *plaques* in the pharynx, or erosions or slight ulcerations in the larynx, inhalations of corrosive sublimate in alcohol and water, as recommended by Demarquay and Schnitzler, are used and highly spoken of. Under this treatment all the least serious of the pharyngeal manifestations quickly disappear; ulcerative processes of any extent will require, in addition, cauterization with nitrate of silver in substance.

In other cases, where secondary symptoms exist, the inhalations must be associated with the internal use of mercury—inunctions are usually employed. In extensive ulceration of the epiglottis and of the larynx, pencillings with a solution of iodine and iodide of potash in glycerine are spoken of as being very efficacions; it is likewise of use in dysphagia caused by ulceration of the epiglottis, new growths and hypertrophies of the mucous membrane, and follicular swellings. Potash, internally, is to be used at the same time.

In perichondritis, if time be allowed, inunction over the larynx of the *ungt. cin.* and internally some preparation of potash—a treatment which not infrequently diminishes the swelling within a day or two. If stenosis of the larynx and urgent dyspnœa are present, tracheotomy is of course a necessity.

Nervous affections of the larynx, sometimes existing with a mild catarrhal inflammation, are best treated by inhalations of chlorate of potash and insufflations
of muriate of morphia.   The galvano-cautery has been used by Schnitzler in several instances to destroy the warty syphilitic outgrowths found in the larynx, and
is recommended where pencilling with the above iodine solution fails.   Finally,
the various forms of stenosis of the larynx, pharynx, and trachea, due either to
polypi or cicatrices, must be relieved by appropriate surgical measures.—*Archives
of Dermatology*, April, 1879.

Castanea Vesca in Whooping-cough.

This paper (Betz's *Memorrbilien*, xxiii. 12), by KOVATSCH, of Laibach,
relates the treatment of several cases of whooping-cough with the extract of *cas-
tanea vesca*, a drug which was brought into notice recently by the late Dr.
Fleischmann, of Vienna, whose conclusions the author gives as follows.   The
drug can be given with the greatest good effect: 1. When, within the first eight
days the number of daily paroxysms does not increase, or does not exceed twenty.
2. In cases of uncomplicated whooping-cough, and where the spasmodic attacks
are well marked.   3. When the catarrhal symptoms are moderate.   4. In anæmic flabby individuals who are free from the scrofulous diathesis.   There is
nothing to expect on the other hand from this drug: 1. When the attacks exceed
twenty in the twenty-four hours in the first eight days after the administration of
the drug.   2. In case of profuse catarrh of the bronchi, complications of capillary
bronchitis, with broncho-pneumonia and extensive collapse of lung. ·3. In cases
of enlargement of the glands in the anterior mediastinum and of the bronchial
glands when such enlargement can be detected by examination.   The results
obtained by the author are summed up as follows: 1. The extract is of no use
given in the first stage of whooping-cough, when the characteristic paroxysms
have not developed.   It does not prevent the development of the second stage,
nor hinder the bronchial inflammation, nor lessen the fever.   2. In the second
stage of the disease, when the paroxysms are well marked, but there are no complications; when the fever is moderate, and there is only bronchial catarrh, not
pneumonia, capillary bronchitis or tuberculosis, the extract often brings about a
rapid diminution in the number of daily paroxysms, but it must be given for at
least a fortnight for the effect to be obvious.   3. When, after a week or a fortnight's exhibition of the extract the attack sinks to about two or three in the day,
but the night attacks remain constant, then it is well to continue the drug.   4.
When there is no dangerous complication, besides a considerable degree of bronchial catarrh; or, in the third stage, when there is always more or less of this
affection, it is well to give the extract with some expectorant, such as ipecacuanha
or senega.—*London Med. Record*, April 15, 1879.

Carbolic Acid in Whooping-cough.

The use of carbolic acid inhalations is recommended strongly by Dr. SEEMAN
(*St. Petersburg Medicin. Wochenschr.*, Jan. 6, 1879); and in order that the
inhalation may have the best effect, he advises that it should be administered
during sleep, as it is difficult to insure that a child should inhale sufficiently long
or enough of the medicament while awake.   Woollen material, saturated with a
5 per cent. solution of the acid, should be hung round the head of the bed.   In
this paper the spasm of the glottis is attributed to an excitation of the centripetal
fibres of the vagus, which is caused by the pressure of the distended vein in the
jugular foramen, with giving way of the intra-jugular ligament, as a sequela of
rickets.   On the ground of this hypothesis, Oppenheimer proposes the name

Asthma Rhachiticum. The occasional occurrence of even fatal convulsions in spasm of the glottis, the author ascribes to excitation of the medulla oblongata by the overloading of the blood with carbonic acid during the stage of apnœa.— *London Med. Record,* April 15, 1879.

———

Treatment of Whooping-cough by Atropia.

Mr. ARTHUR WIGLESWORTH, of Liverpool, began over four years ago to treat all cases of whooping-cough solely with the sulphate of atropia, from infants two months old to the adult. It required some little time to find out the average dose to begin with ; but he now begins with 1-120th of a grain (or one minim in a drachm of water), in children from one to four years of age, either diminishing or increasing the dose as occasion dictates ; and, except in very severe cases, only order it to be given once a day ; but when the nightly paroxysms are very severe, he orders half the dose to be repeated about an hour before bedtime.

The results that follow its administration may be summed up thus : 1st. There is a steady diminution in the *number* of paroxysms. 2d. There is a diminution in the *duration* of the paroxysms. 3d. There is a change in the character of the " whoop," as if the vocal cords were not so closely approximated. Further, if the atropine is withheld the beneficial effects derived from it subside.—*Lancet,* April 12, 1879.

———

Compressed Air-Baths in Whooping-cough.

MOUTARD-MARTIN says (*Union Méd.,* March 11, 1879) that compressed air-baths are very efficient in every stage of whooping-cough. He has treated three patients, aged respectively seven, twelve, and fourteen, with compressed air in the incipient stages of the affection, and in every case it assumed a mild form, and did not last long.—*London Med. Record,* April 15, 1879.

———

The Experimental Pathology of Pleural Effusion.

The influence of the presence in the pleura of air or liquid upon respiration has been studied in an interesting series of experiments by Professors WEIL and THOMA, which they relate in the current number of Virchow's *Archiv.* The special object of the experiments was to study the mechanical influence of these conditions on the respiratory process, with reference especially to the conditions which obtain in similar morbid states in the human subject. The points attended to were, the effect on the frequency and depth of respiration, and the effect on the inspired air. For the production of the conditions of hydrothorax injections of cocoa-butter were employed, which has the advantage that it remains fluid at the temperature of the body, and sets after death. It was found that the quantity of air inspired per minute increased if the injection was of moderate volume, but was diminished if the volume of the injection was very large. The point at which diminution commences was found to vary in different animals, even when the relation of the weight of the injected fluid to the whole body-weight was taken as the standard. As a rule, however, injections which were of less than 1-150th of the body-weight caused an increase, but those of a greater preportion caused a diminution in the volume of air breathed per minute. With large injections the amount of diminution amounted to from 5 to 71 per cent. It corresponded in degree to the quantity of the injected fluid. The alterations in the frequency and depth of breathing were less constant than the changes in the volume of air breathed. Increase in the latter was observed in some cases to coincide with an increase in both frequency and depth ; in others with an increase in the frequency and unchanged or diminished depth of breathing; in others, again, with an increase in the depth of respiration and uniform or diminished frequency. Diminution in the volume of air breathed was due either to a diminution in frequency and depth of respiration, or to diminished frequency with increased depth, or diminished depth with increased frequency. Most frequently, then, the increase of the volume per minute with small injections, and the diminished volume with large injections, corresponded respectively with an increase in the number or a diminution in the depth of the respirations.

The absolute quantity of the carbonic acid exhaled was diminished by large injections in approximate correspondence to the diminution of air breathed per minute. In small and moderate injections, on the other hand, it presented no considerable diminution, and in some cases even a slight increase. The percentage of the carbonic acid in the expired air showed no deviation from the normal. These results corresponded with those which had been obtained by Guttmann in his experiments on the injection of mucilage into the pleural cavity of rabbits. Certain discrepancies may be explained by differences in the mode in which the observations were made.

The increase of the volume of air breathed in the case of slight injections furnishes new evidence of the capability of the organism to compensate for morbid states by increased exertion in the apparatus concerned. On the other hand, the lung must have undergone a certain amount of retraction, compensated for by increased action of the respiratory centre by excessive stimulation of the vagus. This increased action proved, however, insufficient to compensate for the interference produced by large effusions. By them not only is the lung greatly compressed, but the thorax is maintained in a condition of inspiration, only to be overcome in a slight degree by the most energetic action of the respiratory muscles. The diminished excretion of carbonic acid was evidently related to this interference. To ascertain whether there is actually a diminished formation of carbonic acid fresh experiments are necessary.

Another interesting series of similar experiments were made to ascertain the effect on the respiration of pneumothorax, both with the cavity of the pleura closed and with an opening communicating with the external air. Closed pneumothorax caused an increase of every condition observed in the above experiments. The volume of air breathed increased in almost all cases from 3 to 29 per cent., the average increase being 14 per cent. The frequency of respiration increased from 6 to 72 per cent., the average increase being 24 per cent. The depth of respiration also in most cases was increased from 9 to 24 per cent., the average being 10 per cent. Only when the respiratory movements were excessively frequent was their depth lessened. The excretion of carbonic acid, however, was increased in three cases from 17 to 23 per cent., and in one case it was diminished. In the latter case the percentage of the carbonic acid in the expired air was diminished, in the other case it was increased. When an opening to the external air was maintained, however, the results were very different. All the elements in respiration exhibited a diminution, often very considerable. It is not difficult to understand the mechanism of this diminution in the air breathed and carbonic acid expired, since the effect of the respiratory movements in the lungs is, as is well known, greatly lessened in this condition. All the experiments were made on rabbits, and great care was taken to eliminate as far as possible the uncertainties arising from the great variation presented by the respiratory process in these animals under normal conditions.—*Lancet*, April 12, 1879.

Pulmonary Thrombosis as a Cause of Sudden (or Rapid) Death in Certain
Cachexiæ, Tuberculosis, Carcinosis, etc.

Dr. HUCHARD (*L' Union Médicale*, January 23 and 25), after calling attention to the well-known fact that in cachectic diseases, owing to the profound
changes which the composition of the blood undergoes, together with progressive
enfeeblement of the cardiac contractility, the tendency to sanguineous coagulations in the veins of the limbs, the sinuses of the dura mater, and elsewhere, is
great, and fraught with much danger, from the consequent presence of wandering
coagula in the veins, and their arrest in the right side of the heart, or even as
emboli in the pulmonary artery, maintains that in many cases when sudden death
is due to plugging of the pulmonary artery, the plug has been formed at the spot
where it is found, and that we have to do with a thrombus, and not an embolus.
It has been pointed out that in cases of marasmic embolism the plug is usually
formed at spots where there is the greatest tendency to blood stasis, *i. e.*, at the
points furthest removed from the action of the cardiac impulse or the thoracic
aspirations; now the position of the pulmonary artery is little calculated to favour
this tendency to clotting; but, on the other hand, the blood it contains is rich in
carbonic acid and poor in oxygen, two conditions which favour thrombosis; moreover, in pulmonary tuberculosis the right side of the heart may become so feeble
from muscular degeneration, and so much of the respiratory surface of the lung
may be destroyed by the disease, as to afford conditions very favourable to pulmonary thrombosis.

M. Huchard, in support of his view, gives the details of a case of sudden death
in advanced phthisis, where, at the autopsy, a clot was found occupying the left
branch of the pulmonary artery and its bifurcations, and of such a character as
left no doubt that it had been formed at the spot where it was found. M. Charcot had also observed a case of pulmonary tuberculosis, the subject of which was
suddenly seized with extreme dyspnœa, steadily increasing until the death of the
patient, which occurred at the end of three days. Clots were found after death
in the pulmonary arteries, in the right ventricle, and in the veins of the right
lower limb. Examination of the clot in the pulmonary artery showed that it had
been formed where it was found. Other observers have borne testimony to the
occurrence of the same condition as a cause of sudden death in phthisis.

M. Huchard mentions also a case of gastric carcinoma, where the patient died
suddenly from a violent attack of dyspnœa, and where, at the autopsy, consistent
homogeneous plugs were found in the branches of the left pulmonary artery, which
appeared to have been formed at the spot where they were found.

M. Huchard thinks his observations throw a new light on the history of sudden
death in phthisis. He admits that the most common cause of sudden death in
advanced tuberculosis is the simultaneous existence of cerebral anæmia and cardiac paresis. "The brain does not transmit to the heart the necessary nervous
influx. The heart no longer sends to the brain the blood necessary to nourish and
animate it, a vicious, morbid circle, from which the patient cannot escape, and
life is therefore arrested." In such case, death arises from syncope, but there are
other cases in which symptoms of asphyxia are blended with those of syncope; in
these we have to do either with pulmonary embolism or pulmonary thrombosis.
In the latter case death may be less rapid, but it may also be equally sudden if
the thrombus is produced in a lung already greatly affected, and the function of
which is almost entirely destroyed.—*London Med. Record*, April 15, 1879.

Creosote in Phthisis.

Dr. Bonnefontaine (Union Méd., March 11, 1879) has found that consumptive patients who are rather fanciful concerning their food and medicine will easily take creosote in the shape of Dartais' capsules. These are very small globules containing each about five centigrammes of creosote, and quite tasteless. The drug must be taken three times a day, before every meal, in doses of three globules each time, and followed by a cup of chocolate or milk, a glass of wine, or some soup.—London Med. Record, April 15, 1879.

Infusoria in Sputum.

Of six cases of gangrene of the lungs, in which Dr. Kannenberg (Virchow's Archiv for March) has examined the sputum, in five he found not only the forms of fungi which Leyden and Jaffe have shown to be common in sputum (bacteria, leptothrix pulmonalis, and some spirilla), but also infusoria of the family of monads. They were present in the sputum immediately after expectoration, and were in most cases abundant, commonly embedded in plugs of fungus, but readily recognizable by their movement. Two forms were distinguishable, monas lens and cercomonans. The former is a pale spherule, somewhat smaller than a red blood-corpuscle, with a long filament often wrapped around it. The latter is somewhat larger than a lymph-corpuscle, also provided with a filament, often divided dichotomously, and presenting in its hinder part a process, and commonly with a clear nucleus in its interior. At rest, both forms are very similar.

It at first appeared doubtful whether these infusoria were actually expectorated from the lung—whether they might not come from the buccal fluids, or even be developed in the receptacle after expectoration. But their origin in the lung was proved by three facts: (1) The infusoria were found only in putrid plugs, certainly from the lung, and in these they were aggregated in nests, so that sometimes twenty or thirty were found in a single field of the microscope. (2) In sputum just expectorated they were found to present the most active movement, and the longer the sputum was kept the more languid they became. Twenty-four hours after expectoration the monads could no longer be found. (3) They could never be found in the secretion of the mouth, and the repeated cleansing of the mouth by permanganate of potash had no influence on the appearance of the infusoria. In two fatal cases the lungs were carefully examined, in the endeavour to discover the infusoria, but without success. This seems explicable by the fact that in the sputum-pot they ceased to be visible in twenty-four hours.

This appears to be the first published demonstration of the occurrence of infusoria in sputum. They were seen by Leyden in his investigations, but regarded as of extraneous origin. This occurrence seems to be related especially to putrid processes, for they have not been found in cases of abscess of the lung in which micrococci are common. Their germs must be supposed to enter the lung by the inspired air, a favourable nidus for their development being presented by the gangrenous part. It is probable, therefore, that their presence may in some cases afford valuable diagnostic information.—Lancet, May 3, 1879.

Case of Aneurism of the Heart treated Hydrotherapeutically.

Sieffermann reports (Gaz. Méd. de Strasb., February 1, 1879) the patient, aged 25, who presented all the symptoms of a cardiac aneurism. The dulness at the base of the heart was normal, the right ventricle did not appear to be abnormally enlarged, but the dulness of the left ventricle was much extended in all directions, and formed towards its base a tumour which reached almost to the last left floating rib. There was no arching. A continuous purring thrill could be heard over the dulness, being especially loud in the middle. The pulsations of the heart were feeble and irregular. The impulse of the arteries was hardly perceptible, and about 100 a minute. The heart sounds could only be heard at the base of the organ; they were not accompanied by any blowing noises. The patient would become breathless after the least exertion. He was for two months put under hydrotherapeutic treatment, beginning with shower-bath, under very little pressure, all over the body. The pressure was gradually increased, and the stream allowed to play directly on the cardiac region. The patient remained under this treatment for two months, and left the establishment feeling much better and stronger. The purring sound could still be heard at a distance of about four inches from the lowest left floating rib.—*London Med. Record*, April 15, 1879.

Aneurism of the Left Ventricle.

At a recent meeting of the Société des Sciences Médicales (*Lyon Méd.*, January 26, 1879), a very interesting specimen of an aneurism of the left ventricle was presented. The patient had always been healthy, but much addicted to drinking. In April, 1878, the first symptoms of the subsequent affection appeared, anorexia, migrating pains in the groins, and rapid loss of flesh. Subsequently he began to vomit his food, either at night or the next morning. On examination, a hard tumour, which occupied about four square inches, was found in the epigastric region. The patient looked cachectic, but no other disease or trouble could be discovered at the time. In November a very small amount of fluctuation could be felt in the lower portions of the abdomen. In December the tumour could no longer be felt, the patient vomited his food about an hour after taking it, and died on the next day. At the necropsy it was found that the whole of the stomach was filled with alimentary matter. The small curvature was entirely occupied by a hard, fibrous neoplasm, which surrounded the pylorus, constricting it to a considerable extent. This tumour was attached by adhesions to the posterior walls of the abdomen, the pancreas, and spleen; all the parts covered by it were hard. The most interesting object, however, was the heart, which, although of normal weight and size, showed on the outside a tumour of the size of a nut, which, on an incision being made, proved to be an aneurism of the left ventricle. Its walls were rugged, the whole of it was calcified, and blood-clots and fibrine were found between the partitions of the inner walls. An embolus originating from one of the above-mentioned clots must in all probability have been the cause of death. The diagnosis—alcoholic cirrhosis of the liver, had been made previous to the patient's decease.—*London Med. Record*, April 15. 1879.

Treatment of Diarrhœa by the Hot-Water Douche.

SCHORSTEIN advises, in the *Wiener Med. Presse*, No. 49, 1878, the application of a douche of hot water under strong pressure to the umbilical region, in cases of diarrhœa. The temperature is at first 50°, but may be raised to 72°. The duration of the application lasts from three to five minutes; after it the patient takes a hip-bath of 50° to 62°. This treatment is generally repeated not more than twice daily. Dysenteric diarrhœas combined with tenesmus, and dysentery itself, if not inveterate, are treated in the same way. The effect is very rapid, and lasts much longer than opium treatment does; the pain is also calmed very quickly. The author has also found this hot douche answer in cases of colic caused by biliary calculus, and in many kinds of neuralgia, sciatica excepted, where it was desirable to remove renal calculi and gravel, or long accumulated fecal matter.—*London Med. Record*, April 15, 1879.

—

Fatty Change (and Failure) of the Muscular Wall of the Gut, as a direct and indirect Cause of Intestinal Obstruction and Death.

Mr. FURNEAUX JORDAN, Professor of Surgery at Queen's College, Birmingham, makes the following suggestive remarks (*British Med. Journal*, April 26, 1879) on the etiology of intestinal obstruction. He says:—

For several years past, I have from time to time seen cases in which, with, perhaps, no premonitory symptoms, continuous vomiting and tympany, lasting one, two, or more days, have been followed by death. While these symptoms appeared in some cases to come on spontaneously, in others, and I think more frequently, they followed some abdominal or pelvic operation. The cases, as a rule, happened in fat persons, in persons with large abdomens, in persons with signs of degeneration in various organs and with a history of habits which naturally lead to visceral changes. Examination of the bodies disclosed great internal accumulations of fat, and occasionally indications of visceral degeneration, but, curiously, no obvious or recognized cause of intestinal obstruction. In all the cases, the intestinal canal was greatly loaded with fat, and presented a strikingly yellow appearance; in some cases, indeed, it seemed to be simply a tube of fat. In one case, the microscope conclusively showed that the unstriped muscular fibres of the bowel were converted into fat. In observing and reflecting on these cases, of some of which I will speak later, I have arrived at the following conclusions:—

1. The smooth muscular fibres of the bowel are subject to fatty degeneration, which may become more or less complete; and that, consequently, they may, and do in given cases, wholly cease to contract.

2. This fatty change of the essential element of the gut-wall, when it ends in complete cessation of contractility, causes death by intestinal obstruction. Fatty failure of the intestines being in some cases extensive in area and reaching high up towards the stomach, the ensuing obstruction is acute, the vomiting incessant, and death early. In other cases, there may be less complete, or more limited, or irregularly distributed fatty change; and there will follow a slower or more fitful stream of symptoms and a later death.

3. Fatty transformation in the gut is more likely to appear (though perhaps not exclusively) in fat, especially very fat persons; in those who, from habits or natural tendency, are liable to have fatty degeneration of other organs, especially of the heart. Death in heart cases is quick and direct; in intestinal cases, slower and more indirect, but nevertheless very certain.

4. As premonitory syncope or exhaustion may happen from time to time before death from heart-fattiness, so "attacks" of obstruction may run before final obstruction from intestinal fattiness.

5. Failure of the bowel is helped on by continued flatulent distension, however it arises; the altered muscular fibres being so injured by overstretching that they never regain their functional contractility. Herein may be traced a likeness to atony of the bladder, where, it is well known, long-continued distension is, in certain cases, followed by entire loss of contractility; and it is not unlikely that fatty conversion of the muscular wall of the bladder is the basis of certain obscure cases of retention and cystitis coming on after middle age. It is conceivable that healthy gut may become the subject of fatal atony from long-continued stretching; but some, however slight, fatty change would greatly favour such a result.

6. In a limited number of cases, death is due directly to failure of intestinal action, and may come without obvious exciting cause. The muscular fibre is now

no longer muscular. In a larger number of cases, death comes more indirectly from some immediate shock to the abdominal organs. In strangulated hernia, when fatty bowel is present, the blown-out tube never again contracts. The vomiting continues, or returns, and death follows, notwithstanding that reduction has been easy and complete, and that there is no inflammation, or gangrene, or other cause of death. All injuries and operations in persons with failing gut are liable to be followed by vomiting, which ceases only with death. Especially is this so in operations on the abdominal or pelvic organs. Herniotomy and lithotomy are now and then followed by fatal vomiting, and subsequent search brings nothing to light; no injury to the peritoneum, no hemorrhage, no inflammation, no other lesion; nothing but a hugely distended bowel.

The cases which led me to believe that, in certain instances, death begins in the gut from entire cessation of action in the intestinal muscular fibre, and that the cessation was due to fatty degeneration, I now briefly cite.

Several years ago, a lady so stout that she had long been confined to her room —the staircase of her house was also narrow and awkward—without any previous complaint, began to vomit. The vomiting, at first occasional, became incessant and fecal in character, and she sank in two or three days. I examined the body. The intestinal canal was from end to end enormously distended with gas; but there was nowhere any localized obstruction of any kind. The bowel was strikingly yellow in appearance; and the amount of fat, not only on the body, but within the abdomen, could only be described in words that would savour of caricature. After the most careful examination, no other appearances could be found to account for death.

Another case, which made a vivid impression on my mind, was that of an exceedingly stout man. He got out of doors a little in a specially made phaeton with a bottom so low that it just cleared the road, and was reached with one short step. Without injury or premonitory incident of any kind, symptoms of intestinal obstruction (sometimes urgent and sometimes with intervals of ease) set in, and in a few days he died. A very yellow distended bowel was seen; indeed, I remarked in this case, as I have in others, "The bowel seems a tube of fat." The distension was not uniform, but more in some coils than in others. There was, however, no band, or twist, or stricture, or cause of obstruction of any kind. I had not yet concluded that death might be caused by fatty failure of the gut. I was merely suspicious, and afraid that it might be so, or I should have called in the aid of the microscope.

In a case of strangulated hernia in a very stout man, the bowel was reduced easily and with marked gurgling, and for a few hours he seemed better; but vomiting returned, and he died. On examination, no inflammation, or gangrene, or apparently adequate cause for death, was found. The abdominal organs were greatly loaded with fat. The heart was somewhat softer than natural. The extreme yellowness of the bowel so struck me, and my reflections and fears had now taken so clear a shape, that I determined to have a microscopical examination of the muscular fibre of the bowel. This was carefully made for me by an experienced microscopist, Dr. Wood (one of our staff), and left no doubt of the marked fatty change in the suspected structure. Dr. Wood did not content himself with the appearance of the fatty intestine; he examined portions of healthy intestine, and found a striking contrast.

Not long ago, I had two cases of lithotomy, both of which ended fatally within twenty-four hours, after several hours of incessant vomiting. The cases were singularly alike, and a description of one will serve for both. A big fat "drinking" man of sixty had enlarged prostate and a large vesical calculus. There was no tangible evidence of renal or other visceral disease. There was no peculiarity in the operative steps to account for the result. I could not to-day alter any single step in the operation for the better. He was free from hemorrhage or marked shock. His condition for a few hours was quite comfortable; then occasional vomiting set in, and tympany of the abdomen appeared. The vomiting became frequent and was associated with great exhaustion, and ended fatally. In a subsequent examination, a description of the appearances would answer for both bodies. The internal organs were loaded with fat; the heart was somewhat pale and soft; and the kidneys were not healthy. The intestinal canal was singularly and uniformly yellow, and everywhere enormously distended. There were no signs anywhere of inflammation, or peritoneal injury, or extravasation of blood, or infiltration of urine.

I believe the operation here destroyed the vitality, so far as contractility was concerned, of the bowel. Flatulent distension followed, and irretrievably spoiled the gut. This condition, affecting all or a large portion of the canal, and affecting it even to the vicinity of the stomach, was practically a condition of acute, high-up, and complete obstruction.

Here the question naturally arises, What are the customary explanations, now and heretofore, of the causes of death after continuous vomiting which follows the reduction of strangulated hernia, which follows also operations for uncomplicated herniæ, which follows lithotomy and other operations on the pelvis and abdomen. The very variety of the explanations testifies to their improbability. One says shock; another says shock with feeble heart; another says ether or chloroform vomiting; another says rapid septic poisoning; another says incipient peritonitis. I am far from saying that these, or some of them, are inadequate causes of death under certain circumstances; but they do not satisfactorily account for death in the cases I bring forward. In pure shock, with or without cardiac degeneration, vomiting is rare; in cases of, say crushed knee-joint, or amputation at the hip, or even in severe abdominal injury (in healthy persons), nervo-muscular action dwindles down to death without vomiting. That ether or chloroform vomiting should recur after some hours of comfort is at least hypothetical; hypothetical also is rapid septic poisoning without rigor, or rise of temperature, or any other likeness to the known septic state. Peritonitis without the slightest sign of peritonitis is too metaphysical a pathology to grasp. In fatty change and consequent failure of the gut, we have an explanation which is based on clinical and microscopic observation, which clears up all difficulties, and which is consistent with known pathological laws.

—

Hypertrophic Cirrhosis with Jaundice.

M. HANOT (*Progrès Médical*, No. 10) publishes a case of this disease, described by him in his thesis (1875). Patient, a young married woman, 22, had been ill and jaundiced for two years; she had not abused alcohol; she complained of pain in the right side, and frequent bleeding from the nose. The abdomen was much distended; the liver dulness passed from four fingers' breadths below the false ribs to six centimetres (2½ inches) below the clavicle. The spleen was enlarged and painful. The subcutaneous abdominal veins were slightly dilated. No ascites. The pulse was very small, 100, the skin hot, dry. Temp. 39.6° C. (105.2° F.). Heart and lungs normal. Urine contained bile-pigment and albumen. Ascites developed before death, together with general œdema of the lower extremities. At the autopsy, the thoracic organs presented no anomaly, except some serous effusion. The liver weighed 2700 grammes (about 9 lbs.), was large, of woody toughness, and gray; its upper surface was slightly granular; the lower surface more uniform. On section the granulations were better seen.

The microscopical examination made by M. Menu, showed extra- and intra-lobular cirrhosis, with abnormal development of biliary canaliculi.

Influence of Medicinal and Tonic Substances in Producing Glycosuria and Diabetes.

According to CYR's opinion (*Bull. de Thérap.*, December, 1878), arsenic, phosphorus, and mercury may cause persistent diabetes. Substances which are more diffusible, such as alcohol, ether, chloroform, even if used for a long time, do not seem often to produce this disease, but if it should come on, the author would attribute it to the effect of one of these substances on the nervous system. The same remarks are applicable to the abuse of certain drugs which act especially upon the nervous system, such as opium, strychnia, curare, and also bad beer, or when this disease supervenes in horses which have been fed with wet oats. Carbonic oxide may also cause glycosuria. In the latter part of the article the author speaks of telluric poison as a certain cause, not only of glycosuria but also of diabetes; this latter affection may be attributed directly to glycosuria, and indirectly to the disturbing effect of the telluric poisoning upon the chylopoietic apparatus.—*London Med. Record*, April 15, 1879.

Renal Hemorrhage in a Child.

This case was brought by M. COTTIN before the Anatomical Society in Paris. The child, aged $3\frac{1}{2}$ years, died with eclampsia, the attacks of which had lasted five days, and were very violent and almost continuous. At the autopsy, there was proved to be a hemorrhage in the right kidney at its lower end, presenting the form of a clearly limited apoplectic focus. It was about the size of a large nut, and occupied both parts of the kidney, but especially the cortical. In the centre, the section of a considerable-sized vessel was seen whose lumen was completely blocked by a fibrinous plug. The presence of the vessel (the seat of the thrombosis), exactly in the centre of the apoplectic focus, clearly indicates the point of origin and the mechanism of the hemorrhage. The rest of the kidney, as also the corresponding organ, was perfectly normal.—*Gaz. des Hôpitaux*, p. 219, 1879.

Perinephritis and its Literature.

NIEDEN has written an inaugural dissertation (*Ueber Perinephritis Hauptsächlich in Ætiologischer und Diagnosticher Bezichung*, Leipzig, 1878) founded upon six cases which have come more or less under his own observation or knowledge, and upon a laborious collation of various authors, Rosenstein, Ebstein, Rayer, Vogel, Trousseau, Lancereaux, Simon, Hallé, Lecygne, etc., from whose writings, and the various periodical records, a table of 166 cases have been compiled.

The article is a lengthy one, and we can only give the bare conclusions of the author, but it will, as a whole, well repay perusal. The disease consists of an inflammation of the fat capsule surrounding the kidney, and of the connective tissue which is behind the peritoneum, and extends towards the pelvis. For the most part this inflammation leads to the formation of large abscesses, more rarely to small circumscribed ones. The latter condition is more apt to occur when pyelitic or pyelonephritic abscesses make their way slowly outwards. The usual sequel of these cases, if incision be delayed, is that they make their way outwards into the lumbar region or other places, after having burrowed about in the deeper parts. In other less frequent cases the internal organs are perforated, patienlarly the intestine, or thorax, or abdominal cavity, before the abscess makes its way externally. It is but seldom that resolution without suppuration occurs. In eight cases gangrene was noticed, and caused death in two cases. One hundred and two of the cases were males, forty-two females, twenty-two are undetermined. The middle period of life furnishes the largest contingent of cases, but the recorded instances in children have largely increased of late. Etiologically there are two chief groups, which must be distinguished as primary and secondary perinephritis, and these again may be much subdivided. All those cases are primary, which follow some external cause or some general bodily state; those which are secondary owe their origin to the extension of disease from neighbouring organs. Under the former heading are placed perinephritis from wounds and contusions, large effusions of blood, great muscular effort, sudden chill, fever, and blood poisoning of various kinds. As a cause of secondary perinephritis, renal disease ranks first in importance. Thus pyelitis and pyelonephritis, particularly that form dependent upon calculi, may start severe disturbances in the tissues about the kidneys, and, moreover, the inflammation need not of necessity start from the pelvis of the kidney, but may take its origin in any part of the kidney, ureter, or even from the bladder. This may be by secondary suppuration of the kidney, by direct perforation of the ureter or pelvis of the kidney, or even without any perforation, by direct extension. However produced, an extensive circumrenal abscess is the usual result; more seldom there is a circumscribed abscess, or adhesive inflammation only, which may later, by making its way externally, cause contraction of the suppurating area, and the formation of a fistula. By a similar extension of inflammation, chronic catarrh of the bladder, both primary and when resulting from urethral stricture, may lead to perinephritis. To these must be added suppurative nephritis not due to calculus and renal phthisis; new growths; rupturing of serous cysts on the surface of the kidney, and parasitic inflammations due to the presence of echinococci (five cases); strongylus gigax (two cases), etc. Perinephritis, consecutive to disease of neighbouring organs, though less frequent than the previous form, yet embraces a large number of cases. There are records of cases from peritonitis, "inflammation of the entrails," perforation of the colon in one or other of its divisions, from typhlitis and perityphlitis, from inflammation (phlegmon) of the duodenum, from gall-stones, from hepatic abscess, rupture of the liver, and rupture of the gall-bladder, with discharge of gall-stones. From the thoracic viscera come cases where vomicæ in the lungs have opened through the diaphragm, and of pleurisy, which has set up perinephritis (six cases). Another large group comes by means of the continuity of and conduction by the retroperitoneal connective tissue, the kidney being (as in many of the other cases) quite unconnected with the disease. Such are cases originating in spinal caries and psoas abscess (Rosenstein records a case in which the "*ganz intacte Niere schwamm*"); in operation wounds or traumatic wounds of the pelvic viscera, male or female, and puerperal inflammation; the operation of lithotomy; for urethral stricture; extirpation of the rectum and castration receiving special mention. This exhausts all the known causes of perinephritis, but there yet remain many cases which come into none of the before-mentioned groups. There are many other cases where, with a history of a chill only, or general bodily illness, the question must be answered why this particular part has become inflamed. If to this no positive reply can be given, still the fact remains that many credible observers have met with cases in which the symptoms of perinephritis have rapidly developed after a severe chill. It is probable that in these cases there is a feebleness of resistance, perhaps in consequence of some bygone affection, on the part of the connective tissue, which may be called a local predisposition. To the anatomical disposition of the parts is due the fact that the inflammation is progressive in most cases, and almost constantly terminates in suppuration, while the depth and inaccessibility of the inflammation preclude all energetic treatment. A very important factor in the rapid spread of the abscess in all directions is the extension of the perinephritic cellular tissue to the diaphragm, the spine, the hip, the buttock, and all the pelvic organs, and there is still another connecting link between the bladder and perirenal tissues in the ureter and renal pelvis.

Trousseau refers to the possibility of pain giving rise to inflammation and abscess, but the three cases cited by him were cases of obvious and sufficient disease of the pelvic organs, etc., lithotomy, castration, and long-continued disturbance at the neck of the bladder. With such evident pathological conditions, pain only indicates the first symptom of a commencing inflammation. In many other cases, no doubt, a careful clinical and anatomical investigation would make clear the mode of extension of the inflammation, particularly from the pelvic viscera, and so narrow the number of cases which are yet doubtful as to their etiology.

The diagnosis of perinephritis rests chiefly upon three symptoms: tumour, pain, and fever; these, with some other diagnostic points which may accompany them, form together a clinical picture which is easily recognizable.

The first symptom is usually fever, which attacks suddenly with rigors, followed by heat, sweating and then apyrexia, so as to simulate intermittent fever. The usual symptoms of fever are present, and an obstinate constipation, due in part to compression of the colon. The nervous symptoms have been observed by Trousseau to rouse the suspicion of typhus. In the latter part of its course the fever becomes more remittent in type, usually with a severe exacerbation at the onset of the suppuration, and in the process of pointing. Severe nervous symptoms, such as violent delirium or coma, are only present in very acute cases, especially those where gangrene supervenes. Should the fever continue after the pointing or opening of the abscess, either of which is usually associated with a sudden fall of temperature, the hectic type is assumed with the rapid establishment of a general cachexia.

There are other important symptoms. Pain which is usually situated under the false ribs, is dull in character, and changes its position from side to side. It is increased by movement or pressure, and passes for rheumatism or neuralgia. Local swelling is often long delayed, but sooner or later an indistinct resistance to deep palpation appears, which gradually assumes a more definite outline. There is dulness extending over a continually increasing area, so as to press upon the diaphragm, to appear in the thigh, or perhaps an abscess opens into the hip-joint. The tumour is immovable, rounded, and fluctuating. Then the skin becomes infiltrated, hot, and red. Emphysema of the skin has been twice noticed by Trousseau, due to communication of the abscess with the colon. Spencer Wells and Simons have laid stress upon the importance of ascertaining the position of the colon in retroperitoneal tumours. On the left side it lies in front of, on the right inside the tumour. English and American authors have also made much of the position of the corresponding lower extremity. The thigh is flexed at the hip, as in psoitis and coxitis, and should persons so affected attempt to walk, they lean with their arm extended upon the thigh. This position was noticed in twenty-five of the 166 cases. Anæsthesia of the whole extremity or of special regions, and neuralgia, have been noticed. The nature of the pus differs in the case of primary and secondary perinephritis. In the former it is thick and odourless, mixed with dead particles of connective tissue. In the latter it is serous or ichorous, mixed with urine, or offensive from decomposing urine or contact with the neighbouring colon, even though no actual perforation of the intestine has taken place. Calculi may occasionally come through the wound. Not seldom the kidney can be felt by the finger through the wound.

The urine offers nothing characteristic, as a rule, though in special cases there may be special symptoms, such as hæmaturia, pyuria, the passage of echinococci (Case 110), worms (Case 21), and of calcareous particles.

With regard to the abscess, it seldom opens into the peritoneum ; less rare is perforation of the colon (ten cases). The stomach, duodenum, pleura, and lung have all been occasionally involved. The bladder, urethra, and vagina were perforated once each. Externally it may open below Poupart's ligament, in various situations, or about the buttock, or in the lumbar region, the most favourable situation for the patient being the last-named. A permanent urinary fistula remains sometimes.

For differential diagnosis very little need be said. The occasional occurrence of serous cysts, hydatid cysts, and carcinoma of the kidney must be remembered. In the first two named, œdema of the skin is never present ; in the latter the tumour is hard, irregular, and associated with hæmaturia and rapid cachexia.

The distinction between perinephritis and psoitis is often difficult. To determine that point, attention must be directed to whether the pain is more severe in the renal or iliac region ; whether the movements of the thigh are much limited, and whether in sitting down the body is made to rest on the tuber ischii of the unaffected side to relax the so-called "lumbar fold."

Dr. Nieden advocates early incision, and in the majority of cases the prognosis would appear to be favourable.—*London Med. Record,* April 15, 1879.

The Cure of Leprosy.

The official report on the employment of gurjun oil in the treatment of leprosy, at the Leper Asylum, Mahaica, British Guiana, by Mr. John D. Hillis, visiting surgeon, is published. We are glad to learn that this treatment, which was carried out carefully according to the directions of the late lamented Dr. Dougall, has been found by Mr. Hillis to effect results confirmatory of those published by its originator. Of thirty-two patients submitted to this treatment during nine months, a very great improvement in all the symptoms occurred in sixteen of the cases ; eight had their symptoms ameliorated ; and one case so far recovered that he was enabled to return to his family and friends—in all, twenty-five cases out of the thirty-two much benefited. The report contains a concise, but complete, clinical history of the cases before and after treatment, and is completely illustrated by photographs. It forms a contribution of some value to the literature of leprosy. —*British Med Journal,* April 26, 1879.

Surgery.

Chancres of the Eye.

THIRY (*La Presse Médicale Belge,* 4 Août, 1878) believes that the ocular conjunctiva is rarely, if ever, the seat of chancre, and this he seeks to explain by the fact that the tears neutralize the virulent action of the virus. The author relates an interesting case. Patient, a man of 23, had on the margin of the upper lid an ulceration, involving the caruncle and the lachrymal canaliculi. The lid was swollen, and there was serous chemosis. A diagnosis of phagedenic chancre of upper lid was made. The genitals showed no lesion. The patient admitted having been exposed, and remembered that four to five days thereafter he had noticed a painful pustule on the inner canthus of this eye. The ulcer was cauterized with acid nitrate of mercury, and in three weeks it was cicatrized. Later there was swelling of the cervical glands and development of syphilitic cachexia, and for more than a year he was under treatment.

Another case is given of a woman, 56 years old, who presented herself with a binocular iritis, with a papular eruption of the face. On the upper lid was a firm, resistant, and indolent swelling, and beneath it a small and incompletely cicatrized ulcer. The patient admitted that five weeks before there had appeared a small pimple on the upper lid—eight days later the tumour. Fifteen days later still came the affection of the sight. The patient's husband was examined, and found to have a chancre of the lip and others in the mouth. The writer goes on to say that a remarkable fact in favour of the unity of the virus of chancres was that the husband, who had chancres on the mouth and on the lip, showed no trace of syphilitic affection.—*Archives of Dermatology,* April, 1879.

—

Lysis of the Rectus Internus, with Conjugate Deviation of the Eye.

In 1859, Dr. Achille Foville was the first who made the co-ordinations of the eyeball a special object of study, and who postulated the idea, treated at the time as purely hypothetical, that the abductor muscles of one eye, and the adductors of the other, must receive their nervous impulse from the same source. He illustrated his theory by the fact that two horses harnessed together are guided to the right or the left by means of one rein.

Subsequently, Professor Gubler, Dr. Desnos, and Dr. Féréol devoted much care and study to the same subject. M. GRAUX, in his *Thèsis de Paris,* 1878, has availed himself of their observations, and adding some which he had had the opportunity of making, he was enabled to form important conclusions on the subject from anatomical, clinical, and physiological points of view.

Clinically, all the oculists who had studied the paralysis of the motor muscles of the eye, did not go beyond acknowledging and describing, in the eye which was on the non-affected side, a secondary deviation which affected the rectus internus, and produced converging strabismus.

It has, however, now been proved by recent observations that there exists another form of paralysis of the external rectus, in the case where the rectus internus of the opposite eye, instead of moving in the opposite direction to its congeneric muscle, remains associated with it in its movements. Two different anatomical lesions correspond to these two different forms of paralysis of the external rectus. In the first form, which is also the one more commonly met with, the sixth nerve is found to be affected either after it has left the pons, or while it is still within it; in this case, however, the lesion does not affect the origin of the nerve, and only extends to the nerve filaments which run between the origin of the nerve and the spot where it emerges from the pons. A lesion of the origin of the sixth nerve corresponds to the second form of paralysis, which is more seldom met with beneath the floor of the fourth ventricle. If, therefore, in examining a patient with paralysis of the sixth nerve, we should find a conjugate deviation of the right eye, we may be sure that there exists in the pons a lesion (hemorrhage or tumour) which is restricted to the origin of the left sixth nerve. The precision with which this spot has been ascertained is most remarkable, as the lesion does not occupy more than the space of a few millimetres in the pons; and, up to the present time, the anatomical diagnosis has always been verified at the necropsy.

But another still more remarkable fact, which Féréol has been the first to observe, is that, in those cases, the conjugate deviation of the healthy eye only occurs in binocular vision at a distance, because here the healthy internal rectus works in conjunction with its fellow, the paralyzed external rectus ; again, on the other hand, if both eyes are made to converge, looking at a point at a short distance, that is to say, if both internal recti work together, the muscle on the healthy side will have recovered its normal action.

We may, therefore, infer from what has been said, that : 1. The nucleus of the sixth nerve not only supplies the motor nerve to the external rectus of the same side, but also sends a few fibres to the internal rectus on the opposite side, a phenomenon which Dr. Foville has been the first to observe.   2. That the internal rectus, which is evidently supplied with nerve fibres from the blind nerve, either obeys the latter (convergent vision at a short distance), or the fibres which run to it from the sixth nerve on the opposite side (vision at a great distance), as has been observed by Féréol.—*London Med. Record,* April 15, 1879.

Cataract Extraction, with a statement of two hundred and fifty cases.

At a late meeting of the New York Academy of Medicine (*Med. Record,* May 10, 1879), Dr. C. R. AGNEW read a valuable and interesting paper, and offered for the consideration of the Academy a tabular statement of two hundred and fifty consecutive cases of cataract extraction, with such comments as seemed to him to be the fruit of the experience which they afforded.   One hundred and eighteen of the number had already been published, while one hundred and thirty-two had not heretofore been tabulated.   He brought the cases altogether in order that a broader basis might be made for such animadversions and deductions as naturally followed from their consideration.   Of course we all desired to know what was the best method for the removal of a hard cataract, and what was the prognosis in such operative interference.   In considering the question of cataract extraction it was difficult to generalize, unless we did it upon a basis of a very large number of cases.   Ever since von Graefe had given us the method of modified linear extraction, the danger of failure to give improved vision in cataract cases had steadily lessened whenever ophthalmic surgery was intelligently practised.   He thought it might be safely said that the danger of total loss might be stated as being considerably less than *ten* per cent.   In the group of 118 cases already published by him the percentage of failure to restore vision was $9\frac{1}{2}$ per cent.   In the group of 132 cases the percentage of failure to restore vision was $8\frac{11}{33}$ per cent.   Combining the results of the two groups there was a percentage of failure to restore vision of $8\frac{4}{5}$ per cent.   Dr. Agnew thought that the more obvious lessons which those cases taught might not be without value as helping to show us what to do or what not to do in our immediate practice.   The more experience he had, the more his confidence increased in the comparative value of that method for the removal of hard cataract which was known as G*raefe's modified linear method.*   By that he meant the method which consisted essentially in the removal from the eye of the crystalline lens, without its capsule, by making an incision upward in the margin of the cornea, and removing by an iridectomy that opposing portion of the iris which laid in the way of the easy delivery of the lens.   In common with most, if not all surgeons, he made a wound, the edge of which extended about a millimetre back from the margin of the clear cornea, while at least three-fifths of its entire extent was distinctly in the clear cornea, but bordering upon its opaque edge.   The position of the wound differed decidedly from that which Graefe first selected, and for a most excellent reason that it kept away, throughout the greater portion of its extent, from the limbus of the cornea and the ciliary region, thus lessening the danger of disastrous ciliary irritation and inflammation—the danger which Graefe soon discovered and shunned. The knife he used resembled more nearly that sold as Liebreich's than the one employed by Graefe. It was a very narrow, straight bistoury, which, by its narrowness and thinness, could be easily propelled through the corneal tissue, encountering the minimum of resistance, and being most easily directed in the manœuvre necessary to make a sufficiently large and clean corneal wound. To hold the eyelids open he used Graefe's silver-wire speculum. He usually gave the patient ether to profound anæsthesia, taking all precautions to lessen the danger of vomiting. To steady the eyeball he used the ordinary fixation forceps, applying them as closely as possible to the margin of the cornea exactly opposite the place where he intended to make the corneal wound.

Considerable art was required to make the cut just where it should be. He usually divided the cornea into four zones by drawing five imaginary lines. One passed through the centre of the pupillary space, with two above and two below. The upper and the lower lines just grazed the clear corneal edge, while the others were exactly intermediate. He commenced his incision usually about a millimetre from the clear edge of the cornea, upon the intermediate line. The instant the point of the knife entered the anterior chamber he directed it downward and forward until it reached the centre of the field of the pupil, going on in the plane of the iris, but avoiding its tissue. He then passed the knife onward, giving to its point a curved direction upward, and made the counter-puncture on the intermediate line at a point as nearly as possible opposite the wound of entrance or puncture. That manœuvre made the dimensions of the wound in the anterior chamber as large as the outer edge of the cut would seem to indicate, and the ends of it sharp and clean, and less likely to ensnare the cut edges of the iridectomy. As the knife, in making the counter-puncture, emerged beneath the conjunctiva of the limbus, it was well to give it a somewhat quick thrust in order that the aqueous humour might not follow into the subconjunctival space and burrow there before the conjunctiva was pierced. In completing the corneal wound he endeavoured to have three-fifths of its extent distinctly in clear cornea, approaching the opaque edge and yet its central portion, one-half a millimetre at least, from it. He thought that a wound made throughout in the opaque cornea or the limbus did not heal so well; moreover, he had seen ugly and even disastrous trouble set up in the ciliary region by carrying the entire wound in the limbus. He was very imperative on the necessity of having the wound large enough for the easy delivery of the lens. An insufficient wound was the worst possible defect in a cataract operation.

In the iridectomy the iris should be coaxed out of the anterior chamber by a little gentle pressure with the horn-spoon over the upper ciliary region. It was better that the iris should prolapse than that the iris-forceps should be introduced into the anterior chamber. If, however, the desired prolapse of the iris could not be produced in that manner, the forceps could be introduced. Usually the amount required was removed by three snips of the scissors. The aim should be to leave a clean-cut coloboma without jagged edges or any tags of iris in the corneal wound.

The next step in the operation was the laceration of the lens capsule. It had been proposed to deliver the lens capsule and all without laceration, but he had not been so favourably impressed by what he had read and seen as to be induced to try that method. The best that could be said for it was that it did not necessarily always cost a loss of the eye.

With reference to division of the capsule, he thought the practice had commonly been to use the cystotome freely and to break up as much of the anterior capsule as possible without coming in contact with the uveal surface of the iris too

freely.   He had never been able to convince himself that any considerable portion of the anterior capsule could be invariably cut out by any method of concurring
incisions.   He had, therefore, always contented himself with such a free division
of that portion of the anterior capsule as extended from below the axis of the
lens upward to its periphery, and sideways to the edges of the cut iris.   Lately,
acting upon a suggestion made by Dr. Knapp, he had confined his work with the
cystotome more to the mere peripheral portion of the capsule, opening the sac of
the lens along its upper and anterior edge, taking care not to lacerate the suspensory ligament or to open the vitreous chamber.   That operative procedure was
first suggested and done by Dr. Gruening in Morgagnian cataract, and Dr. Agnew
thought the method was a most substantial addition to the extraction manœuvres.
It might be true that a secondary operation might be very frequently necessary
to break a hole in the capsule which would become more or less opaque, but such
a procedure was extremely common after the older method of free division of the
capsule at the time of the operation.

For a year or two he had resorted quite frequently to a preliminary iridectomy,
hoping by so doing to lessen the number of total losses after extraction.   His experience had led him to believe that it was of value in exceptional cases only, or
when we had more than usual reason to dread accidents at the time of the extraction operation, or certain bad after-complications.

At present he was in favour of the preliminary iridectomy : 1. In cases of known
or gravely suspected fluidity of vitreous humour ; 2. In cases of extreme marasmus, when the nutrition of the eye was very doubtful ; 3. In cases in which an
anæsthetic could not be used, and in which the patient had *no* self-control, or
when from extreme deafness the surgeon was unable to command quick obedience
on the part of the patient ; 4. In cases of extensive pterygium or chronic conjunctivitis ; 5. In some cases of synechia, anterior or posterior ; 6. In cases of
partial staphyloma.

Dr. Agnew then referred to certain minute details which he regarded as of the
utmost importance, such as thorough removal of lens crumbs by manipulating the
cornea with partially closed eyelids ; moistening the surface of the cornea if there
was the slightest suspicion that its epithelial covering was growing dry ; aiding
the delivery of the lens by a little pressure on the eyeball, over the upper scleral
lip of the corneal wound ; bringing forward the lens by well-directed pressure
with the horn-spoon, so that the nucleus and critical portion could be delivered
together.   Those difficulties would be at their minimum if the corneal wound was
large enough.

At one time Dr. Agnew thought it best to dilate the pupil with atropia before
extracting the lens, but had discontinued the plan.   He had not seen any reason
for instilling eserine before the extraction, but on the contrary some cogent ones
against its use at that stage—among others, that it now and then induced much
irritation of the eye and active hyperæmia.

Dr. Agnew then gave a somewhat detailed account of the after-treatment of
the patient, such as related to covering the eye, and the general hygienic and
medicinal management of the case.   So long as the tarsal edges of the eyelids
remained natural in appearance, not being in the slightest degree reddened or
swollen, the scleral conjunctiva only moderately injected, the cornea clear, and
the anterior chamber neither muddy on the one hand, nor too clear and too deep
on the other, and the iris changed but little from the color of that in the fellow-
eye, and the reflex from the pupillary field was either clear and black or only a
little milk-and-water looking from the presence of a few thin crumbs of cortical
lens matter, we might remain at ease.   Usually, little after-treatment was required of a surgical kind, however, and we simply had to meet inflammation in

some one of its acute or subacute forms. He felt, however, that after having done a good clean extraction through a sufficiently large corneal wound, we might, as a rule, content ourselves by vigilant inactivity.

His method of applying cold to the eyes was by means of pieces of muslin that had laid for some time upon a block of ice.

When atropia caused irritation, duboisia should be substituted for it.

Statement of Results in the Group of 132 Cases.—By Graefe's method there were 80 successes, 11 partial successes, and 8 failures.

By Graefe's method, with preliminary iridectomy, there were 22 successes, 2 partial successes.

By Liebreich's method there were 6 successes and 2 failures.

By Le Brun's method there was 1 failure.

The successes were $81\frac{1}{3}\frac{7}{3}$ per cent.; partial successes, $9\frac{2}{3}\frac{8}{3}$ per cent.; and the failures, $8\frac{1}{3}\frac{1}{8}$ per cent.

Statement of Results of the whole 250 Cases.—By Graefe's method there were 146 successes, 20 partial successes, 15 failures, and 3 unknown.

By Liebreich's method there were 21 successes, 2 partial successes, and 6 failures.

By Graefe's method, with preliminary iridectomy, there were 22 successes and 2 partial successes.

By Le Brun's method there were 4 successes, 2 partial successes, and 1 failure.

By the flap operation there were 6 successes.

The successes were $79\frac{3}{5}$ per cent.; partial successes, $10\frac{2}{5}$ per cent.; failures, $8\frac{3}{5}$ per cent.; and unknown, $1\frac{1}{5}$ per cent.

Further analysis was read, after which Dr. Agnew gave a detailed report of two cases of unusual interest, and which illustrated the value of certain steps in the operation. Special reference was made to beneficial results following the administration of large doses of calomel [fifteen to twenty grains], when there was reason to believe that the vicinage of the bloodvessels was occupied by lymph-cells.

—

The Semeiological Value of Mydriasis and Myosis.

At his ophthalmological clinic in Paris (*Gazette des Hôpitaux*, No. 18, 1879), M. De Wecker made the following observations:—

The functional changes of the iris, dilatation or contraction, may be of great consequence in the diagnosis of the diseases in which they are met with; and the exact analysis of their details is of importance in relation to the recognition of the causes that have produced them.

Mydriasis is a concomitant symptom of paralysis of the third pair of cranial nerves (the common motor oculi nerve). In these cases, however, it is not complete, for a still greater dilatation may be produced if atropia be dropped into the eye. Mydriasis, therefore, is not solely under the influence of the third pair, complete dilatation of the pupil being the result of paralysis of the common motor oculi, and of stimulation of the fibres of the great sympathetic, which is the dilator of the pupil. Mydriasis may therefore be of a paralytic or of a spasmodic origin. Mydriasis which results from *paralysis* is symptomatic of a cerebral lesion; while *spasmodic* mydriasis appears in affections in which *spinal* irritation plays the principal part. Besides these two quite distinct classes, it often happens that an irritation primarily cerebral may exert its maximum influence on the sympathetic system, while at the commencement of a meningitis there may be apoplectiform attacks. Traumatism, or a blow on the head, may produce both excitation and paralysis; or, in other words, the same and sole cause may induce at the same time paralysis of the common motor oculi, and excitation of

the sympathetic. This variety has been produced a great number of times experimentally on animals. In children mydriasis is very often due to spinal excitation; and it is thus a frequent result of the irritation produced by intestinal
worms, the inveterate practice of onanism, etc. For the same reason, it appears
in the initial stage of hysteria and epileptiform attacks.

The treatment of mydriasis must evidently vary according to whether it is
paralytic or spasmodic. All mydriases of *paralytic* origin are generally accompanied by a paralytic lesion of the ciliary muscle, while *spasmodic* mydriases
ordinarily leave the muscle of accommodation intact. It will, therefore, most
frequently suffice to investigate the *power of accommodation* in order to determine
whether the probable cause of the mydriasis be paralytic or spasmodic. If a
patient, the subject of mydriasis, presents no disturbance of accommodation, we
may declare that the cause of the mydriasis is spinal; while, if the integrity of
this be not preserved, the cause is cerebral. In this latter case the disturbances
of accommodation are easily recognized. Thus, the subject of hypermetropia, not
being able to accommodate the eye regularly, is unable to see distinctly, whether
near or at a distance; in emmetropia there is no longer clear perception of near
objects; and in myopia the faculty of reading is reduced to the vicinity of the
punctum remotum. One or other of these conditions, according to the case, will,
then, indicate a cerebral lesion as the cause of the mydriasis. Of course, all the
subjects of mydriasis, whether paralytic or spasmodic, complain of the dazzling
produced by light, dependent solely on the dilatation of the pupil; but this occurrence will not be confounded with disturbance in accommodation, properly so
called. Mydriasis of *spinal* origin is a symptom of great value in prognosis, and
often so in the diagnosis of these affections. Thus, it is an anticipatory symptom
of locomotor ataxy; and in general paralysis it is also of great value. Still, it
must not be forgotten that in these affections it is only transitory. We should
abandon the modes of treatment formerly employed, the sole admissible indication
seeming to be the dropping into the eye a solution of eserine or pilocarpin made
into a collyrium with five centigrammes of distilled water. After using the collyrium we must observe how long the effect continues, as it is by the duration of
its action in inducing contraction of the pupil that we should be guided—the interval of each instillation being rendered more and more long according to this duration. If, however, no change is observed, it is useless to tease the patient with
an application which is scarcely palliative. Advantage may be derived also from
the continuous electric current.

Myosis presents itself in two forms entirely analogous to those of mydriasis—
a spasmodic form, determining the contraction of the sphincter by the excitation
of the third pair; and a paralytic form, dependent on the sympathetic. The
same effects on the accommodatory apparatus are also observed, the paralysis of
the fibres of the sympathetic not influencing the muscle of accommodation, while
the spasmodic irritation of the common ocular motor nerve gives rise to disturbances of accommodation. Spasmodic myosis is symptomatic of cerebral irritation,
and the paralytic form depends on spinal affections. Paralytic myosis is especially of great value. A patient who as yet has presented no manifest sign of
locomotor ataxy is the subject of very marked myosis. If this be due to ataxy,
a remarkable fact is observable. He is still able to contract the pupil a little
more than it is already. The iris, however, does not contract when the eye is
submitted to an oblique light; but such contraction takes place when the patient,
while looking at distant objects, is desired to regard near ones—that is, when we
have caused him to put his accommodatory power into activity. Paralytic myosis
may also arise from compression of the sympathetic by a gland, a goitre, or a
tumor, and in this case it may be unilateral, ceasing when the compression dis-

appeais. It is obviously of impoitance to be able to make an exact diagnosis of the foim. Unfoitunately, with iegaid to tieatment, theie is not much to be hoped foi, atiopia having a veiy tempoiaiy action. The examination of the patient is especially useful in this sense, that it enables us to foiesee an affection which is not as yet iecognizable by the othei clinical signs that aie oidinaiily pathognomonic, so that by the adoption of appiopiiate tieatment its evolution may be somewhat ietaided.—*Med. Times and Gazette*, May 3, 1879.

Painless Method of Excising the Whole Tongue.

Mr. RICHARD BARWELL, Suigeon to, and Lectuiei on Suigeiy at, Chaiing Cioss Hospital, London, makes (*Lancet*, Apiil 19, 1879) the following iemaiks on a case of a man on whom he peifoimed excision of the whole tongue nine days ago.

The disease was a laige epithelioma situated as fai back in the oigan as the anteiioi pillai of the fauces, occupying chiefly the left side ; that is to say, the tumoui itself and the ulceiation weie confined to that side, yet the condition called ichthyosis extended acioss and some distance on the iight of the iaphe. Now my late colleague, Mr. Faiilie Claike, pointed out some yeais ago (*Med.-Chir. Trans.*, vol. lvii., p. 155) that this moibid state is the immediate pie-cuisoi, or, indeed, the fiist stage of epithelioma. To take away a pait of the tongue and to leave behind an ichthyotic poition would be a giave mistake. It was necessaiy, theiefoie, in this case to iemove the whole bieadth of the oigan fiom a point veiy neai the epiglottis. I desiie to fix youi attention upon the method I adopted, upon its ease both to suigeon and patient, and upon the ab-sence of bleeding or exteinal mutilation ; especially as you will find in woiks on suigeiy, much used by students and piactitioneis, ceitain methods of opeiation desciibed and figuied of which I entiiely disappiove. Foi instance, Regnoli's ope-iation consists in cutting away the whole flooi of the mouth by incisions along the middle line and iound the body of the lowei jaw, then diagging the tongue thiough the opening down upon the fiont of the neck, and seveiing it fiom its base. Anothei method is to slit soft paits and jaw fiom the mouth to the hyoid bone, and by diagging the paits asundei to lay baie the ioot of the tongue. These opeiations cause much hemoiihage, aie veiy dangeious, and pioduce hoi-iible mutilation. I have no hesitation in saying that they should only be men-tioned as I mention them now—namely, as ielics of a past and, in this paiticulai iegion, of a baibaious stage of suigeiy. Even the division of muscles, etc., passing between the jaw, hyoid bone, and the tongue, as suggested by Sii James Paget, so as to enable the suigeon to diag the last-named pait out of the mouth, is quite unnecessaiy, because, as you have seen, the tongue can be iemoved *e situ* with the gieatest ease as fai back, if necessaiy, as the epiglottis ; nay, if it weie desiiable, that valve could, as fai as the meie mechanism of the opeia-tion is conceined, be iemoved with the tongue fiom the hyoid bone.

The method itself is veiy simple. The instiuments iequiied aie a small scal-pel, one or two Liston's needles, and an éciaseui, or bettei, two éciaseuis. When the patient is well undei the influence of the anæsthetic, place a gag be-tween the jaws, diaw the tongue a little foiwaid, and pass thiough the iaphe a stiing, with which the oigan is to be simply contiolled, not diagged out of the mouth, which must be avoided. An incision, about a quaitei oi a thiid of an inch long, is now made fiom the hyoid bone foiwaid, and stiictly in the middle line. Thus fai you will see my opeiation iesembles Nunneley's, except that my incision is fuithei back and shoitei ; but fiom this point the methods diffei, for that surgeon passed by means of a seton-needle the loop of an éciaseui chain into the floor of the mouth through the frenum of the tongue, and then dragged the part to be removed forward through the loop; and, although he could remove considerable parts by these means, he could hardly get at the whole organ, and I think his opening into the mouth too short and direct, nor did he eliminate pain.

By my method, when the raphe of the mylo-hyoid has been divided, the knife is laid aside, the genio-hyoid and genio-hyoglossus muscles are separated from their fellows by the handle of the scalpel or by the finger if the surgeon have a small finger-tip, and the root of the tongue is readily reached; but the mouth is not to be opened here. An armed Liston's needle is now placed in the wound, and the forefinger of the other hand between the diseased side of the tongue and the jaw, as far back as it will go, viz., a little beyond the last molar tooth—and to this point the needle is guided, taking care to keep it rather nearer to the bone than to the side of the tongue; here it pierces the mucous membrane, enters the mouth, and the thread, being released, is withdrawn, a loop of cord being left behind. The same thing is then done for the other side, except that here a loop in the mouth is unnecessary. The écraseur is now taken in hand; it must have one end of the wire detached and bent into a sort of hook at as sharp an angle as the material will bear. Tie an end of the last placed thread in the bend of this hook; then by traction on the other end, that in the mouth, draw the wire along the track of the needle. When the metal appears in the mouth just beyond the last molar tooth, pull the wire gently through till the nozzle of the écraseur is close to the supra-hyoid wound; then detach the thread and pass the wire hook into the loop of twine that enters the mouth on the diseased side of the tongue, and by gentle traction draw the metal from thus far back in the mouth, out at the hyoid wound, and attach it to the body of the instrument. Before screwing the wire tight, pass a finger along the dorsum of the tongue and ascertain its exact position. I am not afraid of its lying too far forward—it might easily, without care, sit too far back, also it might slip away from the desired place as the screw is used; therefore, having fixed the exact line along which the tongue is to be severed, I place my finger where that line intersects the raphe on the dorsum of the tongue; to it I pass the Liston's needle, letting its point project a line or two, and taking care that the wire lies behind it; by this means the écraseur can be guided exactly along the required plane. When the base of the tongue has been cut through, and the wire has come out at the wound, the loop of the same or of another écraseur is passed over the tip of the tongue into the line of incision, and the tissues, small in quantity but very vascular, which attach the tongue to the floor of the mouth, slowly cut through, when the whole organ is severed, and is removed from between the lips.

Now to recall your attention to the man himself. He lost during the operation not more than ten drops of blood, and none since. He has in front of the hyoid bone a very small scar of an already healed wound,[1] and no other external mutilation. He has lost the whole of the tongue, well clear of the disease, as you see by the specimen, and within a line or two of the epiglottis; yet he has no fever, his temperature is normal, and he takes tepid liquids without difficulty. Whenever I have asked him if he is in or has suffered any pain, he invariably answered in the negative. It seems strange, at first sight, that an organ so sensitive as the tongue can be removed without a moment's pain, especially as a good deal of suffering follows the usual modes of excision; yet, when we have considered the matter together, you will see that this is a neces-

---

[1] The very oblique and valvular communication between this wound and the cavity of the mouth renders the passage of fluids along it almost impossible; thus obviating the production of a fistula.

saiy iesult of my method of opeiation.   By avoiding any diagging of the tongue foiwaid, but, on the contiaiy, getting the écraseui wiie aiound it *in situ*, and by keeping that wiie, just pievious to its entiance into the mouth, iathei neai though not close to the iamus of the jaw, I divide the sensoiy neive of the tongue, the lingual-gustatoiy, close to the bone ; it then ietiacts into its gioove, and the whole wound must of necessity be insensible to pain.   Theiefoie the man could immediately aftei the operation take abundance of liquid nouiishment, avoided fevei, and the pait has rapidly healed.   I would suggest, though I have not yet had an oppoitunity of ieducing the pioposal to piactice, that when a less poition of the tongue has to be iemoved the lingual-gustatoiy neive of one or both sides, accoiding to the extent of amputation, might with advantage be divided on the iamus of the jaw.

The Manometer in Thoiacentesis.

One of the gieatest difficulties which aie met with in the piactice of thoiacen-tesis consists in knowing the piopei moment at which to stop in diawing off the fluid.   In oidei to appieciate the modifications which the intiathoiacic tension may undeigo in effusions in the pleuia, M. POTAIN has adapted a manometei to the aspiiatoiy appaiatus which is employed in the opeiation.   The manometei is in constant communication with the effusion, so that the piogiessive diminution of intiapleuial tension is easily peiceived, and one can stop in time to avoid the seiious accidents which iesult fiom a too sudden iemoval of piessuie, such as con-gestion of the lungs, cough, pain, albuminous expectoiation, etc.   The piessuie, which is measuied, is the iesultant of the vaiious concoidant or opposing actions which, in the noimal state, pioduces thoiacic aspiiation.   Fuithei account must be taken of the state of the pleuia and lung, such as thickening of the seious membiane, cainification of the pulmonaiy tissue, etc.   Othei elements which inteivene, and cause the intiapleuial piessuie to vaiy, aie a noimal or less iigid state of the thoiacic walls, the iesistance of the mediastinum, the abundance of the exudation, its height, its weight, etc.   The indications of the manometei should be consulted fiom the commencement of the opeiation, duiing and aftei the outflow.   The initial tension is almost always positive, but exceptionally it may diop to zeio or even below.   Sometimes it iises without the eneigy of the iespiiatoiy movements being foi the moment exaggeiated.   It is impossible to establish a piopoitional ielation between the tension of the fluid and its quantity. In geneial, high piessuies aie obseived with abundant effusions, especially when they aie inflammatoiy and iecent in young and vigoious subjects; while low, initial piessuies are iecognized in the opposite conditions (old effusion, cachectic subject, contiacted lung, etc.).   In a woid, in chionic effusions, the manometei may seive as a guide in appieciating the moment at which it is desiiable to intei-iupt the flow of liquid ; so long as the distuibance is slow and giadual, extiaction of the fluid may in geneial be continued.   It is desiiable to suspend it when, aftei piogiessive loweiing, a *brusque* and notable diminution of piessuie is obseived.   In geneial, a modeiate depiession, coinciding with the evacuation of an abundant collection of fluid, is a favouiable piognosis.   The above subject foims the mateiial of an inteiesting essay, by M. Homolle, in the *Revue Men-suelle de Médecine et de Chiiuigie* for Febiuaiy.—*Biitish Med. Jouinal*, Apiil 19, 1879.

Fiactuie of the Ulna without Displacement or Mobility.

A man, aged sixty-six, came to the Chaiité ten days aftei he had fallen on his hand, complaining that he could not use his iight aim.   He paid little attention to it at fiist, being able to use his aim foi the oidinaiy puiposes of life, but finding himself unable to pursue his employment. A swelling was found just above the wrist, and crepitation could be felt below the middle of the ulna. On making pressure at the two extremities of the bone, so as to cause a separation of the fragments from each other, Prof. GOSSELIN was unable to produce any abnormal mobility of the ulna, and it was only on pressing at the seat of swelling that he felt the bone yield to his finger. This was a case, then, of fracture of the ulna without displacement or mobility ; and it is in consequence of the absence of this mobility that these fractures are so often overlooked during the first days after their occurrence, they usually not being discovered until the eighth or tenth day. This, however, is of little consequence, as an apparatus is not required so soon after the accident. The appearance of swelling at the inner part of the forearm, after a fall on the hand, should always lead us to suspect the nature of the accident. In the prognosis we should bear in mind that the fragments of the bone may be carried towards the radius, and a fusion of the two bones of the arm has to be guarded against. Indeed, the treatment required has only this possibility in view, the chief indication being to press the muscles towards the interosseous space. This is done by means of graduated compresses placed on the anterior and posterior surfaces of the arm, applying over them two splints and a roller. Or, better still, three bands of diachylon may be applied, these not being liable to become loosened, and leaving the integuments exposed in their intervals.— *Med. Times and Gaz.*, April 26, 1879, from *Rév. Méd.*, March 29.

Fatty Embola in Fractures.

At the Société de Biologie (*Le Progrès Médical*, March 1, 1879), M. DEJE-RINE stated that in November last he published two cases of fatty embola follow-ing osseous alterations. Since that time he had observed ten others ; in examin-ing the lungs of each of these cases, he had always observed very plainly the ex-istence of fatty embola in a degree proportional to the intensity and extent of the osseous disturbance. He had also found, as had been seen by other authors, that death supervened shortly after the traumatism. In two cases only, were the fatty embola found in the liver and the kidneys. No opportunity had offered for observing a case where it was general, as had been many times seen in Germany. M. Déjérine had also made experimental researches on this subject, and these were carried out in the laboratory of M. Vulpian on a large number of dogs. By varying the procedure, the fatty embola had been produced in the animals in dif-ferent degrees, varying from a very slight embolon, up to a very abundant amount, such as was seen in man after a large traumatism. The operations undertaken by M. Déjérine consisted at first, in the production of simple fractures without com-munication with the external air. In these instances the embola in the lungs were very slight, and sometimes caused no change. When, on the other hand, the osseous medulla was implicated, either wholly or in part, by the introduction of foreign bodies into its canal, the fatty embola were very manifest, and it was pos-sible to follow the fat in the blood from the veins of the limb to the vessels of the lung. If, instead of introducing into the medullary cavity an inert foreign body, such as a piece of iron, a substance was substituted which was capable of self-dilatation, as for instance the laminaria digitata, then the pulmonary fatty embola were obtained in an extremely considerable quantity, the lungs being literally injected with fat. These experiments confirm those of Bergmann and Hahn. M. Déjérine remarked further that the embola produced by the introduction of pieces of laminaria into the medullary canal were much more pronounced than those obtained by other experimental methods. It appears, therefore, very prob-able that fatty embolon in man follows a rapidly developed osteomyelitis, for by pressure from within outwards the fat penetrates the osseous capillaries, and so enters the venous circulation. In animals it is difficult to produce a true osteo-myelitis, but in introducing a piece of laminaria into the whole length of the medullary canal, M. Déjérine found a persistent irritation of the medulla could be produced, and so an excentric compression of the medullary canal.

At the Société Anatomique (*Le Progrès Médical*, March 8, 1879), M. Duret stated that he had observed when with M. Verneuil, a case, which clearly showed the origin of the fatty embolon. The patient was a man with a fractured tibia, which, in consequence of movements and efforts made to rise, had been converted into a compound injury. Death rapidly took place. At the *post-mortem*, around the wound was found a reddish zone, formed by ruptured blood capillaries; beneath this was a yellowish band, constituted by numerous very fine granulations and small oil globules. These were also found in the veins of the limb, and were similar to those composing the osseous medulla. Besides these, the debris of fatty globules derived from the periarticular tissues were seen. M. Duret thinks it is therefore demonstrated, that the origin of the fatty embolon should be sought for in the veins coming from the injured site.—*Lond. Med. Record*, April 15, 1879.

Case of Neuralgic Osteomyelitis.

At a meeting of the Société de Chirurgie, on January 8, 1879, M. ANGER communicated the following curious fact. The patient, a man aged 54, had one day been out hunting, but did not over-fatigue himself. The next day he suddenly felt a violent pain in the right leg, which prevented him from walking. Nothing could be seen on the member, the tibia was not tender to pressure, or even when struck with some instrument, but the pain was intense whenever the patient's foot touched the ground. During the whole of the following month nothing could be seen on the diseased leg, no swelling, no redness, nothing but the same pain, which came on in paroxysms, without any regular intermittence. The pains were most violent on the calf of the leg, the ankle, and along the course of the anterior tibial nerve. A blister was applied to the inner surface of the tibia, and the gathering subsequently incised down to the periosteum, when it was found that the latter was detached from the bone on a circumference of about a threepenny piece. A few days later a purulent gathering was discovered on the upper third of the bone. Later on, the knee was swollen, which swelling was said to be osteomyelitis of the tibia, which had invaded the knee. The medullary canal of the tibia being filled with pus, a drain was introduced, large incisions made on both sides of the knee, and Lister's treatment adopted. The leg suppurated for about three months, when abscesses appeared on different parts of the body, and the patient died.

We have here a case of spontaneous osteomyelitis, which for a whole month was restricted to the tibia; no particular spot of the bone was ever found to be particularly painful, and during that month there was no swelling. The only peculiar phenomena were spasms and incessant muscular twitching; these may, perhaps, prove useful in future in making a diagnosis. It is evident that the case in question was one of neuralgic osteomyelitis.—*Lond. Med. Record*, April 15, 1879.

Midwifery and Gynæcology.

Ovarian Pain in Pregnant Women.

Dr. Budin, Chef de Clinique d' Accouchements, calls attention (*Progrès Médical*, No. 9) to a vivid pain which is sometimes produced during the latter months of pregnancy, and during labour, by a very moderate amount of pressure made on the abdomen by the ends of the index and medius fingers. The pain is sometimes so sharp that it causes exclamations or tears to start in the eye. It never occurs spontaneously, and its production is confined to the vicinity of a line drawn from the umbilicus to the anterior-superior spine of the ileum, sometimes a little above, and sometimes below this line, and at a distance varying from ten to fifteen centimetres from the umbilicus. At the seat of this pain so excited may be felt a movable body resembling the ovary in shape and size. Its presence is most frequently felt on the left side, the existence of a resisting surface—usually the back of the fœtus—being necessary in order for the body to be felt and the pain to be excited. Sometimes this can only be done during the contraction of the uterus. Dr. Budin thinks it possible that this "ovarian pain" has been confounded with certain neuralgia which several authors have termed rheumatism of the uterus, and with the pain sometimes caused by the pressure of the head on the uterine wall. It is sometimes very easy to distinguish also the round ligament, but pressure on this causes no pain. None of the women upon whom this tenderness has been produced were hysterical.—*Med. Times and Gaz.*, April 26, 1879.

Tubal Gestation.

At a late meeting of the Obstetrical Society of London, Dr. Routh contributed the notes of a case of Tubal Gestation. The patient, aged 22, was admitted into the Samaritan Hospital on January 31, 1878, complaining of pain in the lower abdomen, which had commenced a month previously. The catamenia were regular and profuse, the last period terminating abruptly a few days before admission. On examination an irregular rounded swelling was found occupying the left iliac and hypogastric regions, dull on percussion. Per vaginam a large mass, about the size of a cocoa-nut, filled the entire pelvis, the os uteri being pushed forwards and upwards, and reached with difficulty. The tumour appeared to contain fluid, and large pulsating vessels surrounded it. It was at first believed to be a hæmatocele, but, later, pregnancy was suspected from the discolouration of the genitalia. On February 18th it was tapped per rectum by the aspirator, and a pint of serous fluid was drawn off. This was followed by troublesome hemorrhage, to arrest which a solution of iron was injected, and subsequently withdrawn by the aspirator. No bad symptoms occurred till the 21st, when rigors set in, followed by feverish excitement, and the temperature ran up to 104° F. On examination, the tumour, which had been emptied, was found to be again distended with fluid. A membrane, which proved to be decidua, had passed from the vagina. After consultation surgical interference was negatived. Next day she died. At the autopsy a large thin clot concealed the viscera. On removing this the peritoneal cavity was found to contain a pint of fluid blood, and there were masses of clot in the cellular tissue of the iliac fossæ. A tumour, about the size of a cocoa-nut, lay behind the uterus, extending to the right into the iliac fossa, displacing the cæcum, and backwards against the fifth lumbar vertebra. It was soft, and its surface very vascular. It could be seen even *in situ* to be a dilatation of the right Fallopian tube. On examining the back of the tumour, a small aperture was discovered. On opening the tumour it was found to contain one ounce of blood, a placenta, and a fœtus of about three months' development. The umbilical cord was about four inches long, and attached to the front of the cavity. The remainder of the Fallopian tube was coiled behind the uterus, in Douglas's space, under the left tube. No trace of the opening made through the rectum with the aspirator could be detected. The author then gave the details of a large number of published cases of extra-uterine fœtation, from which he drew the following conclusions : That a discharge of blood resembling the catamenia frequently occurs, but that it varies in intensity, time, and quality ; that the cases of tubal pregnancy, if diagnosed early, should not be left to nature, but should be treated by one of two proceedings—either simply tapped by the aspirator ; or tapped, and subsequently a solution of morphia injected into the amnion.

Dr. PLAYFAIR inquired why the author had limited his discussion of possible methods of treatment to puncture and injection of morphia? Dr. Routh could not be ignorant of Dr. Thomas's well-known successful case in which a similar tumour was opened from the vagina by the galvano-caustic knife, a plan of treatment which seemed to him particularly valuable in such a case, inasmuch as the cautery not only obviated any risk of hemorrhage from division of large vessels, but the sac could be thus easily emptied of its contents. leaving the placenta *in situ*, and subsequently thoroughly drained, and washed out with antiseptics.

Mr. DORAN, who had made the post-mortem examination, exhibited the specimen which he had prepared from it, which showed beautifully the relation of parts   He remarked that the rent whence proceeded the hemorrhage was situate on the upper and posterior aspect of the cyst, and had gastrotomy been performed on the advent of the dangerous symptoms, the cyst could have been easily reached from above, and the laceration detected, the fœtus might have been removed, and the bleeding vessels secured by the cautery.

Dr. BANTOCK believed that gastrotomy offered the best hope of relief in cases of tubal pregnancy. If the fœtus happen to be in the outer part of the tube the sac might even be pediculated, and the pedicle could be ligatured or treated like that of an ovarian tumour.   If near the uterine end the sac could be opened, the fœtus could be removed, and complete drainage could be effected, after securing the edges of the opening to the lips of the abdominal wound, with every probability of success.

Dr. BARNES considered the operation from below of greater value, being more accessible.

Dr. GODSON said that tapping per rectum incurred the risk of fetid gases passing from the bowel into the cyst, and he related the case of a patient upon whom he had operated for retention of menstrual fluid, owing to an imperforate hymen. in which this had occurred.

Dr. GALABIN remarked that with reference to the inference to be drawn from Dr. Routh's case as to the question of treatment, it was of interest to recall the statistics of the late Dr. Parry, who in his monograph had collected a far larger number of cases than any other author. From a review of these he drew the conclusion, that although the treatment of simple puncture might seem at first sight to be so promising and so innocuous, yet it was more dangerous than either leaving the case to nature or evacuating the cyst by a more free opening, a large majority of recorded cases having ended fatally.

Dr. ROGERS, from consideration of this and other cases, advocated gastrotomy and removing the fœtus without the placenta, putting a drainage-tube into the sac, and treating in the usual way ; or if there were a pedicle and no strong adhesions, this might be ligatured, and the whole ovum removed.—*Lancet*, May 3, 1878.

Post-mortem Delivery per Vias Naturales.

Dr. A. THEVENOT (*Ann. de Gynec.*, Oct., Nov., and Dec., 1878), reviews with great care the comparative merits of post-mortem delivery by the Cæsarean operation and by extraction per vias naturales, which latter he calls the Italian method, since what little repute it has thus far obtained is chiefly due to the labours of Rizzoli. Five cases are quoted in which post-mortem delivery was accomplished by version. Two of the children were born alive, and continued to live; the third lived seven hours; the fourth only gave a few signs of life; the fifth probably died during the operation. The author considers that, if a large number of cases should furnish results proportionate to these, nothing could speak more forcibly in favour of the operation. It cannot be denied that post-mortem extraction may present difficulties leading to such loss of time as to involve serious danger to the child. This objection, however, is to a great extent counterbalanced by the promptness with which the proceeding may be undertaken at the very instant of death, or even during the agony, whereas the Cæsarean operation involves hesitation and delay. In regard to the chances of saving the child by the Cæsarean operation performed after the mother's death, the author first quotes Breslau's conclusions from experiments performed on animals, to the effect that (1) when the mother's death has been sudden and violent, there can be no doubt that the human fœtus, as well as those of animals, survives the mother; (2) we may admit that this survival is longer in the human than in other species; (3) the Cæsarean operation is not likely to furnish a living child unless done within fifteen, or at most twenty, minutes after death; (4) if the mother has died of some blood disease, such as cholera, typhus, puerperal fever (during pregnancy or labour), scarlet fever, or smallpox, we cannot hope to save the child, because the conditions necessary to its existence have not been wiped out at a blow, but gradually destroyed. The same is true in cases of poisoning by substances, such as hydrocyanic acid and the like, which cause a very rapid decomposition of the blood; chloroform, which does not appear to enter in substance into the child's circulation, seems to constitute an exception to this rule. Discarding as fabulous the old reports upon the proportion of children saved by post-mortem Cæsarean section, we find that those reported during the present century show only two successful cases in a hundred attempts. If we choose the Cæsarean operation, we must first ask ourselves if the mother be really dead, if we are not about to open a living woman—a doubt which has stayed the hand of more than one physician. Moreover, the operation is such a grave one in itself, that no one would think of doing it without the consent of the family, and the family often hesitate, sometimes refuse, whence an almost unavoidable delay. Brief, too, as may be the necessary preparations, they demand a few instants, for it should be done as carefully as if the woman were living. Several very striking cases are given, in which the death of the mother was only apparent. Apparent death is less rare in women than in men, and least of all during gestation. In one of the cases (by d'Outrepont), the woman recovered consciousness at the very moment that the Cæsarean operation was about to be begun; in two (Peu and Reinhardt), this occurred at the instant that the skin was cut; in two (Budin and Sédillot), consciousness was not recovered until the sutures were being inserted after the operation—both women recovered; in one (Trinchinetti), a per saltum hemorrhage from the arteries of the incised uterus converted apparent into real death; and in one (Baudelocque), delivery was accomplished per vias naturales after the surgeon had opened the uterus—but the woman did not recover. It can scarcely be denied that, in the present state of science, the physician can distinguish actual from apparent death, but the necessary investigation takes time—time which the accoucheur cannot devote to it, for the child's safety demands instant decision. Upon one sign alone can he depend—the absence of the physiological heart-sounds; but Peu, Rigaudeaux, d'Outrepont, and Talinucci found no heart-beats, and Otterbourg explicitly states that auscultation of the chest gave only negative signs. Even admitting Bouchut's opinion that a heart which has been inaudible for twenty minutes cannot resume its functions—the child may die in one-tenth of this time. The harrowing circumstances of such a case, too, may naturally hinder the auscultator from recognizing a few very slow and very feeble heart-beats. It is well, therefore, to treat a woman who dies during advanced pregnancy as if she were only apparently dead. Especially does this hold good in cases of eclampsia. In eight out of seventeen cases of apparent death quoted, the cause of the condition is given, and in six of them it was convulsions. As a rule, a grave disease, an accident, or a profound emotion provokes labour. At the moment of death, especially if it have been slow, it is rare, after the fifth month, that the cervix is not for the most part effaced, and often dilatation has begun. The operation of artificial delivery is, therefore, seldom difficult. After sufficient dilatation of the os uteri with the fingers, aided, if necessary, by a dilating forceps or by slight incisions, the choice of the method of delivery lies between version and the forceps—a question to be settled on general principles.

In addition to post-mortem delivery, the article deals with the matter of inducing and hastening labour during the death agony. Fifteen cases are quoted in which this practice was followed. Thirteen children were born alive, six of whom survived, and seven lived only a very short time. The two that were still-born seemed to have been dead for several days. Of the living children, one was expelled spontaneously after the induction of labour by uterine douches; twelve others were extracted after artificial dilatation of the cervix—eight by version, and four with the forceps, of whom four and two respectively survived; of the six children who survived, four were born of phthisical women; one of a woman attacked with cerebral hemorrhage, and one of a woman affected with a chronic tumour and with hydramnios. Of the seven children who were born alive, but died within a week, four were born of women with cerebral apoplexy, one of a woman with Bright's disease, one of a mother attacked with a bronchial and intestinal disease, and one of a patient with sacro-coxalgia, who was dying of hectic fever. Inasmuch as the temperature of the fœtus is a higher degree than that of the mother, in diseases accompanied by a very high temperature, there is great risk that the child will perish rapidly, and our action should, therefore, be prompt in such cases. The same is true, according to Esterle, in cholera, phthisis, hemorrhage, the acute exanthemata, cerebral inflammation, eclampsia, cancer, syphilis, and lead-poisoning. The operation is to be recommended even in the interest of the mother, for not only does it seem not to shorten her life, but it almost always ameliorates her condition, often prolongs life, and in some instances has been followed by recovery. In all cases subjected to autopsy, the lesions of the genital canal have been found trifling—nothing more than slight lacerations of the cervix; hemorrhage has not been noted in any of the cases, and the uterus has always been found normally contracted. The time to interfere is when the fœtal heart-sounds begin to flag, and delivery should be slow or rapid according to the state of mother and child. The remainder of the article deals chiefly with medico-legal questions.—*American Journal of Obstetrics*, April, 1879.

Death from the Injection of the Perchloride of Iron within the Uterus.

At a late meeting of the Obstetrical Society of London (*Med. Times and Gaz.*, April 5, 1879), Dr. CORY showed the uterus and appendages of a woman aged forty, who died in St. Thomas's Hospital. She had been admitted on account

of uterine hemorrhage, from which she had suffered for ten weeks since the expulsion of a vesicular mole. A fortnight after admission she had such a severe
attack of bleeding that the resident accoucheur injected by means of a Higgin-
son's syringe, a solution of perchloride of iron through a long tube which entered
the uterus through a considerably dilated cervix. The woman became suddenly
collapsed, and died almost before the tube could be removed. At the post-mortem
examination a small quantity of darkish fluid was found in the recto-vaginal
pouch ; this contained a large amount of iron. A portion of vesicular mole still
remained attached to the uterine wall. The fluid appeared to have entered the
peritoneal cavity through the left Fallopian tube.

Dr. Braxton Hicks remarked that probably the astringent action of the injection had caused the os uteri and the cervix to contract on the pipe, preventing
the exit of a portion of the solution ; this being so, the patency of the cervical
canal cannot be relied on alone.

Dr. Barnes called attention to a mode he had before brought under the notice
of the Society, of applying perchloride of iron to cases like this by swabbing, or
by using a tube perforated at the end containing sponges saturated with the styptic
solution, which oozed out under the pressure of a piston. In Dr. Coxy's case
there was evidence of shock. That the mere contact of iron solution with the
peritoneum was not necessarily fatal or dangerous, was certain. He had on more
than one occasion swabbed large surfaces of the peritoneum to restrain hemorrhage from adhesions during ovariotomy, the patients recovering.

Dr. John Brunton suggested the use of a canula for injecting, made after
the manner of the double male catheter in common use, thereby permitting the
solution to escape

Dr. Aveling said that such an apparatus would be useless, as the clots would
stop up the outlet.

Dr. Edis was of the same opinion, and said that an instrument of this kind
had been tried.

———

Removal of an Inverted Uterus by the Elastic Ligature.

M. Chauvel related the following case to the Société de Chirurgie (*L' Union
Méd.*, May 1) : A woman, aged 18, entered the hospital of Orleansville, Algeria,
having been delivered of her first child seven or eight months previously. Great
force was used in removing the placenta, and an inversion of the uterus was
recognized soon after, but, after some ineffectual attempts at reduction had been
made, the case was left to itself. Painful and abundant hemorrhage occurred at
each menstrual period, and was reproduced by the slightest efforts. The patient
was very anæmic, in a good deal of pain, and quite unable to undertake any
work. A careful examination having been made, it was ascertained that a partial
inversion was present, constituting a tumour the size of a medium orange, with a
broad pedicle. All attempts at reduction, or support by means of a Gariel
pessary, only inducing debilitating hemorrhages, an operation was, at the earnest
request of the patient, determined on. On January 7, M. Chauvel, having
assured himself of the continuity of the pedicle of the tumour with the circular
projection formed by the lips of the cervix, passed the metallic noose of a serre-
nœud around the pedicle, making sufficient constriction to arrest the oozing of
blood from the surface of the uterus. Protecting the neighbouring parts with
slips of cardboard, he next traced, by means of a cautery heated to a dull red, a
furrow some millimetres in depth just below the metallic noose. In this furrow
was placed the elastic ligature, formed of a caoutchouc drainage-tube, about four
millimetres in diameter, the ends of which, after sufficient constriction had been

made, weie secuied by a waxed thiead. The *serre-nœud* was then iemoved, not a diop of blood having been lost duiing the opeiation. On Januaiy 16 the tumoui came away, and the patient was dischaiged at the end of the month. She is now able to undeitake the haidest woik without eithei pain oi fatigue.— *Med. Times and Gazette*, May 10, 1879.

Medical Jurisprudence and Toxicology.

Poisoning by Piussic Acid as a Result of the Decomposition of Ferrocyanide of Potassium.

Cases of poisoning by piussic acid aie common enough, but it is iaie to heai of an instance in which the acid has iesulted fiom the decomposition of a feiio-cyanide within the body. One instance has been iecoided by Piofessoi Sonnen-schein, in which the poison was a pioduct of the ieaction of taitaiic acid on the feiiocyanide. In the following ease, ielated by Di. Volz, of Ulm, in the *Viei-teljahrsschrift für gerichtliche Medicin.*, hydiochloiic acid was mixed with the feiiocyanide of potassium. A meichant was found dead in his bed. On a night-table neai the bed theie was a bottle containing a yellow liquid, labelled hydio-chloiic acid, and a cup containing some diops of this liquid. As he had thieatened on seveial occasions to destioy himself, no ciiminal inteifeience was suspected. The body was examined on Apiil 11th, about foity houis aftei death, undei a tempeiatuie of 55° Fahi.

Theie was a cadaveiic iigidity without any sign of putiefaction. The skin was in geneial pale, with a slight violet discoloiation at the back pait of the body. On the iight side, undei the lowei lip, the skin was diy, like paichment, and of a biownish coloui. The inside of the lowei lip was of a biight ied coloui, and the epideimis sepaiated fiom it on contact. The coats of the stomach weie softened, and gave way at the gieatei cuivatuie on the attempt to iemove the oigan. It contained about two ounces of a daik biown liquid, which was col-lected in a glass vessel. The mucous membiane was softened, and of a daik coloui, but red towaids the caidia. The bloodvessels weie goiged with coagu-lated blood, black, and of the consistency of pitch. The duodenum was ied-dened exteinally, and the mucous membiane was softened, with patches of ied-ness scatteied ovei it. The vessels weie stiongly injected, and theie was one small ulceiation in the posteiioi coat. The lungs weie congested, and piesented a numbei of tubeicles. The heait was flabby, and contained daik fluid blood in the iight ventiicle, and a daik colouied clot in the left auiicle. The tongue was of a biownish ied coloui, diy, and iough; the fauces weie blanched. The lining membiane of the œsophagus was softened, and easily bioke down undei the fingei; the bloodvessels weie distended with daik-colouied clotted blood. The mucous membiane of the laiynx and tiachea was of a biight ied coloui. The biain piesented no paiticulaily maiked appeaiance; theie was injection of the pia matei, with some seiosity in the lateial ventiicles.

The condition of the mouth, thioat, laiynx, œsophagus, and stomach, indicated beyond doubt the action of a mineial acid, but it was doubtful whethei this was ieally the cause of death. Theie weie indications of death fiom a moie iapidly acting substance than a mineial acid. A chemical analysis showed that piussic acid was piesent in the contents of the stomach. This was ieadily obtained by distillation, and the saline iesidue was found to contain piussiate of potash.— *London Med. Recoid*, Feb. 15, 1879.

Alcohol as an Antidote to Strychnia.

M. HAMEAU, in the *Gazette Médicale de Bordeaux*, relates several experiments made by him with a view to ascertain the effect of alcohol given hypodermically in cases of poisoning with any salt of strychnine. A rabbit, which had been apparently dead five minutes, had a hypodermic injection of one gramme of alcohol. In less than three minutes the extremities were relaxed, and the convulsions were much feebler, and occurred at longer intervals. In twenty-five minutes the animal was on its feet, had no more convulsions, and could eat. The next day it was perfectly well. The same experiment was repeated several times with the same success, while other rabbits which were poisoned with strychnine, and not treated with alcohol, died. The same quantity of alcohol being injected into a rabbit which had not been treated with strychnine, the animal fell into a sort of stupor, and died the next day.

The question is, whether alcohol may be considered as an antidote of the poison itself, or as a powerful sedative, the effect of which on the cerebro-spinal system is diametrically opposed to the action of strychnine, and would, therefore, be found useful in nervous conditions similar to those produced by the poison. It has accordingly been used in a case of spontaneous and traumatic tetanus, but without any effect. It is only fair to add that the patient was dying.—*London Med. Record*, March 15, 1879.

Iodide of Starch as an Antidote to Various Poisons.

In a paper read before the Medical Society of Florence, Dr. BELLINI recommends the iodide of starch as an antidote to poisons generally. This compound is free from any disagreeable taste, and has not the irritating properties of iodine. Hence he finds that it may be easily administered to patients in large doses. Bellini states as a result of numerous experiments, that at the temperature of the stomach, and in the presence of the gastric juice, the iodide combines with a great number of poisons, forming with some of them insoluble compounds, and with others soluble compounds which are innoxious so long as they are not in too large a quantity. This antidote may be safely employed in all cases in which the nature of the poison is unknown. It will be found most efficient in cases of poisoning by sulphuretted hydrogen gas; by the alkaloids and alkaline sulphides; by caustic alkalies; by ammonia; and especially by those alkaloids with which iodine forms very insoluble compounds. It is preferable in this respect to the ioduretted tincture of iodine. In reference to salts of lead and mercury, it aids the elimination of the poison. In cases of acute poisoning, an emetic should be used soon after its administration.—*London Med. Record*, Feb. 15, 1879.

Hygiene.

Filtration Experiments.

The subject of filtration has lately excited a good deal of attention, and the merits of different methods have been much discussed. A large number of experiments have been made at the Army Medical School at Netley, and we feel sure that no apology will be needed for placing before our readers the results of the investigations of so distinguished an authority as Dr. DE CHAUMONT into the matter. These results may be summarized as follows :—

1. Animal charcoal, in loose fragments, has a very powerful immediate purifying effect ; its action is rapid, and, with a sufficient depth of charcoal, water may be carried through pretty nearly as fast as it will run with a moderate pressure. The charcoal acts better somewhat compressed than quite loose. If the water is to be used immediately, the power of the charcoal will last a considerable time, but it is prudent to clean or renew it frequently. The passing of distilled water through it and the use of potassium permanganate are useful, but the only effectual method of cleaning is reburning.

When water which has been filtered through charcoal is stored for any time it soon begins to show evidence of low forms of life, and after a time a more or less abundant sediment of organisms becomes formed. This takes place even when analysis immediately after filtration shows no appreciable amount of organic matter by the albuminoid ammonia process. This may arise in one of two ways, viz., either very minute germs pass through the charcoal untouched, or the phosphates yielded by the charcoal to the water furnish pabulum to the germs from the atmosphere. When water is allowed to remain in contact with animal charcoal which has been used as a filter, it takes up again in process of time as much organic impurity as it had before, and sometimes even more ; occasionally it becomes distinctly offensive. Hence, it would seem to be dangerous to allow filters to remain permanently in cisterns, as is the practice in some instances ; the charcoal cannot be aërated, and must, therefore, soon get impure.

2. The silicated carbon and similar forms (with the charcoal in porous blocks) are powerful filters at first, but they are apt to clog, and require frequent scraping, especially with impure waters. Water filtered through them and stored shows signs of the formation of low forms of life, but in a less degree than with the loose charcoal. After a time the purifying power becomes diminished in a marked degree, and water left in contact with the filtering medium is apt to take up impurity again, although perhaps in a less degree than is the case with the loose charcoal.

On the whole, the loose charcoal seems to be the more practically useful, as its power lasts longer, it does not tend to clog so easily, and it is more easily cleaned. In neither case, however, is it advisable to store the filtered water or to have water long in contact with the medium. A contact of four minutes is sufficient to purify water with loose charcoal, whereas the solid blocks take a much longer time.

3. Inorganic substances.—Of these the most important at present before the public is the spongy iron. This is a very powerful filtering substance, and is used generally in contact with what is called "prepared sand," a mixture of fine gravel with *pyrolusite*, crude binoxide of manganese. The object of this last substance is to remove the small quantity of iron taken up by the water. The action of spongy iron is slow but complete ; about twenty-two minutes is the time for exposure, and this is usually sufficient to purify all but very impure waters. The water filtered shows no tendency to favour the growth of low forms of life, and may be stored with impunity ; water may also be left in contact with the medium for an indefinite period without undergoing any deterioration. Another inorganic substance is that used in the "Filtre Chamiot," exhibited at the Paris Exhibition. It is finely ground slag (*scorie de fonte*), and is said to purify water well. This filter is so arranged as to compress the air inside, and so aërate the water, as well as clean the filtering medium when required.—*Sanitary Record*, March 28, 1879.

CONTENTS.

Published Monthly, price $2.50 per annum, free of postage.

Also, furnished together with the AMERICAN JOURNAL OF THE MEDICAL SCIENCES *and the* MEDICAL NEWS AND LIBRARY *for* SIX DOLLARS *per annum in advance, the whole free of postage.*

HENRY C. LEA, Philadelphia.

THE MONTHLY ABSTRACT

OF

MEDICAL SCIENCE.

VOL. VI. No. 7.   **For List of Contents see last page.**   JULY, 1879.

Anatomy and Physiology.

Structure of the Lamina Cribrosa.

Dr. E. D. MACKELLAR (*Glasgow Medical Journal*, vol. x., No. 12) considers that, although the proportion differs in different eyes, yet in most cases of the fibres entering into the formation of the lamina cribrosa, those of the choroid are in excess of those derived from the sclerotic, and that, in some eyes, the choroidal fibres are hardly supplemented by the sclerotic at all. He then discusses the bearing of this fact on hypermetropia, and argues as follows: In every eye in which a great amount of accommodation is necessary to obtain clear vision, the choroid is of necessity pulled upon and strained by the action of the ciliary muscle, and if the lamina cribrosa be mainly formed by that tunic, it follows that the disk, the retina, and its vessels, are all exposed to serious disturbance. Whenever the ciliary muscle contracts, the fibres of the choroid, which pass through and support the optic nerve, are put on the stretch, and the retinal vessels and disk suffer; and, whenever that muscle relaxes, the whole fundus becomes abnormally hyperæmic, from the sudden cessation of tension in the lamina cribrosa. In this manner, the author considers many cases of retinitis, abnormal conditions of the vessels of the fundus, and hyperæmia, with subsequent anæmia and atrophy of the disk, are due, not to central changes or primary alterations in the tissues themselves, but to the effects of choroidal irritation.—*London Med. Record*, May 15, 1879.

Axis Cylinder and Ganglion Cells.

SCHULTZE (*Archiv für Anatomie u. Physiologie Anatom. Abth.*, iv., 1878) thus sums up the results of his observations: "I have succeeded," he remarks, "by means of reagents of very different kinds, in demonstrating a fibrillar structure in the axis cylinder of the medullated nerve fibre, and, in some instances, in the abdomen of the ganglion cell in vertebrata; and I therefore hold it as very highly probable that these primitive fibrillæ correspond to pre-existing structure-elements present in the living tissue. I have further seen indications of this fibrillar structure in the living fibre."—*London Med. Record*, May 15, 1879.

Coagulation of the Blood.

C. H. VIERORDT (*Arch. für Heilk.*, Band xix. p. 198) has been engaged upon a series of investigations as to the time which elapses between the shedding and the coagulation of blood in its normal and diseased conditions. The mode of procedure was by puncture of the thoroughly cleansed skin with a needle or lancet, to obtain a drop of blood of moderate size, which was received into a capillary tube of one millimetre in diameter. In the capillary tube was placed a clean horse-hair, which became inclosed in the clot, by coagulation. On watching the hair, it was seen to become covered with an adherent clot so long as the coagulation is going on, whilst the part which is withdrawn after coagulation is ended is free from any such clot. This point is noticed, as well as the time of drawing the blood, and the interval between the two is assumed by M. Vierordt to be the period of coagulation. From 262 individual observations the author has found the mean time of coagulation to be 9.28 minutes, a result which is in close agreement with that given by H. Nasse, who stated that ten minutes is the ordinary time. Venous blood obtained from the finger after a ligature had been applied coagulated much more rapidly, differing from arterial blood by an average time of three minutes. A similar acceleration was found in animals which were starved, or which had been previously bled. Numerous observations on the sick gave as a general result that in diseases which chronically affect nutrition, as phthisis, scurvy, and anæmia, there was an increased rate of blood coagulation; whilst improvement in nutrition frequently caused a more lengthened period to elapse before the coagulation took place, as in convalescence after croupous pneumonia. One set of observations, however, did not agree with this rule, as in convalescence after typhus fever an increase in the time of coagulation was not observed, and this was also the case in the increase of the nutritive powers after gastrectasia.—*London Med. Record*, May 15, 1879.

Physiological Movements of the Membrana Tympani.

M. GELLÉ (Société de Biologie, reported in *Le Progrès Médicale*, Oct. 26, 1878) has studied the movements of the entire tympanum by means of the graphic method. In ordinary deglutition, as in Valsalva's experiment, the tympanum is displaced. M. Gellé has found, however, that the maximum displacement should not amount to more than one-tenth of a millimetre, to prevent damage to the auditory apparatus; for any displacement of greater extent shakes the fenestra rotunda too much, and modifies the apparatus of hearing. From this physiological fact consequences which are useful for the treatment of diseases of the ear may be deduced.—*London Med. Record*, May 15, 1879.

Materia Medica and Therapeutics.

Action of Iodoform.

HÖGYES (*Archiv für Experiment. Pharmakologie*, x. 3 and 4) endeavours to arrive at a permanent settlement of the discrepancies between the statements made by previous inquirers concerning the toxic and narcotic properties of the compound in question; further, to test the statements recently made by Binz with regard to its mode of operation. The following is a summary of the chief results of his inquiry: 1. Iodoform, in adequate doses, is fatal to dogs, cats, and rabbits. Death is caused by a gradual paralysis of the circulation and respiration; it is preceded by wasting of the body, but not by convulsions. 2. After death, we find fatty changes in the liver, kidneys, heart, and voluntary muscles. One or two hemorrhagic extravasations are almost always present in the lower lobes of the lungs. 3. Large doses cause marked drowsiness in the dog and cat; no such effect is witnessed in the rabbit, even after a lethal dose. During the period of somnolence, reflex irritability does not appear to be much interfered with. 4. What changes does iodoform undergo before its absorption? If it is introduced in an undissolved condition, the first step is its solution in whatever fatty matter may be at hand (in the intestines, the oily ingredients of the chyme; in the subcutaneous tissue and the serous cavities, the oily constituents of the tissue-juices and serous liquids). The only solution of iodoform next gives up its iodine to any albuminous principles that may be present; the iodide of albumen thus produced is speedily taken up into the blood, while a few minute coagula and colourless oil-globules are left behind. 5. Precisely the same series of changes occurs when a solution of iodine in oil is injected under the skin or into a serous sac. 6. An iodide of albumen prepared by mixing white of egg with a solution of iodine in sodium iodide, produces narcotic effects in the cat and dog, just like iodoform; like this, moreover, it fails to produce them in the rabbit. 7. Whether we administer iodoform, iodine dissolved in oil, or iodide of albumen, the iodine is gradually eliminated from the system in combination with the alkali-metals. Broadly, we may regard the action of iodoform, locally applied, as equivalent to the prolonged and gradual influence of iodine. Its action on the system after absorption is likewise, in the main, that of iodine, but with some hitherto inexplained peculiarities.—*London Med. Record*, May 15, 1879.

Conine and its Salts.

The *Annuaire de Thérapeutique* for 1879, edited by M. Bouchardat, gives an abstract of an inaugural thesis by TIRYAKIAN, on conin and its salts, which possesses considerable interest. The experiments were performed in the laboratory of M. VULPIAN, and the conclusions arrived at were as follows: Conine or conicine is a very unstable substance. As commonly sold it is very impure, and gives very variable results; when pure it has a powerful irritant and even caustic local action. Its hypodermic use should therefore be a subject of careful consideration, and should not be rashly adopted. It appears to be more active when ingested into the stomach than when injected subcutaneously. In the latter case it does not completely disappear, the channels of absorption being partially destroyed by its local action. Hence it should, as a rule, be administered by the stomach. It acts as a poison, both on man and animals; but the organism speedily tolerates it, and owing to this toleration it is necessary constantly to augment the dose. There is no danger under these circumstances of a cumulative action being exerted, since conin is rapidly eliminated from the system. Five grains of conine injected in divided doses into the veins of a moderate sized dog, are eliminated in the course of two hours, provided any symptoms of asphyxia be removed by artificial respiration. The toxic action of conine may be divided into three stages. The first stage is characterized by depression and a feeling of sadness. General rigors then supervene, which are coincident with the acts of inspiration, and about the same time there is loss of power over the limbs. During the second stage the rigors are more distinctly marked; the respiration is considerably interfered with, becoming incomplete, rapid, and sometimes accompanied by chattering of the teeth; the pulse is quickened; reflex excitability is increased. This period lasts from half an hour to an hour. The third period is characterized by the diminution of the convulsive phenomena, the diminution and abolition of reflex irritability, slowing of the pulse and of the respiration, visual disturbances, and finally profound collapse. A fourth stage might perhaps be added, according to whether the collapse is followed by death or recovery. In the latter case the animal passes through the same phases of intoxication that it had previously presented, only in an inverse order. Sensibility

first returns, violent rigors are then observed, the respiratory and cardiac movements gradually regain their former strength and volume, the animal begins to be
capable of performing spontaneous movements, the locomotive power is recovered, a drunken condition follows, and at length, in the course of an hour or two,
it walks and runs with ease, appearing only to be a little depressed. Conine is
neither a muscular nor a cardiac poison; it acts essentially on the cerebro-spinal
centres. The substance which acts on the peripheral extremities of the motor
nerves is not conine—it is a kind of empyreumatic essential oil, which M. Mourrut has extracted from conine supplied from Germany, and which probably
exists in all commercial specimens of the drug. The chlorhydrate and bromhydrate of conine are stable salts; they induce symptoms which are identical
with those of conine itself, but are more energetic. The fatal effects of a poisonous dose of these substances seem to be due to asphyxia. Physiological antagonism between conine and strychnia is possible, but has not yet been demonstrated.
The convulsions caused by strychnia can, however, be suppressed by conine. To
obtain any sensible effect of the bromhydrate of conine in an adult man, a dose
of at least 1.5 grains is required, and the quantity may be increased to three,
four, or five grains, according to the effects required or the tolerance of the
remedy exhibited by the patient. The bromhydrate is rapidly eliminated by the
skin and lungs, hence the doses should not be too small, nor must too long an interval be allowed to intervene between two doses. As much as fifteen grains of
conine, and perhaps more, may be given in the course of twenty-four hours, in
the form of pills, syrup, or draught, or the same quantity may be administered
subcutaneously, as the bromhydrate does not appear to exert any local stimulant
action. The symptoms in man closely resemble those observed in animals.
They are, briefly—great muscular weakness, lassitude, fatigue, heaviness of the
eyelids, heaviness of the head, difficulty of walking, sleep, or often rather a
state of torpor without sleep. The intellectual faculties are perfectly preserved.
There is no aberration of the sensibility, except sometimes slight hyperæsthesia
and tingling of the fingers and toes, but it is never perverted or diminished.
Vision is sometimes temporarily disturbed, objects being seen as through a fog.
There is no cephalalgia or vertigo. The pupils undergo no alteration. The
pulse remains unchanged. There are no disturbances of the digestive tract;
neither nausea, vomiting, nor diarrhœa. Respiration, secretion, and the temperature of the body are unaltered. Infants at the breast are not affected by
conine when this is administered to the mother, and they bear small doses well.
The author believes that conine will be found to be of service in bronchitis or
phthisical cough, and in nervous cough, in whooping-cough, in epilepsy, in neuralgic and articular pain. It is rationally indicated in cases of hyperæsthesia, in
chorea, convulsion and trembling, and in tetanus.—*Lancet*, April 26, 1879.

—

Action of Quinia.

The action of quinine upon the circulation has been carefully investigated by
Dr. Guido Cavazzani (*Ann. Univers. di Med. Chirurg.*, Milano, Dec. 1878),
who finds that in the frog, small, as well as large, doses of sulphate of quinine
when brought into contact with tissues which have been deprived of their epidermis, occasion a slowing of the heart-beat. The action of quinine upon the
heart is not very marked, but, if it is contracting very rapidly, the muscle becomes pale, the cavity is completely emptied, the heart remains contracted in
systole. The ventricular diastole occurs slowly, so that the auricles impel but
little blood. Quinine causes great constriction of the arterial and venous capillaries, the constriction bearing a definite relation to the amount injected. The
circulation of the blood-corpuscles is hindered in many of the capillaries, but the

author has been unable to decide whether the circulation of the plasma likewise ceases. In moderate doses, quinine may accelerate the peripheral circulation, whilst in larger quantities it impedes, by reason of its constricting action upon the terminal vessels. Quinine has a paralyzing influence upon the respiration. From these observations it may be deduced, *à priori*, that quinine in considerable doses is of use to stimulate the peripheral circulation by limiting the vascular area. In energetic doses it is useful in phlogosis by modifying vasomotor paresis.—*London Med. Record*, April 15, 1879.

Toxic and other disadvantages of Atropia Collyria.

Several cases of poisoning by atropia collyria have come under recent observation, and many of them were discussed at a meeting of the *Soc. de Méd. de Paris*, November 23, 1878. The first case is that of one of the most distinguished chemists in Paris, who had been treated for some time by Dr. LUTAUD for a chronic affection of the respiratory tract. While convalescent he was taken ill with iritis, and consulted an ophthalmologist, who prescribed appropriate treatment, which the patient followed for some days. Suddenly, one night he manifested such violent symptoms, that Dr. Lutaud had to be summoned in haste, and found the patient in a most distressing state. He was delirious, sometimes gay, and at other times furious, his excitement was extreme, and only grew calmer at long intervals. When first seen, he was crouching on his knees and elbows, and uttered long and plaintive moans, as if suffering intensely. Suddenly he would grasp his head with both hands, and become so violent that his attendants could scarcely hold him. He did not recognize any one, could not articulate, and it was utterly impossible to obtain any answer from him. His eyes were prominent, the conjunctivæ injected with livid vessels, and the mydriasis was so strong that the rim of the iris no longer responded to the action of light. He was evidently quite blind. The palpitations of the heart were tumultuous, respiration abrupt, stertorous, irregular, and quick. There was no paralysis, no trembling, no convulsions, the pulse was small, frequent, feeble, and irregular, the skin cool and clammy. Although the pupils were dilated, and Dr. Lutaud knew that his patient had been using sulphate of atropia, yet, as he was ignorant as to the dose of the drug, it did not occur to him to attribute to it these severe symptoms. Dr. Dieulafoy, who was called in half an hour later, was equally at a loss as to their cause. A hypodermic injection of three centigrammes of acetate of morphia was then administered, and soon after the delirium ceased, and a most alarming stupor set in. After a great deal of trouble they succeeded in making the patient swallow a few spoonfuls of strong coffee. It was not till several hours after he had been called in that Dr. Lutaud found out that the patient had the night before suddenly raised the dose of sulphate of atropia from five centigrammes to ten, while the proportion of water remained the same, viz., ten grammes, and that he had used this very strong drug as a lotion every hour, without having previously taken the necessary precautions of compressing for some instants the inferior lacrymal punctum. He then first became slightly comatose, and afterwards delirious, so that there could be no doubt as to the symptoms being due to poisoning with sulphate of atropia. This was also confirmed by the happy effects of the subcutaneous injection of morphia. Eight hours after the first symptoms had shown themselves, the patient could utter a few words, and answer vaguely the questions which were put to him. He was then allowed to sleep for a few hours, and on waking asked his attendants with the greatest calmness what they were doing there; he had not the least remembrance of what had happened, and felt perfectly well, with the exception of a rather quick pulse, a feeling of dryness in the throat, and dilatation of the pupil.

A few days later he could again attend to his business without any further complications. It is one of the characteristic phenomena of atropia poisoning, that the symptoms disappear very rapidly, and Dr. Lutaud quotes several cases where the patients had been taken to the hospital shortly after the symptoms of poisoning had manifested themselves, and awoke very much astonished in finding themselves there. They could not in the least remember what had happened, and were quite well after forty-eight hours.

It appears, from what has been said, that eye-lotions and applications which contain atropia may penetrate into the puncta lacrymalia, and thence into the pharynx and digestive tract, thereby causing very serious toxic symptoms. These accidents, however, do not last long, and are remarkable for the suddenness with which they both appear and disappear. Precautions ought to be taken to avoid them by compressing the puncta lacrymalia during the application, and thereby preventing the liquid from passing into them and thence into the pharynx. The most experienced oculists, such as Desmanes, Galezowski, Meyer, Von Wecker, Abadie, Camuset, Fieuzal, and Gillet de Grandmont, are all of opinion that, as as a rule, poisoning through a collyrium containing neutral sulphate of atropia does not often occur, and then only in the case of old people.

PELTIER in his thesis on the subject (*Thèse de Paris,* 1877), says that the symptoms vary exceedingly in intensity, from a simple heightening of the temperature to a general intoxication, but in every case they must be ascribed to an idiosyncrasy which cannot tolerate atropia. They either appear suddenly after one or more applications of the drug; or after the treatment has been carried out for some time. Another peculiarity is that the accidents are sure to be repeated, even after the treatment has been interrupted for months, and sometimes if only one drop of the one-thousandth part of a solution of sulphate of atropia is dropped into the eye. Mackenzie has observed hallucination in such cases; Testelin attacks of acute delirium. M. Richet had under his care in 1858, at the Hôpital des Cliniques, a patient who had been operated on for cataract, and who every night after atropia had been dropped into his eyes had a violent attack of fever with intense delirium. M. Galezowski quotes the case of a patient who collapsed and lost consciousness after the use of this drug. The following are the characteristic symptoms of atropia poisoning: dryness of the mouth and throat, unquenchable thirst, loss of taste, feeling of numbness in the face, excessive mydriasis, cephalalgia, vertigo, giddiness, photopsia, and delirium. It seems as if in general the anti-atropic idiosyncrasy is determined by the primary affection of the eye, although cases have been observed where it showed itself only after a prolonged treatment, or even suddenly after iridectomy had been performed or the patient operated on for cataract.

M. Peltier quotes in his thesis the following cases where the idiosyncrasy suddenly showed itself after an operation:—

A woman, aged 46, who was suffering from double iritis and interstitial keratitis, had iridectomy performed by M. Galezowski, who prescribed two drops per diem of a collyrium containing one centigramme of neutral sulphate of atropia dissolved in ten grammes of water. On the first day, the patient complained of dryness in the throat and intense headache. The next day, the treatment was continued and the patient complained still more. The collyrium was then stopped, and the symptoms disappeared at once. Two months later, one drop of collyrium containing two centigrammes of the neutral sulphate of atropia in ten grammes of water was given, and as it gave rise to the same symptoms, the treatment had to be given up.

The same phenomena occurred in a man aged 24, after iridectomy, and in another, aged 44, who had been operated upon for granulations of the conjunctivæ.

The first drop of the collyrium caused intense peri-orbitary pains and a violent conjunctivitis. A woman, aged 53, had been operated on for a lachrymal ectropion, three drops daily of collyrium, containing the usual proportion of atropia, were prescribed. The next day the patient complained of violent peri-orbitary pains, photopsia, and sleeplessness, as well as dryness of the mouth and throat. Two days later, the symptoms had increased, and eczema of the eyelids had set in. The atropia was suppressed and the patient recovered. M. Galezowski quotes the following observations in his *Recueil d'Ophthalmologie:* A young girl, aged 24, who was suffering from an abscess in the centre of the right cornea and violent pains in the peri-orbital region, was treated with leeches and a collyrium, containing two centigrammes of atropia. After ten days she felt weak, her arms trembled, her throat was dry, she had high fever and was delirious every night, and saw everything red (a very rare phenomenon). Her principal complaint, however, was a continuous feeling of nausea and giddiness, which only ceased when the treatment had been stopped.

Another case is that of a child, aged 3 years, suffering from hypopyon and a central abscess of the right cornea, who was treated with the usual dose of atropia. For twelve days all went well, when the mother said that her child had been delirious and had had convulsions during the whole of the preceding night, after the atropia had been dropped into her eye. Instead of three drops two were then given, and during the following five nights the child was delirious, asked for something to drink throughout the day, and moaned continuously, pointing to its forehead as if it were painful. The atropia was stopped, and the symptoms suddenly ceased.

Death has been seldom known to follow in those cases of poisoning. Desmanes only quotes one instance of it, where the patient, an infant, aged four months, died of convulsions after the use of a lotion containing the usual dose of atropia. In another case, the patient, an old lady, became violently excited and attempted to destroy herself. Cessation of the treatment immediately restored her to her normal mental condition.

Dr. MEYER, one of the leading oculists of Paris, has recorded the following cases which came under his immediate notice.

A painter had been for some time under Dr. Meyer's treatment for acute iritis of the left eye, and had used a collyrium containing four centigrammes of sulphate of atropia and ten grammes of water. He had been told to use great precautions every time he applied the drug, compressing the puncta lacrymalia, keeping the eyelids closed for a few moments, because movement of the eye tends to increase the action of the lachrymal ducts; also to wash his eye carefully with warm water after opening the eyelids. This treatment had been carried out successfully for more than a month, when suddenly the general state of the patient became alarming; his eye was better, but his temperature was very high, he had no appetite, complained of feeling ill, slept badly, was delirious, and had optic hallucinations. As the pupil of the right eye (the healthy one) was dilated, it was suggested that atropia might possibly be at the bottom of this state of things. The patient being closely questioned, confessed that he had neglected to carry out the doctor's prescriptions during the last week. The drug was not administered, and the patient soon recovered. In some cases atropia may be dispensed with without any detriment to the eye, if such alarming symptoms should appear; but in other cases when it is absolutely necessary that the patient should be treated with atropia, the medical man is placed in rather a dilemma, as, *e. g.*, in cases of iritis. Dr. Meyer has attempted in similar cases to counteract the dangerous effects of atropia by hypodermic injections of morphia, and has always found these answer very well. If the injection is made at night, the patient may use the atropia during the day without experiencing any bad results.

The following case of Dr. Meyer also tends to prove the antagonistic action of morphia towards atropia. The patient had been operated upon for cataract by discision, and used a solution of atropia for the purpose of keeping the pupil dilated while the cortical substance was being absorbed. As he happened at the same time to be taking a solution of arsenic for his general health, he mistook the drug, and one day swallowed by mistake fifteen drops of the atropia solution three times. He was in a most alarming state when seen by Dr. Meyer, had lost his voice, could not swallow, had vertigo, hallucinations, and was tormented by an incessant desire to micturate, which he could not satisfy. An injection of morphia was then given, and twenty-five minutes later the patient was able to pass his water. An hour and a half later on, the symptoms of intoxication reappearing again, a second injection was administered, followed by a third in the course of the night. The next day the patient had completely recovered. The question has naturally arisen whether the poisonous drug is really absorbed through the lachrymal ducts, and subsequently through the mucous membrane of the digestive tube, or if the absorption does not rather take place through the conjunctivæ, which are known to possess very rapid powers of absorption. This question has not yet been answered satisfactorily, and the opinions of authors vary much on the subject.   •

As atropia is apt to give rise to such troublesome and dangerous symptoms, the desire has naturally arisen to discover some other substance which possessed all its efficient properties without its drawbacks, and might be used in its place. Several alkaloids have been suggested, such as daturine, hyoscyamine, eserine, duboisia, gelseminium, and chlorhydrate of pilocarpine.

VON WECKER thinks that eserine will take the place of atropia in the treatment of affections of the cornea, for the following reasons: 1. Eserine lowers the ocular pressure, while atropia increases it by dilating the vessels. 2. Eserine diminishes the secretion of the conjunctivæ by contracting the vessels, while atropia increases it. 3. It reduces diapedesis, but atropia, by pushing the iris back towards the corner of the anterior chamber, is apt to retain in the eye fluids which ought to be allowed to flow out. Meyer and Galezowski have both used duboisia with great success in cases where atropia could not be tolerated. It is, however, a curious fact that in some patients duboisia has produced conjunctivitis, and had to be replaced by atropia, which did not cause any evil results. It has also once or twice given rise to general symptoms of poisoning.

Chlorhydrate of pilocarpine seems to act very much like eserine in affections of the cornea.

SCHROFF, in comparing the therapeutic effects of atropia, daturia, and hyoscyamia, says that the two latter are less apt to produce dryness of the throat and skin, etc., than the first. The delirium caused by atropia is a very violent one, the patient is apt to burst suddenly into fits of uncontrollable laughter and to throw himself about wildly, while the delirium caused by hyoscyamia is of a calmer nature, the patient feeling inclined to sleep and rest. Neither does it cause paralysis of the sphincters of the rectum and the bladder like atropia and daturia, although it acts powerfully upon the sphincter of the iris.

Last, but not least, chlorhydrate of gelseminium may be safely used instead of atropia; it dilates the pupil, and does not paralyze its powers of accommodation for more than thirty hours. This is very convenient for the patient, as he is then enabled to resume his general occupations, and read or write, which is of course entirely out of question after atropia has been dropped into the eye.—*London Med. Record*, May 15, 1879.

Use of Pilocarpinum Muriaticum in Children's Diseases.

WEISS (*Pest. Med. Chir. Presse*, 1879, 2) has had the opportunity of observing the effects of pilocarpine in fourteen cases where the patients were suffering from nephritis, complicated with general dropsy, following scarlatina. In four cases there existed extensive bronchitis, in two diphtheria, and in one pneumonia of the left side of the lung. In each of these cases the results produced by pilocarpine were most favourable, and the patients could all be dismissed as cured. One of the most important properties of pilocarpine is that it prevents the dropsy from increasing, keeping it stationary without implicating the kidneys, till the latter have recovered their power of secreting urine more abundantly. Two different kinds of solutions were used for the hypodermic injections; a 1 per cent. solution for children under four years, and a 2 per cent. one for children above four years. In such young patients, where collapse seemed to threaten from prolonged illness and great weakness, 4 or 5 drops of ether were added to the solution of pilocarpine in the syringe. The author observed, that whenever he used this mixture, the young patients did not present the phenomena which generally followed the injection of a solution of pure pilocarpine, viz., vomiting, nausea, hiccough, pallor, and a feeble pulse. The injections were made once daily into the upper arm, beginning with half a syringeful, and rising to a whole one. The effects of pilocarpine generally appeared after a few minutes, beginning with a slight flush on the face, which, however, gradually increased, and only disappeared when the perspiration had ceased. The latter set in after three to five minutes, beginning on the forehead and face, and gradually spreading over the rest of the body. The duration of the perspiration was different; in one case it lasted for $1\frac{1}{2}$ hours, in another $3\frac{1}{2}$ hours, in a third case, of very considerable universal dropsy, where the amount of urine passed in the 24 hours was only 150 c.c.m., the secretion lasted for 15 hours, after which, the œdematous infiltration decreased considerably. The quantity of fluid secreted in the saliva and the perspiration were in direct proportion to the amount of pilocarpine which had been injected, and to the strength of the solution. Thus, a 2 per cent. solution always called forth a more considerable secretion of perspiration and saliva than a 1 per cent. solution. Two out of the fourteen patients complained of pains in the abdomen after the injection, and four of headache. In eight cases, the pupil was seen to contract; the contraction began at the same time at which perspiration set in, and lasted from 30 to 45 minutes. The temperature was taken in every case both before and after the injection, and in several of them was observed to fall rapidly after the injection; this decrease, however, never lasted longer than from half an hour to three hours, after which time the normal temperature was again reached. Only in one case, where the perspiration had lasted for 16 hours, the temperature, which had been 40.4 deg. Cent. before the injection, fell to 38.6 35 seconds after it, and did not rise again. The pulsations of the radial artery increased in a minute from 12 to 30; the pulse was full and jerking; this acceleration lasted from 15 to 30 minutes, after which time the pulse regained its previous character. In four cases, the patients vomited. The vomited matter consisted mostly of mucus. After the injection, almost all the children coughed very much; in four cases where there was extensive bronchitis, and in a fifth, which had been showing symptoms of œdema of the lungs and uræmia, the lungs were entirely cleared from the secretion which had accumulated in them by the frequent coughing within 48 hours. In nine cases, there was a strong desire to micturate immediately after the injection; and, in three, to evacuate the bowels. The motions were thin and very offensive, and were passed in great quantity. In a case of constipation which had lasted four days, the bowels were moved copiously immediately after the injection.

There was no notable increase in the quantity of urine passed after pilocarpine had been injected; it was of a much lighter colour than before. The following are the author's conclusions:' 1. Pilocarpine has proved to be a very successful remedy for children who suffer from nephritis and scarlatina; 2. In giving it to children, care should be taken to begin at first with small doses, which may later on be gradually increased; 3. If the little patients are very weak and are likely to collapse after the injection, a few drops of ether should be added to the pilo-carpine solution; 4. The drug produces a very copious and lasting secretion of sweat, such as no other drug ever has been known to call forth—it acts quickly; 5. In cases of bronchitis, complicated by dropsy, which often produces dyspnœa in children, the affection of the bronchi vanishes very soon after the remedy has been administered.—*London Med. Record*, May 15, 1879.

Medicine.

Pathology of Addison's Disease.

In the *Archiv de Physiologie Normal et Pathologique*, 1878, Nos. 5 and 6, M. JACQUET arrives at the following conclusions: 1. In Addison's disease, the bronzed skin one finds only as a lesion of the sympathetic system, and pigmentation, without atrophy, of the nervous cells of the ganglia which are in the neighbourhood of the diseased suprarenal glands. 2. The degeneration of a part of the nervous fibres attaching the semilunar ganglia to the nervous centres ought to be regarded as secondary and consecutive to the process of sclerosis which accompanies the tuberculization of the capsules. 3. That lesion is insufficient to serve as the basis of a pathogenic theory of Addison's disease. 4. Hyperpigmentation of the nervous cells of the great sympathetic and of the cerebro-spinal system is a fact of the same order as the hyperpigmentation of the epidermic cells of the Malpighian plexus. 5. This hyperpigmentation renders probable the existence of an altera-tion of the blood by the substances which a suprarenal gland would, in the nor-mal state, be employed in utilizing by transforming them. 6. The alteration of the blood by functional or organic insufficiency of the suprarenal glands is a patho-logical phenomenon analogous to that which exists in chronic uræmia. 7. Along-side of the melanodermia, by alteration of the suprarenal tissue, there seem to exist cases in which the melanodermia is due to the lesion of other blood-making organs. 8. Clinical researches in Addison's disease ought especially to be di-rected to the chemical analysis of the blood and the urine.—*Lond. Med. Record*, April 15, 1879.

Retrogressive Lymphadenomatous Growths.

At a recent meeting of the Pathological Society of London (*Med. Times and Gazette*, May 17, 1879) Dr. COATS, of Glasgow, exhibited for Dr. Gairdner, specimens of tumours taken from a man aged fifty-two, who had been under the care of Drs. Thomson and Norrie, of Dumfries. About twelve or fourteen months before his death, the patient began to observe tumours in his abdominal wall, the tumours appearing and disappearing at intervals, according to his own account. After six or seven months he was seen by Dr. Thomson, who then found a large tumour, four inches by three, in the abdominal wall, near the an-terior-superior spine of the ilium, having the characters, when first seen, of a fatty growth; it was repeatedly examined at short intervals for a week or two, but aftei a few months had passed could not be seen at all when again looked for. Ten months aftei the fiist appeaiance of these swellings the patient's geneial health began to fail, and he suffeied fiom sickness and vomiting. He was now seen by Dr. Gairdner, who found as many as thiity-foui tumouis ovei the body, most of them being situated subcutaneously, though some weie deepei. The patient's sickness and vomiting continued, and death took place soon afteiwaids. Post-moitem theie weie found numeious tumouis, not only in the subcutaneous tissues, but also in the connective tissue of the abdomen. In the fatty capsule of the iight kidney theie weie seveial, quite distinct fiom both the kidney and fiom the supia-ienal capsule. The left supia-ienal body was appaiently involved in a mass of similai tumouis, many of which weie bieaking down like blood-clots. One laige tumoui almost occluded the calibie of the intestine, and theie weie seveial in the mesenteiy. He (Dr. Coats) had found the tumouis composed of a coaise ieticulum, in which theie weie many iound lymphoid cells. The tendeney seen in seveial of them to hemoiihage and bieaking down might possibly explain the absoiption and disappeaiance of those that had vanished duiing the life of the patient. The exhibitoi iequested that the specimens be iefeiied to the Moibid Growths Committee.

Dr. NORMAN MOORE asked whethei any change had been obseived duiing the life of the patient in the condition of the blood. In a iecent case in St. Bartholomew's Hospital, wheie theie had been many tumouis in vaiious paits of the body, among them a laige one neai the kidney, the white blood-coipuscles had been found maikedly incieased, though haidly to the degiee chaiacteiistic of leukæmia. But in that case theie had been no histoiy of absoiption of the tumouis.

Dr. GEORGE THIN had seen a case at Vienna, in the *clinique* of Hebia, exactly similai to the one iepoited by Dr. Coats, only theie was even a gieatei numbei of supeificial tumouis in the foimei than in the lattei case. That one had been unique in Hebia's expeiience, and theie was much discussion as to its ieal natuie. Post-moitem, many giowths had been found in the cellulai tissue of the abdomen, as in Dr. Coats's case. Some of these had been sent to Ranviei of Paiis for examination, and he had declaied them to be lymphoid in chaiactei. He (Dr. Thin) did not see that such giowths should necessaiily be consideied lymphoid, although they weie found to contain lymphoid cells, for any inflammatoiy lesion undei the skin would be attended with the exudation of white blood-coipuscles. Anothei case has just been iepoited by Dr. Duhiing, of Ameiica, undei the name of inflammatoiy neoplasm, which also seemed fiom the micioscopic desciiption to be of a similai natuie.

Sir JAMES PAGET said the iepoit of such a case was useful, and likely to help in the explanation of those iaie instances in which tumouis diagnosed to be canceious had disappeaied aftei a time. He suspected that theie was a gieatei numbei of such cases on iecoid than might be imagined, and the collection of them would be an inteiesting and impoitant undeitaking. Thiee cases of the disappeaiance of tumouis in this way weie known to himself. One was in the peison of a young man, who had suffeied for two oi thiee yeais with what appeaied to be ordinary lymphadenomatous giowths, theie being clusteis of enlaiged glands in the neck, axilla, and gioins. The patient had also paiaplegia—a symptom he had found in anothei case of lymphadenoma. Within a week these tumouis all suddenly disappeaied, but the patient then began to suffer fiom dyspnœa, and soon afteiwaids died, no autopsy being allowed. Anothei case, mentioned in his lectuies at the College of Suigeons, was iegaided as one of multiple medullary cancei (what would now be called small-celled saicoma), and the micioscope corroboiated this diagnosis. The giowths occuiied in the neck and axilla. Theie was also a veiy laige mass ovei one deltoid, which suppuiated and sloughed, duiing

which piocess neaily all the othei giowths disappeaied. The man iecoveied,
and enjoyed good health for some months; but the giowth afteiwaids iecuiied,
and caused death. The thiid case was one which he had diagnosed as medullaiy
cancei of an undescended testis. Theie was a tumoui as laige as two fists, and
he had piesciibed liquoi potassæ and iodide of potassium, undei which tieatment
the mass soon entiiely disappeaied. In eight or ten weeks, howevei, it iecuiied,
but disappeaied again undei the same tieatment. This also happened a thiid
time; but, having iecuiied a fouith time, it was no longei amenable to tieatment, and the patient died. The micioscope confiimed his oiiginal diagnosis as
to the natuie of the giowth.

Dr. WILKS also thought that such cases weie not so veiy iaie as was thought.
Theie was at piesent in Guy's Hospital a giil who had had tumouis of the arm,
shouldei, and gioin. All the tumours had disappeaied except that of the arm.
He had iegaided them as of a lymphoid chaiactei. Many yeais ago he biought
befoie the Society a young woman who piesented at fiist a numbei of soft tumouis
ovei the body, which afteiwaids disappeaied. These weie iegaided at the time
as blood-cysts, but they may have been of the natuie of these lymphoid giowths.

Mr. BUTLIN iecalled the case of a boy he had alieady biought befoie the
Society, in which theie had at fiist been tumouis in the paiotid iegion, and afteiwaids in the testes and abdomen. All the tumouis weie found to be lympho-
saicomatous on micioscopic examination. The left testicle had incieased in size
till death; while the othei had diminished somewhat though not entiiely. He
had found the pelvic glands much moie affected on the iight side than on the
left, and he had a notion that this diffeience was connected with the changes of
the testes, those on the iight side having piobably become moie involved as they
ielieved the testicle of that side of its moibid pioducts, wheieas on the left side
the testicle had gone on uniielieved.

The PRESIDENT mentioned that, in the discussion on lymphadenoma, Sir W.
Gull had stated veiy piominently that he had seen spontaneous disappeaiance of
lymphoid tumouis in this way.

Dr. BARLOW mentioned the case of a boy in which lymphadenomatous tumouis
of the mediastinum, which had deflected the tiachea fiom the middle line, iapidly
disappeaied at that site befoie death. He had seen anothei similai case attended
with consideiable pyiexia. In a thiid case, a patient of Dr. Stephen Mackenzie,
the tumouis had iapidly disappeaied undei aisenic.

Dr. STEPHEN MACKENZIE coiioboiated the last statement. The patient,
aftei taking fifteen diops of liquoi arsenicalis daily for a week, began to impiove,
and aftei a foitnight the swellings diminished so iapidly that the patient declaied
most of the diminution had taken place in a single night. He believed the
patient was now quite cuied. Anothei case, piesenting subcutaneous tumouis
believed to be of syphilitic oiigin, had been tieated with iodide of potassium,
and in thiee weeks the tumouis had entiiely vanished. Syphilitic giowths
weie of couise veiy similai histologically to these lymphadenomatous tumouis,
and when the foimei disappeaied so quickly with iodide of potassium, he thought
it need not be wondeied at if the lattei should also be found to disappeai veiy
iapidly.

Dr. WILKS wished to add his testimony to the gieat value of aisenic in these
cases of lymphadenoma. All the cases he had seen impiove had been tieated
with aisenic.

Dr. COATS, in ieply, could not say whethei the blood had been examined
duiing the life of the patient. The object in view in biinging foiwaid the case
had been alieady in a gieat measuie attained by the inteiesting discussion it had
called foith.

Prevention of Relapses in Typhoid Fever.

IMMERMANN is of opinion (*Centralbl.*, No. 1, 1879) that relapses in cases of typhoid fever are due to the presence of the typhoid poison in the system, except in instances where the patient has committed some error in diet. The latter occurrence can of course be prevented by watching the patient carefully, and the author has endeavoured to prevent the former by putting the convalescent through a systematic process of disinfection. The process consisted in giving the patients daily from 4 to 6 grammes of salicylate of soda for ten or twelve days, beginning from the first day the temperature assumes its normal state. Fifty-one patients were treated in this way, and only two suffered from relapses; one owing to something she had eaten in secret, and the other because, owing to a mistake, the drug had not been given to him immediately after the fever had left him. Fifteen out of sixty-seven patients who had not been treated with salicylate of soda had relapses. The author concludes from these observations, that salicylate of soda is not only a powerful preventive of relapses in cases of typhoid fever, but that it also would prove very useful in procuring immunity from the disease for the nurses and attendants.

Immermann has also observed that patients who had been treated exclusively with cold water showed a greater tendency to relapse than others who had undergone a combined water and quinine, or salicylate of soda treatment.—*London Med. Record*, May 15, 1879.

The Doctrine of Uræmia.

The doctrine of uræmia, in the literal sense, has almost disappeared from theoretical pathology. Frerichs and Gallois are believed to have demonstrated that whatever poison is circulating in the blood it is not urea. Gallois especially maintained that urea injected into the blood of dogs is incapable of causing the symptoms of "uræmia." It cannot, however, be said that the attempts at any other explanation have been more successful. The carbonate of ammonia theory has never received enough evidence to render it even probable, while Bernard demonstrated that this substance is incapable of determining the symptoms which have to be explained. The doctrine that the poison is really urea has been revived by M. Picard, of Lyons, in a recent communication to the Société de Biologie ot Paris. He states that he has succeeded in causing in dogs convulsive attacks by the injection of urea. As an example of these experiments he gives the following: Fifteen grammes of urea were injected in solution into the jugular vein of a dog weighing two kilogrammes and a half. The animal, after some minutes and some attempts at vomiting, presented tremor and then an epileptiform convulsion. The head was thrown back, the jaws champed, and clonic spasm was equally intense in all four limbs. The attack lasted some minutes, and was followed at short intervals by two other identical attacks. After that the animal was motionless, in a state of muscular relaxation, and soon died.

The explanation of the occasional failure of the experiment M. Picard believes to be this. If a sufficient quantity was injected, there coincided with the above symptoms a complete suppression of the urinary secretion. The bladder emptied itself at the commencement, and remained empty till death. On the other hand, if an insufficient quantity was injected, there was an enormous increase in the urinary secretion, and the urea was eliminated as fast as it entered the blood. In this way large quantities of urea could be injected gradually without inducing any other trouble than polyuria.

M. Picard concludes from these experiments that urea is doubtless the cause of the nervous symptoms of renal disease. This is probably an inference hardly warranted by the results obtained. He certainly, however, has demonstrated an important source of fallacy in experiments on this subject, and has shown that the theory of a true uræmia cannot be considered as altogether defunct.—*Lancet*, May 24, 1879.

Meningitis cured by Iodide of Potassium.

M. RODET relates, in the *Lyons Médicale*, a remarkable case of meningitis, which has suggested to him interesting reflections on the subject of the employment of iodide of potassium in this disease. A girl of 18 had reached the eighteenth day of a well-marked acute meningitis, which had produced paralysis of the right arm, when M. Rodet prescribed for her 3 grammes of iodide of potassium every twenty hours. The following night the patient showed slight improvement, and began to recover a little consciousness. Next day the dose was raised to 4 grammes, and, the following day, to 5 grammes, and continued at that for the subsequent days. She improved under this influence, made rapid progress, and, five days afterwards, the patient might be considered as convalescent. The paralysis of the right arm had completely disappeared. M. Rodet observes that this treatment of meningitis has been recommended by several practitioners, and nevertheless may be said to remain almost completely unknown. It was particularly indicated by Dr. Bourrousse of Laforre, who praised it very highly, even declaring it to be an infallible remedy. It is probable that the reason the remedy has not been more generally used, is because physicians who had tried the treatment have given it with too much timidity and in too weak a dose to obtain a curative effect, and thus have been led to think it ineffective. M. Fonssagrives, in his *Treatise on Therapeutics*, mentions the opinions of various other writers on this subject, and concludes that iodide of potassium constitutes an important improvement in the treatment of an affection, the incurability of which is notorious, and that this means cannot be too highly recommended. He adds, however, that this medicine ought to be given from the outset of the disease, before it has produced serious disturbances in the membranes and the brain. M. Rodet thinks, nevertheless, that iodide may render service even at a more advanced period of the disease.—*London Med. Record*, May 15, 1879.

Sclerous Basilary Meningitis.

Dr. LABARRIÈRE has published in his thesis (*Thèse de Paris*, 1878, and *Bulletin Général de Thérapeutique*, December 15, 1878) ten cases of this peculiar affection, which is seldom met with in private practice, and therefore rather difficult to diagnose. The only certain etiology of sclerous basilary meningitis is tertiary syphilis. The plaques compress the cranial nerves, thereby giving frequently rise to paralysis of the motor nerves, and sometimes of the sensory nerves. These paralyses are, with very few exceptions, permanent. This form of meningitis is generally accompanied by encephalic complications, some of which are of a syphilitic origin, and independent of the meningitis, while others result from the latter. In spite of its clearly defined syphilitic character, a specific treatment has very little effect on the meningitic exudation, and the patient seldom recovers from it. The most important point, therefore, in the treatment is to prevent the exudation from forming, and a very energetic antisyphilitic treatment must be at once begun with a patient with a history of syphilis, in whom we find a paralysis of some cranial nerve complicated with persistent headaches. The author strongly recommends in such cases mercurial frictions, combined with iodide and bromide of potassium, taken internally, Van Swieten's liquid, or a seton in the region of the neck, etc.—*London Med. Record*, May 15, 1879.

Contributions to the Pathological Anatomy of Acute Delirium.

JEHN (*Arch. Psych.*, viii. page 594) has had the opportunity of observing and studying four cases : the first patient was ill for twenty-two days, and eight days before he died gangrene of the right leg set in, beginning at the foot, and spreading rapidly over the whole limb. The right forearm, from the hand to the elbow upwards, was also similarly affected. At the necropsy, an unexpected complication was met with in the shape of a hard tumour, of the size of a nut, on the left side of the pons, which seemed to spring from the acoustic nerve ; the ganglia of the sympathetic cardiac plexus were partly degenerated, and the cortex of both kidneys showed fatty degeneration.

The second case lasted for sixteen days ; a few days before death phlegmonous inflammation of the right foot set in, and on the night preceding the end, the patient's back, abdomen, and legs were covered with numerous pustules. At the necropsy the latter were found to communicate with abscesses under the skin. The liver was partly in a state of fatty degeneration, and the capsules of the kidney very adherent, the cortex being of a yellowish tinge.

In the third case, the patient was delirious for twenty-six days ; in the course of the last six days a gangrenous phlegmon of the right leg set in. The liver was swollen, and in a partial condition of fatty degeneration, the cortical layer of the kidneys of a yellowish hue and adhering to the capsules. The author considers this case, as well as the fourth, as being closely allied to acute paralysis.

In the latter, acute delirium set in towards the end of an illness which had lasted four months ; it broke out while the patient was under mercurial treatment for syphilis, and lasted for fourteen days. Here also a gangrenous inflammation was observed, similar to those which have been described above, which broke out in the vicinity of an open syphilitic ulcer on the right thigh. At the *post-mortem* examination, the posterior columns were found in a state of gray degeneration.

In comparing the results of the microscopical examination in all four cases, they were found to be alike in several points. The pia mater was always thick, dark, and of the consistence and appearance of jelly, the vessels, especially in the gray matter, were all more or less in a state of fatty degeneration, and traces of small hemorrhages could be detected in their vicinity. The nervous system seemed to have been affected secondarily, the affection manifesting itself in a fatty degeneration of the cells of the ganglia ; in some cases the former had entirely vanished, and in their place only a large mass of fatty globules could be seen, while in other cells the change had hitherto confined itself to the nucleus, increasing it in size. The author is of opinion that such cases ought to be considered as acute meningo-encephalitis.—*London Med. Record*, May 15, 1879.

—

Ergot in Insanity.

Dr. ENRICO TOSELLI (*Archivio Italiano*, Settembre, 1878) has a long paper on the effects of ergot of rye in the treatment of mental derangement. He thinks that this drug produces cerebral anæmia, its action being the reverse of nitrite of amyle. In fact, he has found by experiment that, contrary to the opinion of Schüller, the cerebral vessels contracted by ergot may be dilated by the inhalation of nitrite of amyle. Brown-Séquard demonstrated that the primary effect of ergot was the contraction of the bloodvessels in all the organs in the body, as well as the contraction of the fibres of the uterus. Vokes obtains favourable results in treating hemicrania ; Silva, in the treatment of cerebral hyperæmia ; Crichton Browne, in the congestive form of mental alienation in recurrent mania, in chronic mania with lucid intervals, and in epileptic mania. Dr. Toselli found it of great use in treating serous diarrhœa, a frequent complication of dementia,

especially in the paralytic form.   In administering it for this purpose he observed
that his patients passed out of the state of sleeplessness, and that their mental faculties were less obtuse.   He either used the aqueous extract of the *Secale cornu-
tum*, or the *ergotin Bonjean*, given twice during the night in doses of from 50
centigrammes up to as much as 4 grammes.   He found that ergotin acted most
quickly and surely in the form of hypodermic injection.   Ergot diminishes the
frequency of the pulse, contracts the vessels, augments the pressure of the blood,
and lowers the temperature.   Digitalis has more power in moderating the action
of the heart, whereas ergotin has a greater effect upon the bloodvessels and in
diminishing the temperature.   Sometimes ergotin acts as a diaphoretic and diuretic.   Sometimes the therapeutic effects have not appeared with a large dose,
and only manifested themselves when it was reduced.   Sometimes the calmative
effect following the use of ergotin lasted as long as a month.   Toselli used the
drug in thirty cases and found the most benefit from it in paralytic insanity, in
chronic mania, and in dementia accompanied by agitation, insomnia, hallucination of the senses, especially when these symptoms accompany melancholia and
hypochondria.   He does not pretend to have cured any case of insanity with ergotin, though he thinks it may arrest the course of general paralysis.—*Brain*, April,
1879.

Pleuritic Epilepsy and Hemiplegia.

In 1875, M. Raymond read before the Société des Hôpitaux two very interesting observations on the subject of patients who were suddenly seized with convulsions and hemiplegia, some time after having been operated upon for empyema, while injections were being made into the pleura.   Several similar facts
have since been observed which M. AUBAIN has, together with a case which had
come under his own observation, worked up very successfully in his thesis (*Thèse
de Paris*, 1878, and *Journal de Médecine et de Chirurgie*, February, 1879).
The *modus operandi* is as follows : A patient who has been suffering from purulent pleurisy, and on whom the operation for empyema has been performed, has
his wound washed out every day with some disinfectant.   He bears these injections without experiencing any inconvenience or pain for a month, six weeks, or
more, when suddenly, without any premonitory warnings, the patient, who is sitting up in bed while the injection is being made as usual, falls backwards in a
state of imminent syncope.   In a very short time convulsive spasms come on ;
they are almost always universal, but generally stronger on the side which corresponds to the empyema.   The patient's teeth are set, the pupils, which have at
first been contracted, are subsequently dilated.   The tonic convulsions are followed by contractions ; the breathing becomes stertorous, the patient foams at the
mouth ; urine and feces are passed involuntarily ; he remains in a state of epileptic coma for half an hour or an hour, when he again recovers consciousness.
Sometimes nothing more occurs, or another similar fit may supervene the same
day, or two or three days later, without any injury to the patient.   But in some
very serious cases the patient does not recover consciousness ; fit follows fit ; the
contractions persist ; in a few cases opisthotonos has been observed, and the patient dies in ten or fifteen hours.   This is termed pleuritic epilepsy.   In some
cases, however, another phenomenon has been observed in connection with those
already mentioned, viz., hemiplegia.   It may affect only one of the lower or superior extremities, or the face, the paralyzed members always being on the side
which corresponds to the empyema.   Motility is seldom entirely abolished, so
that the affection might perhaps rather be defined as a certain degree of paresis,
without any distinct disturbances of the sensibility.   It is transitory, and if the
patient recovers from the attack it also disappears a few days later.   Lastly, there

is a third class, in which the hemiplegia comes on gradually without any preceding convulsions. The symptoms are the same as above, but the affection always
disappears entirely after a certain time. That these accidents are very dangerous
is demonstrated by the fact that four out of the ten cases mentioned by M. Aubain
have terminated fatally. At the necropsy, no cerebral lesion which might account
for the fatal issue could be discovered ; the pathogenesis of the cases is also very
obscure. It is very curious that these accidents should always happen when the
patient is almost convalescent, and at the moment when the injection is being
made. In order to avoid this complication great care should be observed in making
the injections into the pleura. Very small quantities of the liquid must be injected
at the time, and not too much force used in the operation.—*London Med. Record,*
May 15, 1879.

<hr/>

History of Neuritis.

The history of neuritis is not old, and, in spite of numerous researches, its etiology
and nature are still very obscure. Inflammation of the nerve, or more correctly
the nerve string, may be brought on by three different processes. 1. It may be
an acute parenchymatous neuritis, where the nerve tube alone is affected ; 2. It
may be an interstitial neuritis, characterized by a protracted inflammation of their
intra- or perifascicular connective sheaths ; 3. It may be a mixed consecutive
neuritis, or inflammation of the nerve tubes, originating in their being continually
compressed by the increasing growth of their sheaths.

All these lesions are quite clear, and each has its peculiar characteristics, which
have been clearly demonstrated by microscopic examinations. But the symptoms
which correspond to each of them are far from being clearly defined, and M.
Gros (*Lyon Méd.*, March 16, 1879) has passed rapidly over this portion of his
work, contenting himself with merely mentioning muscular atrophy and cutaneous eruptions as being the effects of affections of the trophic nerves.

These inflammations of the nerve cords have the peculiar tendency of advancing occasionally towards the nerve centres, and producing secondary alterations
in them, and a very important point to be noted is that this secondary spinal
affection may manifest itself even when the primary affection has apparently
come to a stop. Thus, at a given moment, a peripheric lesion cannot only give
rise to medullary symptoms, but also to lesions of the spinal cord.

In short, a neuritis which is disseminated over the peripheric nervous system,
can, partly through certain symptoms which are peculiar to it, and partly by extending to the cord, give rise to different syndromi, which clinicists have described
under different names.

The author has collected ten cases in corroboration of his views, and among
them Landry's case of *acute ascending paralysis;* Duménil's case of *ascending
neuritis;* Jaccoud's case of *progressive nervous atrophy;* and Eichorst's case of
progressive acute neuritis. He acknowledges himself that these cases are incomplete, and present only few points of similarity, but he thinks that they may
all be connected by one common symptom, viz., muscular atrophy, which is accompanied by more or less distinct sensory troubles. According to them, there are
three forms of disseminate neuritis. 1. An acute form, which lasts generally
three weeks, during which time muscular atrophy is not sufficiently developed to
be demonstrated clinically, and which ends fatally ; this is "acute ascending
paralysis ;" 2. A subacute form, which lasts from six to twelve months ; in some
cases the patients recover, and the power of movement is restored in certain parts
of the body, while in other cases they die ; 3. A chronic form, which is generally met with, and which may last up to five years.

Vol. VI.—20

All this classification must, however, be considered as mere hypothesis, as it has not yet been sufficiently proved that all the three forms we have mentioned really belong to the same disease. The connecting link between them is muscular atrophy, but when this is wanting, as in the first form, there only remains a very feeble support for the author's theory, viz., an anatomical lesion, the neuritis. It would perhaps hardly be admissible in pathology to found a whole classification on a simple anatomical lesion, while the symptoms produced by it differ widely from each other in many points.—*London Med. Record*, May 15, 1879.

Treatment of Exophthalmic Goitre.

M. SÉE says, in his book on the diagnosis and treatment of cardiac diseases, that the only treatment of exophthalmic goitre which he has found successful is a combination of hydrotherapy with tinct. veratri viridi. He prescribes the latter in doses of from 10, 12, to 20 drops *per diem*, to be taken in four or five doses, and continues this treatment for several weeks and even months. In this way he has succeeded in curing a young woman who had presented all the characteristic symptoms for fifteen years, and a young girl who, at the age of seventeen, began to suffer from palpitations and hypertrophy of the thyroid gland—a case of exophthalmos, with palpitation.—*London Med. Record*, May 15, 1879.

Amygdalitis.

VERNEUIL asserts (*Gazette des Hôpitaux* and *Lyon Médical*, No. 9, March 2, 1879) that the purulent focus which invariably develops during the last stages of amygdalitis is not situated in the interior of the tonsil, but in its vicinity, viz., in the cellular tissue which separates the organ from its groove. The tonsil does not adhere very firmly to this groove, and when tumefied through the inflammation, it bulges out between the anterior and posterior pillars of the velum of the palate, and moves backwards and forwards at every movement of deglutition. This mobility is one of the principal causes of the formation of the abscess. The gland being continually displaced, a serous bag forms in the connective tissue, which stretches between both pillars and occupies the bottom of the groove of the tonsil. In this serous bag the purulent gathering is formed. The abscess is always very deep-seated, and cannot, therefore, easily be reached by a bistoury, as an incision directed in a straight line towards the tumour which the tonsil forms in the isthmus of the larynx would not be able to reach it. To open the abscess it would therefore be necessary to cut through the anterior pillar of the velum of the palate; this pillar, which is much enlarged and protruding, forms the anterior wall of the abscess; but, at the same time, it is highly œdematous, so that in order to pierce it a very deep incision would have to be made, and, in doing this, the carotid artery might easily be injured. It would, therefore, appear that abscesses of the tonsils had better be let alone. They must not be opened, and it is better to wait and allow the pus to make a way for itself through the anterior pillar. Happily the affection never lasts long, and the abscess generally opens spontaneously on the fourth or fifth day.—*London Med. Record*, May 15, 1879.

New Method of Producing Tuberculosis.

TAPPEINER, the author of this interesting article, which was originally published in *Virchow's Archiv*, vol. 74, page 393, is a physician living at Meran, in the Tyrol, and was led to undertake his researches on this subject, from having frequently observed the fact that healthy girls, who belong to healthy families, and had been nursing consumptive patients, became consumptive and died quickly.

He was moie and moie impiessed with the idea that phthisis was contagious, and suspected the contagion was spiead by the attendants or nuises bieathing the air impiegnated by the patient's expectoiations.

His expeiiments weie conducted in the following way : he made animals (dogs, who veiy seldom suffei fiom tubeiculosis) bieath in a space the air of which had been impiegnated, by means of an atomizei, with phthisical sputa that had pieviously been diluted in watei. In eleien cases, with one exception, miliaiy tubeiculosis of both lungs iesulted, most of the animals also had tubeicles in the kidneys, and some in the livei and spleen. The nodules fiist appeaied in the thiid week aftei the fiist inhalation ; a veiy small quantity of sputa is sufficient to pioduce the eiuption. As the disease was not in eveiy case confined to the lungs only, the authoi thinks that the action of the inhaled paiticles is not a mechanical, but a specific one. Identical expeiiments weie undeitaken with calves' biains, which had been piepaied in a similai way to the sputa, for the puipose of veiifying the foimei experiments, and gave a negative iesult.—*Lond. Med. Recoid,* May 15, 1879.

——

Some Peculiaiities in the Night Sweats of Phthisis.

ROUSSELOT (*Revue Médicale de l'Est,* January 15, 1879) iegaids the night sweating of phthisis as entiiely suboidinated to the pyiexia, the vaiiable couise and evolution of which it closely follows ; he looks upon it as an effoit of natuie to modeiate and ieduce the febiile movement by a diveision to the suiface. He also maintains that if, when theie exists a consideiable iise of tempeiatuie, theie be no noctuinal peispiiation, we get a diveision towaids the intestinal surface, and diaiihœa appeais. Moieovei, we often obseive a cuiious alteination of these two phenomena, one appeaiing when the othei disappeais, and *vice veisâ.* Hence, he concludes, that it is not always iight to check the sweatings, especially when they come on at the commencement of phthisis, and accompany a iapid evolution of the pulmonaiy tubeiculization with high fevei and active pulmonaiy congestion. That in such case, to attack the peispiiation is to attack the effect not the cause, and it is not likely, theiefoie, to be attended with success. But when abundant sweatings occui togethei, with a noimal flow of uiine and fiequent diaiihœa, then it is necessaiy to diiect our theiapeutic effoits to aiiest the excessive diain ou the system.—*London Med. Recoid,* May 15, 1879.

——

Treatment of Cardiac Dyspnœa.

M. Séε, in his book on the diagnosis and tieatment of heait-disease, advocates the use of iodide of potassium in cases of continuous caidiac dyspnœa, eithei alone or combined with opium, digitalis, oi chloial, beginning with doses of $1\frac{1}{4}$ giamme, and iising giadually to 2 or 3 giammes, to be continued for some time. Opium is added in doses of fiom 10 to 15 centigiammes, in oidei to counteiact the effects of iodine ; and chloial is useful in cases wheie digitalis is not toleiated. The piesciiption would then be as follows : ℞. gum julep, 120 giammes ; iodide of potassium, 2 giammes ; and hydiate of chloial, 4 giammes. To be taken eveiy two houis duiing the day.—*London Med. Recoid,* May 15, 1879.

——

Milk Diet in Heait Disease.

M. Séε, in his book on the tieatment and diagnosis of heait disease, iegaids milk as a most poweiful diuietic ; he does not appiove of exclusive milk diet, which, in his opinion, ieduces the patient to a state of extieme inanition, but piesciibes a mixed milk diet of about two lities and a half of milk *per diem,* added to the patient's usual food. This does not in the least interfeie with the diuietic

effects of milk. These effects must not be attributed merely to the water contained in the milk, as has been supposed by some authors, because the same quantity of pure water would in no wise produce the same results. It is evident,
therefore, that only the sugar and salts possess the diuretic properties, their action
being similar to that produced by salts of potash and soda by their osmotic power.
These diuretic properties seem to be much more powerful when the milk has not
been boiled; it should, therefore, be taken unboiled and fresh from the cow if
possible, or, at least, lukewarm, as cold milk does not act in the same way. It
seems as if boiling the milk destroyed these properties; nevertheless, it must
never be forgotten that some patients can only digest milk when boiled, so that
the rule is not without exception.

Another curious point in the action of milk is, that it is equally powerful in
cases where the cardiac affection is not combined with dropsy. M. Sée has often
observed that patients who either no longer suffered from dropsy, or never had
suffered from it, were extremely benefited by a mixed milk diet; the action of
the heart became much calmer and more regular, and the palpitations disappeared
altogether. M. Sée entirely disapproves of whey and grape cures for patients
with heart disease.—*London Med. Record*, May 15, 1879.

—

Case of Abdominal Aneurism in a Syphilitic Patient.

M. VALLIN presented, at a recent meeting of the Société Méd. des Hôpitaux
(February 28), several preparations from a patient who died from the rupture of
an aneurism in the abdomen. The patient, aged 45, had spent the greater part
of his life in Cochin China, and had come back in a state of great dyspepsia,
anæmia, and cachexia. He also suffered from violent pains in the lumbar
region, the pains being felt particularly when he walked fast or attempted to
pass from the recumbent position to the upright one. An anæmic murmur could
be heard over his heart, and he complained of palpitations, and entered the
hospital in a state of highly advanced cachexia. There was a history of syphilis,
which dated about fifteen years back, had disappeared under very energetic anti-
syphilitic treatment, but had recurred five or six years later; in fact, a gumma
could be detected on the lower part of the leg, as well as a large exostosis, of the
size of half a pigeon's egg, in the interosseous space of the same limb. M. Vallin,
who ascribed the patient's extreme cachexia and anæmia to syphilitic intoxication, treated him with iodide of potassium and mercurial frictions, which proved
successful, as far as the syphilitic growths were concerned; but the pains still
continuing, and increasing in violence, he could not help suspecting that there
was something else the matter with him besides syphilis. After a close examination he discovered pulsations in the left hypochondriac region, and heard a blowing noise; this could only be caused by an aneurismal dilatation; the pulsations
of the crural artery on this side were not isochronous with those on the right.
The antisyphilitic treatment was nevertheless continued, and the patient left the
hospital, and died suddenly during the act of sitting up in bed. At the necropsy
the peritoneal cavity was found to be filled with a great quantity of blood. There
were no less than four diverticula on the aorta, three of which might safely be
termed aneurisms. The last was situated between the duodenum and the head
of the pancreas, and was the one that had burst.

The question is, whether in this case there existed any relation between syphilis and the aneurism. It is well known that the former affection may cause
sclerosis of the arteries through proliferation of the cells; this naturally would
render some portions of the vessels less resistant to the pressure of the blood, and
thereby greatly favour the formation of aneurismal sacs. Aneurisms have also

been noticed before in syphilitic patients, under circumstances which render it almost certain that a relation exists between the two affections.—*London Med. Record*, May 15, 1879.

Periarteritis Nodosa.

In the first number of Virchow's *Archiv*, Kussmaul and Maier published an account of what they believed to be a "hitherto undescribed peculiar affection of the arteries," to which they gave the name of Periarteritis Nodosa. Their patient was a young man, who, after a somewhat irregular life, was attacked by indefinite illness, the principal symptoms of which were increasing chlorotic marasmus, albuminuria, and progressive general paralysis with muscular pains. On *post-mortem* examination they found diffuse infarction of the kidneys, with extensive ulcerating enteritis, and wide-spread granular degeneration of the voluntary muscles; but the most important appearance was a peculiar thickening of the small arteries, usually circumscribed so as to resemble small knots. The branches as large or less than the coronary arteries were principally affected, in the heart, intestine, stomach, kidneys, spleen, and voluntary muscles; in the liver, cellular tissue and the branches of the brachial and phrenic arteries the lesion was less marked. In consequence of this affection the lumina of the vessels were dilated into small aneurisms in some places, in others narrowed, and there was considerable obstruction to the circulation, so that the changes in the kidneys, intestine and muscles, clearly were secondary to the disease of the circulatory apparatus. In a recent number of the same periodical Dr. P. MEYER describes a very similar case. A sergeant in the army, aged 24, of rather dissipated habits, but who had previously enjoyed excellent health and was of a robust constitution, acquired gonorrhœa and a chancre in the autumn of 1876, followed by constitutional symptoms in January, 1877, for which he was treated by inunction. From this time he never regained his former health, but always remained pale and thin; in August he complained of pains in the neck, loins, and calves of the legs, accompanied by fever and abdominal pain, for which he was admitted. His conjunctivæ were yellow, his pulse and temperature were high, he sweated profusely; there were no physical signs of disease in internal organs. In September, his ankles became œdematous, and in October, albumen appeared in his urine. His chief complaint was of abdominal pain, and there was a small quantity of ascites present. He died rather suddenly on October 22, and at the *post-mortem* examination conditions were found very like those in Kussmaul and Maier's case, with the exception of the ulceration of the intestine, which was absent. The size of these nodules varied from a poppy or hemp seed, the usual dimensions, to being occasionally as large as a bean. The affection was less marked in the extremities, and apparently entirely absent in the brain. The larger vessels, the aorta, carotids, etc., were quite healthy. On microscopical examination, these small nodules were found to be aneurismal sacs communicating with the lumina of the vessels, and with thin walls formed of a delicate connective tissue of recent growth. Some of them were obliterated and filled with completely organized thrombus. The nodules were generally situated at the points of division of the vessel. The connective tissue in the immediate neighbourhood was thickened, very fasciculated, and many capillary vessels could be seen in it. As the artery entered the nodule it became dilated and fusiform. The media and interna could be distinguished at first, but after a short distance the whole vascular wall presented the appearance of a bright homogeneous membrane. When the fenestrated membrane was still recognizable, muscular fibres on its outer side presented this shining appearance, which suggested the notion of amyloid degeneration, but iodine and methylaniline gave negative results. In some cases the change from the normal arterial wall to the homo-

geneous shining membrane was quite abrupt. Another peculiarity was that the
lesion was not always circumscribed, but sometimes so diffused as to convert a
small branch into a stiff yellowish white cylinder. Dr. Meyer believes the disease
commences in the adventitia and next involves the media, which gives way.
Hyaline masses, sometimes seen in the lumina of the vessels, he regards as derived
from the endothelium of the interna. Multiple aneurisms have been described by
Virchow in the pia mater, by Baerensprung in the skin; MM. Charcot and Bouchard's observations on miliary cerebral aneurisms are well known; but these
differ from the cases now under consideration, by their restriction to a special
organ. Cases of multiple aneurism distributed throughout the body have been
placed on record by Pelletau, Rokitansky, and Weichselbaum. Pelletan's case
is given without details; he apparently knew nothing of the clinical history.
Weichselbaum's case is very similar to the others here alluded to; it is to be
found in the *Allgem. Wiener Med. Zeitung* for 1877, No. 28. According to him,
the affection commenced by endarteritis, and he regarded the case as syphilitic,
relying entirely upon Heubner's position that syphilitic endarteritis has characteristic anatomical appearances. We know now that this is a mistake. It is not at
all clear what is to be considered the true etiology of this affection; all the cases
were in young men; two of them had led dissipated lives, and had probably drunk
too much; one certainly had had syphilis. Dr. Meyer thinks the abuse of alcohol
may have directly caused such an increase of blood-pressure as to lead to changes
in bloodvessels predisposed to disease by the cachectic state of the individual,
whether syphilitic or otherwise. The other point of interest in the cases was the
striking resemblance of the symptoms to those of acute trichinosis. Kussmaul
and Maier noticed this, and even thought it possible that the aneurisms might
have a parasitic origin, suggesting the name *Aneurysma verminorum hominis*.
There seems to be no ground whatever for such a hypothesis, and the resemblance
in the symptoms is properly explained by the localization of the affection in the
muscles in both diseases; in both there is more or less disturbance of the nutrition
of the muscular substances, with more or less permanent inflammatory change resulting.

Diarrhœa Adiposa.

SEYDELER publishes the following case in the *Berliner Klinische Wochenschrift*, No. 7, 1879: The patient was a delicate lady of 17, mother of a child
one year old. She had been suffering from catarrh of both apices of the lungs,
consolidation of the apex of the right lung, coughing, and weakness. After
spending the summer in two or three watering places, her health had improved,
with the exception of one symptom, frequent diarrhœa, which was not amenable
to any remedies. When the author first saw his patient, he found her in bed,
looking comparatively well. There was a cavity in the apex of the right lung;
she did not cough very much, neither did she expectorate much. Her principal
complaints were a feeling of lassitude and diarrhœa. The tongue was clean, anorexia prevailed. The posterior wall of the pharynx felt hard to the touch, and
protruded like a tumour; the larynx was free, crepitation and whistling could be
heard over both apices of the lungs, bronchophony, and cracked pot (*pot fêlé*)
sounds. The transverse diameter of the liver was smaller than in the normal
space. The pyloric and right hypogastric regions were tender to pressure, but
no nodules or knots could be felt. The pulse was small, 100–120, the temperature regularly rose in the afternoon. The patient lived principally on beef-tea,
milk, claret, and water. A month later the author, on examining the motions
of the patient, discovered in them large quantities of a whitish fat-like substance.
The patient died soon afterwards in the author's absence, so that he was not able

to verify his diagnosis of multiple tuberculosis. The fatty masses which the author had collected from the motions of the patient were of different sizes, varying from a French bean to a walnut, either round or spindle-shaped, and white both on the in- and outside. They floated on water and crumbled when boiled. If, after having been previously dried for some days, they were heated on a plate of glass, a large quantity of fat escaped, which soon grew solid; the residuum was a brownish granular substance, which burned to a cinder after the fat had been melted out, and smelt strongly of melted butter. Under the microscope, and when treated with cold solutions of caustic potass or ether, peculiar formations could be detected, which Funke has called sebaic acid. The question is, Where did the fat come from in this patient, who lived principally on milk? And how was it that she did not lose more flesh and present a more emaciated appearance after this enormous less of fat? May it not be supposed that in this case tuberculous degeneration, having spread to the organs whose principal function is the digestion of fat, viz., the liver and pancreas, greatly impaired these functions, and that the milk, *sit venia verbo*, having been churned in the stomach and intestines, left the latter in the form of butter?—*London Med. Record*, May 15, 1879.

Histology of Acute Nephritis.

Dr. THADAUS BROWICZ, of Cracow (*Centralblatt für d. Med. Wissenschaft*, March 1st) has induced nephritis by subcutaneous injections of cantharidin in rabbits, in order to determine the changes in respect to the question in dispute as to the primary seat of the lesions. He found the kidneys large and swollen, with their cortical substance stained a deep brown-red, in some places passing into a paler or yellowish colour. The histological changes were restricted to the secreting part of the organs, the labyrinth. The vascular tufts were at first swollen; later on, there was to be seen a layer of hyaline or finely granular material between the tuft and the capsule, which compressed the tuft and stretched the capsular wall. There was no nuclear proliferation to be seen in this. The same material was found in the uriniferous tubes in the shape of tube casts. This finely granular (paraglobulin?) substance, on closer examination, was found to be composed of oval short corpuscles, which cleared and partly disappeared with acetic acid. The epithelium of the narrow urinary tubules was swollen and cloudy, even so as to occlude them. Inside the epithelial layer there were in many places round cells, which resembled in appearance, size, and staining relations those of the interstitial intertubular tissue, and in the absence of any appearance of proliferation of the epithelium were probably wandering cells. The interstitial tissue showed only a small number of colourless corpuscles, which were collected together in little groups. In the straight tubules, besides cloudiness and loosening of the epithelium, there was no change. He concludes, therefore, that the parenchymatous nephritis, described by Virchow, is not secondary and necrotic, as Kelsch thinks, but the consequence of the exudation into the urinary tubules; and interstitial nephritis, the later stage of which is so often found post-mortem, is a distinct process, an analogy being found in the superficial inflammatory affections of the lungs, in which the connective tissue often takes part.—*London Med. Record*, May 15, 1879.

Scleroderma.

At the meeting of the Société Médicale of the Hospitals of Paris on the 13th December, reported in the *Progrès Médical*, 15th March, 1879, M. BLACHEZ presented a patient 34 years old, suffering from scleroderma. After having experienced a feeling of numbness in the hands and nervous disorder for two or three months, he found himself suffering from growing puffiness of the hands and feet. This œdema, temporary at first, soon became permanent, and lasted from four to six months. Then only did the hardening of the skin begin, which manifested itself especially in the hands and feet, then in the legs, the belly, and, later, the face. No trouble showed itself of sensation or of motility. During the last fifteen days only some pigmentary spots had appeared on the hands; meantime, the health remained excellent. To sum up, this man had passed through three distinct phases—first, nerve disorder and numbness; second, a period of œdema and effusions; third, a period of localized induration. Dr. Blachez had employed friction with iodine ineffectually during the first period. He had not used electricity, which had been recommended in certain forms of scleroderma by Dr. Armaingaud. M. Vidal had observed similar phases in persons affected by scleroderma, but the œdema was not a constant phenomenon. Electricity had not given him any good results. Warm douches to the spinal column had appeared to succeed. His treatment was in favour of the opinion which considered scleroderma as a disorder of the nutrition of the nerves. Dr. Blachez had not found any painful point about the spine in his patient. There was no asphyxia of the extremities. The local temperature had not been examined.—*London Med. Record*, May 15, 1879.

Surgery.

Antiseptic Surgery in Paris.

The Society of Surgery has, during several of its last sittings, been occupied with a long debate on antiseptic dressings, in the course of which it has become apparent that the antiseptic system of surgery has established itself triumphantly in Paris, and is indeed in a fair way completely to revolutionize the results hitherto obtained in those hospitals which have from time to time been so notoriously bad as to have become a by-word in Europe. The parable has been taken up in succession by M. Farabœuf, Lucas-Championnière, Panas, and others, and with certainly a crushing result. M. Lucas-Championnière deserves not only the credit of being one of the first of French surgeons thoroughly to study and carefully to appreciate the whole meaning of the theory of antiseptic surgery as well as the practice of it by Mr. Lister. By his writings, and still more by his example in the various surgical services in Paris of which he has from time to time had charge, he has succeeded in demonstrating so completely that results as excellent and as free from mortality may be obtained in French wards as in any others, that it is clearly impossible for French surgeons to hold out much longer against a demonstration so striking. Indeed, the battle may be said, after reading this discussion, to have been already won. The brilliant and striking speech of M. Farabœuf sufficiently shows that among the younger generation of surgeons not only are the Listerian methods fully appreciated, but the principle on which they are based is perfectly apprehended and will not be dropped.

M. Farabœuf was justly merry over the numerous combinations under which the Listerian method is, in England and elsewhere, concealed, parodied, or modified; and in all the debate there is nothing which seems to have been more warmly approved or more thoroughly felt than his powerful statement. But perhaps the most satisfying, because the fullest of facts, is the short speech of M. Panas, towards the close of the discussion, at the meeting on April 2d. This highly distinguished surgeon and recently appointed professor of the faculty said frankly:

"I am one of those who, for the last two years, have very carefully carried out antiseptic surgery. For twenty-five years I have acted as hospital surgeon, and I have employed various dressings. I can, then, compare myself with myself, and my former results with those of to-day. I present to you first a patient who has had his knee laid open by me for a chronic hydrarthrosis of a year's date. This hydrarthrosis had a traumatic cause. There were, therefore, inflammation and fever. It was under these conditions that I opened the joint. I made an incision of six *centimetres*. A yellow fluid mucous with fibrinous flakes flowed out. The synovial membranes were of the thinness of the thumb; there were enormous synovial fringes. The patient was carried back to his bed, and had his limb placed upon a cushion without being immobilized. The cure was complete at the end of six weeks. The synovial membrane has recovered all its physiological suppleness; there is no stiffness. The patient has resumed throughout the year a very hard service on the railway. Except for the cicatrix, this knee is absolutely like the other. This is the fourth knee-joint opened in my wards; the others were opened by M. Lucas-Championnière, one, among others, in a patient whose leg another surgeon wished to amputate. This series of cases shows that the surgery which we now carry out differs from the surgery which we carried out before. I have seen the knee-joint opened under this method for foreign bodies for suppurating arthritis with caries, fever, etc.; so that this operation, which was formerly contraindicated, is now permissible on condition of employing the dressing of Lister. He who would do it by any other method at present, would deserve to incur police penalties (serait peut-être passible de la police correctionnelle").

Notified by the President at this time that so absolute a statement was hardly permissible at a society from which it might go out with considerable notoriety, and might lead to unpleasant consequences to a surgeon who should open a knee-joint under other conditions, M. Panas observed that, of course, that was not his intention; but he wished to point out that with the Lister dressing an articulation might be opened with great safety, whilst in other less perfect dressings it was a great imprudence. He continued:

"I pass to the amputations of the breast. I have performed fourteen amputations, all treated antiseptically (*avec la Lister*). I do not include an old woman of eighty-two, upon whom I was forced to operate, and who died on the fourth day of senile exhaustion. The fourteen others have all recovered. There are patients who recovered in eleven days; others in twelve days; the average was twenty-four days. Whenever I have employed other methods, the patients left the hospital after an average of six weeks. The duration of treatment is, therefore, reduced by half. Another important result is the absolute disappearance of erysipelas from my wards. At St. Antoine, when I commenced my surgical practice in charge of the wards, out of every three patients with amputation of the breast, I had two cases of erysipelas. The scourge of the wards of Nélaton at the Clinical Hospital, and of Velpeau at the Charity, was erysipelas. Of my fourteen cases of amputation of the breast, thirteen recovered without any application. In the fourteenth woman, there was a slight erysipelatoid tendency; but it was at the Lariboisière where all the medical and surgical wards in the hospital were full of erysipelas. During these two years, I have not had in my wards any case of purulent infection. I have operated in very serious cases of strangulated hernia; my patients have recovered without any application. In fourteen operations, I had two deaths; but in one case of crural hernia the woman was already moribund and cold. I had to make her an artificial anus, and she died

without reacting. Another patient died of tetanus after he was cured of his operation. In another patient, when I had operated, a flood of fecal matter made
its exit. The intestine was perforated. Nevertheless, the man recovered. As
to vertebral abscesses (*abcès froid*), they had come to be considered as things not
to be touched. I had been in the habit of recommending my pupils not to touch
these abscesses, by reason of the danger which the operation offered, and also
because sometimes such abscesses healed if left alone. The method of successive
subcutaneous punctures led to grave accidents and caused fistulæ. It was the
same with capillary aspiration. I had arrived at a sort of surgical nihilism. It
was then that I began to employ Lister's dressing. The simple uncomplicated
progress of abscesses thus operated on and thus dressed is what has struck me the
most. In the great amputations, it is certain that the mortality has fallen since
the employment of antiseptic methods. M. A. Guérin is one of our most skilful
operators. During the war, at the Hôpital St. Martin, before the invention of
the cotton-wool dressing, M. Guérin had as many deaths as operations. Two
months later, at the Hôpital St. Louis, during the Commune, on patients much
more exhausted, but with the cotton-wool dressing, M. Guérin had excellent
results. If we, who have seen various dressings and various surgical methods,
have arrived at giving a large preference to the antiseptic dressings, and in particular to Lister's dressing, much more ought this dressing to be accepted from the
outset by the younger generation. The modifications which people have endeavoured to impose on Lister's dressing have not up to this time been happy. Thus
Callender contents himself with carefully washing the limb with carbolic acid
before opening the psoas abscesses; and then, after the incision, he washes the
depths of the cavity with a strong solution of carbolic acid. He covers the wound
with lint dipped in carbolized oil, without employing the other parts of Lister's
dressing. I have tried this dressing once this year in my service in a patient
having a psoas abscess. The results have not been good, and I have returned to
Lister. I never washed out the wound with so-called pure water, as that water
always contains vibriones. For the washing and dressing of eyes on which I operated, I employed a one-per-cent. solution of boracic acid."

Those who know the intelligence, skill, and erudition of M. Panas, and who
have had an opportunity, as we have had, of visiting his wards at a date prior to
the commencement of the antiseptic dressings, and at a time when M. Lucas-
Championnière was first introducing the method into the wards by the example
of a few cases so treated, will appreciate the frank, courageous, and outspoken
declaration of M. Panas, and the effect which such a statement, so conclusive in
itself and so effectually made, cannot fail to produce upon all his colleagues in
the hospitals. He is known to be a surgeon of great skill, of excellent ability,
and large information; and the emphatic indorsement which he has given to the
completely revolutionizing results of the introduction of antiseptic methods is
unanswerable. It reads, on a small scale, like the now historical statements of
Nussbaum of Munich and Volkmann of Halle, which made the Listerian method
universal throughout Germany. The results in English hospital wards can, of
course, never present the same striking contrasts; for the observance of a religious cleanliness and of a quasi-scientific isolation of each individual case has now
for the last quarter of a century given results so good in our English hospitals
after surgical operation, that the perfection of antiseptic methods cannot affect
statistics in the same violently demonstrative manner as it affects the surgical
statistics of France and of Germany, where the results of operation had for the
last twenty years presented a lamentable contrast to those to which we have been
accustomed in our hospitals. Indeed, it is curious, and to an English reader
hardly credible, that, even in the course of this discussion, there still linger the

old remains of disputes as to whether union by primary intention can be attained sufficiently often after amputation to make it justifiable to make that the customary object of all dressings after such operations. Nevertheless, the prevalent custom now making its way in most of our hospitals—nearly all performing under the Listerian precautions certain operations which are beset by particular danger—is of itself a practical tribute hardly less striking than that which M. Panas pays to the value of the antiseptic method. M. Panas said, by a sort of slip of the tongue which he hastened to correct, that to lay open freely a knee-joint in a case of hydrarthrosis or foreign body otherwise than under antiseptic precautions might almost be considered to call for judicial interference. That was, of course, an oratorical exaggeration, which he immediately withdrew. But it is probable that there are few surgeons at the present moment who would not accept the proposition that to do so would be to inflict upon the patient an immense additional risk, and upon a surgeon, in consequence, an additional anxiety of which few would be willing to take the responsibility; and the dressings of Mr. Lister in London, and the remarkable examples which his wards have afforded of the almost incredible immunity with which all the joints, and the pleural cavity itself, may be opened under an antiseptic spray and with antiseptic precautions, have so profoundly impressed the greater number of metropolitan surgeons, that during the last two or three years antiseptic surgery by the Listerian method may be said to have established itself in London as the ultimate resource when it is necessary to perform hazardous operations upon serious cavities, or upon deeply seated parts which till lately would have been considered beyond the reach of the surgeon's knife.—*British Med. Journal*, May 10, 1879.

Trephining for Epilepsy Depending upon Injuries of the Skull.

The statistics of Stephen Smith (*New York Journal of Medicine*, March, 1852), comprising 27 cases; of J. S. Billings (*Cincinnati Lancet*, June, 1861), 72 cases; and, finally, the table of 12 cases operated upon and published by Dr. S. Bontil (*Boston Med. and Surg. Journal*, vol. x., 1872), give irrefragable proofs of the utility of trephining in epilepsy produced by injury of the cranium. Russel (*Brit. Med. Journal*, 1865) collected 78 cases, but without giving the names of the operators, or the bibliographic source. ECHEVERRIA in this communication (*Archives Générales de Médecine*, Dec. 1878) also cites the statistics of Billings, and gives the opinion of Cooper and Copeland as in favour of the trephine, fortified, in their opinion, by the success of Dudley, Guild, and other surgeons. Velpeau did not approve of the operation, except when there existed an œdematous and crepitant cicatrix; Syme and Solly felt the gravity of the operation, but the former thought it well to operate where an open wound communicated with the fractured cranium.

Since that time, the improvements which have been made in the instrument used, and the recent discoveries in cerebral localization, with the success obtained by Broca, Bœckel, Lucas, Championnière, Marraud, Proust, and Terrillon, would seem to indicate that a reaction has set in against the doctrines hostile to the operation.

Dr. Echeverria then gives a table of 145 epileptics who were trephined, the name of the operator, the result of the operation, and the bibliographical source. The results may be briefly given as follows: 93 cures; 18 improvements, 5 in which there was no change, and one where the symptoms were aggravated; the deaths 28; total 145 epileptics, of whom 6 were females. 3 children from seven months to 12 and 13 years, 17 youths, and the remainder adults. Primitive pericranial lesions existed in 32 of these 145 cases.

As to cranial injuries, several reports only indicate the fracture without naming the site. There were, however, specified 15 fractures of the frontal, 11 fronto-parietal, 3 of the temporal, and 6 of the occipital bone; the remaining 26 observations do not state the bone injured. It is worthy of note that the left parietal bone has been most frequently the seat of fracture. The various kinds of fracture in the 113 cases corresponding to the cranial lesion were 16 cases of simple depressions of bone; 13 by firearms, in one of which the projectile remained in the wound seven years; 31 comminuted and complicated; 34 simple fractures; 3 multiple; 5 with external fistulous openings; 1 fracture of the parietal, with traumatic aneurism of the middle meningeal artery; and, lastly, 2 cases in which the fracture was complicated by protrusion of brain matter.

The difference in the mortality between the early and the late operations is not remarkable; 3 deaths occurred amongst 17 of the former, and 25 among 138 of the latter, being a mortality of 17 per cent. for the early and 18 for the late operations. The causes of death amongst the 28 fatal cases were of a very diverse nature.

Suppuration upon the whole surface of the brain; great effusion of blood in the brain under the seat of the operation; gangrene of the membranes and abscess of the brain; hemorrhagic openings into the longitudinal sinus; abscess of the brain in one case, and gangrene after meningitis in another; meningitis and erysipelas; encephalitis by loss of cerebral substance; in the other operated cases death followed a meningitic encephalitis, the immediate consequence of the operation.

Death took place on the 17th day after the operation in the patients of Bell and Heywood; of Bylou's cases, one with abscess of the brain died on the 39th day, the other the 3d day. Warren's patient had continual hemorrhages from the longitudinal sinus during the nine last days; in Adams's patient the fatal symptoms developed themselves on the 14th day in the temporal region. The patients of Gross and Gilmore succumbed rapidly, and the cases of meningo-encephalitis were not less rapid in their course.

In 1864, Henri Charbon repeated the operation 27 times upon the Count Phillip of Nassau, and the result was cure. This number was, however, surpassed by Mebée de la Touche, who, in the space of fifteen months, made 52 applications of the trephine, of which 27 penetrated to the dura mater. Saviard trephined a patient 20 times; Gooch 13 times; Despoites 12; and, finally, at an earlier epoch, Russ and Legendre, surgeons of the King of Navarre, in 1686 elevated nearly the whole of the two parietals, their patient living thirty years, although hemiplegic; results which seem to protest against those who reject the operation on account of its extreme gravity.

The five cases in which no change took place after the operation hardly protest against the very numerous facts which prove that, as a rule, the benefit obtained by the operation in cases of epilepsy due to traumation, is immediate and permanent. Traumation followed by functional troubles indicates sufficiently the treatment by the trephine. And it may be affirmed, on the strength of a long experience, that no epilepsy caused by traumatic lesion of the cranium is ever cured by time. A disease which, apart from its own peculiar dangers, exposes its victim to so many and various accidents, demands that the trepan be employed without hesitation or useless delays, except when fever occurs, immediately on the accident. On the other hand, we may remember that, as a rule, epileptics are exempt from disturbances following the most grave wounds, and also the rapidity with which their wounds cicatrize, circumstances which diminish the risks not only of the trepan in cases of long standing, but also of all surgical operations practised upon epileptics. Except in very well-defined cases of immediate epilepsy, with fever and traumatic meningo-encephalitis, there should be no hesitation in operating each time that the symptoms indicate it. Large portions of bone may be removed, if necessary, and the practice of the American surgeons is not to close the wound until all bleeding has ceased, when it will do well without antiseptic treatment. Galt's instrument is the safest, as it is not liable to wound the dura mater, and is so contrived that when the bone is cut through, the instrument will not cut further.

The principal accidents following the operation in the cases collected above may be shortly named. Five times there were intra-cranial hemorrhages; in one there occurred a traumatic aneurism of the middle meningeal artery, which was quickly arrested by the cautery. In one case there was hemorrhage from a branch of the middle meningeal, which ceased spontaneously. Croft's patient had large clots between the dura mater and the brain, caused by the rupture of a meningeal vessel, wounded by the fractured bone, and there occurred during the operation bleeding from two small arteries of the scalp. Warren's patient had hemorrhage from the longitudinal sinus during the last nine days. In one of Gross's cases there was a large collection of blood from the rupture of a diseased vessel near an exostosis on the internal face of the depressed bone. In one of Dudley's and two of Gilmore's cases there was loss of cerebral substance consecutive to the traumation. The first ended happily, the other two fatally. The patients of Broca and Bœckel, who had hernia cerebri, recovered, in spite of the very serious conditions under which they were trephined. We may conclude that the trepan is the best means for the cure of accidental epilepsy consecutive to traumatisms of the cranium ; that the immediate operation succeeds hardly to the same degree as the late, fever in either case being a serious contraindication to the trepan. Insanity and paralysis are the complications which justify rather than contraindicate the trephining of the cranium in epilepsy produced by traumatic lesions of the head. The operation succeeds equally when syphilitic products in the cranial bones resist specific treatment, or in other cases where they cause epilepsy or serious cerebral attacks.

The statistics of a considerable series of operations show that the mortality of the operation for accidental epilepsy by wound of the head, without taking account of the time of the operation, is 19.30 per cent., the cures 64.13 per cent., the improvements 12.41 per cent., and the cases in which the epileptic attacks have not changed 3.44 per cent.

It is of the first importance for the success of the operation to protect the membranes as far as possible, and to avoid their violent reaction against the slightest injury or foreign body. It is not less necessary to employ the silver suture, and not to unite the edges of the wound until all bleeding has ceased, and, lastly, to prevent suppuration and infiltration of the pericranium and of the brain. There must be no hesitation to promptly clear and set free all pus from the wound. The constant application of ice to the wound, the internal administration of ergot and hemlock (prepared from green fruit), the free action of the bowels by terebinth enemata, with a moderate diet, and especially the placing of the patient in a large area, are the main conditions for obtaining rapid cicatrization of the wound.

It is also prudent to guard the patient, for some time after the operation, under the influence of anti-epileptic treatment, in order to destroy all remains of habit in the nervous system, a tenacious element in epilepsy.—*London Med. Record*, May 15, 1879.

—

Case of Wryneck successfully treated by Division of the Spinal Accessory
Nerve, after Failure of Stretching.

The following interesting case occurred under the care of Professor ANNANDALE at the Royal Infirmary, Edinburgh.

A young woman, aged twenty-four, was admitted into the surgical wards on February 7, 1878. She had passed the three months immediately preceding this date in the medical wards under the care of Professor Grainger Stewart, where trial had been made of all those internal remedies likely to benefit her condition, but without any permanent improvement. The patient was employed in a power-loom factory, where, in order to follow the movements of a shuttle, it was necessary for her to keep continually turning her head from side to side, and as the handle of the machine at which she worked was at her left side, she had occasion to turn most frequently in that direction. After a spell of unusually hard work the patient began to experience a constant sensation of discomfort and uneasiness in the neck, accompanied by occasional twitching movements. The head seemed to be drawn somewhat towards the left side, and on moving it the patient found that additional effort was required to follow the movements of a shuttle, which necessary tended to return it to its former position. The rotation of the head towards the left soon became more marked, and the spasmodic movements increased in violence and frequency.

On admission it was observed that, while at rest, the head assumed the position of rotation to the left, and was depressed towards the left shoulder, which was elevated to meet it. She was generally to be seen sitting with her chin supported on her left hand, looking over her left shoulder. Any movement of the head from this position at once excited the spasmodic movements. These consisted in a series of jerks, becoming more violent as they lasted, by which the head was brought round to the left from any position of rotation towards the right. Though much relief was obtained by avoiding bodily or mental effort, yet it was only during sleep that complete quiet was obtained.

The difficulty of determining the muscles primarily affected was unusually great, yet by observing during the attack the superficial muscles thrown into contraction, the position assumed by the head, and the situation to which the pain was referred, it seemed probable that the following were the groups of muscles chiefly involved: First, the left obliquus inferior, rectus capitis posticus major, and splenius, which rotate the head towards the left; and, secondly, the left sterno-mastoid and trapezius, which depress the head towards the left shoulder and rotate it to the right. The clonic spasms appeared to be due to the alternating action of these two groups of muscles. The case seemed to be one in which overwork had induced a state of, as had been designated by Dr. Poore, "chronic fatigue or irritable weakness" in at least two opposing groups of muscles, those most used by the patient, as a result of which they had become liable to spasmodic action. The most certain means of inducing the clonic spasms was any attempt to perform the habitual movement—in other words, to use either group of affected muscles.

The explanation of the other marked feature of the disease—the permanent deformity—follows from this; it was *assumed* because by it the greatest possible amount of relaxation of both groups of muscles at one time was obtained: the rotation of the head to the left relaxed the first, and the approximation of the head to the shoulder the second group. The adoption of this position was an attempt to abstain from using either group of muscles, and so to avoid the action of the most powerful cause of the spasms.

All this naturally indicated the necessity for more complete rest, such as might be obtained by paralyzing one group of muscles. In order to effect this the following operation was performed: On February 10th Professor Annandale made an incision from below the tip of the mastoid process on the left side, extending downwards for about three inches along the anterior border of the sterno-mastoid muscle. The border of the muscle was cleared, and some of its fibres divided transversely and turned aside. The left spinal accessory nerve was exposed and stretched, and, in case section of it should afterwards be deemed advisable, a silk ligature was applied loosely round it. The wound was then closed, the ends of the ligature being brought out at its lower angle.

No beneficial change whatever followed this procedure; accordingly, on the following day, Professor Annandale removed the stitches from the wound, and by means of the silk ligature brought the nerve within reach, *divided* it, and after separating the divided ends, removed the ligature, and closed the wound. A few hours after section of the nerve had been accomplished, when the patient was able to sit up, it was found that she could move her head slowly round to the right, and could keep her face looking steadily forwards. During the healing of the wound she continued to acquire steadiness and freedom of movement of the head up to the time of her dismissal, on the 16th of March.

The patient was seen in March, 1879, a year after the operation, when she was found to be free from any symptoms of the disease from which she had formerly suffered. The sterno-mastoid and trapezius muscles on the left side were then as well developed as on the right, and the appearance and movements of the neck and shoulders were absolutely normal. In the interval she had resumed her employment, and had only left it on account of her marriage—a circumstance in her social history which testifies to the completeness of the cure.

Three other cases of section of the spinal accessory nerve for spasmodic wryneck are recorded. One of these is the case of Mr. Rivington, of which no particulars have been published.[1] The others, performed by Mr. De Morgan, seem to support the explanation which has been offered of the present case. One was identical with the case now described, but on the opposite side. In it the right spinal accessory nerve was divided with a successful result.[2] In the other the head was rotated to the right also; here the left spinal accessory nerve was divided without curing the disease.[3]—*Lancet*, April 19, 1879.

Luxation of the Left Arytenoid Cartilage.

STOERK brings forward (*Wiener Med. Wochenschrift*, No. 50, 1878) two cases of a most interesting affection, viz., of luxation of an arytenoid cartilage. In both cases there was falsetto voice from early childhood. In one case, the etiology was most likely to be found in cicatricial contraction after diphtheria; in the other no cause at all could be detected. There was in both cases immense tumefaction of the left arytenoid cartilage, which attained in one case three, in the other four times its natural size. In the first case, occurring in a gentleman aged 33, the immobile thickened left cartilage, which was turned in a transverse direction, filled nearly completely the upper aperture of the larynx; its healthy fellow was rendered immobile, too, in consequence of its being pushed backwards by the tumefied neighbour; and thus the vocal cords were permanently in a state of passive tension corresponding to that of the highest falsetto. This gave a simple explanation for the symptom at once attracting attention, viz., for the patient's permanent falsetto voice. Each simple catarrhal inflammation of the narrowed air-passages proved nearly fatal to the patient, bringing on attacks of suffocation. Thus Stoerk resolved in 1868 to relieve this state of things by producing a loss of substance on the posterior and external part of the mucous membrane of the tumefied left arytenoid cartilage, in the hope that the cicatricial contraction would produce a better position. This result was obtained, and the

[1] British Medical Journal, February, 8, 1879.
[2] British and Foreign Medico-Chirurgical Review, July, 1866.
[3] The Lancet, August 3, 1867.

respiration became easier for a short time. Soon, however, the old state of things returned. The operation was again performed a few years later, with the same temporary success. In 1874, the patient went to Schroetter to try his method of gradual dilatation by catheterism of the larynx. Stoerk candidly admits, that this method was accompanied not only by subjective relief, but by an actual dilatation of the upper aperture of the larynx. This fact was ascertained by Stoerk himself, the patient presenting himself repeatedly at his house whilst he was under Schroetter's treatment. In 1876, the patient died suddenly, cause of death unknown.

The second case, also occurring in a strong and healthy man, was very much like the first with regard to the symptoms of phonation and respiration. Here, however, the entire larynx could be seen, the vocal cords remaining close to each other even during deepest inspiration, as in cases of paralysis of the posterior crico-arytenoid muscles. The epiglottis stood quite straight, the right arytenoid cartilage was pushed outwards and backwards by its tumefied left neighbour, the processus vocalis of which occupied the place where the centre of the right ought to have been. In this case, also, catheterism was tried for two years, but without the slightest result.—*London Med. Record,* May 15, 1879.

—

Treatment of Impermeable Stricture of the Urethra.

At a late meeting of the Clinical Society of London (*Lancet,* May 10, 1879), Mr. HULKE read notes of a case of Retention of Urine, caused by Impermeable Urethral Stricture, treated by tapping the bladder above the pubes, and later by external section of the stricture, a catheter passed through the bladder and a staff per penem, as far as the obstruction, being used as guides. The patient, 40 years of age, was admitted into the Middlesex Hospital on November 29th, with retention of twelve hours' standing, the bladder being distended to the umbilicus. He had been treated for stricture twelve years previously. It being found impossible to pass a catheter, Mr. Hulke emptied the bladder by aspiration above the pubes. Twenty-seven hours later, no urine having been passed, a trocar was passed into the bladder above the pubes, and a canula left *in situ;* and on the third day this was substituted for a gum-elastic catheter. During the next few weeks the patient had two attacks of pleurisy. Several unsuccessful attempts were made to pass a catheter per penem, and on January 3d, Mr. Hulke divided the stricture from the perineum, a staff passed through urethra up to the stricture, and a catheter through the prostatic urethra from the bladder down to it being used as guides. The tough fibrous tissue was divided, and the catheter being withdrawn, the staff was guided into the bladder, and, lastly, another catheter passed over the staff into the viscus. The suprapubic aperture was allowed to close, and the case did well. Mr. Hulke remarked that the suprapubic tapping was selected in preference to Hunter's and Cock's method, because of the deviation of the urethra to the left. Not that this operation (first suggested by Hunter, and then practised by Dittel) was intended to supersede puncture through the rectum, but that it was suitable for exceptional cases, such as this. It was not more liable to be followed by urinary extravasation, which did not occur in any of Dittel's cases, nor had Mr. Hulke found it to take place; whilst a provincial surgeon had made the same statement, based on an experience of seventeen cases. It admitted further of antiseptic precautions, and had the advantage of allowing the course of the urethra before and behind the stricture to be made out if division from the perineum became necessary. He had some little difficulty in finding the orifice of the prostatic urethra. The suggestion to use a catheter passed through the external wound as a guide to perineal section is made in a foot note appended to the remarks made by Hunter in the collected edition of his writings.

Mr. MARSH said that in *The Lancet* for 1838, Mr. Hursley records a case of impermeable stricture, where he performed suprapubic tapping, and passing an instrument downwards through the stricture, managed by its means to draw upwards into the bladder a catheter passed per penem. Mr. Hulke's paper was very valuable as affording another means for treating a very difficult class of cases.

—

Remarks on the Production of Cystitis by Contagion through the use of Instruments.

Sir HENRY THOMPSON, in a recent communication to the *British Medical Journal* (May 10, 1879), says: I have long suspected that cystitis is capable of being propagated by the direct transference of inflammatory products from the bladder of one patient to that of another. All are sufficiently familiar with the fact that purulent matter from the vagina, and probably from the uterus also, produces inflammation of the male urethra, and that conjunctivitis may be caused by contact with pus from either source; and I believe it is quite unnecessary to imagine that any specific quality attaches to purulent matter produced in these localities, rendering it more than ordinarily virulent and contagious. Certainly no proof can be adduced that such quality exists; a decision on this point, however, does not necessarily affect the question whether cystitis may be originated or not by contagion.

Every one knows that the operation of sounding the bladder—it may be for stone or for tumour, etc.—is sometimes, although rarely, followed by an attack of inflammation more or less severe. Such an occurrence is, in some circumstances, not unnatural. A delicate organ is mechanically disturbed, and, if force be employed in the process, some inflammation of the mucous membrane is a not improbable result. Hence the extreme importance of adopting a method and instruments which shall accomplish the object in view with the smallest degree of distension and movement; and also of forbearing to make such an exploration, except in circumstances which manifestly indicate its necessity. In my experience of such cases of this kind as have fallen under my observation during many years, I have remarked that the inflammatory attacks which follow sounding occur in two modes, distinct from each other. Thus, in some instances, the patient has a shiver, occurring within three to four hours of the time of the examination; soon afterwards, the urine is passed too frequently and with pain, becomes cloudy, and some general fever sets in. In such, the cause of inflammation is clearly a mechanical one, and, if the patient be healthy, it soon subsides with rest and treatment. But, in a few other instances, no disturbance occurs until the lapse of forty to fifty hours, or thereabout, after the sounding. The subject of the examination has been in all respects well since the sounding took place, and felt, if anything, only slight soreness during the first few hours following the operation. After the interval named, he experiences a little undue frequency of micturition, loses appetite, is chilly or has a shiver; and by degrees symptoms of cystitis appear, and continue a marked course for a few days, with varying persistence according to circumstances. Usually, the patient attributes his condition "to some cold he must have caught the day after the examination," and by no means attributes his troubles to the instrument, as he infallibly does in the circumstances first described.

Why, in certain circumstances, these phenomena should occur so long after the provocation which must have given rise to them, has, as I have already intimated, frequently afforded me an interesting subject of speculation. But a case has recently occurred, which I have been enabled to watch closely, and which seems to throw light on the nature of these examples of the second kind. I shall give the chief particulars in detail.

A medical man, under sixty years of age, having had occasion, as he thought, to pass for himself a silver catheter (No. 10) daily, had a new one made; there was a peculiarity in its construction, the lower or curved portion, about two inches and a half in length, being separate and attached by a screw to the shaft. Such catheters were frequently made formerly for the purpose of packing in a surgical pocket-case. He passed this daily with great ease during some weeks, on no occasion producing irritation. One day, and this was the only occasion on which he used the catheter for another person, he introduced it into the bladder of a patient whose urine was highly muco-purulent, and who was indeed suffering with severe cystitis. He believes that, immediately after using the catheter, he washed it in the ordinary way. Subsequently, on that day, he employed it as usual for himself; and it is somewhat curious that he did not use it the next day—not because he felt any irritation, but, on the contrary, because he was arriving at the conclusion that the instrument was no longer necessary. The next day but one after his last employment of the catheter, about forty-four hours after, he felt chilly, and micturition was slightly painful. Next day he had some fever, no rigor, but increase of temperature; his urine was cloudy and passed frequently. The day after, he was confined to bed; the temperature varied between 102° and 103° for a few days, and the urine was loaded with muco-purulent jelly-like deposit during one or two days. After more than a week's confinement to his room, he gradually improved and soon perfectly recovered, having in his urine now no trace of the attack; he empties his bladder perfectly, and, in relation to the urinary system, has nothing whatever to complain of.

The circumstances of this case will go far, I think, to suggest the strong probability that this attack of cystitis was caused by the transference of infectious matter, by means of the catheter, from the patient for whom it was once used to the subject of our case. I can scarcely doubt that the exceptional formation of the instrument, the screw-attachments which on examination, moreover, appeared to be a little loose, offered a chink, in which matter lodged, especially as this lower part was not detached for cleaning—the eyes of the catheter serving that purpose, as in the ordinary instrument.

It may very naturally be urged: if inflammation be so easily produced through contagion by passing instruments not scrupulously rendered clean, so numerous and varied as these are, and so frequently used, how is it that cystitis is not a very frequent result—for this it certainly is not—of ordinary catheterism?

I think the reason is not far distant, and that it may be found in the action of the catheter itself. The moment the instrument reaches the bladder, the urine rushes through the orifice, and carries off in its current any minute particles which may be adherent to its extremity. In bougies, no opening for the lodgment of adventitious matters exists, and any risk of contagion by their use must be considerably less. Besides, the action of the urethra itself, clinging to the instrument and sweeping off, almost at the external meatus, as it does by that action, most of the lubricating material, is a sort of defence to the internal passages from danger. On the other hand, in examining a bladder, the sound is rarely used as a catheter, and although it has often an eye in its extremity, the handle is closed, and urine seldom passes through it. The various movements of a sound in searching the bladder are calculated to detach, within its cavity, foreign particles, if any such exist, in or about the eye.

The practical question, how to prevent any transference of matter to the bladder and urethra, in employing instruments of any and every kind, presses for solution. It is one of extreme importance to all concerned, and the occurrence of an accident of the kind described, however rare it may be, is one the bare possibility of which cannot be contemplated without extreme repugnance.

After some consideration and some experimental trials, I think the following recommendations will render contagion by instruments impossible.

Firstly: All metal instruments—catheters, sounds, and lithotrites—after use, at any rate in cases of muco-purulent urine, should be plunged for a minute or two into boiling water, to which either a little common soda or a little carbolic acid has been added. If the boiling point of water be not considered absolutely sufficient, a strong solution of chloride of zinc in water may be used. At the strength of twelve per cent. solution, the boiling point is 220° Fahr., or eight above that of boiling water. For some years past, as advised in the last edition of my lectures, I have always placed all gum and other catheters and bougies in a bath of weak carbolic acid immediately after use.

Secondly: I have more recently—that is, since the occurrence described—added a solution of carbolic acid to the oil used for the lubrication of instruments. Oil being the remedial agent for the caustic effects of carbolic acid, there is no danger in applying to the urethra a comparatively strong solution of the acid in oil, since no irritating effect whatever is produced, and the disinfectant influence is unimpaired.

For the last two months, I have used the following formula, and can, therefore, guarantee that it is absolutely uninritating: R Acidi carbolici med. gr. xii; olei olivæ ℥i.

A free use of this as a lubricant to all instruments before using will, I believe, insure, at all events in combination with the modes of cleaning just described, safety from the occurrence of any contagion by means of instrumental treatment.

—

Lithotrity by a Single Operation.

Dr. HENRY J. BIGELOW, in a recent communication to the *Lancet* (May 17, 1879), says that his method is now no novelty in America, and adds the few following recent examples of his operation which was named litholapaxy.

An operation which I performed January 26th, in the case of a medical gentleman, aged sixty-seven years, lasted fifty minutes, and consisted of two crushings, occupying fifteen minutes; three evacuations of fragments, nine minutes; changes and other delay, twenty-six minutes. Two hundred and sixty grains of phosphatic stone were thus removed. The patient had no trouble from the operation, and on the thirteenth day went home to the country well. There were no fragments left in the bladder.

In another case (February 10th), that of a man aged fifty years, one diameter of the stone measured 1⅜ inches. The operation lasted one hour and twenty-one minutes. The crushings occupied twenty minutes, the evacuation of fragments thirty, while the changes, etc., were recorded at thirty-one minutes. Three hundred and two grains of hard oxalic calculus were crushed and drawn out,—with some delay in the operation, due to fragments lodged behind a high prostate. I was unable to break the stone with Charrière's or rather Collin's instrument. The patient had no unfavourable symptoms, hardly a trace of blood, and no fragments were left.

This case, which involves, so far as I know, the largest hard stone yet evacuated at one sitting, is an example of what can be done by the new process. In evacuating such stones, it need only be said that, the smaller the tube the more minutely must the fragments be broken, and the greater will be the liability to obstruction. Small stones, common in these later days of lithotrity, especially soft ones, are not unfrequently crushed at one sitting, by any lithotrite, without ether, and if reduced to sand, may really need no tube to evacuate them.

The following case is as good a test of the new operation as I could wish. The patient, aged thirty-three, entered the hospital October 31st, about four months and a half ago. His condition was so bad that it was thought unadvisable to attempt any operation, even lithotomy. The urine was ammoniacal and fetid, always containing a large quantity of blood, also pus and mucus to the amount sometimes of nearly one-half by measurement. Micturition was very frequent, occurring at intervals of from ten minutes to half an hour, day and night, during much of this time. The straining was excessive, ineffectual, and productive of great suffering. Three unsuccessful attempts having been made on previous days, a sound was first introduced into the bladder, under ether, November 10th. The next day the temperature rose to 103°, and remained thereabouts till the fourth day, when another complication presented itself. The left knee became suddenly inflamed and swollen. It has remained so ever since. During the next two months the temperature ranged from 100° to 102° daily—afterwards slowly receding though the other symptoms did not abate. I saw the case, for the first time, March 7th. With so diseased and irritable a bladder, it was evident that litholapaxy could be considered only as an experiment. It was a last resort, being perhaps better than lithotomy. Should it succeed, it would testify strongly in favour of the new method ; should it fail, it could hardly be counted against it. On the 9th of March I operated. In the neighbourhood of the triangular ligament an obstruction prevented the passage of sounds larger than a No. 15 French calibre. After snipping the meatus, this obstruction was divulsed by Voillemier's instrument, and it then admitted a full-sized lithotrite, and a straight tube 29 French, for which, later in the operation, 30 was substituted. Two hundred and forty grains of stone were now slowly and carefully removed in sixty-eight minutes. An abundance of flocculent and fibrinous material concealed the fragments when lying in a basin, and testified to the inflammation. At 4 P. M., four hours after the operation, the temperature had fallen from 99° to 96°. In eight hours more, at midnight, it had risen to 103°, with a pulse of 130, where it remained through the day, the tongue being red, smooth, and dry. A general pain in the region of the bladder and urethra required opiates. Yet on the third day the tongue became moist, with a light coat, the temperature had fallen to 99°, and the pulse to 84. This improvement still continues. The patient has had no such comfort for many months. During the first week after the operation, he passed his water six times in twenty-four hours almost without pain, and there has been no tenderness over the bladder. The urine contains very little sediment, and, apart from the knee, which remains as it was, the patient is rapidly convalescing.

My new lithotrite proves to be very efficient, and I am recently indebted to London makers (Weiss and Son) for an instrument that works perfectly. It is of a good size for general use ; a smaller one, if preferred, may be used in special cases. The instrument is non-impacting, and keeps clean in the bladder for an indefinite time. Its rounded tip protects the bladder in a protracted operation, as it also does the prostate during introduction. For the old wheel, which hurts the hand in long crushing, the ball is a welcome substitute. And unless the human hand undergoes some modification of what are now its easiest movements, the system of a *right hand lock*, here first employed, must, as I believe, whatever be the size of the lithotrite, supersede in time any previous method of locking.

———

Prolapsing Internal Hemorrhoids.

Professor GOSSELIN referred in a recent clinical lecture (*Gazette des Hôpitaux*, April 29, 1869) to a case in which internal hemorrhoids only descended during defecation, sometimes with bleeding, were difficult of reduction, and attended by considerable pain. There being no contraction of the sphincter, forced dilatation was not required, and the chief indication consisted in diminishing the size of the hemorrhoids, a practice that is preferable, when practicable, to their removal by operation, which is attended with considerable danger. When they are diminished in size they either return spontaneously, or are easily returned without pain by the patient. In this case the diminution was brought about by parenchymatous cauterizations made with Paquelin's thermo-cautery. No loss of blood took place; the eschars were soon eliminated, cicatrization promptly followed, and the diminished hemorrhoids were returned with very great facility after stool. The patient has had to take some aperients, especially rhubarb; and before leaving the hospital he was cautioned not to remain too long at stool, which most persons with prolapsing hemorrhoids are very apt to do, when the efforts made render the hemorrhoids larger, increase the hemorrhage, and prolong the malady. He was also cautioned to avoid strong alcoholic drinks, which increase the size and produce congestion of the hemorrhoids. Finally, he was told to avoid constipation, keeping the bowels freely opened either by rhubarb or enemata, so as to avoid expulsory efforts, and large masses of feces which produce irritation and maintain the hemorrhoids. In these cases of internal hemorrhoids the surgeon should content himself with obtaining these three results—that they do not descend during progression, that they do not bleed, and that when they descend at stool they are easily reduced.—*Med. Times and Gazette*, May 10, 1879.

Operation for the Radical Cure of Congenital Inguinal Hernia in the Child.

Dr. GEORGE BUCHANAN, Professor of Clinical Surgery in the University of Glasgow, in a short communication on this subject to the *British Medical Journal* (May 17, 1879), says:—

Prof. John Wood's operation for the radical cure of inguinal hernia in the adult is, on the whole, so successful and so free from danger, that I am surprised so few of the many hundreds affected with hernia in every community seek the relief it affords. I presume it is because there must always be some hesitation in accepting the present risk, however small, which accompanies an operation; and a hope that the much greater danger of strangulation may never occur. But in the case of young boys the risk arising from an operation is much less. I think it has been shown that the peritoneal cavity, especially under antiseptic precautions, may be opened with impunity. But even this risk is, in Mr. Wood's plan, not encountered; and it seems to me strange that boys who have a congenital hernia which cannot be kept permanently reduced by any apparatus—a state of matters which every hospital surgeon sees repeatedly—should be allowed to grow up with a deformity which prevents them from being useful and happy members of society, and debars them from a great many employments.

I confess, however, that I have been disappointed with the results of my attempts to cure congenital hernia in children by Mr. Wood's operation with pins used subcutaneously. Either I did not succeed in pushing them through the anatomical structures I intended, which is so easy to do in the adult with the strong curved needle, or I failed to lock them and twist them, as it is necessary to do; but, from whatever cause, in the two cases on which I operated the result was unsatisfactory. The hernia came down as soon as the pins were taken out.

I determined, therefore, to perform an operation consisting of opening the sac and obliterating the canal by the introduction of strong sutures. The steps followed will be best understood by the report of a case which formed the subject of a clinical lecture.

Robert Inglis, aged sixteen months, was the subject of congenital inguinal hernia, which was observed shortly after his birth. It was small when first noticed, but soon increased in size; and it had grown with his growth. It was on January 9, 1879, about the size of a turkey's egg, and distended the left side of the scrotum. It could be reduced with ease; but it as easily slipped down, and no apparatus or bandage could retain it in its place. Trusses had been tried at various times; but no sooner did the child move than the hernia came down. On returning it into the abdomen, the finger was readily pushed through the inguinal opening; but even then, unless pushed far up, the bowel slipped down alongside of it.

Before performing any operation, I accustomed the little patient to the pressure of a bandage. I returned the bowel, and applied a large thick pad, which was bandaged very firmly with a figure-of-eight bandage round the groin. This retained the hernia in its place for some hours; but the movements of the child and repeated fits of crying brought it down usually within twenty-four hours.

On January 25, 1879, I performed a radical operation as follows. The patient having been put under the influence of chloroform, the rupture was returned and kept up by the finger of an assistant. A longitudinal incision was made along the whole length of the sac, from opposite the internal ring to the bottom of the scrotum. This divided all the textures down to the peritoneal sac, which, as usual, had been thickened by the presence and movements of the hernia. With the handle of the knife and a few touches of its point, I separated the sac from its superficial structures, leaving the posterior part lying over the cord, which was seen behind. I now divided the sac into two halves by a transverse cut, except at the back, where it was adhering to the cord. One half was folded down over the testicle, so as to form a sort of *tunica vaginalis*. The upper half was rolled into a sort of ball or plug, which I pushed into the internal abdominal ring and had it kept there by the assistant. I now approximated the walls of the inguinal canal much in the same way as in the wire-operation for the radical cure of hernia in the adult. The superficial structures having been previously pushed aside and slightly dissected from off the abdominal aponeurosis, the relations of the rings and the canal could be felt and in great part seen. I took a strong nævus-needle and pushed it through the external pillar of the canal at a spot opposite the internal ring; then, guiding it with the point of my left forefinger lying in the internal ring, I made it lift up the lower border of the internal oblique muscle, and emerge through the internal pillar of the external aponeurosis about half an inch above its lower edge. A strong waxed silk thread was now passed through the hole at the point of the needle, which was then withdrawn, pulling the thread with it. The thread was then tightly tied, including the structures through which the needle had been passed, and so fixing into the internal ring the rolled-up bit of the sac, care being taken that the external raw surface of the sac should be turned outwards toward the integument which was to cover it. A little below the first stitch, a second was introduced in the same direction, care being taken to avoid the structures of the cord, which lay at the bottom of the wound. The edges of the external ring were now drawn together tightly above the cord by a strong silver wire; this was made to take a very strong hold, by passing the needle first through the external pillar, across the ring, and through the internal pillar. In making the internal puncture, I passed the point of the needle so far towards the linea alba as to make it pierce from below the tendon of insertion of the rectus muscle, so as to give a firm hold. When the wire was drawn through with the needle, it was clamped, so as to squeeze together the boundaries of the external ring; and it was retained in that position by a little rod of silver with a hole at its point, through which the two ends of the wire were passed; and, having been drawn tight, they were fixed by a turn round the rod. The silk threads were clipped short; and the wires, with the little clamping rod to which they were fixed, were allowed to hang out at the bottom of the wound. The edges of the incision were now united with thin silver-wire sutures, and the wound dressed with antiseptic precautions. The child was placed on a St. Andrew's cross, the upper arms of which were joined by a sheet of calico on which the body rested; the legs being securely bandaged with strips of adhesive plaster to the lower limbs of the cross. The pelvis and chest were also securely fixed to the apparatus. In this way, the movements of the child were effectually controlled.

Two days after the operation, the scrotum was swollen, as if a portion of hernia had escaped from beneath the bandages; but this proved to be only a soft fluctuant swelling, probably an effusion of serum into the artificial tunica vaginalis, which had been formed by the folding down over the testicle of the lower half of the hernial sac, as described in the operation. In two days, this swelling had disappeared, and the scrotum was in its natural state. On the fourth day after the operation, the wound was dressed. It was found almost united, except in the place where the wires were left hanging out. On the tenth day, the little clamp and wire were removed, and the parts were found quite matted together.

It is unnecessary to detail the further progress. The dressings were changed every two days, and at the end of four weeks cicatrization was practically complete. The child was then freed from restraint; but, for precaution, a bandage was still applied round the groin.

May 1st. At this date, the radical cure of the hernia is perfect. No amount of exertion either of the limbs or on crying has the slightest effect on the inguinal region of the abdominal walls.

The result has exceeded my expectations, and I shall not hesitate to practise the operation in all similar cases, and even to adopt it as a means of accomplishing a radical cure in cases of strangulated hernia in which an operation for the relief of strangulation has become necessary.

—

Spondylitis Deformans.

Dr. ALLEN STURGE, at a recent meeting of the Clinical Society of London (*Lancet*, May 24, 1879). read the notes of a case of spondylitis deformans. The patient, a man aged twenty-six, was an artificial flower maker, who had been under his care at the Royal Free Hospital. The mother suffered very much from rheumatism. One brother had severe chronic rheumatism, and another was said to be subject to gout. The patient's health had been good before the present illness; there was no distinct history of syphilis. Prior to his illness he had been a strong, upright man, and a rapid runner. The present condition began eight years ago, with pain in the back, which had never since quite left him. Gradually the back became stiff, both in the cervical and dorsal regions. When he came under care the spinal column was remarkably fixed throughout. The lumbar and dorsal regions together formed a curve of large radius, with the convexity backwards (spinal lordosis); and the spine, as a whole, was on a plane posterior to that of the sacrum. producing a projection forwards of the abdomen, the legs being carried back in a corresponding degree to catch the centre of gravity of the body. There was no special tenderness of the spine at any part. In bending forwards, the spine, as a whole, remained quite stiff, and flexion appeared to be almost entirely confined to the lower two or three lumbar vertebræ. The cervical part of the spinal column was very stiff. Power of flexion of the head forwards and backwards was very limited, and lateral movement of the head was almost abolished. Power of rotation, though imperfect, was less impaired than the other movements. The thorax was very rigid; breathing was almost wholly abdominal. On drawing a deep breath there was a slight movement of expansion, but scarcely any of elevation. Dr. Sturge remarked that this condition was one of very rare occurrence, and would appear to be rheumatoid in its nature. The post-mortem changes were described a good many years ago by Professor R. W. Smith, of Dublin, and more recently by Dr. von Studen, of Altona. They were like those met with in rheumatoid arthritis of other parts of the body— viz., absorption of the articular cartilages, nodular growths on the articular surfaces of the bones and anchylosis of the adjacent vertebræ, to which must be added absorption of the intervertebral cartilage. It might coincide with rheumatoid affections elsewhere, but in many cases it was confined to the spine or to the spine and costo-sternal articulations. Todd had seen a case in a man aged twenty-five, and Eulenberg had met with it in a girl twelve years old. As a rule, however, bony anchylosis of the vertebræ occurred in old people; but it was doubtful whether the disease in young persons could be looked upon as identical with that which occurred in old people.

Mr. BRYANT referred to a case recorded by Dr. Fagge in the Pathological Transactions (vol. xxviii. p. 201), where there was a general anchylosis of the vertebræ and of the costo-vertebral articulations. The patient died from fracture of the ribs. He had been subject to rheumatism. In reply to the President, he said that in that case there was only slight deformity. To Mr. Barker, he said there was actual synostosis.

Mr. HEATH said that fusion between some of the vertebræ was not so rare. Some anchylosed spines were found in the burying-ground which was excavated during the rebuilding of King's College Hospital; but such instances would hardly have led to the amount of deformity present in Dr. Sturge's case, where the curvature seemed to resemble that of angular curvature.

—

Excision of Papilloma of the Bladder.

At a recent meeting of the Clinical Society of London (*Lancet*, May 24, 1879), Mr. A. T. NORTON read the notes of a case of papilloma of the bladder, excision, death. A female, 34 years of age, was admitted into St. Mary's Hospital, suffering from the effects of long-continued hemorrhage from the bladder. The urine contained also much mucus and phosphates, small portions of phosphates being frequently passed. There was great pain after micturition, and constant desire to pass water. No calculus could be found, but the bladder was thick in the region of the trigone; and a digital examination per urethram under chloroform confirmed the diagnosis of a tumour of the bladder. The growth was one inch square, slightly raised, and coated with phosphatic deposit. Its removal was decided upon, the alternative to the patient lying between the risk of a severe operation and the continued pain, possible early fatal hemorrhage, or blood-poisoning. It was impossible to remove the growth through the urethra, and it was decided to cut away the mass by opening the vagina. It was considered that the growth could not be removed without cutting through the urethra. The spring scissors were inserted, one blade into the bladder nearly up to the tumour, and the other into the vagina, and closed; the front wall of the vagina was then incised centrally to within half an inch of the uterus, and the vaginal wall was dissected from the bladder; the growth was then seized with the vulsellum forceps and drawn forwards, and was then excised by the scissors and removed. Bleeding was arrested by actual cautery, and the lateral flaps of the vagina approximated by sutures. To prevent further hemorrhage, a catheter was inserted, and the bladder compressed by plugging the vagina. No bleeding of importance took place. The temperature remained below normal, and the pulse rose to 120.

Severe vomiting was persistent until the tenth day after the operation, notwith-standing subcutaneous injection of morphia and five-grain doses of quinine adminis-tered frequently by the stomach. After the tenth day she was considered out of danger, was making good progress, took food well, and was cheerful; but two days later, after vomiting, she fell asleep, and died in sleep from syncope. On post-mortem examination the heart was found to be healthy, its left side empty. The blood was mostly fluid. The wound was sloughing on the surface, some phosphatic deposit around it and the orifices of the ureters. Vesical mucous membrane congested, but of normal consistence. No peritonitis, and no throm-bosis. Examination showed that so far as the peritoneum was concerned a tu-mour nearly twice the length and breadth could have been removed through the wound, but the ureters would be included in such an operation. Whether or not such inclusion of the ureters would add to the severity of the operation cannot be proved, but it is probable that the urine would escape without injury to the parts around. A microscopical examination showed the tumour to be a papilloma. Since writing the above case Mr. Norton said that he had operated upon a second case of tumour of the bladder, now in the hospital. This case had completely recovered from the effects of the operation.

Mr. HEATH asked if the growth extended beneath the mucous membrane; for if confined to the surface it might have been removed by scraping.

Mr. KNOWSLEY THORNTON had lately met with a similar case in which he advised operation, but the patient objected. She was an old lady, and had some symptoms of stone. Some large nucleated cells being found in the urine, he dilated the urethra, and found a soft mass projecting into the bladder above the left ureter. It was of the size of a half walnut, and examination of a small shred showed it to be a round-celled sarcoma. At the time he had thought of three methods of removal, viz., through the vagina, as Mr. Norton had done; or by a suprapubic operation; or by opening the bladder through the peritoneum. There would be no great risk in the third of these alternatives, provided the urine were not putrid.

Mr. MORRIS asked whether Mr. Norton had operated on account of the pro-fuse bleeding or on account of the pain endured by the patient; and also whether, in the operation, he had removed the whole thickness of the wall of the bladder? A few years ago he had under his care, at the Middlesex Hospital (the case is recorded in the *Med.-Chir. Transactions*), a woman, 46 years old, who had suffered from vesical hemorrhage for eight or nine years, and for a few years from pain. A small papillary growth was found, and at first strong caustics were applied with temporary relief. Then he removed a large portion of the growth by the écraseur. Although the symptoms were relieved at the time, the patient died ultimately from hydronephrosis, set up by occlusion of the ureters by the growth.

Mr. HULKE asked why the urethra was slit up. He could quite understand that it might be necessary to open the bladder, but he did not see why it was needful to slit up the urethra. Then it appeared that the anterior wall of the bladder and of the vagina were divided, and that much and continuous vomiting followed these severe measures. It was true that after death the orifices of the ureters were found to be free, but then caustic was applied after the removal of the tumour, and the stitches in the wound would drag on the ureters, so that it was quite possible that they were for a time occluded.

Dr. GLOVER asked if any other organ was involved. He mentioned a case of vesical hemorrhage, due to a growth in the bladder, which ended fatally very rapidly, and he urged that, before operating, the constitutional condition of the patient should be considered. None of the neighbouring organs were affected.

Mr. BRYANT asked Mr. Norton why, after having confidence in dilatation of the urethra for the examination of the case, he had not the same confidence in it for operation. For localized growths could well be attacked through the dilated urethra. He had thus removed a sessile growth from the bladder by forceps and écraseur, and in two other cases he had found no difficulty. But he would hesitate long before proposing the severe measures described by Mr. Norton. He was not, however, prepared to say that in Mr. Norton's case the operation was not a justifiable one.

Mr. MARSH agreed with Mr. Bryant up to a certain point. What was the extent to which the urethra could be dilated without leading to incontinence of urine? Mr. Lane recommended that nothing larger than an acorn should be forced through the urethra. The operation of division of the vesico-vaginal septum was rather dangerous and formidable; but Mr. Marsh had seen it done, and had done it himself, for the removal of calculi. He agreed with Mr. Hulke as to the serious character of an operation in which the urethra was laid open in its whole length.

Mr. BRYANT added that by rapid dilatation almost anything might be done. Slow dilatation nearly always led to incontinence.

Mr. NORTON, in reply, said that the growth did not extend beneath the muscular coat. In operating he cut down into the vagina, peeled the vagina from the bladder, seized the bladder, and, dragging it forwards, removed the growth by spring scissors. The danger of hemorrhage, possibly leading to early death, determined him to perform the operation. He did not think that splitting the urethra added much to its gravity. The vomiting he attributed to the operation. Urine flowed freely. No other organs were examined after death. He did not think that the constitutional condition of the patient should be considered when she was dying from the disease; nor did he think he would have succeeded in removing the growth had he attacked it through the urethra.

Midwifery and Gynæcology.

Use of Creasoted Glycerine in Ulcerations of the Neck of the Womb.

MENDESSOHN says (Revue de Thérap. Méd. Chir., Feb. 15, 1879) that he has derived much benefit from painting the ulcerated portions of the neck of the womb with the following solution: ℞, pure creasote 2 grammes; glycerine, 50 grammes; alcohol, 25 grammes. This was applied either every day or every other day, for a length of time varying from twelve to forty days.

Thirty-seven patients in all were treated; twenty-eight were suffering from simple ulcerations or erosions; twenty-six of these recovered, and two improved much in health. Of seven cases of granular and fungoid ulcerations, six recovered and one improved. The mean number of days they were under this treatment was seventeen; only one patient remained under it for forty-four days, as in her case there was a complication arising from a metritis with considerable leucorrhœa.

Two cases of chancrous ulcerations were treated with creasoted glycerine for thirty to forty days, without success, so that the author was obliged to recur to iodoform, which induced speedy recovery.—London Med. Record, May 15, 1879

Statistics of Uterine Fibroid Tumour.

Dr. ÖRUM, in Howitz's *Gynäkol Meddlelelser*, says that fibromata of the uterus have been found in 53 out of 1002 bodies of females examined *post-mortem* in the Communal Hospital of Copenhagen. The state of the uterus was noted in all the cases. No fibromata were found before the tenth year; in women above 20 years of age, they were found 7.75 per cent.; in women above 40, in 9.5 per cent. The tumours were in 28 cases single, in 9 double, and in 16 cases there were several in the same individual. In more than half the cases (28) they were small—as large as a nut. In 19 cases they were interstitial, in 13 subserous, in 5 submucous, and in 8 various forms were found. Fibrocystic degeneration was present in one case. In one case the fibroma gave rise to fatal peritonitis.— *British Med. Journal*, May 31, 1879.

Tubercle of the Cervix Uteri.

M. CORNIL has presented to the Paris Hospital Society two very interesting and rare cases of tubercle of the vagina and uterine cervix. One case occurred to himself, and the other to M. Rigol. His own case was that of a phthisical patient, who presented a localized tumour in the deep part of the pelvic peritoneum, with uterine pains and leucorrhœa. With the speculum, he ascertained a superficial erosion of the cervix uteri at the level of the meatus. This ulceration was about half a *centimètre* in diameter, with sharply cut borders and yellow surface. On one of the borders were three small yellow granules slightly projecting. The ulceration was touched with a brush moistened with tincture of iodine diluted with hot water. Cicatrization was rapid; and three weeks afterwards the patient left the hospital almost completely cured. At the same time, a slight ulceration was noted on the frænum of the tongue; this had also arisen by yellow tuberculous granulations, and rapidly cicatrized. M. Cornil especially drew attention to the rarity of tuberculosis of the uterine cervix and of the vagina. In the necropsy of M. Rigol's patient, general miliary tuberculosis was found. There was a crop of whitish granulations on the cervix uteri and in the wall of the vagina; nothing in the cavity of the cervix. In these two cases, the lesions were clearly marked. M. Cornil gave an account of the microscopic examination of the granulations. M. Fournier, while recognizing the rarity of tubercles of the cervix, had, nevertheless, in eight or ten cases observed on the cervix ulcerations which were certainly not chancres. But these women were tuberculous; and he had asked himself if he ought not to put these ulcerations to the account of the tuberculosis; but he had never yet seen the initial tubercle. The history of tuberculosis of the cervix was still to be studied. Finally, M. Fournier admitted that in scrofulous and phthisical persons ulcerations are found, and that these ulcerations may be regarded as tuberculous. M. Cornil agreed with M. Fournier. He was, however, of opinion that not all the ulcerations of tuberculous persons were tuberculous, and that this was a question deserving of study.—*British Med. Journal*, May 17, 1879.

The Jaundice of New-born Children, and the Proper Time for Tying the Funis.

In an article on the Pathology of the Jaundice of New-born Children, Dr. PORAK (*Annales de Gynécologie*, Sept. and Oct. 1878) supports the view that this disorder, in the great majority of cases, is of hæmic origin, and not dependant on any hepatic obstruction, or any peculiar condition of the hepatic circulation. Under the definition of jaundice, the author includes all those cases in which a yellow coloration of the skin arises spontaneously, and does not limit himself, as some authors have done, in the consideration of the jaundice of the new-born to those cases in which there is a yellow tinge of the conjunctivæ. When the surface of the body is much reddened, and a slightly jaundiced tint of skin is thus rendered difficult to recognize, he finds that the best means of diagnosis is to expel the blood for a moment by firm pressure with the finger upon a limited surface.

In his observations of a large number of children, the author divides cases of jaundice into three degrees. He finds that the affection of the conjunctivæ by itself fails to form a satisfactory distinction, for although their coloration generally coincides with intensity of the general yellow tint of the body, it is quite independent of its extent. The *first degree* of jaundice he calls that in which the chest, the back, and the face are alone affected. The tinge generally commences in the face, but sometimes upon the chest, where it is generally deeper than elsewhere. The conjunctivæ always remain unaffected, and the yellow tinge is always very slight. It generally commences towards the end of the first day, and has completely disappeared by the third or fourth day.

In the *second degree* the jaundice is more extended; the abdomen, and sometimes the upper segment of the limbs are yellow. The hands and feet, and generally the legs and forearms, remain free. The conjunctivæ are generally yellow, but the author has observed several cases of very extensive jaundice in which they remained white. Jaundice of the second degree generally lasts from three to six days, and has completely disappeared by the sixth or seventh day. In the *third degree* the jaundice is general, and the author distinguishes it from the second degree by the coloration of the hands and feet. The author has never found the urine to contain pigment except in a few instances in which the tinge of the skin was not only much deeper than usual, but acquired a greenish tint. In these the jaundice was of much greater duration, and commencing towards the end of the first day, had often not disappeared by the ninth or tenth day. The author considers them to have a different pathology, and to depend on hepatic obstruction, not, like the authors, on a hæmic cause.

Out of 245 children, the author found only 50, or 20.16 per cent., who had no jaundice; 34, or 13.71 per cent., had jaundice of the first degree; 91, or 36.69 per cent., had the second degree; and 73, or 29.50 per cent., had the third degree. No special digestive trouble was found to be associated with the jaundice, and absence of bile in the feces was *never* observed. As to the condition of the urine, the author finds, that while the fœtal urine is pale and clear, that passed for the first few days after birth is rather deeply coloured, and often deposits a sediment. After the third day, the urine generally becomes clear and more abundant. In the case of jaundice, the author did not observe any deviation from these changes, except in the three instances only out of 248. In these it contained bile-pigments, and he regards them as having a different pathology. The author accepts the distinction made by M. Gubler as to the condition of the urine in obstructive jaundice, and that due to a changed blood-pigment, which he calls hæmaphéin—namely, that in the former case the urine is greenish-yellow, stains linen, and gives a play of colours (green, blue, violet, red) with nitric acid, while in the latter case it is pale yellow with a brownish tinge, and with nitric acid gives only a brownish-red tint. In most cases of jaundice of new-born children, even of the third degree, he finds that the careful addition of nitric acid in a test-tube brings out only an extremely thin reddish diaphragm, but in a few instances a much broader dark band was produced above this, showing some pigment not usually present in the urine, which he thinks may be hæmaphéin. Of the three jaundiced children whose urine contained bile-pigment, one died in the hospital, and the other two were lost sight of when they appeared to be in a hopeless state. In all three of these cases the motions were strongly tinged with green, showing that there was no obliteration of the biliary ducts.

As to the pathogeny of the disorder, the author first discusses the theory that it depends upon local or general cutaneous congestion, escape of blood from the vessels, and changes in its colour like those which occur in an ecchymosis. One or other form of this doctrine has been accepted by Breschet, Billard, Valleix, Andral, Weber, West, Zeissl, and others. To this the author objects that, if it were true, the changes of tint ought to be observed which occur in an ecchymosis, but are absent in the jaundice of the new-born ; and further, that it fails to explain the cases in which the conjunctivæ are affected, and those in which the jaundice is limited to the trunk and face. Against the view that the jaundice is obstructive, due to retention of meconium or catarrh of biliary ducts, according to the latter opinion of Virchow, he contends that the character of the urine, so rarely containing any bile-pigment, shows that obstructive jaundice is exceptional in the new-born. Against the view of Frerichs that the cause is a relative excess of pressure in the bile-ducts, due to sudden diminution of pressure in the portal vein, and consequent reabsorption of bile, he argues that numerous cases of pathological obliteration of the portal vein have occurred, and that jaundice has not been the consequence, while the same argument from the state of the urine applies to this as to the last theory.

In favour of the view that the jaundice is of hæmic origin, the author cites the anatomical evidence of Virchow (who at first maintained the hæmic theory, though he has since abandoned it), with reference to the urinary infarctus of new-born children. That author found these small masses in the kidneys to contain a dark pigment, which gave with nitric acid a reaction different from that of bile-pigment, while the same pigment frequently infiltrated the epithelial cells of the kidneys, and their nuclei. Neumann also, in seven cases of jaundiced children who died within the first week, found similar infarctus in the kidney, and also found in various organs both within and without the vessels, small acicular dark-red crystals (hæmatoidin or bilifulvin). In children not jaundiced, who died within the same period, these crystals were not found. Krebs and Orth have also found similar crystals in cases of jaundice of new-born children. Similar crystals are found in macerated fœtuses, whose blood has undergone cadaveric change, and stained their tissues, forming the fœtus sanguinolentus of the Germans. The chemical distinction between hæmatoidin and bilifulvin being still undetermined, the author considers that these crystals must be ascribed to blood-pigment. From observations by Lépine and Hayem, he infers that great changes take place in the first few days of life both in the number and size of blood corpuscles, from which must be inferred a rapid evolution and coincident destruction of them, the pigment resulting from the latter of which processes has to be partly excreted by the kidneys. To anomalies in this process, probably due in part to a deficiency of hepatic activity, the author attributes the production of the hypothetic hæmaphéin, a derivative of the imperfect elaboration of hæmoglobin, and the presence of this in the liquor sanguinis he considers to be the cause of the hæmic form of jaundice in new-born children. With this view agrees the fact that children are more liable to jaundice who are enfeebled, or whose nutrition is deficient, as children in foundling hospitals, twins, or those born prematurely.

The author has also made a number of observations on the progress in weight in infants, to determine the advantage or otherwise of adopting the plan proposed by Budin of not tying the funis until some minutes after birth, when it has ceased to pulsate, in order that the infant may have the benefit of the additional amount of blood which, by this means, is withdrawn from the placenta (see

Obstetiical Jouinal, vol. iv. p. 194). He finds that when the funis has been tied late, the childien do not appeai to thiive bettei than when the old plan has been followed, and that in the foimei case theie is a gieatei loss of weight duiing the fiist day or two. He fuithei finds that when the funis has been tied late, the childien are notably moie subject to jaundice, and he consideis that this effect of an additional quantity of blood in the ciiculation is a fuithei evidence in favoui of the hæmic oiigin of the disoidei.—*Obstetrical Jouinal of Great Biitain,* May, 1879.

Hygiene.

Eiysipelas Caused by Sewei Gas.

Yeais ago, the idea that facial eiysipelas, or indeed that any vaiiety of this diie disease, could be oiiginated by the entiance of sewei-gas into houses, hospitals, or institutions, would have been condemned as too absuid for ciedence. Bittei expeiience, extending ovei a numbei of years, backed by the ieseaiches of Mr. Pridgin Teale and otheis, has, howevei, finally settled the question in dispute. Theie is now no moie doubt that eiysipelas is oiiginated by sewei-gas than that typhoid fevei is due moie often than not to impuie watei. For instance, at the Old Infiimaiy, Lincoln, which was situated on a hill above the city, eiysipelas and sewei-gas weie constantly piesent in the waids. We iemembei seeing twelve or fifteen cases theie some twelve years ago. At that time the hospital diains communicated with the town seweis; and as neithei weie ventilated oi disconnected, the hospital had the benefit of the full piessuie of the sewei-gas of Lincoln, because the hospital lavatoiies and closets occupied the highest points to which any of the sewei connections extended. At Manchestei, as we showed some months ago, sewei-gas had demoialized the health of the staff, and had so incieased the amount of eiysipelas and pyæmia that the suigeons weie afiaid to peifoim even the smallest opeiation. Recently the authorities of a laige London hospital pioceeded to ventilate the whole of the diains and seweis in connection with theii institution. Up to the time these alteiations weie made, pyæmia and eiysipelas had almost diiven the medical staff to despaii. When the whole of the ventilation was completed, and so soon as the piessuie was iemoved fiom the tiaps of the closets and lavatoiies, no fiesh cases weie found to occui. For months the hospital waids weie fiee fiom eiysipelas and pyæmia. Suddenly, howevei, theie was a fiesh outbieak of these diseases, but it was noticed that the epidemic was confined to one of the suigical waids, built apait fiom the main building on the pavilion plan, and having only one stoiy. Close investigation pioved that the ventilation pipe in this wing had been stopped up by a caieless woikman. When this was iemedied, all tiace of the epidemic disappeaied, and for foui yeais this hospital has been almost fiee fiom these diseases. Space will not allow us to quote fuithei evidence on this occasion, but any one who is inteiested in the subject will obtain much useful infoimation fiom Mr. T. P. Teale, of Leeds, who has made this subject almost a special study. We have been led to make the above iemaiks because, duiing the past week, an investigation of gieat inteiest has been conducted by the Someisetshiie Coionei into the causes of a fatal outbieak of eiysipelas at the County Lunatic Asylum. It appeais that fiom Decembei, 1878, to May, 1879, 23 cases of eiysipelas occuried in the female infirmary waid, of which 2 weie fatal. Bad smells had been constantly piesent in this waid, and in othei paits of the building, for many months past. Seveial of the inmates had suffeied fiom seveie diarrhœa, of which one died; soie-thioat, loss of appetite, headache, and nausea attacked most of the patients. On the male side 9 cases of eiysipelas occuiied, 2 of which weie fatal. Heie, then, we find 32 cases of eiysipelas occuiiing in a lunatic asylum in five months, of which 4 pioved fatal. When we iemembei the nausea, headache, soie-thioat, and geneial malaise expeiienced by othei inmates, coupled with the epidemic of diaiihœa and bad smells, it is not difficult to divine that sewei-gas was almost eveiywheie piesent thioughout the institution. This was suspected by the supeiintendent, Dr. Medlicott, and so with the aid of the assist-ant medical officeis, Messis. J. F. Wood and T. S. Sheldon, a seaiching investi-gation was made into the diainage aiiangements. It was then discoveied that none of the soil-pipes weie ventilated; most of them weie of lead, and seveial weie rat-eaten and iiddled with holes. On taking out the pan and siphon of the infirmary closet a veiy bad smell was piesent, which was found to be caused by a hole in the soil-pipe, 3 by $1\frac{1}{2}$ inches. This paiticulai soil-pipe had a diiect com-munication with the main sewei. The main diain outside the infirmary waid—wheie most of the eiysipelas cases occuiied—had been choked moie than once duiing the yeai, and on one occasion it was blocked entiiely to the extent of thiee or foui yaids. In othei paits of the building the fall was insufficient, and in consequence the main diain had been stopped seveial times.

In biief, almost eveiy sanitaiy evil was found to be piesent in this ill-fated institution; feimenting sewage was a constant factoi, and sewei-gas, conveyed fiom the seweis to the waids by the rat-eaten soil-pipes, had committed its fatal iaivages unchecked and unsuspected for at any iate months, and we suspect even for yeais.

The moial is plain to iead, but difficult to get people to iealize. Modein buildings, whethei laige or small, especially wheie they are situated in oi neai towns, must poui theii sewage into the main seweis. As a consequence diain-pipes must, to a gieatei oi less extent, pass inside the houses, and so a iisk oi sewei-gas is incuiied. What is the iemedy? Simply to put an open manhole, with pipe-diains passing thiough it between the sewei and the house, to put a siphon with ventilatoi between the manhole and the sewei, and in eveiy case to caiiy the soil-pipe above the top of the buildings, and to leave it peifectly open at the top. In this way sewei-gas is effectually excluded fiom houses, a constant diaft of fiesh air passes down the open manhole, and thiough eveiy inch of the household diains, and defective tiaps and rat-eaten soil-pipes may piactically be defied. Unless the connection with the sewei is cut outside an inhabited build-ing, and unless eveiy inch of soil-pipe is thoioughly ventilated in the simple way we have desciibed, dangei of blood-poisoning exists. With these piecautions, simple and compaiatively inexpensive as they are, even the oldest buildings may be made not only sweet but peifectly healthy.—*Sanitary Recoid*, June 6, 1879.

CONTENTS. .

Published Monthly, price $2.50 per annum, free of postage.
Also, furnished together with the AMERICAN JOURNAL OF THE MEDICAL
SCIENCES *and the* MEDICAL NEWS AND LIBRARY *for* SIX DOLLARS *per
annum in advance, the whole free of postage.*

HENRY C. LEA, Philadelphia.

THE MONTHLY ABSTRACT

OF

MEDICAL SCIENCE.

VOL. VI. No. 8. **For List of Contents see last page.** AUGUST, 1879.

Anatomy and Physiology.

Physiology of the Secretion of Sweat.

That the secretion of sweat is under the control of the nervous system has been recognized for some years past, LUCHSINGER and others having demonstrated that a copious discharge of this secretion can be induced in the feet of the cat and dog by stimulation of the sciatic and brachial nerves. That it is essentially independent of any changes in the circulatory system is shown by the fact that it can be made to occur in an amputated member, and in limbs the temperature of which is below the normal. The secretion is thus shown not to be a mere transudation, but the result of the activity of special glandular cells, called forth, as in the case of the salivary glands, by the stimulation of certain nerves. The sudoriparous nerves, running in the sciatic nerve, are derived from the abdominal cord of the sympathetic; for if this be divided, and the lower extremity be stimulated, perspiration breaks out on the hind foot, though if the sciatic be first divided, no such secretion is observed. After division of the sympathetic in the abdomen on one side, the animal no longer sweats on that side when exposed to heat. But the fibres do not arise in the great sympathetic; they appear to emerge from the spinal cord by the rami communicantes of the first four lumbar roots, and the last two or three dorsal. Sweating can be induced by reflex action, and also in a very marked and singular manner by jaborandi, and by the active principle of that drug—pilocarpin. In from three to five minutes after the subcutaneous injection of a solution of hydrochlorate of pilicarpin, in man, the flow of saliva increases, perspiration appears, first on the head, and then gradually over the whole body, and lasts about an hour, or, if the patient be in bed, for two or even three hours. This effect Luchsinger considers to be due to the pilocarpin acting as a direct stimulant to the nerve-centres. He tied the abdominal aorta in a cat, and then injected pilocarpin into a vein. Under these conditions the pilocarpin was unable to reach the glands in the posterior extremities; and thus to act as a direct stimulant; nevertheless the feet were soon bathed in sweat. Atropin inhibits the secretion of sweat, for if, after the injection of one one-hundredth of a gramme of pilocarpin, three one-thousandths of a gramme of atropin be injected, the commencing perspiration is arrested in about ten minutes. If now a hundredth of a grain of pilocarpin be injected into one of the feet, beads of sweat burst forth on this foot; but the rest of the body, being still under the influence of atropin, remains dry. The experiments of Luchsinger have been repeated and confirmed by Nawrocki, who satisfied himself that there is a common centre in the medulla for the secretion of sweat in both fore and hind feet. He followed the course of the fibres innervating the glands of the fore limb, and ascertained by means of sections at different points that they leave the spinal cord between the third and fifth cervical vertebræ. These fibres enter the brachial plexus with the thoracic portion of the sympathetic, and are occasionally confined within the sheath of the median nerve, though more frequently they are distributed between the median and ulnar nerves, the median having the larger share. Adamkiewicz, in a more recent publication, finds, like his predecessors, that the secretion of sweat is independent of the circulation, and that it may be induced by artificial or voluntary stimulation of the muscles, or of their nerves, by mental stimuli, as by the imagination; and, lastly, as a reflex act by stimuli applied to the skin. In man the secretion is always bilateral and symmetrical, and is not necessarily eliminated in the immediate vicinity of the point stimulated. Heat excites it, and, indeed, the activity of the secretion seems to stand in direct relation with the temperature of the several parts of the body. His views differ from those of Luchsinger in regard to the nervous apparatus, for he believes that the motor centre of the secretion is situated on the surface of the brain. The nerves pass through the medulla to the spinal cord, and unite at the secretory centres, which are probably placed in the anterior horns of the gray matter. From these horns secretory fibres emanate and leave the cord in connection with motor nerves, whilst others enter the sympathetic at higher points of the cord. Vulpian, in following out these experiments, found that although some of the excito-sudoral fibres may, in the cat, pass from the sympathetic to the sciatic nerve, yet that there are others in considerable number which pass directly from the spinal cord by the seventh lumbar and first sacral—that is to say, by the roots of the sciatic itself. Vulpian points out that an interesting parallel may thus be drawn between the nervous mechanism of the sweat-glands and that of the salivary glands; for it is known that the submaxillary glands receive excito-salivary fibres from the chorda tympani, and other fibres from the cervical portion of the great sympathetic. He is, however, unable to coincide in the view that the filaments for the sweat-glands in the foot and forelimb of the cat pass out from the cord *entirely* with the spinal roots of the superior thoracic ganglion. A large part no doubt do so, but others accompany the roots of the spinal nerves entering into the formation of the brachial plexus. Luchsinger and Truempy have quite recently investigated the chemical properties of sweat. An acid reaction is generally attributed to this secretion, but these observers have ascertained that in man as well as in the cat the reaction is really alkaline, and that the acidity which has been observed is due to the fact that the secretion of the sebaceous glands is ordinarily acid, or rather becomes so in the act of decomposition, to which it is prone. The whole subject has been well analyzed and treated by M. Blanchard in the *Progrès Médicale.—Lancet*, June 14, 1879.

The Movements of the Eyelids.

At a late meeting of the Royal Medical and Chirurgical Society (*Lancet*, June 14, 1879) a paper was read on "The Movements of the Eyelids," by W. R. GOWERS, M.D., of which the following is an abstract:—Under normal conditions the lids leave the cornea approximately uncovered in all positions of the eyeball, moving with it. For these movements and for the voluntary closure and opening of the lids, there are only two muscles, the orbicularis and the levator. These will not explain all movements, and it is probable that the eyeball itself moves the lids, not by the conjunctival connection, but by the pressure of the convexity of the sclerotic, and to a less extent of the cornea, the edges of the lids lying in or near the sclero-corneal sulcus. This effect is greatest on the upper lid, partly because the tarsal cartilages are attached at their extremities below the transverse axis of the eyeball. The eyelids are moulded on the globes, the shape of the palpebral fissure depending on the position of the eyeball, and being curiously altered in some abnormal lateral positions. In closing the eyelids gently the lower lid is raised by the palpebral orbicularis; in rotation up of the globe the lower lid is raised, not by the orbicularis, but by the pressure of the globe, and the movement is slight if the globe is very prominent. Depression of the lower lid in looking down is by pressure of the cornea. The upper lid is maintained in position by the balance of tone between the levator and the orbicularis. If the latter is paralyzed, the lid is a little higher than normal. The descent of the upper lid, in looking down, is not by contraction of the orbicularis (for it is unaffected in facial palsy), but is by the pressure of the sclerotic against the tarsal cartilage. The lid is raised on upward rotation of the globe by the levator, the contraction of which, if sudden, is excessive. With this is associated a synergic action of the frontalis; the latter is sometimes habitual, and then is relaxed with the levator on looking down. The action of the levator associated with that of the superior rectus is beyond voluntary control, and, in the simulated ptosis of hysteria, necessitates a strong contraction of the orbicularis to keep the lid down, if the patient is made to look up. The associated relaxation on looking down prevents almost all voluntary contraction of the levator in that position. Gentle closure of the lids, as in sleep, is by the palpebral orbicularis; the levator being relaxed, the recti passive. Forcible closure is by the whole orbicularis, the levator being released and dissociated from the superior rectus, which contracts, rolling the globe up. Hence, probably, the centre for strong closure of the eyelids is physiologically distinct from that for their gentle closure. If the orbicularis is paralyzed the associated inhibition of the levator still occurs on an attempt to close the lids. But, if the inferior rectus is paralyzed, a fruitless attempt to rotate the eyeball down is not attended with inhibition of the levator. This phenomenon (of which photographs were shown) is difficult to explain. Possibly, this relaxation of the levator is not the result of a central mechanism, but is reflex from the commencing tension on the fibres, and so does not occur if the globe does not move. If so, the fact is of much interest in relation to the mechanism of other movements in the body. Lastly, it is pointed out that the eyelids commonly participate in the movements of the eyeballs in vertical nystagmus. After the reading of the paper, Dr. Gowers exhibited a patient who illustrated well the dissociation of isolated voluntary movements of the upper lid from the action of the superior rectus. She had slight double ptosis, more on right than left side, and had no power to bring the eyelids voluntarily into normal position. When she looks up, however, the levator contracts to full degree in conjunction with the superior rectus.

Dr. BAXTER asked for an explanation of Graefe's phenomena in Graves's disease, when the upper lid fails to accompany the globe in its downward movement, so that a zone of white sclerotic is left between the lower edge of the upper lid and the cornea. Dr. Gowers had pointed out that normally the descent of the eyelid was due to a relaxation of the levator occurring synchronously with contraction of the inferior rectus, the globe dragging the lid down. If there were exophthalmos this mechanism should be even more marked; or it might be that marked exophthalmos would prevent the fall of the lid. But in two cases of Graves's disease Dr. Baxter has now under care, there is no exophthalmos, and yet in both Graefe's phenomenon is marked.

Dr. GOWERS, in reply, said that since his attention had been directed to the subject he had not had the opportunity of examining cases of Graves's disease.

Materia Medica and Therapeutics.

Conchinin as an Antipyretic.

Dr. STRUMPELL has treated fifty cases of intermittent fever, enteric fever, pneumonia, erysipelas, puerperal fever, and phthisis with this drug, which has been strongly recommended by Wunderlich, von Böck, and Ziemssen in malarial, intermittent, and typhoid fever. He gives the results of his treatment in the *Allegemeine Medicin. Central-Zeitung* for May 14th. Conchinin was given in seventeen cases of enteric fever, where the cold-water treatment was not applicable. The patients were, if possible, bathed during the day; and at night, if the temperature were high, they took one or two *grammes* (fifteen or thirty grains) of conchinin, with diluted sulphuric acid and peppermint-water. The effects on the temperature were the same as those obtained by quinine. The fever decreased during the following eight to twelve hours, and at the same time there was a moderate decrease in the frequency of the pulse. Typhoid fever patients vomited, as a rule, from fifteen to thirty minutes after taking the medicine; this, however, did not interfere with its effects, because it had already been absorbed. In a few cases, the patients complained of singing in the ears. Given in the form of an enema, it did not produce satisfactory results. In twenty cases of intermittent fever, conchinin acted in the same way as quinine. A *gramme* and a half or two *grammes* were given in a convenient vehicle from six to twelve hours before the time when the attack was expected, and the same dose, or perhaps a smaller one, shortly before the next attack. Later on, half a *gramme* to one *gramme* of conchinin was given for several days in the form of pills or capsules; and this treatment was in every case attended by the best results. Conchinin has proved equally efficient in erysipelas and croupous pneumonia, but it has little or no effect on the remittent or intermittent hectic fever often met with in phthisis.—*British Medical Journal*, June 21, 1879.

—

Iodoform as an External Antipyretic.

In an article in the *Deutsche Medicin. Wochenschrift* for June 7th, Dr. COLS-FELD, of Bremen, describes a case in which he accidently found that the external application of iodoform was followed by a lowering of temperature. The subject was a phthisical patient, whose temperature had risen to 103.4 deg. Fahr. He complained of troublesome ill-defined pain in the left front of the chest, for the relief of which, other means having failed, iodoform collodion (having a strength of 33.3 per cent.) was applied. The next day the temperature had fallen to 98.6 deg. Fahr., and the pain in the chest had entirely disappeared. The iodoform was then omitted, and the temperature again arose; but it fell when the iodoform collodion was reapplied, the strength now used being ten per cent. The odour being unpleasant, the patient discontinued the application for two days; but the febrile symptoms set in so energetically that he again had recourse to it, with marked relief. Dr. Colsfeld says that he did not observe any ill effects to be produced by the application of the iodoform, but he thinks that the expectoration was reduced in quantity. He does not pretend to say that the application would be useful in reducing the febrile process in the purely pulmonary affections of the lungs, pleura, peritoneum, etc.; but he suggests that it might be tried. The author refers to the observations of Binz, who found that the internal administration of iodoform had the effect of reducing the respiration, pulse, and temperature in a cat.—*British Medical Journal*, June 21, 1879.

Antiseptic Dressings with Boric Acid.

SOLGER says (*Berl. Klin. Woch.*, 1878, No. 42) that he uses boric acid in the antiseptic treatment of wounds in the following way. The cotton-wool which is going to be used for the dressing is plunged into a 10 per cent. water solution of borie acid, which is warmed to a temperature of 50 deg. R., then taken out and allowed to cool down to 35 or 40 deg. R., put on the wound, which has been previously thoroughly disinfected, and kept in its position by another layer of dry cotton-wool and a bandage. The high temperature of the dressing has a hæmostatic effect on the wound. According to the manner in which it is used, boric acid will either increase or lessen the property of cotton-wool, allowing the secretions of wounds to filter through it. If a plug of cotton-wool be soaked in a 15 to 20 per cent. solution of borie acid at a temperature of 60 deg. R. and above, then allowed to cool down to 35 deg., and spread out over the surface of a suppurating wound or abscess, or a fresh wound, and fastened by means of dry wool and bandages, the boric acid forms on evaporating a large quantity of boric acid crystals, at the same time the wool adheres so firmly to the skin that it entirely excludes the air and remains thus for months. On the contrary, the wool will allow the secretions to filter through it if it has been soaked in a mixture of borie and carbolic acid (five parts of borie and two parts of carbolic acid, and 100 parts of water). Boric acid dressings will be found very useful in the minor surgical operations.—*Lond. Med. Record*, June 15, 1879.

—

Glycerine as a Food.

Some years ago glycerine was proposed as a supplementary food, capable, it was even said, of taking the place of cod-liver oil in the nutrition of the invalid. The recommendation was made upon theoretical grounds, and received little confirmation from experience. Careful observations which were made, especially by the late Dr. Cotton, at the Hospital for Consumption, failed to show that it produces any effect on nutrition such as results from the administration of cod-liver oil. The opinion was thus formed that glycerine possesses little or no claim to be regarded as a food. The question has not, however, until now received much scientific investigation. To some researches by Catillon and others we directed our readers' attention on a previous occasion.[1] The effect of glycerine on the interchange of material in the organism—*i. e.*, its value as a food—has lately been further studied by Dr. Immanuel Munk, in a series of experimental inquiries undertaken at Berlin, the results of which are published in the current number of Virchow's *Archiv*. The question is of interest not merely because glycerine has been proposed for the purpose above stated, and is occasionally administered as a vehicle for certain drugs, or to the diabetic as a substitute for sugar, but also because it is, in one sense, a constant article of diet. It is known that fat is decomposed in part in the alimentary canal, under the influence of the intestinal mucus, into its fatty acid and glycerine, and the amount of this decomposition is at present unknown. Again, all wines contain a certain quantity of glycerine, which is one of the products of the alcoholic fermentation of sugar. Pasteur says that natural wines contain from six to eight grammes of glycerine per litre, while Neubauer puts the amount in the same volume at seven to eleven grammes. Moreover it has been proposed to use glycerine as a preservative agent. Munk has shown that the addition of two or three per cent. of glycerine to milk will postpone the lactic-acid fermentation for from eighteen to twenty-four hours. It is, therefore, important to know what influence is exerted by this substance on the vital processes. Of the toxic effect of large doses we possess

[1] The Lancet, vol. ii. 1877, p. 322.

information; the experiments of Munk have reference to the effect of the digestion of small quantities. Whether any nutritive value can be ascribed to glycerine, and what quantity may be taken without interference with the processes of the body, are the points specially considered.

Any substance introduced into the economy may influence the decomposition of material in two ways—by increasing or diminishing, on the one hand, the destruction of the nitrogenous material, or the exchange of albumen, and on the other the excretion of carbonic acid and absorption of oxygen. The effect of glycerine on the latter has been already studied by Scheremetjewski. But it is to the former point, the effect on the albuminates, that attention must especially be directed to determine the food-value of any substance. This is indicated by the effect on the excretion of nitrogen, and in the case of man and the carnivora the nitrogen passing away by the urine and feces affords the necessary information. The value of the observations of Catillon on this point is lessened by the fact that the diet of the animals experimented on was not strictly regulated.

It has been found that large quantities of glycerine produce hæmoglobinuria and also diarrhœa, both of which disturb the accuracy of observation. It was necessary therefore to give such doses of glycerine as should not produce these effects, and in the case of dogs not to exceed twenty-five to thirty grammes daily. These quantities were found by Munk in no way to modify the excretion of nitrogen. Any influence of glycerine, at least in medicinal doses, on the exchange of albumen may thus be put aside. According to the ordinary definition of a food, glycerine does not possess any nutritive value. If, however, the urine only is examined, there is found a slight diminution in the amount of nitrogen, as observed by Catillon. This is quite compensated for by the increased excretion by the bowel.

What is the fate of glycerine introduced into the economy? Is it decomposed or excreted?—and if the latter, in what form? When large doses are given so as to produce hæmoglobinuria, the urine contains a substance which readily reduces copper, but has been said, on the ground of its effects on polarized light, not to be sugar, but to be probably a decomposition, or transformation product of glycerine. According to Plosz, moreover, it is not capable of fermentation. It is very difficult to say whether any unaltered glycerine passes away, since the detection of a small quantity in the urine is a matter of great difficulty. It seems certain, however, that the greater part, if not all, is decomposed in the organism, and that when moderate quantities only are given the decomposition is complete. It was observed by Weiss that the quantity of glycogen in the liver is increased by the administration of glycerine. From the analogy with other substances which have a similar effect, such as albumen, gums, etc., Munk suggests that the glycerine absorbed from the intestine and carried by the portal vein to the liver is not itself transformed into glycogen, but rather, by its quick decomposition, limits the use of the liver glycogen, or furthers its formation from other materials. However this may be, the glycerine undergoes decomposition without its products having any influence on the changes in albumen, such as the carbo-hydrates exert. With reference to this, it may be remembered that glycerine has no chemical connection with the carbo-hydrates, but is rather to be regarded as an alcohol—the tertiary alcohol of the propyl series.

The solubility of glycerine renders it highly probable that the greater part of that which is taken into the stomach passes rapidly into the blood. A small part may be unabsorbed, and in the lower part of the intestine may undergo fermentation and reduction, with the formation of butyric acid, carbonic acid, etc., although this decomposition can take place only in a neutral liquid—a condition not easy to obtain in the intestine. Gorup-Besanez has also shown that in an alka-

line solution, the action of oxygen in an active state breaks glycerine up into formic, propionic, and perhaps acrylic acids. There is some probability that, in the
tissues, where similar conditions obtain, the same decomposition may occur; and
the intermediate products, propionic and formic acids, may be further oxidized
to their ultimate products, carbonic acid and water. Scheremetjewski showed
that the ingestion of glycerine causes an increase in the excretion of carbonic acid,
which Catillon has affirmed may amount to 7 per cent. This increase in the
production of carbonic acid must be accompanied by the liberation of its equivalent of heat, and so the generation of heat should be increased by the administration of glycerine. Hence there is the highest probability that glycerine may be
of service in this respect, but that it is of no value as a tissue-food.—*Lancet*,
June 7, 1879.

Medicine.

On the Use of Benzoate of Soda in Diphtheria.

LETZERICH says (*Beil. Klin. Woch.*, No. 1, 1879) that he has repeatedly
given this drug in diphtheria, and has always found it to answer very well. He
attributes his success to the antiseptic properties of the drug, by which the development of the diphtheritic bacteriæ is arrested. He also points out that it is a
most effective remedy in infantile, gastric, and intestinal catarrh, and in mycotic
catarrh of the bladder. In short, he fully corroborates Professor Klebs's statement when he says, that in benzoate of soda we possess a very powerful remedy
in all affections arising from the presence of contagious matter in the system. The
following is the author's method of administering the drug : R. Natr. benz. pur.
5 grammes, solve in aqua destillat. ; aq. menth. pip., āā 40 grammes; syr. cort.
leur., 10 grammes. Infants under one year were given a dessertspoonful every
hour. Children from one to three years old, must take a larger dose, viz., a
tablespoonful every hour, the proportion of the benzoate of soda being also increased from 5 to 7 or 8 grammes. To patients from three to seven years old, 8
to 10 grammes are given; those over seven, from 10 to 15 grammes. Adults
should take from 15 to 25 grammes in the same solution, the proportion of the
solvents and the syrup remaining the same. The diphtheritic membranes were
powdered with benzoate of soda, in severe cases once in three hours, in lighter
cases from two to three times daily. A solution of the strength of 5 per cent.
forms a very efficient gargle for older children.—*Lond. Med. Record*, June 15,
1879.

On the Effect of Cold Air in Measles.

KACZOROWSKI says (*Przelad Lek.*, Nos. 6 and 7, 1878) that cold air is one of
the most efficient remedies in eruptive affections. He happened to discover this
interesting fact by mere chance in the case of a smallpox patient who escaped into
the courtyard on a cold winter's day. The next day the pustules, which were
already filled with pus, were dried up. Another case is that of a man who, while
suffering from an abscess on his thigh, suddenly took measles, accompanied by a
troublesome feeling of itching and burning of the skin. He was carried into a
room without a fire, and, within a few hours, the itching subsided, the eruption
disappeared, and the patient recovered from the measles on the third day.

The author has also found that in gangrenous affections of the lungs, or in inveterate fetid catarrhs of the trachea, cold air is a very efficient remedy. He

does not attempt to explain the fact, but says that he prefers cold air to cold baths in acute feverish affections.—*London Med. Record*, May 15, 1879.

Nitrite of Amyl in Sea-sickness.

Mr. Crochley Clapham, to whom is distinctly due the credit of introducing this remedy to the notice of the profession, again writes reminding us of the fact, and remarking that "with due attention to details he looks upon the drug as curative in at least 90 per cent. of all cases treated." By a reference to his first article on the subject, published in the *Lancet* of Aug. 21st, 1875, it appears that during several trips across the Pacific, Mr. Clapham treated altogether 124 cases. In 121 of these, he tells us, success was evident and complete. The drug was administered by inhalation, three drops of the nitrite being poured on a handkerchief held close to the nose of the patient, the inhalation being conducted rapidly. A caution is added, to the effect that not more than three drops should be used in the absence of medical advice. In July, 1878, we published an article on the same subject by Dr. J. Rudd Leeson, who was successful in about three-fourths of the cases treated, the remaining fourth complaining of a feeling of sickness, but without vomiting. One or two cases did not improve in any way. Dr. Leeson thinks that three drops for women and five for men is the minimum dose, but that caution is required. Dr. Clapham says it is not a dangerous drug, except of course in cases where the arterial system is more or less rigid from osseous deposits. In August last Mr. Clapham and Dr. R. Leeson each contributed a letter to our columns, in which the former quotes some favourable experiences of Dr. Crichton Browne in crossing to Sweden, and Dr. Leeson gives a very emphatic proof of the comparative harmlessness of that drug, for the particulars of which we must refer our readers to the *Lancet* of August 10th, 1878. On the 3d inst. Mr. Dingle, surgeon to the Peninsular and Oriental Company's ship Mirzapore, gives a favourable account of the remedy, saying that in one day he administered it in at least a dozen cases, and that in all the effect was markedly successful, though in some instances it was necessary to repeat the dose, which he limited to three drops. But one of Dr. Dingle's patients has written to us, and says that, according to his observation on the occasion referred to, the drug ought to be administered with very great caution *and always under medical supervision*. Later, as our readers will have observed, one or more favourable reports have appeared in these columns. Under such circumstances, and with such an accumulation of evidence, we consider it right, as Mr. Clapham suggests, to draw the attention of those who often "go down to the sea in ships" to the remedy. And we should recommend ship surgeons to take Mr. Clapham's standard—as a rule, to limit the dose to three drops, and not to take it except under medical advice. He also recommends that the patients when under treatment, should be in bed, because a good sleep is generally the first result, from which the person awakes wanting to eat. It is usually better to allow one fit of vomiting to occur before the treatment is commenced, "to insure the *bona fide* character of the seizure." Some, however, do not vomit at all, but are very ill, and with these, he considers the nitrite to be equally successful.—*Lancet*, June 7, 1879.

Intracranial Aneurism in a Boy.

Dr. Von Unge relates in *Hygeia* (abstract in *Nordiskt Medicin. Arkiv.*, Bandet xi, 1st Häftet) the case of a boy aged 15, who had good health up to the age of 5, when he had measles. After this, it was said, he had constant headache, pain in the stomach, impaired appetite, and often diarrhœa with palpitation. At the age of 13, the headache became more troublesome, and was referred to a point immediately under the crown of the head, somewhat towards the forehead. He often had pain in the legs. In the spring of 1878, he frequently had obstinate hiccough. In the beginning of June, 1878, he became worse, and a high fever set in. On the 17th, he had a convulsive attack affecting the whole body, followed by unconsciousness; this occurred twice in the day. On the 19th, he was admitted into the Serefina Hospital, where he died on the 23d in a state of coma. There was ptosis of the left eyelid; the temperature was 102° to 104° Fah.; there was no albumen in the urine; the heart's action was much quickened, and the first sound was followed by a blowing murmur at the apex. At the necropsy, the subarachnoid space at the apex was found moderately full of a clear fluid; at the base and sides of the brain it was distended with coagula and a small quantity of blood-coloured fluid. On the left posterior cerebral artery immediately after the bifurcation of the basilar artery, was an aneurism of the size of a cherry. No change had been produced in the surrounding parts by the pressure of the aneurism. Where the aneurismal sac came off from the vessel, the lumen of the latter was filled by a thrombus. In several parts of the brain there were capillary hemorrhages. The aorta presented nothing remarkable. The muscular tissue of the heart was fragile; on the borders of the mitral valve were some excrescences of gelatinous consistence.—*British Med. Journal,* June 7, 1879.

Contributions to the Etiology of Hemorrhages in the Brain.

The following are the conclusions at which EICHLER has arrived (*Deut. Archiv für Kl. Med.,* Bd. 22, Heft 1; and *Med. Chir. Rundschau,* April, 1879): 1. Primary idiopathic cerebral hemorrhage is caused by the bursting of miliary aneurisms. 2. Miliary aneurisms are in reality true spontaneous aneurisms. 3. They owe their existence to chronic endarteritis, which is identical with arterial sclerosis. 4. Both miliary aneurisms and arterial sclerosis are an essentially senile affection. 5. Dissociating aneurisms must be carefully distinguished from miliary aneurisms. They are simply hæmatomata of the coat of the vessel, and never the cause but the result of a hemorrhage. 6. Similarly capillary ectasies must be separated from miliary aneurisms. The former may be compared to the telangiectasis which occurs in other places; both affections may be congenital. 7. The walls of the intracerebral arteries consist only of three layers; the inner and middle layer, and an external layer which is separated from the muscular layer by a lymphatic space.—*London Med. Record,* June 15, 1879.

Ophthalmoscopic Appearances in the Tubercular Meningitis of Children.

The following is an abstract of a paper on this subject, which was read by Dr. GEORGE GARLICK, at a late meeting of the Royal Medical and Chirurgical Society (*Lancet,* June 14, 1879). The ophthalmoscope discloses changes in the optic discs of about 80 per cent. of the children who die of tubercular meningitis. These changes fall under one of two heads—viz., optic neuritis or distension of the retinal veins alone. As the discs vary physiologically in different individuals and even in the same person, the two are often not alike; progressive change is better evidence than can be obtained from a single examination. In a small proportion of cases the optic changes occur very early in the course of the disease, and enable a diagnosis to be made when the symptoms are equivocal; this is the case when the meningitis is seated chiefly about the optic commissure. But the ophthalmoscopic changes are an important factor in the diagnosis in a much larger number of cases. The two forms of disc change—viz., the optic neuritis and distension of the veins—appear related respectively to meningeal inflamma-

tion and pressure. The intracranial pressure may result from excess of ventricular or of subarachnoid fluid, and gives evidence of its presence in the anæmia
of the cranial contents. The palsy of the limbs is mostly found on the side
opposite to that hemisphere of the brain which presents that greatest meningeal
affection. No such definite relation exists with regard to the optic discs. In
many cases of tubercular meningitis which run an indefinite course, especially
those which are secondary to some other advanced disease, the optic changes
share the indistinctness of the other symptoms. The ophthalmoscope counte-
nances the idea that some cases of tubercular meningitis recover, and even in
fatal cases a temporary improvement may occur in the discs. Tubercles of the
choroid appear to be an uncommon complication.

Dr. COUPLAND confirmed from his own experience the statement as to the
rarity of choroidal tubercle. In upwards of five years at the Middlesex Hospital
he had not met with it more than four times, two cases occurring in 1874 being
recorded by him in the Path. Soc. Trans. This did not bear out Cohnheim's
belief as to the frequency of choroidal tubercle in goneral tuberculosis.

Dr. GOWERS testified to the extreme exactness of Dr. Garlick's observations,
which proved how much could be learned by careful and continuous observation
from day to day. Many depended too much upon a single examination, but Dr.
Garlick had shown that the progressive changes were a chief feature in the diagnosis. His observation as to the distension of the optic sheath with subarachnoid
fluid confirmed Graefe's statement that the optic neuritis of tubercular meningitis
was always descending, a statement which has been disputed by many. It was
true that Cohnheim's observations have not been confirmed in this country, but
Cohnheim himself stated that choroidal tubercle occurred less frequently in connection with cases of tuberculosis with meningitis than in those without it.

Dr. BARLOW also bore testimony to the value of the careful and continuous
observations of Dr. Garlick, and the truth of the fact stated that it was necessary
to watch the cases from day to day in order to arrive at just conclusions. The
separation of the changes into two distinct forms was a considerable advance.
Dr. Barlow thought that the mechanical theory of optic neuritis would have to be
abandoned, and that the condition should be looked upon in the light of affections
of homologous tissues, the retina being only a prolongation of the brain. The
great frequency of softening of the brain-substance in tubercular meningitis, as
compared with simple meningitis, pointed to changes in brain-tissue itself in the
former disease. He had specimens of six cases of tubercle of the choroid ; and
he would be inclined to associate the choroidal affection with the disease of the
pia mater, and the optic neuritis with cerebritis.

Mr. PARKER asked if there was a history of injury in each of the cases of recovery. In all the instances of recovery from so-called "tubercular meningitis,"
injury had been the starting-point. Dr. Barlow's remarks interested him, because
for some time he had thought that cases of tubercular meningitis should more
properly be styled "cerebritis." In microscopical examination of one case he
had found both brain and spinal cord the seat of extensive small-celled infiltration, without any marked change to the naked eye.

Dr. GARLICK, in reply, said there was a history of slight injury in one of the
cases of recovery, but too much weight should not be placed upon histories of
injury. In the other three there was no such history ; in one there had been
previous otitis.

—

Acute Meningitis Treated by Doses of Iodide of Potassium.

M. RODET records, in the *Lyon Médical*, 1878, No. 52, the case of a young
girl aged 19, suffering from very acute meningitis (fever, vomiting, delirium,

sleeplessness, outcries, dilated pupils). The treatment was by antispasmodics and sedatives. At the end of two days, her state was aggravated with loss of consciousness, obstinate constipation, and monplegia of the right upper limb. Death seemed imminent. The use of antispasmodics was continued, and there was further prescribed a flying blister to the nape of the neck, and three *grammes* of iodide of potassium (equal to forty-six grains and a half), in twenty-four hours. The next morning there was a slight amelioration, especially in the intellectual condition; the same state of paralysis. A purgative enema produced abundant evacuation. The improvement made sensible progress; the paralysis began to diminish on the third day of the employment of the iodide of potassium; on the eighth day it had completely disappeared, and the patient was convalescent. The treatment was continued. The iodide was carried on the first day to as high a dose as four *grammes*, on the third to five *grammes*, and continued at that dose up to the eighth day, and then progressively diminished. This case deserves attention in respect to the successful treatment of so severe an affection as acute meningitis. M. Rodet follows his report by mentioning a certain number of cases cured by iodide of potassium, and cites the opinion of Fonssagrives. He lays great stress on the largeness of the dose of iodide of potassium.—*British Medical Journal*, June 21, 1879.

Treatment of Epilepsy.

Dr. A. HUGHES BENNETT, Physician to the Hospital for Epilepsy and Paralysis, Regent's Park, records (*British Med. Journal*, June 7, 1879) an analysis of the results of treatment of one hundred cases of epilepsy by the bromide of potassium or ammonium. The following he finds a convenient and efficacious prescription: R. Potassii bromidi gr. xx; ammonii bromidi gr. x; spiritus ammon. aromat. ℥ss; aquam ad ℥j. Fiat haustus ter in die sumendus.

The first dose was taken before getting out of bed in the morning, the second in the middle of the day on an empty stomach, and the third the last thing at night. If, in the course of a fortnight, the attacks continued, the dose was increased week by week, till there was some obvious modification in their severity or frequency; and this has been, if required, gradually increased to from sixty to ninety grains, three times a day. In the event of the first or any subsequent dose proving efficacious in warding off the seizures, it was continued for about a couple of months; that is, assuming no really dangerous signs of poisoning presented themselves. The fact of the bromide rash or moderate constitutional weakness being developed was found of no great importance, if the attacks were in abeyance. At the end of from two to three months, according to circumstances, the dose was gradually diminished, till the smallest possible amount necessary to materially modify the paroxysms was found; and this, when ascertained, was, the health remaining good, continued for many months.

Of the hundred cases treated in this way, it may be stated in general terms that, with only one or two exceptions, the bromides have had the effect of materially modifying the frequency and severity of the epileptic seizures. At the same time, opportunity was not afforded in all of these to test the efficacy of the treatment for a sufficient length of time.

Not only do the bromides materially modify the frequency of epileptic attacks, but they often diminish the severity of those which occur. They also improve in many respects the general health, and persons who suffered from headache, nervousness, and other ailments, are often greatly relieved in these respects.

The administration of the drugs may arrest the seizures for many months, and the moment they are discontinued, the attacks at once return, indicating that it is these agents which keep the paroxysms in abeyance, and that their action is not permanent.

What effects has a prolonged use of the bromides on the general health? Of the forty cases, which for a period of at least six months were continuously under the influence of these drugs, the following gives a general idea of the result.

In 62.5 per cent. of cases, the prolonged use of the bromides, sufficient to ward off or greatly modify the epileptic attacks, did not produce any physiological effects, or in any way influence the general health. In 35 per cent., some symptoms of bromism were produced; namely, in 25 per cent., there were weakness and languor of body, loss of appetite, and the usual physical symptoms; in 20 per cent., there were depression of the mental faculties into dulness, apathy, tendency to sleep, and so on; and in 15 per cent., there were well-marked signs of the bromide rash. One patient died while taking large doses, but whether as a result of the remedy or of the disease it is very difficult to determine. As a rule, however, the symptoms of bromism were slight, and their effects very temporary, and rapidly disappeared on discontinuing the drug for a time.

It may be said in conclusion that, in the bromide of potassium, we possess a valuable agent for suppressing the most dangerous symptoms of one of the most terrible maladies to which human flesh is heir, and further experience may enable us, through its influence, to effect a complete cure of the disease itself.

Contributions to the Study of Tuberculous Spinal Meningitis.

CHATEAUFORT, after having summed up the few cases of this special form of tuberculous meningitis which have been published, arrives at the following conclusions (*Thèse de Paris*, 1878): Lesions of the spinal meninges are met with in the majority of, if not in every case of tuberculous meningitis. Generally the cerebral meningitis is the predominant affection, and the spinal meningitis is an epiphenomenon which is seldom recognized; in some cases, however, the spinal accidents precede the cerebral symptoms. From an anatomical point of view, both cases are identical with the tuberculous infiltrations of the coats of the brain, which cause a softening of the convolutions. To these correspond analogous infiltrations which give rise to diffuse or circumscribed myelitis. The following are the symptoms which have been most frequently observed in this affection; disturbances of the sensibility, characterized by radiating pains, cutaneous hyperæsthesia alternating with disseminated anæsthetic spots. At the same time, or a little later, there occur motor troubles, spasms, and contractions, ultimately succeeded by paresis or true paraplegia. As in cases of paraplegia due to transverse myelitis, we here meet troubles of micturition, retention or incontinence of urine, constipation, or escharæ. Although it is often very difficult to discern in the course of tuberculous meningitis to what extent the brain and spinal cord are affected, still it is possible in some cases to be sure of the existence of granulations on the spinal marrow, and in almost every case to suspect it. Tuberculous spinal meningitis has no peculiar etiology, nor does it differ from cerebral meningitis in its evolution; it is almost always accompanied by cerebro-spinal tuberculosis. Hitherto this affection does not seem ever to have been cured; it is, however, probable that spinal meningitis, as well as cerebral meningitis, may be arrested in its development.— *London Med. Recovd*, June 15, 1879.

Curative Influence of Mania on other Bodily Disturbances.

SNELL quotes a case of severe icterus (*Allg. Zietschr, f. Psych.*, xxxv., p. 446) in which the patient, who was almost reduced to a hopeless condition, rapidly recovered, after having gone through an attack of acute mania. These attacks were repeated three times, and every time left the patient stronger and better than before. The author has observed similar curative effects of maniacal excitement in a series of chronic affections, such as the initial stage of phthisis pulmonum, chronic disease of the liver, gout, rheumatism, digestive troubles, and different functional nervous troubles. This effect cannot be ascribed solely to increased muscular activity, as the patient mentioned above was quite unable to move during the first stage of mania, on account of her extremities being much swollen. The author tries to explain this fact by assuming that nervous power is much increased during those times, as evidenced by the rapid absorption of exudations and similar processes.—*London Med. Record*, June 15, 1879.

Neuropathological Affections.

BERNHARDT publishes the result of his researches during the last two years, on peripheric paralysis, in the *Deut. Arch. f. Klin. Med.*, xxii., page 362. Among the several cases of saturnine paralysis quoted by him, the most interesting are: 1. A typical case of paralysis of the extensor muscles on the left hand of a left-handed patient. 2. A case of affection of the supinator muscles. 3. A case of paralysis in a painter, which might easily have been mistaken for saturnine paralysis. A case of paralysis of the radial nerve is also mentioned which was caused by a violent stretching of the muscles ; and a case of paralysis of the ulnar nerve, which came on after typhoid fever. He then quotes a case in which all the nerves of the arm were paralyzed ; two cases of paralysis of the sciatic nerve and its branches which followed after a neuritis of the nerve, and goes on to speak of the nature of inveterate serious or cured paralysis of the facial nerve. Concerning the accompanying twitching, which is often observed in old cases of paralysis of the facial nerve, the author strongly opposes Hitzig's views on the subject. Hitzig believes that the division of certain peripheric motor nerves causes a peculiar condition of irritation in corresponding motor parts of the central nervous system. Bernhardt attributes that condition of irritation to a propagation of the stimulus from the nervous centres to the neighbouring ganglionic centres of the other muscles of the same region.—*London Med. Record*, June 15, 1879.

Good Effects of Ammoniacal Sulphate of Copper in Neuralgia of the Fifth Nerve (Tic Douloureux).

Dr. FÉRÉOL having found several times obstinate cases of neuralgia of the fifth nerve, which had resisted a variety of other means, rapidly and completely cured by the administration of ammoniacal sulphate of copper, reports to the Académie de Médécine (April 1st, 1879) on the subject (*La France Médicale*, April 5th). The first case is that of a strong man, aged 32, who had suffered so atrociously from terrible neuralgic crisis, that on some days he was scarcely free for a few minutes at a time. Six teeth had been vainly extracted, and anti-neuralgic medication exhausted. He then tried ammoniacal sulphate of copper. The amelioration was considerable on the first day ; on the second, the patient slept all night for the first time in two months ; and, at the end of ten days, he left the hospital cured. A second case of supra-orbital neuralgia in a strong young man, occurring every morning and ceasing at noon, had been vainly treated by leeching, blistering, and full doses of quinine. The ammoniacal sulphate of copper, given in a dose first of all of 0.10, and then 0.15 centigrammes daily, produced an immediate amelioration of pain, and the patient described himself as cured. The medication was continued for a week, and the neuralgia did not return. Similar effects were obtained by M. Féréol in a lady aged 43, delicate, nervous, but not hysterical, suffering from persistent right hemicrania, with atrocious pain in the fifth pair of nerves, which drove her almost wild, and for which she had vainly tried quinine, aconite, morphia, hypodermic injections, etc. Similar results were obtained in an old man, aged 60, suffering for eighteen months from a horribly painful neuralgia, starting from the nasal branch of the fifth, and in whom local and general treatment by the oldest of anodynes and anti-periodics, had been vainly tried. In this case, the results were not permanent; the patient, having an invincible dislike to the sense of nausea produced by the sulphate of copper. The formula employed is the following: distilled water, 100 grammes; syrup of orange flower or peppermint, 30 grammes; ammoniacal sulphate of copper, 0.10 to 0.15 centigrammes, to be taken in the course of twenty-four hours, especially during food, in order to avoid irritating the stomach. In one patient, the dose was raised to 60 centigrammes a day without any other inconvenience than slight gastric pain, and a little diarrhœa. The medium dose was 0.10 to 0.15 centigrammes, which should be continued for from ten to fifteen days, even after the complete disappearance of the pains.—*Lond. Med. Record*, June 15, 1879.

Case of Co-ordinative Disturbance of the Muscles of Speech.

AUFRECHT reports (*Deut. Med. Woch.*, February 22, 1879) the following case :—

N. L., joiner's apprentice, had become overheated turning a grinding stone in a stooping position, when suddenly a stream of cold water was poured from a pipe above him over the back of his head and neck. Half an hour later he noticed that he could no longer speak. A few days later he came with his mother to consult the author. She stated that the lad had always been well, with the exception of measles and scarlet fever, which he had in his infancy, but that she herself had suffered from repeated attacks of melancholy, which lasted each time about five months. She had, however, been well for the last three years. The patient is 17 years old, well built and fairly nourished, no abnormal conditions can be detected in any of the vital organs; he swallows well, the tongue is protruded without any deviation to the right or left. When asked to speak, he makes the following remarkable efforts to utter a word. He opens his mouth wide, so that the lower lip protrudes over the lower dental arch, the tongue is thrust forth so that its tip touches the mucous membrane of the under lip, and squeezes between the latter and the dental arch of the lower jaw, assuming, at the same time, a more convex shape. Simultaneously, both the sterno-cleido-mastoid muscles contract and jerk the head forwards ; both they and the whole of the dorsal surface of the tongue are very hard and rigid to the touch in such moments. Not before all these movements have been accomplished simultaneously, the patient utters the required word. He tells his whole history in a clear and lucid way, but has to go through the same manœuvres at every word, or sometimes after two or three words. When asked to count if possible without stopping, he does not get beyond number six ; but, between the numbers, the mouth is kept open, the sterno-cleido-mastoid muscles remain contracted during the whole of the time, and the head is thrust forward.

He was treated with bromide of potassium, and a blister applied to the neck ; eight days later, he had so far improved as to be able to speak more coherently, and, though the above described symptoms still occurred after several words, the action of the muscles was less energetic than before. Four weeks later he was able to speak without the least apparent abnormity ; but when asked to count without stopping to take breath, he would go on till eighteen, then stop to draw a long breath, and execute the same manœuvres with the head and tongue though only slightly. If, however, told to inspire frequently while counting, so that wind does not fail him, no disturbance ever occurs. A fortnight later he was dismissed from treatment as being quite well, and has remained so ever since.

Two similar cases have come under observation before; one is quoted by Panthel in *Deutsche Klinik*, 1855, p. 451; and the other by Fleury in the *Gaz. Hebd.*, Nos. 15, 16, April 14, 20, 1865. Panthel's case was a boy of 12 years who fell down in a swoon at his father's funeral, and, when restored to consciousness a quarter of an hour later, was unable to speak. All his other functions were perfectly normal. This state lasted three days, and, during the whole of the time, whenever the boy attempted to speak, the muscles of the pharynx, which are innervated by the hypoglossus, were in a state of continual vibration, which only lasted as long as the boy had the intention to speak. If the muscles were compressed externally, the spasm ceased, and the boy was able to speak as long as the compression lasted. A fortnight later, the same state recurred after a slight fright and lasted two days; also, a few weeks later, when it passed over after a few hours.

In Fleury's case, the patient was a man aged 33, who had had one tonsil extirpated. This operation was followed by serious disturbances of sensibility and the sense of taste, aphonia, congestion of the brain, and epileptiform fits; at the same time, he had lost the power of speech, whenever he attempted to speak, his tongue would curve upwards, pressing on the palate, and there remain immovable. There was no affection of the tongue or lips, as he could smoke, whistle, etc. Neither was his intellect affected in any way; he could read, write, etc., and communicate with his surroundings by means of a pencil and writing tablets. After fifteen months of antiphlogistic treatment he regained the power of speech, but he remained epileptic.

Reflections.—It is clear from the history of the case that the muscles of speech could not have been affected; the lesion, therefore, was confined to the nerves which innervate them, the hypoglossus and the accessories. The term lesion is too strong to be used here, as we cannot speak of an anatomical lesion as occurring either in the origin or the course of the nerve, because, if this were the case, the nerves would be incapable of working their respective muscles, and we see that here the functions of the latter were in no wise disturbed. It is difficult to find a satisfactory explanation for this curious phenomenon. The author's theory is that, through some unknown agent, the roots of the hypoglossus and accessories, which exercised every effort to articulate the word ready in the brain, were so extensively excited that instead of inducing speech they impeded it, causing what might be termed ataxy of the speech.—*Lond. Med. Record*, June 15, 1879.

Hyperæsthesia of the Pharynx and Larynx.

GANGHOFNER gives an account of eight cases of purely nervous hyperæsthesia of the pharynx and larynx (*Prag. Med. Woch.*, 1878, Nos. 38, 40). They are mostly such as come often under the notice of specialists, and are a source of much trouble and annoyance both to them and their patients on account of their pertinacity. In by far the greater number of the cases, even the most scrupulous examination failed to detect any anatomical cause by which to explain the troubles; in others, there were minute pathological affections, small erosions in the pharynx, etc., which were, however, too insignificant to account for the sufferings of the patient. In a few cases, Ganghofner observed other nervous troubles, such as cardialgia, neuralgic pains, etc., nervous dysphagia, and œsophagismus.

The troubles caused by the disease are a feeling of burning, pressure, pricking, and dryness in the pharynx or larynx, sometimes in both organs at once; at the same time, the patients sometimes complain of a feeling as if their throat were being forcibly compressed, or as if they had a foreign body in the throat; in some cases, the pain extends as far as the tip of the nose or the tongue. If the larynx is affected, spasms of the glottis occasionally ensue, or a purely nervous spasmodic cough without any expectoration; the latter sometimes as often as thirty or forty times daily, but, as a rule, not quite so often. These phenomena are either persistent, or they only appear periodically, and are then provoked by much speaking, irritating food, or mental emotions.

Among the 24 cases observed by the author were 15 female patients and 9 male, averaging in age from 8 (boy) to 57 years. The etiology of this affection is not clear. It has often been ascribed to anæmia, but anæmia did not exist in every case. It was generally preceded by inflammation of the organs of the throat, simple anginas, etc. It often occurs in hysterical patients, but has also been met with in cases where no other hysterical symptom was manifest. The author has frequently observed that several individuals in the same family have successively been affected by it, so that he is inclined to think that there may be a hereditary disposition to this affection. Affections of the genital organs also seem to have some influence on its development.

Ganghofner discriminates two forms of the affection—one due to a continuous irritation of the peripheric terminations of the nerves in the mucous membrane, and another purely central, and not caused by any external influence. In treating this affection, it must always be borne in mind that there is a great tendency to frequent relapses, and that it is a very stubborn disease. The treatment consists in cold baths, sea-bathing, change of air, milk cures, mountain air, etc., or in the use of the galvanic current. Painting the throat with solutions of bromide of potassium, tannin, glycerine, morphine, inhalations of weak solutions of salt, etc. In some cases, it will be found advisable to give bromide of potassium internally, or even to administer hypodermic injections of morphia.—*Lond. Med. Record*, June 15, 1879.

Retro-Sternal Suffocative Goître.

M. DUPLAY recently (*Gaz. des Hôp.*, May 6 and 8) delivered at the St. Louis a clinical lecture on this subject. A woman, fifty-eight years of age, had observed for more than twenty years a small indolent tumour at the right side of her neck just above the sternum. About six months ago, while still continuing indolent, the tumour rapidly increased in size, and gave rise to such difficulty of respiration as to induce her to come to the hospital. When admitted the tumour was found to be about the size of an egg, and covered by the infra-hyoidean muscles. It was not adherent to these and the skin, but some prolongations which extended into the mediastinum had contracted adhesions. It was hard and without fluctuation. It participated in the movements of elevation and depression of the larynx, but this organ as well as the œsophagus was unaffected. Great dyspnœa was induced without any exertion, and even without this the respiration was considerably embarrassed. The tumour was pronounced to be due to an enlargement of the right lobe of the thyroid gland. On account of the age of the patient, and family antecedents, the tumour was deemed to be possibly scirrhus; but cancer supervening on slight hypertrophy of the thyroid of so many years' standing is a rare occurrence. The uniform solid consistency of the tumour, and especially its absolute indolence, also militated against the idea of malignancy, as cancer of the thyroid is remarkable for the severity of the neuralgic pains which extend to the cervical region and to the arms. The woman, moreover, was in good health and not emaciated.

The disturbance of the respiratory organs observed in suffocative goître may depend upon different anatomical conditions. The gland, in place of being situated at the anterior part of the neck, may embrace the larynx and trachea like a ring, so that when it exerts fibrous retraction consequent on hypertrophy, the laryngo-tracheal tube may become constricted as by a ligature. But this is a rare occurrence. Another form, of which this patient seems to offer an example, and which is described as *goître plongeant*—internal goitre, or, more properly, retrosternal goitre—is sometimes very difficult of diagnosis, in consequence of the whole of the tumour being placed behind the sternum. But ordinarily, as in the present case, the tumor is to a certain extent apparent above the sternum and sterno-clavicular articulation, sending a prolongation behind the sternum. It may be asked how so small a tumour, and so little fixed and immovable, can give rise to such serious functional disturbance by the compression it exercises on the neighbouring organs ; and, in fact, in small retro-sternal goitre this is a phenomenon somewhat difficult of interpretation, even with the aid of an autopsy. The most probable supposition seems to be that, when the goitre is situated quite at the upper extremity of the thorax, it tends, by virtue of a kind of aspiration which takes place at the moment of inspiration, to insinuate itself into the anterior mediastinum, where, opposed by the sternum as a barrier, it presses on the trachea, producing permanent disturbance of respiration, which is increased when the respiratory movements are multiplied. This disturbance may suddenly acquire great gravity, and even prove rapidly fatal. But this accident, instead of being attributed to the production of congestion of the glottis, as it sometimes has been, is more probably due to the compression exerted either on the recurrent nerves, especially the right, or on the pneumogastric itself.

The prognosis of the affection is of great importance. In this case, in which the tumour only determines moderate dyspnœa, the patient may yet be carried off very rapidly, without the tumour having increased in size, or having undergone any modification whatever. A vivid moral emotion might determine a suffocative paroxysm, although such a termination is a rare one. What is more common is to find the dyspnœa progressively increasing, and then, after awhile, to see suffocative paroxysms supervene, which, after having recurred a certain number of times, finish by proving fatal. And even if the suffocative paroxysms are delayed, we may find, if the tumour continues to increase, other functional disturbances produced in connection with the œsophagus, the vessels, or nerves.

Before speaking of the treatment which should be adopted in these cases, Dr. Duplay cautioned his hearers against the dangers which result from a too ready surgical intervention in tumours of the thyroid body. Whatever the diagnosis may be that has been formed, these affections must not be meddled with until absolutely forced to it by the progress of the disease or the instances of the patient. Slight as the operation may be that is performed in this region—even a simple puncture with the exploratory trocar—the patient may be killed by it. Of this M. Duplay has seen numerous instances. In the present case, in which the accidents have not acquired a very great intensity, general treatment may be first tried, this consisting chiefly in the employment of preparations of iodine. Most excellent results are obtainable from these in young subjects, and when the affection has been treated by them from the first. When the symptoms become more menacing, surgical interference must be resorted to. Some surgeons, especially Bonnet, regarding the dyspnœa as due to the constriction produced by the infra-hyoidean muscles, have divided these, but with no satisfactory results. Another operation by Bonnet, which sometimes succeeds, consists in the displacement of the thyroid and cauterization. The object of this operation is the raising the tumonr and the prevention of its exercising compression on the trachea during the aspiration which accompanies inspiration. Bonnet passed three or four solid pins under the skin immediately behind the sternum, transfixed the corresponding portion of the hypertrophied thyroid, and brought out the points of the needles

on the opposite side, curving them so as to fix the tumour in a permanent manner.
To maintain it thus he applied the Vienna caustic, which destroyed the skin, subcutaneous cellular tissue, and even a small portion of the tumour. During cicatrization, cohesion took place between the hypertrophied thyroid and the integuments. The interstitial injection of tincture of iodine, without being more
dangerous than the preceding method, has the inconvenience of inducing primary
inflammatory augmentation of the dimensions of the tissues before their eventual
retraction can be secured. The removal of the thyroid, heretofore reputed so
dangerous an operation, has been revived in England, Germany, and America
with considerable success, the mean mortality only being one in three.—*Med.
Times and Gaz.*, June 28, 1879.

Atelectasis Pulmonum.

After a very thorough critical review of the different hypotheses which have
prevailed on the etiology of acquired atelectasis, LICHTHEIM details his own
experiments (*Arch. f. Exp. Path. and Pharm.*, Band x, and *Prager Med.
Woch.*, March 26, 1879). They were undertaken in accordance with Traube's
directions, with the exception that the author replaced the rolls of paper used by
Traube for the purpose of stopping up the alveoli by small tents of laminaria,
which he introduced into a bronchus through the tracheal wound, as he considered them more effectual in keeping out the air. After the operation, the
circumscribed portion of the lung was found to be quite atelectatic, the animals
dying in the course of the following twenty-four or forty-eight hours with all the
symptoms of acute dyspnœa, which had set in immediately after the operation,
and was owing to the acute compensatory inflation of the remainder of the lung,
which in some cases even caused pneumothorax by the bursting of some alveoli.

In a second series of experiments, where one of the bronchi was ligatured in
the pleuritic cavity, the animals lived longer, the lung was atelectatic, presented
inflammatory changes, and was imbedded in a layer of tough pus.

For the purpose of elucidating the question whether the air contained in a
portion of the lung which had thus been circumscribed could be absorbed by the
blood or not, Lichtheim ligatured the corresponding pulmonary artery and veins.
He thought that absorption could only be carried out as long as the circulation
remained uninterrupted, but he was disappointed in finding that, twenty-four
hours after the operation, the lung had increased in size, and contained a great
quantity of frothy serum, slightly tinged with blood. The blood could only have
penetrated into the lungs through the branches which the art. med. pericard. and
the art. œsophag. send to this organ. This unexpected difficulty in entirely
suspending the circulation in one lung made Lichtheim try another method. He
decided no longer to submit the absorbing fluid, but the absorbing gas, to voluntary alterations. This experiment was preceded by another, by which he endeavoured to ascertain the rapidity with which the air was absorbed by the portion
of the lung which had been thus separated. He found that the mean time of
absorption was about three hours, the shortest time was two and a half hours,
and the longest four hours. In a similar way he tried to calculate how much
time was needed for the absorption of each of the constituents of the atmospheric
air. This was done by introducing a canula into one bronchus of the lung in
question, thus bringing the gas which was being experimented with into contact
with the lung, while the other half of the organ was left undisturbed. It was
then found that the oxygen and carbonic acid disappeared much more rapidly
than atmospheric air, and nitrogen much more slowly than the latter, from the
circumscribed portion of the lung. In order to explain one of the principal conditions of absorption, viz., the increased tension of the gas during the process

within the separated lung, Lichtheim assumes "that the elasticity of the pulmonary tissue cannot be satisfied until the last air vesicle has been expelled." Lichtheim ascribes the atelectatic condition of the lung which is often met with, both while the organ is still within the thorax and after it has been removed, to an exchange of gas, which takes place through the wall of the alveoli between the air contained in the latter and the outer atmosphere; here the tension of the air in the lungs, which is heightened through the elasticity of the alveoli, plays a most important part.

In the last part of his work the author tries to explain in what way the atelectatic condition of the human lung is brought about. This condition is met with in children suffering from bronchitis, where one portion of the lung is often rendered atelectatic through the accumulation of mucus in the bronchi, and debility of the respiratory muscles; or, in croup, where the bronchi are always found filled with mucus and fibrinous clots at the post-mortem examinations. Lichtheim also classifies under the head of atelectasis that form of the affection which is observed in pleuritic exudations and restricted to that part of the lung which is beneath the level of the liquid. It must, however, be borne in mind, that this is only the case in less voluminous exudations and transudations, where, although the pressure exercised on the fluid can be much lower than the atmospheric pressure, yet the portion of the lung which dips into it is empty of air, tough, not bloodless, but of a dark colour. Here we cannot speak of a compression as we would in the case of exudations that are under high pressure; but this condition of the lung is simply owing to the fact that the air contained in the portion of the lung which is beneath the level of the liquid, can no longer be renewed, as the lung no longer is able to follow the inspiratory movements of the thorax, and it must, therefore, be absorbed.—*London Med. Record*, June 15, 1879.

On the Pulmonary Complications of Typhoid Fever.

The following are the conclusions to which GUILLETMET has arrived (*Thése de Paris*, 1878): 1. The symptoms of typhoid fever may be classed under two heads, as derived from congestive or destructive lesions. 2. The congestive symptoms are particularly marked in the skin, the intestines, the brain, the lungs, and in other viscera. 3. The lungs are always congested in typhoid fever. These congestions are not stationary in the first stages of the disease, but may easily be drawn to some other place; therefore counterirritants applied to the skin will always prove useful. 4. Later on the pulmonary congestion is caused by stasis, which frequently originates in degeneration of the heart. 5. The stasis in its turn causes enlargement of the spleen, acute œdema, and bloody infiltration of the lungs. The enlargement of the spleen is complicated with catarrh of the bronchi, which gives rise to the emphysema that is occasionally observed. 7. Inflammation of the lung occurs sometimes, generally in the shape of lobular, lobar, or interstitial pneumonia 8. True pneumonia is very rare in typhoid fever, it is almost always a pseudo-pneumonia. If true pneumonia, complicated with hepatization, should come under notice, it will always be on the fourteenth day of the illness, and during convalescence. 9. Tuberculosis has often been observed following in the rear of typhoid fever. 10. The complications of typhoid fever which do not often come under observation, are primitive pneumonia, pleurisy, hæmoptysis without tubercles, pneumothorax, infarcta, and gangrene of the lungs. 11. Primitive pneumonia in typhoid fever is a rarely occurring affection, and it is often difficult to prove that the fever was the primary affection. 12. Pleurisy occurs very seldom without inflammation of the lungs; it generally develops towards the end of the illness or during convalescence. The exudation may be very considerable, and have no tendency to be reabsorbed. 13. Hæmoptysis has sometimes been observed; it is mostly a symptom of a pulmonary apoplexy, but may also be caused by the patient's having taken cold. 14. Pneumothorax has once come under observation in the course of typhoid fever, though there were no lesions of the lungs sufficiently considerable to explain their rupture. 15. Infarcta have often been found in the lungs of typhoid fever patients. 16. Infarcta are often the cause of secondary inflammations of the lungs of the pleura. 17. Infarcta on a whole originate in the decreasing energy of the cardiac action, through which coagulations form, and thereby give rise to emboli. At other times these emboli come from some gangrenous or purulent part of the organism, when they have a typhoid character. 18. In the same way the gangrenous affections of the lungs may be explained. 19. If an embolus should be thrown into the principal trunk of the pulmonary artery, or into one of its principal branches, death is rapidly caused by asphyxia.—*Lond. Med. Record*, June 15, 1879.

—

Nervous Dyspnœa in Nephritis.

ORTILLE (*Bull. Général de Therap.*, No. 6, March 30) has divided this interesting pamphlet into two parts. The first is devoted to the clinical side of the question. Dyspnœa is one of the symptoms of uræmia, it occurs in a twofold form: an acute form, characterized by attacks which often cause death, and a chronic form, which is complicated by paroxysms. The former is evidently of nervous origin. The second has been attributed to cardio-pulmonary troubles; this explanation is unsatisfactory, because the intensity of dyspnœa does not depend upon lesions of the heart and the lungs; another explanation given was the asphyctic state of the blood, but the experiments related in the second part of this work, show that the blood is not asphyctic. It results, therefore, that in these two forms of dyspnœa, the nervous element is the principal, if not the only cause of the respiratory troubles. This nervous dyspnœa is recognized: 1. By the frequent occurrence of uræmic vomiting. 2. By the negative results obtained by auscultation of the lungs and the heart. 3. By its intensity. 4. By the constant fall of the temperature. 5. By the presence of albumen in the urine. The following are the therapeutic indications: sub-cutaneous injections of chlorhydrate of morphia will prove useful in paroxysms of dyspnœa; against the uræmic intoxication, the author recommends diaphoretics, especially chlorhydrate of pilocarpine, in subcutaneous injections of $2\frac{1}{2}$ centigrammes, and diuretics, among which phosphate of zinc has proved particularly efficient. In the second part, the author describes his experiments. By cutting out the kidneys in dogs, or by tying their ureters, they were placed in the conditions favourable to the development of uræmia, and all the characteristic symptoms of this affection were subsequently observed in them. The blood of these animals having been analyzed at different times, the results were as follows: It contained a normal proportion of oxygen and carbonic acid, and could, therefore, not be said to be asphyctic; neither could it be the cause of the uræmic dyspnœa. Ammonia was constantly present in the intestines, but not always in the blood; this would prove that when it is found in the blood it is only there secondarily, and not as Frerichs would have it, the cause of uræmic accidents. As neither the amount of urea, nor the excess of extractive matter contained in the blood, suffices to explain the symptoms of uræmia, its explanation must be sought in the state of the tissues. The blood, which has not been sufficiently purified, does not adequately nourish the tissues of the body, the result being a state of starvation, which manifests itself in the nervous system by special functional troubles, such as dyspnœa, coma, delirium, convulsions—in short, all the symptoms of uræmia. The latter, should, therefore, no longer be considered as a laxed state, but as cachexia.—*London Med. Record*, June 15, 1879.

Chondrosis of the Auricle.

An interesting case in veterinary pathology, and which has an important bearing on human physiology, is recorded by Mr. HUGUES in the *Journal de Médecine de Bruxelles.* The right auricle of a horse aged six years was found to be completely cartilaginous, being composed of three pieces of cartilage closely united to one another by fibrous ligaments. The largest had the curvature of the corresponding ventricle, the outer surface being convex and the inner concave; it measured 14 centimetres by 9; the second piece measured 7 centimetres by 4. In no part could any trace of muscular fibres be discovered. The horse died of acute pleurisy, myocarditis, and pericarditis, consequent on a long drive after a journey, and until the commencement of the illness, a few days before its death, it appeared to be in perfect health. Mr. Hugues points out very pertinently that the case strikingly illustrates the passive rôle of the auricles in the action of the heart.—*Lancet,* June 14, 1879.

—

A Case of complete Obliteration of the Arteria Anonyma, and nearly complete Obliteration of the Left Carotid and Subclavian Artery, complicated with an Aneurism of the Aorta and Cancer of the Œsophagus.

This title sufficiently indicates the different lesions met with at the autopsy of this case, reported by PREISENDORFER. The patient (*Arch. f. Path. Anat. und Phys.*, vol. lxxiii. page 594), aged 45, had complained chiefly of difficulties in deglutition, owing to a cancer in the œsophagus, from which he died; the other lesions not having caused him any special inconvenience. The physical examination had, however, revealed three suspicious symptoms: dulness of the superior sternal region, a slight bruit along the sternum, and a remarkably small pulse of the upper compared to that of the lower extremities; but still these symptoms were not grave enough to admit of a positive diagnosis, or to lead to suspicion of the remarkable obliterations of the arteries mentioned above. These cases are very rare, and must probably be ascribed either to a congenital vitium or to an obliterating arteriosclerosis. A similar preparation exists in the museum at Cologne, and Riegel also met with a patient who was suffering from the same affection.—*London Med. Record,* June 15, 1879.

—

Case of Atresia of the Pulmonary Artery with Atrophy of the Right Ventricle.

RAUB (*Med. Jahr.*, Heft 3, 1878) observed a remarkable anomaly of the right heart in a female child, aged 29 days, who showed symptoms of cyanosis. The right auricle is considerably dilated, the auriculo-ventricular opening is very narrow, and the valves are rudimentary and fixed to the wall of the ventricle. The right ventricle is exceedingly atrophic, and could scarcely hold a small lentil in its cavity. It contains a depression of the size of a millet grain, which is the rudimentary infundibulum. There is complete atresia of the pulmonary artery; and the valves of the latter vessel, which is very narrow at its opening, are only indicated by almost invisible folds. The left auricle is normal, and the ventricle comparatively voluminous. The intraventricular partition exists, the foramen Botalli is of normal dimension; a little underneath is a small opening of the size of a pin's head. The arterial duct springs from the left branch of the pulmonary artery, about 4 millimetres beyond the bifurcation. The most remarkable point in this case is the absence of the lesions which have often been observed coincidently with strictures or atresiæ of the pulmonary artery. Another fact which deserves to be noticed is the atrophy of the right ventricle. The blood of the

venæ cavæ met with an obstacle on entering the ventricle on a level with the
strictured auriculo-ventricular opening; it succeeded in dilating the right auricle
thereby penetrating into the left heart through the foramen Botalli. Rokitansky
was the first to describe this mechanism, and to show that the inverted conditions
produce the dilatation of the right ventricle which is generally met with in atresia
of the pulmonary artery.—*London Med. Record*, June 15, 1879.

The Genesis of the Double Sound in the Crural Artery.

PREISENDÖRFER draws attention (*Berl. Klin. Woch.*, 1879; and *Med. Chir.
Rundschau*, April, 1879) to one of the causes of a purely arterial double sound,
which has hitherto escaped observation. He noticed it in a man, aged 44, who
was suffering from cardiac insufficiency, while the valves of the heart had remained
healthy. A regular series of strong pulsations, alternating with weaker ones, could
be felt at the radial artery (pulsus bigeminus); the frequency being sixty-four
double pulsations in a minute. If the crural artery was auscultated without
pressing upon it, a distinct double sound could be heard, which corresponded to
the radial pulsations, and changed into a distinct double bruit when the artery
was pressed down with the stethoscope. The patient left the hospital after a six
weeks' stay, apparently much better, but came back in a fortnight in a very bad
condition. The pulse still remained regular, in spite of the increased venous
symptoms; but the double sound on the crural artery could not be heard this
time. It would result from this observation that a pulsus bigeminus is able to
give rise to the phenomenon of double sound in the crural artery, which phenomenon proves that the vascular walls still possess a comparatively normal elasticity, and that the pulsations are still relatively rapid and strong. It is clear that
these double sounds may occur in the most various rhythms, and that many cases
of double sounds in the crural artery could be explained in the same manner.—
London Med. Record, June 15, 1879.

On Thrombosis.

In some lectures given at the Hôpital des Enfants-Maladies, M. BOUCHUT
(*Gaz. des Hôpitaux*, March 13, 20, April 3, 1879) dwells on the subject of
thrombosis of veins in cachectic and chronic maladies; a subject which he first
wrote on in 1844. Instances of this are very numerous; not only do they occur
in the lower limbs, but in the iliac veins, the portal vein, the jugular, the pulmonary arteries, the sinuses of the dura mater, and in the right cavities of the
heart. The symptoms of this thrombosis of course differ with its seat: thus, in
the pelvis, it may cause swelling and pain in the lower limbs; in the vena cava,
intestinal hemorrhage; in the brachio-cephalic and the jugular, hæmoptysis. So
in the sinuses of the dura mater this cachectic thrombosis produces convulsions in
the child and delirium in the adult. M. Bouchut gives a *résumé* of 68 cases in
illustration of this last statement, in all of which *post-mortem* examinations were
made. He admits with Lancereaux that there are thromboses of inflammatory
origin, and those due to retarded circulation; but confines himself to those of the
latter class, which he has had an opportunity of observing frequently and carefully in children. The affection begins at the end of acute diseases, and in the
course of chronic ones, with sudden convulsions of short duration, or with delirium
of a more or less marked kind, announcing the approach of death. Convulsions
are seen in these cases up to the age of about seven years; while delirium is met
with only in older children and adults. In the 38 observations of final convulsions in children affected with different cachectic diseases, 35 had thrombosis of
the sinuses, and three overfilling with blood and encephalitis. The cases occurred

under the following heads. Final convulsions from thrombosis of sinuses, 35 cases; chronic enteritis, 5; measles (catarrhal pneumonia), 2; chronic pneumonia, 5; phthisis, 8; anasarca without albuminuria, 1; chronic albuminuria, 2; whooping-cough and pneumonia, 7; scrofulous cachexia and tubercle of the bones, the lungs, and the intestine, 1; gangrene of the mouth, 1; diphtheria, 2—35. Convulsions, with stases of blood in the sinuses without thrombosis: chronic pneumonia, 1; whooping-cough, 2—38.—*London Med. Record*, June 15, 1879.

On Hysterical Attacks of Gastric Origin.

Ν. DALLY communicated to the Société de Thérapeutique at a recent meeting (February 12) the following two interesting cases which had come under his observation. The first was that of a young girl who was always taken with paroxysms of hysteriform clonic convulsions during the act of swallowing her food, principally of a solid nature. A slight touch or pressure on the stomach would also invariably cause a paroxysm, which would increase in violence if the pressure was greater. Besides those cases where the attacks were brought on by external causes, he noticed that these phenomena were always in some way connected with the passage of food through the pylorus. Ν. Dally treated the patient with electricity, applying the constant current to the region of the stomach; this at first brought on most violent attacks, lasting from four to five hours; but the treatment having been continued with the addition of "douches," the patient rapidly improved in health.

In the other case, the paroxysms were less violent, and never lasted more than three to five minutes. The patient was a lad of 13, in whom they also were caused by the passage of food through the pylorus. He was treated in the same way as the girl, and recovered rapidly. Both cases present a great resemblance to each other; perhaps the only difference being that in the girl the paroxysms were evidently of the kind noticed in hysteria major, whilst, in the boy, they resembled the twitching of St. Vitus's dance.—*London Med. Record*, June 15, 1879.

Intussusception of Ileum into Cæcum associated with Polypoid Tumour.

At a late meeting of the Clinical Society of London (*Lancet*, June 7, 1879) Dr. COUPLAND read notes of a case communicated by himself and Νr. HULKE, of Intussusception of the Ileum into the Cæcum through the Ileo-cæcal Valve, associated with a Polypoid Tumour; laparotomy on the fifth day; great immediate relief; death on the seventeenth day. The case was that of a spare, old-looking blonde, sixteen years of age, of highly hysterical temperament, who was admitted into the Middlesex Hospital on March 11, 1879, having been seized the previous day with colicky pains and vomiting. She had just recovered from a similar attack, lasting a few days, and was said to have suffered in the same way some two years before. The bowels had been moved naturally that morning, but no blood had been passed. On admission the paroxysmal abdominal pain was the chief symptom, but there existed a prominent cylindrical swelling in the upper part of the right iliac region, and an area of dulness below this. There was no general abdominal distension, and no constitutional disturbance. The case being regarded as one of fecal accumulation and typhlitis, sedatives were given and enemata administered—the latter without effect. The vomiting, however, continued, being provoked by anything she took. The pain, less severe on account of the opiates, still remained, and no change took place in the swelling or extent of dulness. On the 14th she was obviously weaker, the vomiting was

' bilious" in character, the abdomen more tympanitic.   A large soap-and-water injection to the amount of four pints was returned discoloured and with a peculiar penetrating odour.   The question of intussusception (between which and the former diagnosis the case had always seemed to lie) was now seriously entertained, and Mr. Hulke was consulted.   He found nothing on rectal and vaginal examination, and after a further consultation with Mr. Nunn and Dr. Cayley, it was decided (seeing the patient's critical state) that the abdomen should be explored. Laparotomy was accordingly performed, and Mr. Hulke detected an intussusception of the ileum through its lower end into the cæcum.   Reduction being found impossible, the ileum immediately above was secured to the lower angle of the wound and opened.   Great relief followed, the vomiting and pain entirely ceasing, and the pulse gaining in force ; but thirty-six hours after the operation the patient sank from the peritonitis which was present at the time of operation. The post-mortem examination revealed an intussusception of fully three feet of ileum, though its lowermost six inches and through the valve, the invagination extending for a distance of twelve inches into the colon.   The lips of the valve and the surface of the gut included between them were deeply ulcerated ; much lymph occurred between the serous layers of the invagination, whilst the central tube was filled with blood-clot, except for its upper three inches, which was occupied by a firm fleshy cylindrical polypoid mass, about the size of the little finger. There was slight general recent peritonitis.   The other organs were healthy. The obscurity in the diagnosis, the absence of melæna, the time that elapsed before the symptoms became severe enough to point to complete obstruction, and the fact that the vomiting never became stercoraceous, were dwelt on.   It was pointed out that this variety of intussusception was of comparatively rare occurrence.   The coexistence of a polypoid growth (it was lipomatous in character), and its situation at that part of the gut which was the last to become invaginated, were also points of interest ; the presence of the tumour doubtless preventing reduction as well as hastening the ulcerative process.—Mr. Marsh asked whether there were any cases of fecal obstruction on record producing such symptoms as this case presented ; for it was plain that owing to the error in diagnosis much valuable time was lost, and when surgical aid was invoked the case had passed beyond the time when such interference would have succeeded in effecting a reduction of the intussusception.   Mr. Hulke had done all that could be done ; but it seemed as if physicians should seek for surer signs of diagnosis, so as to call in surgical aid early.

Mr. Bryant said the case was of great interest, but he confessed on hearing it that he felt much as Mr. Marsh did as to the question of diagnosis.   It did not appear to him that the symptoms were such as characterize fecal obstruction. The patient was seized with an acute abdominal attack, which subsided and then recurred ; and then unfortunately, when the diagnosis was made, Mr. Hulke had but little chance of doing good.   The history of the case was peculiar.   There was absence of tenesmus or discharge of blood-stained mucus, and possibly this might have led to the discarding the idea of intussusception.   The presence of a polypus was very interesting ; the invagination was clearly produced by an effort of nature to get rid of the growth.   He referred to a preparation in St. George's Hospital Museum, where a growth similarly caused intussusception.   He had thought that ileal intussusception through the ileo-cæcal valve was one of the most usual forms ; and he remarked that blood was found in abundance in the invaginated gut, and yet did not appear externally.

Mr. Hulke, in reply, said that hemorrhage from the bowel when present was a valuable sign, but he had frequently found cases where there was no passage of blood.   When, as in this case, the obstruction and strangulation of the gut are very acute, he should not expect that blood would have escaped. The wonderful rally the patient made after the operation from her deeply collapsed condition before operation was very interesting.

Dr. Coupland replied that the evidence in favour of intussusception when the patient was admitted was too slight to warrant his calling in the aid of the surgeon. The case lay between that and fecal accumulation with typhlitis, and no one regretted more than he did that in taking the simpler ground he had diminished the chances of recovery from early surgical interference, to the importance of which he was fully alive. At the same time, looking to the extremely strangulated condition of the bowel, and the position of the growth, firmly fixed as it was between the lips of the valve, he doubted if reduction could have been effected even if such interference had been made at the outset. Statistics show that this form of intussusception was by far the rarest of all forms, the commonest being that where, commencing at the valve, the invaginating cæcum drags the ileum after it into the colon.

———

Simulation of Ascites in Intestinal Obstruction.

Dr. MARKHAM SKERRITT, at a recent meeting of the Clinical Society of London (*Lancet,* June 7, 1879), related two cases to show that dulness in the dependent parts of the abdomen, changing its site with alterations in the position of the patient, which is commonly regarded as the most reliable sign of ascites, may exist when there is no fluid in the peritoneal cavity. The first case, fully reported to the Society on Feb. 14th, was that of a patient admitted into the Bristol General Hospital with intestinal obstruction from what proved to be a plug of fibrinous exudation. When the patient lay on his back there was dulness in both flanks as high as the anterior superior iliac spines; but when he turned on either side the uppermost flank became resonant. Post-mortem, the small intestine was found to be greatly distended with liquid feces and gas, and there was no fluid in the peritoneal cavity. The second case was that of a boy aged sixteen, admitted into the Bristol General Hospital five days after the onset of symptoms of intestinal obstruction. Here also there was dulness in both flanks when the patient lay on his back, and there was resonance in the uppermost flank when he lay on his side. At the post-mortem examination a coil of small intestine was found to be bound down by tough adhesions; the gut above was greatly distended with fluid feces and gas, and there was no fluid in the peritoneal cavity. The following explanation was given of the simulation of the physical signs of ascites in these cases: The gas and the liquid feces in each coil of intestine necessarily obeyed the same physical laws as did the gas-containing intestines and the free fluid in ascites; that is, in each coil of intestine the gas would rise to the top in whatever position the patient lay, and the feces would sink to the bottom; and this was appreciable to percussion on account of the great distension of the individual coils, and also of the large proportion of fluid feces contained in them. According to this theory, when the patient lay on his back the dulness in each flank was the sum of the dulnesses due to the liquid feces in the individual coils, and when he lay on either side the resonance in the uppermost flank was the sum of the resonances produced by the gas in the same individual coils. The existence of this physical sign in the absence of ascites had apparently not been before described, and the fact was of some practical importance, because this source of fallacy in the diagnosis of ascites would be met with in cases where the presence of peritoneal fluid would be of considerable diagnostic value: it would present itself only where there was arrest of passage of feces. This stasis might be due either to a mechanical obstacle or to enteritis or peritonitis simply; and the apparent presence of a small quantity of peritoneal fluid would in such a case be stiongly in favoui of the existence of peiitonitis, and theiefoie against the utility of suigical inteifeience. It was theiefoie necessaiy to iemembei that in cases wheie theie was gieat distension of the intestines with liquid feces, the common physical sign of ascites might exist when theie was no fluid in the peiitoneal cavity.

Dr. COUPLAND mentioned a case of acute intestinal obstiuction (fiom volvulus due to a Meckel's diveiticulum) iecently undei Dr. Cayley's caie in the Middle-sex Hospital, wheie the gieatly distended ideal coils weie so full of flatus and fluid feces that the signs of peiitoneal effusion weie piesent duiing life.

Dr. TAYLOR asked whethei the sign of fluctuation-wave acioss the abdomen was yielded in these cases; still the shifting of dulness of the flanks fiom change in position was one of the suiest signs of peiitoneal effusion.

Dr. SCERRITT ieplied that no fluctuation-wave was obtained, but that sign was fiequently absent in cases of ascites when theie was yet sufficient fluid to yield dulness in the flanks.

—

Gas in Peiitoneal Cavity in Typhoid Fever.

At a late meeting of the Clinical Society of London (*Lancet*, June 7, 1879), Mi. G. BROWN iead notes of a case of gas in the peiitoneal cavity in typhoid fevei ielieved by puncture. The patient, a young man, aged twenty-one, came undei Mi. Biown's caie for typhoid fevei in Octobei last. The tempeiatuie was high thioughout, ianging fiom 102° to 105.2° duiing the height of the fevei. The case was complicated with double pneumonia. In the thiid week of the fevei tympanites developed, at fiist localized to the intestines, but a few days latei the physical signs indicated that gas had escaped fiom the intestine into the peiitoneal cavity, or was being geneiated in the cavity itself. The distension of the abdominal wall giadually became moie and moie extieme, the tympanitic note entirely masking the hepatic and splenic dulness, and it could be elicited ovei the steinum as high as the aiticulations of the fouith costal caitilages. Thiough upwaid piessuie on the diaphiagm theie was uigent dyspnœa, the in-spiiations ieaching as high as fifty pei minute, and the heait was displaced up-waids and outwaids, so that the apex beat was half an inch outside the nipple, and in a line with it. Mi. Biown pieiced the abdominal wall with a small aspi-iatoi tiocai an inch below the umbilicus, and on withdiawing the canula a iush of gas took place, which continued for seveial seconds. The gas was odouiless. The ielief was immediate; the heait iegained its noimal situation, and in a few minutes the iespiiations fell fiom fifty to thiity-six pei minute. No ill effects followed the opeiation. The patient succumbed, howevei, fiom the lung com-plications thiity-six houis aftei. As to the souice of the gas, Mi. Biown dis-missed the idea of peifoiation of the intestine on the following giounds, viz.: 1st, the giadual development of the gas in the peiitoneal cavity; 2d, absence of symptoms of collapse, which might have been expected had peifoiation taken place; 3d, the fact that the tympanitic condition of the colon and small intestine was unielieved by the opeiation (had the peifoiation existed, gas would piobably have continued to escape into the peiitoneal cavity aftei the opeiation, but of this theie was no evidence, although the patient lived thirty-six houis afteiwaids); 4th, the fact that the gas was odouiless. Mi. Biown advanced two theoiies as to piobable souices of the gas—1st, the gas might have passed by diffusion thiough the intestinal wall: or 2d, it might have been deiived diiectly fiom the blood by exosmosis thiough the delicate walls of the peiitoneal capillaiies; and this was the moie piobable fiom the fact that for seveial days pievious to the distension taking place the blood was highly chaiged with caibonic acid gas, in consequence of impeifect aeiation in the lungs. Mi. Biown said he was unable to decide this point, and prefered to merely record the case in the hope that other observers would be able to throw more light upon the subject, should similar cases occur in their practice.

—

Diffuse Inflammation of the Liver from Phosphorus.

In a paper reprinted from the *Deutsches Archiv für Klinische Medecin*, Dr. ANSPECHT describes experiments made upon rabbits by injecting a solution of phosphorized oil (one in eighty) into the subcutaneous tissue of the back. Three milligrammes was the dose thus administered at each injection. Twenty-one animals were experimented upon; and of these, thirteen died after one injection, two after two, three after three, and the rest after four, five, and nine. The conclusion arrived at is this. Phosphorus, or some modification of it produced in the blood, leads to a series of chemical changes in the liver-cells, with the formation of albuminoid granules and fat-grains in their protoplasm, but the liver-cells are not destroyed. If the subject of the experiment do not die in consequence of these changes, then the liver-cells become completely restored. If the phosphorus be administered in too frequently repeated doses, the albuminoid grains and fat-granules are no longer formed, but the cells become pale and glassy, with distinct nucleus, and the interstitial tissue becomes diseased. The changes observed are compared with those which ensue in the kidney when the ureter is ligatured, and are found to be very similar. The conclusion derived from a review of both sets of experiments is that in either case a parenchymatous inflammation is the primary change; that when the obnoxious element causing this, which may be of various kinds, is at work sufficiently long or sufficiently often to hinder the speedy resolution of the inflammation, secondary changes follow in the interstitial tissue, and an intestinal inflammation is started.—*British Med. Journal*, June 7, 1879.

—

Urinary Phthisis.

TAPRET (*Arch. Gén de Med.*, May and July, 1878) considers urinary phthisis as belonging to the class of affections which Pidoux designated under the name of anomalous phthisis. He thinks that the symptoms by which it shows itself are sufficiently characteristic to enable the practitioner to make a correct diagnosis, and consequently to adopt a rational treatment. So far as regards the etiology of the disease, urinary tuberculosis is essentially an affection of adult age; it seldom occurs in females, but appears in males between the age of 20 and 45. The symptoms present some interesting variations, according as the processus is principally confined to the kidneys, the bladder, the prostatic gland, or the urethra.

Primary or Isolated Tuberculosis of the Kidney.—The symptoms of this affection (hæmaturia, albuminuria, pus in the urine, combined or not with polyuria, spontaneous pains, or pains caused only by pressure on the lumbar region) are not characteristic, and might as well be attributed to other renal affections, such as interstitial nephritis, gravel, etc., thus rendering the diagnosis very difficult. The progress of this affection is generally slow, except in cases where the tubercles develop more rapidly, when death occurs generally at the end of a few months. The patient dies of uræmia, owing to the destruction of the renal tissue.

Primary or Isolated Tuberculosis of the Bladder.—M. Tapret thinks that there really exists a tuberculous cystitis, which has hitherto escaped observation, because attention had been principally directed to the kidneys, and the general opinion was that lesions of the bladder occurred only in very exceptional cases or in the last stages of the disease. The characteristic symptoms of this cystitis are: hæmaturia, appearing at an early stage, so-called premonitory hæmaturia, polyuria, which only shows itself at irregular intervals, and owing to divers causes;

pains in the region of the neck of the bladder and a peculiar tenderness of the bladder, the latter being almost always irritable, and in a permanent state of contraction. In the few cases where it has retained its normal capacity, it is sometimes possible, by passing a sound into the bladder, or rectal examination, to feel a hardened spot on the fundus of the organ. This tuberculous cystitis generally progresses very slowly, and ends in consumption or urinary phthisis, unless some local accident should bring on a cachectic state more rapidly.

Primary or Isolated Tuberculosis of the Prostatic Gland.—This embraces two distinct clinical forms of the affection, a rectal or circumferential form and an urethral or urethro-cystic form. The latter presents the symptoms which are generally attributed to cystitis or tuberculous urethritis, pains during micturition, and while the catheter is being used, blennorhagia, prostatorrhœa, spasmodic retention of urine. During the latter stages of this affection, fistulas generally form, opening from the prostatic gland into the urethra, the rectum, or the perineum. According to N. Tapret's opinion, all those various symptoms of the presence of tubercles in the genito-urinary organs only acquire importance after the urinary tracts, and especially the neck of the bladder, have been invaded by tubercles. When the neck of the bladder has been reached, the disease assumes a characteristic appearance, which is typical, and may be thus briefly defined. An individual, aged from 20 to 40, who has hitherto enjoyed good health, suddenly sees hæmaturias appear without any special cause, and without pain; these are followed after an interval of time, varying according to the individual, by retention of urine, which, however, is easily overcome; then the desire to micturate begins to grow more and more frequent and imperious. The act itself is very painful; the patient passes, with a great deal of pain and trouble, a few drops of urine leaving a deposit of blood-streaked pus in the vessel. At intervals the urine is more abundant, clear, almost normal (nervous urine), or dusky and discoloured (in deeply-seated diseases of the kidney). There is also blennorrhœa of the deep parts of the urethra; the bladder is either small or dilated, the neck painful, the fundus hardened; no traces of any foreign bodies; the renal region is tender to the touch, and the prostatic gland presents a knotted appearance. The general state of health of the patient remains for a long time satisfactory. His temperature is hardly ever raised or his digestion impaired. The principal complaint is that he cannot stand upright without suffering. The progress of the affection is, though slow, yet sure to be fatal, and death is due either to the urinary phthisis or to a complication with acute pulmonary phthisis. All these phenomena, however, are far from having the same semeiological importance, and the most important are: difficulty in micturition, modifications occurring in the character of the urine, and urethral discharges.

1. Difficulty in micturition. There is frequent desire to micturate during the night, accompanied by painful or painless contractions of the bladder, neck of the bladder and urethra. The character of the pain varies, according to whether it occurs in the intervals between micturating or during the act itself. In the first case the patient complains of a feeling of pressure behind the os pubis, at other times there is a burning sensation, which radiates towards the umbilicus, the perineum, and the rectum, or the pain comes on in paroxysms, like renal colics. The patients are melancholy and despair of improvement. The pain during micturition presents generally the following characteristics.

1. The desire to micturate is accompanied by an intense feeling of pain.

2. The pain is only experienced during the first stage of the act, and dies away later on.

3. The pain is experienced towards the end of the act, when the bladder con-

tracts, to expel the last drops of urine. The patients compare it to a sensation of burning heat and stricture of the neck of the bladder.

Modification in the Character of the Urine.—Here we meet with either hæmaturia, polyuria, or pus in the urine. Transitory hæmaturia originates from the kidneys, persistent from the bladder; if only appearing at the end of the act of micturition, it is due to a lesion of the bladder. It has been observed at different stages of urinary tuberculosis. So-called premonitory hæmaturia often occurs when the patient is apparently in good health, and it is either very profuse or very slight. The author has given them the characteristic name of urethral epistaxis, and attaches little or no importance to them. Later on, the hæmaturia is generally very painful, and not very abundant. The blood is not mixed thoroughly with the urine, and is precipitated on the bottom of the vessel, together with the muco-purulent detritus. Considered from a diagnostic point of view, hæmaturia in this stage may be considered as equivalent to hæmoptysis in pulmonary tuberculosis. Polyuria appears either at an early stage of the disease or towards the end, when the kidney is entirely degenerated. In the first case it is transitory, the urine is pale, clear, and does not contain albumen, but varies much as to quantity and quality. In the second case the urine is thick, whitish, changes colour immediately after it has been passed, and deposits a muco-purulent or bloody precipitate, without, however, becoming any clearer. It is generally called renal urine. The presence of pus in the urine is often one of the first symptoms of urinary phthisis. It often continues unnoticed for months or years, while in other cases the patient happens to notice it by chance. It is not a very favourable symptom, as it proves the individual to be under the influence of some diathesis, which is on the point of manifesting itself more clearly and pronouncedly.

Urethral Discharge.—This symptom only appears when the urethral duct itself has been affected by the disease. If the lesion is situated in front of the anterior sphincter, the discharge is incessant, and may be compared to blenorrhagia, but if the prostatic part is the seat of the affection, the discharge merely consists of a few drops of a muco-purulent fluid, which appear before and after micturition.— *London Med. Record,* May 15, 1879.

Prurigo Formicans.

Dr. HILLAIRET, lecturing at the St. Louis Hospital (*Rév. Méd.,* May 3) on a case of prurigo formicans, occurring in a youth of twenty who had been tormented with it since he was six years of age, observed that he could not agree with Professors Bazin and Hardy in believing that this inveterate form of prurigo is curable. In all the cases which he has met with that have commenced at an early period of life, every means that has been tried has failed in effecting a cure, although temporary alleviation may be obtained. The treatment which he has found most successful in attaining this latter object, although a painful and disagreeable one, succeeds in giving relief, which may last two or three months. It is that employed for the rapid treatment of itch. First, the whole of the body is thoroughly washed with "black soap," and immediately afterwards a prolonged bath is taken. On leaving the bath the patient is thoroughly rubbed with sulphur ointment. Next day the same treatment is repeated. It is then suspended for two days, when it is again put into force for the last time.—*Medical Times and Gaz.,* June 14, 1879.

Surgery.

Surgical Carbolism.

Dr. KUSTER has published in Langenbeck's *Archiv*, vol. xxiii, the results of his experiments on poisoning with carbolic acid. The animals (dogs) were poisoned by injecting the drug into their veins in a few cases by subcutaneous injection. When the first method was used, a dose equalling 0.036 to 0.076 per cent. of the weight of the animal proved fatal. The characteristic symptoms of the poisoning were general muscular trembling, alternating with clonic convulsions, sensory troubles, and high temperature. The latter rose either during the operation, if the acid had been introduced into the system by transfusion, or immediately after, if it had been subcutaneously injected; but varied much according to the dose. If small or medium doses were given, the temperature rose constantly (.9 or 1.8° Fahr.) during the hours following the administration of the drug, and fell the next day. If large doses were administered very gradually, the temperature rose suddenly at first and then sank again : but, if they were given at once, the temperature first sank considerably and then rose. These changes of temperature are regarded by the author as being the characteristic effects of carbolic acid. The symptoms of carbolic acid poisoning in man have been classified in three different stages, according to the severity of the case. In the first stage, often the only symptom of poisoning is the change in the aspect of the urine. In the second stage, the digestion is impaired, the pupils move with difficulty, and the temperature is high. This last symptom is regarded by the author as being almost identical with the fever described by Volkmann under the name of aseptic fever. He explains chronic carbolic acid intoxication by supposing that large quantities of the drug, being repeatedly at short intervals introduced in the system, continually deprive the tissues of sulphuric acid by absorbing it, and thus impoverish them. The third and most severe stage of poisoning is characterized by the well known brain-symptoms. Occasionally, muscular trembling and convulsions have also been observed in man, but only to a slight degree. The following conditions seem to predispose the system to carbolic acid intoxication :—1. Anæmia; 2. Septic and pyæmic fevers, and other weakening agents; 3. Infancy; 4. A peculiar individual idiosyncrasy; 5. The spot where the acid has been introduced into the organism. Husemann holds that it is most apt to produce poisoning when introduced into the circulation, less so if given hypodermically, still less if given in the form of enemata, or rubbed into the skin, or applied to internal surfaces, and finally if inhaled. Sulphate of soda has often been recommended as an antidote to carbolic acid, but Dr. Küster has not found it to answer in severe cases. In order to avoid intoxication, he advises to wash out large cavities with an 8 per cent. solution of chloride of zinc, instead of carbolic acid. A 2 per cent. solution of the latter may, however, be used without danger for children and for operations in the abdominal cavity.—*British Med. Journal*, June 7, 1879.

Phosphaturia in Surgery.

N. VERNEUIL has called attention to the fact that N. Tessier, junior, of Lyons, in his Thesis of 1876, says that he had noted the curious coincidence of various affections of the eye, of cataract in particular, with phosphatic diabetes. He related the history of various phosphaturic patients in whom the extraction of the lens had been followed by disastrous effects ; he showed also the influence of phosphaturia on the formation of callus in fractures. These facts had much impiessed Ν. Veineuil, when some chaiacteiistic cases came undei his notice. In 1877, he iemoved a small fibioid tumoui fiom a young lady. Stiuck by the slowness of the cicatiization and the geneially bad state of the patient, he iecognized, on examination, that she eliminated eveiy day by the uiine a consideiable quantity of phosphates. Ν. Tessiei had also obseived extieme slowness in the foimation of callus, aftei a fiactuie of the humeius, in a lady also suffeiing fiom phosphatic diabetes. Ν. Veineuil is not indisposed to believe that theie exists a ceitain ielation between phosphatic diabetes and the oiange-yellow coloui of the pus of ceitain wounds. In 1877, Ν. Veineuil had in his seivice a young man aged 17, who had fiactuied his aim by a ielatively slight effoit; and this man piesented polyuiia and phosphatuiia. Ν. Veineuil cites two othei cases of affections of bone coinciding with phosphatic diabetes.—*Biitish Medical Jouinal*, Νay 24, 1879.

—

Nystagmic Movements of the Eyes caused by Auial Affection.

Dr. PFLÜGER publishes in the *Deutsche Zeitschr für Pract. Med.*, 1878, Νo. 35, and *Centralblatt für die Medicin. Wissensch.*, Νay 31st, 1879, a ease of polyp in the eai, complicated with a chionic puiulent cataih of the middle eai, wheie nystagmic movements of the eyes and tendency to falling invaiiably appeared when the loop that had been put iound the polyp was diawn lightei or even pulled. The authoi explains this case by assuming that the peculiai movements of the eyes weie due to the fact that the iiiitation was piopagated fiom the polyp to ceitain peiipheiic poitions of the biain. This asseition is suppoited by the situation of the polyp, its basis occupying a laige poition of the ioof of the exteinal ioof of the lateial meatus, especially the tegmen tympani, and being immediately in fiont of the tympanum. Hitzig and Curchmann have proved that theie exist in the biain seveial spots which, when stimulated, cause nystagmus.— *Biitish Medical Jouinal*, June 21, 1879.

—

Resection of Seveial Ribs for Enchondioma.

At the last meeting of the Society of Geiman Suigeons, Dr. KOLACZEκ of Bieslau showed a woman aged 40, in whom a gieat pait of the left anteiioi wall of the thoiax had been iemoved by opeiation, so that a laige poition of the lung and of the heart weie only coveied by skin. The inspiiatoiy and expiiatoiy movements of the lung, and the contiactions of the heait, could be seen even at a distance; the contiactions of the left auiicle and ventiicle could be distinctly felt with the hand. The patient was admitted into the hospital at Bieslau last yeai, on account of a tumoui occupying the left fiont of the chest. It was an enchondioma as laige as a man's head, and was intimately connected with the iibs, fiom which it spiang. Extiipation was commenced by a veitical incision ovei the gieatei ciicumfeience of the tumoui. The skin was intact, and was easily dissected off. The iibs weie now divided on each side by bone-foiceps; the costal pleuia, which was intimately adheient opposite the tumoui, was of necessity iemoved. Theie was thus left in the chest-wall an opening moie than a handbieadth in size, extending fiom the thiid to the sixth iib, in which the lung and the peiicaidium with the pulsating heait lay exposed. The opening was coveied with the skin; diainage-tubes weie placed in the uppei and lowei angles of the wound, and a thiid was intioduced into an opening made in the posteiioi pait of the thoiax. The opeiation was done undei antiseptic piecautions. The pleuia was washed out with a two pei cent. solution of caibolic acid, and Listei's diessing was applied. The healing piocess was uninteiiupted; and at the end of foui weeks the patient was dischaiged with only a small fistulous opening at the uppei angle of the wound. The lung was remarkably collapsed, so that the integument was drawn in towards the cavity of the chest; it was only when the patient coughed that it rose to the level of the chest-wall. The heart was not displaced. The woman was in good health, and able to work; but unfortunately there was indication of a return of the disease in the end of one of the ribs.—Professor von Langenbeck said that he had met with a similar case. It was one of sarcoma of the thoracic wall. After extirpation, the patient at first appeared to be doing well; but she died at the end of six months. He attributed the death to chronic poisoning with carbolic acid.—*British Med. Journal*, June 14, 1879.

Successful Gastrostomy.

At the recent meeting of the Society of German Surgeons in Berlin, Prof. TRENDELENBERG, of Rostock, showed a boy aged 12, in whom an artificial opening into the stomach had been made on account of stricture of the œsophagus from swallowing sulphuric acid. The case was shown for the purpose of demonstrating the good condition of the lad, and the manner in which he took food. Into the gastric fistula a conical horn cannula was introduced, and this was closed by a common cork. In taking food, the cork was removed, and an India-rubber tube, a finger-breadth in diameter, and long enough to reach the mouth, was introduced into the cannula. The boy took the food into his mouth, and chewed and swallowed it; but, as it could not pass down the œsophagus, it was regurgitated, and was pressed down through the India-rubber tube into the stomach. Dr. Trendelenburg has done gastrostomy in two other cases, for cancer of the œsophagus. One proved fatal in fourteen days; the other in ten weeks.—*British Med. Journal*, June 14, 1879.

Enteroraphy.

In a report of a clinical lecture by Prof. N. SCHEDE (*Deutsche Medicinische Wochenschrift*, No. 19, 1879), details are given of three cases—one of artificial anus and two of fecal fistula, in which, as cure could not be effected through the usual means, the portion of intestine involved in the disease was removed, and enteroraphy performed. This report is of much interest as a contribution to the statistics of an operation to which much attention has recently been directed by German surgeons, and also as describing certain modifications in the operative method, and in the after-treatment, applied by the author in dealing with his three cases. The operative treatment in each case was carried out with strict attention to antiseptic precautions. In two of these cases complete cure was promptly attained. In the third case a favourable progress towards recovery was suddenly arrested through pulmonary embolism.

The subject of the first case was a very feeble woman, aged forty-three, who, three weeks before she came under the notice of Professor Schede, had suffered from strangulation of a femoral hernia on the left side. An operation performed for the relief of this condition had exposed a coil of gangrenous intestine, and resulted in the establishing of an artificial anus. In the left inguinal region was an opening into which the little finger could be passed, and from which there was a constant discharge of fluid feces. No fecal matter was discharged by the anus. There was a free opening into the portion of intestine above the opening in the groin, but neither the finger, nor even a probe, could be passed into the lower segment. After the patient had for two days been subjected to a preliminary treatment, consisting in evacuation of the portion of bowel above the false anus, in exclusive feeding by clysters, and in frequent administration of opium, the following operation was performed: A vertical incision was first made through the abdominal wall. commencing just above the upper margin of the false anus and carried upwards for a distance of about three inches. The portion of intestine above the opening was then exposed, drawn outwards through the wound, and inclosed temporarily in a stout catgut ligature in order to prevent any flow of intestinal contents during the subsequent steps of the operation. The short piece of intestinal canal between this ligature and the artificial anus having been washed with a 5 per cent. solution of carbolic acid, the upper margin of the outer orifice was cut through and the adhesions of the upper segment of gut were carefully divided. The contracted extremity of the lower segment of gut was then dissected out of a bed of cicatricial tissue and also secured by a ligature of catgut. A wedge-shaped portion of mesentery, corresponding to the interspace between the portions of gut, having been excised, the edges of this membrane were first brought together and fixed by sutures, and afterwards the margins of the two portions of intestinal canal. The catgut ligatures were now removed. These had served their purpose so well that not a drop of fecal fluid had been observed during the operation. Fearing that there might result a failure of uninterrupted primary union between the two applied portions of intestine, and, in order to prevent any discharge of intestinal fluid into the abdominal cavity and consequent fatal peritonitis, Prof. Schede did not at once return the sutured portion of the intestinal canal. The upper and lower portions of the external wound having been closed by sutures, this portion of gut was retained without the middle portion of the wound, and prevented from slipping inwards by a large bent needle passed through the mesentery and the opposite margins of abdominal wall. This exposed portion of gut and the whole seat of the operation were then covered by Lister's dressing. No indications of febrile reaction were manifested during the subsequent progress of this case. The patient vomited soon after the operation, but only once. The dressing was changed on the second day, and again on the sixth day. On the fifth day there was a free discharge of fluid feces by the anus. Subsequently, defecation was regular and normal. On the tenth day the bent needle was removed, and the exposed coil of intestine, then covered by healthy granulations, allowed to fall back into the abdominal cavity. At the end of the fifth week the patient was discharged as cured.

In the second case, a woman aged sixty-two presented a very large irreducible umbilical hernia of ten years' standing. The skin stretched over this swelling was very thin and smooth, and at the most prominent part was a large ulcer, which, at its middle, led down to intestine. Near this ulcer were two small fistulæ, through which almost the whole of the fecal matter was discharged, but a very small portion being passed by the anus. As spontaneous cure was not to be expected in this case, Prof. Schede decided on operative treatment. After incision of the thin and tense skin over the hernia, and exposure and careful separation by dissection of the portions of intestine below the ulcer, two provisional catgut ligatures were applied, as in the former case, and about four inches of intestinal canal cut away, together with a wedge-shaped piece of mesentery. The two portions of intestine were then brought together and united by sutures. A large portion of prolapsed omentum, having been tied in three portions, was next removed. The sutured portion was, as in the first case, retained without the abdominal wound by means of a large bent needle. The patient suffered severely from vomiting on the day of operation, and afterwards progressed favourably until the fourth day, when she died suddenly from embolism of the pulmonary artery. At the *post-mortem* examination the edges of the applied portions of intestine were found to have completely and firmly united. The peritoneum was quite free from traces of peritonitis.

The third case was one of artificial anus in a woman aged fifty-eight. This had resulted from strangulation of a hernia through the linea alba, a little below the navel. It was thought very probable that a portion of jejunum was the part affected, since solid food passed from the artificial anus within one hour after deglutition, and fluids within twenty minutes, the discharged matter being mixed with much unaltered bile. The strength of the patient had been supported by the injection of peptones into the peripheral portion of intestine. A large portion of the feces was discharged at the anus. After unsuccessful trials of all usual means of relief, it was decided to perform enteroraphy. The fistulous opening, which was situated a little below and to the right side of the navel, was included between two curved incisions through the abdominal wall. The knife was then carried upwards and downwards in a vertical direction, so as to enlarge the wound and expose the extremities of the upper and lower segments of intestine. The two portions of intestine were then brought together and united by sutures, as in the first and second cases, but, in consequence of close adhesion of each extremity to the surrounding parts, it was found impossible to draw the sutured coil outwards through the wound. The edges of the incision in the abdominal wall were then brought together and fixed by sutures. This patient made a speedy recovery, and, during the subsequent progress of the case, the temperature remained normal. There was normal defecation by the anus on the fourth day.

The author points out the advantage of temporary deligation of the intestine in the operation of enteroraphy. The proceeding he holds is quite free from danger, and undoubtedly assists the operator and prevents effusion of intestinal contents into the peritoneal cavity and over the raw surfaces. It remains doubtful, he acknowledges, whether any advantage attends the practice of retaining for a time outside the abdomen the sutured portion of intestinal canal. The applied edges of intestine speedily unite by primary adhesion, and effusion of fecal fluid may be prevented through the apposition of other peritoneal surfaces. That the plan is not a dangerous one is proved by the good results in the first ease.—*London Med. Record*, June 15, 1879.

Contributions to the Study of Tuberculous Cystitis.

These contributions of GUEBHARDT (*Etude sur la Cystite Tuberculeuse*, Paris, 1878, A. Delahaye) are based on the study of 33 cases of tuberculous cystitis which, for the greater part, were made at the hospital Necker under Professor Guyon. The author holds that there exist two principal classes of tuberculous cystitis: a primary one, which is not preceded by tubercles in any other organ; and a secondary one, which follows immediately upon tuberculosis of the lungs or the genital organs, and hastens the end. The first class can often remain confined for a certain time to the bladder without spreading to the rest of the organism, and then attack either the genito-urinary tract, or any other organ. The author insists especially on the difference between what is termed urinary tuberculosis, and genito-urinary tuberculosis. The latter is often met with, while the former is more rare and localized in the bladder, urethra, and the kidneys, without spreading to the genital organs. At the *post-mortem* examinations, granulations, which are first gray, then yellow, are always found in the bladder, as well as characteristic ulcerations, either isolated or in groups, of various sizes. These lesions always begin at the neck of the bladder, and spread thence into the urethra, the prostatic gland, the ureters, and the kidneys. The pain is sometimes almost excruciating, and often takes the form of neuralgia; other symptoms are urethral and vesical spasms and hæmaturia. Although these phenomena are not pathognomonic, still they may often help towards making a diagnosis in most of the cases. The treatment consists in painting the neck of the bladder with a weak solution of nitrate of silver.—*London Med. Record*, June 15, 1879.

Use of Chloral in a Case of Retention of the Urine.

TIDD reports (*Archives Méd. Belges*) a case of a young woman in the eighth month of pregnancy, who thought that she had been in labour for twenty-four hours, and had not passed urine during the whole time. The bladder was enormously distended, and protruded far above the os pubis and into the vagina, so that it was impossible to reach the neck of the uterus with the finger. The external genital organs were considerably swollen, and the pain most violent. Unsuccessful attempts were made repeatedly to introduce the catheter, but the organs were so swollen that it was impossible to pass any sound into the bladder. It was then proposed to puncture the bladder, fearing it might burst, but as this was objected to, Dr. Tidd resolved to try chloral, which had been used successfully by some surgeons in similar cases. Accordingly, a solution was prescribed, consisting of ten grammes of chloral dissolved in sixty grammes of water, and given by teaspoonfuls first every half hour, and then after two hours. The patient soon fell into a deep sleep, during which she passed unconsciously an enormous quantity of urine. Seven days later she gave birth to a healthy child, and has not since suffered from retention of urine.—*London Med. Record*, May 15, 1879.

—

Osteomyelitis during Growth.

In the *Revue Médicale de l'Est* for April 15, 1879, p. 226, there is a somewhat interesting discussion on a work of M. Lannelongue on *Osteomyelitis during the period of Growth*, which shows, at any rate, how far the French pathologists are from uniformity of opinion on the subject. "In the opinion of some," as the reporter, M. Heydenreich, says, "the affection always begins with the periosteum and thence invades the other parts of the bone; others think that the medulla is always first attacked; whilst there are, finally, eclectic authors who think that the affection may begin with one or the other of these elements." The author of the work in question, M. Lannelongue, believes that the disease always begins in the medulla, and, therefore, proposes the trephining of the bone as the only means of stopping its course; whilst M. Gosselin denies this proposition, and says that, in many cases, even when the superficial layers of the bone are attacked, the central parts are unaffected. He prefers, therefore, the term "osteitis," whilst he nevertheless admits the advisability of trephining as being always innocuous. So that he would trephine the bone as an exploratory measure, and if medullary cavity is found infiltrated with pus, then enlarge the opening. In some apparent opposition to this teaching, M. Gosselin says that the suppuration in the medullary portion of the bone is a consequence of the superficial suppuration, and takes place chiefly in cases where the free incision necessary to evacuate the matter thus situated has been neglected. M. A. Guérin supports the latter view of the case, and dwells still more strongly on the necessity of freely incising the periosteum, and even prolonging the incision into the spongy tissue of the bone, which, in these cases, is generally softened. M. Lannelongue's view was supported on anatomical grounds by M. Panas, who describes medullary tissue as existing, not only in the central canal of the bone and its neighbourhood, but also in the deeper layer of the periosteum and in the Haversian canals. In accordance with this alleged anatomical fact, M. Trélat points out that the affection in question is most common at the time that the medulla is in greatest abundance, and is most perceptible in the situations where it is in greatest quantity. M. Gosselin, however, denies the anatomical fact, asserting the absence of medulla in the Haversian canals and under the periosteum. The embryonic cells (osteoblasts) have, as he asserts, no histological connection with the medulla of the central canal. Such embryonic cells may, indeed, be found in abundance in inflammatory affections, but they should not be confounded with medulla, or with any proliferation or modification of medulla. And the clinical aspect of the case shows the same thing, according to him : there are in ordinary cases two periods—one of acute fever, in which there are no reasons for thinking that the central parts of the bone are affected ; and the second period, that of suppuration, in which also the pus is in almost all cases confined to the periosteal and superficial parts of the bone ; though there are instances in which the medullary canal is found affected at this period of the disease.

As far as our own experience goes, we think M. Gosselin's pathological and clinical description extremely accurate. As to pathological anatomy, we have had frequent opportunities of proving by dissection that the ordinary acute periostitis of early life does not as a rule affect the central parts of the bone at all, and, in such cases, we cannot support the proposal to trephine the bone (if at least it is proposed to do this at an early stage of the disease), or regard the operation as being in the least degree innocuous. At a later period, when the bone is dead, it would no doubt be safe to trephine it, but it would also be useless. In small bones which have no distinct medullary canal, it is possible that a trephine might give adequate exit to matter ; but, in most of such cases, the total removal of the bone or of the part would probably be the more feasible and the more rational step. To trephine a long bone, such as the tibia or femur in an early stage of acute periostitis (as we generally style the disease) would only complicate the case, and, as it would seem, render inflammation of the central parts more probable. In fact in the experience of the present writer, it is only a very small proportion of cases of acute periostitis in which the medullary membrane or medullary canal are implicated, and, when this is the case, the central inflammation is too diffused to be relieved by anything short of extirpation.

We need not say, then, that we differ materially from the opinion expressed by M. Heydenreich in the following words : "We cannot but be struck by this pathological fact that the periosteum, bone, and medulla, present a kind of solidarity when attacked by the same causes of disease, and are generally simultaneously affected, though in different degrees." True as we hold this to be of the periosteum, and the bone which lies directly beneath it and derives its nutrition exclusively from it, it does not seem to us either true or probable with respect to the medulla, which has quite different anatomical and physiological relations. In fact, we have often been struck in examining cases where acute periostitis has run its fatal course rapidly to see how perfectly unaffected have been the central portions of the bone and the medullary canal. Examined later on, these parts will have perhaps perished along with all the rest of the shaft of the bone ; but this is obviously only a secondary or incidental result of a disease which at first was quite confined to the superficial facts. The point is a very important one when a proposal to trephine the bone is under discussion.

Acute osteomyelitis, as far as we have been able to observe, is a different affection, caused almost always by penetrating wounds, not amenable to treatment by external incision, as acute periostitis very often is, nor in fact to any known treatment short of complete removal.—*London Med. Record*, June 15, 1879.

———

On the Treatment of Gunshot Wounds of the Knee-Joint in time of War.

BERGMANN, who was consulting-surgeon in the Russian army on the Danube (*Centralbl.*, No. 18, May 13), had ample opportunity of testing the superiority of the new methods of treating wounds during the war. He confines himself, however, to speaking of gunshot wounds of the knee-joint, which have hitherto yielded very unsatisfactory results. Thus, during the American war, out of 1000 gunshot wounds of the elbow-joint, 194 proved fatal, while 837 out of 1000 gunshot wounds in the knee-joint, were followed by the same result. The author was soon obliged to abstain from a strict antiseptic treatment, as all the conditions necessary to make this treatment successful were wanting; there were hardly any beds to be had, and the wounded lay mostly on the floor. Herr Bergmann therefore restricted himself to the most simple process of antiseptic dressing, using antiseptic material for the purpose of absorbing the secretions of the wound. This was done in the following way: as soon as possible after the wound had been inflicted, the vicinity of the spot where the shot had penetrated was cleansed, then the whole limb was wrapped in a thick layer of antiseptic cotton-wool, the latter firmly pressed down by means of an elastic bandage, and the whole. including the ankle and hip-joint, imbedded in plaster-of-Paris, and allowed to remain undisturbed for a fortnight or more. In some cases the first application of this dressing sufficed to promote the healing of the cutaneous wounds. The author's pamphlet (published in Stuttgart, 1878) also contains two tables of gunshot wounds in the knee; the first contains all the lesions of the knee which were received into the hospitals at Piätra and Simnitzelli, fifty-nine cases in all, thirty of which were cured, two only after a secondary amputation, five were dismissed with doubtful results as to their being cured, and twenty-four died (44.5 per cent.). This is a by far better result than has been obtained in former wars under much better conditions. If we analyze the cases, we find that out of the twenty-eight cases which were cured without amputation, only in one a considerable suppuration set in, whilst all the others were healed almost without suppuration. Wherever the latter set in, the chances of recovery decreased very rapidly, whether the limb was amputated or not; although it was in nowise strictly limited to the severer wounds. In five cases out of twenty-three which healed rapidly, the capsules had been affected; in several of the other cases, other bones had suffered. Two of the patients who had been cured, died sometime after of intercurrent diseases. At the necropsy, it was found that in one case a fragment of bone had grown into the insertion of the crucial ligaments, and several small pieces of cloth were found in the other patient's wounds. This mode of treatment of smaller gunshot wounds, by keeping the limb immovable, and allowing the wound to heal under the eschar, will be followed by more favourable results if the wound has come under treatment at an early stage, and before the sanguineous infiltrations which have penetrated into the intermuscular connective tissue begin to decompose. The second table contains a list of fifteen cases which were treated in this way, only one of which died of pyæmia (6.6 per cent.). These favourable results speak for themselves, and there can be no doubt, that this method of treatment will hereafter take a prominent place in field surgery.—*London Med. Record*, June 15, 1879.

—

Ligature of the Ischiatic Artery.

M. TILLAUX related (*L'nion Méd.*, May 20), at the Société de Chirurgie, the case of a mason, aged twenty, who, having fallen from a scaffold, was brought to the Beaujon in a state of collapse. There was a fracture of the thigh, with a wound, which, however, did not seem to communicate with the fracture. During the first fortnight all seemed going on well, when a very painful swelling became developed behind the great trochanter. There was fluctuation, but neither pulsation nor *bruit-de-souffle* in the tumour; and, under the belief that it was a subentaneous abscess, a vertical incision was made into it, which was followed by a formidable jet of blood. An aneurism being thus the cause of the tumefaction, a large horizontal incision was at once carried through the gluteus to the ischiatic notch, where the artery was found divided as it left the pelvis. A bony splinter, apparently proceeding from the edge of the sacrum, and to which the production of the false aneurism was doubtless due, and could be felt. The artery was cut through close to the pelvis, and the hemorrhage instantly arrested by a hæmostatic forceps applied to the central end. This was left *in situ* for forty-eight hours. The patient entirely recovered, *forcipressure* here having been of great service, seeing the difficulty of applying the ligature or torsion. M. Tillaux drew attention to the singularity that so large an aneurism should have remained twenty days without its existence having been suspected.—*Med. Times and Gaz.*, June 21, 1879.

On Nerve-Stretching.

A case of convulsions of the face, which was cured by stretching the facial nerve, is related in No. 40 of the *Berl. Klin. Woch.*, 1878, by Dr. BAUM. The patient, a woman, aged 35, who had previously had a few epileptiform attacks, became subject to convulsive twitchings of the muscles of the left side of her face. They lasted generally for one minute at a time, and were repeated every two or three minutes. Finding that all the remedies used, and even the galvanic current, were of no avail, the author resolved to try whether nerve-stretching would prove successful. He accordingly laid bare the facial nerve near the stylomastoid foramen, and, seizing it roughly with a pair of forceps, he lifted the nerve from the surrounding tissue. The left side of the face was paralyzed for about half an hour, after which sensibility had returned, and the convulsions disappeared. The author ascribes a part of his success to the squeezing of the nerve, and points out that there is no danger of paralysis, as the latter, even if it should occur, is transitory.—*London Med. Record*, June 15, 1879.

Epileptiform Neuralgia, Treated by Nerve-stretching.

Dr. T. GRAINGER STEWART, Professor of Practice of Physic in University of Edinburgh, makes the following remarks (*British Med. Journal*, May 31, 1879) on a case of this kind:—

On returning from my autumn holiday, last year, I found among the patients under treatment, in my department in the Royal Infirmary, one who had been sent up from the surgical wards, suffering from epileptiform neuralgia. He was a man of seventy years, and was employed as a station-master on one of the railways of Cumberland. There was no evidence of hereditary predisposition to nervous disease; he was a temperate man, and his surroundings had been for the most part favourable. In his railway work, he had naturally been somewhat exposed to the weather, and a good deal to draughts, but never in any extraordinary degree. He had been perfectly healthy till the year 1862, when he was seized with facial neuralgia. At first, the pain was of a burning character, and it gradually increased in severity, the paroxysms becoming, as time went on, more frequent and intense, until at last his life was almost intolerable to him; indeed, had it not been for the remissions during which the pain was easier, and the periods of immunity during which he was entirely well, it would have been so. These periods of immunity varied in length—sometimes six weeks, sometimes three months, and on one occasion a whole year; but, sooner or later, the attacks returned, and for six or eight weeks he had little freedom from agony, and never for a moment a feeling of security. The attack from which he was suffering at the time of his admission to my wards had lasted from the end of April, and showed no signs of abatement up to the time I saw him. He was a short man, rather thin, but not emaciated, and said he had lost during the past year about a couple of stone in weight; still there was nothing wrong with him, excepting the neuralgia, and often that was not severe. When a paroxysm occurred, his face would suddenly change ; twitching of its muscles on the right side set in, leading to the strangest grimaces ; the agony began simultaneously with the movement, and was most intense in the lines of distribution of the middle branch of the fifth nerve on the right side. The patient would seize his head with his hands and press the painful part with the utmost violence ; would drive his knuckles into the space beneath the malar bone ; would slap his face, tear his hair, twist his body in all directions, and sometimes lose all self-control and shout out in his agony. This would continue for a few seconds, or perhaps a minute or two ; then the pain and other symptoms would subside. The paroxysms might recur almost immediately or not for hours ; generally, they were most severe in the evening and during the night. They were induced easily by touching the skin or pulling the hairs of any part of the area of distribution of the affected nerve, or by touching the gums or tongue. Mastication had thus become impossible, and all food had to be taken in the liquid form ; and no effort was spared, by the use of tubes or other contrivance, to smuggle it past the sensitive region. Nine of the teeth had been extracted in the hope of obtaining relief, but without benefit.

It was clear that the case afforded a typical example of the malady which Trousseau has described as epileptiform neuralgia. No doubt, many of you are familiar with that classical description, and will remember that it includes two varieties : the more common, one in which there is pain without spasm ; the more rare, in which pain and spasm coexist.

A few years of practice had sufficed to satisfy Trousseau that the disease was quite different from ordinary neuralgia of the face, and one of the features was its utter incurability. This feature, along with its suddenness of appearance and disappearance, led him to associate it with epilepsy, and to employ the name now in general use. He sketches several cases with his wonted vividness, of which the following may serve as an example :—

" This poor patient had for many years been subject to the convulsive form of neuralgia. His paroxysms lasted sometimes a few seconds only, and sometimes a minute ; they recurred whenever he spoke, drank, or ate, or whenever one touched with the tip of a finger the few teeth which he had left. The pain was seated in all the branches of the trifacial nerve of one side, but chiefly in the infraorbital division. Several of the nerve-trunks had been divided already ; but the relief had only been temporary, and the pain had always obstinately returned after an interval of from a few weeks to a few months. The extraction of his last remaining teeth gave him no relief. Prolonged applications of a solution of cyanide of potassium did some good ; but, the pain still returning, as awful and as unbearable as ever, I decided upon dividing the infra-orbital branch. Bonnet performed the operation with great skill. The patient was relieved instantly, and remained free from pain for several months. The following year, I saw him again, suffering in the same way in the course of another nerve of the face, and with the same convulsions. Professor Roux, as far as I can remember, again divided several nerves. Lastly, in 1841, Dr. Piedagnel saw in his ward at La Pitié this same individual, whom he had known thirty years previously, when house-physician at the St. Antoine Hospital. The poor man's face was scarred from the surgical operations which he had undergone ; for, whenever the pain became intolerable, he implored the help of the knife, for this at least gave him relief for a few days, and sometimes a few months."

Our poor patient had like Trousseau's, submitted to many plans of treatment, but with a like want of relief. He had had many teeth extracted, as we have seen ; had opium by the mouth, and morphia subcutaneously ; had croton-chloral and other sedatives, quinine and iron, all without result ; and, after a further trial

of many of these, the question arose whether we should dismiss him as incurable
or try yet other remedies.   Experience seemed to show that Trousseau's gloomy
prognosis was better warranted by facts than the brighter one maintained by Dr.
Anstie ; and we certainly could not look with hopefulness to any of the ordinary
methods.   Section of the nerve, or neurotomy, might have been tried ; but the
advantage obtained in former cases had been merely temporary, the pain reappearing as soon as the nerve had healed, or even sooner, or, even at the best, not
being long deferred.   Excision of a piece of the nerve, or neurectomy, had not
produced results conspicuously better.   Neither of these methods, then, commended itself for adoption in this case ; but it seemed to me possible that the
plan of nerve-stretching introduced by Nussbaum, and which had proved so
markedly useful in some similar conditions, might be tried with advantage.   My
first personal experience of that plan of treatment was in 1876, when a patient was
admitted to my wards complaining of various nervous symptoms, and, above all,
of very agonizing pain in the line of the sciatic nerve.   As none of the sedatives
usually helpful afforded any relief, I thought that Nussbaum's plan might be
tried ; and, after consultation with Professor Lister, it was arranged that he should
operate.   He did so with the use of antiseptic precautions, and the operation was
followed by extraordinary relief.   Since that time, it has taken its place in Edinburgh, and has been successfully performed by Mr. Chiene and several other of
our surgeons.

In the absence of Professor Annandale, Dr. Bishop, who was in charge of the
clinical surgical wards, proceeded on October 22d to operate.   With the usual
antiseptic precautions, he cut down upon the infra-orbital nerve at its point of
emergence from the bone ; and, having isolated the nerve, stretched it as vigorously as its size seemed to warrant.   In the course of that day, there were several
severe attacks, and for some time the pain occasionally recurred ; but it speedily
abated, and for a month thereafter there was almost complete immunity.   At the
end of that time, paroxysms recurred ; and on November 28th another attempt
was made to stretch the nerve.   In consequence of the matting of the tissue in
the cicatrix, the nerve was cut through, and the parts became anæsthetic for the
time.   Still the pain continued, and it was soon clear that little or nothing had
been gained by the second operation.   However, on examining the patient closely,
I found that the points of origin and of maximum intensity of the pain were
different from what they had been at first ; that the pain now mainly originated
in the mental branch of the third division of the fifth, instead of in the labial
branch of the middle division ; and I then regretted that I had not had the mental
nerve stretched as well as the infra-orbital.

On December 18th Dr. Bishop proceeded to operate upon it also.   The operation afforded instantaneous relief, and from that day to this there has been no return of the pain.   Last week, I received a letter stating that he had never had a
twinge of pain since the last operation was performed.

Considering that the disease has hitherto yielded to no treatment, it seems that
this case is of considerable value.   It is true that it is but one case, and the practice may not prove equally successful in others.   It is also true that the relief may
not prove permanent.   It is only five months since the last operation was performed, and the patient has had at least one period of immunity as long during
the course of his illness.   But it cannot reasonably be doubted that the present
immunity is due to the operation ; and till evidence turn up to prove its failure,
I think the treatment deserves a trial in every such case.   Indeed, I would say
that, even should the pain recur, the plan of treatment is entitled to take the
foremost place among the remedies for the disease.   With regard to the operation,
there are two points on which I should like to insist : 1. That all the branches

affected should be stretched, and not merely the one in which the disease is chiefly localized ; and 2. That, the nerve being grasped, not merely should traction be made upon the proximal part, but upon the distal also, the lip and cheek being seized and pulled downwards while the nerve is held at the point of emergence.

The case affords an illustration of the associated sympathetic or reflex pain. I think we may conclude that after the first operation there was no paroxysm originating in the infra-orbital nerve, but pain was felt there in association with the morbid action in the line of the third division. I have known of a member of the profession getting, as he said, the whole anatomy of the fifth nerve flashed upon his consciousness by the acute pain produced as he was having a nasal polypus extracted ; and as there was pain felt in all the branches when the one was irritated, so here the pain was irradiated along the nerves which had so long been the seat of morbid action.

As to the *modus operandi* of the procedure, it is impossible to speak positively ; but there is apparently only one condition which such a procedure could relieve, viz., a shrinking or shortening of the nerve from thickening of its fibrous tissue ; but whether this be the correct explanation or not, its utility is beyond question.

—

On Neuralgia of the Infraorbital Branch of the Trifacial Nerve Cured by Lücke's Operation.

The following case was published in the *Deutsche Zeitschr. f. Chir.*, Band xi, Heft 1 and 2, by Dr. AEPLI. The patient, a stonemason, aged 68, had been suffering for fourteen years from facial neuralgia, which he attributed to a violent cold. The pain was principally located in the region of the left infraorbital nerve; it lasted generally from 30 to 60 seconds, and vanished suddenly, to reappear after a longer or shorter interval. The patient's health was generally good. The paroxysms of pain recurred more and more frequently ; sometimes ninety times in twenty-four hours, and became so intense, in spite of all the remedies employed, that it was decided to make the resection of the left infraorbital nerve (Wagner's method). The piece which had been excised was four centimetres long, and the sensibility in the region between the eye and the mouth was totally extinct on that side. Eight months later the patient again presented himself, this time suffering from neuralgia of the right infraorbital nerve, the left side having remained free from pain. Neurectomy was afterwards performed on the right side, but the second operation did not prove as successful as the first, as the patient began to complain of the pain two months subsequently in both sides of the face. It was then decided to attempt a third operation, this time by Lücke's method, i. e., temporary resection of the zygomatic bone. In consequence, however, of the previous operations, it was not easy to find the nerve, so that only small pieces could be excised. The wound was treated antiseptically, and a drainage-tube put in ; on the fourth day, the patient had a few slight attacks, after which, he was completely cured.—*Lond. Med. Record*, June 15, 1879.

—

Treatment of Intercostal Neuralgia by Surgical Operation.

The following case was described by Professor von NUSSBAUM in the course of a clinical lecture delivered at Munich in December last, and reported in the *Aerztliches Intelligenz Blatt*, No. 53, 1878. The patient was a gentleman who during a period of twenty years had suffered from severe and obstinate intercostal neuralgia. In the early stages of the affection there had been only occasional attacks at long intervals. Subsequently these attacks became more frequent, and sometimes lasted for months, and finally the patient suffered very severely from neuralgic pains, coming often in the course of each day, and lasting at times for two or three hours. No relief could be afforded in this case by the subcutaneous injection of morphia. Pressure over the affected region increased the patient's suffering during a paroxysm, but did not excite pain during an interval of ease. The chief seat of the pain was the region between the xiphoid process and the umbilicus; and the patient during each paroxysm suffered from a feeling of constriction around the body at this level.

In consequence of the urgent request of this patient for some therapeutical measure that might possibly give relief, Professor von Nussbaum took into consideration the anatomical conditions of the case in their bearing on the operation of nerve-stretching. The affected nerves were clearly the terminal abdominal branches of the eighth, ninth, and tenth intercostal nerves on each side. It was necessary to find two spots where, without dangerous wounding, these nerves could be exposed and manipulated. The conclusion was finally arrived at that the most suitable wounds for the purpose would be two vertical incisions in the epigastric region, one on each side, and at the distance of a hand's breadth from the outer margin of each rectus muscle. It was regarded as an impracticable operation to reach the affected nerves near the spinal column, and then to expose them to such an extent as to permit the manipulations necessary for stretching.

On November 3d, chloroform having been administered and antiseptic precautions taken, an incision eight centimetres in length was made in the epigastric region on the left side. The soft parts having been divided almost as far as the peritoneum, the three intercostal nerves were exposed. Each nerve was then taken between the thumb and index finger, and then slowly and forcibly stretched. The wound having been closed and covered by antiseptic dressings, a similar incision was made on the right side. Here was some difficulty in exposing the nerves, and in the course of the dissection the peritoneum was wounded. A small portion of omentum that protruded from this accidental wound having been replaced, and the edges of the peritoneum having been brought together by fine catgut, the three nerves were stretched, and the incised parts dressed antiseptically, like that on the opposite side.

During the after-treatment this patient remained free from fever. The wounds were almost quite closed on the twentieth day after the operation, and on the twenty-fifth day the patient returned to his home, having been quite free from neuralgic pains during the whole of this interval. From the last report received from the patient, Professor von Nussbaum learnt that there had been no indications after his return of any recurrence of the neuralgic affection.—*London Med. Record*, March 15, 1879.

Syphilitic Inoculation.

In a lecture upon this subject, delivered at the St. Louis (*Gaz. des Hôp.*, April 8), M. FOURNIER delivered some observations, of which the following is an abstract:—

When a successful inoculation is made, a simple chancre, a special and pathognomonic lesion, is produced, which is easily recognizable at the end of twenty-four or forty-eight hours. It consists of a pustule which, when it has burst, leaves a hollow ulcer with abrupt and incised edges and a yellowish fundus, and is surrounded by an extensive areola, which in a few days may attain considerable dimensions. In relation to diagnosis of syphilis, what is the assistance we derive from inoculation? It renders service to the surgeon by producing the two following results—(1) It enables him to differentiate a simple chancre from a venereal infecting chancre; and (2) to differentiate ulcerated syphilides from simple chancre.

1. *Inoculation serves to distinguish Simple Non-infecting Chancre from Syphilitic Chancre.*—This law reposes on these two considerations—(1) Syphilitic chancre cannot be inoculated on the subject of it; (2) simple chancre can always be inoculated on the subject of it—it is anti-inoculable. Simple chancre is a "strong pus," as it was formerly called, and takes invariably and indefinitely. Liebmann inoculated himself 2700 times with simple chancre, the last chancres being as positive as the first. In a great number of cases we are unable to diagnosticate the quality of a chancre. But the diagnosis of chancre is one concerning which patients are in great haste to be assured. Dismayed, they rush in indescribable anxiety to the surgeon, and desire to be informed at once, yes or no, whether they are the subjects of pox. Whenever, therefore, the objective signs do not suffice to inform the practititioner, inoculation will prove useful in giving precision to his diagnosis.

2. *Inoculation serves to distinguish Simple Chancre from certain Ulcerated Syphilides.*—Some ulcerated syphilides are located on the genital organs, and nowhere else; and then risk being mistaken for simple chancres, from the characters of which they are but slightly distinguished. Their differential diagnosis constitutes one of the greatest difficulties in the diagnosis of syphilis, and the question can only be settled by inoculation. Simple chancre will positively reply to inoculation, while the inoculation of syphilides will prove negative; so that, where there is doubt, inoculation should be performed. In some cases it may render the greatest service. A patient came from the country to consult me, who had been under treatment for more than two years for supposed simple chancres, ulceration having "decorticated" the corpus cavernosum. He absolutely denied having had syphilis, and refused inoculation or even an anti-syphilitic treatment. Returning two months later, the ravages of the phagedæna having increased, he consented to inoculation, which, practised on two successive occasions, proved negative, demonstrating the syphilitic nature of the ulcers. He underwent specific treatment, and the ulceration, which had lasted during twenty-eight months, and was continually extending, became arrested immediately, and in two months had undergone complete reparation, the recovery confirming the diagnosis.

Such are the results which are furnished by inoculation, but it supplies no others, and more need not be sought from it. It will remain mute if we seek for the differentiation of the accidents of the primary period from those of the tertiary period of syphilis. The pus derived from the ulcers of either of these periods will always furnish only negative results. But, even so restrained, the results of inoculation have their value, and more than this cannot be exacted.

Practice, Surveillance, and Treatment of Inoculation.—1. First of all, an absolute precept must be laid down. Inoculation must never be practised except in the interest of the patient. It is morally indispensable that it should never be resorted to unless a practical necessity for it exists. It should never degenerate into an experiment *in anima vile*. If it is a mere question of pure science, the practitioner should experiment upon himself, and not upon his patients. 2. Inoculation should only be practised when a serious indication exists, the importance of which renders the operation legitimate. It should be known, in fact, that inoculation is attended with some danger—the danger, in fact, of a simple chancre which may take on an ulcerative and extensive form, and lead to detachment, lymphangitis, erysipelas, and even phagedæna. No doubt such cases are rare, but they are authentic. I have seen and opened, several times, buboes in the axilla consequent on inoculations practised on the arm; and an example is recorded of phagedæna invading the integument of the thigh, and even placing the patient's life in peril. The practitioner is responsible for the inoculation and the chancre with its consequences that may ensue ; and this he should never forget. Unfortunately inoculations have placed some practitioners in most uncomfortable and painful positions. As a general rule, therefore, we must be discreet in its application, only resorting to it when a serious indication authorizes its employment. 3. Inoculation should never be done except with the full and free consent of the patient, who ought to be informed of what we are about to do, the intention of the procedure, and even the dangers that may attend it. I formally condemn inoculations " by surprise," practised on unconscious patients, thus transformed into subjects of experiment. Medical dignity prohibits such unjustifiable procedures. 4. Where should inoculation be performed? The choice of the region is of no great importance, but preference may be given to that of the deltoid. For the upper extremity being less exposed than the lower to fatigue, the danger of bubo is less ; the cicatrix is covered by the dress, and, being in the vicinity of the vaccine cicatrices, its nature is not observable. 5. A sharp and grooved vaccine lancet is the best instrument for inoculation, being very superior to the needle, pin, etc. Charged with pus from the doubtful ulcer, without scratching or causing bleeding, the lancet is passed into the skin to the depth of one or two millimetres at the most. It should be directed horizontally, parallel to the surface of the skin, as without this precaution it may penetrate too deeply, becoming dangerous and yet less demonstrative. The inoculation should be protected by covering it with a watch-glass, which is fastened on by several circular strips of diachylon. In this way the pustule is allowed its full development without risk of irritation. When a simple chancre is the result of the inoculation it must be treated and healed as rapidly as possible, bringing it to an end while still small. The best means for this purpose is the application of Ricord's carbo-sulphuric paste, made of such proportions of carbon and sulphuric acid as to allow the mixture to attain the consistence of blacking-paste. A small portion is applied to the chancre and kept on its place by wadding. The paste produces a black crust adherent to the tissues, which slowly dries in two or three weeks. It is very rare for this cauterization to fail in its object. Inoculation, thus practised and treated, is an inoffensive practice, exempt from danger, and one that is authorized for the establisment of the diagnosis, and consequently the prognosis, in doubtful cases.—*Medical Times and Gazette*, June 21, 1879.

Midwifery and Gynæcology.

On the Duration of Life of the Fœtus in Utero after the Mother's Death.

This question has been carefully investigated by C. GAREZKY, in his inaugural dissertation, St. Petersburg, 1878 (and *Wien. Med. Woch.*, No. 22, 1879). He has collected 379 cases, in which the Cæsarean operation was performed after death ; 308 infants were extracted dead, 37 showed signs of life, 34 were born alive ; but of these, only five remained alive for some time. The author then gives a sketch of Breslau's experiments on animals, and sums his conclusions up as follows. 1. The fœtus undoubtedly survives the sudden death of the mother. 2. If it can be extracted in the course of the first six minutes, it may be born alive. 3. Six to ten minutes after the mother's death, the child may still be alive, though slightly asphyxiated. 4. Ten to twenty minutes after death, the infant is highly asphyxiated. 5. In a great many cases, the infants are either highly asphyxiated or dead after the first minute. 6. The shorter the time is which elapses between the cause of the mother's death and the ceasing of the cardiac action, the longer the fœtus remains alive. 7. If the mother's death has been caused by some quickly acting poison, the chances for the child's life are greater than when it has been brought on by some other cause.—*British Med. Journal*, June 14, 1879.

—

Spontaneous Delivery After Death, with Extrusion of the Uterus.

Dr. OSTMANN relates the following case in the *Vierteljahrschrift für Gerichtliche Medicin*, Baud xxviii, p. 228. Madame S., who had been married about five months, was suddenly seized with rigors, headache, and vomiting. For about a week, she had been exposed to ill-treatment by her husband, but she had continued her daily work without appearing to suffer from any particular illness. She died suddenly without having experienced any abdominal pain, and without any symptom indicative of abortion. The body was examined twenty-four hours after death. There was a dark discoloration about the abdomen, which was greatly distended. There was no sanguineous discharge from the genital organs; but, at the time of raising the body to place it in a coffin, it was found that a fœtus, with its umbilical cord and placenta had escaped from the vagina. There were no marks of violence on the skin, nor any appearance of wounds or other injuries internally or externally. Putrefaction was far advanced. Between the labia and the inner surface of the thighs, there was a knuckle of intestine about eight inches long, as well as a membranous sac. The mucous membrane of the vagina was of a reddish-brown colour, and at the upper end the canal was laid open, but there was no effused blood. The uterus was found in the membranous sac above described. It was of a dark color; its walls were thin and soft; and its inner surface had a dirty red colour; at the point of insertion of the placenta, it was of a brownish-red. The fœtus presented nothing unusual in appearance. The genital organs were carefully examined. There was no mark of wounding or other mechanical injury upon them, and there was no effused blood. On these facts, the experts who examined the body came to the conclusion that abortion had taken place after the death of the woman. They concluded that if it had taken place during life, there would have been copious hemorrhage. Putrefaction had taken place with great rapidity; the gases evolved had accumulated in large quantity in the intestines and the cavity of the abdomen. The pressure produced by these gases had caused an expulsion of the fœtus, followed by that of the uterus and intestine. According to the observations of Hollmann, the pressure produced by the gases evolved in putrefaction is sufficiently great to lead to a rupture of the genital organs and the extrusion of the intestines. The rapid putrefaction of the body had caused in this case, by gaseous pressure, an annular rupture of the uterus and the expulsion of this organ.—*British Med. Journal*, June 7, 1879.

———

Medical Jurisprudence and Toxicology.

Infanticide: Destruction of the Child During Delivery.

The following case is narrated by Dr. EBERTZ in the *Vierteljahrschrift für Gerichtliche Medicin*, Band xxviii, page 215. A maid-servant, H., became pregnant by her master. The girl slept with her mother, aged 71, who had formerly been a midwife, but had long ceased to practice. She was delivered during the night, but the delivery was kept secret. Two days afterwards, the authorities discovered that the girl had been recently delivered. The dead body of the child was found under the bed; the left arm being separated from the body. An inspection showed that the child had not breathed after delivery, and

that it had died either before or during labour.   The skin had a grayish blanched
appearance.   The left half of the thorax, the left shoulder, and the soft parts
about the left arm had a reddish-brown colour.   Blood, partly liquid, was diffused
in the cellular tissue and in the muscles.   The tissues had been cleanly cut in a
circular form ;   the forearm found with the body fitting evenly into the wound.
The left clavicle was dislocated.   The experts came to the conclusion that death
had taken place from hemorrhage.   The skin was pallid.   There were no cadaveric spots and no patches of lividity, the internal organs were generally pale, the
cerebral sinuses empty, and the heart bloodless.   The hemorrhage had been
caused by a wound of the brachial artery in the separation of the arm by a cutting instrument.   No information could be procured of the mode in which the
delivery had been effected.   The old midwife, who had died five weeks after her
confinement in prison, had stated that it was a breech-presentation, that the child
had come into the world dead, and with its body in the state in which it was
found.   The accused, H., admitted that her mother had assisted in the delivery,
but that her sufferings were too acute to allow her to form an idea of what she
had done.   She further stated that an arm had presented itself, and that the
body of the child did not pass until about a quarter of an hour afterwards.   From
these facts, the experts concluded that there had been a presentation of the left
shoulder, and that the dislocation of the clavicle proved that there had been very
forcible traction of the arm ;   further, that the tearing off of the arm had been
effected during life.   This could not have been done by the girl herself, because
the arm of the child was in the vagina.   The midwife had therefore used criminal
violence during delivery, a fact proved by the extravasations of blood in the soft
parts.   They also inferred that the midwife, finding that a shoulder presented,
endeavoured to turn it, and, from ignorance, used undue force by pulling the
hand.   This led to extravasation of blood and dislocation of the clavicle.   It
was at this time that the arm was cut off, and after this delivery was accomplished.
Dr. Spillman, who reports the case, observes that it is of some importance as
showing, in reference to a child which has not breathed and which has not lived
after birth, that such violence may be inflicted on it as to cause its death during
delivery and while still within the body of the mother.   The extravasations of
blood in and about the tissues of the shoulder manifestly proved, in spite of the
absence of the signs of respiration, that the child was living when this violence
was applied to it, and that its death was owing to these injuries.   [There can be
no doubt of the correctness of this opinion.   Although the lungs did not furnish
any evidence of life from the establishment of respiration, the evidence that the
child was living is sufficiently proved by the condition of the body ;   this showed
that there was a free circulation going on at the time when the violence was inflicted.   In England, this case would have been dismissed, as there would have
been no proof of the child having been born alive ;   and without that proof, under
the present state of the English law, the destruction of a child during delivery
or in the act of birth is not murder.   In the above case, the killing of the child
appeared to arise more from blundering ignorance than from any intentional
act ;   hence it must be regarded as rather a case of manslaughter than of murder.]
—*Brit. Med. Journ.*, June 28, 1879.

Hygiene.

Experiments on Disinfection.

Two sets of important researches on disinfection have been lately going on at
Berlin.   In both, the test of the efficacy of the particular disinfectant used has

been the effect produced by it either in destroying bacteria and vibriones in putrid fluids exposed to its action, or in preventing their development in a form of "Pasteur's fluid," in which the objects that had undergone disinfection in various degrees were immersed.

The first experiments, those of Dr. MEHLHAUSEN, Director of the Charité Hospital, refer chiefly to the disinfection of rooms in which scarlet fever and other infectious cases have been. The result arrived at is that the most energetic and the cheapest disinfectant is sulphurous acid. Chlorine gas has the disadvantage of destroying clothes and furniture exposed to it, while it is less easy to manipulate, and four or five times as expensive as sulphurous acid. Twenty grammes of sulphur per cubic metre of space destroy, when burnt in a closed room, all bacterial life in sixteen hours. Besides blocking up the doors and windows, Mehlhausen advises that the room shall be previously warmed, if the weather is cold, in order to prevent the gas finding its way into the neighbouring apartments. It is also advisable to damp the floor before lighting the sulphur, so as to profit by the great solubility of sulphurous acid in water. Eight hours is long enough to keep the room shut up after the sulphur begins to burn, and at the end of that time any clothes or bedding in it will be effectually disinfected. Mere free exposure of an infected room to the air by allowing the windows to stay open several days is not enough to disinfect it. This has been practically proved at the Charité Hospital after scarlet fever and measles in several instances.

The second series of experiments were made by Dr. WERNICH, of Breslau, in the chemical laboratory of the Berlin Pathological Institute (*Centralblatt Med. Wiss.*, No. 13, 1877), upon the disinfecting power of sulphurous acid and of dry heat. The method adopted consisted in preparing an "infecting material" by steeping woollen threads, pieces of linen-rag, and cotton-wool, previously proved to be free from atmospheric organisms, in putrid solutions of fæces or meat, and gently drying them. These substances were then tested for their capability of producing bacteria by means of the modified Pasteur's fluid above mentioned, which consisted of distilled water 100 parts, cane-sugar 10 parts, ammonium tartrate 0.5 part, and 0.1 part potassium phosphate. This solution was freshly prepared before each set of experiments, filtered, boiled for half an hour, and immediately poured into the test-glasses and preserved with the usual precautions. To test the effect of disinfection, the wool or wadding, after exposure for a definite time to a definite degree of heat in an oven, or to a measureable volume of sulphurous acid in a bell-glass, was immediately transferred to the Pasteur's fluid, and the efficacy of the disinfectant was estimated by the rapidity of development of bacteria if such appeared, or by their complete absence, as indicated by the fluid remaining perfectly cloudless. It was thus found that 3.3 per cent. of sulphurous acid by volume failed even after many hours to prevent the development of bacteria, but that if the amount of gas reached from 4.0 to 7.15 per cent. by volume of the contents of the bell-jar, and the process had gone on for at least six hours, no bacteria at all developed. On the other hand, while exposure to a temperature of 110° to 118° Cent. even for twenty-four hours failed to destroy the bacterial germs, five minutes' exposure to one of 125° to 150° Cent. invariably succeeded, and the test fluid remained clear even for eleven days or longer. Dr. Wernich specially reminds us that his results must not be taken as applicable to all forms of bacteria, some of which probably require severer measures for their complete destruction. He also points out that it is easier to disinfect wool than linen, and that cotton wadding is the most difficult of all to free from infectious germs.—*Med. Times and Gaz.*, June 7, 1879.

CONTENTS.

Published Monthly, price $2.50 per annum, free of postage.
Also, furnished together with the AMERICAN JOURNAL OF THE MEDICAL
SCIENCES *and the* MEDICAL NEWS AND LIBRARY *for* SIX DOLLARS *per
annum in advance, the whole free of postage.*

HENRY C. LEA, Philadelphia.

THE MONTHLY ABSTRACT

OF

MEDICAL SCIENCE.

VOL. VI. No. 9.   **For List of Contents see last page.**   SEPTEMBER, 1879.
Entered at the Post-Office at Philadelphia as Second-class matter.

Anatomy and Physiology.

The Structure of Brunner's Glands.

A few years ago it was generally accepted that the special glands found in the duodenum—the glands of Brunner—belonged to the same type as, and probably subserved, functions similar to, the salivary glands and pancreas. They were considered to belong to the type of compound racemose glands until, in 1872, Schwalbe showed that many of them also conformed to the type of compound tubular glands; and now we find M. RENAUT, one of the pupils of Ranvier at the College of France, declaring that none of them partake of the racemose structure, but that all may fall under the head of compound tubular glands. He develops this in a brief article in a recent number of the *Progrès Médical;* and as it involves some facts of interest in histology it may be worth while to reproduce the gist of his remarks in this place.

At the commencement of his paper M. Renaut gives a brief description of an ordinary racemose gland—*e. g.*, the parotid. It consists of a number of poly-hedral acini, composed of secreting gland-cells, which empty their contents into an *intralobular* collecting tube from which the acini of a lobule depend like grapes upon their pedicles. These canals are lined by striated cylindrical epithe-lium containing large oval nuclei, seated on a delicate basement membrane. They open into a series of larger ducts, the *interlobular*, the epithelium of which is often stratified, whilst the wall on which it is placed is more or less lamellated. These tubes in turn open into the main excretory duct, the *interlobular*, typified by the ducts named after Steno and Wharton in the salivary glands, the epi-thelium of which consists of cylindrical and calciform mucus-secreting cells.

Now the duodenal glands do not conform to this acinous type. They may be divided into two groups: the inner or superficial, which are lodged within the muscularis mucosæ; and the outer group, which lies in the lax submucous tissue outside the muscularis mucosæ. The first group forms a very distinct layer visible beneath the villi and the crypts of Lieberkühn. When closely examined, they are seen to be composed of multifid cul-de-sacs—comparable to much-divided fingers of a glove,—a central canal from which lateral diverticula spring, without any change in calibre, the connective tissue at the point of entrance forming a spur-shaped prominence, so that if deprived of its epithelium the interior of the ramified glandular cavity would present a villous appearance. The surface of a section may present many circular spaces, as in acinous glands; but if the section have traversed the tubes in their long axis, the true character of the diverticula is seen, and the projections at their points of attachment to the collecting tubes are rendered manifest. Each gland-lobule is composed of some fifteen to twenty cul-de-sacs, opening into one another, all lined by the same kind of epithelium. There is no change in type of the epithelium as in an acinous gland; for it consists, in the main tubes as in the branches, of translucent prismatic cells, having flattened nuclei at their bases; they are somewhat columnar, and are filled with mucus, as in the muciparous glands of the œsophagus, bronchi, and pylorus. A protoplasmic process can generally be seen passing from the base of each cell to anastomose with similar processes from its neighbours, forming thus a delicate meshwork on which the cells are seated. There is no subepithelial endothelium, the underlying fixed connective-tissue corpuscles being separated from the epithelial layer by a thin, translucent, non-nucleated membrane. The secondary and tertiary diverticula all open into the same larger collecting tubes, of which the epithelium, although more flattened, has the same mucoid contents. The main collecting tube or duct passes vertically upwards to open by itself on the surface of the mucous membrane at the bottom of a deep linear sulcus, or else opens into a Lieberkühnian gland. In the latter case the transition of the epithelium is very distinct, the character of the Lieberkühnian cells being columnar with striated free border, and granular contents, intercalated with calciform cells. This fact, that Lieberkühn's crypts frequently serve as excretory ducts to Brunner's glands, has not been hitherto noted.

The outer, submucous, or intermuscular group of Brunner's glands do not form a regular series, but are grouped in voluminous lobulated masses, which in general configuration simulate the racemose type. But here, just as with the inner group, they are composed of multifid digitate tubes, but arranged on so complex a plan as to give the appearance of acini when divided transversely; where the section has divided them longitudinally their real conformation is apparent. The excretory tubes passing from this deeper group may receive accessions from the glands of the superficial group on their way through the muscularis mucosæ; whilst some open directly on the surface, others terminate in a Lieberkünian crypt. From this it will be seen that M. Renaut proves that Brunner's glands pertain all to the compound tubular type, and not to the racemose; he compares their disposition to a fasciculated root, rather than to a bunch of grapes. He further believes that these glands are differentiated for the secretion of a peculiar kind of mucus; holding that the absence of any granular material in the cells shows that they do not possess the characters of cells which secrete a special ferment as well as mucus; and he points out that the true mucous glands of the œsophagus and bronchi have a similar fundamental structure. His paper concludes by pointing out the pathological fact that a diffuse papillary growth may conceivably arise in the seats of such glands under the influence of chronic inflammatory processes, the spur-like projections at the points of connection between the cœca and the collecting tubes giving rise to such papillary outbuds. He thinks this is to be very commonly seen at the site of laryngeal mucous glands in the neighbourhood of tubercular or syphilitic ulceration, but it has not been noticed in the duodenum. We may add that possibly the rare occurrence of cylindrical epithelioma of the duodenum may also take its rise in these glands.

M. Renaut's observations have been made on the human subject, and under peculiarly favourable conditions. He has been enabled to remove the first portion of the duodenum from the body of a decapitated criminal, about thirty minutes after death, when the heart could still be made to contract by mechanical irritation. The portions removed were hardened in alcohol, and in solutions of gum and alcohol; and the microscopical sections variously stained with purpurine, picrocarmine, and a new reagent, which he terms "primérose hæmatoxylique," prepared by mixing a solution of eosin with hæmatoxylin solution.—*Lancet,* August 2, 1879.

Action of the Succus Entericus in Man.

Dr. BERNHARD DEMANT (*Centralblatt f. d. Med. Wissenschaften*, Feb. 15, 1879) has had an opportunity of studying the secretion and action of the succus entericus in the human subject. The patient, who had been badly operated on for hernia, had a large fistula at the lower part of his small intestine, which was so situated that the alimentary canal was completely divided into two parts; of these, the upper portion communicated with the stomach, whilst the lower part, which secreted the pure juice, terminated as usual in the rectum. With the succus entericus thus obtained, the author has performed many artificial digestions with the following results. The secretion obtained from the intestine of man is a thin clear fluid with a strongly alkaline reaction. Its secretion generally takes place in small quantities; during digestion, however, more is formed than at other times, and at night it ceases to be secreted. Aperients have no influence upon the secretion, either as regards its nature or its digestive power. The succus entericus contains no peptic (albumin digesting) ferment, and it has no influence upon the various forms of proteid materials, such as boiled fibrin and albumen, casein, vegetable fibrin, and legumin. Starch is converted by it into grape sugar; cane sugar is changed into grape sugar. Inulin, however, which has been proposed for diabetic patients as a substitute for bread, is not converted, by digesting with this juice, into grape sugar. Fats containing free fatty acids are emulsified, but neutral fats remain unacted upon. Dr. Demant promises to publish a further account of these important researches into the nature of a secretion which has given rise to so much controversy, in a future number of Virchow's *Archiv.*

Cerebral Localization.

M. BROWN-SEQUARD has communicated to the Société de Biologie of Paris a series of facts in support of his views regarding cerebral localization and of his objections to current theories, and an abstract of his communication has been published in the *Gazette Médicale.* He divided, in a rabbit, the left lateral half of the pons, with the effect of causing complete anæsthesia of the left paw. Dividing then the posterior columns of the cord at the level of the tenth dorsal vertebra—a section which is usually followed by hyperæsthesia of the posterior extremities—he found that the anæsthesia persisted on the left side, hyperæsthesia being present on the right. He then completed the hemisection of the cord by dividing the rest of the left half; on this side the anæsthesia gave place to hyperæsthesia, while the insensibility was transferred to the other. Hence M. Brown-Séquard draws the conclusion that in lesions of the brain the anæsthesia does not depend on the damage to the conducting fibres, but on an influence exerted at a distance upon the spinal cord.

In another series of experiments he divided the right corpus striatum, and in most cases the result was a paralysis of both left limbs. Having then divided the pons upon the same side, the left-sided paralysis disappeared, and a paralysis of the right side came on. Thus the crossed paralysis was replaced by a direct paralysis. Hence he concludes from these facts that identical results can be obtained experimentally for both motion and sensation, and that it is possible, by suitable sections, to transfer the paralysis from one side to the other.

In a third series of experiments M. Brown-Séquard found that if, in a dog, for example, the excito-motor zone of the brain be exposed, galvanization of this region will readily excite movements in the opposite limbs. If then the corresponding half of the pons be divided, the movements caused by galvanization, instead of being lessened, are rather increased, unless the animal is in a state of syncope. Hemisections of the crus and of the motor regions of the medulla have given similar results with a few exceptions. In an animal in which the right motor half of the pons had been imperfectly divided, the left half of the medulla was afterwards divided. There remained then, as means of communication between the two tracts, only a small portion of the anterior longitudinal fibres of the right side. But in this case galvanization of the motor centres on the right side and on the left produced exactly the same movements in the limbs on the opposite side to the centres galvanized. This experiment, repeated a certain number of times, has always given the same results.

M. Brown-Séquard has promised to furnish soon the complementary proof from experimental lesions of the motor centres. At present he believes himself authorized to declare that a somewhat profound lesion of these centres determines, not a true paralysis, but motor disorders with an alteration of the muscular sense ("pseudo-paralysis"). The complete removal of the motor centre produces the same effect. On the other hand, if this motor centre is removed by an incision beyond its limits, so as not to irritate or injure it, slight functional disorders may be observed during the first few minutes, but even the "pseudo-paralysis" ultimately disappears. These experiments are, we need not say, of the highest importance, and no doubt will receive the attention they certainly deserve.—*Lancet,* June 28, 1879.

Materia Medica and Therapeutics.

The Antifebrile Effects of Cold Enemata.

In the *St. Petersburg Med. Woch.* of June 14, M. LAPIN, one of the *internes* of Prof. Manassein's clinic, gives an account of the trials that have been made there of cold clysters as an antipyretic means. After noticing the few observations upon the subject which have already been recorded, he gives an account of the fifty observations which he has made in Prof. Manassein's wards. Of these he has published a detailed account in a Russian journal, confining himself in the present communication to a general statement of the results.

Prior to the administration of the clyster the temperature of the patient was taken, while lying on his back, in the axilla, the hypogastric region, and the rectum. The temperature of the litre of water employed varied from 5° C. to 10° C. (41° F. to 50° F.), and Hegar's apparatus at a pressure of two feet was used for the administration. After the water had been discharged the temperature was again taken in the same localities. Of the fifty trials, twenty-six were made on fever patients, twelve on patients with non-febrile diseases, and twelve on persons in health. From these trials the following conclusions are drawn— 1. Cold clysters form a practical means of reducing temperature, the influence of which continues for a considerable time. After clysters at 10° C. the temperature scarcely reaches its former height in the axilla for from thirty to forty minutes, in the hypogastrium after an hour, and in the rectum after an hour and a half. With clysters at 5° C. the cooling in the axilla lasts for forty or fifty minutes, but in the hypogastrium and rectum it lasts a much longer time than when water at 10° C. is used, so that the prior high temperature has never been observed to be regained until from two to two and a half hours after. 2. The clysters at 10° C. are well borne in all cases without exception, sometimes leaving behind them a pleasant sense of coolness extending over the whole body. Those at 5° C. are by some just as well borne, but in others they induce unpleasant sensations in the abdomen. In recurrent fever even shivering may be produced. 3. The depression of temperature is more considerable in cases of fever than in non-febrile affections, and in the healthy. (In the fever patients the fall of temperature varied from 0.60° to 0.40° in the axilla, from 1.50° in the hypogastrium, and from 5° to 1.70° in the rectum. In non-febrile cases it varied from 0.40° to 0.30° in the axilla, from 1.40° to 1.10° in the hypogastrium, and from 1.60° to 1.30° in the rectum. In healthy persons it varied from 0.60° to 0.30° in the axilla, from 1.30° in the hypogastrium, and from 2.60° to 1.40° in the rectum.) 4. Not only is the temperature diminished, but also the number of the pulse and respiration to a small extent. 5. The greatest diminution of temperature takes place in the rectum ; next in the hypogastrium, and least in the axilla. 6. An advantage of the cold clysters as an adjuvant of other energetic antipyretic means consists in their fulfilling other indications besides the depression of temperature : *a.* They remove the accumulation of masses of feces, which so frequently occurs in fevers; *b.* They diminish meteorism by contributing to the removal of gases ; *c.* In this way they render possible greater freedom in the movements of the diaphragm, and remove a source of self-poisoning of the economy by means of the gases; *d.* To a certain extent, they diminish the afflux of blood to the organs in the vicinity of the rectum, especially the uterus and bladder. 7. Stools follow the use of the clysters at different times in different individuals, varying from a quarter of a minute to two minutes and a half. 8. There can be no doubt that, when a clyster is also indicated in non-febrile cases, the cold clyster should be preferred to the warm in all those cases in which, besides the emptying of the intestine, it is desired to produce a tonic effect on the canal, or to diminish the amount of blood in the pelvic organs.—*Med. Times and Gazette*, July 19, 1879.

Pilocarpine and its Action in Ocular Therapeutics.

GALEZOWSKI'S experiences, confirmed by others, have demonstrated (*Ann. di Opthal. Zunglind*, Ann. 7, Fascie. 4) that pilocarpine instilled into the eye has a myotic action stronger than eserine. He has remarked, also, that nitrate of pilocarpine acts less actively than chloral hydrate. He adds that pilocarpine can be very usefully employed when the prolonged use of eserine has provoked irritation in the conjunctiva. M. Rasupoldi has remarked that every time he has instilled a drop of pilocarpine into the eye of a cat, a very abundant salivation has been produced in about ten minutes. He has seen hypodermic injections of pilocarpine diminish very sensibly the urinary secretions in cases of insipid diabetes. In affections of the iris, or kerato-conjunctivitis, he has obtained very good results by employing either an infusion of jaborandi, or hypodermic infusions of pilocarpine.—*London Med. Record*, July 15, 1879.

Silkworm-gut Sutures.

Mr. J. HOPKINS WALTERS recommends (*Medical Times and Gazette*, June 28, 1879) silkworm- or fishing-gut as a material for sutures, its chief excellence consisting in its causing little or no irritation when embedded in the tissues. The way in which the latter tolerate its presence is wonderful, far surpassing either fine silk or silver wire, and, being perfectly soft while contained in moist structures, it remains pliable, admitting of, and participating in, the movements of these, instead of being stiff and resisting like wire. Another valuable quality is its comparative indestructibility, in this greatly differing from catgut, which, after a few hours, becomes completely softened and disintegrated, and finally incorporated with the surrounding tissue.

Fishing-gut maintains its integrity for many weeks, its strength seeming in no

way impaired after removal. Its peculiar structure seems to render it almost as
incapable as wire of becoming impregnated with the discharges from wounds which
so often make silk injurious, if not absolutely dangerous. When Mr. Walters
first used this material he always steeped it for a minute or so in glycerine of carbolic acid, but he has neglected to do so for a long time past and does not find
that it makes any difference.

Medicine.

Giuntoli on Acute Rheumatism in Infants.

This affection, strange to say, was entirely unknown to the ancients. It is
never mentioned by them in any of their writings (*Lo Sperimentale*, Nos. 11 and
12, 1878, and *Med. Chir. Rundschau*, No. 3, March 1879). In 1837, Berton,
speaking of it, says that it is a comparatively rare occurrence ; but since his time
many authors have given a great deal of attention to the subject. Although it
may be said that no age is safe from this affection, still it is seldom met with
before puberty, and only in very exceptional cases before the age of five. In
England, however, it seems to occur more frequently than in other countries
probably owing to the dampness of the climate.

Chomel says that he only met with two cases in infants and seventy-two in
adults. Roger is more fortunate in this respect, as he sees on the average twelve
cases in infants in a year. The progress of the disease on the whole is about the
same as in adults, except that neither the fever pains nor sweating attain the same
height ; the subacute form is the one most frequently here met with. The disease
does not always manifest itself at first by pains in the joints ; in a great many
cases the prodromi consist in pains in the muscles, a general feeling of prostration,
and headache, or a slight angina ; this state sometimes lasts for a week or more.
The temperature seldom rises beyond 100.4, except in cases of severe complications. The patients suffer a good deal from gastric and intestinal troubles, and
from profuse epistaxis ; sudamina never appear. Notwithstanding the tendency
to delirium peculiar to children, they are seldom delirious except in cases of cere-
bral-rheumatism. The pains are generally restricted to the joints of the lower
extremities, and seldom spread to the hands ; in very few cases are they sufficiently severe to prevent sleep. The skin is never discoloured, even if there
should be considerable swelling ; the number of joints affected varies very much,
but the affection very rarely confines itself to only one joint. According to the
majority of authors on this subject, the affection seldom lasts longer than 8 to 15
days, which is shorter by a week than in adults; during convalescence the patients are generally very anæmic, and suffer from excessive prostration.

A simple articular rheumatism very seldom ends fatally, except if new complications should arise, but the child, even if once cured, is never safe from new and
repeated attacks ; it might indeed be said that they are quite the rule. In most
cases the heart is also affected, and either remains diseased, or a rheumatic diathesis is gradually developed, which later on manifests itself in a new form with
choreiform movements. In some cases even suppuration has been known to
occur. Affection of the heart and pleura in rheumatism must never be regarded
as a complication, but merely as a spreading of the disease to other serous membranes ; the nervous system is also much exposed to rheumatic attacks, evidenced
by the frequent cases of chorea and cerebro-spinal meningitis, affections designated by Giuntoli under the felicitous name of visceral rheumatism. That the

heart should remain free is quite an exception, as in three-fourths of all the cases where the heart is not affected from the very first, it is sure to suffer later on.

Another phenomenon which has been observed more frequently in infants than in adults, is that the cardiac affection precedes the articular affection. According to Roger, endocarditis is the most common complication, endo-pericarditis is not quite so frequently met with, and pericarditis still less so. The former is not always recognized in its first stages, as the symptoms under which it generally manifests itself are a slight fever, pains in the region of the heart, and occasionally very severe dyspnœa. Often the only symptom betokening the affection of the cardiac valves, consists in a slight blowing murmur, which is strongest at the apex of the heart, and accompanies the ventricular systole. The prolonged existence of the cardiac bruits is one of the surest diagnostic symptoms by which the organic bruit may be distinguished from the anæmic murmur which so frequently occurs in rheumatism ; the former is also always restricted to the base, and does not extend in the direction of the large vessels. As a cardiac complication is not always accompanied by fever, and might therefore easily be overlooked, it is of great importance never to omit making a thorough examination of the heart. Whether ulcerous endocarditis ever occurs in rheumatism has not yet been sufficiently proved. Slight affections of the endocardium often pass away entirely after several months, without leaving any traces (Trousseau) ; in other cases some pathognomonic symptom appears much later ; but frequently the heart struggles painfully for years against the obstacles which exist near the valves. Palpitations and troubles in breathing appear next, and sooner or later, spontaneously or by means of some intercurrent affection or a relapse of rheumatism, the circulation is more and more disturbed, dropsy and other organic diseases appear and multiply, and the patient succumbs often many years after the appearance of primary endocarditis to cardiac cachexia. Bouillaud mentions the case of a woman, aged twenty-nine, in whom the existing cardiac disease was evidently due to an acute attack of rheumatism, which had occurred in her tenth year. Guersant and Bamberger mention other cases which ended fatally after a much shorter duration. Pleuritis has been considered by all authors as a frequent complication of rheumatism. Roger even asserts that he has met with it more often in infants than in adults. Bilateral pleuritis complicated with cardiac affection is considered very dangerous ; there is nothing characteristic in its course, as it is often latent and not accompanied by pain. Rheumatic pneumonia is, according to Grisolle, a very rare disease, which he has only observed once in a girl aged seventeen. Fuller says that this complication is more frequently met with, and he accordingly mentions two cases of girls, aged respectively twelve and fourteen ; they both ended fatally. Claisse had a boy, aged eight years, under his treatment, who was suffering from a complication of acute rheumatism with endocarditis and broncho-pneumonia ; a few days later a second complication arose, in the shape of bilateral pleuritis and pericarditis ; but notwithstanding this series of complications, the patient recovered after eighteen days. The nervous system is very frequently the seat of rheumatic manifestations. Cerebral and spinal affections have been observed in children as often as in adults, but the most frequent form under which they manifest themselves is chorea, which is a characteristic symptom of the latter affection in infancy.

Cerebral rheumatism, which Bouchut has never observed, has been met with in children in all the forms which are peculiar to adults. The author reckons among these delirium, which he does not consider as a reflex, but as a diathetic symptom. He also mentions a case in which, two days after the first manifestation of articular pains, opisthotonos and grave cerebral symptoms set in, and death ensued on the fourth day. As a rule, however, this affection always seems

to accompany other complications. Chorea St. Viti has been very frequently
met with in rheumatism. Roger regards it as a necessary concomitant of cerebral rheumatism. Trousseau records several cases where cerebral rheumatism
and chorea apparently mutually compensated. That both affections should be
so frequently combined is a phenomenon peculiar to infancy. A more or less
considerable intellectual disturbance has often been also noticed in the course of
rheumatism; it varies considerably in duration, and is generally combined with
chorea (Griesinger's prolonged form of encephalopatia rheumatica and Mesneti's
folie rheumatique). The apoplectic form of cerebral rheumatism is as rare an
occurrence as the foregoing one. According to Roger, the prognosis of cerebral
rheumatism in children is less unfavourable than in adults, and may even be said
to be favourable if chorea or delirium are the only complications which arise.
In 1850 Professor Sée was the first to point out the frequent coincidence of chorea
with articular rheumatism; to-day no one doubts that they are connected. Trousseau mentions seventy-one cases in which chorea occurred, either together with
articular rheumatism or cardiac affections, or alternating with them; he regards
both the latter as expressions of the rheumatic principle. In most cases chorea
complicates only a more advanced and less severe stage of rheumatism; it appears
less frequently in the acme or at the beginning of the disease, and has only been
known in very few cases to precede the affection, as noticed by Sée in five cases
out of forty-two. At other times it appears only at the second or third attack,
and often alternates with the latter.

It is principally the slight and subacute form of rheumatism which is complicated with muscular disturbances, and as if both affections intended to balance
each other, the chorea is very slight in grave cases of rheumatism or cardiac affection, while a simple torticollis is often followed by a most serious attack of St.
Vitus's dance. Patients, suffering from a complication of rheumatism with
chorea, generally present some cardiac disease, either endocarditis or endoperi-
carditis. While Roger looks upon chorea cardiaca and chorea rheumatico-car-
diaca as manifestations of a rheumatic diathesis, Giuntoli is of opinion that chorea
ought not to be considered as a complication of rheumatism in cases of pale
cachectic children, where the cardiac bruits are not restricted merely to the apex
of the heart, but extend over the base and the large vessels. He quotes the history of a child of ten, who had chorea and cardiac bruits, although no articular
pains had been observed. Two weeks later acute articular rheumatism broke
out, which later on was complicated with endocarditis and a relapse of chorea.

The reason why all cases of rheumatism are not complicated with chorea has
been ascribed to a disposition which is peculiar to infancy, and especially to girls.
It seldom appears in children under eight years, and relapses frequently occur
till the twentieth year. A sudden fright is often said to be the cause of it; and,
as we have said before, the prognosis is generally a favourable one.

The connection between chorea and rheumatism is not only peculiar to infancy,
but can often be traced in hereditary dispositions. Patients suffering from chorea
frequently are the descendants of people who have suffered from rheumatism.
Sée was able in eight cases to verify this phenomenon in the same family, and
Trousseau often predicted chorea in cases of rheumatism. Thus chorea appears
as a manifestation of a rheumatic affection of the nerve centres. Fifty years ago
Copland opposed the theory that these convulsions were of a reflex character,
saying that rheumatism had a tendency to spread from the articular regions to
internal fibrous membranes, the pericardium and the pia mater of the spinal
cord. Both the pathological anatomy of the disease, as well as the symptoms
observed *intra vitam*, tend to affirm the assertion that both affections are connected. So far as the anatomy is concerned, it must be admitted that the *post-*

mortem results have not always been the same, but in every case the cord or its membranes have been the seat of the manifestation. Both chorea and rheumatism, whether they both occur together or separately, always produce the same phenomena; from our present point of knowledge we must still, however, maintain that rheumatism has a strong tendency to attack the nervous system, especially the spinal system, and to produce muscular spasms in individuals who are so predisposed. Still, although a rheumatic chorea exists, and cannot be denied without deliberately refusing to recognize positive facts, yet it would be just as unreasonable and hasty to assert that chorea is merely of rheumatic origin.

So far as other nervous phenomena occurring in the course of rheumatism are concerned, it is still doubtful whether it is in any way connected with contractions or tetanic rigor of the extremities, as the latter are generally met with during the first years of life only, when muscular rheumatism is almost unknown; neither has it as yet been positively proved that it is in any way connected with esssential infantile paralysis. Rheumatic, as well as other neuralgias, are very rarely met with in children.

The author never observed a case of erythema nodosum and papulosum, and he even doubts the existence of a purpura rheumatica.

Muscular rheumatism is of rare occurrence in infancy, and Giuntoli has never observed it apart from affections of the joints, so that it should be regarded as a symptom of rheumatism, especially as it often appears in connection with chorea and cardiac affections. The etiology of rheumatism in infants is the same as in adults; perhaps the hereditary predisposition is more pronounced too; *e. g.*, Taccaud says that acquired rheumatism, which is much more frequent than the inherited, generally appears at a more advanced period of life, generally between the twentieth and fortieth year. Chomel even goes so far as to consider rheumatism in children merely as an exceptional phenomenon due to hereditary predisposition. Concerning the question as to whether there is a more marked tendency to this affection in males than in females, or *vice versâ*, the various authors differ much in their opinions. Vogel has even discovered a special relation between the age of the patient and the seat of the disease, which he defines as follows: in children the upper extremities, and the organs of the head and thorax are always affected by rheumatism, and the lower extremities and abdominal viscera in adults. This is partly true, as far as the viscera are concerned.

One of the most frequent causes of rheumatism is cold, and principally damp cold; the opinion has for a long time prevailed that scarlatina often produces it also; but as both affections are peculiar to infancy, it has not yet been proved beyond doubt that there really exists some internal connection between them. In the course of scarlatina, the joints often become very painful; this symptom lasts sometimes for one or two days, and then disappears without leaving any traces, while at other times the articulations become inflamed and suppuration ensues. Purulent pleuritis and pericarditis often occur in scarlet fever, but cardiac affections belong to the rare complications. *Endocarditis scarlatinosa* has never been known to end fatally. Trousseau admits the existence of a scarlatinous rheumatism, and points out that scarlatina is often followed by chorea; and Hughes, Ogle, Fuller, Long, and Roger record similar cases. It seems as if scarlatina had the power to rouse the latent tendency to rheumatism in individuals who are under the influence of a hereditary predisposition, without, however, giving to the latter a peculiar *cachet*. The complications of scarlatina have a tendency to suppuration, and that may be the reason why the complications of rheumatism which arise in the van of scarlet fever take the same turn. The relation which exists between both affections is, however, still an open question, which further investigations will doubtless solve. The diagnosis of rheumatism

is easy, but unfortunately slight pains in the joints are too often regarded as
growing pains, and too little attention is given to the heart in such cases.   Acute
attacks of rachitis are apt to produce symptoms not at all unlike those caused by
rheumatism ; but the extreme youth of the patient, together with the characteri-
istic deformity which soon follows, prevent the error in the diagnosis.   Diffuse
phlegmonous periostitis often first appears in infancy in the form of rheumatism,
as either one or several joints become exceedingly painful ; but in this case also
the fact that the swelling is either above or below the joint, and never on the
joint itself, the general state of the patient and the formation of large purulent
foci, help to make the differential diagnosis.   Roger draws the attention to the
fact that vertebral rheumatism might easily be mistaken for spinal méningitis,
seeing that in both affections the patient presents the characteristic position of
lying in bed with his head thrown backwards, and his back arched and stiff. He,
however, points out that the age of the patient will prevent the mistake in children under three years of age, as rheumatism very seldom occurs before this
epoch ; and that at a more advanced age, affections of the central nervous system and its membranes would easily be detected by troubles of the motility and
sensibility.   In no case of chorea must the repeated auscultation of the heart be
neglected.

The author strongly advocates the use of opium in rheumatism, in doses of
three to five centigrammes every three to four hours, or Dover's powders in doses
of from two to six decigrammes.   In cases where opium should fail, chloral hydrate and bromide of potassium must be given, and the patient during convalescence be kept under a stimulating and strengthening treatment.   It is remarkable
that Giuntoli should have entirely overlooked the powerful remedy for rheumatism which we possess, in the shape of salicylic acid, and we are entirely at a
loss as to what special reason of the author this neglect should be attributed. Its
efficiency is entirely beyond all doubt, and the drug might at least have been
mentioned among the others.   Cardiac complications are treated by painting the
cardiac region with iodine, and applying blisters ; bleeding or leeches are only
indicated in cases of much pain and dyspnœa.   Cerebral symptoms must be
energetically treated, by applying leeches to the mastoid processes, and giving
large doses of opium and chloral, as well as purgatives internally ; but, notwithstanding all efforts, the complication is apt to end fatally.   Children who have
once suffered from rheumatism must be very carefully protected by prophylactic
means from relapses.   Cold water cures, mountain air, sea bathing, etc., will
prove beneficial in strengthening their constitutions and preventing repeated attacks of the affection.—*London Med. Record*, June 15, 1879.

—

Transfusion in Acute Leukæmia.

This case occurred in the wards of M. Gubler at the Hospital Beaujon.   The
patient was a baker's boy, aged 24.   He had been ill two months with general
malaise and extreme weakness.   He was very pale.   The spleen and liver were
much hypertrophied, and the lymphatic glands in several parts were also large.
The blood contained one white globule to five or six red.   He was treated with
ferruginous tonics, arsenic, and hydrotherapy, but the disease made rapid progress,
the spleen augmenting in size with surprising rapidity.   Hemorrhages from the
nose now commenced, and his eyesight became impaired, and a second examination of the blood showed that there were as many white as red globules.   In the
presence of this galloping leukæmia, transfusion was resorted to.   The brother
supplied 100 grammes of blood, and sixty were injected.   During the transfusion
the patient experienced a feeling of warmth in the arm, then in the shoulder, and

some seconds afterwards he was seized with a dry cough. Five minutes after the operation the pulse was 104°, the same rate as before it, but the sphygmographic tracing showed that the up stroke now approached the vertical. There was an immediate rise of temperature in the axilla from 38° to 38.4° C. He was much improved for three days, when fresh epistaxis occurred, and, desirous of returning home, left the hospital.—*London Med. Record*, July 15, 1879.

Diphtheria treated with Inhalations of Oleum Eucalypti.

MOSLER draws attention (*Berl. Klin. Woch.* May 26, 1879) to the fact that the fatal accidents which are so liable to occur in diphtheria are frequently due to mismanagement. It is a great mistake to go on reducing the organism which has already lost much of its power of resistance by a strict diet, antiphlogistic treatment, and emetics. The latter are especially dangerous in increasing the tendency to failure of the heart's action, and thereby inducing death. The author has obtained very favourable results by submitting his patients to a stimulating and tonic treatment, and thus diminishing the liability to paralysis. Concerning the local treatment of the affection, Herr Mosler is a strong advocate of the views of Waldenburg and Oertel, who have lately pointed out that the use of caustics in the treatment of the local affection is apt to give rise to ulcerations in the throat, and that this danger could be avoided, and equally good results obtained, by inhaling disinfecting substances. The author has made a great number of experiments concerning the efficacy of the different substances which are generally used for the purpose. He has found that the usual disinfectants, such as carbolic acid, salicylic acid, permanganate of potash, etc., are apt to cause symptoms of irritation in the bronchi. A very useful remedy in diminishing the tendency to repeated attacks of diphtheria is a strong solution of sea-salt, mixed with the water which is used for the purpose of inhaling. Herr Mosler has also obtained very good results by adding a dose of the oil made from the leaves of the eucalyptus tree to the water contained in the glass cup of the inhaler. He gives the history of a case which was treated in this way. The patient, a girl, aged 20, was suffering from a severe attack of diphtheria. Both tonsils, the uvula and the arches of the palate, were covered with thick whitish patches. There were also a few ulcerations of irregular form and ragged edges. Inhalations of twenty minutes duration were ordered to be made every hour. Ten grammes of the ol. eneal. e foliis was mixed with the same amount of spirit of wine, and ten drops of this mixture added to the water. At the same time she took, every half hour, five drops of a mixture of ten grammes of sesquichloride of iron and the same quantity of water in claret. This treatment was kept up for three days, during which the symptoms remained the same, and the patient had high fever. On the fourth day she became worse; a teaspoonful of the mixture of oil of eucalyptus and spirit was then added to the water, and the inhalation kept up during the night. On the next day the temperature began to sink, and the diphtheritic membranes had been partially expectorated. The patient then continued steadily to improve, and the number of inhalations was reduced to three or four daily. She left the hospital after a stay of three weeks.—*London Med. Record*, July 15, 1879.

Early Syphilitic Affections of the Nervous System.

Prof. MAURIAC closes a long and able paper (*Annales de Dermatol. et de Syphilig.*, vol. x., No. 3) on this subject, with the following deductions from the facts and researches at his command :—

1. Syphilis may attack the nervous centres at a very early period after the initial lesion.

2. The early cerebro-spinal lesions are those which develop during the virulent period of the malady, that is to say, during the first two or three years.

3. There are degrees in this precocity of the cerebro-spinal syphiloses : the first include those which set in within the first twelve months ; the second those which develop in the second or third year of the constitutional malady. Statistics seem to show that those of the first degree are more common than those of the second.

4. Among the early visceral localizations of syphilis, those in the cerebro-spinal system are incomparably the most numerous.

5. They are also the most dangerous. Their gravity does not increase with their diathetic age; those which develop during the first months of syphilis are as formidable as those which belong to the more advanced stages of the malady.

6. All the forms, all the degrees, all the phenomenal combinations that constitute the symptomatology and the processes of the localizations of syphilis in the neural system, are met with in the early as well as in the late cerebro-spinal syphiloses.

7. Certain symptomatic complexes, however, seem to predominate. The most frequent are those which consist in an attack of hemiplegia, involving the whole of one side of the body.

8. Among the attacks of hemiplegia, the syndroma comprising the right hemiplegia and aphasia is the most common.

9. The paralytic forms are much more common than the convulsive or epileptic, in the early cerebral syphiloses.

10. In the cerebro-spinal syphiloses the psychical troubles and the incoördinations of movements are never systematized as they are in mania, general paralysis, and locomotor ataxia.

11. The absence of systematization in the cerebro-spinal syphiloses must be regarded as one of their chief characteristics. The only exception is in the case of the syndroma of right hemiplegia and aphasia.

12. Early localizations of syphilis in the spinal cord are much less common than in the encephalon.

13 The lesions which seem to belong to the early cerebro-spinal syphiloses are diffuse or, more frequently, circumscribed hyperplastic effusions into the cortical layer of the brain and the pia mater, and changes in the Sylvian arteries with consecutive ischæmic softening.

14. In some cases of early cerebro-spinal syphiloses that terminated fatally, no lesion was found, but at that time the existence of arterial syphilis had not been recognized. It may be presumed that death had resulted from sudden anæmia of the nervous centres that are essential to life.

15. With regard to the etiology of the early cerebro-spinal syphiloses, only very vague conjectures can be advanced. In most of the cases, the initial lesion as well as the consecutive cutaneous and mucous manifestations were very mild in character.

16. The general cause of the constitutional malady is not modified by the appearance of early localizations in the nervous centres. The other manifestations develop before, during, and after the localization in the neural system, without presenting any deviations from their usual forms, degrees, course, or topography.

17. The precocity of the cerebro-spinal syphiloses furnishes no special indication with regard to treatment. Whatever may be the age of the constitutional malady, the localizations in the nervous centres demand the same specific medication. The peculiar conditions of each case furnish the secondary indications relative to the choice, doses, and combinations of the two specific agents.—*Med. Record*, Aug. 16, 1879.

Spasms of the Phrenic Nerve treated with Ether-spray.

Dr. REGONI reports (*Memorab.*, 5, 1879) the following case : The patient had for eight days previous to his admission to the hospital been suffering from a continuous and very violent hiccough, which he attributed to having eaten a large quantity of vegetables and macaroni. The hiccough had began an hour after the meal, and had increased in violence, so that the patient could neither eat nor sleep, and was very weak. Every attempt to take food, or even water, increased his sufferings, and was followed by bilious vomiting. While examining the patient, the author was struck by the violent and incessant movements of the diaphragm, the thorax being comparatively quiet. The patient complained of dyspnœa, and was slightly cyanotic. The stomach was much dilated and tympanitic on percussion. Pulse and heart were normal. The diagnosis, "spasm of the phrenic nerve," having been made, a spray of sulphuric ether was directed for ten minutes, first to the epigastrium, then for five minutes on both sides of the throat. During the *séance* the hiccough decreased in violence and frequency ; another application was made in the course of the forenoon, after which the patient slept for two hours. The treatment was repeated several times in the course of this day and the next, and the patient recovered.—*London Med. Record*, July 15, 1879.

—

Sea Water in Treatment of Chronic Catarrh of the Throat.

Professor MOSLER, of Griefswald, says in the *Berlin. Klinische Wochenschrift*, June 2, 1879, that he has for some years most successfully treated patients with chronic catarrh of the throat by gargling with sea water. Special rooms for gargling have been erected on the seashore in some watering places, according to his directions. It is, however, essential that the patients should be given special directions how to gargle. As the affection is generally located in the naso-pharyngeal space, it is necessary that part of the water should come in contact with the nasal cavity. In order to attain this, the gargling movements must be confined with movements of deglutition. A marked improvement in the state of the patient follows as soon as the latter has acquired this particular art of gargling. Patients who suffer from chronic pharyngitis, and who are exposed to much fatigue through singing, preaching, etc., have been completely cured by gargling twice a day for many months with a tumbler of cold water, to which are added from one to three tablespoonfuls of a twenty or twenty-five per cent. solution of sea-salt. To protect the teeth from the influence of the salt water, they must be cleaned immediately after the gargling with a tincture prepared by the author. Another of the advantages of this method is that the disposition to relapse gradually decreases, especially if the patients be directed to wash their face, neck, and forearms with cold water, and rub them dry before gargling in the morning and at night. After this has been kept up for some time, the mucous membrane of the nasal cavity and the pharynx changes entirely, and the disposition to diphtheria which predominates in certain families is greatly diminished.—*British Med. Journal*, Aug. 2, 1879.

—

Syphilis of the Trachea and Bronchial Tubes.

VIERLING has collected, *Deutsch Archiv f. Klin. Med.*, p. 326, 1878, 46 cases of syphilitic disease of the air-passages, from which he draws the following conclusions. When syphilis attacks the trachea, ulceration always occurs, and tends generally to cicatrization and consequent narrowing of the tube ; but sometimes the ulcer extends so deeply as to perforate the tracheal wall and give rise to an abscess. In two cases of ulceiation of the left bionchus, the left bianch of the pulmonaiy aiteiy was opened. In 30 cases, theie was concomitant syphilitic affection of the phaiynx; in 36, the tiachea was attacked, with or without implication of the bionchi as well; fi\e times the bionchi alone suffeied. Bionchial syphilis is iaie beyond the two bionchi. Age and sex ha\e no paiticulai influence on the de\elopment of the disease. Fi\e or six cases weie attiibuted to heieditaiy syphilis.

The piincipal symptoms are cough, puiulent expectoiation, piogiessi\e dyspnœa, and, wheie the phaiynx is also affected, hoaiseness, and subsequently, aphonia. The piognosis is most unfa\ouiable. Tiacheotomy has been peifoimed in 14 cases of tiacheal stenosis, but only twice successfully.—*London Med. Record*, July 15, 1879.

—

Chancres of the Tonsils and the Buccal Cavity.

M. SPILLMANN has published in the *Revue Médicale de l' Est*, two cases of chancie which aie \eiy iemaikable, both for the peculiai ciicumstances attending the infection, and for the difficulty of making a diagnosis.

The fiist was that of a lady, aged 59, whose position in life was such as to exclude all suspicion of syphilitic infection. She consulted M. Spillmann for a slight soie thioat which she had had for about a foitnight, the pain being moie \iolent duiing the act of swallowing. Theie was also a consideiable swelling of the glands at the angle of the iight maxilla. On examination of the throat, a wound of the size of a threepennypiece was seen on the suiface of the iight tonsil, slightly depiessed, and of a giayish hue. The mucous membiane aiound it was œdematous, and the paiotid glands enlaiged and tendei to piessuie. No othei lesion could be disco\eied eithei in the mouth or thioat, nor was theie any exteinal iedness of the skin. The patient heiself did not complain of any particulai feeling of ill health, and seemed to considei hei disease as a \eiy tiifling mattei. M. Spillmann, who was well acquainted with his patient's way of li\ing, could not concei\e the existence of syphilis; but, a few days latei, the chaiacteiistic syphilitic iash bioke out, so that theie could be no doubt as to the natuie of the affection. The only difficulty to sol\e was the etiology of the case, and, aftei a gieat deal of tiouble, it was disco\eied that the patient had adopted a baby which she was biinging up by hand, and that, in oidei to see if the tempeiatuie of the milk in the feeding-bottle was iight, she often used to tiy it by diinking fiom the iubbei mouthpiece. The infant being examined, was found to be suffering fiom heieditaiy syphilis, with ulceiations of the mouth and the genital paits.

The second case is not less inteiesting iespecting the way in which the infection had been communicated. An upholsteiei's appientice, aged 13, had had for some days pie\ious to his consulting M. Spillmann, a small ied patch of the size of a threepennypiece on the lowei lip; this patch was induiated at the base, the glands weie enlaiged—in shoit, it was an undoubted chancie of the lip. It seemed impossible at fiist to disco\ei the cause, when it was disco\eied that the boy used to woik with a man who was suffeiing fiom syphilis, and took his nails fiom the same bag as this man. Upholsteieis, it seems, aie in the habit of putting into theii mouths handfuls of the small nails which they use for theii woik, putting back the suiplus nails into the bag. The woikman was examined and found to ha\e syphilitic patches in the mouth, and theie can, theiefoie, be no doubt that the boy was infected by putting into his mouth nails which weie impregnated with the sali\a of this man.—*London Med. Record*, July 15, 1879.

The Etiology of Paralysis of the Cryco-Arytenoid Posterior Muscles.

OTT contributes (*Prog. Med. Woch.*, No. 15, 1879) an interesting case of paralysis of the posterior crico-arytenoid muscles, which was due to pressure of the posterior crico-arytenoid nerves. A man, aged 57, had swallowed a large piece of meat, which had stuck in his throat for twenty-four hours, and resisted all his attempts to dislodge it. He had no pain, only slight dyspnœa, and was unable to swallow even a drop of water. The next day he consulted a physician, who pushed down the piece of meat with a sound. The patient felt better directly, could breathe more freely, and was able to swallow. This state of things, however, did not last long; he again began to suffer from difficulty in breathing and swallowing, and was obliged to take only liquid food. The voice had remained unaltered; but the patient was obliged to speak in short abrupt sentences, from want of air. When examined by the writer, it was found that the false vocal cords were slightly swelled, and red; there was a space of four millimetres between the arytenoid cartilages. The rimi glottidis was partly covered by the vocal cords during inspiration and expiration; only an irregular triangular opening could be seen at its posterior end. The left vocal cord was wider than the right, and did not move at all, while the right moved sluggishly. During inspiration, the vocal cords were approximated. The arytenoid cartilages did not move either during respiration or phonation. The mucous membrane of the incisura inter-arytenoidea was swelled and pale, and the colour of the vocal cords a dingy yellow. The treatment consisted at first in faradization of the larynx, but it afforded no relief to the patient. The dyspnœa increased, and became most severe even when the patient was perfectly quiet. It was noticed that the rima glottidis had become much narrower, the left vocal cord having advanced to the middle of the fissure; the right arytenoid cartilage was partly hidden by the left. As the patient could only swallow with difficulty, it was necessary to feed him through the tube. He lost his appetite, and was very much wasted, and reduced in strength. At last the dyspnœa became so intense, that tracheotomy had to be performed, to save the man's life. Immediately after the operation, the patient was able to swallow without any trouble, and continued to do so henceforth. The larynx presented the same changes as before the operation. The patient had still great difficulty in breathing; the thorax was immovable during respiration, and the intercostal spaces were drawn in. The vocal cords were immovable, and during phonation a space of about three millimetres remained open in the back part of the fissure. For this reason, the patient had to be dismissed with the canula in his throat, to prevent asphyxia. The author attributes the paralysis of the muscles which open the glottis to the pressure which the large piece of meat that was firmly wedged in the pharynx during twenty-four hours, must have exercised on the crico-arytenoid posterior muscles and their nerves. His assertion is based upon the well-known fact that the conducting function of a nerve is entirely destroyed by pressure. Thus, in the present case, the nerve having lost all control over the muscle it governs, the latter became paralyzed, and gave rise to the phenomena we have described. The difficulty in swallowing, which increased whenever the dyspnœa became worse, decreased when the sound was introduced, and finally disappeared after tracheotomy, can only be explained by assuming the existence of a spasmodic stricture of the œsophagus.— *London Med. Record*, July 15, 1879.

—

Agaricum in the Night-Sweats of Consumptive Patients.

Professor PETER says, in his lectures on the treatment of tuberculosis (*Bull. Gén. de Thérap.*, March 30, 1879), that agaricum is one of the most efficient drugs for curing the debilitating night-sweats of tuberculosis. The drug is not new ; it was first mentioned by De Haen, and Andral experimented with it in the Hôpital de la Pitié. He proved that it has the power of preventing the sweating, and that it may be given in doses of two grammes without provoking any digestive trouble ; a dose of three grammes induced an attack of diarrhœa. He used to give it in doses of 20 centigrammes. Trousseau ordered the same dose to be taken two hours before bedtime, and always found it answer very well, except in cases of very great cachexia, where the sweating was much reduced, though not entirely suppressed. Peter gives it in doses of from 20 to 30 centigrammes with good effect. He illustrates its power by several cases in which it has proved efficient, of which we here quote the case of a young man who suffered from consumption, and had very profuse night-sweats. After entering the Pitié, these sweats continued during the day time also, and the patient was much reduced by them. Twenty centigrammes of agaricus were given him, and the night-sweats disappeared. The treatment was continued, and, six weeks later, the patient had regained flesh, felt much better, and left the hospital.—*London Med. Record*, July 15, 1879.

—

The Use of Iron in Certain Stages of Cardiac Disease, and the Advantage of Combining Chloride of Ammonium with Iron.

In a very interesting and instructive paper (*Practitioner*, August, 1879) Dr. T. GRAINGER STEWART, Prof. of Practice of Physic in the University of Edinburgh, draws attention to two points. First, that in certain cardiac cases, particularly those in which the aortic valves are diseased, a peculiar condition sometimes arises which demands for its treatment large doses of iron. Second, that in some cases, both belonging to the above group and of other kinds, the reception of iron by the system is greatly facilitated if chloride of ammonium be administered along with it.

In illustration of both points he cites the following case:—

Neil McLeod, a seaman, 33 years of age, was admitted to the Royal Infirmary on the 23d October, 1877, complaining of breathlessness on exertion, giddiness, palpitation and pain in the region of the heart. In 1867 he had suffered from rheumatic fever, but was not aware that any cardiac complication had then existed. In 1875 he observed that his strength was failing, that he had become breathless on exertion, was apt to cough, and often had passing fits of giddiness. These symptoms rapidly increased, and he soon felt himself unfit for duty.

At different times he was under treatment in the infirmary at Calcutta, and in Greenwich Hospital, and although he made each time a temporary rally, he soon fell back, and on the whole the debility, breathlessness, and pain were gradually increasing.

The exacerbation of illness which led him to seek admission to the infirmary, had been induced partly by hard work while employed in a coasting vessel scarcely seaworthy, and partly by intemperance.

On admission his face was pale, his expression anxious, his eyes were somewhat staring, his lips slightly livid. His temperature was normal, and beyond flabbiness of tongue and some feebleness of digestion, there was no disease of the alimentary system. The liver dulness was increased, measuring seven inches in the mammillary line, and the organ was tender on pressure. There was some bulging in the præcordial region. The apex beat of the heart was felt strong and diffused, the area of dulness of the heart was increased. On auscultation in the mitral area, a loud, harsh, systolic bruit was heard, propagated towards the axilla and inferior angle of the scapula. There was also a slight diastolic murmur. In the tricuspid area there was a short systolic murmur, and a prolonged diastolic.

In the aortic area the first sound was weak and impure, there was also a loud high-pitched diastolic murmur propagated down the sternum to the ensiform cartilage. In the pulmonary area the second sound was accentuated. The pulse was forty-six per minute, weak and compressible, and even in this condition presented something of the water-hammer character, although much less distinctly than it did at a later period in the history of the case. There was no dropsy, and the urine was natural.

There could be little doubt that the valvular lesions had originated in connection with the rheumatic fever, and it was clear that these lesions were incompetence of the aortic and mitral valves, with impairment of the muscular power of the heart. All the other symptoms, the general poverty of blood, the cerebral anæmia, giddiness, and general distress, were secondary to these. The indications for treatment were to obtain rest, to support the strength, and in particular to strengthen the heart and improve the condition of the blood. If these indications could be met, it seemed likely that the symptoms due to anæmia and deficient nutrition of the brain would disappear, and that on their disappearance the patient would be comparatively well. With the view of meeting the first indication, the patient was directed to remain in bed; the second, food rich in nitrogen, and in quantities small at a time but frequently repeated, was ordered; and the third, perchloride of iron in full doses was prescribed. At first twenty minims of the tincture were given three times a day, but the doses were gradually given more frequently until he was taking five or six in the twenty-four hours. It was at once apparent that these measures were doing good. The pallor became less marked, the giddiness and headache less troublesome. But some functional derangement of the stomach and liver set in, the tongue became furred, the appetite impaired, the liver somewhat more enlarged from increased congestion, and the headache became again more severe; the patient's condition thus continued to be manifestly perilous. In these circumstances, instead of abandoning perchloride of iron, I added to it chloride of ammonium in doses of half a grain to each minim of the tincture. This was followed by the best results, for the gastric and hepatic symptoms rapidly disappeared, and for a considerable time the patient went on taking the mixture six times a day, so that he used two drachms of the tincture of perchloride of iron daily, without exhibiting the slightest sign of gastric or hepatic disturbance.

As a result of this treatment, to quote the words of Mr. Henry Handford, M.B., the clinical clerk, "a gradual but marked improvement in his general condition took place. His face lost its anxious expression, the palpitations became less distressing, the action of the heart less tumultuous, although still not quite regular. The pulse became much stronger and more frequent—seventy in the minute—and more characteristic of aortic regurgitation. The aortic diastolic murmur became less loud, but nevertheless was quite distinct. The mitral symptoms remained unaltered. The congestion of the liver was not so great, as shown by a decrease in the vertical dulness. The transverse dulness of the heart was unaltered." It may be added that the pallor and the signs of cerebral anæmia became less marked, and the patient left the infirmary in a condition which enabled him to resume his occupation.

This case afforded an example of a condition by no means uncommon, but of which Dr. Stewart has been unable to find a satisfactory description in books. The first glance at the patient leads one to notice the pallor, the very anxious expression, the restlessness, the pale lividity of the lips, the throbbing of the carotids, and perhaps of the temporal arteries; whilst the patient complains of giddiness, perhaps of headache, certainly of breathlessness, and of a debility that amounts at times to faintness. He is somewhat relieved by food, and unless there is some dropsical effusion to prevent it, he is easier in the recumbent position. But he obtains very little sleep. The explanation of his various symptoms is readily found. The pallor and the head symptoms are due in part to anæmic deterioration of the blood and partly to imperfect filling of the arteries supplying the face and brain. The throbbing is due to the ill-filled condition of the arteries, contrasting with their sudden temporary filling during the ventricular systole; while the breathlessness and the lividity are connected with the dilatation and the partial failure of the heart's action. Sometimes the distress is aggravated by the existence of dropsical effusion, and it seems to be specially severe when the pericardium is its seat. Such cases sometimes prove rapidly fatal by sudden syncope, and sometimes death follows upon a long agony, characterized mainly by symptoms of cerebral anæmia. These cases do not seem ever to recover spontaneously.

Treatment by the administration of cardiac tonics, and especially of iron, leads in many cases to decided improvement. The form which Dr. Stewart finds best is the tincture of perchloride, but it must be given in large quantity. He has gradually been led to give it in larger doses; sometimes even to the amount of twenty minims every two hours, more frequently every four hours, continuing its use for days together. In many cases the patients speedily experience relief, and before long there is manifest improvement. As in the patient whose history is given, they are enabled after a time to leave the hospital and return to work.

But there is great difficulty in carrying out this plan of treatment from the gastric and hepatic derangement which so frequently follows upon the use of iron. During the past two years Dr. Stewart has sought to meet this difficulty by combining chloride of ammonium with the iron, according to the suggestion of a medical officer of the Indian service, to the members of which we are so much indebted for our knowledge of the value of that salt in hepatic affections. During that time he has repeatedly been thus enabled to administer iron in large doses in combination with chloride, to patients who otherwise could scarcely have used iron. It will be observed that in the case now recorded, the iron speedily led to dyspeptic symptoms, so that it was impossible to persevere with its use. But the addition of the chloride both relieved the existing dyspepsia and enabled us to continue to administer the iron in large doses, and for a considerable time. So far as he can judge, iron is the only remedy which could have saved the life of the patient at the time, and but for this effect of the chloride of ammonium, he does not know how he could have administered iron so freely as to suffice.

But the combination of perchloride of iron and chloride of ammonium is useful not in cardiac cases only.

Dr. Stewart narrates two cases, of which notes have been given him by his friend, Dr. James Ritchie.

A lady, aged 62, suffering from carcinoma uteri, had frequent attacks of metrorrhagia which had produced profound anæmia. The tincture of perchloride of iron was prescribed, but it produced so much gastric irritation that it had to be discontinued. After the stomach had recovered she was again ordered tincture of perchloride, with the addition of ten grains of the chloride of ammonium to every twenty minims of the tincture. This mixture was well received by the stomach, and was continued for some weeks without the slightest disturbance of digestion.

Again, a boy of 13, of feeble and rather strumous constitution, suffered from sore throat, gastro-intestinal disturbance, headache, giddiness, and almost daily epistaxis. The liver was enlarged so as to extend down nearly to the umbilicus, was tender, and had an uneven surface. The spleen also was enlarged, and projected three inches beyond the costal cartilages. Microscopic examination of the blood showed marked increase of the white corpuscles, with great diminution of the red, and an unusual amount of granular material. In this case it seemed highly probable that the iron alone could not be received, and accordingly the combination of iron and chloride was administered. The medicines were well borne, and speedy improvement of the general condition took place.

<hr />

Cardiac Complications in Gonorrhœa.

M. MOREL states (*Rev. des Sciences Méd.*) that he has collected all the cases hitherto published—13 in number—of heart-affection occurring during the course of gonorrhœa. Of the 13 cases, two are examples of pericarditis, and 11 of endocarditis. All the valves of the left side of the heart have been found affected, but the aortic most frequently so. The cardiac affection is usually mild in character, and only revealed by slight symptoms, which may be easily overlooked. Two cases, however (Obs. de Lorain et de Desnos, mitral endocarditis), ended fatally. The affection generally shows itself during the course of gonorrhœal rheumatism ; but, in two cases (Lacassagne, Marly), it is expressly stated that there was no rheumatism. In five cases, the first manifestation of joint affection appeared during an attack of gonorrhœa. In five cases, the antecedents of the patient are not mentioned ; three only are noted as having suffered from rheumatism previous to any urethral discharge. Age does not appear to influence the development of cardiac complication ; in these cases, the youngest patient was 23, and the oldest 50. All were males.—*London Med. Record*, July 15, 1879.

<hr />

Cardiac Neuritis.

Attention has recently been called by some Continental physicians to a pathological condition of considerable clinical interest and importance, especially in connection with some forms of angina pectoris. Dr. Peter, the eminent physician of La Pitié, and well known as the editor of the last edition of Trousseau's *Lectures*, has been especially concerned in endeavouring to give prominence to the theory that, when symptoms of angina pectoris accompany disease of the coats of the aorta (aortitis) with dilatation of that vessel, the peculiar clinical phenomena observed are due to an inflammation of the nerves of the cardiac plexus : an inflammation which extends from the arterial tunics to the branches of the cardiac plexus in contact therewith. Several cases have been reported and analyzed in support of this view. In one case observed and reported by Dr. Bazey, the cardiac plexus was carefully dissected at the necropsy, and the nerves composing it were found thickened and presenting moniliform swellings along their course. It has been noticed that in these cases, in contradistinction to others which are purely neuralgic, the pain is permanent instead of intermittent, or at any rate, there are certain points which remain always painful on compression with the finger, especially, for example, the intercostal spaces along the left border of the sternum. In some of these cases, compression of the left vagus in the neck would at once induce pain in the region of the cardiac plexus, and the pain would radiate along the course of the branches of the pneumogastric ; as for instance, along the back of the sternum, in the stomach which becomes distended with gas, and in the region of the pulmonary plexus. M. Bucquoy has also noticed, at the termination of such attacks, severe pain in the hepatic region, which he refers to a participation in the disturbances of the terminal ramifications of the vagus on the right side. M. Peter maintains that the aortic insufficiency which frequently coexists in such cases must be regarded simply as a " contingent fact," and as quite incapable of itself to excite the paroxysms of angina. He, however, is especially urgent in calling attention to the far more serious significance of aortic insufficiency when it arises from an affection of the arteries, when disease of the aorta extends to and implicates the sigmoid valves, than of aortic insufficiency of endocardial origin: since the former condition commonly leads to a cardiac neu- ritis with all the grave phenomena of angina pectoris. M. Huchard has also in- sisted on the fact that the gastro-hepatic disturbance which he has observed in several cases of cardiac disease is exclusively dependent on a phlegmasia of the cardiac plexus ; such as severe pain after food, enormous distension of the stom- ach with gas, pyrosis, anorexia, and vomiting.   Hence in cardiac neuritis we may encounter a great variety of symptoms, according to which of the numerous ramifications of the pneumogastric are especially involved ; disturbance of cardiac rhythm and syncope if the cardiac branches themselves be chiefly involved; or gastro-hepatic symptoms or pulmonary symptoms, if the branches going to the digestive or respiratory organs be mainly implicated.

The morbid anatomy of the nerves of the cardiac plexus has been specially ex- amined by Putiatin of St. Petersburg, who has found in some cases, after death from cardiac paralysis, in which no coarse changes in the cardiac structures could be discovered, a diseased condition of the cardiac ganglia limited to distension of their vessels, and an intermixture of granulation-cells with the nerve-fibres and corpuscles. In older cases, where organic disease of the heart also existed, more decided pathological changes were observed, consisting chiefly in increase of inter- stitial connective tissue and atrophy and granulation of the nerve-cells.

This is a somewhat neglected branch of cardiac pathology, to which we would especially direct the attention of our many able and industrious morbid anato- mists.—*Brit. Med. Journ.*, July 12, 1879.

Treatment of Infantile Diarrhœa.

At a late meeting of the Medical Society of the County of New York (*Med. Record*, July 26, 1879) Dr. A. JACOBI read an instructive paper on the above subject, from which the following extract is made.

The preventive treatment of diarrhœa, depending on defective alimentation, consisted in so changing and arranging the milk used for babies that the casein would not coagulate in large lumps, and thus become more digestible. That object could be obtained by adding such farinaceous food as did not contain much starch. It consists in diluting the boiled and skimmed milk with barley-water or oatmeal gruel. It must be boiled to check its tendency to become sour, to re- move a portion, though small, of its casein and fat, and to expel the gas con- tained in the raw milk to the amount of three per cent.

Of the two, he preferred barley for general use. He recommended that the barleycorn which was employed for infant diet should be ground as thoroughly as possible in a coffee-mill, both in order to diminish the period necessary for cook- ing it, and also in order to retain the gluten. *It was even preferable, for very young infants, to cook the barley whole for hours*, thereby to burst the outer layers of cells, empty their contents, and then, by straining, to get rid of the larger part of the starch which was found toward the centre. There was no danger to which little children were so liable as that which arose from their ten- dency to diarrhœa. His advice, therefore, was to administer barley to children who manifested a tendency to diarrhœa, and oatmeal to those having a tendency to constipation, and, whenever a change occurred in the intestinal functions, to give one or the other, according as constipation or diarrhœa predominated.

He held that mixture to be the *conditio sine quâ non* of the thorough digestion of the milk. It only would insure the proper nourishment of the infant. With that food alone he had seen children endure the heat of summer without any attack of illness whatever. He had occasion again and again to be convinced of the reliability of the mixture. It had the advantage, too, that it necessitated no dependence upon the honesty or competence of the apothecary or manufacturer, but could be prepared by any one, however poorly situated. Should a slight diarrhœa occur, or a little casein be vomited (a rare accident, to be sure), or casein occur in the stools, then all that was necessary was to diminish the proportion of milk. It might sometimes be necessary, though very seldom, to withdraw the milk entirely for a time, but only in cases of real illness. If the physician or attendants had properly apportioned the ingredients of the mixture, we might be rather sure that the child's digestion and assimilation would be regular and normal. Infants that were partly nourished at the breast almost invariably thrived well with the addition of his mixture. Children, from their fourth or fifth month and upward, might often be fed with it exclusively, and not unfrequently nothing else was given from the day of the birth.

The addition of barley or oatmeal for the purpose of rendering milk digestible was not, however, absolutely indispensable, though he had learned to prefer them. For, gum arabic and gelatine were also very valuable ingredients, indeed, of infant foods. Dr. Jacobi then dwelt at some length upon the changes which gum arabic and gelatine undergo when put into the stomach.

Curative Treatment.—The amount of food should not be larger than we had reason to expect could be easily digested. At all events, either lengthen the intervals between the meals or reduce the quantity of food given at one time, or both. When diarrhœa made its appearance in infants who had been weaned, it was desirable to return them to the breast. Those who never had breast-milk might be given the breast if they could be induced to take it, but only rarely would that be found possible. Whenever a child at the breast was taken with diarrhœa, the passages from the bowels should be studied as to their contents. If a certain amount of curd was found in them, the least that was to be done was to mix the breast-milk with barley-water. That might be done in such a manner that, each time before nursing, one or two teaspoonfuls of barley-water was given the child, so that the farinaceous food and the breast-milk mixed in the stomach. Or, it might be found advisable to alternate breast-milk and barley-water. In bad cases, particularly when the milk was found to be white and heavy, and contained a great deal of casein, it would be found necessary to deprive the child *altogether* of its usual food. In such cases, the child would do better on barley-water alone (that to be continued for one or two days), than to expose it to the injury which would certainly follow the continuation of the casein food.

When diarrhœa occurred in children who had been fed alone upon cow's milk, unmixed or mixed, it was necessary to reduce the quantity of cow's milk in the mixture. As a rule, we had to remember that cow's milk alone was apt to produce diarrhœa, and it should be considered as a maxim that, whenever diarrhœa made its appearance, the amount of cow's milk given to the child should be reduced. When a mere reduction of the quantity did not suffice, it was very much better to deprive the child of milk food altogether. Not infrequently the removal of milk from the bill of fare was the only thing which would restore the child to health. It was possible that a mixture, such as recommended by Dr. Rudish, already mentioned, would be found digestible, even in such cases. In many cases, as a dietetic measure, it would be found advisable to add one or two tablespoonfuls of lime-water to each bottle of food with which the child was supplied.

In those cases in which barley-water did not seem to suffice as a nutriment, or where it would be dangerous to allow children to lose strength, a mixture which he had used to great advantage was the following: Mix the white of one egg

with foui or six ounces of bailey-watei, and add a small quantity of table salt
and sugai, just sufficient to make the mixtuie palatable. The child could take
this eithei in laige or small quantities, accoiding to the case.

In those cases in which the stomach was iiiitable, and \omiting had occuiied,
it was now and then bettei togi\e a small quantity, e\en one or two teaspoonfuls,
and iepeat the dose e\eiy ten, fifteen, or twenty minutes, than to gi\e laigei
quantities at longei inteivals.

In those cases in which the stiength of the child has suffeied gieatly, he recommended the addition of biandy to the mixtuie in such quantity that the child
would take fiom one diachm to one ounce (grms. 4.0 to 30.0), moie or less, in
the couise of twenty-foui houis.

In those extieme cases in which the intestinal cataiih was complicated with
gastiic cataiih, wheie the passages weie numeious and copious, and \omiting
constant, wheie both medicines and food weie iejected, theie was fiequently but
one way to sa\e the patients, and that was to depii\e them *absolutely* of e\eiy-
thing in the foim of eithei diink or food or medicine. It was tiue that such
babies would suffei gieatly fiom thiist for an houi or two, but it was a fact that,
aftei two or thiee houis, those childien would look bettei than befoie the abstemious tieatment was commenced. Not infiequently foui or five houis of total
abstinence would suffice to quiet the stomach and diminish both the secietion and
the peiistaltic mo\ement of the intestinal tiact. In some cases *six* or *eight* houis
of complete abstinence would be iequiied ; or such childien might be staived for
e\en *twelve* or *sixteen* houis, with final good iesults. The first meals afteiwaid
must be quite small, and they would be ietained, and, as a iule, such childien
would subsequently do well.

Di. Jacobi heie enfoiced the necessity of supplying the patient with as much
cool fiesh air as possible. The woist out-dooi aii was bettei than close in-dooi
aii. If possible, the childien should be sent immediately to the countiy and into
the mountain air.

The second indication consisted in the iemo\al of undigested masses ietained
in the intestinal tiact. Not only in cases in which the diaiihœa had iesulted
fiom pie\ious eiiois in diet of the child, but also in those cases dependent upon
sudden changes of tempeiatuie and exposuie, it was desiiable to empty the intestinal tiact. For that puipose castoi oil, calcined magnesia, or calomel might be
used.

Thiid. Nothing should be gi\en that contained salts in any soit of concentia-
tion. Thus, beef-tea should be a\oided. It must be iemembeied that that foim
of meat-extiact contained a \eiy laige amount of salts, and that the diiect effect
of those upon the intestinal canal might be pioducti\e of \eiy unpleasant consequences. If the people insisted upon gi\ing it, and theie was no special contia-
indication to its use in a gi\en case, it should be administeied only in connection
with some well-cooked faiinaceous \ehicle, and the best of all foi that puipose
was bailey-watei ; or it might be mixed with beaten white of egg, but no moie
chloiide of sodium should be added. For the main dangei in beef-tea was the
concentiated foim in which its salts weie gi\en.

Fouith. E\eiything should be a\oided that incieased peiistaltic motion. Thus,
caibonic acid and ice inteinally.

Fifth. A\oid whate\ei thieatened to inciease the amount of acid in the stomach and intestinal tiact. Theie was so much acid in the noimal, and still moie
in the abnoimal stomach and intestinal tiact, that it was absolutely necessaiy to
neutialize it. For that puipose it was safei to iesoit to piepaiations of calcium
than of sodium or magnesium. So fai as lime-watei was conceined, its adminis-

tration, ceitainly, was coiiect chemically. But we should not place too much ieliance upon that populai iemedy. We should not foiget that it contained about one pait of lime to eight hundied of watei, and that it was necessaiy to swallow at least *two* ounces of the fluid in oidei to obtain a single giain of lime.

A fuithei indication was, *the necessity of destioying feiments.* For that puipose most metallic piepaiations would do faii seiiice. One which had been extensively used was *calomel*, and now in *small doses* fiequently iepeated—$\frac{1}{16}$, $\frac{1}{4}$, or $\frac{1}{2}$ a giain eieiy *two* or *thiee* houis. As to its effect as an antifeimentatiie, theie could be no doubt.

Nitiate of silvei, when giien foi the same puipose, should be *laigely diluted*. Fiom $\frac{1}{30}$ to $\frac{1}{15}$ of a giain dissoliêd in a teaspoonful or tablespoonful of watei, might be giien eieiy *two* oi *thiee* houis, and not infiequently with faii iesult. That was especially impoitant with iegaid to injections of nitiate of silvei into the iectum, wheie it was apt to do as much haim as good. Whenever it was to be giien in that way, the solution should be mild and laigely diluted, or the anus and its neighbouihood should be washed with salt watei befoie the injection was administeied.

Bismuth acted ieiy faiouiably. Modeiate cases of diaiihœa would usually show its effect ieiy soon. Doses of fiom $\frac{1}{2}$ to 2 or 3 giains, giien eieiy *two* or *thiee* houis, would act ieiy faiouiably indeed. In those cases in which the diaiihœa had lasted foi a long time, the doses of bismuth should be laige in oidei to be ceitain of immediate contact of the diug with the soie suiface.

A final indication was the depiession of the hyperæsthesia of the geneial system and of the intestinal tiact in paiticulai. Theie had been authois who condemned the use of opium altogethei, which, ceitainly, was incoiiect. The doses should be *small*, and they might be iepeated fiequently. Administeied in that mannei, opium could be used with peifect safety both inteinally and in an enema. One of the iules foi giiing opium was that the child should not be waked up foi the puipose of taking the medicine. Whenever theie was feai of collapse, it was safei to giie $\frac{1}{200}$ of a giain eieiy half houi or houi, than to administei $\frac{1}{50}$ of a giain eieiy two houis.

Alcohol.—Small and fiequent doses would ceitainly stimulate the neiious system, digestion, and ciiculation, and they also stimulated the skin and incieased peispiiation. Alcohol, giien in that mannei, ceitainly aiiested feimentation. Moieoiei, it took the place of food, and acted faiouiably as food when no solid caibo-hydiates weie toleiated by the intestinal tiact. As it was absoibed in the stomach, so did it piotect the intestinal tiact.

Finally, it is necessaiy to ieduce the amount of secietion taking place fiom the suiface of the intestinal tiact. For that puipose astiingents might be used, such as alum, lead, tannic acid, peinitiate of iion, and, what had alieady been spoken of, nitiate of silvei. In all those cases in which the stomach paiticipated in the piocess to any consideiable extent, almost any astiingent would pioie ineffectiie. To fulfil seieial indications at the same time, it was often good piactice to combine iemedies.

The main indications weie to neutialize acids, to ieduce neiious iiiitability, to aiiest secietion, and to change the condition of the suiface of the cataiihal mucous membiane.

For that puipose, in the geneiality of cases, he combiiied bismuth, opium, and chalk, accoiding to the following foimula: ℞. Bismuth subnit., gi. i; Piepaied chalk, gis. ij; Doiei's powdei, gi. $\frac{1}{2}$.

That combination was suitable foi a baby *ten* or *tweive* months of age, and the dose could be iepeated eieiy two houis. In all those cases in which acid was very abundant, it was necessary to increase the doses of antacids without necessarily giving large doses of opium.

Hot bathing was especially serviceable in those cases in which the surface was cool and the temperature of the body, measured in the rectum, was pretty high. To relieve intestinal pain, plain warm fomentations; to relieve heat, cold applications were sufficient.

Camphor stimulated the heart, and reduced temperature, and might be used internally or subcutaneously according to the necessities in the case. For subcutaneous injections it might be dissolved in either oil or alcohol. The effect derived from camphor as a stimulant was not permanent, but very much more so than that produced by carbonate of ammonia. The dose might be from $\frac{1}{4}$ to $\frac{1}{2}$ a grain every hour or two, when only a moderate stimulation was required. In urgent cases it might be given in doses of from *five* to *ten* grains in the course of an hour, and usually the effect would be favourable. It was, however, only in cases in which real collapse was present that doses of five or ten grains would be required.

There was no remedy that would act more favourably in conditions of great debility and collapse than *musk*. It might be given in doses of five or ten grains, and repeated every half hour or hour. More than two or three such doses would not be required to yield a result.

———

Pathological Anatomy of Muscular Atrophy.

HAYEM (Paris, 1877) has endeavoured to draw up the anatomo-pathological history of muscular atrophy, independent of the different pathological causes. He includes under the name of muscular atrophy all those muscular affections in which the striated fibres have either entirely disappeared or only become much reduced in size. In the first chapter of his book he enters fully into the structure of the normal muscular tissue and the modifications which the striated substance is apt to present under certain conditions. We have given a short *resumé* of the conclusions at which he has arrived in his researches on the influence of traumatic lesions or certain chemical agents on the formation of vitreous deposits, and on the changes which the muscle undergoes in the dead body. 1. The vitreous transformation of the muscular fibres is not merely a modification caused by death, but a change peculiar to living fibres, probably due for the greater part to the contractile power of the fibres. 2. The loss of vitality of the muscular fibres can be anatomically recognized by a peculiar change which takes place in the striated substance, and by the fact that certain fluids no longer possess the power of transforming it into the vitreous substance. 3. The muscular fibres resist the process of decomposition for a certain length of time. When putrefaction has finally set in, the changes produced in the fibres are such that they cannot be mistaken for pathological alterations, except in the frog, where the changes wrought by putrefaction do not differ much from changes which would take place in degenerated *intra vitam*. The second chapter contains the anatomo-pathological history of the muscular tissue. It begins by a general survey of the lesions of the striated substance (modification of the striæ, loss of transparency, simply atrophy, diverse degenerations), of the muscular cells (tumefaction, multiplication, neoformation, atrophy, degeneration), of the sarcolemma, the perimysium of the vessels and intra-muscular nerves. The author then proceeds to describe the changes occurring in the muscles, which correspond to the various causes of muscular atrophy. Atrophies caused by some nervous affection are most frequently met with. In cases where the atrophy is merely the consequence of a simple suppression of voluntary stimulation (hemiplegia originating in some cerebral affection, prolonged inactivity, etc.), the muscular lesions are not very important. A few fibres have become atrophic, and the rest have retained their original size, and merely undergone a very slight degree of granulo-pigmentary degeneration, which gives the muscle a brownish colouring, that has long ago been pointed out by M. Charcot. When the atrophy is caused by some destructive lesions of the cells of the anterior horns of the spinal cord, the affection assumes a greater importance. In acute central myelitis, of which three cases have come under the author's notice, the muscular fibres undergo an acute fatty degeneration, they become opaque and their nuclei are swelled. In infantile paralysis, and in chronic affections of the spinal cord (progressive muscular atrophy, sclerosis, partial myelitis, etc.), the muscular fibres present numerous modifications. Some are merely atrophic, with occasional proliferation of their nuclei; others are undergoing a granular degeneration, which is attended during its first stages by a considerable multiplication of the nuclei, and, during the latter stages, by atrophy of the same. In a third class, the fibres are infiltrated with pigmentary granulations, or present certain modifications in the structure of their striæ. The existence of vitreous degeneration in amyatrophias due to some spinal affection has not yet been sufficiently proved. As the muscular fibres become atrophic, the connective tissue becomes thicker, and is covered with a layer of fat cells. Similar changes have been observed in amyotrophia, following the lesions of nerves (neuralgia, neuritis, traumatic lesions, etc.). After having stated and criticised the different opinions which have been emitted by various authors on the pathological physiology of these muscular atrophies, which are closely allied to changes in the spinal cord or the nerves, the author ranges himself among the partisans of the theory of the trophic effects. He admits that the cells of the anterior horns of the gray substance of the medulla exercise both a motor and trophic influence on the corresponding muscles, and that this effect is transmitted by the medium of the motor nerves. It results from this, that any change which is capable of suppressing or diminishing the influence of the medullary cells on the muscles, will be followed by paralysis and atrophy. In one of the most remarkable portions of his work, the author exposes his views on atrophy of the muscles resulting from dyscrasia; acute starvation does not produce any notable alterations in the muscles, but acute marasmus always gives rise to very considerable lesions. The muscles are semi-transparent and of a purplish colouring; they are soft, viscous, sticky; their vessels are filled with blood; every trace of interstitial fat has disappeared. If the fibres are examined while yet fresh, they seem to have grown thinner, they are semi-opaque, and present the appearance of having been covered with dust. Some of them consist apparently of a semi-liquid grayish substance, in which hardly any traces of striation are left; others are undergoing fatty or granulo-pigmentary degeneration. The muscular cells are not increased in number, some of them have assumed the appearance of small vesicles. These changes in the muscular tissue attack all the muscles of the body, including the heart. The changes wrought by chronic marasmus do not vary much from those which have just been described. The wasted muscles are of a pinky gray tint covered with yellow lines and spots; they are soft and flabby. The microscope lesions are diffused over the whole muscle, and may be described as simple atrophy, the striation still existing, granular degeneration, fatty degeneration, or pigmentary degeneration. Small hemorrhages and accumulations of interstitial adipose tissue are frequently found in the perimysium. Muscular atrophy resulting from acute affections complicated with changes in the blood, presents altogether a different appearance. It may be limited to one particular region or be diffused over the whole system. In the latter case, the alterations in the muscular tissue resemble more or less those observed in acute marasmus; the muscles are con-

gested, the striation appears blurred and indistinct, and the sarcolemma is in a
state of partial degeneration. The circumscribed lesions, on the contrary, have
all the characteristic symptoms of inflammatory lesions ; they are the principal
cause of symptomatic myositis with its host of complications, such as hemorrhage,
suppuration, etc. The author winds up with a short sketch of muscular atrophy,
due to poisoning with certain substances, or to primary affections of the muscles.
—*London Med. Record*, July 15, 1879.

—

Generalized Scleroderma, with Bronzing of the Skin and Punctate Vitiligo
(Leucoderma).

The patient, a man, aged 43, had always had a brown skin, but twenty months
before he came under notice, he somewhat suddenly became as brown as a
mulatto. At the same time he was seized with violent itching all over the body,
and scratched and rubbed himself till the blood flowed. Not only the exposed
parts became tinted, but also the skin of the back and abdomen. M. Féréol
describes the colour as one of yellow-brown, or sepia, very like, at first sight, the
coloration of Addison's disease. The abdomen was most affected ; the genitals
and extremities less so. A stroke with the finger nail upon the skin produced a
persistent white streak, due to the elevation of the epidermis, mapping out a dull
white upon the deep black of the pigmented derma. The mucous surfaces of the
mouth, etc., presented no pigmentation, except a very pale tattoo upon the lower
lip, opposite some carious teeth. The bronzing was in some parts uniform ; in
others granite-like from two tints. Besides this feature, there were a number of
white patches distributed symmetrically, and occupying all those parts where the
bones made prominences. Almost at the same time that the change of colour
commenced, the patient perceived that his skin became hard and inextensible,
seeming to fit tightly to the deeper parts. This was particularly so with the
hands, the trunk, and the face, so as to hinder his work and even impede mastication. The description of the case by M. Féréol is one of typical scleroderma,
affecting the hands, as well as other parts, producing contraction of the palmar
fascia, and showing also superficial scars of a former necrotic process, such as is
known to occur in some cases of scleroderma. He experienced considerable impediment in his movement ; he could not dress himself, and walking fatigued him.
He breathed well, notwithstanding the thoracic sclerosis. There was grating in
some of his joints. His antecedents are also important. His mother, though
still living, is very nervous. In his youth he was strumous, suffered thrice from
pneumonia, and after that, being a looking-glass maker, he suffered from mercurial poisoning. He subsequently suffered from a long attack of rheumatism,
which attacked all his joints, and crippled him considerably for a long period.
M. Féréol insists much on this rheumatic attack as determining the development
of the scleroderma. but it is also worthy of discussion whether Addison's disease
is not coexistent with scleroderma, or whether the coloration is anything more
than an excessive development of the pigment, which is usually present in excess
in leucoderma, in parts which are not leucodermic. All things considered, M.
Féréol inclines to the opinion that the case is not one of Addison's disease with
scleroderma, but that the coloration and scleroderma are both determined by some
common cause.—*London Med. Record*, July 15, 1879.

Surgery.

Analysis of Three hundred and fifteen Cases in which Foreign Bodies were lodged in the Brain.

Dr. H. R. WHARTON analyzes (*Phila. Med. Times*, July 19, 1879) three hundred and fifteen cases in which foreign bodies were lodged in the brain, of which one hundred and sixty recovered, while one hundred and fifty-six died.

In one hundred and six cases the foreign body was removed, death following in thirty-four cases, recovery in seventy-two cases.

In two hundred and ten cases no attempt was made to remove the foreign body, death following in one hundred and twenty-two cases, recovery in eighty-eight cases. It should be here stated that some ten patients who recovered sufficiently to attend to their regular occupations, but ultimately died at periods varying from three to fifteen years from the effects of their injuries, have been classed as having recovered.

Considering the severity of the injury, the proportion of recoveries is large, but on examination of the cases it will be observed that many of the recoveries were not complete, the patients afterwards suffering from epilepsy, vertigo, impairment of mind, incapacity for physical exertion, paralysis, loss of sight and hearing. In one hundred and eleven of the cases of recovery the above-named symptoms were wanting, while they were present in forty-nine cases.

In the one hundred and eleven cases that recovered without bad symptoms, the foreign body was removed in fifty-six cases and allowed to remain in forty-five cases. The question of interference for removal of foreign bodies is one which has caused much discussion, but on which Dr. W. thinks authorities are now generally agreed. In the following collection of cases the results of its removal were not only most satisfactory as regards recovery, but also as regards the completeness of the recovery. There can be no doubt that the presence of the foreign body increases the gravity of the injury, and that when its position can be clearly located, and when its removal is not accompanied with too great a destruction of tissue, it should be attempted. The difficulty of locating the foreign body is seen to be great, for when it has once passed out of sight the surgeon has no means of discovering its position, except by the probe. Extreme care should be exercised in passing a probe along the track of a foreign body in a wound of this nature, as little force is required to cause the probe to pass through the unresisting brain structure in a course different from that taken by the vulnerating body, and the surgeon may add other wounds to an already most serious injury. On the other hand, where the body cannot be accurately located, all attempts to find it by frequent probing should be desisted from, for, as has been shown, a large number of cases have recovered where it has not been removed, and there is a possibility of its becoming encysted, and of recovery taking place in this way or of life at least being prolonged.

Dr. W. thinks that Prof. Thomas Longmore, in his article on trephining in injuries of the head, expresses the opinion of the best surgeons of the present day. He says, " If the site of lodgment of the projectile is obvious, it should be removed with as little disturbance as possible, but trephining for its extraction when the place of its lodgment is not definitely known, but where the projectile is only supposed by inference to be lodged in a particular spot beneath the cranium, is an unwarrantable operation."[1] The presence of the foreign body in the brain in many cases excites inflammatory action, which may be either rapid or slow in its

---

[1] Holmes's System of Surgery, vol. ii. p. 181.

progress, sometimes destroying large amounts of brain-tissue before the case ends fatally. That cerebral abscess is a frequent cause of death is clearly shown by the fact that it was present in at least fifty-three of the fatal cases where post-mortem examinations were made ; in many other cases the examination was made solely with reference to the location of the foreign body, and the condition of the surrounding tissues is not stated.

Apoplexy is also shown to be a cause of death in these injuries, but much less frequently than abscess. Pressure of the foreign body on the venous branches, interfering with the return of blood, causing effusion into the cavities of the brain, and this effusion by its pressure interfering with the function of the nerves which have their origin from the base of the brain, is also noted as a cause of death. Convulsions and coma, also resulting from this interference with the circulation of the blood in the brain, are frequently noted. A tendency to coma, it might be here stated, as in all head injuries, is a most unfavourable symptom, nearly every one of these cases in which it was marked proving fatal.

The presence of the foreign body in the brain seems to predispose to inflammatory action ; in some cases of recovery where the foreign body remained in the brain, the cases progressed favourably until some cerebral excitement was experienced ; five cases are recorded where death took place suddenly after excessive drinking, in one case during the excitement of a game of cards, in another after a slight injury of the head.

Seven cases were complicated with hernia cerebri ; three of these proved fatal, four ending in recovery.

In quite a number of cases the foreign body remained in the brain for some time without causing any unfavourable symptoms, when suddenly cerebral symptoms were developed and death quickly followed. Dr. W. thinks that the experiments of M. Flourens will help to explain these cases. He introduced leaden bullets into the brains of rabbits and dogs. The balls were placed on different parts of the upper region of the encephalon and on the lobes of the cerebellum. The balls left to the action of their own weight, penetrated by degrees the substance of the brain, and ultimately stopped at the base of the cranium, the passage made by the balls healing after them.[1] This fact that bodies were found to change their position may account for the sudden deaths in cases where their presence had previously occasioned little trouble.

Brodie's opinion that recovery is more apt to follow wounds of the anterior portion of the brain is strengthened by examination of the cases where the foreign body penetrated the frontal bone, of which there were one hundred and thirty-two, followed by death in fifty-eight cases and recovery in seventy-four cases.

There were fifty-eight cases of penetration of the parietal bones, followed by twenty-seven deaths and thirty-one recoveries.

The occipital bone was penetrated in twenty-three cases, with sixteen deaths and seven recoveries.

The temporal bones were penetrated in thirty-one cases, with twelve deaths and nineteen recoveries.

Wounds of the orbit were by far the most fatal, eighteen in number, followed by seventeen deaths and one recovery, although the persons were in many cases unconscious of the injury, and the unfavourable symptoms developed suddenly.

The sphenoid bone was penetrated in five cases, with four deaths and one recovery.

In forty-nine cases where the wound of entrance was not definitely stated, there were twenty-two deaths and twenty-seven recoveries.

---

[1] Dublin Med. Press, July to December, 1862.

Glycosuric Ocular Affections.

(i) Dr. GALEZOWSKI makes a communication (*Recueil d' Opthalmologie*, 3d series, No. 2, Feb. 1879) upon a new affection of the eye, glycosuric keratitis. Three cases are reported. One of these presented some phenomena of a corroding ulcerous nature; the other two of diffuse keratitis. One of the most characteristic symptoms of these affections is complete anæsthesia of the cornea, in spite of photophobia more or less intense, and peri-orbital pains. Glycosuric keratitis presents itself under two forms—*a.* Corroding ulcer; *b.* Diffuse superficial kera-titis. It yields readily under the influence of a severe anti-glycosuric regimen, with warm water douches to the eyelids, administered regularly two or three times a day, and with alternate instillation of atropine and eserine. A case is reported where this treatment gave good results. (ii) *Paralysis of the Third, Fourth, and Sixth Pair of a Glycosuric Nature.* The author's researches have shown that of 100 patients afflicted with paralysis of the sixth pair, glycosuria was traced as the cause in eight cases. It was not so with paralysis of the third pair. This is explained, in the author's opinion, by the original position of the two motor nerves. (iii) *Glycosuric Amblyopia without Lesion.* This malady very often resembles alcoholic amblyopia. It declares itself rapidly, and causes a certain degree of weakness of vision; it remains stationary for months and even years, but is susceptible of amelioration and complete cure under the influence of a simple dietetic regimen. The difference between glycosuria and alcoholic amblyopia may be known by the following signs. (i) The affection generally attacks but one eye, while in alcoholic amblyopia it is binocular. (ii) In glycosuric ambly-opia, the patient often distinguishes, although by a great effort, the typographical character number 2. In alcoholism he cannot do so. (iii) Alcoholic amblyopia is often accompanied with a perversion of the chromatic faculty. This phenomenon never exists in glycosuric amblyopia; but there does exist often in both a partial colour blindness. (iv) When alcoholic amblyopia has lasted some months, the papilla is observed to become anæmic, resembling a progressive atrophy of this nerve. In a glycosuric amblyopia, the papilla remains always red, and even with an appearance of congestion. A case is given of amblyopia of a glycosuric nature, with an analysis of the urine, made by M. Mehu, of which the following is the result. Urine, 11.2 gr.; uric acid, 0.27 gr.; sugar, 48.7 gr.; mineral salts, 7.3 gr.; organic matter, 4.98 gr.; water, 927.55 gr.—*London Med. Record*, June 15, 1879.

Excision of Cancerous Stricture from the Rectum.

At a late meeting of the Royal Medical and Chirurgical Society (*Lancet*, June 28, 1879), Mr. JOHN GUY read a paper in abstract on this subject. The patient, a lady aged thirty-seven, was conscious of having suffered for twelve months from symptoms which were clearly those of cancerous stricture of the rectum. She consulted the author of the paper in 1878, when he discovered a moderately tight stricture, formed of cancerous tissue, ulcerated on its internal surface, about two inches and a half from the anus, occupying the seat of what is known as "Houston's third ligament," just above the tip of the coccyx. Defecation had become difficult, and was often attended with violent straining and the passage of blood or discoloured and offensive sanious fluid. As her sufferings increased, and the necessity for colotomy became imminent, Mr. Gay, with the concurrence of Mr. Worley, of De Beauvoir-square, whose patient she was, after ascertain-ing that the stricture mass had formed no connections or adhesions with sur-rounding parts, but was movable amongst them, advised its removal, to which the patient gladly assented. This was done on the 4th of November, with Mr.

Harrison Cripps' and Mr. Worley's assistance, in the following manner : It was at first deemed possible to carry out this object somewhat after the manner that Nature casts off portions of bowel—viz., by invagination, and, with this purpose in view, the operation was begun. The rectum was slit up behind to the coccyx, by means of a strong bistoury (the patient having been placed under the influence of an anæsthetic by Mr. Cumberbatch), and the bowel reached below the stricture by cutting through the levator ani, fascia, and its other investments. The morbid growth was then detached from its surroundings by tearing, as well as a ring of healthy bowel both above and below.   An attempt was now made to invaginate the diseased bowel into the healthy portion below, but the absence of sufficient elasticity and mobility on the part of the textures concerned stood in the way of its accomplishment.   Excision was then the only alternative, and this was done by cutting across the healthy bowel, first below and then above the disease, partly by the knife, and in other parts by the benzine cautery ; some vessels required tying, and other bleeding was stopped by searing.   No attempts were made to bring the edges of the wounds together by force ; they were simply laid together, and the whole dressed antiseptically.   The patient had a very good night's rest after the operation, and was sensibly conscious of having been re- lieved of the source of her suffering.   Nothing untoward occurred for the first fortnight but vesical retention for two or three days, which called for the catheter, and fecal incontinence, unaccompanied by any pain. . From that period to the 10th of May, the date of the last report, her course was chequered.   In Decem- ber she had an acute attack of cystitis ; when this had passed away she suffered from frequent and irregularly recurring attacks of abdominal spasms, with or without distension or obstruction, which terminated in severe rectal tenesmus. Under the influence of opiates and hot fomentations these subsided, and for a time passed off, but they did not finally cease until the vertical cleft in the bowel had healed.   The surfaces of the cut sphincter were exceedingly sensitive, and it was supposed that these spasms were in some way connected with their rawness. After that some folds of skin at the verge of the anus became ulcerated by fecal irritation, and had to be removed.   In the month of January it was found that a diaphragm had formed by the thickening of submucous areolar tissue in the neighbourhood of the internal sphincter, with an aperture that allowed the intro- duction of the forefinger.   As the aperture did not appear inclined to become narrower, the barrier was not intentionally interfered with, for with its formation the fecal incontinence lessened, and the alvine discharges became consistent, and, at times, hard, so that it was accredited with the design of supplementing the suspended action of the sphincters.   In April the patient began to fall away, and symptoms showed themselves which were only consistent with a recurrence of the disease, and, on examination, cancerous nodules were found on the os uteri and adjoining vaginal tissue against the intestinal cicatrix, and no doubt could be felt but that they had formed in the cicatricial tissue as well.   In May, however, her condition had improved in some respects. She was free from pain, the abdomen was soft, the motions more under control than they had previously been, and she took her food.   Pain and difficulty in micturition, from which she had suffered during a part of the previous month, had also passed away.   The local symptoms, however, were unchanged.   The author did not claim this as a successful case, but thought it deserving the consideration of the Fellows, inas- much as it gave grounds for hoping that the surgery of the rectum had not been exhausted.   It showed, first, that the system was more tolerant of severe injury to the rectum than had been suspected, for it bore without resentment the re- moval of a considerable and an entire cylinder from that part of the bowel which closely adjoined the peritoneal cavity.   The temperature did not exceed 100° at any time subsequent to the operation, and only rose to that point for two or three hours on the fifth day. And, secondly, that nature is quite adequate to the process of repair. It is admitted, too, that the recovery was protracted and attended with great suffering, but on reviewing its steps and stages by the side of the painful symptoms with which it was accompanied, it is clear, the author thinks, that the troubles were due to the fact that, throughout, nature was deprived of the assistance of art. Had the sundered portions of bowel been brought more closely into apposition, the cleft in the sphincters been immediately reunited, and all portions of superfluous skin removed from the anus, the suffering must have been much ameliorated, the healing less protracted, and the chance of recurrence of the disease, to a corresponding degree, lessened. The author offered some suggestions for utilizing the rectum, by slitting it up, in cases in which nearer access is needed for surgical purposes, or even exploration to the higher portion of the rectum, such, for instance, as cases of intussusception, impaction, fistulous passages, polypoid and other growths, ulcers, etc. ; and, moreover, that in cases of imperforate anus, taking the coccyx as the "landmark," and assuming that the cul de sac reaches as far as that bone or below it, the bowel might without danger be entered at that point, and an opening made from within. The author concluded by trusting that this case, although incomplete and, in point of aim, in all probability, unsuccessful, might give confidence for future proceedings in the direction indicated, and that, if so, it might, by its relation, conduce to mitigate suffering and to prolong if not to save life.

The PRESIDENT doubted whether excision of true cancer of the rectum were a preferable operation to colotomy, owing to the certainty of speedy recurrence of the disease.

Mr. CRIPPS said that all the specimens he had examined had not been examples of cancer properly so called. The disease began as an adenoid growth in the submucous tissue, proceeding to ulceration and cicatrization, so that the floor of the ulcer becomes dense and scirrhus-like. In a case of his own he had removed a recurrence four months after the primary operation, and since then (about two years) the patient had remained quite well. Her condition was better than if colotomy had been performed. Another patient operated on by Sir James Paget three years ago was now in good health and attending to business.

Mr. HOLMES thought the operation performed by Mr. Gay was not only novel, but, on anatomical and surgical grounds, was dangerous. He knew of cases where, after removal of portions of the rectum, death had ensued from cellulitis and peritonitis, without the peritoneum being injured at the operation. The danger would be increased by slitting up the bowel and removing a zone of it, as Mr. Gay had done. At the same time he thought excision might be of advantage in selected cases ; and he agreed with Mr. Cripps that all the cases are not true cancers. He had excised the lower end of the rectum for an adenoid growth eighteen months ago, and the patient remained well, but had no control over the bowel, the sphincters having been freely removed. Mr. Gay's patient was still in a position to have colotomy performed.

Mr. CRIPPS had notes of thirteen cases (five under his own care) with two deaths ; one from peritonitis, where the peritoneum had been specially wounded.

Mr. HULKE said that several years ago Mr. C. Moore, at the Middlesex Hospital, had performed excision of the rectum for cancer in four or five cases, and Mr. De Morgan in two. All these patients succumbed in three or four days from diffuse pelvic inflammation. Still, in select cases the operation was justifiable ; and he had done it himself. If the disease were beyond reach then colotomy was preferable.

Case in which Sixteen Inches of a Varicose Vein of the Leg were successfully Excised with Antiseptic Treatment.

Mr. THOMAS ANNANDALE reports (*British Med. Journ.*, June 21, 1879) the following case :—

James S., aged 21, a joiner, was admitted to the Royal Infirmary on January 13th, 1879. The patient, who was a great athlete, stated that, four years ago, he strained his leg whilst attempting a high jump. The accident was followed by considerable pain in the part, and by swelling of one of the veins on the anterior aspect of the left leg. Before this time, he had never suffered from any varicosity of the veins.

On admission, the patient was found to have a large single tortuous vein, of about the breadth of one's little finger, running directly upwards from the external malleolus of the ankle-joint for about ten inches along the anterior surface of the left leg ; then crossing the tibia obliquely for about three inches, it continued upwards for six inches on the internal aspect of the leg, terminating opposite the inner tuberosity of the tibia.

Operation.—The patient being young and healthy, and the general venous system, with the exception of the part above described, being unaffected, Professor Annandale thought right to attempt a radical cure by excision of the diseased vessel. Accordingly, on January 17th, he made an incision over the lower part of the vein, exposed the branches entering it, tied them with catgut, and then cut them through, in this way separating the affected vein from the surrounding textures. He then ligatured the vein above and below, and cut it out, in this way removing the lower ten inches of the diseased vessel. He next treated the upper six inches in a like manner, but left the middle oblique portion *in situ*, being unwilling to cause a cicatrix over the anterior aspect of the tibia ; and hoping that this portion, being ligatured at both ends, would become obliterated. The operation was carried out, and the wound dressed, with antiseptic precaution. During the operation, an elastic bandage was placed round the lower part of the thigh, to keep the diseased vein prominent.

January 18. The wounds were dressed ; they looked very well, and quite free from irritation. The blood in the middle oblique portion was found to be coagulating.

On the 22d, 25th, and 27th of January, the wounds were dressed under the carbolic spray ; and on February 2d, the wounds being quite superficial, the carbolic dressing was discontinued, and boracic ointment substituted for it. This dressing was applied daily till February 6th, when the wounds were found to be healed.

A day or two afterwards, the patient was dismissed from the hospital, being instructed to wear an elastic bandage lightly applied whilst at his work.

March 4. The patient returned from the country to-day, and stated that he had been at his work ever since leaving the hospital, and that he had not felt any inconvenience from the effects of the operation. On inspection the wounds were found to be firmly healed ; there was no return of varicosity in the limb, and the middle part of the vein, which had been ligatured and left *in situ*, had completely disappeared.

In his remarks on the case, Mr. Annandale says the case was most favourable for operative interference. The healthy condition of the patient, the limitation of the varicosity to one principal vein, and the failure of ordinary treatment to relieve the symptoms, made the case in his opinion a perfect illustration of the class of this affection which is best suited for operation. Until the introduction of Lister's antiseptics, his experience of the different methods of operative interference foi the ielief of vaiicose veins of the lowei limb was not encouiaging; but when the value of catgut ligatuie and othei antiseptic details had been fully and piactically tested and pioved, he felt convinced that the most piomising pioceeding was the antiseptic excision of a gieatei oi less poition of the affected vein.

On Novembei 7th, 1874, a veiy aggiavated case of vaiicocele came undei his caie; and as all the usual tieatment had failed, he cut down upon the speimatic veins, exposed the laigest of them, and cut out fully two inches of it, having fiist ligatuied the vein with catgut above and below the points of its division. The iesult in this case was a complete cuie. About six months afteiwaids, his patient maiiied; and, in the yeais that have since elapsed, seveial childien have been boin to him. A note of this case was published in the *Biitish Medical Jouinal* of Januaiy 30th, 1875. In the Jouinal of the 23d of Januaiy of the same yeai, Mr. John Maishall published the abstiact of a clinical lectuie in which he advocated a similai opeiation, and iciated a case in which he had iemoved successfully about nine inches of a vaiicose vein of the leg. Mr. Chailes Steele, in a papei in the Jouinal of Januaiy 30th, 1875, advocated the iemoval, without the application of a ligatuie, of small poitions, about an inch, of vaiicose veins, and iepoited seveial cases in which he successfully caiiied out this plan.

In the case of vaiicocele iefeiied to, and in the piesent case, the opeiation was peifoimed without any complication of compiessing the veins by pins above and below the poition to be iemoved, as in Mr. Maishall's opeiation. The veins weie exposed by dissection, any bianches passing into them being ligatuied and divided in the piogiess of the dissection. When the poition of the vein to be iemoved had in this way sepaiated fiom the suiiounding tissues, a catgut ligatuie was applied at both ends of the sepaiated vessel, which was then cut away. In the case of the opeiation on the leg, an elastic bandage was applied iound the lowei pait of the thigh, so as to keep the affected vein piominent.

It is inteiesting to note that the poition of vein lying ovei the tibia, and which was not interfeied with, in oidei to avoid a cicatiix ovei this bone, became oblite-iated; and theiefoie the entiie affected poition of vein, measuiing about nineteen inches in length, was effectually iemoved by the opeiation.

Elephantiasis Aiabum of the Leg, treated by Ligature of the Femoial Aitery.

Mr. Ciosby Leonaid, Consulting Suigeon to the Biistol Royal Infiimaiy, iepoits (*Biitish Med. Jouinal,* June 21, 1879) the following case :—

Alfied R., aged 19, was admitted into No. 14 Waid of the Biistol Royal Infirmary, on May 4th, 1868, with elephantiasis of the iight lowei limb. He was of daik complexion, small make, only foui feet and a half in height, looked pale and weakly, had a caiewoin expiession, but said that he had not had any seiious illness, that his appetite was good, and that he felt well. He had been neaily all his life in Biistol. His fathei died of phthisis; otheiwise his family histoiy was good. He had been at school until eight months ago, when he was appienticed to an engiavei. When thiee months old, his mothei noticed that the iight leg was shoitei than the left, and it giadually incieased in size dispiopoitionately to the left, not being painful, but giving iise to a peculiai gait. Thiee months ago, the enlaigement began to inciease moie iapidly—accounted foi piobably by the fact that, for five months pieviously, he had been woiking at his tiade, which necessitated much standing, sometimes foi houis consecutively. He had not suffeied much pain or constitutional distuibance; but, at inteivals, pain of an aching chaiactei, and chiefly in the calf of the leg, would come on suddenly, lasting about thiee days, and often accompanied with sickness and feveiishness. These attacks did not appeai to follow any unusual exeition, oi to be dependent on any extei-

nal cause. Although much inconvenienced by the size and weight of the limb, he could walk three or four miles at a stretch.

The whole of the right lower limb was hypertrophied, and felt hard and firm; the hypertrophy extended to the nates, the greatest enlargement being between the knee and ankle. There was a marked constriction at the ankle, and a prominent mass of hypertrophied tissue on the dorsum of the foot and on two of the toes. The skin on the foot and posterior surface of the leg was rough and thickened, and of a brownish colour. He had hydrocele on the right side, and thickening of the skin and subcutaneous tissue of the scrotum. The following were the measurements of the limbs, taken when in the horizontal position.

	Right.	Left.
Middle of thigh . . .	19½ inches.	15 inches.
Knee	16 "	12 "
Middle of leg	23½ "	10½ "
Middle of foot . . .	13¼ ..	8½ '
Base of toes	11¼ ..	—

May 9. He was ordered to remain in bed, with the leg and foot raised on an inclined plane.

20th. The foot and leg had considerably diminished in size, and the whole limb felt less hard; but the circumference of the thigh had increased, and there was more enlargement about the nates. The measurements now were: middle of thigh, 20 inches; knee, 16 inches; middle of leg, 17 inches; middle of foot, 12 inches; base of toes, 10½ inches. He was ordered up on the 22d, and on the 28th the increase in size of the thigh and nates had disappeared, and the leg was returning to its original condition of hardness. I proposed to ligature the femoral artery; and, on consultation with my colleagues, this was agreed to.

20th. The patient being under the influence of ether and chloroform, I placed a ligature of whipcord round the femoral artery, just above the sartorius. The skin and subcutaneous tissue were about an inch in thickness, looking like condensed fat and cellular tissue, infiltrated with a serous fluid, which exuded freely. The artery was small, and its pulsation could not be felt until the sheath was opened. The wound was brought together with horse-hair sutures and adhesive plaster; the entire limb was bandaged with a flannel roller and enveloped in cotton-wool. On removal to his bed, a tin of hot water was applied to the foot and one on each side of the leg, with a blanket over all. No unfavourable symptoms followed the operation; there was sickness and some febrile disturbance for three days. On the fourth day, I removed the central sutures, and purulent fluid escaped freely.

June 5. He was well in himself. The leg was rebandaged, its temperature and appearance being satisfactory. The purulent discharge from the wound was slight.

11th. The ligature came away yesterday; the wound was healing. The limb was obviously smaller. An ordinary bandage was firmly applied from the toes upwards, to be readjusted when necessary.

17th. He was allowed to get up. The wound had been healed for several days. The hydrocele had disappeared, and he said that he was quite well.

He was discharged on September 1st, and ordered to wear an elastic apparatus on the foot and leg.

The following are the measurements taken subsequently to the operation:—

	Middle of Thigh.	Middle of Leg.	Middle of Foot.	Base of Toes.
June 5. . .	19 inches.	17½ inches.	11¾ inches.	11½ inches.
" 11. . .	17¾ "	14½ "	11½ "	—
" 18. . .	17½ "	14 "	11½ "	—
July 3. . .	18 ..	13½ "	11¾ "	10½ "
" 13. . .	18½ ..	12¼ "	11¼ "	—
" 20. . .	18½ ..	12⅛ "	11 "	—
" 27. . .	17½ ..	12 "	11 "	—
Aug. 8. . .	17½ ..	11½ "	10½ "	9¾
" 17. . .	17½ ..	10¼ "	10½ "	—
" 29. . .	17 ..	10¼ "	10½ "	9¾ ..

1871.—*January* 17. He called on me, looking stouter, and said that he had continued in good health and suffered but very little inconvenience from his leg; that for many months he had been travelling with a troup of Christy Minstrels, and taking the dancing part of the performance. His right leg measured: middle of thigh, 19 inches; middle of leg, 11¼ inches; middle of foot, 10¼ inches. Unfortunately, the left leg was not measured, so that the relative proportion of the two limbs is unknown.

In September, 1876, I met him in Liverpool. He said that his leg was much the same, and that he was still performing with the Christy Minstrels.

The result of this case is satisfactory. The progress of the disease was arrested, the hypertrophied condition of the limb much diminished, and the man has enjoyed good health and been enabled to lead an active life. I have found statistics of sixty-nine cases of elephantiasis Arabum, treated on Dr. Carnochan's principle; of these, forty were cured (three of them by digital compression of the artery); thirteen improved (three temporarily); and sixteen were unsuccessful.

Case of Complete Dislocation of the Head of the Radius forwards, successfully reduced twenty-four days after its Occurrence.

Dr. J. C. OGILVIE WILL, Surgeon to the Aberdeen Royal Infirmary, reports (*Lancet*, June 7, 1879) the following case of a comparatively rare injury, in which an excellent result was obtained under peculiarly unfavourable circumstances:—

A. B——, aged five, when running at school, fell over a form on March 22d, 1878. On her return home she complained of pain in her left elbow, but no attention was paid to it until the following Sunday, when, on her arm being suddenly seized by one of her parents, she cried loudly, and seemed to be much hurt. No advice was sought until the 29th March, when my friend Dr. James Brander was called in. He found great inflammatory swelling of the left elbow-joint, with some œdema of the hand and forearm. The inflammatory symptoms were so marked that, although he felt satisfied, from the very evident malposition of the limb, that the patient was the subject of severe injury of the joint, he did not feel justified in manipulating the parts so as to ascertain the exact nature of the case. Soothing applications were prescribed, and strict rest enjoined. The swelling of the tissues in the neighbourhood of the joint persisted, the skin became brawny-red, and the œdema of the hand remained undiminished. On April 8th he kindly requested me to visit the child in consultation with him, when the presence of the luxation was ascertained; but, on account of the inflamed state of the parts, it was not considered prudent to attempt reduction at the time, and we agreed to delay operations for a few days. On April 17th, inflammation having greatly subsided, I again visited the child, and, after chloroform had been administered, the following appearances were elicited: Forearm semi-pronated,

midway between complete extension and semi-flexion, with well-marked inclination outwards; external border of forearm slightly shortened; an unnatural
vacuity behind and below the external condyle in the situation normally occupied
by the head of the radius; an alteration in the direction of the long axis of the
radius, which, when followed with the fingers, led to a point in front of the external condyle, where the head of the bone could be distinctly felt.   On attempting
to flex the forearm it was found impossible to bend it to a greater degree than a
right angle, a feeling of locking being very manifest.   Complete extension was
readily achieved, and there was an abnormal degree of lateral motion.

Reduction was effected with some difficulty by extension and counter-extension,
and thumb-pressure applied to the head of the radius.   A rectangular splint was
applied.   Ten days afterwards Dr. Bransby commenced passive motion of the
joint; and on May 17th, when I next saw the patient, recovery was complete,
the motions of the joint being in every way perfect.

Remarks.—Considerable diversity of opinion seems to exist regarding the com-
monness or rarity of dislocation of the radius forwards, Hutchinson[1] stating that
it is not uncommon, and Erichsen[2] that it is the most usual of the three dislocations of the radius alone; while Boyer[3] wrote: "Mais on ne connaît pas d'observation bien authentique de la luxation de l'extrémité supérieure de cet os en
devant. . . . . Nous doutons que cette luxation puisse avoir lieu sans une
complication de fracture. . . . . On ne peut donc, dans l'état présent de nos
connaissances, admettre une luxation de l'extrémité supérieure du radius en devant."   Boyer's statement that this dislocation cannot occur without fracture has
been completely refuted, but the paucity of cases recorded by writers of surgical
works would lead to the belief that it is rare.   Sir Astley Cooper[4] only met with
it six times.   Malgaigne[5] met with three uncomplicated cases.   Hamilton[6] saw it
nine times.   Chelius,[7] Bransby Cooper,[8] and Pirrie[9] have each placed two cases
upon record.   Many other isolated examples have been recorded, but I only cite
the names of a few surgeons who have had great experience in this department
of surgery as indicative of the comparative rarity of the lesion under notice.
Apart from its frequency or infrequency the case possesses features of interest.
The symptoms presented by it were those generally described, but the only one
to which I would direct attention is the oblique inclination of the forearm outwards, which, as I have already stated, was well marked, and which was certainly
most striking.   To Malgaigne must be ascribed the credit of first describing it,
and he speaks of it as "unphénomène essentiel," notwithstanding which, with
the exception of Hamilton, Lane,[10] and Nélaton[11] (who gives "l'inclinaison de
l'avant-bras en dehors" as one of the diagnostic signs between complete and incomplete dislocation forwards, it seems to have escaped the observation of other
writers on the subject), some of whom give figures representing the appearance
accurately enough, and who, while detailing all the other symptoms at length,
yet omit to even notice the one to which Malgaigne has so forcibly alluded.   In
the case now under notice it was the first symptom observed, and one of the most

---

[1] Med. Times and Gazette, vol. i. 1866, p. 410.
[2] Science and Art of Surgery, 7th ed., vol. i. p. 486.
[3] Traité des Maladies Chirurgicales, 2de, éd., tom. iv., p. 239.
[4] Dislocations and Fractures (edited by Bransby Cooper), p. 452 et seq.
[5] Traité des Fractures et des Luxations, tom. ii. p. 655.
[6] A Treatise on Fractures and Dislocations, 4th ed., p. 579.
[7] Chelius's Surgery (edited by South), vol. i. p. 791.
[8] Loc. cit., p. 457.
[9] Principles and Practice of Surgery, 3d ed., p. 395.
[10] Cooper's Surgical Dictionary, 8th ed., vol. i. p. 540.
[11] Pathologie Chirurgicale, tom. iii. p. 184.

telling of any of the signs elicited; it therefore seems to be well worthy of note, and deserving of more attention that it has yet received.

The next point of interest is the reduction of the luxation at so distant a period from its occurrence as twenty-four days. The difficulty of reducing even a recent dislocation of the kind is universally acknowledged, and has been well put by Nélaton in the following sentence: "Pour la luxation complète, la difficulté de la réduction, déjà signalée par Hippocrate, semble prouvée par la proportion des pièces pathologiques recueillies, comparée aux faits observés sur le vivant." Sir Astley Cooper failed in two cases, and Hamilton in one, on the seventh day, and in Malgaigne's collection of twenty-five cases, excluding six which had been unrecognized, manipulation failed in eleven, only eight of the entire number ever being reduced. The only case with which I am acquainted where reduction was successfully accomplished at a late period was one under the care of Gosset,[1] who succeeded in effecting replacement three weeks after injury. Hutchinson reduced one at a still later date, but reluxation followed. The case now recorded is, so far as I have been able to ascertain, the only one on record where manipulation was followed by permanent reposition of the bone at so distant a period as twenty-four days.

The last point worthy of mention is the after-treatment of the case, which, so far as the time of commencing passive motion of the joint is concerned, differed from that generally inculcated. The danger of reluxation taking place has been so universally admitted that it has been laid down as a rule that the injured joint should be kept perfectly immobile for a period of from four to five weeks (Chelius, etc.). In this case, however, I ventured to take a different course, for I feared that if this injunction were obeyed we would never be able to overcome the resulting stiffness of the articulation, and that immobility would be permanent, for the child was timid in the extreme, and not one likely to make use of, or to allow that interference with, her arm which would have been requisite for the restoration of the functions of the injured member. On this account I suggested to her medical attendant the advisability of practising passive movement at the end of ten days, first once a day, and then oftener, the splint being replaced immediately afterwards. Dr. Brander, agreeing with this view, and finding that all inflammatory symptoms had disappeared, and that there was no tendency to reluxation, carried out the treatment so successfully that when I next visited the patient, four weeks after the dislocation was reduced, I found that she had regained the full use of the joint, and that she could move it as easily and perfectly as she did its fellow—a result which far exceeded my fondest anticipations, and which certainly justified the departure from the hard and fast line drawn by surgical authorities when dealing with the after-treatment of dislocation of the head of the radius forwards.

Midwifery and Gynæcology.

The Discussion on the Forceps.

The discussion on "the Use of the Forceps and its Alternatives in Lingering Labour," which was opened by Dr. BARNES at the meeting of the Obstetrical Society in May, has come to a close, and we think that the result of that discussion will be to place the employment of the forceps in midwifery on a better and

---

[1] Cooper, loc. cit., p. 458.

more scientific basis than it has hitherto occupied. The opening address of Dr. Barnes was characterized by a moderation and breadth of view such as to make it one of the most important papers on the subject. The value of the observations of many others of the speakers upon this question cannot be overestimated, for a great number of the best-known and most experienced of English and Irish obstetricians took part in the debate.

The result seems to be in the main to support the propositions laid down by Dr. Barnes at the conclusion of his opening speech, that in almost all circumstances the forceps is preferable to its alternatives ; that forceps may be not infrequently used with advantage when the head is in the pelvis and the os dilated, but that in proportion as the head is high in the pelvis and the os undilated, the necessity, utility, and safety of the forceps become less frequent. There was on the whole a marked unanimity with regard to the use of the forceps when the head is in the pelvis or on the perineum, and the opinion of almost all the speakers was in favour of a moderately frequent, as against an infrequent or very frequent, recourse to the instrument under these circumstances. Discussion chiefly took place with regard to the high operation, and the use of the instrument before the os uteri is dilated, as practised and recommended by Dr. George Johnston. It is a matter of regret that Dr. Johnston did not come over to take part in the debate, for his practice was made the subject of keen criticism and his statistics of careful sifting. Dr. Kidd pointed out some curious results which followed from Dr. Johnston's statistics with regard to the employment of the forceps before the os is dilated, but it was left for Dr. Roper to show from those statistics the grave results of the practice advocated by the late Master of the Rotunda.

It was laid down emphatically in the course of the discussion that the forceps is an instrument the use of which is to save maternal and fœtal life, and it is by the results of different modes of practice that we must judge of their fitness or desirability. Forceps statistics, as a rule, are of little value, because factors play a part in one practice which are absent in another, and *vice versâ*, such as difference of nationality, different external circumstances, etc. ; but in the reports of the Rotunda Hospital we find statistics which may apparently be fairly compared, because the practice has been carried on in the same building for many years, and amongst the same people. And it is this comparability that gives to the reports of the institution their perhaps chiefest value. Dr. Collins was Master of the Rotunda from 1826 to 1833 ; he used the forceps but very rarely. Dr. George Johnston was Master from 1868 to 1875; he used the forceps very frequently. Both these gentlemen have published the results of their practice while Masters of the institution.

During the Mastership of Dr. Collins there were 16,414 deliveries. During Dr. Johnston's period there were less than half that number, 7862. From this fact alone it may fairly be expected that the hygienic conditions of the hospital were much better during Dr. Johnston's term of office than during that of Dr. Collins ; for if the building were moderately full during the former period, it must have been greatly overcrowded during the latter. And such we find to have been actually the case for during Dr. Collins's mastership there was an epidemic of puerperal fever, which carried off fifty-six patients, while there was no epidemic of any kind during Dr. Johnston's mastership.

Dr. Collins used the forceps or vectis 27 times ; Dr. Johnston in 752 cases—that is, in the same number of deliveries, sixty times as frequently. Here is what may be fairly characterized as the practice of two extreme views of the use of the forceps, carried out under apparently similar circumstances (with the exception already stated—overcrowding), and it is by the result to mothers and children they should be judged. In treating statistics and drawing inferences from them, there are certain errors into which we are liable to fall, and in dealing with forceps statistics this error is not uncommon.   To compare the proportion of maternal or fœtal deaths in forceps deliveries is to compare the incomparable, and arrive at enormous inferences, for the frequency of the operation is not taken into account.   The way to reduce mortality in forceps operations to a minimum would be to use the instrument in every case, or in simple cases only, avoiding difficult ones.   What is wanted is not only a small proportion of deaths in forceps deliveries, but a small one in total deliveries, and this should be the object of recourse to the forceps.   Now Dr. Collins lost 4 women of his forceps deliveries— that is, 1 in 6 or 7.   Dr. Johnston lost 58, or 1 in 13 only; but though Dr. Johnston's proportion of deaths in forceps deliveries is only one-half that of Dr. Collins, yet in the same number of deliveries the former lost 39 women by forceps for each one lost by the latter.

Passing on to the total maternal mortality from all causes—forceps included— we inquire, How does the frequent use of the forceps affect this, as shown by the practice of Drs. Collins and Johnston?   And we find that, out of 16,414 delivered by Collins, 164 died; and of the 7862 delivered by Johnston, 169 died— that is, in Johnston's practice rather more than two women died for each one that died in Collins's.   Here it should be observed, that of the 164 women who died in Collins's time, 56 perished in an epidemic of puerperal fever.

The next important point for consideration is the amount of the fœtal mortality under the two systems.   The saving of fœtal life is a strong reason and motive for frequent use of forceps.   Now it is a remarkable fact that, while Dr. Johnston had recourse to the forceps in many cases with a view of saving fœtal life, yet his reports do not contain any data whereby the total fœtal mortality can be calculated; this is a strange omission in the reports, and one of which we have, by reason of its importance in coming to a correct conclusion about Dr. Johnston's practice, a right to complain.   It is found that, of the 752 children born by the aid of forceps under Dr. Johnston, 54 were still-born, of which 4 were putrid. Of the 24 born by the aid of forceps under Dr. Collins, 8 were still-born—that is, a mortality five times as great as in Dr. Johnston's practice if we regard the proportion to the number of forceps cases alone, but only one-twelfth as great in an equal number of deliveries.

With regard to the number of still-births in the total number of deliveries, we find that, exclusive of premature births (before or at the sixth month), there were 1009, or nearly 6.2 per cent., under Dr. Collins.   According to Dr. Barnes, the proportion of still-births to total deliveries during Dr. Johnston's mastership was 6.1 per cent. ; so that in this respect a very frequent use appears to have a very slight advantage over a very rare use of the forceps.

It would be expected that with such rare use of the forceps Collins would have had frequent recourse to the perforator; and we do find that it was used by him 118 times, or 1 in 141 cases; while by Johnston it was used 28 times, or 1 in 281 cases.   That is, Collins used the perforator twice as often as Johnston, and in this way probably destroyed some children which might have been saved had he possessed and had recourse to the improved forceps of the present day.   A more frequent recourse to forceps would perhaps have diminished Collins's mortality, as Ramsbotham's and Roper's statistics (which are fairly comparable) at the Royal Maternity Charity appear to show; yet very frequent recourse to the instrument appears, on the other hand, to increase greatly the maternal mortality. It is impossible, while reading the reports of the Rotunda Hospital under the two systems—that of very rare and that of very frequent use of the forceps—not to be struck with the terrible maternal mortality under the latter, and it is difficult to avoid the conclusion that the grave results were the direct effects of the practice.—*Lancet,* July 19, 1879.

The Anatomical Proof of the Persistency of the Cervix in Pregnancy.

Dr. M. SÄNGER, of Leipzig, is the author of a long and excellent article on this subject in the *Archiv für Gynäkologie,* Bd. xiv., in which, after an elaborate historical criticism of this vexed subject, in the course of which the writer controverts with great ability the views of Bandl and Küstner on this subject, he gives an account of the condition of the cervix uteri in the case of a patient who had died suddenly in a convulsive seizure about the end of the ninth month of utero-gestation. Cesarean section was performed immediately after death by Professor Credé, and the state of the uterus, and especially of the cervix was carefully determined by Dr. Sänger. It was found that the plicæ palmatæ of the mucous membrane of the cervix were perfectly intact, and that the membranes covered with the decidua ran closely down to the edge of the cervical mucous membrane. It was impossible to doubt where the cervix ended, and where the lower uterine segment began. There was no intermediate space, as is insisted upon by Bandl and Küstner, between what they call the inner os and ring of Müller. The anatomical evidence of the case, more especially when subjected to microscopical examination, in the most emphatic manner supports the view of the persistency of the cervix during the whole course of pregnancy until near delivery, and contradicts flatly the view, that in any sense the cervix is used up in such a manner as to amplify the lower uterine segment. In Dr. Sänger's case there was no elevated ring at the junction of the cervix and lower segment of the body, as in Müller's case (lately given in this Journal, p. 595, vol. xxiv.), but the cervix and body of the uterus ran directly the one into the other in the same plane. Dr. Sänger thinks that though anatomical evidence is the most reliable in deciding this question, careful clinical observations, taking care that the soft cervix is not shortened unnoticed during the exploration, is also of great value as corroborative evidence of the persistency of the cervix. The dimensions of the vaginal portion of the cervix in Dr. Sänger's case are as follows: " Anterior wall, 1.5 centimetres, = .6 inch; posterior wall, 2 centimetres, = .8 inch; the breadth of its base at the highest part of the vaginal end, 2.5 centimetres, = 1.0 inch.—*Edinburgh Med. Journal,* Aug. 1879.

Cæsarean Section, with Temporary Ligature of the Cervix by Esmarch's Bandage, on Account of Threatened Rupture of Uterus in a Case of Extreme Pelvic Contraction and Rigid Cervix.

In No. 12 of the *Centralblatt für Gynäkologie,* for 1879, a case is recorded by LITZMANN, of Kiel, in which this method of controlling hemorrhage at the operation was adopted without removing the uterus, as Porro recommends. Strict antiseptic precautions were observed. The uterine wound was sewed with catgut ligatures. The abdominal wound was sewed with silk stitches. The child was saved in this case. The mother died eighty-five hours after the operation under symptoms of protracted shock. Litzmann makes the following observations in conclusion upon this case: 1. The temporary ligature of the cervix had neither injured the child nor diminished the contractile power of the uterus. 2. The closure of the uterine wound by a suture had sufficiently fulfilled the means of arrest of hemorrhage, notwithstanding the subsequent loosening of the knots. The loosening of the knots was due not to the material, but to defective tying of them (a granny instead of a reef-knot). The force of resistance of a catgut ligature tied in a reef-knot was subsequently sufficiently established by us in an experiment with thick tangle-tents laid in water after tying them. 3. According to the clinical symptoms, which enable us to recognize essentially a persistently increasing paralysis of heart and bowel muscle, as well as according to the results of post-mortem examination, the fatal issue is to be considered as due to severe shock of the nervous system, brought about partly by the enormous distension and tension of the cervical wall antecedent to the operation, partly by the operation itself. In regard to the latter, the great cooling of and unavoidable mechanical interference with the bowels in connection with the prolapse of the intestines, which was only reduced slowly with considerable force, must be considered as specially important factors.—*Edinburgh Med. Journal*, Aug. 1879.

The Uses of the Hot-water Douche in Parturition.

Dr. ALBERT H. SMITH, in a paper read before the Philadelphia County Medical Society (*Phila. Med. Times*, Aug. 16, 1879), claims as facts proven by experience that the hot-water douche (110° to 115°) thrown upon the cervix uteri or the rim of the undilated os will stimulate contraction of the longitudinal and oblique muscular fibres of the uterus into an expulsive effort, while the circular fibres surrounding the os relax under its influence; 2d, that a similar douche thrown into the cavity of the relaxed and bleeding uterus, after the expulsion of the fœtus or the placenta, will produce prompt and vigorous condensation of the uterine walls, with an immediate closure of the sinuses; and, 3d, that a like application to a bleeding surface from laceration in the passage of the child through the pelvic canal will arrest the hemorrhage at any point, whether it be from a tear of the circular artery in the cervix, or from rupture of the vascular tissues upon the anterior margin of the vulva about the vestibule, or from the furrows upon the posterior wall and the labia.

Dr. Smith has found the application to the cervix of the hot douche thoroughly and rapidly effectual in the first stage of normal labour at full time, almost equally rapid in a rigid condition in an accidental premature labour, and more slowly— though with ultimate effect—in the induction of labour in a quiescent uterus. The method of application is simple. The patient should lie upon her back, with a bed-pan placed far under her sacrum, so that there should be no danger of the water getting upon her clothing.

The injection should be thrown into the vagina with a syringe with a rubber tube and metal nozzle with a large hole in the end, and Dr. Smith prefers the Davidson bulb-syringe, as the stream can be driven with more force, and with the intermittent action necessary with that instrument. A quart to three pints of water medicated with ʒij of 90 per cent. solution of carbolic acid, or ʒss of Labarraque's solution should be thrown into the vagina. The pipe being directed *against* the cervix, not into it. The douche may be repeated every hour or two, according to the demands of the case, or the violence of its results.

The condition in which we get the most signal effects from the douche is that of uterine inertia after the placental delivery, and in this condition Dr. Smith is inclined to think that we have an absolutely reliable agent to control bleeding—an agent which may reduce the terrors of post-partum hemorrhage, and make its fatal termination an almost impossible event if applied at any time while power of reaction is not entirely exhausted.

The nozzle should be carried on the index finger into the vagina, while the opposite hand grasps firmly the uterine globe. The fingers in the vagina may be moved about freely to break up clots rapidly, there being sometimes a complete distension of the vagina with firm, hard coagula. The stream is kept up continuously, washing out as fast as the clots are loosened; the nozzle is to be carried to the os uteri, and directed into the orifice. If the coagula in the uterus are loose and not abundant, the force of the stream may be sufficient without carrying the finger into the uterine cavity, but if the hemorrhage has been great, and the uterus largely distended, it is better boldly to introduce the pipe, guarded by the finger, and, moving it around gently, let it, with the aid of the stream, detach from the intra-uterine surface all shreds of membrane or small coagula which may be found adherent to the surface, and which, if not removed, will act as centres of coagulation. While this is going on, the hand upon the uterine tumour feels it steadily and, generally, instantly contracting, condensing itself into a firm, hard mass, receding completely into the pelvic cavity below the brim. The water passing from the vulva is soon observed to be free from colour, and the hemorrhage is arrested. A uterus after such accident ought to be carefully watched and compressed in the hand of the accoucheur or of an assistant until all probability of secondary relaxation is over.

Finding the use of the douche so successful in controlling hemorrhage, it has naturally followed to adopt it as a preventive, and for nearly two years past Dr. Smith has been resorting to its use habitually (or at least wherever at all easily practicable) in every case of labour. The apparatus is made ready during the latter stages of labour, and so soon as the placenta is delivered, the douche is administered precisely as just directed for the relief of hemorrhage, except that it will rarely be necessary to carry the finger and the pipe farther than to the os uteri (the *internal* os, the external os, and cervical cavity being expanded at this stage). The vagina is thus cleansed and disinfected by the water—medicated as before—the clots are washed from the lower segment of the uterus, and the organ stimulated to contract—which it does firmly, rarely showing a disposition to relax, and often remaining low down in the pelvic cavity below the brim for twenty-four hours; and in no case so far, where satisfactorily done, has any flooding occurred after it. After-pains are diminished greatly, and the lochia but slightly abundant.

As to any danger from the absorption of the carbolized solution, it seems almost impossible, where the outlet of the uterus is so patulous as it is after labour, that any fluid could be retained in its cavity long enough to be absorbed; but the recent statements of so reliable an authority as Fritsch, that serious consequences have followed its use in some cases, would make it desirable that every precaution should be taken against such retention.

The Behaviour of Spermatozoa in the Vagina and Uterus.

Dr. D. HAUSMAN, of Berlin, in a pamphlet on this subject, gives the result of a considerable number of selected observations, made with all suitable precautions, with regard to the duration of the life of the spermatozoa in the vaginal mucus, and in that of the cervix uteri. He records seventeen observations of the cervical mucus, and twenty of that from the cervix uteri, obtained in cases in which he could rely upon the account as given as to the time of the last coitus; and in which no vaginal injections had been used, either shortly before or since the coitus. Out of a much larger number which he has made, he has rejected the greater part, because the data in these respects were not absolutely certain. These observations agree with those of Marion Sims and others, in showing that the spermatozoa perish quickly in the vagina, but retain their life and activity for a much longer period within the cervix. So soon as four hours after coitus, he found that the great majority of spermatozoa in the vagina had been seen to move, although a considerable number retained their vitality. In five cases in which the last coitus had occurred about twelve hours before the examination, the spermatozoa were found to be all dead, except in one instance, in which a few were seen to be moving amongst a large number which were motionless. The case was one in which an acute anteflexion existed, which would hinder the advance of the spermatozoa towards the uterus, while the widely patulous external os would allow them readily to escape from the uterus into the vagina. In six examinations of vaginal mucus about fifteen hours after coitus, the spermatozoa were found abundantly present in all, but none of them showed signs of life. Four examinations were made from thirty to thirty-eight hours after coitus. In one of these the vaginal mucus, which was mixed with urine, showed no spermatozoa; in two, they were abundant but dead.

In one case, however, in which coitus had taken place thirty-eight hours previously, and menstruation had commenced twelve hours later, living spermatozoa were found in the mixture of vaginal mucus and menstrual blood. The author entertains no doubt that these had penetrated into the uterus, and had been washed down again in the menstrual flow. In a case examined forty-six hours after coitus no spermatozoa could be detected in the vagina, although they were present in the cervix uteri.

In no case, even when the examination was made within an hour after coitus, was the reaction of the vaginal mucus changed from acid to alkaline, by the addition of the alkaline seminal fluid.

The general conclusion is that the great majority of the spermatozoa perish in the vagina very shortly after their deposition there, and that none of them retain their motion there, beyond twelve hours at the outside, unless menstruation has come on in the meanwhile.

To obtain the cervical mucus for examination, the author exposes the os by the speculum, wipes away from it first all adhesive vaginal secretion, taking care to brush it away from and not towards the os, and then obtains a drop of mucus from the cervical canal, by means of dry forceps, sound, or Braun's syringe. In order to obtain the secretion from the body of the uterus, he first thoroughly cleanses the whole of the cervical canal from all the secretion which it contains. As to the presence of spermatozoa in cervical mucus, the results are the following: In six observations on cases in which the external os was normal in size and position, and its secretion almost normal, at various times up to a week after coitus spermatozoa were *always* found. In ten similar cases, in which the observations were made eight and fourteen days after coitus, spermatozoa were absent. In four observations, made within a week after coitus, with the os uteri normal in size, and with normal secretions, but somewhat deviating from its normal position, spermatozoa were always found. In one observation on a similar case, made seven and half days after coitus, into case of normally patent os uteri, but decided uterine catarrh, no spermatozoa were found. In two observations on the same case, in which the external os was moderately constricted, and deviated somewhat to one side, in one instance, one and half hours after coitus spermatozoa were found, in another four hours after coitus none were found. In four observations on cases of great constriction of the external os, spermatozoa were absent in all.

The author concludes from these facts that normally, as Marion Sims also holds, the spermatozoa are not merely deposited in the vagina and left to make their own way into the uterus, but that they are impelled into the cervix at the moment of ejaculation. He attributes this in the main to the pressure of ejaculation, although he does not assume any exact apposition between the os uteri and the orifice of the male urethra. This view is confirmed by two of his observations in the case of women accustomed to use twice a day with an irrigator a vaginal injection of a litre of a solution in the one case of sulphate of copper, in the other of carbolic acid (1 in 50), both of which are well known to destroy spermatozoa immediately. Although these injections had been used shortly before coitus, abundant living spermatozoa were found in the cervical mucus within six hours after that act. He also quotes in favour of his view the success of the practice of preventing the occurrence of pregnancy by placing a tampon against the cervix uteri. He concludes that the occurrence of conception through the migration of spermatozoa from the vagina, or from more external parts, into the uterus, by their own activity, must be regarded as an exceptional chance; and believes also that even if they should make their way into the cervix after some interval, their vitality and power of surviving many days would probably be impaired by their sojourn in the vaginal mucus, which so quickly destroys them.   He infers further, that by even a moderate contraction of the external os the penetration of the spermatozoa into the cervix is rendered uncertain, that by a considerable contraction it is prevented as a rule, and that therefore the operation of incising a narrow external os for the cure of sterility is a justifiable one.

In the vaginal mucus the proportion of spermatozoa was always considerably less than in a remaining drop of semen removed from the male urethra after coitus and before the first micturition.   In the cervical mucus their number was relatively very few, and the author concludes that only a very small proportion of them normally reach the interior of the uterus.   Besides the living spermatozoa found in the cervical mucus, a considerable number of dead ones was always found also.   The longest period after coitus at which living spermatozoa were found was seven and a half days, a period exceeded in an observation of Percy, who found them alive after eight and a half days.   The longer the interval after coitus the less active were the movements of the spermatozoa, and the sooner did they cease to move after removal from the body.   The author concludes that it is probable that they may retain their vitality for as much as ten days before reaching the ovum.   That stringy cervical mucus is not necessarily fatal to spermatozoa was proved by an observation in which living ones were found in abundance in a plug of such mucus.

The author rejects the plan of intra-uterine injections of semen for the cure of sterility, believing that normally only a few of the spermatozoa themselves reach the body of the uterus by their own activity, leaving behind the other constituents of the semen.   In cases, however, of stenosis of the internal os, or of flexion causing a narrowing of the canal near that situation, the secretions being healthy, he proposes, within the first twelve hours after coitus, to pass a large sound into the uterus, in the hope of thus carrying on beyond the point of obstruction some of the spermatozoa containing cervical mucus.   He does not, however, report any result obtained in one case in which he repeatedly tried this measure.—*Obstet. Journ. of Great Britain*, August, 1879.

—

The Treatment of Obstinate Retroflexion of the Uterus.

Dr. SCHULTZE proposes (*Centralblatt für Gynäkologie*, No. 3, 1879), a plan for the cure of obstinate retroflexion based upon the behaviour of the uterus in involution after delivery or abortion.   He has observed that the uterus in such cases, if it is kept by a pessary in normal position during the process of involution, will afterwards retain its position unaided, even though the flexion may have been of old standing, owing to the renovation of the whole tissue which has taken place.   He proposes, therefore, to institute a process in some degree analogous to involution, by first of all dilating fully the cervix by laminaria tents, and then repeatedly injecting a solution of carbolic acid, or a dilute solution of perchloride of iron, the effect of which is to excite uterine contractions resembling those of labour.   After full dilatation of the cervix the finger is first introduced into the uterus fully up to the fundus, and by its means reduction is effected more safely than by the sound.   Moreover, if any adhesions exist, tethering the fundus backward, their existence and position can thus be clearly made out.   During the process of reaction the uterus is kept in place by the author's figure-of-eight pessary, and he finds that, in this way, it becomes sensibly reduced in size, and that the pessary may eventually be dispensed with.   The author considers that dilatation by laminaria tents is quite free from danger if the precautions recommended by him (*Centralbl. fur Gynak.*, 1873, No. 7) be taken. In very nearly 400 cases of their use within a single year he has seen not a single one of parametritis of temperature over 38° C., or of any other abnormal reaction.—*Obstet. Journ. of Great Britain*, Aug. 1879.

—

Ovariotomy.

J. Boye gives in the *Gynäkolog. og Obstetr. Meddelelser*, Band 11, an account of twenty-three cases of ovariotomy performed by him in 1876–78, five of which were followed by death. Among the recoveries were several especially difficult operations, and cases in which the patients' condition was very miserable : but the author has become more and more convinced that, so long as the patient is not nearly or actually moribund, neither her condition nor the operative difficulties of the case present any certain contraindications to ovariotomy. Among the five deaths, three occurred from tetanus, in patients operated on in different places and at intervals of several months. In seeking for the cause of the tetanus, the author directed his attention especially to the management of the pedicle. In the first case of tetanus he used the clamp ; he then left off the extraperitoneal treatment of the pedicle, and used the catgut ligature : the cautery, he says, requires too long a time, and is unsafe. In the next eight cases the catgut ligature was used : but one of these died of tetanus. In this case, which was believed to be one of double ovarian tumour, one of the tumours was found to be a gravid uterus, much distended with hydramnios ; it was punctured, and the operation was completed. A drainage-tube was placed between the edges of the abdominal wound. Abortion at the third month took place four days afterwards ; the patient went on till the tenth day, when she was seized with tetanus, and died five days later. This mishap led Boye to desist from applying the drainage-tube immediately after the completion of the operation. In the third case of tetanus, the author was obliged to apply the clamp quickly to end the operation, as the needle-punctures in the pedicle, which was thick and vascular, continued to bleed after the ligatures were tied. The patient made very favourable progress for some days ; but tetanus then set in. The author has endeavoured to discover a method of ligature which will not disappoint, so that the pedicle can be returned into the abdomen with safety, and the operation ended as rapidly as with the clamp. In the next five cases, he used silver thread ; the course of the cases was favourable, but the application required too long a time, and two of the patients had pelvic abscess. He then used, in the next six operations, a caoutchouc drainage-tube ; one of these cases ended fatally, but the patient was already in a hopeless state before the operation. A caoutchouc tube dipped in a solution of carbolic acid was introduced by means of a strong curette, by which, in order to prevent it from slipping, it was brought through a fold of peritoneum, along the two opposite sides of the pedicle. The ends of the tube lay parallel with each other beyond the pedicle, and were drawn as tight as possible with the fingers, while an assistant tied them together with silk thread. If the pedicle were very thick, or absent, the tube was carried across through the pedicle or base of the tumour, and was tied on both sides. In one of these cases, peritoneal abscess occurred ; but the author thinks that this may have been due to other circumstances. The advantages of this method are these. 1. It can be carried out quickly, nearly as quickly as the application of the clamp. 2. It is very secure. 3. In the cases in which it is used, it was generally not followed by reaction. The first seven cases were operated on without antiseptics ; and one died of tetanus ; the other sixteen cases were operated on under the spray. Regarding the insertion of a diainage-tube immediately after operation, the author thinks that it is not of any use, as it quickly becomes encapsuled with exudation, so that large quantities of fluid may remain in the abdomen without being able to escape through the tube. The author attaches much importance to bandaging the abdomen as firmly as possible. He treats pelvic abscesses by opening them as early as possible, either by means of a trocar through the rectum, or, if the pus again collect, by making an opening from the vagina and inserting a drainage-tube.—*British Med. Journal*, July 12, 1879, from *Nordiskt Med. Arkiv.*, Band. xi.

Medical Jurisprudence and Toxicology.

Case of Death from Chloroform.

Geh. Med.-Rath Prof. Dr. BARDELEBEN observes (*Deutsche Med. Woch.*, June 7) that until the year 1876 he had had the good fortune never to have met with a death from chloroform, although he had witnessed and participated in its administration in more than 30,000 cases. During the ten years that he has directed the surgical clinic at the Berlin Charité, anæsthesia by chloroform has been induced at least 1200 times per annum ; and at his former clinic at Greifswald (1849–68) the average number of cases was more rather than less than 1000. No notice is taken here of his cases in private practice. But in 1876 there occurred in his clinic four cases of death from chloroform, which were published by his assistant, Dr. Koehler, in the third volume of the new series of the Charité *Annalen*. In three of these cases, other circumstances besides the administration of chloroform might have contributed to the production of the sudden death. However, the resolution was at once taken, in order to be certain that only quite pure chloroform was employed, to use exclusively the chloral-chloroform, prepared with the greatest care in Schering's factory. This chloral-chloroform (to which, on the advice of O. Liebreich, one per cent. of pure alcohol is added on first opening the bottle, in order to guard against any possible decomposition) has ever since then been employed at the Charité, as it was in the case to be related. In fact, the chloroform used in this case was taken from the bottle which was employed in a whole series of cases, and the conviction was so strong that the mishap arose, not from any impurity of the chloroform, but from individual conditions which we have not yet mastered, that this same preparation has continued to be employed. How advantageously this chloral-chloroform differs from ordinary chloroform may be recognized without any aid from chemistry. If we drop some drops into the palm of the hand and rub this powerfully, either no smell at all remains or only that of chloroform, while if we do the same with ordinary chloroform there is not uncommonly an unpleasant smell left, resembling that of fusel oil.

The case to be now related is one of especial signification, because it is in every respect so uncomplicated. The chloroform was quite pure, and only twenty-two grammes of it were employed. The patient exhibited no organic defect that could have contributed to sudden death ; the operation (stretching a contracted knee) was unattended with violence, wounding, or interference with the respiratory or circulatory organs ; all precautionary rules were observed—the patient lying in the horizontal position, without compressive clothing, his stomach being empty. Suddenly the heart stops ; and the most energetic procedures, instituted immediately, fail to recall life. The patient, a scrofulous lad, aged twelve, was admitted on account of a white swelling of the knee, with contraction to an acute angle. As it was deemed proper to stretch the limb, the lad was placed under chloroform two days after his admission—all the organs on examination being found in a normal condition. While Prof. Bardeleben was describing the case to the class, seven grammes of chloroform were administered under the direction of his assistant by means of the Esmarch mask. Like all children, he resisted at first, so that it is certain that all the chloroform did not reach the air-passage. When he had become more quiet, Junker's apparatus was substituted for that of Esmarch. This, especially intended for bichloride of methylene, Prof. Bardeleben finds very convenient and economical for chloroform, but employs it seldom at the commencement, owing to the relatively longer time (especially in restless children) which is required to produce insensibility with it. With this fifteen grammes more of chloroform were used—making twenty-two grammes in the whole, at the most. When the muscles began to relax the rectification of the joint was easily accomplished. A small chondroma was discovered attached to the upper part of the bones of the leg, and while this was being examined there occurred slight contractions of the flexor muscles, and the lad by screaming showed that he had become sensitive to pain. While about to resort to more chloroform during the application of the gypsum bandage it was found that the heart had ceased to act. A few seconds later the respiratory movements also ceased. The tongue was at once drawn out of the mouth, and an electrode of an inductive apparatus was applied to the region of the phrenic nerve in the neck, in alternation with the employment of artificial respiration by the postural method. Scarcely had two minutes elapsed when the lad again cried out, the respiratory movements recommenced, and the pulse could again be felt; so that it was believed that the application of the bandage was possible. The hope of this was soon dissipated, for the pulse and respiration speedily ceased again. The effects were actively resumed; and when compression of the thorax and faradization of the phrenics were found to exert no influence on the diaphragm, rhythmical compression of the thorax, with alternate insufflation of air, was substituted. The autopsy proved how instrumental these combined means were in forcing air into the lungs, these appearing of a bright-red colour, while all the other organs were filled with dark-coloured blood. After all these efforts had been pursued for half an hour without effect, and the body had become considerably cooled, all present pronounced the boy absolutely dead. Although in this stage of the case it would have been of no avail to make trial of the hypodermic injection of nitrate of strychnia, yet Prof. Bardeleben feels strongly convinced that in cases like this, in which death evidently takes place from primary paralysis of the heart, and not from asphyxia, besides every care being taken to keep the air-passages free, and to employ artificial respiration, the hypodermic injection of strychnia should also be practised, its efficacy as an antidote to chloroform having been made known to the Berlin Medical Society ten years since by Prof. O. Liebreich.

At the autopsy the principal circumstance observed was the great fluidity and dark colour of the blood. The veins and sinuses of the brain contained a great deal of blood, as did the tela and choroid plexus; and the vessels of the substance of the brain were also in a lesser degree distended. All the cavities of the heart, of which only the left ventricle was contracted, contained a considerable quantity of this dark fluid blood, not a trace of coagulum existing. None of the organs exhibited any diseased appearances.—*Med. Times and Gazette*, Aug. 2, 1879.

CONTENTS.

Published Monthly, price $2.50 per annum, free of postage.
Also, furnished together with the AMERICAN JOURNAL OF THE MEDICAL SCIENCES *and the* MEDICAL NEWS AND LIBRARY *for* SIX DOLLARS *per annum in advance, the whole free of postage.*

HENRY C. LEA, Philadelphia.

THE MONTHLY ABSTRACT

OF

MEDICAL SCIENCE.

VOL. VI. No. 10.   **For List of Contents see last page.**   OCTOBER, 1879.

Entered at the Post-Office at Philadelphia as Second-class matter.

Anatomy and Physiology.

On the Physiology of the Liver.

M. PICARD, of Lyons, communicated (*Le Progrès Méd.*, May 3, 1879) some experiments which appear to show that section of the nerves going to the liver does not cause diabetes. The nerves supplying the liver do not exercise any great influence upon the circulation in the organ. In a previous communication, he showed that section of the nerves supplying the liver did not cause any increase in the amount of urea in the blood. M. Picard finds that dogs survive the section of the nerves, and that in animals which have undergone this operation the amount of sugar in the urine, and the quantity of bile secreted, are nearly the same as in the normal individual. The liver appears, therefore, to be to a certain extent independent of that part of the nervous system which directly enervates it. The blood appears to lose in the liver a portion of its hæmoglobin. After section of the nerves of the liver, subsequent stimulation shows that they have only a dull sensibility, whilst excitation of their distal extremities produces no immediate or marked effects. The flow of blood through the gland does not, so far as can be determined, depend upon the nervous supply, but it is more abundant during expiration. Prolonged stimulation of the peripheral extremities of the hepatic nerves causes a change in the urine, which becomes diabetic. In brief, therefore, the experiments of M. Picard have afforded the following results: The liver probably contains secretory fibres, such as is shown by the fact that there are nerves which bring about the appearance of sugar in the urine. It receives but few sensory and vaso-motor fibres, and its functional activity is in opposition to the reflex action exerted by other organs whose circulation is to some extent correlative to its own. Digestion, which increases the functional activity of the glands, stomach, etc., and causes a congestion of the intestine, produces a more active circulation in the portal vein and liver, and gives an impulse to the functions of the whole organ. The glycosuria, on the other hand, appears to be directly dependent upon the hepatic nervous system, through which it may be called into increased activity.—*London Med. Record*, August 15, 1879.

—

On Fecundity and Sexuality.

M. GAETAN DELAUNAY, in a recent communication (*Le Progrès Médical*, May 31, 1879) states that fertility, which is unlimited in the lowest classes, decreases as the human race is approached. The inferior races are more fruitful than the superior; the black, yellow, and other races being more fertile than the white. Amongst Europeans, the Russians, Spaniards, and Italians, i. e., the nations which are the least advanced in civilization, are the most fertile; whilst the least fertile are those furthest advanced in the scale of evolution, viz., the

Fieneh and Swiss. It has been stated that the relative sterility of France was voluntary, but M. Delaunay refutes this accusation. Fertility diminishes in a nation as it becomes more highly civilized. Intellectual persons, and those who live in towns, have a smaller number of children than the ignorant and labouring classes. The young and the old are more fertile than adults, and the same is true of the weak as opposed to the vigorous. Athletes and persons who perform much brain work have but few children, as has been shown by Dr. Drysdale. The lower tissues reproduce themselves more readily than the higher ones. A plant or animal which receives too great a supply of food becomes infertile. Thus, dogs belonging to the poor produce more offspring than others of the same race which belong to the richer class. The wretched and badly fed are more fruitful than the wealthier, and, therefore, fertility has no relation to the means of livelihood. Summer and warm climates increase the fertility. In short, therefore, fertility being at its maximum in those least advanced upon the path of evolution, and at its minimum in those furthest advanced in the same scale, it may be regarded as being in an inverse ratio to the evolution. *Sexuality.*—The lower races produce more females and the higher nations more males. Young and old animals bear more females than males. From the age of thirty-five onwards a man begets more girls than boys. The vigorous produce boys, and the weakly girls. Under the first empire, when all adult males were serving in the wars, a very large majority of girls were born. Years of dearth favour the pro- creation of girls, and years of abundance of boys. Idleness tends to cause the birth of females. Persons who perform much mental labour are more liable to produce girls than boys. A majority of girls are born in summer and in warm years, and of boys in winter and cold years. In short, therefore, an individual of a less high degree of evolution produces girls, of a higher degree boys, whilst, at a still higher degree, he again begets girls. In the same way, one who is fed too little or too much produces girls, boys being born when he is simply well fed. Upon this communication M. Galippe remarked that the biological law laid down by M. Delaunay was wrong, inasmuch as it was unsupported by conclusive facts. It was, moreover, entirely incorrect in regard to England, the English being cer- tainly far advanced in the scale of evolution, whilst they produce a large number of children.—*London Medical Record*, August 15, 1879.

—

The Transformation of Glycogen.

Dr. SEEGEN has published, in Pfluger's *Archiv für die gesammte Physiologie,* Band xviii., a series of experiments on the influence which saliva and pancreatic juice exercise on glycogen. It has been believed till now that saliva, pancreatic juice, and diastase are able to convert glycogen entirely into grape-sugar. Dr. Seegen's experiments gave results which differ widely from the opinion before mentioned. He sums them up in the following paragraphs. 1. As soon as saliva or pancreatic juice comes into contact with a solution of glycogen, transformation into sugar begins. In about thirty or forty minutes, the glycogen has disappeared; the opalescent solution has become quite clear. The glycogen at this moment is transformed into sugar and into Brücke's achroodextrin. The transformation of a part of the dextrin continues for twenty-four to forty-eight hours. 2. The quantity of sugar finally formed does not correspond to the quantity of glycogen used. With the aid of Fehling's copper solution, one is able to discover only forty or fifty per cent. of the quantity of sugar which ought to be found if the whole bulk of glycogen has undergone transformation. 3. The sugar formed is not grape-sugar. Its power of reducing oxide of copper is about two-thirds of the reducing power of grape-sugar, and its power of turning the plane of polarization to the right is nearly three times as great as that of grape-sugar. 4. Diastase acts in the same way on glycogen. 5. Starch also is not entirely transformed into sugar by the action of ferments. The sugar formed is not grape-sugar. Its power of reduction is one-third less and its power of rotation much greater than that of grape-sugar. 6. Dr. Seegen proposes to call the sugar produced by the action of ferments on starch and glycogen ferment-sugar. 7. Glycogen boiled with acids is changed into grape-sugar, but only about 75 per cent. of the glycogen is transformed into sugar. Only by boiling glycogen with acids in hermetically closed glass tubes for thirty-six to forty-eight hours, the whole bulk of glycogen is transformed into grape-sugar. 8. When the action of ferments or acids on glycogen is at an end, there remains in solution, besides sugar, a sort of dextrin, which differs from Brücke's achroodextrin in various ways. It is very soluble in alcohol, and ferments are unable to turn it into sugar. Considering the resistance it opposes to the action of ferments and acids, Seegen proposes to call it dystropodextrin. 9. The sugar found in the liver is grape-sugar. Dr. Seegen refers to a paper which he has lately published in Pflüger's *Archiv*, Band xix, and in which he states that it has as yet been impossible to isolate a liver-ferment. What has been found by Wittich's or Bernard's process has been glycogen containing a trace of a fermenting substance. The same component has been extracted out of a boiled liver, where the ferment, if it had existed, would have been destroyed by the boiling process. Such traces of ferment, or rather such a minimal fermenting action, belongs to nearly all the albuminous tissues; and Seegen has found that even albumen obtained in the laboratory from blood exercises the same diastatic action, which in its intensity cannot be compared to the action of a ferment. Considering that a real ferment has not yet been found in the liver, and considering that the sugar of the liver differs from the sugar formed by real ferments, Seegen thinks a doubt might be justified whether the formation of sugar in the liver is to be attributed to the action of a ferment.—*British Med. Journal*, June 21, 1879.

Materia Medica and Therapeutics.

On the Physiological Action of Salicylate of Soda.

M. OLTRAMARE (*Le Progrès Médical*, June 14, 1879) a pupil of Professor Chavean, has made a large number of experiments upon animals for the purpose of determining the physiological action of salicylate of soda. When introduced directly into the veins, the drug constantly increases the pressure, the number of pulsations, and the systolic force of the heart; this effect is transitory, and is due to a direct stimulation of the heart, and probably, also, of the motor centres. At the same time, the rapidity of the current of blood, as measured by means of the hæmodromograph constructed by Professor Chauveau, increases gradually; this second effect, being due to a dilatation of the bloodvessels, is much more persistent than the previous one. Under the influence of repeated injections, the irritability of the heart is diminished, and when the poisonous dose is reached, that is to say, one gramme per kilogramme of the body weight for the dog, ass, and horse, irregularities of the pulse occur, it becomes intermittent, the blood-pressure falls rapidly, and the heart ceases to beat. The animal dies from paralysis of the heart, and not, as has been stated, from asphyxia. The examination after death shows that the abdominal viscera, in relation with the vascular phenomena observed during life, are intensely congested. If the medulla be divided, a very marked condition of anæmia succeeds the hyperæmia; it therefore appears, according to M. Oltramare, that salicylate of soda acts upon the vaso-motor centre in the medulla. If a parallel be established between the anatomico-pathological processes of acute articular rheumatism, the physiological effects of salicylate of soda and its therapeutic properties are incontestable. M. Oltramare believes that he can prove that this remedy acts by substituting a state of general dilatation of the capillaries for a localized hyperæmia. So long as the rheumatic lesions are of a purely vascular nature, salicylate of soda appears to possess a therapeutic value, but when disorders of nutrition intervene, it is of necessity inefficacious. It is for this reason that salicylate of soda is useless in the subacute or chronic forms of rheumatism, and this want of success in such cases seems to support the theory here advanced.—*London Med. Record,* Aug. 16, 1879.

Experimental and Clinical Study of Conia and its Salts.

M. TIRYAKEN has studied (*Le Progrès Médical,* June 14, 1879) the alkaloid which forms the active principle of Conium maculatum. He finds that the conia whose action has hitherto been investigated is not a pure alkaloid, for it is mingled with an empyreumatic substance, whose effects, comparable with those of urari, have contributed to the belief that conia was possessed of much more intensely poisonous properties than is really the case. Conia has, however, a local irritant action which prevents its being administered by hypodermic injection. In poisoning by conia three phases can be distinguished. The first is characterized by depression and lowness of spirits, rapidly succeeded by paralysis of motion, and moaning during inspiration. During the second stage the moaning becomes gradually louder, whilst the respiration becomes feeble, incomplete, and hurried, the pulse-rate and the reflex irritability being at the same time increased. This stage is followed by one of collapse, accompanied by slowing of the pulse and respiratory rhythm, and ultimate death or recovery according as the elimination of the poison is impeded or hastened. From these observations it is concluded that conia acts upon the central nervous system, and is not a muscular or cardiac poison. M. Tiryaken has also studied the action of the hydrobromate and hydrochlorate of conia. He finds that the action of these salts is comparable with that of the alkaloid, but that they are so feeble that he is able to prescribe a gram of the hydrobromate in 3–5 doses in twenty-four hours. This remedy may be employed with advantage in neuroses, and in the spasmodic affections of chronic bronchitis.—*Practitioner,* September, 1879.

On the Physiological Facts in regard to Anæsthesia.

M. SIMONIN believes (*Le Progrès Médical,* May 3, 1879) that of the various symptoms of etherization three appear to predominate. By means of these symptoms a diagnosis of the various degrees of etherization may be made, and by them the surgeon may be guided in the administration of an anæsthetic, and may obtain the full effect without risk of accident. The symptoms alluded to are, firstly, the manifestation of peripheral insensibility, markedly in the temples and cornea; secondly, the condition of the muscles of the lower jaw; thirdly, the state of the pupils, more especially in regard to their contraction, and to the relaxation of the iris. The conclusion of the author in regard to these points is, that when the peripheral insensibility sets in, the patient is in a fit state for the surgeon. The patient is in no danger so long as the jaws remain closed. Lastly, the contraction of the iris is a nearly constant symptom of the surgical period of etherization, and the maintenance of the contraction shows that the anæsthetized patient is not in any danger. But dilatation of the pupil should cause uneasiness, or at any rate should provoke the greatest attention on the part of the surgeon to the state of his patient.—*London Med. Record,* Aug. 15, 1879.

The Effect of Anæsthetics on the Circulation.

The comparative effect on the circulation of intravenous injections of chloral, chloroform, and ether, has recently been studied by M. ARLOING, and an account of his researches has been communicated to the Académie des Sciences. A solution of chloral was employed of the strength of 1 in 5, and a mixture of chloroform and ether with twenty volumes of water. Large animals (horses or dogs) were employed for the experiments. The needful dose was given in divided portions, and injected slowly into a vein far from the heart. Cardiographic tracings with the apparatus of MM. Chauveau and Marey show that the three substances do not all produce the same effects. All cause an acceleration of the cardiac pulsations, but this is more considerable, and occurs more promptly, with chloroform than with others. Chloral produces, first, a retardation. Both chloral and ether lower the pressure in the right ventricle, while chloroform increases it. Chloroform and ether augment the force of the heart's contractions, while chloral lessens it. Hence it seems legitimate to conclude that the pulmonary circulation is quickened by chloral and by ether, and is retarded by chloroform.

By means of a new hæmodromograph of M. Chauveau the modifications in the pressure and in the rapidity of movement of the blood in the arteries have been recorded. Injections of chloral cause, first, a slight increase in the intra-arterial pressure, as well as in the quickness of the cardiac systole, and a diminution in the frequency of the heart's action—*i. e.*, an increase in the diastolic pause. Soon a fall in pressure and an increase in frequency result, and these continue as long as the anæsthesia. Chloroform often causes, at the outset, a slight dilatation of the vessels, soon replaced by a still stronger contraction, which makes itself evident in spite of the increase in the force of the cardiac systole. During the third period of chloroformization the vaso-constrictive action lessens, but does not give way to an opposite action—at least, unless the dose of chloroform is poisonous. Ether affects the arterial circulation in the same way as chloral: in extreme etherization the accelerated pulsations present a marked dicrotism; and there is a retrograde movement at each pulsation, as if the column of blood oscillates in the large arteries.

The venous pressure during chloralization is increased, and the tracing obtained may present arterial pulsation. With chloroform the venous pressure varies, just as does the arterial pressure. In etherization the two at first vary in the same manner, but later the venous pressure is increased, just as in the administration of chloral.

The conclusion from these facts is that the movement of blood in the capillaries lessens slightly at the commencement of chloralization and of etherization, and undergoes subsequently a considerable increase. The capillary flow first suffers a temporary augmentation by the influence of chloroform, and quickly lessens, to increase slowly at a later period, but without attaining always the normal rapidity.

·Of the state of the cerebral circulation during the sleep of anæsthesia little is known. According to some observers there is at first hyperæmia, and, when sleep is well established, there is anæmia. According to others, even the profound sleep is accompanied by cerebral hyperæmia. The means of observation hitherto employed have been either insufficient or have been liable to error. The best method is to study the changes in the rate of movement of the blood in the artery which carries it to the brain, leaving the cranium intact, and to compare these changes with those in the pressure within the vessel and in the corresponding vein. Such an investigation shows (1) that all anæsthetics do not produce the same effect on the capillary system, and that it is impossible to reason from one anæsthetic to the others; (2) that sleep from chloroform is accompanied by anæmia, sleep by chloral and ether by hyperæmia of the brain. Hence the conclusion seems to be inevitable that the modifications in the cerebral circulation are not essential to the anæsthetic sleep, and therefore cannot be regarded as its cause. It is probable, from a comparison of the results of ophthalmoscopic examinations with these observations, that the sleep induced by chloroform is that which presents the greatest analogy with natural sleep.—*Lancet*, Sept. 6, 1879.

The Effects of Koumiss on the Urine in Health and Disease.

At a recent meeting of the British Medical Association (*British Med. Journal,* Aug. 23, 1879) Dr. V. JAGIELSKI gave a description of koumiss, its character and composition; its constantly changing nature, with the different varieties thus created; and their several denominations, according to consistency and age. He then enumerated the various solid constituents of koumiss—as casein, fat, albumen, lacto-protein—and considered separately the products of fermentation, as—first, carbonic acid; secondly, lactic acid; and thirdly, alcohol; and commented upon the physiological effects of each, particularly upon the brain, heart, and kidneys; showing the changes which occur in the urine of a healthy subject during a course of koumiss, in regard to quantity, colour, and specific gravity, whereby a tolerably close estimate may be made of the percentage of solids and normal constituents contained in the secretions of a healthy kidney—when the conditions of pressure under which they are developed are at the same time adequately considered. The author stated that with those who drink koumiss freely, the diuresis is augmented (on an average, 1800 c. c. of urine voided in twenty-four hours; in some cases, about 1500 only), the desire to micturate becomes more frequent, and there exists a certain sensation of weight and pressure in the region of the bladder; but these symptoms disappear after a lapse of two or three days, leaving the urine clear and its reaction sour. The density or specific gravity of the urine increases, too, on the average to from 1019 to 1022 c. c., notwithstanding the increase in quantity voided. The urates, phosphates, and sulphates show an increase under koumiss; whilst the proportion of uric acid to urea diminishes. Dr. Biele estimated the elimination of uric acid, in a case where koumiss was beneficially taken for fifty days, as proportionate to each ten *kilogrammes* of bodily weight; and, according to Palubienski, about fifty-seven *grammes* of solids were obtained from the urine of one patient within twenty-four hours. The chloride of sodium varied greatly, individual idiosyncrasies determining the individual urinary capacity. The diseases in which koumiss is generally useful, and in which the urine is found to be of low specific gravity, are not necessarily those of the kidneys, but may also arise from the condition of the blood and the state of general nutrition, or of the nervous system. Dr. Jagielski classified—1. Diseases with increased secretion of urine of *low* specific gravity; 2. Diseases with increased secretion of urine of *high* specific gravity; 3. Normal secretion and sediment in urine; 4. Diminished secretion; 5. Complete suppression of urine. The *quality* of the blood increases the *quantity* of the urine secreted; but it is advisable to ascertain the individual standard in each case before treatment by koumiss, so that subsequent changes may be clearly evidenced. In cases of anæmia, where the specific gravity of the urine was 1008 to 1012 before taking koumiss, it rose, after fourteen days, to 1018–1019. In chlorosis, all the symptoms improve with the appearance of a higher specific gravity, consequent upon three or four weeks' use of koumiss; the amount of urine and its colour becoming normal. The low specific gravity of chronic albuminuria advances under koumiss from 1010 or 1012 to 1018–1020. Dr. Jagielski believed the nervous influence to perform an important part, especially in cases of great weakness, in which fear or alarm may stimulate the flow of urine. This nervousness, however, with its effect upon the urine, is readily amenable to the action of koumiss, and disappears with the increase of the bodily weight. As the solid constituents of the urine march *pari passu* with the gain of flesh, their specific gravity becomes of the highest diagnostic importance. Dr. Jagielski illustrated these views by several cases in his own practice, and by others published in the medical journals. The low specific gravity indicates relative decrease of the normal solid constituents, especially urea, uric acid, and extractive matters. The amount of albumen may vary considerably at first; but, with the exclusive use of koumiss for a day or two, both the volume of the urine and its solids augment with the increase of bodily weight as the albumen disappears. In œdema and anasarca, koumiss often assists in diminishing or removing dropsical accumulations, increases the heart's action, and promotes the general return of strength. Amongst the diseases with increase of urine and of its specific gravity, Dr. Jagielski mentioned several cases of diabetes mellitus in which both quantity and specific gravity diminished, whilst bodily weight increased and strength returned—notably, in those instances in which gastric derangements prevailed to the extent of vomiting any other food. In diseases of the kidneys, such as hyperæmia, hæmaturia, acute nephritis, etc., the use of koumiss had, even in very desperate cases, been effectual in saving life; in all of these, the secretion was either considerably diminished, or for hours altogether suppressed, headache and stupor were manifested, and the urine loaded with blood and albumen to complete coagulation on boiling in a test-tube. Where milk and all other food was rejected by the stomach, koumiss was retained, and from the first afforded hopes of recovery which could not previously be entertained. In smallpox and scarlet and typhoid fevers, where similar conditions exist, equally beneficial results had been obtained. The great diuretic power of koumiss, together with its easy digestibility and nourishing properties, render it available and useful even in those cases which otherwise may fairly be pronounced hopeless.

—

The Use of Duboisia.

At the recent meeting of the British Medical Association, Mr. NETTLESHIP, of London, stated that he had employed a four-grain solution of sulphate of duboisin in a few cases, and had repeatedly got well-marked toxic effects resembling belladonna poisoning. In more than one case there had been considerable delirium. These effects had followed sometimes from the use of only a drop or two or three to the conjunctiva. Mr. Nettleship attributed this to the fact that his duboisia was an extremely pure and therefore potent solution, made from a dry crystalline sample. Isolated cases had been reported by others, but these formed an almost continuous series.

Mr. SWANZY thought it right to mention that in one case, that of a boy aged 12, where duboisin had produced symptoms of poisoning, including delirium, the patient died within a few weeks of meningitis. No head-symptoms had shown themselves until the duboisin had been used. Only a few drops in all of a four-grain solution had been instilled.—*British Med. Journal*, Aug. 30, 1879.

—

Cases of Toxic Symptoms from the Use of Duboisia Drops.

In the following cases, under the care of Mr. NETTLESHIP, at St. Thomas's Hospital, constitutional symptoms, varying in severity from slight transient giddiness to violent delirium, followed the use of this new mydriatic. It may be stated that the preparation was a perfectly clear, colourless solution of sulphate of duboisin, four grains to the ounce, very carefully made by Mr. Plowman, the apothecary to the hospital, from a dry crystalline sample supplied by Messrs. Corbyn & Co. In Case 8 the solution was obtained from Mr. Martindale. The preparations, therefore, may be taken as quite pure. When the supply of the pure alkaloid becomes large enough to insure uniformity of strength in the solutions made by different chemists, it may be unsafe to prescribe a four-grain solution of sulphate of duboisin, and the use of the drug for rapidly dilating the pupil or paralyzing the accommodation in the out-patient or in the consulting-room may not be free from disadvantage. It remains to be seen whether a solution of duboisin, weak enough to be free from risk, will have any advantages over atropine :—

Case 1. E. H., aged seventy-six, male, with cataracts, was admitted on March 25th. Two atropine drops (four grains to ounce) were put into his eyes ; half an hour later, the pupils not being widely dilated, four drops of duboisin solution were used (single drops from a very small pipette). Half an hour afterwards the man was taken from his seat to go into the dark room, when he seemed drowsy, staggered, and said he felt giddy. After waiting a few minutes another attempt was made to remove him, with the same result ; he staggered over to his right side, and had evidently lost power in his legs, the right being the weaker ; he was then taken to the ward. When seen by Mr. Nettleship one hour later he was delirious, constantly picking at things and talking of home, and had been struggling and requiring two nurses to hold him. During the night he became more violent. Next day he was much better ; could stand, but felt weak, and complained of his fingers feeling numb.

March 27th. Almost well again.

He remained in the hospital for three months, and complained to the last that his fingers were numbed ; "they were all right till I came here," he said. Whilst delirious he was seen by Dr. Sharkey, resident assistant-physician, who found the urine free from albumen. He was a feeble old farm labourer. A four-grain solution of sulphate of atropine was used three times a day for many days after the extraction of his cataract without any symptoms showing themselves.

Case 2. H. L., aged sixty-seven, carpenter, was admitted for injury to the left eye nineteen days before. The globe was enucleated. Three weeks after the excision iritis came on in the right eye, and, as the pupil would not fully dilate with atropine, duboisin solution was ordered to be used every two hours (as an out-patient). It was begun on April 9th, in the afternoon. Next day he was admitted as an in-patient at 4 P. M., and duboisin was continued every two hours from that time. The patient was very restless all night, but he calmed towards morning. At 10 P. M. on the following day he became restless and partly delirious, pulling the clothes, and required to be watched all night. Duboisin was stopped at 2 A. M. on the morning of the 12th. At noon of the same day he was not delirious, but answered questions incorrectly, and forgot he had taken his breakfast. There was no special dryness of mouth. Duboisin was used twice again, after which he became delirious, and in the night required a porter to watch him.

At 2 A. M. on the 13th he had morphia subcutaneously injected, and also a small opium draught. He slept from 5 A. M. to 6 A. M. Gradually improved. He slept well that night, and next morning was quiet and rational. He did not remember what had happened. Sulphate of atropine (four grains to the ounce) was used from this date several times daily for more than a week, without producing any toxic symptoms.

Case 3. E. T., aged seventy-five, female, May 6th, attended as out-patient with cataracts. One small drop of duboisin to each eye quickly caused very wide mydriasis. In two or three hours after instillation she staggered in walking, and said "she felt as she had never felt before;" there was slight incoherence of speech; no absolute delirium. She was admitted to the ward, and next morning was herself again.

Case 4. R. B., aged sixteen, female, had ulcer of cornea. On May 10th atropine was ordered three times a day; increased next day to every two hours. In the afternoon of the 12th the pupils were only half dilated, and duboisin was ordered six times a day. The patient was restless all night, having slept well before. In the morning she complained of giddiness and dryness of throat; duboisin was used twice more (five times altogether). The pupils were fully dilated, and duboisin discontinued. The symptoms quickly disappeared.

Case 5. C. H. N., aged twenty-five, a medical student, used duboisin in order to try the rapidity with which it paralyzed the accommodation. A drop of solution of duboisin was applied at 2 P. M., and repeated twice at intervals of half an hour. At 4 P. M. he felt dizzy and made some inaccurate remarks, which he did not afterwards remember. One or two hours afterwards he was able to go home without assistance, and felt quite well next day.

Case 6. A. S., aged twenty-eight, female with ulcers of cornea. At first used duboisin six times a day, and after two days thrice a day; the sixth day it was used only once, and then discontinued because the patient felt dizzy and complained of dryness of the mouth.

Case 7. J. E., aged thirty-six, male, had traumatic cataract of some years' standing. Duboisin was used for examination. The patient said it made him feel "tipsy," and he became very pale, and could not walk straight. No tendency to delirium. He was soon quite well.

Case 8. Mrs. ——, aged thirty-five; myopic astigmatism. Two single drops of duboisin solution were applied to the right eye. After waiting half an hour she felt uncomfortably giddy, and had difficulty in walking quite straight. There was no dryness of throat. After examination she rested for an hour, but was still giddy when she left. On her way home she felt as if she did not know where she was going, and on that and several succeeding days her head felt vacant, and she found herself not understanding or not hearing what people said. She is tall, pale, nervous, and not in strong health.—*Lancet*, Sept. 6, 1879.

Intravenous Injection of Milk.

Mr. A. S. MELDON reports (*British Med. Journal*, Aug. 30, 1879) five cases of intravenous injection of milk. The first was one of exhaustion after typhoid fever. The second and fifth were patients in the last stage of phthisis, and in both life was considerably prolonged by the operation. The third and fourth were cases of anæmia, in both of which life was saved by the transfusion of milk. In the last three cases, goat's milk was used, to which was added carbonate of ammonia.

On the Prolonged Antiseptic Bath.

In an article in the *Archives Générales* for July and August, Prof. VERNEUIL observes that this mode of treating wounds is not now much resorted to, and is suitable only for a small number of cases; but for them it is of such utility, and so superior to all other means of local treatment, that it deserves a very high place as a therapeutic agent, and he the more readily refers to it that surgeons of the present day, in their enthusiasm for new modes of dressing, seem to have forgotten its existence. Prolonged—or as at that time they were employed, permanent—local baths have been used since 1854 by Valette, Langenbeck, Zeiss, and others, after amputations and for wounds of the extremities, and some excellent results have been obtained; and in 1856 Prof. Verneuil commenced his trials with them. In one case of a fracture of the forearm, the limb was retained in the bath uninterruptedly for twenty-eight days, and in many cases of wounds of the hand and forearm the bath was continued for from four to twelve days. This mode of treatment superseded that of continuous irrigation, which, so useful in contused wounds of those parts conveniently placed for its adoption, proves of little avail in those with which the water cannot come in direct contact. In the bath every part of every kind of wound is accessible. In later times, however, Prof. Verneuil has greatly modified this means. For the cumbrous apparatus formerly in use he has substituted ordinary vessels for the reception of the hand and arm, and instead of the permanent bath, which was most inconvenient in application, especially during the night, he now uses simply a bath prolonged for two or three hours only, and repeated two or three times a day. It was found also that this prolonged bath could not be conveniently applied for wounds of the lower extremities, and of late years it has been entirely confined in its application to those of the hand and arm.

The patient may take the bath in bed, either in the sitting position or with his shoulders propped up; or, if strong enough, he may sit in a chair. The water should be of a medium temperature, which may be left to the patient to regulate in such a manner that it feels to him neither too cold nor too warm. Of late years Prof. Verneuil has added disinfecting liquids to the bath, viz., solutions of either the chloride of soda of Labarraque, carbolic acid, or hydrate of chloral, and employing from 10 to 20 per cent. of the chloride, and from 1 to 2 per cent. of carbolic acid and of chloral—varying the doses of the antiseptic according to the effects desired to be produced and the duration of the immersion. Thus, with an infected wound, with gangrene, a more concentrated bath of short duration is employed, as also when the weakness of the patient prevents too prolonged or too frequent baths. Less strong doses are employed when the primary putridity is destroyed, and when the patient is able to continue the bath for four or five hours together. Prof. Verneuil habitually employs carbolic acid, but for those to whom its smell is repugnant he substitutes the hydrate of chloral. Labarraque's liquor is especially useful when gangrene is present, as it has singular power in aiding the elimination of eschars. But many persons can ill bear the smell of the chlorine, and the unpleasantness from this can be greatly diminished by covering the bath with thick cloths, or closing it by a cover. The bath of carbolic acid shows the error of those who regard this substance as an irritant. Over and over again the hand and forearm have continued in a 1 per cent., or stronger, solution for two hours, and almost always the patients have declared that they felt considerable relief from it. In the interval of the baths, the limb, immobilized or not, according to the nature of the case, is conveniently placed on a support, and covered by a compress of muslin folded several times and wetted with the liquid of the bath. A layer of wadding, and over this some oiled silk, complete the dressing. Prolonged immersion gives to the wounds, and especially recent ones, a somewhat pale aspect, but this appearance is of short duration, and in general, when the cleansing of the wound is over, the granulations have an excellent appearance, and assume a vermilion colour scarcely an hour after leaving the bath. The quantity of pus secreted is generally small, and it is especially remarkable for the absence of odour, which is also the case with the eschars. In one of the cases related there was suppuration of the whole hand, and gangrene of the index finger; and yet, although the patient lay in a very small room, when the limb was exposed not the slightest odour could be perceived beyond that of the carbolic acid. Whatever may be the sinuous dis-

positions of the wound, the pus and mortified tissues are so thoroughly disinfected, that neither injections into these cavities nor pressure for the expulsion
of the pus are required. "I have only to quietly wait until the eschars are
detached of their own accord. In a word, I apply here that calculated abstention,
that absence of all meddling with the parts, which I so earnestly recommend for
all wounds in general." Nothing is easier than to keep in a state of the ex-
tremest cleanliness wounds which pass two or three hours in tepid water—its
sufficing to let fall a streamlet of the water from a sponge on the injured parts
and the orifices of any fistulous tracks, gently wiping the neighbouring uninjured
parts. It is not possible to say beforehand how long these prolonged antiseptic
baths ought to be continued. They must at least be used for a sufficient time to
produce the complete cleansing of recent wounds, and the absolute and durable
disinfection of old wounds. But so easy is the means in its application, and so
great is the relief which it generally procures, that its use may be continued for a
long period. Ordinarily, and that even in the most serious cases, the baths are
not required after the fifteenth or twentieth day, when, if it be deemed desirable,
the wadding bandages may be applied, as these enable the patient to take exercise more easily.

Prof. Verneuil relates several illustrative cases, and terminates his paper with
the following conclusions —:

"The prolonged and repeated antiseptic bath is of great utility in a great
number of surgical affections of the hand, forearm, and elbow. It prevents traumatic fever almost certainly in cases of recent accidental or operative wounds
seated in healthy tissue, and in this respect rivals the classical continuous irrigation and the wadding dresses. It possesses the same preventive property in cases
of operations practised in the midst of more or less old morbid centres (*foyers*)
impregnated with purulent and putrid substances, and thus renders more innocent
excisions and extirpations of bones, amputations in gangrene, drainage, counter-
openings, etc. In this respect it is very superior to rival modes of dressing.
Finally, it possesses still more than these the inestimable power of arresting acute
or chronic septicæmia by so modifying recent or old pathological centres that the
production or the penetration of the septic poison is prevented, or at least impeded. The preventive or curative action of the antiseptic bath on surgical
fevers enables us to study with care and profit the qualities and actions of the
poison concealed in wounds, and to dissipate some of the obscurity which still
prevails in the doctrine of septicæmia.—*Med. Times and Gaz.*, Sept. 6, 1879.

Medicine.

On Local Temperatures in Disease.

Professor PÉTÉR (*Revue des Sciences Médicales*, No. 27) has for some time
been studying, by a long series of researches, morbid local temperatures. In his
first communication to the Academy (*Bulletin de l'Académie de Médecine*, 2d
series, vol. vii. No. 8), he occupied himself exclusively with the temperature of
the chest in cases of acute pleurisy, and variations of the temperature, according
to certain fixed conditions.

In his experiments, Dr. Pétér employs the ordinary medical thermometer,
which he places successively in the same intercostal space of the diseased side and
the healthy side, and then in the axilla of the healthy side. The following are

the principal results obtained by this method : First—outside of the pleurisy the parietal temperature is always higher than the average temperature. The local excess of heat is from five-tenths of a degree to upwards of two degrees, and sometimes exceeds this figure. Second—the elevation of the temperature increases with the effusion ; that is to say, the greatest elevation of local temperature corresponds to the period of secretory activity of the inflamed pleura. This hyperthermia amounts sometimes to from two and a half to three degrees. Third—the elevation of parietal temperature decreases in the statical period of the effusion ; that is to say, when the level of the fluid remains stationary, or in other words, when secretion is not going on. The temperature, however, still exceeds that of the sound side by from half a degree to one and a half degrees. Fourth—pleurisy not only raises the parietal temperature of the side on which it is seated, but it raises also that of the opposite side. The parietal temperature, however, of the diseased side is always higher than that of the healthy. Fifth—the parietal temperature drops gradually when the effusion is spontaneously absorbed, still remaining higher than that of the healthy side. This excess of heat lasts for some time, and should not be neglected. It explains, indeed, the possibility of relapse, since it indicates the persistence of the anatomical conditions which preside over the formation of the effusion. Sixth—in pleurisies without effusion, the local excess of heat is less than when there is effusion. The return to the normal temperature also occurs more rapidly. Seventh—the absolute elevation of the local temperature on the diseased side is more considerable than the absolute elevation of the axillary temperature.

What, then, happens when thoracentesis is performed ? Immediately the parietal temperature rises on the punctured side. If the effusion is not reproduced the hyperthermia may still increase by some tenths of a degree ; but this excess only lasts for some hours. Then the parietal temperature decreases, returns to the figure which it had before the puncture, continues to decrease, and finally returns to the normal figure. If the effusion is reproduced, to be again reabsorbed, the local temperature rises after the puncture during some days, then progressively decreases under the influence of medical treatment. If, on the contrary, a fresh puncture is rendered necessary, there results a local, and then a general hyperthermia, the temperature remains stationary with the effusion reproduced, and at each new puncture the same series of phenomena is produced.

According to Dr. Pétér, the local hyperthermia consecutive to the puncture must be considered as a consequence of *hyperæmia a vacuo*. This quite mechanical hyperæmia is necessarily additional phlegmasie hyperæmia. There are thus two congestions of blood in lieu of one, whence occurs augmentation of tension in the vessels of the still inflamed pleura ; and whence also greater richness of the new fluids in leucocytes. Thus the possibility of a purulent transformation of the effusion is comprehensible in the cases where the puncture has been made in the highly febrile period of the pleurisy. The syncope, pulmonary congestion, albuminous expectoration, pain and oppression, which have been noted as the sequel of too sudden depletions of the pleura, are not less easily explicable.

In a further paper on the local temperatures and pulmonary phthisis (*Bull. de l'Académie de Médecine*, 2d series, vol. vii. No. 37), Dr. Pétér endeavours to demonstrate that so soon as tubercles occur at any point, the local temperature rises there. Thus, in cases of pulmonary tuberculization which are still dubious, when it is only by the aid of the most minute investigation that one perceives a slight difference of the tensility and the elasticity of the region, and a little dryness of the vesicular murmur, with respiratory emphasis, the thermometer already shows an elevation of temperature, which may extend from three-tenths of a degree to one degree. The average local temperature of the thoracic wall being in a healthy subject about thirty-six degrees centigrade; this temperature reaches, in the cases referred to, 36.2, 36.3, 36.5, 36.8 degrees. Moreover, this hyperthermia is in general proportioned to the intensity of the local morbid signs. If, for example, the temperature of 36.2 degrees is found outside of the chest where there can scarcely be observed a slight modification of the sound and rhythm of the respiration, there will always be found several tenths more outside where the respiratory roughness is very evident, the emphasis more marked, and the dulness more pronounced. Thus the thermometric method would permit the establishment of a diagnosis in cases where the most experienced practitioners would, up to the present time, have hesitated. Who does not know, for example, how much the symptoms of chlorosis resemble those of tuberculosis at the outset? Now, in chlorosis the temperature of the upper intercostal spaces remains at about 36 degrees, and is in all cases equal on both sides for the same space; whilst in pulmonary tuberculization, the temperature there is always superior to the average by several tenths of a degree to one degree, and the hyperthermia is unequal on one side compared with the other, as are the lesions. Moreover, the investigation of the local temperature of the superior intercostal spaces may serve to fix the diagnosis, in cases in which it is necessary to determine whether a dyspepsia with wasting is idiopathic or symptomatic of commencing tuberculization. M. Pétér cites various interesting observations of cases in which the employment of this method has permitted him to arrive at the truth.

It is especially the disparity in the local hyperthermia of the summits of the chest which constitutes an affirmatory sign of the existence of a local lesion. This disparity is indeed necessarily associated with the actually differing anatomical and physiological conditions of usually similar parts of the organism, the temperature of which ought to be normally equal, and to rise or fall simultaneously, and in parallel lines, it the thermic modifications arise from a general cause. On the other hand, if the figures are dissimilar or too homologous in identical spaces, it is because the conditions which generate heat are changed there; and, under the circumstances, they can hardly be so, except by the tuberculization, which is almost always simultaneously developed at the same points of the summits of the lungs, without being habitually symmetrical there, either in the number, the depth, or the extent of the lesions.

Dr. Pétér has investigated the influence of hæmoptyses on the local temperature. He has found that it rises at the moment of the bleeding; that it remains high while the bleeding lasts, and then drops as it passes off. The variations of local temperature may even extend to the general temperature. In caseous pneumonia the hyperthermia is yet more considerable than in ordinary tuberculosis. It may amount to three or even four degrees.

Thus in all the phases of pulmonary tuberculization, there is a local elevation of the temperature which cannot be conceived without a concomitant and generating hyperæmia. In the first phases of the disease, this hyperæmia would be, according to the expression of Dr. Pétér, "trophica-tuberculous," or tuberculizing; necessary to the development of the tubercle, and circumscribed to the very points at which the tubercle is in course of germination. Later on, the hyperæmia would radiate from the tubercle formed at the intact points of the parenchyma, so as to engender there congestion, hemorrhage, or inflammation. The practical and therapeutical conclusion to be deduced from this view is that it is important to modify and to prevent trophic hyperæmia, whilst it is only localized, from radiating and from disordering the distant parenchyma. That is the part which is played by revulsive treatment—Lister's counter-irritating plasters, cupping points, cauterization, etc.

In these, as in his previous researches, Dr. Pétér employed only the ordinary clinical thermometer in daily use in hospitals. Dr. Decaisne, who analyzes in the *Revue Médicale* the elaborate memoirs of Dr. Pétér, adds the personal researches of Dr. VIDAL, of Hyères, which fully confirm the results of M. Pétér. He finds (*Bulletin de l'Académie*, vol. vii. No. 38) that as soon as a nucleus of tubercles commences evolution, a corresponding augmentation of temperature may be observed on the local surface of the skin. This disappears with the inflammatory period, whether that has been cut short or has given place to the destructive period. Indeed, according to this author, the rise in temperature of the skin corresponds so well to the internal inflammation, that it is possible to exactly draw in the thermometer the outlines of a cavity when the pericavernous tubercles in their turn enter upon evolution. When the local temperature rises, the pulse is always quickened. This is especially seen in galloping consumption. According to M. Vidal, the rise in temperature seems to be caused, not so much by the bulk of blood which flows towards an organ, as by the difficulty which the blood finds in returning from the periphery to the centre of circulation. It would seem that whenever the arterial blood is obstructed in its circulation through the capillaries, heat is given out.—*London Med. Record*, Aug. 15, 1879.

Treatment of Yellow Fever.

Dr. F. PEYRE PORCHER, of Charleston, S. C., advocates (*Louisville Med. News*, August 30, 1879) the following treatment of yellow fever:—

1. Sponge the head, hands, and arms assiduously with ice-cold water at the *very commencement* of the attack, not losing an hour. This is to be repeated at intervals whenever the temperature rises, cold ice-water being quite capable of reducing the temperature. Towels soaked in ice-water are preferable to sponging. Fifteen to twenty minutes generally suffice for each application, its necessity being determined by the existence of pyrexia. Few perform this simple but *essential* procedure as they should do. Prof. T. O. Summers, of Nashville, was perfectly correct when he stated recently that "cold water is the remedy in yellow fever."

2. Give immediately *and but once* Blair's calomel gr. xx, quinine gr. xx, diminishing the dose for children. The quinine may not be essential, though I greatly favour its use for several reasons, and have never seen it produce a single ill effect.

3. Follow in three or four hours with a saline cathartic, which is cooling and antiphlogistic.

4. Apply mustard plasters to the entire abdomen, and place the feet in a hot mustard foot-bath from the beginning of the attack, and repeat them frequently. These may be followed by a blister to the abdomen (which certainly does no injury) in case there is nausea or irritability of the stomach.

5. After the salts have acted give an effervescing or antacid mixture of this nature (which was much used by the late Prof. E. Geddings, of this city): R. Acetate of potash, ʒj ; bicarb. of potash, ʒj ; morphia, gr. j ; water, ℥vj. A teaspoonful to a dessertspoonful every two or three hours to quiet irritation and act as a mild antacid and diuretic.

No other treatment or active measures are required, save the continuance of the cold water and pellet of ice given internally, if desired. The administration of food must be watched with the greatest care throughout the disease.

Doubtless a few drops of tinct. of aconite might prove serviceable, added to the mixture above mentioned or given separately, if the pulse or temperature is with difficulty reduced.

Delirium Tremens.

The *Centralblatt f. d. Med. Wiss.*, No. 25, 1879, contains an interesting résumé of observations on delirium tremens made on a large scale in the hospitals of Dantzic and Königsberg, by Dr. P. Nächke, of Dresden. He finds that this affection is infinitely more common among brandy (*Schnaps*) than among wine and beer drinkers; hence its prevalence in Russia and America. The most dangerous spirit is that distilled from potatoes, probably because it contains more amylic alcohol in the form of fusel oil. Persons who habitually drink several kinds of spirits seem more liable to be attacked than those who restrict themselves to one sort only. In a very large number of cases the attack is determined by a severe fit of intoxication or an epileptic seizure. The influences of race, climate, social relations, etc., are difficult to state accurately. Women suffer less often than men: among the latter, those who are much exposed to weather, and have much outdoor work, or else those whose occupation brings them much in contact with spirits, are most often attacked. The period when delirium tremens is most frequent is from thirty to fifty, the largest number of cases occurring between thirty-five and forty. The youngest patient Dr. Näcke met with was eighteen years old. The most favourable season (for North Germany) is late autumn, and next to that the summer time.

Dr. Näcke finds that 5 per cent. of the cases (at any rate at Königsberg) are only abortive forms, *delirium tremens incipiens*, which may be regarded as the disease limited to its initial stage. This form is the rule with women. He also describes a *delirium tremens chronicum*, lasting weeks or months, and consisting of a series of abortive outbreaks, with more or less well-marked intervals, and succeeding a decided attack of the ordinary disease.

Delirium tremens has a premonitory stage of two to four days. Increased perspiration and thirst are often observed in the course of the attack. The gastric symptoms are very important in forming a prognosis.

In one-third of his cases Dr. Näcke observed slight feverishness, not exceeding 38.8° Cent. (101.8° Fahr.). A temperature higher than the latter points to internal inflammation, especially of pneumonic character. The ordinary fever only occurs in the evening.

Albuminuria occurred in 82 per cent. of the cases, kidney and heart diseases being excluded, and the amount of albumen ranged from minute traces up to enormous quantities. This albuminuria ordinarily disappeared with recovery from the delirium. In one-fourth of the cases it was accompanied with fever, and the two rose simultaneously, but the fever was not always proportioned to the intensity of the delirium.

Some chemical analyses seem to prove that the excretion of phosphorus is diminished at the commencement of the delirium, probably from impaired tissue-change in the great nervous centres. The hallucinations of delirium tremens are all perversions of external sensations, generally of those received through the eye and ear. They are all characterized by depression. Dr. Näcke only noticed illusions connected with animals in one-third of a very large number of cases, and they were not restricted to small animals, but referred also to large ones. In any case the animals are always supposed to be alive and active. All the symptoms usually get worse at night. They do not nearly always disappear completely after the first good sleep, but crop up in different forms for some time longer.

The mortality varies at different times even in the same locality. Dr. Näeko found that, of 860 cases at Königsberg, 24.2 per cent. died. The number of complications also varies very much. The first attack is always the most dangerous. In fatal cases, Näcke, like others before him, failed to find any characteristic morbid changes. The best treatment seems to consist in narcotics given from the first in moderate doses. Three to five grammes of chloral in two doses generally were found to induce sufficient sleep, but the dose required to be pretty frequently repeated later on. Mechanical restraints should be avoided if possible, especially as they give rise to many illusions.—*Med. Times and Gazette,* Sept. 6, 1879.

How to Stop a Cold.

HORACE DOBELL, in his little work on "Coughs, Colds, and Consumption," gives the following plan for stopping a cold. If employed sufficiently early it is said to be almost infallible : 1. Give five grains of sesquicarb. of ammonia and five minims of liquor morphine in an ounce of almond emulsion every three hours. 2. At night give iss of liq. ammon. acetatis in a tumbler of cold water, after the patient has got into bed and been covered with several extra blankets. Cold water should be drunk freely during the night should the patient be thirsty. 3. In the morning the extra blankets should be removed, so as to allow the skin to cool down before getting up. 4. Let him get up as usual and take his usual diet, but continue the ammonia and morphia mixture every four hours. 5. At bed time the second night give a compound colocynth pill. No more than twelve doses of the mixture from the first to the last need be taken as a rule ; but should the catarrh seem disposed to come back after leaving off the medicine for a day, another six doses may be taken and another pill. During the treatment the patient should live a little better than usual, and on leaving it off should take an extra glass of wine for a day or two.—*London Medical Record,* Aug. 15' 1879.

On Erysipelatous Pneumonia.

At a recent meeting of the Société des Hôpitals in Paris, M. STRAUSS reported (*Bull. Gén. de Therap.,* July 15, 1879) a case of erysipelas of the lungs and bronchi. The patient, a healthy strong-built man, aged 26, had entered the hospital on March 14, 1879, with facial erysipelas. Previous history good. On the 20th the erysipelas of the face was nearly gone, when suddenly the pharynx, tonsils, and tongue were observed to be very red (pharyngeal and buccal erysipelas). On the 23d the fever and general symptoms had become much more intense. The patient complained of a slight pain in his right side ; no rigors. He coughed a little ; no laryngeal phenomena. Pneumonia of the base of the right lung was diagnosed. In less than four days the pneumonia had spread over the whole of the right lung, and, on the 28th, the patient died. The *post-mortem* examination revealed some very important lesions of the respiratory apparatus ; the mucous membrane of the larynx and the ary-epiglottic folds were of a normal colouring, which contrasted strongly with the purplish tint of the pharynx and the palate. The mucous membrane on the three upper rings of the trachea was also of a normal colour, but, beyond this, the whole of the trachea was of a deep scarlet hue, which extended over the whole of the large right bronchus and its branches. The left bronchus was again normal. The greater part of the right lung, viz., the entire middle lobe, two-thirds of the upper lobe, and the upper three-quarters of the lower lobe, had been transformed into a hepatized mass, the upper part of which was of a pinkish hue, the rest gray. On making a transverse section, a grayish sero-purulent fluid oozed out. On microscopic examination, the fluid which was obtained by scraping the sections of the lung contained nothing but leucocytes ; no fibrinous casts of the alveoli. Some portions of the lungs were carefully hardened, but, on making new sections, the alveoli were found to be filled with white blood-corpuscles without a trace or fibrine. In discussing the histological changes in the tissue of the lungs which he had just described, M. Strauss said that it was evident that they were very similar to those histological changes which Vulpian, Steudner, and Volkmann had described as the characteristic symptoms of cutaneous erysipelas. He thence concluded that the pneumonia which he had just observed exhibited certain clinical and histological peculiarities which distinguished it from other similar affections. The clinical characteristics were: the occurrence of pneumonia in an individual who was suffering from erysipelas of the face and throat, and had not caught cold; the peculiar way in which the affection began (no rigors, and only a slight pain in the side); the rapid progress of the affection. *Histological Characteristics.*—General gray hepatization, the leucocytes in the alveoli, no trace of fibrinous casts, analogy between the lesions which were observed in the present case and those which occur in cutaneous erysipelas. M. Strauss, therefore, thinks himself justified in asserting the existence of a peculiar form of pneumonia, to which he gives the name of erysipelatous pneumonia, and which was designated by the ancients erysipelas of the lungs.—*London Medical Record,* August 15, 1879.

Pulmonary Tubercle.

Professor Péter thus concludes a long series of papers (*Bull. Générale de Thérap.*) on pulmonary tuberculosis:—

1. The *chronic* is much the most common form of the affection.

2. Of the chronic forms the most common, fortunately, is the *apyretic.*

3. Some chronic cases are at times distinctly *febrile,* with more or less prolonged periods of remission.

4. In another variety of tubercular disease of the lung the fever is *continuous,* presenting no period of remission.

5. The pyretic form of the affection may be *primary* or may *succeed* the apyretic variety; in the latter case the disease is decidedly less dangerous than when it is febrile from the outset.

6. Galloping phthisis and acute phthisis are perfectly uncontrollable by any of the therapeutical measures at our command.

7. Of the four chief varieties mentioned, the first two are more common in private practice than in hospital. In these, which are to some extent amenable to treatment, the double aim which must always be kept before the mind is to *attend carefully to the digestive organs* and to *combat the febrile symptoms.*

8. Tubercle, indeed, and this is no paradox, shows a natural tendency to cure —(1) by softening and expulsion, a process which does some damage to the lung by producing excavation, but which may safely end in cicatrization; (2) by fibroid degeneration of the affected part; (3) by calcification.

9. It is stated above that tubercle may be cured; it would be nearer the truth to say that its evolution is arrested, that it ceases to exist, that it *dies*

10. The grand problem, therefore, in the treatment of the tuberculous, is to *enable the patient to outlive his tubercles,* a problem which, in a great many cases, is certainly not insoluble.—*Glasgow Medical Journal,* September, 1879.

Treatment of Cough in Tuberculosis.

Péter (*Bull. de Thérap.,* April 15, 1879) is a strong advocate of the combination of opium and belladonna in treating the cough of tuberculous patients. He begins by giving 1 to 2 pills, containing each 1 centigramme of extract of thebaicum and 5 milligrammes of extract of belladonna. A mixture of equal parts of syrup of tolu and syrup of turpentine diminishes the secretion and soothes the cough. M. Pétér thinks that the vomiting which often follows a fit of coughing is caused by a morbid hyperæsthesia of the stomach. The food which reaches the stomach irritates the gastric branches of the vagus nerve, and thereby causes both coughing and vomiting. In order to prevent this, he gives immediately before the meal some soothing drug, such as a drop of laudanum in a teaspoonful of water; or a solution of morphia (1 milligramme in a teaspoonful of water). The dyspepsia of tuberculous patients, which manifests itself by a feeling of heaviness in the stomach, is treated with hydrochloric acid (3 drops at the end of each meal in three spoonfuls of water). In cases of gastralgia, a small blister will be found useful. If it has no effect, hypodermic injection of morphia must be given.—*London Medical Record*, August 15, 1879.

—

Hypodermic Injections of Morphia in Dyspnœa caused by Albuminuria.

Dr. ORTILLE has obtained (*Lyon Méd.* No. 27, 1879) good results in cases of albuminurie dyspnœa, which were not complicated with pulmonary œdema or heart disease, by injecting hypodermically five milligrammes of morphia. In cases where the albuminuria has caused œdematous swellings, he recommends from two to three grammes per dose of infusion of jaborandi by the mouth, or to inject hypodermically two centigrammes of the chlorhydrate or nitrate of pilo-carpine. If the patient is very weak and death seems imminent, a dose of from one to two milligrammes of phosphate of zinc is given to stimulate the nervous system.—*London Med. Record*, Aug. 15, 1879.

—

Treatment of Cardiac Dyspnœa.

Professor SÉE says (*Concours Méd.*, July 12, 1879) that in all cases of continuous cardiac dyspnœa he has found iodide of potassium answer very well, especially where the dyspnœic symptoms were combined with a lesion of the tissue of the heart. It is equally useful in valvular lesions. Even if the diagnostic error of mistaking a simple cardiac dyspnœa for true asthma should be committed, the use of iodide of potassium would not be followed by any evil results, as it is an exceedingly useful drug in asthma. The direct effect of iodine in such cases is the promotion or rather liquefaction of the bronchial secretion. This greatly facilitates respiration. The dose given by M. Sée is 1.25 grammes per day; this is gradually increased to from 2 to 3 grammes, and is made as follows : ℞. Iodide of potassium, 10 grammes; Syr. cort. aurant, 200 grammes; 2 to 4 tablespoonfuls per day. Each spoonful must be dissolved in a tumbler of water. Patients suffering from heart disease take iodide of potassium very well—better than other patients. The following are the drawbacks of this drug : 1. Bleeding from the buccal mucous membrane, or bronchitis and hæmoptysis in tuberculous patients. (Phthisis is therefore a counter-indication for the use of iodide of potassium.) 2. Loss of flesh : in fat individuals this is to be regarded as a favourable symptom. 3. Loss of strength: in such cases the treatment must be suspended at once. 4. Loss of appetite. Opium may be added to iodine, in order to prevent the evil effects of iodine. ℞. Iodide of potass., 10 grammes; Syr. cort. aurant, 200 grammes; Extr. thebaic, 0.10 to 0.15 gramme. From 2 to 4 spoonfuls per day. For the extr. theb. the syr. papaveris may be substituted (50 grammes). Opium is given here with a view of making the iodine more easily tolerated, and of diminishing the cough, which greatly inconveniences the patient. Another very useful combination is that of digitalis with iodine, as the one has a soothing influence on the dyspnœa by acting on the lungs, and the other increases the action of the heart and modifies the arterial tension. The following formula will be found to answer well: ℞. Julep gommeux 100 grammes; Iod. of potass., 2 grammes; Tinct.

digit., g. 40; or the following formula: Extr. gent., 0.10 gramme; Pulv. fol.
dig., 0.15 gramme. To take one pill three times daily, together with the sol. of
iodine, which we have mentioned above. In cases where patients cannot take
digitalis, chloral will be found to be a good substitute. Thus, e. g., Julep gommeux,
120 grammes; iod. of potass., 2 grammes; chloral-hydrate, 4 grammes. To be
taken every two hours during the day.—*London Med. Record*, Aug. 15, 1859.

Intra-Vascular Tumour and its Import.

The manner in which general tuberculosis is disseminated from a local caseous
focus has not yet been so thoroughly worked out as has been the development of
secondary cancer; for, although few would be found now to deny that acute
miliary tuberculosis is the result of infection of the organism from a local starting-
point, yet we have hardly got beyond the general assertion that this infection
takes place through the bloodvessels and the lymphatics. Facts, indeed, point
to both these paths of transmission; and, as regards the lymphatic system (with
which tubercle seems to have special affinities), anatomical research has fairly
well established the doctrine of its special infection. We have examples of this
in the local infection of serous membranes—*e. g.*, the perineum—from contiguous
tubercular or caseating foci; and as the lymphatic glands are *par excellence* the
seat of caseous (or "tubercular") inflammation, the existence of lymphatic
tubercle, perivascular tubercle, etc., is readily explained. But observations upon
the actual infection of the lining membrane of bloodvessels, similar to the infection of other endothelia, still afford scope for investigation. It is for the demonstration of this point that Dr. Muegge, pathological assistant of Gottingen,
contributes a paper in a recent number of Virchow's *Archiv*, his observations
being limited to the pulmonary bloodvessels in ten cases of disseminated tubercle
of the lungs. He points out that Rokitansky's dictum that the lining membrane
of bloodvessels enjoys complete immunity from tuberculosis is incorrect, and he
refers to facts recorded by Weigert and Klebs in support of this, to which his
own observations lend further confirmation. Weigert met with miliary tubercle
in the pulmonary vessels in a case of hæmoptysis, and also describes two cases of
acute tuberculosis in which giant-celled tubercle was found in the larger pulmonary veins. Klebs found tubercles in the pulmonary vessels in experiments
on rabbits, and also records the occurrence of miliary nodules in the interior of
the larger pulmonary vessels in a case of human miliary tuberculosis. The inquiry
undertaken by Muegge at the suggestion of Professor Orth was simple enough.
By merely laying open the bloodvessels in tubercular lungs he found in all the
cases he examined some granulations growing from the lining membrane. The
number of these intravascular nodules was in proportion to the number of
granulations scattered in the interlobular and interalveolar tissue of the lungs.
They occurred far most extensively in the veins, and in the smaller tributaries
more than in the larger trunks, their chief seat being at the point of entrance of
one vein into another. Of spheroidal shape and well-defined margin, they project
into the lumen of the vessel, sometimes being barely visible, sometimes as large
as pins' heads; the smaller granulations being grayish and translucent, the larger
yellowish throughout or yellowish in the centre and gray at the margins. Often
in close proximity to tubercle in the surrounding tissues, they occurred also in
parts removed from such.

It is important not to confound these granulations with localized inflammatory
thickenings of the lining membrane, or with organized thrombi in the vessels.
The microscope may be necessary to distinguish between these forms of intra-
vascular change. Simple inflammatory formations are differentiated by the fact

that they do not rise abruptly from the surface of the intima, that they are more
flattened than the tubercles, that they occur in ridges, and in structure are composed of wavy interlacing bundles of delicate fibrous and spindle-celled tissue
between the endothelium and the undulating fenestrated membrane. Small
thrombi, composed mainly of leucocytes and fibrin, are less easy to distinguish,
but even here the presence of the endothelium between the thrombus and the
vessel wall would suffice to distinguish them. Sometimes such a thrombus may
overlie a tubercular granulation.

Microscopical preparations exhibit the granulation as a spheroidal body springing from the lining membrane of the vessel, and composed of closely-packed cells
as large as or larger than white blood-corpuscles. The cells contain one or more
nuclei within granular protoplasm, and a fine reticulum binds the cells together.
Only rarely are giant-cells to be found ; and the larger granulations are either
entirely caseous or else caseous in the centre with a periphery of cells. The elements of inflammatory thickenings are not only round, but spindle-shaped, and
do not form the whole mass of the nodule ; whilst the leucocytes embedded in a
thrombus are less plainly differentiated. The relations of the thrombus to the
endothelium, however, help to distinguish it from a tubercular granulation. The
tubercle is a growth of the intima ; the characteristic wavy line of the fenestrated
membrane bounds it beneath ; and frequently the subjacent muscularis and adventitia show no change whatever. Sometimes, however, both the outer and
middle coats of the vessel are the seats of tubercular growth, in which case there
are generally pneumonic and tuberculous foci in the lung-tissue adjacent. So
that sometimes—just as granulations spring up on the serous surface of the intestine corresponding to tubercular ulceration—the adventitia and muscularis are the
seat of tubercle infected by the growth in the intima. The author admits here
that the question as to which was primary—the growth in the outer or that in the
inner wall of the bloodvessel—cannot always be determined. The relation of the
endothelium to the tubercular granulation is not readily made out, owing to the
great delicacy of the former. Here and there Muegge succeeded in preserving
the endothelial layer passing over the tubercle. In one fortunate specimen a
thrombus surmounted the granulation, and the line of the endothelium divided
the clot from the tubercle. In most specimens the endothelium could be seen
mounting up the sides of the granulation, but it was rarely preserved over its
summit ; and sometimes not only the endothelium, but a portion of the second
layer of the intima lay over the tubercle. It would seem, then, that the latter
was developed, not from endothelium (as in other serous membranes), but in the
subendothelial tissue, from growth of connective-tissue cells, aided possibly by
migrant leucocytes from the vasa vasorum, or from the blood circulating in the
vessel itself. Each of these sources is open to objection—the former that tubercle of
the intima occurs often unassociated with tubercle of the adventitia or muscularis ;
the latter that the tubercle grows in arteries, which, according to Cohnheim, are
never the seat of cell-migration, even in the most intense inflammation. On the
whole, then, it is simpler to conclude that the tubercle is developed from proliferation of connective-tissue cells alone.

The import of this research, if well grounded, is simply this : It proves that in
tuberculous subjects the blood may be, and is, infected with the poison. It proves
that just as in the case of lymphatics leading from the seats of tuberculous change,
and becoming themselves the seat of fresh tubercular growth, so here the bloodvessels themselves may bear witness to their contaminated contents. There is no
strained analogy between this and the ulceration of the air passages in a phthisical
lung by the passage of tuberculous material over them. Both may be regarded
as examples of local infection of tubercle. The rapidity with which the blood-

current flows in the arteries renders these vessels far less prone to such infection than the capillaries and the veins. The capillaries may be the chief seats of the development of granulations disseminated throughout the lung, and much of the poison may be arrested there, but not all; for the occurrence of the granulations in the veins testifies to its passage onwards; and it is interesting to note the comparatively larger number of granulations in the veins than in the arteries, a difference probably due to the difference in the rate of the blood-stream. The main meaning of it all is that it is as strictly correct to speak of the blood as it is to speak of the lymphatic system being the medium for the dissemination of tubercle.—*Lancet,* Aug. 23, 1879.

Simple Dilatation of the Stomach and its Treatment.

In a paper read before the British Medical Association (*British Med. Journal,* Aug. 23, 1879) Dr. T. CLIFFORD ALLBUTT and Mr. E. H. JACOB urged that simple dilatation of the stomach apart from pyloric obstruction is not rare, and yet is not generally recognized by the profession in England. Dr. Allbutt's attention was drawn first to the subject by Kussmaul, in a paper published in 1869, and since that time he had had frequent opportunities of verifying the truth of Kussmaul's statements. Niemeyer, Leube, and others had published similar statements at subsequent dates. Among its chief causes, he referred to gluttonous eating, or the use of much slop or of aerated drinks acting upon the healthy stomach, and to the effects of ordinary ingesta upon the stomach weakened by anæmia or such debilitating diseases as phthisis, acute rheumatism, and the like. Deficiency of peptic secretion in the stomach, if neglected, may lead to the same result. Cases of ulcer or catarrh of the stomach, do not readily lead to dilatation, owing to the intolerance of accumulating contents and to the early and frequent vomiting thus induced. The symptoms and physical signs of dilatation of the stomach were detailed somewhat fully. The absence of pyloric obstruction in many cases must be taken upon an inference drawn from all the circumstances, an inference not always a certain one. Prognosis depends greatly upon such an inference, but treatment is not much affected by it. Treatment by regimen and certain drugs was touched upon, but the author said that, as in dilatation of the bladder, the direct method was to be found in systematic catheterism. This method he had found difficult in private practice, but more easy in the hospital, and in this part of his subject he was greatly indebted to Dr. Jacob's aid. Dr. Jacob had treated several cases for him and his colleagues by means of the stomach-siphon, and these cases were reported and commented upon by Dr. Jacob. The instrument used, and the mode of its application, were described.

Measurement of the Temperature of the Stomach.

Dr. WINTERNITZ, of Vienna, describes, in the *Centralblatt f. d. Med. Wiss.* (No. 24, 1879), a simple method for ascertaining the temperature of the human stomach. He uses thermometers six centimetres (2.4 inches) long, slightly bent in their lower third so as to pass more readily over the base of the tongue and the entrance to the larynx. The scale reaches from 35° to 42° Cent., and each degree is divided into tenths. The thermometer has a small glass ring blown on its upper end, and through this a strong thread is passed, carried up through the sound used for its introduction into the stomach, and secured. The instrument is also further fixed by its upper end being cemented into the hollow of the sound with a solution of gutta-percha. Preliminary experiments showed that no error could arise from the temperature of the parts which the thermometer had to pass through before reaching the stomach, as this passage lasts, at the outside, ten seconds, and the mercury does not begin to rise for about fifteen or twenty seconds. The maximum temperature is reached in four or five minutes. If the act of introduction is delayed by the irritability of the larynx or œsophagus, it is only necessary to cool the thermometer in ice, and thus the mercury will be prevented rising for nearly two minutes. Dr. Winternitz has made use of this method to examine the effect of cold irrigation of the rectum on the temperature of the stomach. Thus injected, 1000 cubic centimetres of water at 11° Cent. reduced it 0.9 Cent., or nearly one degree, in thirty minutes. The most interesting fact, however, brought out by the experiment is that the temperature of the stomach was reduced more than that of the axilla, the former having fallen from 37.15° to 36.25° Cent., and the latter from 37.05° to 36.70° during the irrigation. Dr. Winternitz claims this fact of the greater cooling of the internal organs than of the skin by cold applied to the rectum as a new discovery. He suggests its importance in controlling hyperæmia and inflammation of the stomach, liver, and other abdominal organs.—*Med. Times and Gaz.*, Aug. 23, 1879.

Bowel Obstruction.

EPSTEIN reports (*Centralb. f. d. Med. Wiss.*, April 26) a case of stenosis of the bowel from twisting of the mesentery in a child eight days old. On the fourth day after birth, the child was restless; on the fifth it vomited immediately after each time it sucked, and had thin fluid mucus-containing, but not bloody, stools. The epigastric region was on admission markedly blown out; the lower curvature of the stomach clearly made out through the abdominal walls, below which the belly was sunken and boat-shaped, and the coils of intestine were to be felt loosely rolled up like a ball. The superficial abdominal veins were very full. The vomited matters contained no blood, but bilirubin, and were tenacious and stringy. The motions were frequent, but not copious, and were very pale. On the second day after admission the child died. The whole mesentery of the small intestine was twisted spirally half a turn from right to left upon itself; the duodenum was much dilated in its first two portions; the inferior horizontal portion twisted upon its own axis by the twisting of the mesentery, so that at the part where the perpendicular portion passes into the horizontal, there was complete closure. The cæcum and colon were not in their normal places. There were no signs of old inflammation, so that any twisting of the intestinal axis in the fœtal condition is not to be thought of. The reporter of the case inclines to the view that the torsion took place during the act of birth, which was very sudden; the child nearly falling on the floor.—*Lond. Med. Record*, Aug. 15, 1879.

An Inquiry into Certain Points Connected with Albuminuria.

Recent observations on the frequency with which albuminuria is found in the urine of persons who otherwise present no symptoms of renal disease, and who are free from those general or local conditions with which its presence has been long recognized, make it necessary to reconsider the diagnostic value of this appearance as an indication of kidney-disease. The first question which naturally arises in connection with these observations is, whether there is not some fallacy —whether the substance is always the same identical serum-albumen. Dr. ROBERT SAUNDBY has endeavoured to answer this question in a paper already published in the *Birmingham Medical Review* (July, 1879), in which he tried to show that, *à priori*, it was possible that paraglobulin might be present and give similar reactions to albumen, as paraglobulin diffuses very readily, is soluble in a solution of sodium-chloride such as urine, and coagulates at about 70° Cent. (158° Fahr.). In order to settle this point, he proceeded to precipitate the paraglobulin in all cases of albuminous urine, and then repeated the test for albumen. At first, he used sodium chloride and carbon-dioxide as precipitants; but afterwards, on the advice of Professor Hoppe-Seyler, he used magnesium sulphate. The result of forty-two observations was that, in one case of dyspepsia, the entire albuminous body was on one occasion removed by magnesium sulphate; but a subsequent experiment with the urine of the same case did not have a similar result. In one other case, of phthisis, magnesium sulphate altogether or almost removed the albuminous substance. The second subject discussed was, whether this albuminuria may be accounted for by differences in the diffusibility of certain kinds of albumen. The urine of twenty-one cases of albuminuria occurring under different clinical conditions was submitted to diffusion through vegetable parchment for forty-eight hours in each case. The result showed only slight differences, such as were accounted for by the varying acidity of the urines. The author next pointed out that the albuminuria of young persons is not always completely removed by rest in bed and milk diet. The last part of the paper related to the doctrine of food-albuminuria. The author contended that the quality of the food does not produce a constant and uniform effect on the quantity of albumen excreted, as it would if Parkes and Pavy were right in thinking the increase after food to be due to the passage into the urine of a highly diffusible modification of the albumen of the food. Moreover, the albumen excreted after food does not diffuse more readily than that excreted before food, any occasional differences being explained by the increased acidity of the urine after food.—*British Med. Journal*, Aug. 23, 1879.

——

Cardiac Hypertrophy and Renal Disease.

Professor Buhl, of Munich, whose name is familiar to us from his researches on tuberculosis, has published a paper on the connection between renal disease (granular kidney) and cardiac hypertrophy, which, judging from the abstract of it in *Centralblatt f. d. Med. Wiss.*, 1878, page 668, is likely to set the pathological world a-thinking. The original paper is entitled, "Mittheilungen aus dem pathologischen Institut zu München, 1878."

Von Buhl rejects both the theories of Traube, and of Gull and Sutton, as to the causation of the hypertrophy of the heart in Bright's disease, and, though it is not so stated, it is clear that, in part at least, Dr. G. Johnson's view, as well as Ewald's, lately referred to in this journal would also be set aside.

The following points are urged against Traube's theory—(1) The occurrence of eccentric hypertrophy of the left, or of both ventricles without the presence of granular kidney; (2) the occurrence of well-marked granular atrophy of the kidneys without hypertrophy or dilatation of the left ventricle; (3) the occasional existence of left ventricular hypertrophy without dilatation; (4) the complete absence of signs of a dilated arterial system, which would be the necessary consequence of increased arterial tension; (5) the absence of cardiac hypertrophy in other forms of renal atrophy. Von Buhl further points out (6) that Traube's theory does not explain the hypertrophy of the right ventricle, which coexists with that of the left in 70.8 per cent. of the cases; and that (7) the hypertrophy of the left ventricle is often present *before* the kidneys are atrophied. .

Gull and Sutton's view, that the hypertrophy is due to a general fibrosis of the arterio-capillary system, is met by some of the objections raised above, and also by the facts that at the commencement of the renal affection the fibroid change in the arteries and capillaries is not present, and that it is rare for any other organ except the kidneys to be decidedly shrunken, whereas in a general fibrosis we should expect all highly vascular organs to suffer. .

One general objection to all theories of increased arterial tension as a cause of

the cardiac hypertrophy, and especially to Traube's theory, is the development
of a *collateral circulation* in the kidney itself, by which the place of the constricted vessels is taken by others. According to Von Buhl, on the one hand,
the vessels of the fat capsule, and the fibrous coat of the kidney, and the capillary
network of the cortex, dilate; and on the other, the blood is diverted into the
vasa recta, which run in parallel bundles from the boundary line between the cortical and tubular substance into the latter. The lateral pressure in these vessels
is much raised, and their diameter becomes doubled or trebled. The resistance
of the vasa efferentia becomes of no importance, the blood enters the veins more
freely, and the increase of pressure in the dilated vessels is relieved by increased
excretion of water. The real connection between renal atrophy and cardiac
hypertrophy, according to Von Buhl, is as follows, and it will be at once evident
how much his hypothesis differs from the ordinary explanations of these phenomena. He asserts (1) that kidney and heart are simultaneously affected, but that
the hypertrophy of the heart is due to myocarditis, the result of inflammation of
the pericardium, the valves, and the heart-muscle itself, some form of which is
present in 65.7 per cent. of the cases he has examined. The time when this inflammatory process occurs is the commencement of the renal affection. Now,
the myocarditis may either leave the heart atrophied at once, or more commonly
be followed by dilatation, owing to the diminished resisting power of the diseased
muscle to the blood-pressure, and afterwards by atrophy.

As a fact not previously noticed, Von Buhl describes *a relative contraction of
the aorta* in these cases, which intensifies the hypertrophy of the left ventricle.
Hence he explains the increased arterial pressure and cardiac hypertrophy, not
by granular atrophy of the kidneys nor by a general arterio-capillary fibrosis, but
by the hypertrophy of the left ventricle and the ·relative constriction of the
aorta.

The other changes in the arterial system are sequelæ of the heart disease.
The arterial fibrosis of the kidneys is also secondary. Lastly, it is possible that
excessive muscular exertion, and especially that of the cardiac muscles, may lead
to myocarditis, eccentric hypertrophy of the heart, and other pathological changes
met with in Bright's disease. Thus, these conditions may be a not infrequent
cause of this form of disease.

This short sketch of Von Buhl's new views necessarily excludes the data on
which they rely for support, but his eminence as a pathologist must at any rate
enforce their consideration, even though they deal roughly with current ideas.—
Med. Times and Gaz., June 14, 1879.

Increase of Albuminoid Matter in the Saliva of Albuminuric Patients.

M. VULPIAN has noticed that the saliva of individuals suffering from Bright's
disease of the kidneys, and who were treated with injections of chlorhydrate of
pilocarpine, contained a greater quantity of substances which were precipitated
by nitric acid and heat than the saliva of healthy people. He subsequently asked
M. STRAUSS to investigate the matter in his hospital. M. Strauss arrived at the
same results. M. Vulpian's patient was suffering from a compound renal disease,
the symptoms exhibited being partly of parenchymatous, and partly of interstitial, nephritis. He had been suffering from it for some time. One of M. Strauss's
patients was a man aged 40, who had entered the Hôpital Tenon for a parenchymatous nephritis, of about six months' standing. His urine contained a considerable amount of albumen. Two subcutaneous injections of chlorhydrate of
pilocarpine and one of nitrate of pilocarpine were given to the patient at intervals of several days between each injection. Each time M. Strauss noticed that
by heating the saliva which had been secreted under the influence of pilocarpine,

and adding to it a few drops of nitric acid, it became turbid. The mucus contained in the saliva had been first removed by treating it with acetic acid, and then filtering it. It was found that 1000 grammes of the saliva contained 0.253 gramme of mucine, and 0.182 gramme of albuminous matter, which is precipitated by heat and nitric acid. Another patient on whom the same experiment was tried, and who had also albuminuria, was a man 41 years of age, suffering from insufficiency of the mitral valve. Two subcutaneous injections of pilocarpine, of 2 centigrammes of nitrate of pilocarpine each, were made at an interval of nine days. The saliva presented the same changes as recorded above, and was found to contain 0.45 gramme of mucine and 0.145 gramme of albumen in 1000 grammes of filtered saliva. The saliva of a patient who was not affected with albuminuria was then tested in the same way, and contained 0.330 gramme of mucine and 0.50 gramme of albumen in 1000 grammes of filtered saliva. It results from these experiments that, in patients affected with albuminuria, the saliva is liable to contain a greater amount of albuminoid matter than in the normal state. This interesting fact may perhaps be explained by assuming that the salivary glands are infiltrated by the serous elements of the œdema. If this should not prove to be true, the cause might perhaps be found in an alteration of the epithelium of the salivary glands, or in a modification of the albuminoid constituents of the blood or of the infiltrated fluids.—*London Medical Record*, Aug. 15, 1879, from *Bull. Gén. de Thérap.*, July 15, 1879.

Syphilitic Albuminuria.

In a paper on this subject read at the recent meeting of the British Medical Association (*British Med. Journal*, Aug. 23, 1879) Dr. DRYSDALE alleged that after the brain and the liver, he was inclined to believe that the kidneys were perhaps most frequently of all the internal organs affected with syphilitic inflammation or neoplasms. M. Rayer and M. Ricord had, in 1840 and 1851, given distinct evidence that syphilis attacks the kidneys; and, although it was somewhat rare to find this admitted by professed writers on albuminuria, he (Dr. Drysdale) was convinced, from personal observation, that a large number of cases of that disease among adults were due to this often unsuspected cause. No matter what treatment had been made use of, he had found that, in certain cases of syphilis, a fatal termination occurred by the insidious commencement of nephritis, usually far on in the disease, but occasionally arising precociously, or within a year after infection. The latter was, however, very rare indeed. The morbid anatomy of syphilitic albuminuria may consist of diffuse inflammation of the cellular elements of the kidney, which, as in the case of syphilitic cirrhosis of the liver, spinal cord, etc., leads to the destruction of the secreting cells, and ultimately to fatty degeneration of the organ. In some cases, circumscribed gummy inflammation forms small tumours in the substance of the kidney. The disease usually commences silently, is accompanied by anasarca, and may end in death from asthenia or in coma. The diagnosis is made out by the history of the case, and is often quite clear; but even when the history is indistinct, assistance may be gained by noticing whether there are any scars on the liver after death. Dr. Drysdale gave the clinical history of an acute case of syphilitic nephritis occurring in a young man, aged 28, with large rupial sores recently cicatrized, and with a short history of infection ten months before. He rapidly sank and died. He referred to several other cases which he had to treat in adults, some more chronic in character, and others acute, mostly occurring in the tertiary epoch and associated with gummy tumours of the soft parts or with bone-disease. His experience was that the iodide of potassium sometimes, though rarely, was useful in such cases; and that the prognosis was usually very bad.

Pigmentation of the Face in Abdominal Tuberculosis and other Chronic
Abdominal Affections.

Dr. N. Gueneau de Mussy (*Revue Médicale*, Feb. 1879) says that, twenty
years ago, in a work on the cause and treatment of phthisis, he pointed out the
coexistence of pigmentary patches on the face with abdominal tubercle.   Since
then, the two conditions have been so constantly associated, that he now regards
the one as the sign of the other.   Tubercular disease of the abdominal viscera is
usually indicated by functional troubles which deprive the pigmentation of any
diagnostic importance, but not always ; and this pigmentation may become of
value.   It forms bronzed patches, which usually commence in the temporal fossa,
and then spread over the forehead, where they may cover the greater part, or lose
themselves in a diffused coloration, like that of mulattoes.   Sometimes they
invade other parts—the nose or the malar region ; and they may even appear on
other parts of the body, particularly the backs of the hands, and are sometimes so
extensive as to constitute a species of Addison's disease.   Pigmentation is found
in other abdominal affections besides tuberculosis.   Dr. Gueneau de Mussy has
met with it in four cases of cirrhosis with ascites, and in a case of cancer of the
stomach ; it is present also in the well-known pigmentation of pregnant women,
and may last several months after confinement should anything interfere with
restoration to health.   It is to be distinguished, however, though often coupled
with it, from the greenish-yellow tint not uncommon in abdominal phthisis, and
which appears to be associated with fatty degeneration of the liver ; and if by its
objective character this pigmentation put on the aspect of the melanoderma described by Addison—if in some cases, by its extent, it take this disease as its
model, and appears in, indeed, an early stage—it may well be asked if it have
not some pathogenic connections with Addison's disease, if it do not own the same
cause, acting with less energy.   Dr. Gueneau de Mussy then passes in quick
review the causes of Addison's disease, and concludes that all excess of pigment
is developed under the same pathogenic condition ; and this is a lesion or irritation of the nervous threads which form part of the suprarenal capsules, and form
plexuses in their vicinity.   All irritation or lesion of these nerves, in whatever
part of the abdomen they commence, will end in the same result.   Clinical observation is in accord with this induction.   It has been seen that the most different
affections situated in all parts of the abdomen are associated with the melanoderma
of Addison's disease, or with the partial pigmentation now more particularly in
question.   And an irritation which is physiological and not habitual, such as that
which results from enlargement and congestion of the uterus in gestation, produces
the same effect, and explains the formation of the pigmentary mass which is characteristic of the pregnant state.—*British Med. Journal*, June 7, 1879.

—

Spontaneous Production of Urticaria.

Dr. Dujardin-Beaumetz (*Gaz. Hebd.*, July 25) exhibited at the Société
Médicale des Hôpitaux an hysterical woman, who presented a peculiarity of which
he knew of no other example.   When a word is traced on any part of the body,
in a few minutes an elevation of the skin is produced absolutely resembling urticaria, the inscription remaining thus marked for four or five hours, the temperature of the skin being also raised at these points.   Neither urticaria nor any other
eruption exists on any other part of the body.   Prof. Vulpian has also met with
a case, in a non-hysterical youth, in which elevations of the skin, like those observed on this patient, could be induced 'in the same manner ; and in another
patient Dr. Dujardin-Beaumetz was able to produce erythema at any point to

which he applied a magnet. Dr. Besnier observed that in persons liable to
urticaria this eruption can often be induced whenever the skin is scratched.—
Med. Times and Gaz., Aug. 23, 1879.

The Use of Arsenic in Skin Diseases.

At the recent meeting of the British Medical Association, Dr. ROBERT FAR-
QUHARSON read a paper on this subject, in which he said : About thirty years
ago, the British Medical Association issued a series of queries to its members,
with reference to the use of arsenic in skin disease; and, considering the somewhat haphazard way in which the drug was then used, it was no doubt necessary
to reassure the public mind, as was effectually done by the replies, that its use
was at all events attended with danger. We know now much more precisely in
what cases to prescribe the remedy with good effect; and the question naturally
arises: How do we explain the undoubted fact that, while arsenic frequently relieves and even cures certain forms of cutaneous disorders, at other times it appears
to be inert or even to do harm? It has been supposed by some authorities that,
following up the analogy of the vesicular and pustular eruptions, which form an
occasional, though rare, part of its physiological action, it simply acts as a cutaneous irritant, by stimulating sluggish processes of repair; or, again, we may hold
that it effects some alteration in the blood, through a general influence on cell-
growth; or, thirdly, and most suggestively, we may seek for our clue in the regions of nervous pathology. We know that eczema and psoriasis and lichen, etc.,
often show their neurotic origin in heredity and symmetry, and itching and tingling; they not uncommonly appear in connection with mental shock and depression; and may alternate with, or accompany, such undoubtedly nervous disorders as chorea. Arsenic is generally held to be a nervine tonic, and, speaking
generally, we find it to be an useful and reliable remedy in all the skin affections
of the dartrous class (Clifford Allbutt). In pemphigus, it acts almost as a true
specific (Hutchinson). It is most valuable in lichen ruber, and has been recommended as an antidote to bromide acne; although the question might arise,
whether the arsenic in any way lessens the restraining influence of the bromide
over the epileptic fits. Over impetigo, strumous and syphilitic diseases, it has
no influence; and it would be interesting to note its effect on herpes zoster, which
has been reported as occasionally following its administration. Concerning the
mode of administration, the author preferred to begin with a full dose of ten
minims to fifteen minims, and push boldly on, believing that, as with quinine and
iodide of potassium, troublesome physiological symptoms are here more likely to
follow small quantities than large. Some authorities strongly insist upon the
necessity for producing some conjunctival and gastric irritation before we can obtain the full curative influence of the drug; but the author was opposed to this,
believing these symptoms to be an unnecessary addition to the discomfort of the
patient. When they do arise, they need not cause any alarm; but the sickness which sometimes follows each dose of the medicine is quite a fatal obstacle
to its use. It is important to see that the natural elimination of the drug is not
checked by any renal obstruction; and Dr. McCall Anderson warns us that patients, under the influence of arsenic, are specially susceptible to cold. May it not
be, however, that the bronchial irritation occasionally observed may really be due
to the curative influence of the remedy causing metastasis to the pulmonary mucous membrane? The liquor arsenicalis seems to be, on the whole, the best preparation; the liquor sodæ arsenitis being, in the author's experience, in no degree
less irritating. Children will bear large doses with impunity; and although it is
generally held that girls can take more than boys, the only case in early childhood
in which it had been found seriously to disagree belonged to the female sex.

Finally, it may be asked: Can we really *cure* chronic disease with arsenic? and the answer must be in the affirmative, if we get our case early, treat it systematically and carefully, continue the use of the drug for some time after the skin has become clear; and remember the importance of good food and air, and mental and bodily rest.—*British Med. Journal*, Aug. 23, 1872.

Chrysophanic Acid in Skin Diseases.

In the *Wiener Med. Presse* (1878, Nos. 37–40), Dr. J. NEUMANN records his further experience of this remedy in skin affections. He finds it useful not only in psoriasis and parasitic diseases (such as pityriasis versicolor, herpes tonsurans, eczema marginatum), but also in chloasma uterinum; treated with chrysophanic acid, the latter disfiguring affection may be caused to disappear in a very short time. It exercises a favourable influence also on syphilitic skin diseases and lupus, and its effectiveness seems to be considerably increased by the addition of thymol.—*Glasgow Medical Journal*, September, 1879.

Carbolic Acid as a Remedy against Bee Stings.

Dr. KLAMANN publishes, in the *Allgemeine Medicin Central-Zeitung*, a case of bee-sting, followed by acute symptoms of poisoning, which was relieved within a very short time by a subcutaneous injection of carbolic acid. The patient—a robust, strongly built young woman—was stung in the lower lip by a bee. Soon afterwards she vomited; her face became flushed; the right half of the face began to swell, and the swelling soon spread over the whole face. The woman fainted, and was laid on her bed. When Dr. Klamann saw her soon afterwards, he found her unconscious; the face was dark-red, and much swollen: the sclerotics were injected, the lips cyanotic, the lids œdematous, the fingers and toes pale and cold. The patient did not answer when spoken to; the pulse was 72, hardly perceptible; respirations 24. Nothing abnormal could be detected in the heart, but the impulse was weak. The extremities were immovable. Cold compresses were immediately applied to her head, and five *milligrammes* of carbolic acid in solution were injected under the skin, near the spot where she had been stung. At the same time sal volatile was held to her nose. In about a quarter of an hour the swelling at the lips and eyelids began to abate visibly; consciousness returned gradually; and the mouth could be opened. The tongue was somewhat swollen, but the patient could swallow without much difficulty. In the course of three-quarters of an hour the patient had three attacks of convulsive trembling of the whole body, together with violent twitchings of the muscles of the face. During each of these attacks the patient was very restless; her face became flushed, and she threw her head about. After each attack her face became suddenly pale, the skin of her whole body grew cool, and the pulse could hardly be felt. Gradually, however, the symptoms of poisoning disappeared, and the patient could open her mouth and swallow a few drops of spirit of sal volatile in water. She passed a good night, and the next day went about her work as usual. The lower lip remained slightly swollen during the next few days. A fortnight before the accident she had been stung by a bee in the left forearm; after which the whole limb became swollen, and urticaria broke out over the whole body. The arm was still swollen when she was stung in the lip; and the injection of carbolic acid appeared to exercise a favourable influence on the arm, which, on the next day, had recovered its natural size.—*British Medical Journal*, August 16, 1879.

Surgery.

Sympathetic Ophthalmia.

In a lectuie deliveied at his ophthalmic clinic, D1. DE WEC(ER, (*Gaz. des Hôp.*, June 5) made the following obseivations :—

Sympathetic ophthalmia is a foim of iiido-choioiditis chaiacteiized by a peculiai plastic tendency. Fiom the commencement the exudations tend iapidly to attach the iiis to the ciystalline. In an oidinaiy iiido-choioiditis such adhesion takes place only at the edge, the iest of the iiis being fiee; but in this foim the iiis is applied to the whole suiface of the lens by veiy adheient exudations. Again, the exudative masses which foim with the choioid have a special tendency to ietiact. The anteiioi chambei then, in place of piesenting the shape of a funnel, assumes, in consequence of these ietiactions, an inveise foim, so that the anteio-posteiioi becomes its smallest diametei. As a consequence of its numeious and intimate adhesions with the ciystalline, the iiis becomes gieatly distended and vasculaṛ. This iiido-choioiditis most fiequently aiises in consequence of injuiy done to the othei eye, the accidents which most expose to it being those which affect the anteiioi poition of the ciliaiy body, the impaction of the iiis, and the impaction of a fiagment of the ciystalloid. In its piogiess sympathetic iiido-choioiditis leads to the sepaiation of the pericornean zone, the choioid becoming sometimes entiiely detached fiom the scleiotic owing to the gieat ietraction of the adhesions. This is iapidly followed by the softening of the eye, an essential phthisis. In young subjects the inflammation may pass away, and the masses of exudation become absoibed, so that the anteiioi poition of the eye is sufficiently cleai to allow of the fundus being seen. Veiy little vision, howevei, ietuins, and the affection is fiequently piopagated to the ietina and optic neive.

Sympathetic ophthalmia, for the most pait, appeais in the peiiod between the seventh and the foitieth day. Duiing the fiist week aftei the injuiy of one of the eyes it is not to be feaied, and aftei the sixth week the gieatest dangei is ovei. Neveitheless, D1. De Weckei has published a case in which the iiiitation did not supeivene until twenty-six yeais aftei the piimaiy lesion. The diffeience of time at which it appeais may depend upon numeious causes—on lesions of the inteiioi of the eye, oi on effusions of blood which may supeivene; or a bony oi calcaieous mass, having penetiated the eye without pioducing any giave occuiienees, and iemaining theie immobolized foi a long time, may fiom some cause undeigo displacement, giving iise to new tiaumatism that does not piove so indolent as the fiist, and induces a sympathetic iiritation of the othei eye. Sympathetic ophthalmia sometimes assumes a seiious foim; but this is iaie, and is fai less dangeious than the tiue plastic iiido-choioiditis. The lattei is so dangeious that it is of gieat impoitance to iecognize it fiom its outset. Not infiequently it appeais suddenly; but when theie aie premonitoiy symptoms they also implicate the ciliaiy neives of the othei eye. Vision becomes easily fatigued; theie is pain; the amplitude of accommodation is diminished; and the eyes become iapidly injected, especially aftei sleep. These symptoms should put the practitioner on his guaid, foi sympathetic ophthalmia may iapidly appeai.

Some twenty yeais ago the London school especially numbeied aident paitisans of enucleation, eveiy lost eye being condemned to be iemoved. This piactice, howevei, is not sufficiently justified, especially in young subjects. It is a consideiable opeiation, and we should iemembei that a patient who can pieseive an eye that is still neaily iegulai in foim is in a diffeient position to one fiom whom the globe has been iemoved. In old peisons, about the age of sixty, the question is more simple, as sympathetic accidents are less to be feared. Enucleation should be practised when there are premonitory symptoms of irritation, fatigue of the eyes, peri-keratitic injection, and slight precipitates in the aqueous or vitreous humours. We should not hesitate to operate, even when the other eye has as yet exhibited no symptom, when we suspect that a foreign body may be encysted in the eye, and when this eye is still sensitive, and when retracted cicatrices cause redness of the eye from time to time. When the eyes remain painful, and if palpation of an injured eye induces attacks of pain in it, enucleation is also justified. "Here are indications enough to show that I do not refuse to practise this operation: but with regard to an indolent eye I have my reserves, and I reject it, because I fear exposing the patient uselessly to a sympathetic ophthalmia."

A surgeon finds himself in a very embarrassing position in a case in which vision is already lost in the eye that is the subject of the sympathetic ophthalmia, while a passable vision yet remains in the injured eye. What is he to do? The question of enucleation cannot be raised here. It has been proposed to divide the channels of transmission, the ciliary nerves, by penetrating the sclerotic at the level of the seat of injury. Dr. De Wecker considers it preferable not to divide the ciliary nerves in the interior of the globe, because such incisions are always dangerous when the object is to preserve the eye, but to perform their section at the exterior of the globe, around the optic nerve. Contrary to Graefe, he recommends that all operations on the eye attacked with sympathetic ophthalmia should be entirely abstained from. It is in no case possible to detach the iris from the crystalline and the ciliary processes; and the operation for artificial pupil has always furnished unfortunate results. It is to medical treatment we should have recourse at the commencement of a sympathetic ophthalmia, and this should be the same as in plastic and parenchymatous iritis, having as its basis the most energetic mercurialization. After a certain time occlusion of the pupil results from the various anatomical changes that have taken place; but here also no operation should be performed on the iris. Sometimes, however, we may feel compelled to resort to an operation at the earnest instances of patients who still retain a good perception of light over a sufficient field of vision. But even in these cases we should not allow ourselves to be persuaded unless the patient has been free from all accidents for several years. The operation should be performed as in Graefe's operation for cataract.

Irido-choroiditis may occur *spontaneously*, and it is often observed in young girls at the period of puberty and in women who have reached the menopause. The lesion is connected with the irregularity in the functions of the uterus which occur at these two epochs; and in cases of dysmenorrhœa it should especially be attended to. When menstruation has become regular the affection of the eye is rapidly cured; and, moreover, surgical intervention is not attended with the same danger as in traumatic irido-choroiditis. The sole precaution to observe is the employment of instillations of eserine before and after the operation, in order to prevent the impaction of the iris, which might induce sympathetic ophthalmia.— *Med. Times and Gazette*, Aug. 9, 1879.

Extraction of Metallic Chips from the Eye by the Magnet.

Dr. M'KEOWN records (*Lancet*, Aug. 1878, p. 253), two cases where the eye was saved from destruction by the early use of the magnet to extract deeply seated pieces of iron chips. Dawson B., aged 24, wounded his right eye, three days previously to being seen, with a small piece of metal. The iris was attached to the lens by recent lymph, and a small clean metallic body was sticking at the margin of the adherent pupil. The body was seized by a fine pair of forceps introduced through the cornea, but slipped out of the grasp. A small pointed magnet was then introduced through the wound, which instantly attracted the metal and easily withdrew it. Recovery was rapid.

In the second case, a millwright, aged 32, wounded his eye with a chip of steel, three-quarters of an hour before being seen. A wound about a line in length, was seen in the ciliary region, but no foreign body was visible. A pointed magnet, cautiously introduced, detected the presence of metal which was soon exposed sufficiently to be seized by the forceps and withdrawn. In a fortnight the eye was quite well.

Dr. M'Keown refers to a paper read before the Clinical Society last March by Mr. Hardy. In the case reported a chip of steel was withdrawn by a magnet after having been lodged for seventy-two hours upon the anterior surface of the lens.—*Lond. Med. Record*, Aug. 15, 1879.

Tobacco and Alcoholic Amblyopia.

Dr. HIRSCHBERG, of Berlin, opened the discussion on this subject at the recent meeting of the British Medical Association (*British Med. Journal*, Aug. 30, 1879). He said that much attention has been devoted to it since amaurosis from smoking was described by Mackenzie; and there has been, both in England and abroad, much difference of opinion regarding the share to be assigned to tobacco in the causation of certain well-known and common cases of failure of sight. Whilst von Gräfe and many of his followers in Germany were drawing out the symptomatic differences between progressive atrophy and benign amblyopia, other observers, especially Hutchinson and others in England, worked at the natural history of the latter class of affections, and established the fact that abstinence from tobacco was followed by cure in most cases. Förster, uniting these two points of view, has given much greater definition to the subject, and shown that tobacco causes a symmetrical defect in the central part of each visual field, which accounts for all the symptoms, and which disappears partially or entirely when smoking is abandoned. The speaker had confirmed and amplified Förster's observations. He maintained strongly that tobacco is the cause of the majority of cases of amblyopia which present the following features: failure of both eyes alike, with nearly central scotoma and corresponding defect of colour-perception, without any contraction of the visual field, never passing on to complete blindness, accompanied often by other symptoms of chronic nicotism, and improving or disappearing when tobacco is relinquished. In a minority of cases, alcohol alone appears to be the cause; but the defect of the field in these is thought to be more truly central than in the tobacco-cases. In a very few cases, symptoms exactly like those from tobacco and alcohol occur without the operation of either of these causes.

A case of Tobacco-Amblyopia reported by Professor COHN, of Breslau, was read, in which the importance of considering the quantity of nicotine contained in the cigars consumed, as well as the number of cigars, was prominently brought forward.

Mr. SWANZY (Dublin) thought the amount of nicotine and other deleterious substances contained in various tobaccos had been greatly lost sight of in explaining the difference of opinion which existed in different countries as to the frequency of tobacco-amblyopia. In Germany, although smoking was almost universal, and indulged in excessively, this affection was rare, because the tobacco was light. In Turkey, the same fact might explain an observation of Mr. Brudeuell Carter. In Ireland, amongst the lower orders, tobacco-amblyopia was very common, the tobacco smoked being Limerick twist, an intensely black and moist tobacco, which probably contained large quantities of poisonous matters.

Mr. NETTLESHIP, of London, was of opinion that tobacco-amblyopia certainly did exist, but he did not think that alcohol gave rise to an amblyopia similar to that of tobacco. Tobacco never caused complete blindness. The amblyopia came on in both eyes simultaneously, but the ophthalmoscope never revealed anything approaching neuritis in this affection. Chewing tobacco was even more liable to cause amblyopia than smoking. In confirmation of Förster's observations, the speaker had found a central defect in the field for green and red. He considered mere abstinence the only essential point in the treatment.

Colour Blindness.

At the same meeting, Mr. H. R. SWANZY, of Dublin, opened a discussion on colour-blindness. He said that a good test for the colour-sense should fulfil the following desiderata. 1. It should be capable of rapidly detecting the existence and nature of the anomaly. 2. It should make the least possible demand upon the intelligence of the patient. 3. It should render deception, whether intentional or unintentional, impossible. Hence every method which depends upon the correct name being given to a colour is bad. 4. The possibility of any interference of the judgment must be excluded in order that the sensation to be tested may alone come into play. The spectroscope employed alone does not answer any of the above requirements, and can only be employed in conjunction with other methods. The method by means of coloured shadows, an application of an old experiment, as suggested by Dr. Stilling, is very beautiful, and goes far as an argument in favour of Harvey's theory of perception of colour. Dr. Stilling's pseudo-isochromatic tables have not met with universal favour. They consist of figures and letters in red and brown upon a brown background. Red and brown appear to the red-green blind as similar colours, consequently in such cases the figures and letters should not be distinguishable. Dana, of Kagerö, has published a table with coloured wools arranged in rows, which are to be recognized by the persons examined as being composed of similar or of different colours. The method of Professor Holmgren, of Upsala, has received the greatest meed of popularity. It is conducted by means of coloured wools, which are to be sorted according to a system, the two chief tests being by a skein of pale green wool and one of purple wool. By this means, the colour-sense of an individual may be tested in the space of a minute or a minute and a half, while no word need be uttered on either side, and a large roomful of other people about to be tested may look on without vitiating the tests. There is also a method much in use in these countries upon railways, etc. ; it consists in a card with four coloured squares, red, green, yellow, and blue, to which the correct names are to be given. This is a bad method, for colour-blind persons are often able to name colours correctly by virtue of a certain brightness which one colour possesses as compared with another. Again, some uneducated people are not familiar with the names of colours, and in this way many seem, with such a test, to be colour-blind when not so. Holmgren, Cohn, Magnus, and Joy Jeffries have been the principal observers of late as to the frequency of colour-blindness. Donders, Fontenoy, and others have also examined large numbers. The percentages given by these observers was, amongst men, from 2.87 to 6.6. Amongst women, colour-blindness is extremely rare. The highest percentage for them is given by Dr. Minder at 1.3. Cohn, in 1061 females, did not find one colour blind ; Magnus only one in 2216 ; and Joy Jeffries four in 7942. Mr. Swanzy had examined 1320 persons by Holmgren's method ; of these, ninety were women, and none of them were colour-blind. Of the 1230 males, eighty-two were more or less colour-blind, or a percentage of 6.6. He hoped to add to these numbers, and to make his investigations more complete, especially as regards blue-yellow blindness. It is to be regretted that the above-mentioned observers have not sought more carefully for the latter interesting, although apparently rare, form of colour-blindness. The practical importance of colour-blindness is as great as its physiological interest. It would be most desirable that the various railway companies and the Board of Trade should be induced to adopt Holmgren's test.

Dr. WOLFE (Glasgow) had examined two thousand persons, and found about the same proportion of colour-blindness as Mr. Swanzy. He did not explain his method. He thought that an efficient examination of all sailors and railway servants should be compulsory.

Dr. HIRSCHBERG (Berlin) agreed with Mr. Swanzy that Holmgren's wool-test was the best for clinical purposes. The spectrum was the best means for scientific investigation of the defective perception on which colour-blindness depended. Red- and green-blindness were not the same.

Mr. NETTLESHIP (London) had used several of the tests mentioned by Mr. Swanzy, and was strongly in favour of Holmgren's test as most reliable, and easily used for clinical work.

Mr. SWANZY agreed with Dr. Wolfe, that provision was much needed for the compulsory examination of seamen and railway officials.—*British Med. Journal*, Aug. 30, 1879.

———

On the Etiology of Aural Exostoses, and on their Removal by a New Operation.

Dr. J. P. CASSELLS, of Glasgow, at the recent meeting of the British Medical Association, expressed his belief that difficulties had been caused by regarding all bony tumours in the auditory canal as exostoses. There were two kinds of bony tumours in this situation, exostosis and hyperostosis, the former consisting of new growth, the latter of hyperplasia of the osseous tissue of the meatus. Dr. Cassells believed that the origin and development of an aural exostosis were as follows: A subperiosteal abscess formed over the mastoid, made its way out in the line of least resistance, and discharged; from and around the opening vascular granular growths sprouted up, and increased in size, becoming at the same time changed into bony tissue from the conversion of their cells into bone-cells. The new method of treatment advised for these cases of exostosis consisted in first passing a loop of wire over the tumour, and twisting it upon itself so as to grasp the pedicle firmly. Chloroform being administered, a sharp gouge with a curve carefully adjusted to that of the auditory canal was carried down to the base of the tumour, and, being firmly held there, two or three smart blows with a mallet effected the separation of the bony mass, which was drawn from the meatus by the wire attached. The patient on whom Dr. Cassells operated thus recovered without a bad symptom; and he believed that every aural exostosis might be easily removed in this way.—*British Med. Journal*, Aug. 30, 1879.

———

The Treatment of Non-Suppurative Hypertrophic Catarrh of the Middle Ear.

In a paper on this subject, read at the recent meeting of the British Medical Association (*British Med. Journal*, Aug. 30, 1879) Mr. LENNOX BROWNE said that he preferred to treat the subject in its broad aspect, because he feared that the discussion of the subject of intratympanic injections might give to many the idea that such was the treatment *par excellence* for chronic middle ear disease. He quoted from authorities to show how many aurists had abandoned this measure, and how many more had found it necessary to either greatly limit the cases in which they pursued it, or to reduce to a minimum the strength of the fluids used. He then proceeded to show objections to the procedure alike on physical, anatomical, physiological, and practical grounds. Quoting at length from Wreden, of St. Petersburg, who had made most complete experiments on models, as well as on the dead body and on the living subject, it was urged that, to send fluids in the forms of drops or as sprays, it was necessary to pass the instrument through which they were introduced quite within the tympanum, a proceeding of great danger, being liable to injure the ossicles and certain to set up suppurative inflammation of the drum ; or at least to pass the instrument far beyond the isthmus. But fluids could be driven *en masse* by great force, this also being a measure only more dangerous than the other. The anatomical relations of the tympanum were pointed out, and it was shown how much danger there was of cerebral inflammation, of jugular phlebitis, of mastoid or labyrinthine suppuration, or of facial paralysis, if an acute catarrh were induced. Stating how invariably severe were the symptoms when fluid really entered the tympanum, Mr. Lennox Browne expressed his belief that, when authors reported that they had never had a bad result, such an experience showed that the injected fluid had never passed beyond the isthmus of the Eustachian tube. Again, there was the physiological objection. The tympanum was an air-cavity, whose office was impaired by the presence of a very little mucous fluid, when such was effused as a result of disease. It was often very difficult to disperse this fluid, and there was a great tendency for the lining of the cavity to become thickened, and, as a natural consequence, for its absorptive properties to become diminished. Why should one expect medicated fluids (necessarily, for safety, of very feeble quality) to have a good effect, and why not a bad one, considering the injury done by simple water when it entered the tympanum, as in bathing or on use of Weber's douche ? And supposing these fluids were not absorbed, nothing but harm could result, as many authors, Kramer and Bonnafont among the number, had agreed. When one considered the intimate relation of the mucous membrane of the throat and middle ear, and how frequently topical applications of strong mineral solutions failed to cure hypertrophic inflammatory conditions in the former region, what right had we to suppose that these feeble fluids would do good to similar affections of the middle ear ? On all grounds, therefore, Mr. Browne objected to this treatment. He stated that after their use he had never, on subsidence of the increase of bad symptoms—in his belief the only proof of entry of fluid into the tympanic cavity—found the slightest gain of hearing power. On the other hand, he had often seen most alarming inflammation induced. If, therefore, they were to be employed at all, he would limit their use to suppurative cases in which there was already a pervious tympanic membrane, or he would, at the time of making them, perforate the membrane, a procedure now established as free from danger. The speaker concluded by pointing out that, by means of inhalations, Valsalvan, Politzer, and catheteric inflations, with either pure air or medicated vapours, by use of the post-nasal douche, by faradization, by use of the exhausting speculum (an improvement of Siegel's instrument being exhibited) and lastly, by careful attention to the constitutional diathesis of each individual case, it was possible to greatly alleviate— he doubted if they were ever cured—the conditions under consideration.

Intratympanic Injections.

Dr. WEBER-LIEL'S experience of sixteen years of aural practice, has forced him to give up the idea that it might be possible to cure inveterate catarrh of the tympanic cavity by means of intratympanic injections of medicated fluids. 1. The symptoms of catarrh of the tympanum may depend upon extension of a simple catarrh from the Eustachian tube and the pharyngo-nasal cavity ; then the latter only must be the object of treatment. In this treatment, injections of

stiong nitiate of silvei solutions into the mouth of the Eustachian tube, followed
foui days afteiwaids by the use of the aii-douche, will be found of the best effect
in ieducing the catainhal symptoms. But in oidei to avoid inflammation of the
tympanum, not moie than a few diops of the solution must be blown in with
foice by means of the Eustachian cathetei; and the patient must be foibidden to
blow his nose till foui houis after the injection. 2. Or, secondly, the symptoms
of the intiatympanic catainh are due not only to a catainh of the tube, but to a
collapse of the walls of the Eustachian canal, dependent on insufficient or paialyzed action of the Eustachian tube muscles. In such cases, not intiatympanic
injections, but the awakening of the activity in the tubal muscles by intiatubal
electiicity, must be the tieatment, to cause the disappeaiance of the symptoms of
the secondaiy intiatympanic vasculai stasis and catainh. 3. Symptoms of congestions and catainh of the tympanic cavity may aiise fiom alteiations of the
vaso-motoi and tiophic neives and of the sympathetic supplying the tympanic
cavity. Di. Webei-Liel has found solutions of nitiate of silvei, coinosive sublimate, and common salt, to pioduce inflammation and peifoiation of the membiana
tympani. Caibonate of soda, howevei, has not this effect. Mucus, incrusted
and transuded puiulent mattei, may be diminished by it. Tissue (false bands,
foi instance) and intiatympanic adhesions may be softened by it; so that it may
become moie easy to loosen intiatympanic adhesions by means of the aii-douche,
and to cause absoiption of haidened masses. For this kind of catainhal affection
he has found intiatympanic injections to have a ieally good iesult. The injections, combined with aii-piessuie, weie effected by means of his phaimaco-
koniontron.—*Biitish Med. Jouinal,* Aug. 30, 1879.

Removal of the whole of Right Paiietal, and half the Fiontal Bones, the iesult
of Buins; Skin Grafted on Suiface of Duia Matei; Recovery.

At the iecent meeting of the Biitish Medical Association (*Biitish Med. Jouinal,*
Aug. 30, 1879) Di. J. R. Hayes ielated the following iemarkable case:—

On May 24, 1874, Di. Hayes was called to see Mrs. S., aged 32, who was
found insensible, lying with hei head and face on the heaith, wheie a turf fiie
had been buint out. The uppei pait of the cheek and eyelids of the iight side
weie vesicated; the foiehead and side of the head also suffered; a small poition
of the skin ovei the paiietal bone appeaied chained. She was quite unconscious,
and continued so until the following moining. For thiee or foui days, she was
gieatly depiessed, but fiee fiom pain. Reaction having set in, she suffered veiy
much fiom pain and sleeplessness, which was ielieved by full doses of opium.
She appeaied to impiove until about the sixteenth day, when suddenly she became
slightly deliiious, and suffeied fiom nausea and occasional vomiting, with paialysis
of the left side. The face was not engaged. Those symptoms passed off in ten
days, and hei health giadually impioved. The injuied pait of the face and uppei
poition of the ear, which had sloughed away, cicatiized, and she was able to go
about doing hei household woik. About Octobei 1st, the bones had sepaiated
at the sutuies in a line extending fiom the mastoid poition of the tempoial to the
posteiioi angle of the paiietal, along the lambdoid and sagittal sutuies to the su-
perciliary iidge, and outwaids to the outei angle of the fiontal bone. On Octobei 3, Di. Hayes iemoved the bones included (the whole paiietal and half the
fiontal). The undei surface of the bone was coveied with a thick cuidy mattei;
the depiessions foi the aiteiies, etc., weie obliteiated. No pulsation could be
felt ovei the meningeal aiteiies, and a quantity of fetid pus welled up fiom between the hemispheies. The duia matei, which was coveied with gianulations,
continued to seciete pus fieely. Finding the ulceiated suiface was not cicatiizing,

about December 2d, Dr. Hayes grafted skin on four places on the dura mater; three of them took, and cicatrization commenced from these points, and covered the whole of the exposed surface, the skin-grafts acting successfully. During the whole time, and up to the present, she has not suffered from any brain-symptoms, except that, when the skin-grafts were put on, he placed a pad of lint over them, and bound it with a strip of adhesive plaster. The following day, her left side, including the face, was paralyzed; this continued for four days, when the pad was removed, and the symptoms immediately passed away. She has been since, and is at present doing her ordinary work, and carries a heavy basket on her arm for a great part of the day. Her general health is excellent.

—

On the Treatment of Fistulæ and Scars of the Cheek.

In a short communication to the *Lancet* (July 19, 1879) on this subject, Mr. EDWARD BELLAMY says it is, in the first place, all-important to find out exactly the course taken by the fistula or fistulæ—a matter of considerable difficulty sometimes; and the following classification may have its value in diagnosis: 1. Those opening into the cheek, with a track above the level of the buccal or labial mucous membrane, and which usually discharge saliva only. 2. Those whose track lies below this level, and which discharge pus and muco-purulent fluid and no saliva. 3. A complication of both forms, and which discharge both pus and saliva. With regard to the accurate detection of their course, an ordinary probe frequently gives merely a general idea of the direction without passing into the offsets. Mr. B. has always found that a fine filiform bougie, or, better still, a fine India-rubber French bougie, is more useful than anything else. After having determined the course, irritating cause, and condition of the fistula, in order to avoid further scar, the dead bone, if there be any, is to be removed by delicate but strong forceps or gouge, and afterwards the track should be washed out with a very strong solution of sulphuric acid, which has the effect of completely destroying the fistulous track ; or by the introduction of minute crystals of nitrate of silver, until the granulations appear at the orifice, gentle pressure being maintained. A cicatrix, however carefully the treatment be carried out, is sure to remain, unsightly always and often troublesome, appearing as a "pucker," or adhesion to the underlying bone ; and with regard to its treatment, Mr. Bellamy states, from his own experience, that two methods are open to the surgeon, dependent on the extent or strength of these adhesions. The first consists in introducing a fine blunt-pointed tenotome through the tissue of the cicatrix—laminating it, as it were—taking great care to leave it in free communication with the integument adjacent to it; next, to introduce between the split surfaces a thin strip of sheet-lead, which should be kept in, to prevent the adhesion of the surfaces divided by the tenotome. After a few days, the superficial lamina of the cicatrix may be subjected to gentle movement over the lower lamina, which the patient may conduct himself; this prevents adhesion, and renders the tissue pliant and assimilative. This may be termed the "passive movement" of the cicatrix. The second plan, if the former fails—or indeed it may be advisable at first—consists in dissecting away the adherent tissue entirely, vivifying the edges of the cicatrix and bringing them together by means of fine entomological pins, and so gaining a mere linear scar at worst, care being taken, by movement, to prevent permanent adhesion. The great elasticity of the cheek structure permits of this without any deformity resulting as regards expression. Manipulative skill is necessary for success, but results appear so satisfactory that Mr. Bellamy thinks that, in cases where it is important, for the sake of the patient's looks, operative proceedings should be undertaken, the above suggestions may be of use.

A Case of Long-continued Priapism accompanying Leukæmia.

Dr. SALZER, of Worms, reports (*Med.-Chir. Rundschau,* June, 1879) the case of a man, 46 years of age, who suffered for seven weeks from persistent priapism. He had previously suffered from intermittent fever, but was at this time in apparent good health. One morning he was awakened by an intensely painful erection of the penis, that proved utterly rebellious to treatment. Leeches, warm fomentations, chloral hydrate, and even chloroform narcosis were tried in turn, but all without success. The urine was passed with difficulty, usually in short jets, and most readily in the knee-elbow position. Physical examination revealed only *marked enlargement of the spleen.* Finally, after the penis had been kept for three weeks constantly enveloped in strongly camphorated narcotic poultices, opium and camphor being administered internally at the same time, the priapism gradually disappeared, having persisted fully seven weeks. During the week preceding this attack, the patient had had two attacks of priapism, one of which lasted only a few hours, and the other twenty-four hours. After the appearance of the priapism the patient rapidly lost strength and acquired a cachectic appearance, and the spleen progressively increased in size. Two months after the priapism disappeared there was complete loss of sexual power, and the patient died about eight months afterward. The blood was not examined microscopically, and an autopsy was not permitted.

Dr. Salzer collates from medical literature eight cases of priapism occurring in connection with leukæmia. Various theories have been brought forward to account for the priapism in these cases. Kremme ascribed it to extravasation of blood into the corpora cavernosa, and Longuet to impeded circulation in the smaller vessels and the formation of thrombi, resulting from the altered condition of the blood, while Neidhardt thought that irritation of the nerves might possibly be the exciting cause. Dr. Salzer thinks that the rapid disappearance of the priapism in the two first attacks in the above case argues against the occurrence of an extravasation of blood. He believes that both the temporary and the persistent attacks of priapism were due to irritation of the nervi errigentes. It is well known that priapism may be produced both by peripheral and by central irritation of these nerves. As examples of the former, he adduces the erections accompanying inflammation of the urethra or of the neck of the bladder, swelling of the prostate, etc.; and, as examples of the latter, the erections of insane persons, or that follow injuries of the spinal cord. The priapism of leukæmia, he claims, differs from these varieties chiefly in its longer duration, and hence for its development some special cause must be sought. This may possibly be found either in the presence of anatomical changes in the nervi errigentes, or in pressure on them by swollen lumbar glands.—*Med. Record,* Sept. 6, 1879.

———

Triple Amputation.

An *employé* on the Brest Railway fell from a carriage while in motion, dislocating his elbow, and two other carriages passed over his legs. He was taken to the hospital in a state of syncope, when it was found that the right leg was only held to the thigh by a few slips of muscle and the skin, the femur having been cleanly severed just above the knee and the femoral divided—hemorrhage being arrested by the instant formation of a clot. The left foot and ankle-joint were broken up into a confused mass. Dr. Léscléue, surgeon to the Brest Hospital, amputated at once the right thigh, having only to shape into regularity the musculo-cutaneous strips; but he did not remove the left leg until about fifteen hours afterwards, reaction having by this time taken place. Gangrene having invaded the forearm of the left side, on which the dislocation of the elbow had taken place, amputation was performed on the seventeenth day. The patient did very well, having been cured long since, and is now able, by means of apparatus, to walk. M. Rochard brought the case before the Academy of Medicine as a unique example of a patient having survived a triple amputation performed for the same injury. Baron Larrey, however, observed that the case was not unique, for he had seen a man at the Invalides who had undergone amputation of the four limbs; and he had also seen a young Arab in Algeria, who had recovered after having had the four extremities divided by a train.—*Med. Times and Gaz.*, Aug. 23, 1879, from *Gaz. Hebd.*, Aug. 8.

—

Case of Fracture of the Vertebral Arch of the Fourth Lumbar Vertebra.

GEMMEL reports (*Allg. Med. Cent. Zeit.*, No. 52, 1879) the case of a workman who had fallen from a height of fifty-three feet through the giving way of a scaffolding. When first seen, he was in a state of imminent collapse, so that it was thought advisable to put off the examination till the next day. In the mean time, wine and camphor were given. At the examination, the patient complained of pain in the region of the fourth lumbar vertebra, the tuber ischii, and the right tibia, about six centimetres below the knee. He was not able to move his legs. He had not micturated since his accident, neither had his bowels been moved. The skin over the painful spots showed numerous wounds, which were partly superficial, partly profound, especially on the right tibia, and seemed to have been caused by falling bricks. The processus spinalis of the spinal column was painful to pressure, especially in the region of the fourth lumbar vertebra. The spinal process of this vertebra was dislocated; pressure on the muscles of the back to the right of the processus was very painful; crepitation could not be distinctly heard. The patient could only lie on the left side; the bladder was full, and the urine had to be drawn off by means of a catheter. The patient said afterwards that he had not felt the catheter when it was introduced into the urethra. Cutaneous sensibility of the right leg was absent, the sensibility of the left leg was much weakened. Both legs were powerless, though the muscles of the left extremity could be made to contract by a strong faradic current. The internal organs were normal. *Treatment.*—Extension of the spine. Application of ice to the affected part. Clysmata. Stimulating medicines. The next day the patient was able to move the toes of the left leg; sensibility was also partly restored. The bladder and rectum were still paralyzed, so that the patient passed his motions in bed. He objected to the extension of the spine, as it caused too much pain. He was treated with the faradic current, one pole being applied above the injured spot, and the other moved along the muscles of the legs. Three weeks later he could move the left leg freely; he was conscious of being touched with a pin, but could not say whether the point or the head had been applied to him. The right leg and foot were anæsthetic, with the exception of the inner side of the thigh and fore leg, the anterior surface of the thigh and the tibia, the big, second, and third toes. The patient could move his legs, but not without great exertions. The bladder and rectum were still paralyzed; the urine had a strong ammoniacal odour, and left a muddy sediment. The pain in the spine was so great that the patient could only sit up by resting his body on both arms. The treatment consisted in the application of the electric current, both as before and to the bladder. Thirty-one days later the bladder and rectum were still paralyzed. The cystitis had disappeared. The bowels never moved without an enema in spite of the faradization of the rectum. The patient passed his urine and feces in bed. He could sit up without pain. The right leg could be freely moved, with the exception of the foot. Twenty-seven days later the patient could walk with the aid of a stick. His state was much the same as before. The skin was anæsthetic in the right gluteal region near the anus, on the planta pedis, the region of the musculus peroneus, and the external portion of the thigh. He complained of a sensation of numbness in both legs and feet, saying, "I feel as if my legs were covered with thick woollen stockings." The temperature was raised on the injured leg. When told to walk, he complained of a feeling of weakness in the knees, which bent under him. His gait presented the characteristic symptoms of tabes dorsalis. He kept looking straight before him, threw his legs about and raised them without removing them from the floor. He walked with his legs wide apart. When attempting to stand, his knees bent under him. If told to put his feet together, set his stick aside, and close his eyes, he began to vacillate, and ended by falling forwards. He was unable to turn round briskly. The patient was dismissed after a stay of seven months in the hospital. His condition had remained much the same, with the exception that the temperature of the injured leg was lower than that of the other extremity. The following are the noteworthy points in this case: 1 The rarity of fracture of a vertebra; 2. The permanent paralysis of the bladder and rectum; 3. The sensory disturbance of the rectum, anal region, right gluteal region, bladder, and urethra; 4. The circumstance that the affection assumed the characteristic appearance of tabes dorsalis; 5. The feeling of numbness in the right planta pedis, which region was also anæsthetic. The patient had always enjoyed good health before his accident, and the family history was good.—*London Med. Record*, Aug. 15, 1879.

—

On the Cause of Eversion of the Limb after Fracture of the Neck of the Femur.

At the late meeting of the British Medical Association Mr. EDWARD OWEN read a paper in which he showed that the mechanical explanation of the eversion of the limb after fracture of the neck of the femur was quite sufficient, without bringing in the question of muscular action. Sir Astley Cooper attributed the eversion to the superior strength of the muscles of external rotation; and his views, which have afforded an excellent working hypothesis, have been generally adopted by subsequent writers. Mr. Owen asserted that the thick mass of muscles of internal rotation, which filled up the deep fossa between the front of the iliac crest and the great trochanter, are more powerful than the muscles of external rotation, though the latter are much more numerous. This important fact he had ascertained by testing the relative power of the two groups of muscles by means of a specially arranged spring-balance and indicator. The muscles of internal rotation are the tensor fasciæ femoris, the anterior-two-thirds of the glutæus medius, and the front part of the glutæus minimus. The pyriformis and company would probably be rendered useless as external rotators when, after fracture of the neck of the femur, the great trochanter had fallen towards the great sacro-sciatic notch. Some time since, an old woman came under treatment, who, three months previously, had broken the neck of her thigh-bone. There had been no attempt at union, and the limb lay persistently on the whole length of its outer side : but, on being instructed, the patient could roll it inwards until the foot was at right angles to the surface of the bed. She could not have done this if the characteristic eversion had been due to the superior strength of the external rotators. The posterior surface of the thigh of a man lying supine on a flat surface hardly touches that surface, the weight being transmitted partly by the pelvis, partly by the calf. The centre of gravity of the limb is well to the outer side of a straight line connecting the middle of the acetabulum and the heel. In its search for stable equilibrium, the sound limb rolls outwards until further eversion is checked by the front of the capsular ligament being rendered tense. In this position we find the limb in sleep, after paralysis, and in death. In the mortuary, rigor mortis having passed off, division of the front of the capsule is followed by still further eversion; or, the neck of the femur being divided inside the capsule, the limb will roll over on to its outer side. Similarly, when the neck of the living femur is broken, the limb "tumbles" into the position of eversion; muscular action has nothing to do with it. The administration of chloroform is never followed by a righting of the limb. Those rare cases of fracture of the neck with inversion are to be explained by the fact of the limb having been left in a position of inversion by the violence which caused the fracture; if the fragments are unhitched, eversion at once declares itself and persists. When the femur is fractured below the level of the lesser trochanter, eversion is still a most characteristic feature of the lesion.—*British Medical Journal*, Aug. 30, 1879.

—

Osteotomy in Genu Valgum.

At the late meeting of the British Medical Association (*British Med. Journal*, Aug. 30, 1879) Dr. W. MACEWEN said that there were several points, in addition to those already published, concerning the operation which he had advanced for the rectification of genu valgum by the transverse incision through the femoral diaphyses, which he considered worthy of attention. The first related to the direction of the osseous incision, which ought to be made so as to avoid the external condyle, which may be effected by cutting parallel to the condyles, or by commencing the incision a short distance above a line drawn from the upper margin of the external condyle across the limb to the inner side, the incision commencing from the inner side of the limb. The exact seat of the incision in the soft parts ought to be noticed, with the intention of showing that an incision may be made which would cut no vessel requiring a ligature. This may be done if a point be selected where the two following lines meet each other: a line drawn transversely from the upper border of the patella when the limb is in the extended position; and a line drawn longitudinally, about half an inch anterior to the spine, for the insertion of the adductor magnus tendon. That position is below and anterior to the anastomotica magna, and above the superior internal articular artery; and by making an incision half an inch in length directly to the bone at this point, it is impossible to touch any normal distribution of these branches. The extent of the transverse osseous incision depends upon the nature of the case: in young persons, fully two-thirds of the bone is divided; in old persons with hard brittle bones, the whole bone up to the external dense layer is cut, and force is never applied in bending or breaking the limb to a greater extent than what may be easily done by taking the limbs in the surgeon's hands, and using the one as a fulcrum, the other as a lever. This femoral incision neither impairs nor arrests the growth of the bone, as the experience of the last three years has pointed out; those operated on being increased in height as an immediate result of the operation, and the limbs have grown proportionately since. One or two remarks regarding the pathology of genu valgum may be mentioned, as they have a practical bearing. In genu valgum, there is a lowering of the internal condyle in all cases. Secondly, this lowering may be due to a bend in the lower third of the femur, to a lowering of the internal part of the diaphyses, or to an actual increase in the length of the internal condyle. A slight increase in the length of the tibial diaphyses toward the inner side is also in some cases present; but, in the great majority, not to a sufficient extent to require operative interference. Generally, the

knock-knee is made up from several of the above pathological conditions. Regarding the tibial incision in knock-knee, in by far the greater majority of cases it is
not required in any way ; even the most aggravated cases have been rectified
without it ; but, in some aggravated cases, it may be justifiable, and may contribute slightly to the restoration of the symmetry of the limb. The division of the
tendon of the biceps often does more good than a tibial division. The division
of the femur from the external surface has many disadvantages, and not one single
merit. Regarding anterior tibial curves and their correction, where a single osteotomy can be performed, it is to be preferred ; but where a series of osteotomies
is required, a wedge of bone is more easily removed, and is more satisfactory.

—

Subcutaneous Osteotomy in Young Children.

In a discussion at the last meeting of the British Medical Association on
the subject of subcutaneous osteotomy, Mr. ROBERT WILLIAM PARKER said
that the East London Hospital for Children had afforded him considerable
scope for the performance of osteotomy, and out of a large number of osteotomies performed on children varying in age from three to thirteen, he had never
lost a case ; and in only one instance had there been any suppuration. This
one exception had been a severe case of erysipelatous œdema, which, however,
yielded to treatment, and the boy finally made a good recovery. It was now
generally admitted that the cause of genu valgum lay in a hypertrophic length-
cuing of the internal condyle of the femur ; and although this fact had long
been known, it had never occurred to surgeons to utilize the knowledge for the
correction of the deformity. Mr. Parker thought that a special acknowledgment
was due to Dr. Ogston for having thought out this treatment, and for his boldness
and success in putting it into practice. It was no doubt the first step in the right
direction in the treatment of this disease. Personally, however, he had not
adopted Ogston's operation, but the modification of it first performed by his colleague, Mr. Reeves, and described by the latter gentleman in the British Medical
Journal as "subcutaneous extra-articular osteotomy."[1] This operation was a less
serious one than Ogston's, and just as effective. He (Mr. Parker) believed that
in children the operation could be performed without entering the joint ; for the
layer of encrusting cartilage, together with its synovial lining, would stretch
rather than crack sharply off, as was probably the case in adults. Fortunately
for his patients, he had had no opportunity of putting this opinion to the test of
the post-mortem room. But clinical facts bore him out. Thus, out of about
twenty-five operations, in three or four there had been slight effusion into the
knee-joint. In one case, this effusion had been especially distinct, and was anticipated at the time of the operation ; for, in using the chisel, owing to the
extreme softness of the condyle, it had accidentally entered the joint, a fact of
which he was well conscious. He believed, therefore, that the extra-articular
operation was feasible in children, and that it was merely a matter of operative
dexterity. If, six or eight days after the operation, on removing the first dressing, the joint was found to be normal in size, and capable of being spontaneously
flexed to about two-thirds of its extent, he did not see what more could be wanted
in support of the belief that the joint had not been entered. Mr. Parker had
been gradually led to the present plan of removing the dressings about the fourth
day ; for he found that the wound was generally closed by this time. He was of
opinion that, in children and young adults, this (Reeves's) operation was the
best, because : (1) it is a subcutaneous one ; (2) it is (almost always) extra-arti-

---

[1] See Monthly Abstract for July, 1878, p. 323.

cular; (3) it counteracts exactly the pathological condition which causes the genu valgum; (4) because of the short time necessary for complete recovery.—*British Med. Journal,* Aug. 30, 1879.

Midwifery and Gynæcology.

The Prevention and Treatment of Post-Partum Hemorrhage.

In a discussion on this subject at the late meeting of the British Medical Association (*British Med. Journal,* Sept. 6, 1879) Dr. THOMAS MORE MADDEN, of Dublin, discussed *seriatim* the causes of *post-partum* hemorrhage, and the treatment required by each of these. Having dwelt on the constitutional conditions predisposing to flooding, and the preventive measures by which this might be warded off, even in those who had been habitually subject to this accident on former occasions, he considered the causes of flooding and the management of labour, so as to prevent subsequent inertia or irregular contraction of the uterus. The ill effect, in this respect, of the premature application of the forceps before the full dilatation of the os uteri, and also the production of hemorrhage as the result of undue delay in the second stage, were next referred to. During labour, when there was any reason to anticipate flooding, the preventive measures recommended by the author were: the rupture of the membranes in the first stage; the use of stimulating enemata of a strong infusion of ergot, or the hypodermic injection of ergotine, in the second stage; and a firm unremitting manual pressure over the fundus uteri, from the time the child's head escaped from the vulva until the completion of the third stage, which should never be hastened by traction on the cord, and the permanent contraction of the uterus was secured. In nineteen cases of flooding, the solution of perchloride of iron was resorted to; in eighteen of these, the hemorrhage was thus arrested, and in one instance it failed. Dr. Madden, however, considered that the ordinary mode of using this styptic—viz., by a syringe passed up to the fundus uteri—was a very hazardous proceeding, and exposed the patient to great and needless twofold danger of death from embolism or from peritonitis. He, therefore, recommended instead the direct application of the strong liquor ferri perchloridi to the bleeding vessels by a sponge soaked in this fluid, and carried up by the hand into the uterus, and retained there until a firm contraction was produced. Some cases were referred to in which hemorrhage, that had resisted all other treatment, was thus arrested; and Dr. Madden, therefore, regarded this as the most effectual method of treating flooding. At the same time, he admitted that it was not free from danger, or even to be adopted without grave necessity. Some of the other remedies employed in the treatment of *post-partum* hemorrhage, including the hypodermic use of ergotine, galvanism, and cold and hot injections, were referred to.

Dr. WILLIAM WALTER, of Manchester, said, that since the method of treating *post-partum* hemorrhage by the injection of hot water was brought under notice by Dr. Atthill early in 1878, he had treated in this way eleven cases in the Manchester and Salford Lying-in Hospital. The temperature of the water used ranged from 110° to 120° Fahr.; and the utmost care was taken that the tube (Hayes's) reached well up to the fundus; and that there was afterwards no impediment to the escape of the water from the uterus. The results in the eleven cases—particulars of which were given—led Dr. Walter to the conclusion that the hot-water treatment offered some advantages, in being generally accessible and not disagreeable to the patient; but that, as a means of contracting the uterus, it was, in his experience, not to be relied on. Nevertheless, he hoped to continue the method; and he advised that the temperature of the water should be ascertained by the thermometer in every case. The recent researches of Dr. Max Runge tended to show that, if success was to follow the hot-water treatment of *post-partum* hemorrhage, the temperature of the water must not be so high as it was in his (Dr. Walter's) cases. In all the cases but one, the injection was followed by relaxation and dilatation of the entire uterus; if contraction occurred, it was but temporary; but, when the temperature of the water did not exceed 104° F., the uterus contracted without being afterwards paralyzed. No appreciable effect was produced on the pulse and general condition of the system. After the failure of the injection, the application of the induced current was successful in several of the cases.

Dr. ATTHILL, of Dublin, confined his remarks to the use of the four principal agents used for the arrest of *post-partum* hemorrhage; namely, ergot, cold water, warm water, and the perchloride of iron. Ergot was most unreliable; it took time to act, and, though valuable if administered to anticipate hemorrhage, was nearly useless at the time, even if injected under the skin. Cold was perhaps the most efficient of all agents, if used in the proper cases and at the right time; that is, while the patient was warm, and reaction consequently followed. If its use were prolonged, or the patient were cold and exhausted, it was worse than useless. It was at this stage that hot water came in with advantage, not to supersede the use of cold. Dr. Walter recorded cases in which it failed, or did actual harm; but he used it too hot, namely, at 120°, instead of 100°; and the experiments referred to at the conclusion of his paper showed that hot water was efficient in causing contraction of the uterine muscular tissue. If used at the proper temperature, hot water was far from being an absolutely efficient agent, but it was valuable; it would not replace the use of perchloride of iron, but it must sometimes render it unnecessary. Perchloride of iron was in some cases absolutely demanded, and was the most certain means of checking *post-partum* hemorrhage. It had, in Dr. Atthill's hands, saved several lives; but, like all other remedies, it was not absolutely safe. He knew of one case in which it seemed to cause instantaneous death; but he had known death to follow in a few moments from the simple act of syringing the vagina; air entered the uterus and caused death. Might this not have also been the cause of death when the perchloride was used?

—

Pilocarpin in the Œdema of Pregnancy.

Dr. BIDDER related (*St. Petersburg Med. Woch.*, Aug. 16) at the St. Petersburg Society of Physicians the following case, which he treated in the way described, having from previous experience assured himself that pilocarpin does not induce pains during labour: A primipara, aged twenty-five, was admitted into the lying-in hospital in her eighth month of pregnancy, suffering from considerable œdema of the face, extremities, and external genitals—the small labia forming shining tumours as large as a fist. The urine contained a considerable quantity of albumen. Various remedies having been tried in vain, and one of the labia threatening to become gangrenous, a Pravaz syringeful of a solution (20 per cent.) of pilocarpin was injected twice on the 1st of the month, salivation following shortly after, and somewhat later profuse sweating. The œdema had already become much less by the next day, and on the third another injection was employed. By the 12th all œdema had disappeared, and the albumen of the urine had greatly diminished. No uterine pains were induced during this tieatment, and when hei full time aiiived the woman had an easy delivery of a laige child.—*Med. Times and Gazette*, Sept. 6, 1879.

Muriate of Pilocaipine in Eclampsia.

Di. BRAUN ielates, in the *Beilin. Klin. Wochenschiift* for June 16th, a case of pueipeial convulsions successfully tieated by subcutaneous injections of pilo-caipine. The patient was a iobust, healthy, young woman, who had been re-cently deliveied of hei fiist child. About an houi aftei the child's biith, violent convulsions set in and weie fiequently repeated. When seen by the authoi, five houis aftei delivery, she piesented all the symptoms of a seveie attack of eclamp-sia. The convulsions followed each othei iapidly, and duiing the inteivals the patient was insensible. The bladdei was empty ; no uiine had been passed since hei delivery. Laige doses of chloial-hydiate weie piesciibed, and a subcutane-ous injection of two *centigiammes* of moiphia made; but without effect. Dui-ing the next twenty-foui houis, the patient's state assumed almost a hopeless aspect ; when it occuiied to Di. Biaun that, as the eclampsia of pueipeial women is caused by uiæmic intoxication, a diaphoietic diug would diminish the tension in the aiteiial system and fiee the blood of toxic mattei. He accoidingly made a hypodeimic injection of thiee *centigiammes* of muiiate of pilocaipine. This was followed by veiy piofuse peispiiation and salivation. Duiing the next half-houi, the muscles of the eye and the face twitched a few times. No moie eclamptic fits came on, and the patient iecoveied quickly.—*Brit. Med. Jouin.*, Aug. 9, 1879.

Auscultation in Uteiine Hemoriliage.

Piof. DEPAUL, in a clinical lectuie (*Gaz. des Hôp.*, Aug. 26), obseives that when hemoriliage occuis duiing labuii, it will geneially be found to aiise fiom paitial detachment of the placenta, the coid being too shoit. "I iemembei," he said, "the case of a young woman whose delivery had gone on veiy well, when, as the head was appioaching the vulva, two oi thiee spoonfuls of blood suddenly ap-peared between hei thighs. I immediately piactised auscultation, and found the fœtal heait beating iiiegulaily. It was evident that the infant was suffeiing, and that it was dangeious to await the natuial teimination of the labuii, which might last two or thiee houis longei. Dilatation was complete; and easily peisuading the mothei of the necessity of teiminating the labuii iapidly, I applied the for-ceps. Immediately aftei the child was extiacted theie followed five or six enoi-mous clots, weighing about a couple of pounds. The child was boin iespiiing with difficulty, but soon quite iecoveied. Nevei forget, then, whenevei you meet with a flow of blood, to assuie youiself by auscultation as to the state of the infant, and when dilatation has taken place, hasten to inteifeie whenever life seems in dangei."—*Med. Times and Gaz.*, Sept. 6, 1879.

Eigot in the Tieatment of Fibroid Tumours of the Uteius.

Di. W. H. BYFORD, of Chicago, in a papei iead at the late meeting of the Biitish Medical Association (*Biitish Med. Jouinal*, Sept. 6, 1879), laid down the following piopositions, and offeied aiguments in suppoit of them. 1. When piopeily administered, ergot fiequently veiy gieatly amelioiates some of the tioublesome and even dangeious conditions of fibioid tumouis of the uteius, *c. g.*, hemoriliage and copious leucoiihœa. 2. It often aiiests theii giowth, and checks hemoriliage. 3. In many instances it causes the absoiption of the tumoui ; occa-sionally without giving the patient any inconvenience ; while, at othei times, the iemoval of the tumoui by absoiption is attended by painful contiactions and tenderness of the uterus. 4. By inducing uterine contraction, it causes the expulsion of the polypoid variety of the submucous tumour. 5. In the same way, it causes the disruption and discharge of the intramural tumour. He said that, in administering ergot in cases of fibrous tumour, the action of the drug would depend on the degree of development of the fibres of the uterus, and on the position of the tumour with reference to the serous or the mucous surfaces: the nearer the mucous surface, the better the effect. A good result might be expected under the following conditions: smoothness of contour of the tumour, denoting uniform development; hemorrhage; a lengthened uterine cavity; and elasticity of the tumour. He would expect large fibro-cystic tumours to resist the action of ergot; and a good result was not to be expected in cases of uneven nodulated tumour, absence of hemorrhage, shortness of the uterine cavity, and hardness of the tumour. It was not essential to give ergot hypodermically, though this was a very efficacious method; it might be given by the mouth, in suppositories, etc. If the object were to cause painless absorption of the tumour, the dose should be moderate, and not too frequently repeated; if it were desired to have the tumour expelled, full and increasing doses should be given often, and continued till the object was attained. The preparation which he used was Squibb's fluid extract of ergot. He said, in conclusion, that he disclaimed any expectation that ergot would supplant all other modes of treatment.

—

Extirpation of a Cancerous Uterus.

Dr. Von Massari relates a case of extirpation of the cancerous uterus followed by a fatal result. The patient was fifty-three years old, the mother of nine children. Menstruation had ceased at the age of forty-three. A vaginal discharge had existed for two years, for six months irregular hemorrhage had occurred, and the discharge had become offensive. There was no pain, and the general condition was good. The cancerous cervix was hollowed out into an ulcerated cavity which admitted the finger, bled readily on touching, and from which a scanty offensive discharge flowed. The uterus was quite freely movable, and no trace of the disease could be discovered in the pelvis.

The operation was performed on February 1, 1879, in a room disinfected by thymol spray, and the patient was placed with her head towards the window, the thighs flexed and abducted. A mixture of chloroform 100 parts, ether 30, and alcohol 20, was used for anæsthesia. The vagina was syringed with 5 per cent. solution of carbolic acid. An incision having been made from umbilicus to pubes, the author succeeded with difficulty in pressing the intestines and omentum up into the upper part of the abdomen by means of compresses dipped in warm thymol solution. The edges of the wound were then held apart by means of a kind of clamp invented by the author, so as to allow a free view into the pelvis.

The operator then placed himself between the patient's knees, and introducing the left hand into the vagina, introduced the lowest loop of the sutures for the broad ligament at each side in a manner similar to that adopted by Freund, the needle being inserted at a point 1 cm. from the lateral border of the lip of the cervix, and entering successively the anterior and posterior pouches of peritoneum at a point 1 cm. from the border of the uterus. The first loop at each side inclosed the lower third of the broad ligament, and two more loops secured its middle and upper thirds respectively, the uppermost loop being placed outside the ovary. In closing the wound the author adopted a different method from that of Freund. Three sutures were passed from the vagina into the peritoneal cavity, between bladder and uterus, and a similar number of loops were passed fiom vagina into pouch of Douglas, intended to diaw down the ends of the sutuies after iemoval of the uteius, and so complete the loops, to be tied in the vagina, and so unite the anteiioi and posteiioi cut suifaces. Two of these loops, howevei, weie cut in sepaiating the uteius, and the two coiiesponding sutuies had afteiwaids to be passed by a stiaight needle fiom above into the vagina. Duiing the sepaiation of the uteius, the fundus was diawn upwaids, or to the side, by means of Luei's foiceps. As soon as it was cut away, the pelvis filled iapidly with blood, and the uteiine and some smallei aiteiies weie found to be spiiting, and to iequiie ligatuie. The cut suifaces weie then biought togethei by the sutuies befoie mentioned, and inteimediate gut-sutuies weie inseited, and tied on the peiitoneal side. The peiitoneal cavity was sponged out, and foui diainage tubes inseited, antiseptic diessings being applied. The opeiation lasted an houi and a quaitei, and, at the end of it, the patient's condition was good; pulse 96. In the evening the pulse had iisen to 118; tempeiatuie 38.3 C., and vomiting had occuiied once. On the second moining, tempeiatuie 38.6 C., pulse 120; evening, tempeiatuie 39.3 C., pulse 140. Theie was now fiequent vomiting of wateiy fluid, and the featuies had become diawn. On the thiid evening, tempeiatuie had iisen to 41 C., pulse could not be counted. Death occuiied about midnight.

At the autopsy, the peiitoneal cavity was found to contain about ten c. c. of semi-puiulent fluid, and the peiitoneum was coated thinly with lymph. The iight uietei was found to have been cut acioss about thiee cm. above its opening into the bladdei, and its uppei poition was included in one of the ligatuies. The pelvis, and calices of the iight kidney, as well as the uietei, weie slightly dilated. In the iemoved uterus the innei two-thiids of the wall of the ceivical canal was found to be infiltiated with medullaiy caicinoma.

To avoid the iisk of wounding the uieteis, the authoi pioposes, in futuie, to pass bougies into them, as a pieliminaiy to the opeiation. He finds, howevei, that Simon's method of sounding the uieteis is too difficult and unceitain, and theiefoie pioposes to dilate the uiethia, pass into the bladdei Simon's uiethial speculum, and by its aid to sound the uieteis. In one tiial, he has found this easy to accomplish with the aid of an oidinaiy lamp light and reflector.—*Central-blätt für Gynäk.*, May 24, 1879.

Di. F. J. KOCHS, of Bonn, in the *Archiv für Gynäkologie*, B. xiv. H. 2, ielates a successful case of extiipation of the canceious uteius. The patient was thiity-nine yeais old, the mothei of two childien. She was in good health, and menstiuation was iegulai up to Januaiy, 1878. Aftei the menstiual peiiod of that month, a dischaige commenced. Occasional hemoiihage, but not to any consideiable degiee, had also taken place, and but little pain had been felt. When she came undei the authoi's obseivation, at the beginning of the following Apiil, the ceivix was found to be hollowed out into a deep ciatei, and enlaiged by malignant giowth, which ieached up to about one cm. fiom the vaginal insertion, but nowheie oveipassed that boundaiy. The uteius was about as much enlaiged as it would be in acute metiitis, and was movable, although not quite fieely so. Micioscopic examination of a small poition of the giowth showed it to be caicinoma. The tendency to hemoiihage was consideiable.

Menstiuation came on on Apiil 19th, lasting seven days; and on Apiil 28th, the opeiation for extiipation was undeitaken. The patient was placed with hei head towaids the window, and lowei than the pelvis. The anæsthetic was chloroform, given by Junkei's inhalei; and caie had been taken to administei purgatives for seveial days pieviously. Caibolic spiay of a stiength of one pei cent. was used at the opeiation. The incision was made fiom the mons veneiis to about two finger-bieadths above the umbilicus, and the edges of the wound weie held apart by retractors. It was found possible to hold back the intestines in the upper part of the abdomen by means of a handkerchief dipped in carbolic solution. The three loops of strong silk ligature were placed on the broad ligaments at each side, from above downwards, the last loop entering the vagina. Each loop was doubled, so that the innermost thread was close to the uterus, and the outer one about one cm. from it. The threads of the inner loops were cut short. A simple long, slightly curved needle was used in passing all the ligatures. The lowest loops became slack after division of the upper part of the broad ligaments, and had to be replaced. The lowest loop on the left side had again to be replaced after complete separation of the uterus from the right broad ligament, and from the bladder and rectum. In passing the loops, in order to avoid lesion of the bladder, the finger was passed into that viscus, after dilatation of the urethra. The ovaries were removed, the mes ovaria being tied with silk. A supplementary ovary was noticed on the left side, situated from one to two cm. within the left ovary. This was removed in like manner. The bladder was separated from the uterus by using the scalpel from above, guided by the finger within the bladder. The knife was also used to pierce the vagina from the pouch of Douglas, and the opening so made was enlarged to either side. The ends of the ligatures were drawn down into the vagina, after Freund's method, and the wound of the peritoneum was brought together in a transverse line by six fine sutures. The vagina was finally washed out with carbolic solution, but no tampon placed in it.

Some vomiting occurred the same evening, and it was necessary to use the catheter about ten o'clock, no incontinence of urine having followed the dilatation of the urethra. Temperature 38.2° C.; pulse 120: On the second day, temperature was 37°; pulse 140. The same evening the pulse rose to 160, but after this improvement took place, although vomiting was frequent for several days. On the fifth day the pulse had fallen to 96; temperature 37.8° C. From this day the vagina was washed out with carbolic solution by means of a speculum. On the eighth day, on the removal of one of the sutures, a small collection of pus was evacuated from the neighbourhood of the puncture. Convalescence went on undisturbed till May 24th, the twenty-seventh day, when rigours came on, followed by febrile symptoms. On the 26th, a considerable discharge of pus took place by the vagina. Recovery was steady from this time. At the last examination reported, which was made on June 6th, a funnel-shaped depression remained at the summit of the vagina, with some small protuberances; but these did not show, microscopically, any sign of cancer. There had been no recurrence of menstrual molimen.

To simplify the operation, and avoid the difficult process of placing the lowest loops of the sutures which are to secure the uterine arteries, the author proposes, in future, before placing these loops, to separate the uterus from the bladder and the pouch of Douglas, which will not, he thinks, cause much bleeding. The loops of suture can then be easily carried by a long, strongly curved needle, like an aneurism-needle, from the pouch of Douglas into the vagina, and thence into the anterior pouch of peritoneum through the opening so made.—*Obstetrical Journal of Great Britain*, Sept. 1879.

CONTENTS.

Published Monthly, price $2.50 per annum, free of postage.

Also, furnished together with the AMERICAN JOURNAL OF THE MEDICAL
SCIENCES *and the* MEDICAL NEWS AND LIBRARY *for* SIX DOLLARS *per
annum in advance, the whole free of postage.*

HENRY C. LEA, Philadelphia.

THE MONTHLY ABSTRACT

OF

MEDICAL SCIENCE.

Vol. VI. No. 11. **For List of Contents see last page.** NOVEMBER, 1879.

Entered at the Post-Office at Philadelphia as Second-class matter.

Anatomy and Physiology.

Supernumerary Nipples and Mammæ.

Dr. J. MITCHELL BRUCE, Assistant Physician to Charing Cross Hospital, has made an investigation of this subject (*Journal of Anatomy and Physiology*, July, 1879) based upon the study of 165 cases of supernumerary nipple discovered during the physical examination of the chests of the out-patients attending at the Hospital for Consumption, Brompton, under the care of the writer. The general results may be summarized as follows:—

1. That 65 cases of supernumerary nipple were observed within a period of three years.

2. That of 315 individuals taken indiscriminately and in succession, 7.619 per cent. presented supernumerary nipple.

3. That 9.11 per cent. of 207 men examined in succession presented supernumerary nipple; and 4.807 per cent. of 104 women.

4. That in the great majority of instances the supernumerary nipple was single; but it was without exception situated on the front of the trunk below and within the ordinary nipple; and more frequently on the left side than on the right.

5. That the distance of supernumerary nipple from the ordinary nipple was very various, and that from the measurements of these distances a series of numbers may be obtained which may possibly suggest the unit of distance between the successive pairs of nipples in the original type.

6. That a supernumerary nipple, though frequently well marked, is more frequently small or deficient in one or more of its elements—papilla, areola, follicles, or hairs.

7. That in no case was the supernumerary organ physiologically active; but that in a few cases supernumerary glands appeared to be present (in single women).

8. That inheritance was not traced in any instance.

9. That in more than one instance the anterior abdominal wall was the seat of the abnormality.

—

The Sensory Centres of the Brain.

The position of the sensory centres in the cerebral convolutions has been the subject of a series of experiments by LUCIANI and TAMBURINI, who have arrived at the following conclusions. The visual centres in the dog correspond to an elongated area of the second outer convolution, including the region to which Ferrier assigns the centre for the closure of the opposite eye, and that which he found to be related to movement of the eyes to the opposite side. In the monkey the visual centre includes, not only the angular gyrus, but also a large part, if not the whole, of the convexity of the posterior lobe. The centre for hearing in the dog is found in the upper and hinder part of the third outer convolution; that of the monkey is probably to be found in the homologous region—i. e., in a zone lying immediately below the visual centre, in the upper and middle temporo-sphenoidal convolution. Both these centres are excitable with electricity in the dog and the monkey, but the effect varies according to the position, degree, and form of the stimulus. It seems to the experimenters most probable that the effects are due to the irritation of special motor centres which are included within the sensory zone, although there is no absolute proof that they may not be reflex effects of the stimulation of the centres, caused by subjective visual or auditory impressions. Unilateral destruction of the visual centre causes, almost invariably, complete amaurosis of the opposite eye, and amblyopia of the eye of the same side. Unilateral destruction of the visual centre in monkeys causes bilateral hemiopia of that half of the retinæ which corresponds to the hemisphere operated on. Hence we may infer that there is an incomplete decussation of the fibres of the optic nerve in the dog, and a semi-decussation in the monkey, whether the crossing is completed in the chiasma or in the corpora quadrigemina. In the retina of the dog the fibres from two hemispheres are blended at their termination, but in the monkey they are separated. The blindness which results from extirpation of the cortical centres is not only psychical, but consists in a more or less complete abolition of the power of perceiving the retinal images; there is no winking on objects being suddenly brought before the eye, and the action of the pupil to light is lessened. No ophthalmoscopic changes were visible. Bilateral extensive destruction of the visual centres of the dog produces immediately complete bilateral blindness. The complete destruction of the centres in the monkey causes bilateral hemiopia. A similar result follows the extirpation of one or both auditory centres of the dog: in the former case the ear on the opposite side is completely deaf, that on the same side being much less impaired; in the latter case there is absolute bilateral deafness. Amaurosis, amblyopia, hemiopia, and deafness, are, as consequences of cerebral lesions, transient effects, their degree varying according to the extent of the lesion and the time which has elapsed. The effects of unilateral lesion pass away more rapidly than those of bilateral partial lesions, although these may disappear after eight weeks. Whether complete compensation occurs cannot be stated. The compensation after a unilateral lesion is by means of the centres of the opposite side. If, for instance, the interference with sight and hearing on the right side, which has been produced by a lesion on the left side of the brain, has passed away, the destruction of the right centres abolishes the function, not only on the left side, but also that which had been restored on the right side. The compensation after incomplete bilateral destruction is by means of the portions remaining intact. Should further investigations demonstrate the possibility of complete or incomplete compensation after bilateral complete extirpation, the power must be ascribed to the basal ganglia, thalamus opticus, and corpora quadrigemina—just as, according to the authors, psycho-motor centres may be compensated for.—*Lancet*, Oct. 4, 1879.

Materia Medica and Therapeutics.

The Physiological Action of Chloride of Pilocarpin.

Dr. SMOLENSKI has recently investigated (*Warsaw Medical Archiv*) the physiological action of chloride of pilocarpin. He injected this substance subcutaneously, in doses varying from 0.01 to 0.02 gramme, in thirty-four cases, with the following results: 1. In regard to the circulatory apparatus, within a period varying from one to ten minutes after such injection, and usually antecedently to salivation and sweating, a sensation of fulness and heaviness in the head was experienced; the face became redder, and dilatation of all the visible vessels, whether arterial or venous, was observed. In five of the cases dilatation of the vessels of the retina was observed under the ophthalmoscope. 2. The frequency of the pulse, also antecedently to salivation, was increased. The pulse became not only fuller and larger, but softer and almost invariably dicrotous. The changes in the pulse were always investigated by means of Sommerbrodt's sphygmograph, and the sphygmograms obtained pointed to a condition of diminished elasticity of the coats of the vessels; no elastic vibrations were visible. 3. The next constant symptom was salivation, which reached its acme in the course of twenty or twenty-five minutes after the injection, and disappeared after the lapse of an hour. The quantity of saliva secreted stood in a direct relation to the quantity of the drug injected. Its sp. gr. varied from 1.004 to 1.015. Traces of sulphocyanide of potassium were found. 4. The salivation was constantly accompanied by sweating. The acme of increased perspiration coincided with the acme of salivation. 5. Pilocarpin had no influence either on the quantity or the specific gravity of the urine. 6. Smolenski distinguishes two stages in the influence of pilocarpin on the temperature of the body, a primary and secondary. Immediately after the injection the temperature rose 0.1° to 0.4° C., but subsequently fell 0.2° to 1.2° C. 7. The presence of fever does not change or modify the above-mentioned effects of pilocarpin. No perceptible influence is exerted on the eye when the drug is subcutaneously injected, but after the introduction of a drop of a solution into the conjunctival sac a moderate degree of myosis is induced, which disappears in the course of from two to four hours. In this respect, however, pilocarpin is less powerful than eserine. 8. Amongst the accidental symptoms observed were nausea, headache, sensation of fatigue, drowsiness, and in one case rigours and general convulsions. 9. Atropine acts as an antagonist to pilocarpin, and nitrite of amyl prevents the occurrence of some of the occasional symptoms observed after the use of pilocarpin. The effects on the circulatory apparatus Smolenski ascribes to diminished irritability of the vagus nerve caused by decrease of blood pressure; the diaphoretic action of pilocarpine he attributes to peripheric irritation of the perspiratory nerves in accordance with Luchsinger's experiments. The sialogogue properties he also attributes to a peripheric irritation of the nerves of the salivary glands, because the section of the chorda tympani, or of the cervical part of the sympathetic, does not prevent the occurrence of the salivation. All the experiments were performed under the supervision of Professor Korczynski.—*Lancet*, Aug. 23, 1879.

———

Is Pilocarpin an Oxytocic?

In the *London Medical Record* for January, 1879, there is an account of the experiments of Dr. Hyernaux with this drug upon pregnant rabbits. The results arrived at were that the drug produced no symptom of labour, but, when persevered in, reduced the animal to a moribund condition. In these experiments the drug was administered by hypodermic injection. The results obtained by Dr. Hyernaux on pregnant women were similar. He administered the drug by hypodermic injections to two women. In the first woman labour resulted, but she had already been subjected to warm water enemas, and warm hip-baths, which had excited the commencement of labour. In the case of the second woman, who was subjected to the action of pilocarpin alone, labour did not result. The constitutional symptoms, however, which were produced were marked. Imme-diately after the subcutaneous injection of three-tenths of a grain of chlorohy-drate of pilocarpin, the patient's eyes became brilliant, then humid and tearful, the sight was obscured without great alteration of the pupil, the face became covered with sweat, which poured off in large drops. The pulse rose to 160 per minute, the respiration to 30. The whole body was bathed in sweat. The hands and feet were cold and sticky. There was profuse ptyalism, accompanied by watery vomit and diarrhœa. The urine was abundant. Lastly, it is stated that the patient felt very ill. Not the slightest symptom of labour resulted from all this suffering, although this patient received three injections. In the *Medical Record* for February a case is reported by Dr. Kleinwachter, in which three in-jections were given, and labour resulted at the end of three days. The lying-in was attended by symptoms of metritis, but the patient recovered. In the same number of the same journal is reported a case in which Mr. Clay, of Birming-ham, induced labour by pilocarpin. Eight injections were given, and by the *fourth day* the os uteri was dilated to the size a halfpenny, but was still rigid. The constitutional symptoms as seen in Hyernaux's cases were present, and it is stated that at the end of six minutes after the first injection the pulse was 62, and hardly perceptible. *The collapse was so great that it was feared she would not rally.* The dilatation was eventually effected by Barnes's bags, and a living child delivered by the forceps.

Parisi, of Verona, relates, in the *Gazette Medica Italiana delle Provincie Venette*, a case in which the pilocarpin failed. Bergesio read an account, at the Congress of the Italian Medical Association, of two cases in which it was necessary to resort to Krause's method of inducing labour to aid the action of the pilocar-pin. Dr. Cuzzi, of Milan, also failed in two cases to induce labour by means of the alkaloid. Whether or not pilocarpin may be of use in combating the uræ-mic complications of eclampsia remains to be seen. Possibly, its diaphoretic and sialogogic properties may be turned to account in the treatment of puerperal con-vulsions. It is in this direction that future trials should be made. The rapid action of the drug upon the skin and salivary glands must be an important point in its favour in dealing with eclampsia.

Clearly the term oxytocic (hastener of labour) cannot be applied to a drug the effects of which are, after days of misery and dangerous illness, to reduce the patient's health and strength to the lowest ebb, while, perhaps, dilating the os to the size of a halfpenny, and most likely not changing it in the smallest degree. Whatever the value of the drug may be, it is not oxytocic. Professor Demme, of Berne, says that pilocarpin is an efficacious diaphoretic and sialogogue in the treatment of certain diseases of young children. In appropriate doses, it is well borne by the youngest patients. Unpleasant symptoms are very rare, and can probably be altogether prevented by small doses of brandy before the injection. The cases in which it seems especially suitable are the parenchymatous inflamma-tions of the kidney, with dropsy, following scarlatina and diphtheria. The ages of the patients have been between nine months and twelve years. The doses ad-ministered have been from five *milligrammes* to two *centigrammes.—British Medical Journal*, Sept. 27, 1879.

Physiological Action of Carbolic Acid on the Nervous System.

Dr. J. SUMNER STONE, of Wheeling, West Virginia, as the result of an ex-perimental inquiry (*Phila. Med. Times*, Sept. 27, 1879), finds that in large doses carbolic acid may cause immediate paralysis through spinal depression. Smaller doses cause clonic convulsions of spinal origin. Convulsions and paralysis may exist at the same time in one animal, the posterior extremities being paralyzed first.

Neither motor nor sensory nerves nor muscles are affected by carbolic acid.

Reflex action with small doses is first diminished through irritation of Setschenow's centre; it is then increased through its subsequent paralysis, the irritation explaining the ordinary occurrence of *apparent* muscular weakness in the early stage of the poisoning, while the convulsions follow its paralysis. Larger doses may paralyze Setschenow's centre immediately.

It is probable that the spinal action of carbolic acid is confined to the motor columns.

The Action of Ferments employed as Digestive Agents.

M. VULPIAN (*Le Progrès Médical*, Aug. 16, 1879), on the reading of a paper of M. Mourrut, upon artificial digestion, contributed the following note in regard to the action of the digestive ferments employed in the treatment of dyspepsia. In the lecture at the School of Medicine, delivered last session, M. Vulpian had occasion to discuss the normal and pathological secretions, and was led when considering the secretions which promote digestion to speak of dyspeptics, and of the various means which are employed to relieve them. Foremost amongst the remedies of this kind are the digestive ferments pepsin and pancreatin, to which may be added the vegetable diastase, for various observers have attributed to this ferment the power of assisting the saliva and pancreatic juice in digesting starchy materials. M. Vulpian has made a number of experiments in regard to the action of these substances. He has asked whether the ferment action is exerted freely under the conditions in which the ferments are placed in the stomach ; and whether they manifest the same activity under whatever pharmaceutical form they are ingested. By means of artificial digestions, he has readily proved that the pepsins sold by different chemists have not all the same digestive power. In some cases the cooked albumen undergoes a slow but slight change. The addition of alcohol to an acidified solution of pepsin or to normal gastric juice, however, hinders the digestion. Relying upon these negative results, M. Vulpian is of opinion that it is useless to prescribe wines and elixirs of pepsin. Diastase and pancreatin also, when mixed with natural or artificial pancreatic juice, are far from exercising upon starchy materials such active properties as when they are brought into contact with them by means of simple water.—*Practitioner*, Oct. 1879.

Experiments with Diuretics.

Dr. MAUREL, a naval surgeon, communicated a paper to the Société de Thérapeutique (*Jour. de Thérap.*, September 10), giving an account of a number of careful experiments which he had performed upon healthy individuals in order to ascertain and compare the effects of various reputed diuretics. His general conclusion is that the practitioner can rely only on three of the diuretics among those which have been under investigation, viz., chlorate of potash, salicylate of soda, and digitalis, the first two even of these having but a feeble activity. The other medicinal substances reputed as diuretics—nitrate and acetate of potash, iodide of potassium, squill, and colchicum—are either devoid of action or produce effects of no importance. The reporter, commenting upon this conclusion, observes that he cannot agree with it, having no doubt that nitrate and acetate of potash and squill are energetic diuretics, from what he has observed when they have been employed in suitable cases. The indication for their employment is the point of importance. If, in place of experimenting upon healthy men, Dr.

Manuel had given some of these diuretics, which he accuses of inertia, to subjects infiltrated with serosity, and having abundant collections of water (collections whence the circulation might largely draw to produce abundant diuresis), he would have been less positive in his conclusions, and would have admitted that these substances are excellent diuretics in certain cases of dropsy, when there are no hyperæmic or inflammatory lesions of the kidneys. The reporter terminates with a remark which is often lost sight of by those who are content to draw their conclusions solely from experiments on healthy men and animals. If, he observes, the study of medicinal agents, etc., on healthy men has its great value, it does not suffice for giving a complete measure of their therapeutical power. It is still essentially necessary that clinical observation should intervene in order to obtain a complete history of these substances.—*Med. Times and Gaz.*, Oct. 4, 1879.

Medicine.

The Production of Hæmoglobinuria by Glycerine.

A remarkable difference in the action of glycerine, according as it is injected into a vein or under the skin, has lately been pointed out by SCHWAHN (*Eckhardt's Beitrage*, viii., *Centralblatt*, No. 33, 1879). If glycerine diluted with from 50 to 60 per cent. of water be injected into the subcutaneous cellular tissue, or into the stomach of dogs or rabbits, hæmoglobin is absolutely certain to appear in the urine ; whereas, if an equal quantity be injected into a vein, this phenomenon does not occur. In the same way the blood corpuscles in a mixture of glycerine and blood are unaltered in form or colour. Hence Schwahn regards the hæmoglobinuria after subcutaneous injection of glycerine as the result of diffusion ; certain bodies, especially the metallic chlorides and sulphates, on whose presence the integrity of the blood corpuscles depends, passing out towards the glycerine, so that cellular dissolution follows. Schwahn has found that, if the renal arteries are tied after the subcutaneous injection of glycerine, both bloodplasma and lymph become coloured red by the dissolved hæmoglobin.—*Med. Times and Gazette*, Sept. 20, 1879.

Vaccinating with Thymolized Lymph.

Dr. EMIL STERN, Medical Officer of the Royal Vaccine Institute in Breslau, gives in the *Breslaue ärtzliche Zeitschrift*, No. 8, 1879, an account of some observations which he has made with vaccine matter subjected to the action of thymol. He says that last year Kobert stated that the addition of a one per mille aqueous solution of thymol to humanized lymph in no way injured it, but, on the other hand, afforded a means of preserving it. On repeating the experiments with vaccine matter in the Breslau Institute, he found that the use of lymph mingled with glycerine, salicylic acid, or carbolic acid, gave almost always negative results ; while the aqueous solution of thymol, while it resisted decomposition, did not destroy the specific action of the lymph. Hiller has already shown that the addition of carbolic acid destroyed the action of vaccine matter. Dr. Stern followed Kobert's method of blowing the fresh lymph from a capillary tube on to a watchglass, filling the tube with a one per mille solution of thymol, and blowing this also on the watch-glass. The vaccine matter and the thymol solution are then stirred together, and the mixture is drawn into a clean capillary tube, leaving

behind fibrinous coagula, blood-corpuscles, and accidental admixtures, such as
broken threads, etc. The mixed lymph is always perfectly clear and transparent.
Köhler is said to have never failed in vaccination with the thymolized lymph;
but Dr. Stein has not been able to obtain such success. Of twenty-nine children
vaccinated thus for the first time, characteristic pustules were produced in twenty,
while the operation failed in 9 (31 per cent.). It must, however, be remembered
that nearly one-fifth of the vaccinations with ordinary lymph that has been preserved in capillary tubes fail. As with ordinary lymph, the activity of the thymolized lymph varies with its age. The pustules following vaccination with
thymolized lymph had the specific vaccine character, as was shown by the lymph
obtained from them producing ordinary vaccine pustules when used for vaccination. The latter pustules, however, had only small areola, and there was no
inflammatory reaction; nor was there erysipelas or any phlegmonous process.
Dr. Stein has had no opportunity of testing the thymolized lymph in revaccina-
tion. He says that further observations are required; but that, so far as his observations have gone, they show that the mixture of humanized lymph with a
one per mille solution of thymol does not destroy its activity, that the mixture is
not more irritating than ordinary vaccine matter, and that the addition of the
thymol presents advantages in regard to preservation.—*British Medical Journal*,
Sept. 6, 1879.

Patellar Tendon Reflex.

At a late meeting of the Medico-Chirugical Society of Edinburgh, Dr. BYROM
BRAMWELL read a paper on this subject. After referring to the previous observations of Erb, Westphal, Grainger Stewart, Buzzard, Gowers, etc., the
author proceeded to consider the physiology of the subject. He gave reasons
for supposing, firstly, that the movement of the foot, which follows a sharp blow
upon the ligamentum patellæ when the knee is semiflexed and the leg at rest, is
not mechanical, but is due to a contraction of the quadriceps extensor femoris;
secondly, that this contraction is a reflex phenomenon. He concluded that in
the normal condition of things, the sensory nerves which receive the impression
and convey it to the centre (lumbar portion of spinal cord) are situated in the
ligamentum patellæ itself, but that in some cases of disease—where the phenomena is greatly exaggerated—the reflex may originate in the muscular fibres
of the quadriceps; in the periosteum, as when a contraction follows a blow on
the front of the tibia; or possibly in the skin over the patellar tendon. Two
cases were detailed in support of the possibility of the skin origin of the reflex;
in one the phenomenon followed a blow upon a pinched-up portion of skin, notwithstanding that every care was taken to prevent any dragging on the tendon;
in the other the phenomenon was greatly lessened after freezing. The patellar
tendon reflex, like the ordinary skin reflex, varied greatly in extent in different
individuals; but the author had not seen any case in which it was completely
absent in health; several cases, however, had been met with by Gowers and
others. The writer then considered the alterations of the phenomenon which
are met with in disease, dividing these cases into two classes: (1) Those in which
the phenomenon is absent; (2) Those in which it is exaggerated. Anything
which impairs the integrity of the nervous arc will prevent the occurrence of the
reflex. Diseases or injury of—(1) the sensory nerve fibres, conveying the impression from the surface to the centre; (2) of the nerve centre (lumbar portion
of spinal cord); (3) of the motor nerve, which conveys the impression from the
centre to the muscle, by causing an arrest of the reflex, will prevent the phenomenon. Practically, the arrest generally occurs in the centre (lumbar portion
of cord), for disease and injury of the cord are of every-day occurrence, while

disease of the nerve trunks and anterior roots is rare. All lesions of the lumbar portion of the cord will not prevent the phenomenon—that particular portion of the cord through which the reflex travels must be injured or diseased. The author then referred in detail to individual diseases in which the phenomenon is absent. He stated that in the great majority of cases of locomotor ataxy the phenomenon was absent. In that disease the arrest must either take place in the posterior root fibres or in the posterior horns of gray matter. The posterior columns are outside the reflex tract; the lesion of the posterior columns cannot, therefore, cause the arrest. In the great majority of cases of locomotor ataxy the lumbar portion of the spinal cord is diseased, hence the frequency with which the patellar tendon reflex is absent in that affection. Cases in which the patellar tendon reflex is exaggerated were next considered. Increase in the extent of the phenomenon may depend upon—(1) increased excitability of the gray matter of the cord ; (2) disease or injury of the cord interfering with the fibres which transmit the inhibitory impressions from the brain. These inhibitory fibres of reflex impulses are supposed to be contained, in part at least, in the lateral columns. Disease or injury of these (the lateral) columns will, therefore, be associated with increased patellar tendon reflex.

Professor GRAINGER STEWART said that he had met with no undoubted case of locomotor ataxia in which the " tendon reflex" was retained, but one or two in which some of the symptoms existed while it was retained. He had not been able as yet to satisfy himself of the value of the loss of tendon reflex as an early symptom. He supposed that its disappearance depended upon lesion of the portion of the spinal cord which was the *centre* for that reflex movement, and that the symptoms might appear early or late according to the distribution of degeneration in the cord. He had, however, met with one or two cases in which full confidence in this symptom would have or might have led into error. In the case of a gentleman, which had been some years ago narrated to the Society as an example of malarious paraplegia (see *Ed. Med. Journ.* 1876), a relapse had occurred during the last summer, and some symptoms resembling those of locomotor ataxia had been developed. The patellar tendon reflex was found completely absent in both legs, but in the course of a few weeks improvement set in, and the tendon reflex was restored. In this case adherence to Westphal's diagnostic rule would have led to a diagnosis of locomotor ataxia. He had seen the same condition also in the case of an Irish lady who had few other symptoms of locomotor ataxia, and absolute loss of the symptom had been observed in a well-marked case of polio myelitis anterior subacuta, which had been carefully demonstrated to the clinical class. As to the second group of cases—those in which the function was increased—he had seen it very marked in cases of secondary degeneration of the cord following upon cerebral lesion, as well as in cases of primary lateral sclerosis. Further, in one well-marked case of spastic paralysis following upon Pott's disease of the vertebræ, he had found it greatly exaggerated. Sometimes the exaggeration led to prolonged exhaustion, when the tendon was repeatedly tapped ; and sometimes the traction upon the flexors led to a spasmodic contraction. He agreed with Dr. Bramwell as to the point of origin of the peripheral irritation being in the tendon, and remarked that some parts of the tendon were more sensitive than others.—*Edinburgh Med. Journal*, Sept. 1879.

A Unique Case of Complete Pharyngeal Stricture of Specific Origin.

Dr. JOSEPH MEYERS, Ex-House-Physician to Charity Hospital, New York, reports (*Med. Record*, August 23, 1879), with Prof. Oertel's permission, the following remarkable case which came to his clinic at Munich :—

A man, thirty-three years of age, had a chancre three years ago, followed by eruptions of secondary syphilis, which got well under mercurial treatment. For the past year he had no specific trouble of any kind, and no treatment, until Dec. 25th. He then began to complain of a sore throat, which, with ordinary remedies, got no better, but rapidly worse. On the 10th of January he presented himself to Prof. Oertel at his clinic, when, upon examination, the posterior wall of the pharynx and sides of the pharynx and uvula were inflamed, reddened, and infiltrated; on the uvula beginning ulcerations were noticed, also on the surface of the tonsils. At this time a gargle was ordered, and he was asked to call again in a few days. Prof. Oertel having been called out of town on the 13th of January, the patient did not again present himself till the 15th, when he was brought into the hospital in a dying condition, almost suffocated, with intense dyspnœa, breathing long and wheezing, inspirations 10–12 per minute, pulse almost imperceptible, surface of body cold, face and hands cyanosed, and almost voiceless and speechless. Examination by Professor Nussbaum gave little satisfaction, simply showing an occlusion of the laryngo-pharyngeal space by a stricture, ulceration of posterior pharyngeal wall in a reparative condition, uvula drawn to right pillar of pharynx and there attached; and perforation of soft palate. What condition the larynx was in could not be determined; opening through which he breathed could not be seen. It was supposed that the ulcerative process had destroyed the epiglottis, and closed the upper portion of the larynx. The indication was tracheotomy, which was immediately performed by Professor Nussbaum, with prompt relief to the patient, so that he was able to leave the hospital in a few days, after having been put on mixed treatment. On the 25th of January he again presented himself to Professor Oertel for further treatment. Examination showed an almost complete stricture of the pharynx, extending from the base of the tongue to the sides and posterior wall of the pharynx, a small opening, not even admitting a probe, a little to the left of the centre of the stricture, which formed a sort of lid over the larynx and œsophagus. Through this small opening the patient took food and breathed. Posterior wall of pharynx of an ash-gray colour, presenting an arch-like appearance. No more ulcerations; soft palate perforated and uvula attached to right side of pharynx. Patient wore a tracheal tube; now only had occasional attacks of dyspnœa, with an occasional choking and coughing when he attempted to swallow quickly. He could only take liquid food, but sufficient to sustain him. Opinion of Professor Oertel was same as that of Professor Nussbaum, that epiglottis was destroyed and upper portion of larynx was closed by the stricture. Condition of vocal cords not known; how larynx closed during deglutition—for food and air passed through the same small opening—was not known. I thought, and Professor Oertel agreed with me, that during the act of deglutition the base was lifted and drawn backward in such a way as to approach post-pharyngeal wall, bringing the small aperture over the œsophagus, at the same time closing the larynx, the closure being aided by the aryteno-epiglottidean folds, which, although they could not be seen, were supposed present, and cases of complete destruction of the epiglottis, reported by Bruns, Türck, etc. Its function was known to be replaced by those folds, and in my opinion aided by the tongue (base) approaching the pharyngeal wall. Professor Oertel proposed to operate; to dilate the opening with a knife. Sounds were passed every other day to get the patient used to an instrument, till February 10th, when the first operation was performed. An incision was made forward toward the tongue; bleeding was slight; he was ordered to gargle with cold water. At this time it was noticed that he could gargle much easier. When he was asked if it pained him, he said "only a little" so distinct that everybody present understood him, he having been almost voiceless and en-

tirely speechless. This operation was followed by two more on the 13th and 18th
of February, two lateral incisions then having been made ; opening would then
admit a finger. Examination after second operation showed, to the astonishment
of all present, that the larynx was perfectly intact, epiglottis was entire, vocal
cords were normal. He could now breathe without the tracheal tube, deglutition
was no more interfered with, and the patient rejoiced in the fact that he was
again able to drink lager beer.

The principal points of interest in this case are the completeness of the stricture, its seat, the rapidity of the ulcerative process, the rapidity of the reparative
process at the time without specific treatment, and the larynx being perfectly
intact.

—

Etiology of Paralysis of the Crico-Arytenoid Posterior Muscles.

OTT contributes (*Prag. Med. Wochensch.*, No. 15, 1879) an interesting case
of paralysis of the posterior crico-arytenoid muscles, which was due to pressure
of the posterior crico-arytenoid nerves. A man, aged fifty-seven, had swallowed
a large piece of meat, which had stuck in his throat for twenty-four hours, and
resisted all his attempts to dislodge it. He had no pain, only slight dyspnœa,
and was unable to swallow even a drop of water. The next day he consulted a
physician, who pushed down the piece of meat with a sound. The patient felt
better directly, could breathe more freely, and was able to swallow. This state
of things, however, did not last long ; he again began to suffer from difficulty in
breathing and swallowing, and was obliged to take only liquid food. The voice
had remained unaltered ; but the patient was obliged to speak in short abrupt
sentences, from want of air. When examined by the writer, it was found that
the false vocal cords were slightly swelled, and red ; there was a space of four
millimetres between the arytenoid cartilages. The rima glottidis was partly
covered by the vocal cords during inspiration and expiration ; only an irregular
triangular opening could be seen at its posterior end. The left vocal cord was
wider than the right, and did not move at all, while the right moved sluggishly.
During inspiration, the vocal cords were approximated. The arytenoid cartilages
did not move either during respiration or phonation. The mucous membrane of
the incisura inter-arytenoidea was swelled and pale, and the color of the vocal
cords a dingy yellow. The treatment consisted at first in faradization of the
larynx, but it afforded no relief to the patient. The dyspnœa increased, and became most severe even when the patient was perfectly quiet. It was noticed that
the rima glottidis had become much narrower, the left vocal cord having advanced
to the middle of the fissure ; the right arytenoid cartilage was partly hidden by
the left. As the patient could only swallow with difficulty, it was necessary to
feed him through the tube. He lost his appetite, and was very much wasted, and
reduced in strength. At last the dyspnœa became so intense that tracheotomy
had to be performed, to save the man's life. Immediately after the operation,
the patient was able to swallow without any trouble, and continued to do so
henceforth. The larynx presented the same changes as before the operation.
The patient had still great difficulty in breathing ; the thorax was immovable
during respiration, and the intercostal spaces were drawn in. The vocal cords
were immovable, and during phonation a space of about three millimetres remained open in the back part of the fissure. For this reason, the patient had to
be dismissed with the canula in his throat, to prevent asphyxia. The author attributes the paralysis of the muscles which open the glottis to the pressure which
the large piece of meat, that was firmly wedged in the pharynx during twenty-
four hours, must have exercised on the crico-arytenoid posterior muscles and their
nerves. His assertion is based upon the well-known fact that the conducting

function of a nerve is entirely destroyed by pressure. Thus, in the present case, the nerve having lost all control over the muscle it governs, the latter became paralyzed, and gave rise to the phenomena we have described. The difficulty in swallowing, which increased whenever the dyspnœa became worse, decreased when the sound was introduced, and finally disappeared after tracheotomy, can only be explained by assuming the existence of a spasmodic stricture of the œsophagus.—*New York Med. Journal*, Oct. 1879.

A Rare Form of Diphtheritic Paralysis.

Dr. DAHLERUP describes (*Ugeskrift for Läger*, 3d series, vol. xxvi) the case of a boy aged 12, who, ten or twelve days after recovering from an attack of diphtheritic angina, was seized with difficulty of breathing, which increased to severe dyspnœa at the end of fourteen days. On examination, there was found to be orthopnœa, cyanosis, œdema of the feet, and moderate œdema of the lungs. The heart-beat was somewhat quickened, irregular, and very weak; the area of cardiac dulness was not increased. The heart-sounds were distinct. The pulse was rather feeble. The urine contained a large quantity of albumen. Under the use of digitalis and stimulants, there was slight improvement at the end of a week; the dyspnœa then increased, as did also the œdema of the extremities and lungs; and the patient became collapsed, and died. The temperature at no time of this illness rose above 98.6° Fahr. Dr. Dahlerup believes the case to have been one of progressive diphtheritic paralysis of the heart.—*British Medical Journal*, Sept. 27, 1879.

Intestinal Obstruction successfully treated by Puncture of the Small Intestine.

Dr. W. H. BROADBENT, Physician to St. Mary's Hospital, reports (*British Med. Journal*, Sept. 27, 1879), the following interesting case :—

In February, 1877, I was called by Mr. Rayner to a maiden lady, aged about 60, who presented the usual symptoms of intestinal obstruction—severe tormina, vomiting, and great distension of the abdomen. The seat of the obstruction was made out to be in the neighbourhood of the cæcum, the transverse and descending colon being empty. Opium and belladonna were given, food withheld, and enemata administered; and, the pain and vomiting being quieted, an examination of the rectum was made at a subsequent consultation, when a solid mass was felt pressing down into the pelvis on the right side. It was pushed up as far as possible, and very shortly flatus and feces began to pass. It was ascertained, on inquiry after the examination, that about nine or ten years previously, the patient had been tapped, and that the contents of a suppurating ovarian cyst had been withdrawn. The shrivelled cyst had formed a tumour in the right inguinal region, where she had been accustomed to feel it, and where it was found after the attack. The obstruction was attributed to displacement of this tumour downwards, giving rise either to pressure upon the bowel, or more probably to dragging by adhesion.

There was a slight return of obstruction in March, and again in June, brought on by imprudent exertion; in the autumn, she had a more severe and prolonged attack while at the seaside.

On May 14, 1878, I was again called to this lady by Mr. Rayner. She had then been suffering from complete obstruction of the bowel for several days, which persisted in spite of the treatment which had on the several previous occasions been successful. The tumour formed by the old cyst could now be indistinctly felt in the right inguinal region notwithstanding the great distension of the abdomen, and was only just reached by the rectum; the rectum was held open

by adhesions, so that on passing the sphincter ani the finger moved freely in all
directions in a large cavity. A vaginal examination was impracticable, on account of the contracted state of this passage.

The treatment was continued : in addition to the opium (gr. j) and belladonna
(gr. ⅓) pill taken every three or four hours, and poultices with opium and belladonna over the abdomen, morphia was injected hypodermically. No food was
given by the mouth, but enemata of beef-tea and brandy were administered
every three or four hours, while once a day a copious enema of water or gruel
was employed, for the double purpose of contributing to the relief of the obstruction and of washing out the rectum and removing particles deposited from
the beef-tea, these being liable to become acid and set up irritation which causes
the nutrient injections to be expelled.

No good result was obtained ; and at length, after nearly a fortnight of anxious
watching, and when complete obstruction had lasted three weeks, the intestine
was punctured by a long aspirator-needle. The aspirator was used at first, but
was found to be unnecessary ; an enormous amount of gas gradually escaped, the
tension of the abdominal walls, which had seemed ready to split, was relieved,
and two days later (May 29th) feces and flatus began to pass naturally.

Another attack came on in January, 1879, and when I saw the patient with
Mr. Bridges on January 4th, complete obstruction had existed for several days.
The attempt was made to procure relief by enemata, hypodermic injections of morphia, external applications of opium and belladonna on poultices, and in effect by
treatment similar to that already described, but in vain. Ice also was applied
over the right iliac region ; it gave relief from suffering, but did not set the
bowels free. The patient begged from the first that the gas might be drawn off,
as in the previous attack ; and, as there was no improvement, this was done,
without waiting for the same length of time, on January 8th. The distension
was removed, and during the following night a copious evacuation from the
bowels put an end to the danger.

At this time, indistinct fluid vibration was detected in the right inguinal region
instead of the solid-feeling tumour, and, on the subsidence of the abdominal distension, it was well marked. It was accordingly determined that on any recurrence of obstruction an attempt should be made to remove the cause by aspiration of the cyst, which was evidently refilling after an unusually long interval.
The recurrence happened in May of this year, and I was called to the patient on
the 7th by Mr. Gawith, to whose care she had been transferred. She had been
suffering from bronchitis, and still had a severe cough. There were all the indications of obstruction ; the signs of fluid in the right inguinal region were more
distinct ; and, on examination *per rectum*, an elastic tumour could be felt high in
the pelvis, from the surface of which projected two or three small secondary
cysts. On the 9th, a moderate sized aspirator-needle was plunged into the cyst,
and about six pints of dark brown fluid were drawn off without any unfavourable
results. At first, it seemed as if the desired effect was about to follow : a little
flatus was said to escape when the enemata were used, and a small quantity of
fecal matter was felt in the rectum on examination. This promise was, however, illusory, and, as the distress increased, the intestine was once more punctured on May 20th. A considerable amount of gas had escaped ; and the extreme distension was relieved, though not to the degree required, when, in the
act of coughing, the coil in which the needle was planted was suddenly displaced
to the left and slightly downwards, carrying with it the needle, which now lay flat
on the abdominal wall. It was immediately withdrawn ; but this was followed
by a free escape of gas, which first issued with a hissing sound from the aperture
in the skin, but soon rushed into the subcutaneous cellular tissue, and produced

emphysema, which rapidly spread. This was circumscribed by pressure made by the hands, which also had the effect of directing any gas which had escaped into the peritoneal cavity to the internal opening in the abdominal wall. Another needle was at once plunged into a neighbouring coil of intestine, to take off pressure and prevent gas from passing into the coil from which it had escaped after withdrawal of the needle. Finally, when all issue of gas from the intestine appeared to have ceased, the subcutaneous emphysema was removed by squeezing towards and out of a puncture made by a lancet.

Strange to say, no bad effects of any kind followed; but the pressure had not been sufficiently reduced to permit of the removal of the obstruction. The distension soon became as great as ever; and, with considerable hesitation, the operation was repeated four days later. More gas escaped; the abdomen became soft and yielding, almost flaccid; when exactly the same accident occurred again: the patient coughed and displaced the intestine, the needle had to be hastily withdrawn, it was followed, as before, by gas which escaped from the puncture and rapidly diffused itself under the skin, where its progress could be both seen and felt. Similar precautions were taken, and happily no inflammation followed, but, on the contrary, a copious stool, and the bowels have since continued to act.

Since the above was written the patient has again suffered from obstruction, which was not relieved till the intestine had been punctured. This was done on August 1st with the same fortunate result as before.

I have recommended and practised puncture of the intestine several times in intestinal obstruction, and have never seen injurious effects. The precautions which I consider necessary are the following:—

1. To secure, if possible, absolute freedom from peristaltic action of the bowel. This is done by giving an extra dose of opium by the mouth, or a considerable hypodermic injection of morphia, or both, three or four hours beforehand. No food of any kind should have been taken for some time.

2. To select, if possible, a coil of intestine which shall contain only gas, and not liquid. This will be in the jejunum, and is to be found above the umbilicus rather than below it. An indispensable condition is, that scarcely any food shall have been taken during the entire attack.

3. To pierce the coil exactly at its most convex part. The abdomen should be carefully watched for some time at every visit, and especially before the operation. In some cases, where the walls are thin, the outlines of various coils may be traced even in repose; but this will be more distinct when peristalsis is provoked by pressure, friction, or manipulation of one kind or another; it will be seen also which coils shift and which keep the same position when contracting. The spot chosen for the puncture should be as nearly as possible over the centre of a coil which does not roll about, and by preference in the linea alba. If the needle happen to hit the line of contact between two coils, it may tear both.

4. To exercise great care and patience during the escape of the gas. The needle should be held lightly, but rather firmly, perpendicular to the abdominal wall, and should not be allowed to follow too readily any movement of the intestine. Under the circumstances of obstruction, the respiratory movements are not great. As the gas escapes from the coil selected for puncture, it will collapse under pressure from neighbouring coils, and the flow through the needle will cease; very soon, however, the air in the intestine will distribute itself and enter the empty portion, when it will again escape. This may be aided by gentle manipulation and pressure; but they should not be hastily resorted to: nothing is gained by hurry. Should the tube get blocked, aspiration may free it; but it is safer to drive a little air through the tube into the bowel than to exert powerful suction, which may draw the mucous membrane against the sharp needle.

It is better not to put on a bandage after the operation.

Puncture of the intestine can relieve obstruction only very rarely, and under exceptional circumstances. In the case related, in which there was reason to suppose that the cause of obstruction was external to the bowel, and was due to pressure by the tumour, or by adhesion, or to displacement and dragging of a portion of intestine, it was hoped that removal of distension might permit the parts to return to their previous condition and situation; and other conditions may be imagined in which this might occur, but it could have no effect on a stricture or intussusception. My own experience, however, would lead me to recommend puncture as a palliative; and though I have no experience to guide me, I should think it might be a useful preliminary to inflation, manipulation, suspension head downwards, or other procedures in intussusception, twisting, or imprisonment of the bowel by adhesions.

Anthrax Intestinalis.

At a meeting of the German Medical Society in St. Petersburg (*St. Petersb. Med. Wochens.*, No. 27), the following case was reported by Dr. KADE: A girl aged 17, a seamstress, presented the following symptoms when received into the hospital: Her skin was livid; she was very restless and threw herself about; the heart-sounds were very loud; the throat and lower jaw were œdematous; the glands could be felt only with difficulty both here and in the groin; the abdomen was meteoric and painful; the bladder empty. On being spoken to in a loud voice, she answered slowly and sensibly. There was an excoriated patch on her forehead, and a similar one on the inner condyle of the right femur, where the patient said she had had a pustule before. She had been taken ill three days ago with dysphagia, for which she had taken a dose of castor-oil. On the second and third days, she had felt comparatively well. On entering the hospital, she vomited once, and died three hours later. At the *post-mortem* examination the subcutaneous cellular tissue in the abdominal walls was found to be hemorrhagically infiltrated; the abdominal cavity contained a serous liquid. The mesenteric and inguinal glands also presented a bloody infiltration. The whole of the intestinal tract was injected. In the duodenum several semiglobular swellings were found, which became fewer in number in the small intestine, and disappeared in the large intestine. The spleen was soft, little enlarged; the liver was not enlarged, and was soft. Punctiform extravasations were found in the pelvis of one of the kidneys. Several bloody pustules, partly degenerated, were found on the ary-epiglottic ligaments. In the apex of the right lung was a fresh infarct of the size of a walnut. The longitudinal sinus of the dura mater was filled with fluid blood. Minute extravasations of blood were on the external lamella of the sinus. The blood itself contained numerous bacteria.—*British Medical Journal*, Sept. 27, 1879.

Heroic Treatment of Tapeworm.

Dr. CARL BETTELHEIM (Volkmann's *Sammlung Klinische Vorträge*, No. 166), after carefully summing up our present knowledge of the natural history of the various species of tapeworm, offers some remarks on a speedy method of removing tænia from the intestine, which are well worthy of attention. He asserts that by the plan he adopts he can expel the worm, head and all, in from three-quarters of an hour to less than four hours and a half. The "cure" consists first in an absolute preliminary fast of from eighteen to twenty-four hours' duration, during which the patient is allowed nothing but water, and has his bowels cleared out with three or four tablespoonful doses of castor oil. During this time the druggist is preparing the decoction of pomegranate bark—the anthelmintic which Dr. Bettelheim prefers, and which takes thirty hours to make properly. The following is the formula for it: ℞. Granati rad. corticis, 300.0–400.0 grammes: macera per 24 horas. Deinde coque c. aqua dest. 500.0–600.0 ad remanentiam 200.0–300.0. Such a decoction should be a clear, dark, almost black-brown liquid. The secret of success in the second stage of the cure is to introduce this jorum into the patient's stomach, if possible, in a single dose. This Dr. Bettelheim effects by passing a flexible tube down his œsophagus, and pouring the fluid through it with a glass funnel. Patients generally submit to the tube when told that they must otherwise drink off the medicine at one draught. With some sensitive persons, however, even under its use it may be necessary to divide the dose into three or four portions, and to give them at short intervals of from a quarter of an hour to an hour. The greatest obstacle to this method is the vomiting so often caused by the pomegranate bark, but if the medicine can be kept down for half an hour or an hour the cure generally succeeds in spite of it. The patient should remain absolutely still after his dose, as the best chance of avoiding sickness. Drugs are almost useless to prevent it. Citric acid and ice are the most effectual remedies. If the sickness immediately follows the exhibition of the decoction, as it does sometimes, the extract of male fern must be tried at once, in moderate doses, every hour or half-hour. We may here add a word or two drawn from Dr. Bettelheim's experience, as to the effect of these tapeworm "cures" on the patient, and as to the contra-indications to them. Vomiting has been already mentioned as a troublesome sequela, and severe diarrhœa, faintness, cramps in the calves and forearms, may be caused by the medicine; or merely a feeling of weariness, sleepiness, numbness, or oppression of the chest may be experienced. In all cases, however, the patients have completely recovered either by the evening of the same day, or at any rate by the next morning. A plan of treatment like the above is contra-indicated by the concomitant presence of ulcer of the stomach, or of any other severe gastric derangement not dependent on the tapeworm itself, and by severe illness, and all febrile affections. Wet-nurses, convalescents, and menstruating or pregnant women should not be subjected to a "cure" unless, as rarely happens, the worm is a great annoyance to them; nor should very old people undergo it, nor children who have been already treated once unsuccessfully and have proved very refractory. No "cure" should ever be begun unless the medical attendant has had definite proof that tapeworm segments have been passed by his patients within a day or two. He should preside over the cure himself, and make absolutely certain of the presence of the worm's head in the dejections. This, by following Bettelheim's method, involves little loss of time. The worm often comes away with the first motion, about an hour and a half after injection of the decoction. If the bowels are not moved as soon as that, a dose of castor oil may be given. Should the first "cure" fail, it may be repeated in two or three days' time, but this is rarely necessary.—*Med. Times and Gaz.*, Oct. 4, 1879.

Death caused by an Ascaris Lumbricoides in the Upper Air-Passages.

Dr. Furst has published, in the *Wiener Med. Wochenschrift* for 1879, a summary of twenty-four cases of immigration of ascarides into the upper air-passages, from which we quote the following case: A girl, aged 4, had been received into Professor Billroth's hospital for congenital ectopy of the bladder. One evening, she suddenly had an attack of suffocation. Thinking that she must have aspirated some foreign body, the author explored the larynx without any result, and then performed tracheotomy, as she had suddenly ceased to breathe. As no canula was at hand, a male catheter was introduced into the wound, but met with some obstacle. It was drawn out and then pushed in again, when it went in quite smoothly. Artificial respiration was then resorted to, but the child died. Two hours after death, a female live ascaris, about nine-tenths of an inch long, was seen hanging out of the nostril. It is evident that the catheter had been prevented from penetrating into the trachea by the worm, which probably then changed its position and wandered upwards. The *post-mortem* examination revealed a male *Ascaris lumbricoides*, nearly half an inch long, in the jejunum. The author gives the following clinical sketch of the *modus operandi* of the immigration of ascarides into the air-passages. As far as concerns the etiology, vomiting, fever (as a high temperature always quickens considerably the movements of the ascarides), purgatives, abstinence from food—may all be looked upon as favouring the immigration into the larynx. Children are more liable to it than adults. The symptoms are not always the same; sometimes the worm sticks in the glottis, and such cases naturally invariably end fatally within a very short time. At other times, the worm passes the rima glottidis, when the patient dies of bronchitis in the course of a few days. The majority of the cases that have hitherto come under observation belong to the first class. The patients become aphonic and asphyctic; occasionally these symptoms are preceded by hoarseness during a few moments. Then comes a stage of great excitement, anxiety, and profuse sweating, which is followed by loss of consciousness. In cases of the second class, the patients feel much better after the worm has passed through the rima glottidis; but they do not recover their voice, and complain of pain in the anterior part of the throat. The diagnosis is very difficult and uncertain. In young children, the fits of suffocation are often completely masked by convulsions. If laryngitis, croup, diphtheria, spasm and œdema of the glottis, perforation of cold abscesses, or affections of the lungs may be with safety excluded, one is justified in supposing that a foreign body has penetrated into the pharynx or larynx. Then if it can be proved with certainty that no foreign body has been aspirated, and, moreover, if the patients are troubled with ascarides, it may be concluded that the foreign body in the trachea is an ascaris. This supposition will be rendered still more plausible if, after the worm has passed beyond the glottis, the asphyxia decrease and the trachea becomes painful. If it be not possible to extract the worm, either with the hand or by emetics and expectorants, tracheotomy must be performed. It has been resorted to in three cases out of the twenty-five, but each time with fatal issue. At the necropsy, the worm is generally found in the place where it evidently resided, judging by the symptoms during the patient's life. These places generally bear marks of inflammation, which have been produced either by the mere presence of the foreign body, or by its movements, or else by its peculiar irritating properties. The mucous membrane is red and injected, covered with bloody froth, and in some places eroded. Pneumonia of a circumscribed portion of the lung is sometimes caused by the protracted presence of the worm in one of the bronchi. The inflammatory symptoms are manifested principally in the arytenoid cartilages, as they are much affected by the migrations of this worm from the œsophagus. The usual symptoms of death by asphyxia are also always met with, as well as a certain number of ascarides in the intestines.— *British Medical Journal*, Sept. 27, 1879.

Bright's Disease.

At the late International Medical Congress at Amsterdam the following note was presented by Professor SEMMOLA. It comprised a *résumé* of the communication made by Dr. Semmola to the International Medical Congress at Brussels, on different kinds of albuminuria, which was reported in the *Gaz. Méd. de Paris*,

1875; also a résumé of further researches made by Professor Semmola, and communicated to the present International Congress of Amsterdam. He said:—

1. My first researches were conducted as far back as 1850. I think that I was the first to show the classic influence of alimentation and diet on the quantity of urine which is secreted in Bright's disease. (See Jaccoud's work, *Manual of Internal Pathology*, Paris, 1873, vol. ii. p. 685.)

2. This influence of diet on the increase or decrease of albumen in the urine, according to the greater or less amount of nitrogenous elements in the food, was the starting-point of all my researches. It led me to conclude that it is absolutely necessary to direct our attention not only to the renal lesions, but also to general nutritive disturbances in which the albuminoid bodies are either not at all, or only imperfectly, assimilated and consumed.

3. This idea, which I have always endeavoured to develop concerning the etiology of Bright's disease, has, to my mind, been confirmed by another classical fact which has hitherto remained completely misunderstood. I mean the considerable and progressive decrease in the quantity of urea which is formed in the organism from the first stages of chronic Bright's disease. (See note at the end.)

4. I have always insisted on this classical and fundamental point, and have repeatedly made communications on the subject to the Academie de Médecine of Paris and to that of Naples. I especially insisted on this point in Paris (1867) and in Brussels (1875), and have convinced myself by the study of three hundred clinical cases that the decrease of the urea from the first stages of Bright's disease is owing to a defective oxidation of the albuminoid matter.

I find that in all books authors speak of the defective excretion of urea; but I have never yet been able to discover anything about the defective formation, which I am sure is a principal and fundamental fact: a characteristic phenomenon of Bright's disease.

5. It is caused by the total or partial absence of the cutaneous functions. In consequence of this suppression of the respiratory functions of the skin, two chemical disturbances arise, which are closely united from a biological point of view—viz., the alteration and inassimilability of the albuminoid substances, and defective combustion, *i. e.*, a decrease in the formation of urea. I leave it to experimental physiology to elucidate the part which the cutaneous functions play in the assimilation and combustion of albuminoid matter. I shall merely restrict myself to pointing out the intimate connection between the two which has been revealed by the pathological condition; and I foresee that it will lead to the solution of a problem which is of great importance both for physiology and pathology. As I have said before, this is a capital and fundamental fact, that can be repeated experimentally by varnishing to a certain extent the skin of a dog. It proves that the real chronic Bright's disease is a general affection, a defect in nutrition, in which the changes that take place in the kidneys (beginning with hyperæmia and ending with cirrhosis and atrophy) do not constitute the primary cause of the principal symptoms of the disease. Physiology fails to explain by what mechanism a morbid process, which has been confined to the kidneys from its very beginning—that is to say, at an epoch when they still fulfil their duty as purifying apparatus—could have had any effect on the production of urea, and thus act on the whole system. I beg my honourable colleagues to direct their attention to this point of renal pathology. It is a most important point, that has hitherto remained unobserved, because it can only be studied in the first stages of the disease, which only in rare cases come under notice in hospitals and clinics.

In all other cases of albuminuria that are not instances of true Bright's albuminuria, this decrease in the production of urea which runs parallel with the increase of albumen is not found. Consequently, it is of the highest importance to distinguish carefully between these different kinds of albuminuria so as to avoid a mistake that is often made and is dangerous, both clinically and therapeutically. The cause, the mechanism, the evolution, in short the *cachet* of the general chemical process of nutrition, combined with the decrease in the production of urea, and last but not least, the pathological alterations which take place in both kidneys, form a harmonious *tout ensemble*, which is always the same and constitutes the true type of Bright's disease properly so called.

6. The decrease in the production of urea which takes place in other cases of albuminuria is not in any way connected with albuminous filtration. It may exist in some cases, but varies very much according to the particular disease that has produced the albuminuria, and at the same time created disturbances in the general process of nutrition (heart disease, etc.). Here, however, the decrease in the production of urea is not connected with the phenomena of albuminuria; its progress takes place in an entirely different way, and it is not till the last stage of those various affections, *i. e.*, when the kidneys have become thoroughly diseased (amyloid degeneration, etc.), that a very considerable decrease takes place in the secretion of urea in the urine for want of filtration. It results from the aforesaid, that this decrease is a mechanical effect which gives rise to the accumulation of urea in the blood with all its fatal consequences.

7. In Bright's disease, properly so called, there are two causes for the decrease of urea in the urine. In the first stage of the disease the decrease is caused by incomplete combustion, a defective nutrition, combined with changes in the albuminoid, which is gradually developed, owing to the suppression of the cutaneous functions. Later on, that is to say, when the affection of the kidneys has reached a further stage, a second decrease of the urea takes place in the urine owing to defective secretion.

8. The tendency to exaggerate the anatomical point of view of the affection has led to neglect of the chemical and more universal aspect of it, thereby producing a conclusion which is perfectly paradoxical so far as regards scientific pathology, *i. e.*, "clinical unity" and "anatomical plurality" (large white kidney, amyloid degeneration, etc.). It is impossible to perceive in what way a general alteration, which shows itself with the same symptoms and consequently must spring from the same causes, can bring forth different anatomical results. The final difference in the lesion shows that there has been a difference in the nature of the preceding morbid processes. By combining all the conditions under which the symptoms constituting the clinical aspect can exist, the successive evolution of the process, and the constant relation between it and its special causes, we shall succeed in reconstructing the edifice of true Bright's disease, and in distinguishing it as a peculiar pathological species which differs from other species of albuminuria.

9. The passage of albumen into the urine may take place through the three physiological factors that preside over the renal functions; viz., *a.* chemical constitution of the blood; *b.* degree of pressure; *c.* condition of the histological elements of the filtering apparatus.

10 Consequently, there are three classes of albuminuria, viz.: *a.* dyscrasic albuminuria (caused by excess of presence of the albuminoid constituents of the blood or by the alterations occurring in them); *b.* mechanical albuminuria; *c.* albuminuria produced by irritation, *i. e.*, by some local histological cause existing in the kidney. This species is caused by the irritating effect of all the agents that penetrate into the kidney, either from without or that are formed in the organism.

Diagram of Classes of Albuminuria.

Variety of Albuminuria.	Causes.	Condition of Kidney.	Urea in the Blood and in the Urine.
a. Chemical conditions of the blood. Dyscrasic albuminuria.	Presence in the blood of an excess of albumen, owing to the diet.	Normal kidney.	The maximum of urea, sulphates, and phosphates contained in the urine varies according to the individual.
	An excess of the albuminoid constituents of the blood, owing to defective combustion.	Irritative hyperæmia, which is more or less intense according to the organ or apparatus whose functions are affected: the cutaneous surface, lung-disease, etc.	Progressive decrease of the urea in the urine, though it is not accumulated in the blood. Want of production.
	A change in the chemical constitution of the albuminoid bodies which circulate in the blood. This change renders them incapable of being assimilated, etc. (cachexia).	Fatty degeneration. Amyloid degeneration.	*Idem* owing to the gravity of the case which causes cachexia.
b. Degree of pressure of the current of the blood. Mechanical albuminuria.	Various neuropathic affections having a direct or indirect effect on the vaso-motor system.	More or less transitory renal stasis.	Amount of urea almost normal, within the limits of physiological oscillations.
	Pregnancy: in short, every kind of pressure exercised on the inferior vena cava or the renal veins.	*Idem*, but occasionally the stasis becomes permanent, owing to the general conditions of the organism, or to organic causes that produce the lesion.	Amount of urea not depending on the pregnancy or the organic causes that produce pressure.
	Cardiac diseases that have not yet reached the stage of compensation.	Persistent stasis, cyanosed kidney, cardiac kidney.	Amount of urea decreases in proportion as the affection of the heart increases.
c. Histological alterations take place in the kidneys. Irritative albuminuria.	All the irritative processes in the kidneys, from their first stage up to complete nephritis.	All the anatomical consequences of inflammation beginning at the first stage, and the degeneration of the different kinds of epithelium up to renal sclerosis and atrophy.	Amount of urea is normal or slightly increased, owing to the fever (acute stage).
	The albuminous filtration is more or less considerable in proportion to the rôle and effect that the inflamed elements may have in the mechanism of the urinary filtration.		Decrease in the production of urea, though there is no increase in the blood, owing to general disturbances in the combustion.
		This depends on the special histological seat of the inflammation and its particular course.	Decrease in the production of urea owing to defective filtration, and consequently accumulation in the blood.

These three classes of albuminuria are closely related to different anatomical conditions of the kidney. If each one of these three conditions have been only transitory, the anatomical structure of the kidney may remain in its normal condition and no albuminous filtration will take place (as in series a). In other cases it may be modified by a transitory morbid process, and then regain its previous normal condition. Finally, if the pathological condition that has given rise to albuminuria be persistent, the anatomical structure of the kidney undergoes a gradual change, and causes a particular defined lesion which differs according to the cause, and is in relation with each of the three factors which have modified the renal function so as to determine the filtration of the albumen. This will be more clearly shown by reference to the above diagram.

If we look at the clinical history of Bright's disease properly so called, with a view to classifying it among one of the preceding groups, we find that it cannot be placed exclusively under either of these heads. It is a mixed albuminuria, i. e., its complicated etiological mechanism contains all the other three mechanisms of the other classes of albuminuria, and it forms a pathological specialty that has nothing whatever to do with the other classes of this affection. Analyzed in this way, Bright's disease reveals a constant evolution and a harmonious relation between the nature of the cause, the etiological mechanism, the chemical and anatomical alterations, and the clinical form. The *modus operandi* is as follows: a. The gradual effect of moist cold on the skin. The gradual action of moist cold is the only cause of true Bright's disease. Other causes produce albuminuria and lesions that differ from the true type. b. The respiratory functions of the skin decrease gradually, till they cease completely. Their absence gives rise to the following disturbances, which appear at the same time, and are closely connected with each other: 1. Cutaneous ischæmia; 2. Accumulation in the blood of matter which ought to have been excreted by the skin; 3. Alteration of the albuminoid bodies, so that those which originate from the peptones are not assimilated; 4. Decrease in the combustion of the albuminoid bodies, and consequently in the production of urea.

If it were possible to arrest for a moment the harmonic solidarity of all the organs and apparatus, the kidneys might be excluded, as it were, for a certain time, during which first period they would be in no way connected with the true pathology of Bright's disease. But a similar abstraction can only be conceived in order to show that the anatomical lesions of the kidney are only a secondary process, and do not constitute the initial lesion of Bright's disease.

The four aforesaid causes produce the following effects upon the kidneys:—

1. Renal hyperæmia. (Increase of pressure.)

2. Irritating effect of the said hyperæmia, owing to the accumulation in the blood of substances that ought to have been excreted by the skin, and its dyscrasic condition in consequence. (Inflammatory effects.)

3. Elimination of the albumen through the kidneys (the depuratory organs *par excellence*), because, the constitution of the albumen being altered, owing to paralysis of the respiratory functions of the skin, it has become an useless substance, and may almost be regarded as a foreign body in the organism.

4. The progressive decrease of the urea in the urine is the result of the decrease in its production.

Thus we have a twofold series of effects, that are closely connected with and complement each other, i. e., 1. The general nutritive lesions, with all their characteristic consequences; 2. The anatomical development of the inflammatory process of both kidneys, from the first stage to the last. These two series of disturbances constitute Bright's disease, or Bright's albuminuria.

The differences which exist in the clinical form of other albuminurias, and the combination of various final anatomical lesions existing in the same kidneys, depend entirely on special etiological causes (alcoholism, gout, syphilis, etc.), which modify the general condition of the individual, and consequently add to the renal lesions that are peculiar to the inflammatory chronic process other elements that vary according to either the nature of the alteration, or to their seat being more or less confined to one or the other of the different histological elements which constitute the kidneys. It follows that true Bright's disease has nothing to do either anatomically or clinically with any of the other species of albuminuria, whatever may be their origin. I also believe that it is not at all true, though affirmed by several authors, that Bright's disease may be caused by alcoholism, gout, etc. Whether considered from a scientific or a practical point of view, this appears false; because it is a well-known clinical fact that there is such a thing as albuminuria caused by gout, alcohol, etc. And each one of these affections corresponds to general nutritive alterations, which differ not only according to their etiology, but also are represented anatomically by considerable alterations in the kidneys, which in some cases are due to nephritis. These alterations, however, vary very much, so far as regards the affected spots; sometimes they are restricted to one kidney alone (embolic nephritis, pyelitis, stone, syphilis, etc.). If both kidneys be affected, we always find that there exists a secondary disease, in which predominates an inflammatory condition either of the elements of the parenchyma or of the connective tissue, and which is either due to the irritating effect of a foreign body that passes through the kidneys (alcohol, resinous matter, cantharides, etc.), or to the presence of a deposit of urea that irritates and inflames the neighbouring tissues. In cases of degeneration (fatty, amyloid, etc.), the kidneys are as much affected as many other organs (liver, spleen, etc.); and it would be absurd to regard these cases as belonging to Bright's disease. I repeat it again and again, I am justified by my researches in concluding that true Bright's disease is a constant clinical type, a pathological specialty the characteristics of which *intra vitam* are albuminuria, absence of urea, cachexia, and a peculiar anasarca. The anatomical changes consist in an inflammatory process of both kidneys, which progresses very slowly, and extends gradually over the whole of the organ. These changes, however, are not quite the same for all the elements of the kidneys, but differ according to the physiological part that each element plays in the discharge of the renal function. All the exclusively histological localizations that have been held up as special forms of Bright's disease do not exist in nature in an isolated condition. They may only predominate in some elements that are more affected than others. That this renal affection is always a bilateral one I have already mentioned. I believe that this constant bilaterality constitutes, from an anatomical point of view, the peculiar characteristic or the final control of true Bright's disease, thereby adding a new proof to what I have said, viz., that there exists a profound universal deterioration of the system, which precedes the outbreak of the disease, and must necessarily act on both kidneys at the same time, though with characteristic slowness.

According to my opinion, this constant renal alteration ought alone to be called "Bright's kidney," for the following reasons, viz.: It is caused by the effect of moist cold; the dyscrasia following it is of a particular nature; and finally it develops gradually from a simply hyperæmic state till it becomes atrophic. It may occasionally reveal somewhat different symptoms; but this only takes place when another cause (alcoholism, gout, etc.) is superadded to the action of moist cold. Thus we have a series of complicated effects, both in the clinical form *intra vitam*, and in the nature of the alterations which are found in the kidneys and other organs after death.

POSTSCRIPT.—It is true, that several authors acknowledge that there is a more or less considerable decrease in the production of urea from the onset of the disease; but they ascribe it to the anæmic condition of the patient. Now, this decrease in the section of urea dates from the first time that albumen appeared in the urine, that is, from an epoch when it is impossible to admit that an anæmic condition has been induced by the want of albumen in the blood.

I repeat it, and it is a most important fact, the decrease in the combustion of the albuminoid bodies is caused by an alteration which takes place in them after the suppression of the cutaneous respiration. The decrease of urea and elimination of albumen are two facts which are closely connected with each other from the first moment of the affection.—*British Med. Journal*, Sept. 27, 1879.

Mycosis in Man.

Dr. J. ISRAEL has published, in Virchow's *Archiv*, Band lxxiv., a recent observation on this affection. The patient, a woman aged 39, had had, ten months previously, a fall, striking her chest against the bed-post. Three months later, she had pains in her limbs and daily repeated attacks of fever, and entered the hospital in a state of great prostration. Her appearance was suggestive of general septic infection. The whole body was covered with marks and scars of old abscesses as well as with fresh ones; there was a particularly large one on the left side of the thorax opening into a fistula, through which large quantities of fetid pus were voided. The pus was of a green colour, and covered with small yellow corpuscles of the size of a pin's head or larger, which could easily be taken out with the point of a needle. When examined under the microscope, these corpuscles were found to consist in the centre of a thick mass of fungi, from which long thread-like appendices issued, branching off in every direction. The space between the latter was filled up with pus corpuscles which had undergone fatty degeneration. There were three different classes of fungi: delicate threads of mycelium, micrococci, and a third form pear-shaped and brilliant. The same constituents were found in the other abscesses. The woman died three weeks after entering the hospital. The necropsy showed that the large abscess in the thorax communicated with a large cavity filled with pus in the left lung. The liver, spleen, intestines, and kidneys, were covered with purulent foci varying in size from a lentil to an apple, and containing the same species of fungi. In the kidneys the convoluted tubes were found in several places to contain embola formed of fungi, though there was as yet no suppuration in their vicinity. There could be no doubt as to the abscesses having been caused directly by the parasites, although it was impossible in this case to find the primary source of infection. The author, however, has offered the following hypothesis: He had noticed before that, in cases of caries of the teeth which had given rise to abscesses in the gums, the pus of the abscesses contained fungi which bore a close resemblance to those which he discovered in this case of pyæmia or septicæmia; this led him to suppose that the patient in question had a carious tooth, whence the fungi might have been aspirated into the lungs, and by some chance into a pneumonic focus which had been caused by the fall, and ultimately have been carried through the system through the medium of the circulation.—*British Medical Journal*, Sept. 27, 1879.

Surgery.

Influence of the Atmosphere on Operations.

Professor Trélat, in a recent clinical lecture, drew attention to some facts which seem to prove that the condition of the atmosphere exercises a certain influence on traumatic lesions. He pointed out that the older surgeons, and even those of a more recent period, always put off operations that were not very urgent till certain seasons of the year. Roux, who operated on a large number of cataracts, always kept the operations for the spring; and this tradition was probably based on observation. All the cases of acute septicæmia observed by M. Trélat occurred in June, in hot and sultry days. One case was that of a very healthy woman in her fourth confinement, all her labours having been remarkably easy. She began to feel ill on the first day, and was worse the second day; on the third day the case was hopeless, and she died on the fourth. At the same time, M. Trélat had been operating upon a man suffering from cataract in both eyes. Everything had gone well, and the operation promised to be a very successful one, but during the night the patient suffered much from the heat, and was very restless; the eye grew worse, and a few days later suppuration set in. Another case was that of a woman in whom he operated for cancer of the breast during June. For the first four days all seemed to go well, but on the night of the fifth day the patient suffered intensely from the sultry weather, and passed a bad night. Next day the sore presented a very bad aspect; the patient became slightly delirious towards night, erysipelas set in, and she died on the eighth day. A patient was suffering from multiple fistula and stricture of the rectum. M. Trélat performed rectotomy by means of the galvano-caustic loop. The patient did not loose a drop of blood, and the operation was done under excellent conditions. Towards night, however, he felt a little restless; during the night a profuse fetid diarrhœa set in; and the temperature in the axilla rose to 102.2°. These symptoms grew worse the following days; and on the fourth day the patient died of acute septicæmia. Three years ago, M. Trélat was called upon to perform perineoraphy on a young woman in whom the perineum had been lacerated during parturition. The operation had, against his will, been put off from April to June. It happened to take place on a very hot day, but everything went on so smoothly that the best hopes were entertained, till at night, when the patient became flushed, restless, and died of septicæmia four days after the operation. M. Trélat particularly insisted on these facts, because, although they all took place in different years, yet they occurred at the same season and under the same atmospherical conditions. He also compared them to the remarkable results at which M. Davaine has recently arrived. He found that a very small quantity of septicæmic blood, when injected under the skin of guinea-pigs, caused death within thirty hours if the operation was performed in summer at a temperature of 82° to 86° Fahrenheit. When the experiment was repeated in the winter, not one of the animals died as long as the dose remained the same as in summer. M. Davaine concluded from his experiments that the two-thousandth part of the septicæmie matter needed in the cold season was sufficient to kill a guinea-pig in summer. Another curious fact is, that the seasons seem to exercise no influence on rabbits, who die both in winter and in summer from the same doses. However, M. Trélat thought it impossible not to trace a connection between these experiments and the facts which he had observed, especially as the latter were not isolated. Thus M. Cauchois, in his thesis on the etiology of hemorrhages, mentions that a few years ago, on a very hot day in June, more than a hundred cases of secondary hemorrhage were observed in the hospitals in Paris. It must be added that M. Cauchois shares M. Verneuil's views as to the fact that most secondary hemorrhages are of septicæmic origin. It may therefore be admitted that in these cases we meet with septicæmic accidents which have been caused by the influence of the temperature. M. Tiélat has also shown long ago that the seasons have a great influence on the mortality in the lying-in hospitals. The practical conclusions which may be drawn from these facts is that, so far as operations are concerned, the summer season itself is not to be dreaded so much as the sultry days, or the great heat which often comes on suddenly and unexpectedly. Therefore, it will be safer to avoid as much as possible performing any operations during this season.—*British Med. Journal*, Sept. 6, 1879.

Retro-Pharyngeal Sarcoma.

At the late meeting of the American Laryngological Society (*St. Louis Med. and Surg. Journal*, Sept. 1879), Dr. F. I. KNIGHT, of Boston, reported the following rare case which he saw in consultation with Dr. CHAS. HOMANS.

A lady, thirty-six years of age, had had a hacking cough much of the time for four or five years, and hawking and raising of phlegm, with sensation of strangling in the morning, for the previous year. She had been subject to sore throat, always pronounced "tonsillitis," for four years. She had been subject to dyspnœa on exertion for two years.

In January, 1877, having taken a severe cold, the cough was much exaggerated, she became debilitated, and was ordered to go South, and while at the South she first experienced a feeling of suffocation at night, which was several times afterwards repeated. She had had some dysphagia, but no pain in the throat. The voice was not affected. There was no family history of tumours. On her way North the throat was examined laryngoscopically for the first time by Dr. Samuel Johnston, of Baltimore, who discovered the large neoplasm, to be described. As the patient was unable to remain in Baltimore long enough to submit to treatment from Dr. Johnston, she returned to Boston, and came under my observation, as before mentioned.

On examination of the pharynx in the ordinary manner, nothing abnormal could be seen. With the laryngeal mirror a large tumour came into view, almost completely filling the upper cavity of the larynx. It was round, pretty smooth, rather soft to the touch, covered with congested mucous membrane, in which several vessels could be distinctly traced, and attached broadly in its posterior portion, exactly where, whether to the arytenoid region of the larynx, or to the posterior wall of the lower pharynx, could not be determined at that time. There was no ulceration, and no enlargement of lymphatic glands.

The situation of the growth was almost identical with that of a "fibroid" reported by Voltolini,[1] which also had a broad attachment, and which apparently did not recur after removal by the galvano-caustic loop. It was decided to remove the growth in our case by the same means, after preliminary tracheotomy. Dr. Homans did tracheotomy the next day. Instead of using a simple platinum loop, I had the extremity of Mackenzie's "guarded wheel écraseur" fitted to Voltolini's handle, and protected on the posterior aspect by hard rubber.

Nothing could have been more satisfactory than the operation, the growth being quickly removed close to the pharyngeal wall with but little hemorrhage. It was of the size of a small horse-chestnut, encapsulated, and its cut surface about half an inch in diameter. We had hoped that, notwithstanding its rather

---

[1] Die Anwendung der Galvanocaustik, etc., 2 te., Aufl. Wien, 1872, p. 226.

soft feeling, it, like Voltolini's, would prove a fibroid. But it was pronounced by Dr. Cutler, and afterwards by Dr. Fitz. to be a small-celled spindle sarcoma.

Dr. Cutler's report of the microscopic appearance of the growth after hardening was as follows: "It was composed of moderately small spindle cells, lying singly in a very small amount of intercellular substance. These cells were in many places arranged in bundles, which intersected each other in all directions. In a few places large numbers of round cells of medium size were found, and occasionally star-shaped cells were met with. By far the greater number of cells were spindle shaped. The growth was a spindle-celled sarcoma.

In a few days it had grown to almost its original size, and so it has remained for nearly two years, with a certain amount of shrinkage in the past year. The patient has continued to wear the tracheal tube, has had no difficulty in swallowing, and in fact little annoyance but from the tube, excepting occasional aphonia when she has taken cold. Ordinarily the voice has been very good when the tracheal tube was stopped. Both Dr. Homans and myself felt that it was better to wait for some urgent symptoms before undertaking a radical operation, which would not only endanger life, but involve the risk (with a growth so liable to recur, if life were saved), of increasing the discomfort of the patient.

I have been interested in looking up records of similar pharyngeal growths, and have made brief abstracts of cases found.

Arnott[1] reports the case of a female nineteen years of age, who had noticed a lump in her throat three months. Dysphagia and impaired speech (from obstructed nares) had existed longer. On examination a round tumor was seen filling the upper part of the pharynx, arising apparently from below. It was of the color of the surrounding parts, but its surface was rough and irregular. It was somewhat movable, and seemed attached by a pedicle to the posterior wall of the pharynx below the sight. It was removed by ligature and evulsion. There was no hemorrhage, and the patient left the hospital in a few days. Examination of the tumor showed it to be of the "size of a green walnut," with a narrow pedicle. The surface was mulberry-like. On section it was firm, of uniform character, and "corresponded with what has been called albuminous sarcoma." On microscopic examination there were found caudate, nucleated cells, and a thin layer of epithelial cells on its surface,

Arnott[2] reports another case, that of a female forty years of age, who received a blow from a man's fist on the left jaw. She suffered pain in this region till at the end of a month a suffocative attack at night led to the discovery of a small hard swelling of about the size of a hazelnut in the left fauces. When seen by Arnott a year and a half later she complained of attacks of suffocation and dyspnœa. She could swallow liquids or fine solids without difficulty. On examination a globular tumor projected from left of fauces two-thirds across the isthmus. It was smooth, covered by mucous membrane, had a broad base, and no trace of tonsil or posterior pillar of palate could be seen on the affected side. The mucous membrane was divided, then a layer of muscular fibre, and then a cyst, the walls of which having been pushed back, a ligature was applied, the growth sloughed, and potassa fusa was applied to the stump. At the end of three months the only evidences of disease were granulations arising from the projecting and everted edge of the contracted cyst. This was also called "albuminous sarcoma."

Busch[3] gives three cases of what he designates as "retro-pharyngeal tumors." The first case was that of a man thirty-four years of age, whose voice had been modified for fourteen years. He had had dyspnœa for six months, with suffoca-

---

[1] Lond. Med. Gaz., N. S. 1845, vol. I, p. 530.   [2] L. c. p. 531.
[3] Annalen des Charite-Krankenhausse, Jahrg. 8, hft. 1, p. 89, 1857.

tive attacks in his sleep. There is no mention of dysphagia. On examination a tumor as large as a goose egg, with somewhat uneven surface, was found to extend from the level of the epiglottis up behind the soft palate, which it pushed forward on the left side. The mucous membrane covering it was livid. The tonsil was seen in the middle of the tumor. The external carotid, having been seen to be dilated, was tied previous to the operation on the growth, in order to diminish hemorrhage. An incision was made in the soft palate and mucous membrane covering the tumor, which was then peeled out with the fingers and scalpel. It was so large that, notwithstanding the patient's front teeth were missing, it was with difficulty brought out of the mouth. It was pronounced a sarcoma in a firm connective tissue capsule. There was severe pharyngeal inflammation for a few days, after which the patient was declared cured.

The second case was that of a man aged seventy, who had felt a small bunch in his throat a year before admission to the hospital. On admission deglutition was very difficult. On examination a tumor was found coming from the left, which filled the pharynx. On swallowing, the food passed through a narrow ulcerated slit. The operation was the same as in the preceding case. The carotid, however, was not ligated. As the ulceration prevented the preservation of the mucous membrane intact, a crucial incision was made in it. Severe inflammation followed for a few days. The patient was discharged cured. The growth was stated to be morphologically like that of the preceding case, but with a great preponderance of unripe cell elements.

The third case reported by Busch is that of a man whose age is not stated, who had a growth of the size of a hen's egg, apparently similar to the preceding, arising from the right side of the pharynx. It did not cause him sufficient annoyance to induce him to consent to an operation.

Röser[1] reports a case which occurred in his practice in 1826. The patient's symptoms were dysphagia of six months' duration, extreme at time of examination, dangerous dyspnœa, nausea and vomiting, and hoarseness.

On ordinary inspection of the fauces nothing could be seen, but when the patient was made to gag, a smooth, soft, round, bright-red tumor came into view. By the finger it seemed to be attached to the posterior wall of the pharynx, low down. It was torn out with the forceps used for extracting stone from the bladder. It was two and a half inches in diameter, and covered with mucous membrane except at the place of attachment, which was as large as a "thaler." It looked like an ordinary fibroid, but was softer and more elastic. The microscope was not then in use. As the growth was softer and more elastic than an ordinary fibroid, it may have been sarcomatous. There was very slight hemorrhage after the operation.

Wagner (of Königsberg)[2] gives the case of a man twenty-six years of age, who for twelve years had noticed a small, movable tumor under left angle of lower jaw. This began to increase rather rapidly, and at the same time pain on swallowing was experienced. Some swelling was detected about the left tonsil. About seven months after this he was admitted to the hospital. Ten days before his admission severe pain running up the ear and brow had set in, and the growth increased so much that he could not swallow solids at all, and he swallowed liquids with difficulty. Several times suffocative attacks had occurred in his sleep, and quite considerable hemorrhage. On examination, there was found a tumor of the size of a pigeon's egg under left angle of jaw; inside, the left arches of palate

[1] Medicinisches Correspondenz-blatt des Würtembergischen Aerzlitchen Vereins. bd. 29, S. 161, 1869.

[2] Deutsche Klinik, 1861, p. 61.

and pharyngeal wall were pushed out by a tumor, which was elastic, firm, and smooth, and which seemed strongly attached to the bony wall of the pharynx. The left tonsil was not seen; where it naturally would have been. the tumor was ulcerated. The arcus palato-glossus and mucous membrane of the pharynx were incised, and the tumor dissected out with the fingers, scalpel, etc. It was apparently thoroughly removed. The external tumor was found to be quite distinct. and also removed. The inner growth arose from the retropharyngeal connective tissue of the spine, which was itself sound ; it was of the size of the fist and extended from the base of the skull to the hyoid bone. It was pronounced a soft sarcoma. There was a speedy recurrence, frequent partial removal for relief, and finally death, five months after entrance, the patient having been choked by a piece of the tumor falling upon the larynx.

Larondelle[1] reports the case of a woman, twenty-eight years of age, who had had dysphagia sixteen months. For six months she had been unable to swallow solids, and had sometimes regurgitated liquids through the nose. Her voice was thick, hoarse, and nasal. She had severe paroxysms of cough, and suffocation ; also nausea and vomiting. On examination a large, round, smooth tumor, reddish in color, was seen filling the space between the base of the tongue, the posterior wall of the pharynx, and the larynx. It was attached by a short pedicle (about two centimetres thick) to the left lateral wall of the pharynx below the tonsil. It was removed by the écraseur. It measured seven by four centimetres. It consisted of connective and elastic tissue surrounding alveoli filled with fat cells. Adipose tissue very abundant. It was called sarcoma. Perhaps it should have been classed rather as a lipoma. The pedicle seemed to consist only of mucous membrane. There had been no recurrence at the end of seven months.

Rosenbach[2] reports a case operated on by Prof Baum, of Göttingen. A man, forty-five years of age, was sent to the hospital on account of dysphagia and dyspnœa, with suffocative attacks, which had been developing for six months or more. He had coughed up a piece of new growth half as large as the terminal phalanx of the thumb. On examination of fauces, a large reddish tumor was discovered. It was soft, and its surface was uneven, presenting large and small projections. It was adherent to the pharynx on the right of the hyoid bone. It measured one centimetre horizontally, more vertically. There was no lymphatic enlargement. Tracheotomy was done. Trendelenburg's canula was introduced, and then sub-hyoid pharyngotomy was performed. The growth was torn away with the fingers, and ligatures put upon the adherent stump. The growth was pronounced a round-cell sarcoma. The patient was discharged cured, but there was no subsequent report from him.

Venturini[3] reports the case of a boy, twelve years of age. A year before seen by V. he had had otorrhœa of the right ear, and some enlargement of the cervical glands of the same side. At this time he had some inconvenience in swallowing. When seen by Venturini he was emaciated and livid, and had three large glandular swellings of the right side of the neck.

On examination of the fauces, a large tumor was discovered attached by an extremely short pedicle to the right posterior pillar of the pharynx. On moving it, the patient was threatened with suffocation. It was removed at once by the largest sized wire écraseur. There was but little hemorrhage. The wound healed quickly, and the glandular swellings diminished. The tumor was of the size of a small apple, of a rosy color, nearly round, smooth, elastic, and of a soft, meaty consistence.

[1] Bulletin L'Academie de Médicine de Belgique III Serie. Tome 4, p. 183. 1870.
[2] Berliner Klinische Wochenschrift, 1875, p. 519.
[3] L'Ippocratico, 1871, vol. xix., 3 Ser. p. 39.

On section it had a lardaceous appearance, and on scraping, a reddish-yellow fluid was exuded. The vessels from the pedicle ramified freely in the tumour. On microscopic examination were found uniform round cells, and a granular protoplasm nucleated and contained in a scanty amorphous cellular substance. All the surface of the tumour was covered with pavement epithelium, which connected with it by fibres of connective tissue. The patient was seen three months after the operation. He looked well, and there was no appearance of the reproduction of the tumour. There was still a trace of the operation, and the right tonsil was somewhat atrophied.

Billroth[1] reports the removal by the écraseur of a fibro-sarcomatous polypus of the size of a hen's egg from the pharynx. After nearly six years the patient, who was a man of fifty years, showed no signs of recurrence.

Mr. Syme[2] reports a case of "Fibrous Tumor of the Fauces," which Busch thinks was more likely a retiopharyngeal sarcoma. A man, of thirty-eight years, presented himself, having a large, round, firm tumour, somewhat nodulated, in the region of the left tonsil. It was somewhat movable. It was as large as a small potato. The mucous membrane was divided, and the growth dissected out. The subsequent history as to recurrence is not given.

J. Carreno[3] gives the history of a rather remarkable case. Twenty-one years before his visit to Carreno, the patient, who was then a man of forty-nine years, had noticed in his throat one day while shaving himself a few bodies resembling hairs or straws, which terminated at their ends in little balls about the size of lentils. When Carreno saw him he had terrible dyspnœa, and dysphagia, and stated that during an attack of vomiting, a tumour had protruded an inch outside of the mouth. On examination two large tumors were seen in the fauces, pedicellated, one measuring four inches in length and two and one-half inches in thickness, with a thick and long pedicle, the other three and one-half inches in length, and more than four inches in thickness, its pedicle being thick and short, somewhat resembling cartilage. Their color was that of raw meat. The first was ligated and removed with the bistoury. The second was ligated and removed with a lithotome and curved scissors. The removal of these two revealed the existence of two other pedicellated growths rising from the bases of the preceding ones, and these were ligated several days after. There was much hemorrhage, and danger of suffocation from loosening of a ligature, which was controlled by another. The growths were pronounced fibro-cellular, and contained in their interior a tallow-like, concrete substance, ramified with vessels. They originated in the submucous cellular tissue.

Dr. S. H. Chapman[4] reports a case of "Sarcoma of the Inferior Constrictor of the Pharynx and Inlet of the Œsophagus," which, however, belonged more to the œsophagus, than pharynx, and so does not much concern us at the present time.

Dr. Busch,[5] of Bonn, at the sixth Congress of the Society of German Surgeons, showed several retropharyngeal tumors, one of them a lipoma of the size of the fist. He said that these tumors were rather frequently met with in Bonn. They were lymphomata, fibromata, sarcomata, and rarely lipomata; generally encapsuled and easily removed. Their removal was, however, rendered difficult by the previous employment of electrolysis, the galvano-cautery, etc., which led to the destruction of the capsular limitation and to cicatricial induration between

---

[1] Langenbeck's Archiv für Klinische Chirurgie, Bd. x S. 207.
[2] London Lancet, 1856, vol. i. p. 51.
[3] Observacions de cuatro polipos situados en el centro de la faringe Decados de Med. y Cir. pract. Madrid, 1828, vol. xvii. p. 217.
[4] The American Journal of the Medical Sciences, Oct. 1877.
[5] London Medical Record, Oct. 15, 1877.

the sheath of the carotid, the bucco-pharyngeal fascia, and the surface of the tumor rendering the separation of the latter from the carotid a difficult and dangerous proceeding.

Dr. Cohen[1] refers to a case of round-celled sarcoma of the pharynx, with extensive attachments, which had been attending the surgical clinics at Jefferson Medical College for two years, in which tracheotomy was performed, and large masses removed from time to time for several months subsequently; Dr. Cohen remarks that it is quite likely that the patient would not have survived as long had a radical operation been performed when he first presented himself.

It will suggest itself at once that the facts given do not warrant us in classifying all of these cases under the head of sarcomata. There is no doubt, further more, that other cases which have been recorded as fibroid, belong to this class. It will be seen also that the nature of the growths, properly classed as sarcomata, is very varied, so that we cannot rightly compare even them for the sake of making any deduction as to their clinical history, i. e., time and mode of development, liability to recurrence, etc.

They are interesting, because rare, and with reference to practical procedure. The pedicellated growths are easily disposed of, by ligature, écraseur, snare, scissors, etc. Those with a broad base are much harder to deal with. Few would be as successful as Rösei, in tearing out such a growth with forceps. If it is situated high in the pharynx, it may be dissected out, as in the cases of Arnott (2d case), Busch, and Wagner. But even in this case, if the tumor is situated at the side of the pharynx, which, as we have seen, occurs in many instances, the proximity of the carotid artery and its branches may render the operation very embarrassing, and we have seen that Busch took the precaution to tie the external carotid in one case, having found that vessel to be dilated.

If the growth of the broad base is situated low in the pharynx, there seems little hope from any operation but pharyngotomy. Sub-hyoid pharyngotomy has been performed twice for the removal of tumors of the pharynx, once successfully and once with a fatal result. The fatal case was the well-known one of Langenbeck,[2] in which the operation was performed for the removal of a fibroma of the size of a Bordsdorff apple. Twenty-five ligatures were required, there was much hemorrhage, both primary and secondary, and the patient died on the second day after the operation. The successful case was that of Prof. Baum, reported by Rosenbach, to which we have already made reference.

The propriety of performing this serious and certainly hazardous operation, upon a growth liable to recurrence, before urgent symptoms demand it, I should like to make the subject of discussion by the Association.

Dr. COHEN, of Philadelphia, said that where the symptoms produced by sarcoma were not urgent or could be combated by other resources and the growth was not rapid, he would certainly hesitate in advising an operation. Where symptoms were urgent, or where the growth was rapid, the propriety of evulsion would depend upon a sufficiently limited extent of implication of tissue to justify a hope that the entire mass might be eradicated, with a certain amount of surrounding tissue apparently still healthy. When the attachments of a sarcoma were sufficiently extensive to preclude a hope of removing the entire mass, the only justification for operative procedure would be the desire of averting immediate or approximately immediate death, and thus prolonging the life of the individual for a brief period.

Dr. LEFFERTS, of New York, said Dr. Knight has raised the question as to the propriety of removing the tumor in his case, through an incision in the thyro-

[1] Diseases of the Throat and Nasal Passages, 2d Ed. New York, 1879, p. 252.
[2] Allg. Central-Zeit, 1870, January 29.

hyoid space, and as to the danger of the operation. "Sub-hyoidean laryngotomy," or perhaps more correctly, "pharyngotomy," has been performed but
once in this country, and then by myself, for the removal of a foreign body impacted for years in the upper parts of the larynx. No accident happened during
it, no difficulty was met with, and I should, from my experience of operations in
general, regard this as a very easy and safe one, as far as the operation itself is
concerned. The results, as recorded when it has been performed for the removal
of pharyngeal growths, have not been favourable; results attributable, I believe,
to the nature and location of the neoplasm, and not to the operation *per se*.
Whether or not it be indicated in Dr. Knight's case, which the nature and location
of the tumour make a serious one, that is to say, whether he will be able to best
reach the growth by this means, he must judge, his repeated examinations fitting
him for the task. He has other operations at his disposal, such as dividing the
lower jaw in the median line and separating its halves, a procedure which increases most markedly our opportunity of reaching and working in the lower
pharynx. Finally the question presents itself whether we shall, in such a case as
that of Dr. Knight's (the growth being known to be sarcomatous, and therefore,
in all probability recurrent in its nature, the symptoms not at this date urgent,
certainly not dangerous, and the operation which best perhaps presents a feasible
hope of reaching the mass so thoroughly as to remove it entire, being one where
results, when undertaken for this particular purpose, are not good) operate at
once or wait for more urgent surgical indications. Here, again, individual experience and peculiar views must decide. I should be in favour, in the *present
instance*, of waiting at least for a time if my interpretations of the signs as I have
heard them read be correct; but there is likewise much to be said, probably, by
the advocates of early extirpation.

—

Enterotomy.

At a meeting of the Medical Society in Marburg, held last year, Professor
Röser related (*Berliner Klin. Wochenschrift*, June 30th) a case of enterotomy
for stricture of the bowel, and made some remarks on the subject. In the case
referred to, the sloughing and separation of an invaginated portion of the small
intestine was preceded by the formation of a cicatricial stricture; and an attempt
was made to relieve the patient by enterotomy and the division of the cicatricial
tissue. The patient died of peritonitis. Dr. Röser concluded his communication
with the following remarks on enterotomy. 1. After opening the abdomen, the
best plan, as a rule, is to introduce the hand as far as the cæcum, and thence
trace upwards from the lower end of the small intestine; provided, of course,
that there be no reason for believing the stricture to be in the large intestine or in
any other special part. 2. When it is necessary to make an incision into and to
empty a portion of intestine that is very full, it is safest to draw this portion of
bowel forward and to lay the patient on his side, in order to prevent the escape
of the contents of the bowel into the abdominal cavity. 3. In these circumstances, the escape of the intestinal contents is at first impetuous and explosive,
afterwards intermittent. The first outflow is caused by elastic resiliency; that
which follows, by the peristaltic action of the muscles. 4. In order to restrain
this secondary escape, it may be of advantage to apply provisional sutures to the
opening in the bowel, and to fasten the intestine by the threads to the wound in
the abdominal wall. After this, the sutures may be loosened when necessary,
and the contents of the intestine allowed to escape. This is in accordance with
Nélaton's teaching, that in many cases only a temporary opening of the bowel is
necessary, and not a permanent artificial anus. 5. A temporary opening of the

intestine is especially indicated in cases of valvular stricture, where the portion of bowel above the valve is much distended.   6. Among the forms of intestinal stricture demanding enterotomy, that which follows local peritonitis after the successful application of taxis for hernia merits special attention. If, some weeks after the reduction of a strangulated hernia, symptoms of ileus appear, there is reason for suspecting the presence of inflammatory adhesion and contraction. This suspicion was confirmed in a case which had recently occurred, in which enterotomy was performed, too late, on the twenty-third day after symptoms of obstruction appeared.—*British Med. Journal*, Sept. 27, 1879.

Cancer of the Rectum treated by Excision.

Mr. W. H. Cripps, Surgeon to the Great Northern Hospital, reports (*British Med. Journal*, Sept. 27, 1879) two cases of cancer of rectum in which excision was successfully performed. He says excision of the diseased portion of the bowel for cancer of the rectum has, since the time of Lisfranc, found much favour with foreign surgeons. The operation had, however, fallen into disfavour in this country, and has only been revived during the past few years. In cases judiciously selected, this method of treatment is of the greatest value, both as regards relief from suffering and prolongation of life. But to suppose that it is applicable as a method of treatment in every case of rectal cancer is as unreasonable as the assumption that cancer should be removed by operation whersoever situated. The operation cannot be considered in any way to rival or supersede colotomy, for as a rule it is applicable as a method of treatment for cases in which colotomy is scarcely admissible. Colotomy is a most valuable operation when the cancer is situated higher and causes obstruction or intense pain; while, on the other hand, for excision to be successful, the disease must strictly be confined to the lower part of the bowel. No operation should be attempted unless there be a fair prospect of removing the whole disease; and this cannot be done unless the upper limit of the growth be fairly defined with the finger. Again, the disease must not have invaded the neighbouring tissues to an extent likely to interfere with its complete extirpation. Rather longer portions of the bowel can be removed from women than from men. As a rule, however, four inches is the limit that can be safely removed.

Rectal cancer almost invariably begins as an adenoid deposit in the submucous tissue. The microscopic structure of the growth bears an exact resemblance to the natural Lieberkühn's follicles in the superjacent tissue. If the growth be slow, this resemblance in structure is very perfect; if more rapid, the general plan of an adenoid structure can be traced, but neither the epithelium lining the follicles nor the retiform tissue in the interfollicular spaces can be well defined; there is no regularity in the shape of the epithelial cells, indeed, they rather resemble strips of protoplasm with longitudinal striæ than distinct columnar cells. Again, the fibrous element of the retiform tissue is represented by spindle- or oat-shaped cells rather than by the distinct fibrous structure found in more chronic growths. At first, the mucous membrane is intact over the growth, which can be felt like a foreign body beneath it. It commonly spreads as a thin layer between the mucous and muscular coats; and not uncommonly will the disease thus spread under several square inches of mucous membrane, while its thickness scarcely exceeds one-fifth of an inch; at other times, but more rarely, the disease increases more rapidly in thickness, pushing the mucous membrane inwards, producing a distinct tumour in the cavity of the bowel. Sooner or later, ulcerative action sets in. At first, the mucous membrane over the centre of the mass is destroyed, exposing the subjacent growth. Now, if this subjacent growth exist as a thin layer, it also is destroyed by a continuation of the ulcerative action. It thus not uncommonly happens that a deep ulceration is produced, the base of which, towards its centre, is composed of the remains of the hypertrophied muscular coat blended into a dense cicatricial tissue with the fibrous element of the part. Towards the margin of the ulcer the growth is again apparent, forming a prominent overlapping margin. From points of this margin fungating masses will in time project into the rectum, in which condition the disease usually comes under observation. Space, unfortunately, forbids a minute description of the histological appearance of these growths. The so-called scirrhous, medullary, and epithelial growths are merely "conditions" of adenoid disease, and can be accounted for by taking into consideration the time the growth has been in existence and the particular tissue affected. The appearance commonly regarded as indicative of scirrhous, medullary, or epithelial disease can all be found in various parts of the same specimen.

My experience of the operation of extirpation is too limited to express an opinion as to the rate of mortality likely to follow; and in the majority of cases the operation has been too recently performed to judge of the liability of the disease to return. In five cases in which I have operated, no death has occurred; while in nine operations at which I have assisted, two deaths resulted: one from peritonitis, one from collapse. The best result with which I am conversant is a case in which a well-marked cylindrical cancer was removed nearly three years ago; the patient still remains perfectly well. The two following cases may perhaps serve as examples of what may be expected from the operation. A successful and an unsuccessful case have purposely been selected as illustrations.

CASE I.—A. M., aged 61, being kindly sent to me by my friend Mr. Doran, was admitted under my care at the Great Northern Hospital in April, 1878. She was very thin and emaciated, and for some time had been unable to follow her occupation as a laundress. For more than a year, she had suffered discomfort in the rectum, and had lost blood from time to time, a mucopurent discharge being persistent. During the last few months, the pain had greatly increased, her nights were sleepless, she was tormented with a constant desire to go to stool. She suffered from alternate attacks of diarrhœa and constipation, and could not retain her feces when liquid. On examination with the finger, commencing just within the anus and extending upwards a couple of inches, an ulcerated mass of cancer was felt. This did not completely surround the bowel, a small portion of the anterior wall being free. The patient being placed under chloroform, and in the lithotomy position, a curved bistoury guided by the finger was introduced into the rectum, the point then thrust through the posterior rectal wall, and made to emerge at the tip of coccyx; the tissues intervening between this point and the margin of the anus were cut through with a clean sweep. The sides of the wound being held apart by the folds of the nates being forcibly drawn outwards, a semilunar incision was made at right angles to the first cut; this, the second incision, was just within the margin of the anus, and extending completely round the bowel, while in depth the point of the knife was carried well into the fat of the ischiorectal fossa. The lateral and posterior attachments of the bowel were separated by the forefinger with the sparing use of the cautery and the knife. The dissection of the anterior wall was made more carefully and entirely with the knife. The free portion of the bowel was now seized and drawn down with a moderate amount of force, and cut through just above the disease by means of the benzoline cautery. No attempt was made to draw down the bowel, neither were any sutures or dressings used. The patient made a quick recovery, leaving the hospital in three weeks free from all pain, with some control over her motions, and her general health greatly improved. Three months after this operation, she had complete control over the motions, except when she had diarrhœa, at which times her linen would be a little stained. She complained of no pain, but of a slight itching sensation. Upon examining the parts, there was found a small rose-coloured elevation, of the size of a split pea, upon the anterior margin of the mucous membrane. This was snipped off pretty freely with scissors. Since then, the patient has been frequently seen; she suffers no pain whatever, has not the slightest symptom of any return of the disease, and states that she enjoys better health now (June 16th, 1879) than for many years past. When she has diarrhœa, however, she has to wear a diaper; this causes her no inconvenience. It is now one year and two months since the operation.

CASE II.—A. G., aged 54, a small emaciated woman, with a dark complexion, was admitted into the Royal Free Hospital, November 7th. She has six children living, in good health, and has lost none. The father and mother died at advanced ages; there was no family history of tumours or phthisis. The patient had good health until two years ago, but has always been subject to constipation, for which she has taken castor-oil in considerable quantities. Two years ago, she began to suffer from pain and a feeling of weight in the rectum. Eighteen months ago, she first noticed a discharge of blood and mucus from the bowel. During the past year, she has lost flesh rapidly, having formerly been very stout. She had been for some months in a London hospital, but obtained no relief. Her sufferings were very great; she had lost control over the sphincter, the feces escaping without her knowledge. Upon examination, the parts were found to be very tender, with a growth extending almost to the margin of the anus, about which the skin was œdematous and excoriated. A considerable mass of the disease occupied the lower three inches of the bowel, taking the form of a large irregular ulceration with a hard base and fungating margins. At one point, the disease extended somewhat higher than three inches. The recto-vaginal septum was implicated, but the mucous membrane on the vaginal aspect appeared sound.

Considering the length of time that the disease had existed, and the extent to which it had encroached on the anterior wall of the rectum, it did not seem a very favourable case for operation. The patient, however, was exceedingly anxious to have an attempt made to remove it, having been recommended to consult me for that purpose by my friend and colleague Mr. Macready. The operation was performed in an almost precisely similar manner to that in the previous case. There was no difficulty in detaching the bowel from its posterior and lateral connections, but it required some time and caution to dissect through the recto-vaginal septum; this was done by keeping as near as possible to the mucous lining of the vagina; but even at the time there appeared a suspicion that the disease at this part had not been thoroughly removed. Whilst detaching the upper anterior part of the rectum, the peritoneal membrane was distinctly seen. The diseased bowel being drawn down was cut off with a wire écraseur a little more than three inches from the anus. Upon detaching the portion, a small coil of intestine was seen in the upper part of the wound, but it was not known at what period of the operation the peritoneal membrane had been opened. The knuckle of the bowel was gently pressed up by the finger and disappeared. The wound was treated in the ordinary way, without any dressings or sutures, and kept thoroughly free from all discharge by frequent syringing with warm carbolic lotion. The patient never had a symptom of peritonitis, recovered quickly, and left the hospital at the end of the month free from all pain and much stronger and more comfortable than she had been for a long time; she had no pain on passing her motions, over which she had a fair amount of control. She appeared well and comfortable for three months; she then complained of some irritation about the part, and upon examination a soft fungating nodule could be felt springing from the anterior wall of the rectum. She suffered little pain. A month later, the disease had greatly increased, forming a considerable fungoid mass, blocking up the lower end of the rectum, causing some difficulty in passing her motions. It did not seem advisable to make any further attempt by a cutting operation; but, acting as other surgeons have done in these circumstances, as far as I could with the finger-nail and a blunt gouge, I scraped away the cauliflower mass down to its hard base. The growth was very soft, but did not bleed much. She was greatly relieved by this proceeding, the motions again passing with comparative ease. A rapid return is, however, inevitable.

The microscopic appearances of the growths in both the cases narrated were identical, the difference in result being probably due to a more thorough extirpation being possible in the first case.

Various methods of performing the operation of extirpation of the rectum have been practised. The ligature, the cautery, and the *écraseur*, either singly or combined, all have their advocates. From my own experience, however, these various adjuncts appear to be unnecessary. They greatly prolong and complicate an otherwise simple operation. The free and quick use of the knife for all the first part of the operation, reserving the wire *écraseur* for the final separation of the bowel, appears to me to be the best plan of operating. The preliminary posterior incision of Denonvilliers is of the greatest service during the operation, and completely unfolds the parts and gives plenty of room for dealing with hemorrhage, while it subsequently affords perfect drainage to the wound. No good results from the drawing down of the cut bowel and stitching it to the cutaneous surface; the stitches always give way, and until they do so are a source of danger, by allowing matter to be pent up behind the bowel. I use no dressing nor sutures of any kind whatever; for anything that hinders free discharge is deleterious, owing to the near neighbourhood of the peritoneum and the rapid decomposition that takes place in this part of the body. A frequent gentle and thorough syringing, so as to prevent any accumulation in the wound, is probably the best way of preventing peritonitis.

—

Abscess communicating with the Bladder and Rectum.

M. DUCHAUSSAY related the following interesting fact at the meeting of a medical society (*France Médicale*, No. 103): A gentleman aged 55 was suddenly taken ill during the night with excruciating pains in the abdomen, vomiting, and rigor. One physician diagnosed an attack of nephritic colic; another attributed it to gravel, but did not find any on passing a sound into the bladder. M. Duchaussay thought that there might be some obstruction in the intestine not far from the bladder, and attempted to remove it by an injection of water. Three days later the patient passed pus with his urine and through the rectum. This showed that an abscess must have burst somewhere between the bladder and the rectum, communicating with both. Fecal matter was passed through the bladder. Disinfecting injections of a solution of carbolic acid, etc., were daily used, and the patient bathed frequently. The inflammation was not considerable. There was myelitis, and gradually the feces ceased to be passed through the bladder, except in particles not larger than grains of sand. The patient could take a little food, was sent to a watering-place, and soon recovered. This happened eighteen months before the case was reported. For the last three months the communication between the bladder and rectum had been closed; the patient passed a little glairy matter from the bowels; and, two weeks ago, two pieces of fleshy matter escaped. On examining the intestine it was found that there existed a contraction about five inches from the bladder; the mucous membrane was red and inflamed. The patient was taking twice a week an injection of two pints of water, and a small one daily. To prevent the intestine from being entirely closed, a bougie No. 30 had first been used, and afterwards an ordinary rectal bougie had been inserted into the intestine to keep it open. The cause of this affection is not clear; but in all probability it was due to some small foreign body which had in some way become imbedded into the mucous membrane, thereby causing an abscess.—*British Med. Journal*, Oct. 4, 1879.

Symmetrical Gangrene of the Extremities.

Under this title Dr. J. COLLINS WARREN reports (*Boston Med. and Surg. Journal*, January 16, 1879) the following very interesting case with remarks:—

The patient, a rather feeble person, and of spare habit, presented herself at the Massachusetts General Hospital on June 27, 1878, with a peculiar condition of the tips of all the fingers and toes. She was a native of Scotland, a weaver, unmarried, and twenty-five years of age. The affection was of a character to arrest the attention at the first glance, and differed from anything hitherto observed by many who saw her. The seat of the disease was confined to the pulps of the fingers and toes, usually extending around the edge of the nail to the opposite side. Another striking feature was the colour. The borders of the affected area resembled the semi-transparent purple of a hot-house grape. There was none of the reddish tint seen in intestine at certain stages of strangulation. The lightest shades were always essentially purple in colour. As the centre was approached the hue deepened, until it was difficult to determine whether or not the tissue had assumed the characteristic colour and condition of gangrene. The patient did not complain of much pain, but had become totally incapacitated for work, owing to the condition of her hands. She had been in good health until four months previously, at which time she suffered from frequent nose-bleed during two weeks. Soon after this she noticed that the tips of the fingers and toes became red. She had had a slight cough, and had been losing flesh, but emaciation was not marked, nor did she consider herself as suffering in any other way than from the condition of her hands and feet. An examination of the chest showed some dullness and râles at the apex of the left lung; the heart sounds were normal. There was no history of syphilis. A more careful examination of the finger tips disclosed the fact that the centres of one or two of these purple patches were gangrenous. This became more marked in a few days, and eventually several dry, black eschars, the largest of which was not larger than a ten-cent piece, came away, leaving a healthy granulating surface. In no case was the bone affected. The treatment consisted of the administration of iron internally, good food, and the application of resin cerate to the parts. On July 16th the record states that all but two of the fingers have had sloughs, and these two look as if they were going to slough. The toes have recovered their normal appearance. Although no complaint of pain was made, the patient always held the hands in an elevated position, as if this gave most relief. On August 15th, when she left the hospital, the granulating surfaces had all healed, and the fingers presented a red and shriveled look. There was no gangrene of the toes. The general condition at time of discharge was good.

Symmetrical gangrene, as described by Maurice Raynaud,[1] is a variety of dry gangrene characterized by two prominent features, the absence of any anatomical lesions of the bloodvessels, and the symmetrical development of the disease in the two halves of the body. It may be found in both upper or both lower extremities, or in all four; occasionally the ears and nose are affected.

The earliest change seen in the diseased part is that termed "local syncope," a condition, however, perfectly compatible with health. The patient, generally a woman, perceives a pallor and coldness of one or more fingers. This change,

---

[1] Nouveau Dictionnaire de Médecine et de Chirurgie, vol. xv., page 636.

known as "dead fingers," may last a few minutes or several hours. The exciting cause appears to be an exposure to cold, although but a slight lowering of the
temperature is sufficient to produce it. It appears, however, sometimes to be
emotional in character. The skin is apparently deprived of its blood, and its
temperature is below normal. The reaction which follows is frequently quite
painful. A more advanced condition is known as "local asphyxia;" the pallor
is followed by a cyanotic colour of varying degrees of intensity. On pressure the
colour disappears, and returns very slowly, showing great feebleness in the circulation. The pain is now almost continuous, and in some cases may be compared
to that accompanying onychia, particularly when reaction sets in. This condition resembles that seen in cyanosis, but in the latter affection we find organic
disease, and there is no pain and no reaction. The clubbed finger nails of
cyanosis, erroneously attributed by some authors to phthisis alone, is never seen
in local asphyxia.

In the outset the disease is sometimes mistaken for chilblains, but the deepening colour and pain soon set all doubt at rest. The fingers may become almost
black, and minute blisters appear, particularly on the little finger, later on others,
and situated generally at the extremity. The blister becomes filled with a sero-
purulent fluid, breaks, and leaves an excoriation which may remain several days.
The colour begins now to return, the excoriation heals, and a little conical tubercle is left just beneath the edge of the nail. The improvement is, however, only
temporary; the same changes recur, and may be repeated during a period lasting
one or two years. In an advanced stage the ends of the fingers are covered with
a number of little white scars, the skin is indurated, and they have a thin, sharp,
withered look, as if they had been pinched in a vice, and had preserved the shape
thus given to them.

If gangrene sets in at once there are no vesicles. A third or one-half of the
ungual phalanx may come away.

During the height of the disease the growth of the nail stops temporarily, and
the interval is subsequently indicated by a grooved depression in the nail. The
disease has not been known to terminate in gangrene when situated in the nose
and ears. Cases cited below show this statement to be incorrect. Beyond the
severe pain, upon which Raynaud dwells as a very striking symptom, we find
little else to notice in the condition of the patient. No cardiac disease is found;
possibly a slight souffle may be heard, but not of sufficient strength to indicate
valvular lesions.

In well-marked cases the disease occupies a period varying from a few days to
a month in developing; it remains at its height for about ten days, and convalescence may be fully established at the end of from three weeks to several months.
In no case does death seem to have been caused directly by the disease. Occasionally, after one or two attacks, the condition becomes a more or less permanent one, and the part affected is continually cold and torpid. At times the skin
of the back of the hands and fingers becomes thickened and rigid, and is not
movable on the subjacent parts. The fingers are held semiflexed and anchylosed. The two affections most likely to be mistaken for this disease are chilblains and senile gangrene. In the former we are not likely to find all extremities
affected at an unusual time of the year. Senile gangrene is rarely bilateral; it
extends much further; the characteristic condition of the arteries is usually present. It is easily distinguished from cyanosis depending on cardiac disease.
Owing to the predominance of pain it has sometimes been mistaken for gout.
The prognosis is favourable. If the stage of gangrene develops itself at the end
of a week or ten days, it is probable that a complete recovery will follow the
separation of the eschars. If, however, the disease does not reach this point,

but comes and goes, there is danger that it will settle down into a chronic condition.

In four-fifths of the cases the disease is found in women. In the great majority of cases it occurs between the ages of eighteen and thirty years.

As a low temperature is an exciting cause, we find it most frequently on the approach of the winter months. Not infrequently there may be premonitory symptoms for one or two winters, with return to health in the summer season, and a final termination in gangrene. In one case the disease was found to coexist with diabetes mellitus. Ordinarily we observe no special predisposing cause in the general condition of the patient. How are we to explain these peculiar changes in the vascular system?

It is well known that the quantity of blood in circulation in a given spot increases when the capillary walls are relaxed; that it is diminished, on the other hand, when the walls are contracted; and, when the cavity of the vessel is obliterated, the blood disappears from the part.

This *algidity* may terminate in reaction,—relaxation of the muscular fibres of the vessels,—or it may continue until gangrene takes place.

Symmetrical gangrene begins with a spasm of the capillaries, which may go back as far as arteries of considerable size (radial pulse).

In the simplest cases of spasm we have the "*dead finger*," a passing condition in which the circulation is re-established after a more or less painful period of reaction. This is "*local syncope.*" The veins probably are contracted also. The phrase "*local asphyxia*" is used to denote a more advanced condition. The reaction which follows spasm is here incomplete. The veins having the smallest amount of muscular fibres relax first, and the venous blood flows back into the capillaries, but stops here, as the arteries are still contracted. It will be noticed that this change does not bring about that deep colour which we find in an extremity which has been violently constricted. In the latter case the venous blood is forced back into the arterial system. As in local asphyxia, the reflux stops at the capillaries. There is more transparency in the colour, a mixture of cyanosis and pallor, as it were. There is, of course, as the result of this condition, a certain amount of stagnation in the large veins, and sometimes slight œdema.

On one occasion the author had actual proof of this arterial spasm in a case where temporary disturbance of vision occurred during the attacks; the ophthalmoscope showed a well-marked contraction of the central artery of the retina.

If the condition becomes a permanent one gangrene occurs. Other portions of the body are affected, of course, with this muscular spasm of the arteries, but it is only in the extremities which present a large surface in proportion to their calibre, and consequently readily lose heat, that the conditions are favourable for the death of the part.

How shall we explain the symmetrical character of the lesions? A consideration of the mode of origin, distribution, and action of the vaso-motor nerves may serve to throw light upon this point.

We now no longer look upon the sympathetic as an independent nerve having no communication with the cord. We find filaments of this nerve emerging from the cord in the anterior branches. The same phenomena of congestion which Bernard obtained by division of the sympathetic above the superior cervical ganglion can be obtained by certain sections in different portions of the cord. Experiments have shown that there exists a series of genuine vaso-motor centres ranged up and down the spinal axis. The actual origin of the vaso-motor nerves of given portions of the body has been determined with tolerable accuracy. Starting from this point the fibres in question follow those of the grand sympathetic, or, as in some cases, the cerebro-spinal trunks.

An experiment by Brown-Séquard throws light upon the special action of this
nerve which is brought into play in the present disease. A section of one-half
of the spinal cord near the medulla is followed by a paralysis of the bloodvessels
on the same side, and a permanent spasmodic contraction of the on the opposite
side. There are also corresponding changes of temperature. It is clear that the
vaso-motors on the divided side, having lost connection with their point of origin,
are paralyzed, and a passive congestion takes place in the corresponding part,
while the lesion of the cord, being a source of irritation to the adjacent vaso-
motors of the opposite side, produces a spasmodic contraction of the vessels on
that side. It is known that an intimate communication exists between the fibres
of this set of nerves as well as in the fibres of nerves of voluntary motion.

Let us suppose now that an irritation is created in the central portion of the
cord ; it is easy to conceive how it would reach the vaso-motor fibres symmetrically disposed on each side of the spinal axis. If this excitation becomes permanent, if it go to the point of tetanization, the phenomena of algidity occur ; one
step further and the symmetrical gangrene is produced.

In order to understand how this algidity may be confined to one set of vessels
—for instance, those of the upper or lower limbs—it is only necessary to suppose
a central irritation occurring at a single point in the cord from which the vaso-
motors of the particular region affected happen to emerge. This may be limited
to a single finger of each side. It now remains to determine the way in which
this irritation is supposed to act. The vaso-motor nerves are affected not only
by direct irritation, as in the experiment alluded to, but may be also susceptible
to reflex action. An example of this is the contraction of the vessels of one hand
when the other is suddenly plunged into very cold water. A similar action is
the sudden pallor produced in the face by severe pain inflicted upon some distant
point. In the disease we are now considering it is probable that a similar chain of
events takes place.

Inasmuch as this disease appears after confinements, or may show itself periodically at the menstrual epoch, it is but reasonable to suppose that the reflex irritation may take its origin in the uterus. In a later article[1] on the subject, Raynaud defines this disease as " a neurosis characterized by an exaggeration of the
excito-motor power of the cord presiding over the vaso-motor nerves," and he
advises the application of "constant descending currents" to the spine. The
excito-motor power of the cord is thus weakened, and the reflex contractions of
the vessels are in consequence diminished.

A consideration of the reflex origin of this vaso-motor disturbance would suggest occasional phenomena, such, for instance, as are observed in traumatic inflammations, supposed to be due to reflex actions brought about by irritation of
the cerebro-spinal nerves, and, in fact, we find this to be the case. Vulpian[2] has
described, in connection with the above disease, a symmetrical congestion of the
extremities which he considers as similar to the congestion of the skin seen in
certain cases of neuralgia. It is possible, he thinks, that a sort of symmetrical
neurosis of the peripheral nerves of the extremities occurs, causing by reflex
action dilatation of the vessels of the parts. In using the term vaso-motor neurosis we must accept it in this sense only. The seat of the pain is in the sensitive nerves or in the tissue occupied by them, and the dilatation of the vessels
secondary. Based on this mode of action is the theory of one observer[3] that
neuralgia of the ilio-lumbar nerve brings on congestion of the uterus and its
appendages, and that metrorrhagia and leucorrhœa may thus be produced.

---

[1] Archives Générales de Médecine, 1874, page 5.
[2] Leçons sur l'Appareil vaso-moteur. Vulpian. Paris. 1875.
[3] Cahier des Nevroses vaso-motrices (Archives Générales de Médecine, 1863).

This view is certainly plausible, and the supposition had already occurred to me whether certain fleeting and capricious uterine pains, brought on frequently by emotional perturbations solely, might not be explained by a vaso-motor disturbance of the uterine vessels. The changes seen in the tongue in Dr. Mills's case, presently to be mentioned, are suggestive of such possibilities.

Billroth[1] had seen but one case:—

"A young, very anæmic man, without apparent cause, had first gangrene of the tip of the nose, then of both feet. After suffering for months he died; as on the patient, so on the cadaver, I could find nothing morbid beyond the excessive, inexplicable anæmia." Recently Dr. Medopil[2] reported a case under Billroth's care. The patient was a female, nineteen years of age. She was first seen by Dr. Billroth in September of the year previous. She then noticed that the fingers became dead and pale after washing in cold water. The tip of the index finger of the right hand soon became very painful, remained hard for a time, and finally mortified. The gangrene terminated in necrosis of the ungual phalanx. The middle finger of the same hand was next attacked with inflammation resembling paronychia, which did not extend beyond the radial half of the bed of the nail, and terminated in the exfoliation of small, dry, parchment-like crusts. A year later the index and middle fingers of the left hand were similarly affected, at this time all the fingers of each hand being cold and pale.

Dr. Charles K. Mills[3] reports a case of "vaso-motor and trophic affection of the fingers," which evidently belongs to the chronic and recurrent form of "local asphyxia," and which he believes to be unique.

Under the head of Chronic Vaso-Motor Hyper-Irritation, Dr. A. M. Hamilton[4] describes an affection due to a "temporary spasm of the muscular coats of the small vessels of some limited spot, the site being usually a part of the hand." "The peculiarity is the limited blanching and coldness coming on without assignable cause, and finally subsiding, to reappear perhaps after an uncertain interval," the fingers being chiefly affected—"evidently our local syncope."

Dr. S. Weir Mitchell[5] gives a collection of cases illustrating a form of vaso-motor neurosis of the extremities, to which he gives the name erythromelegia.

A case quoted from Sir James Paget is evidently one of local asphyxia, brought on apparently by excessive use of cold baths.

It is quite evident that many of Dr. Mitchell's cases belong to the group of "local asphyxias," and that some are, on the other hand, "symmetrical congestions."

Dr. T. A. McBride reported last spring to the New York Neurological Society a case of digiti mortui, and is the only American writer whom I have consulted who distinctly recognizes the relation of this affection to local asphyxia and symmetrical gangrene.

Fischer[6] report two cases, one following intermittent fever. The cheeks, ears, and nose were the parts affected. The patient was a man forty-two years old. A second case followed an attack of typhus fever. The writer gives several theories as to the origin of the disease, but inclines to that of Raynaud. A case, reported by Christian, of gangrene of both feet, following malarial fever, deserves to be mentioned in connection with these cases.

Drs. Stewart and Holton[7] report a case of symmetrical gangrene caused by

[1] Wiener medizinische Wochenschrift, No. 23, 1878.
[2] Surgical Pathology, page 302, first American edition.
[3] American Journal of the Medical Sciences, October, 1878.
[4] New York Medical Journal, 1874.
[5] American Journal of the Medical Sciences, July, 1878.
[6] Medical Record, May 11, 1878.
[7] Chicago Medical Journal and Examiner, December, 1878.

chronic endarteritis, the name being obtained from Ziemssen's Cyclopædia, vol. vi. page 383, evidently not due to local asphyxia.

Dr. Bernard Henry describes a case of idiopathic gangrene of the four extremities, which, if not a specimen of the symmetrical disease of Raynaud, certainly merits mention here:—

The patient was a widow, forty-two years of age. She had led a very dissipated life, and had been treated for syphilis ; had given birth to nine children, besides having had frequent abortions intentionally produced. She first noticed after washing a stinging sensation in the hands and feet. They were rendered more painful by scratching, and soon assumed a dusky red colour. When first seen the disease was thought to be purpura. In the course of two weeks the affected parts turned black and mortified. These were the hands and forearms for about a third of their length, and the lower third of the legs and feet. The tip of the nose and the skin over both patellæ and the cartilages of the ears were of a dark hue, and finally sloughed. There was great aversion to warm coverings. The gangrenous portions became mummified. The parts separated, and some were removed, but the patient died at the end of about two months. At the autopsy it was thought that there was some tendency to fatty degeneration of the heart, and apparently mitral stenosis ; there was commencing cirrhosis.

A case very similar to this is reported by Dr. Thomas Camp[1] under the title, A Case of Supposed Ergotism. Both legs, all the fingers, the ala of the right nostril, and the upper part of the helix of each ear were the parts affected. There was a peculiar eruption coming and going on different parts of the body. The patient eventually recovered. Ergotism was suspected in both of these cases, but there was no direct proof.

Midwifery and Gynæcology.

When should we Ligature the Umbilical Cord?

A great deal has been written of late on this subject—the question being first raised by Dr. BUDIN, in a series of communications to Le Progrès Médicale, for 1875–76, in which he stated that tying the cord immediately after the child is born deprives the latter on an average of 92.6 grammes of blood (more than 6 ozs.), which it would have received from the placenta if the ligature had not been applied till two or three minutes after all pulsation in the cord had ceased and the child had cried out lustily. Since the publication of these papers a number of experiments have been made with a view of proving or disproving this very startling statement. SCHÜCKING published the results of his observations in the Berlin. klin. Wochenschrift, 1877, Nos. 1 and 2. He thinks that almost the whole of the blood that is contained in the fœtal portion of the placenta is finally transferred to the infant. This transfer is effected by the pressure exerted by the uterine contractions on the placenta, and not by any aspiration caused by the expansion of the infant's thorax. Schücking estimated the amount of this "reserve blood," as he calls it, at from 70–150 grammes, and the time requisite for the transfer varies from a few to several minutes, being determined by the amount of pressure exerted by the uterus on the placenta. Hence he argues that unless we wish to deprive the fœtus of nearly half of its proper supply of blood, we will

    [1] British and Foreign Medico-Chirurgical Review, July, 1855.

not apply the ligature to the cord till some minutes after the child has been born; and if from any cause, such as *post-partum* hemorrhage, we are obliged to press off the placenta immediately, we should afterwards expel the blood from the placenta into the fœtal circulation by compressing the placenta between the hands. He, at the same time, protests most strongly against treating the asphyxia of newly-born children by allowing some hemorrhage to take place from the cord. This treatment is founded on the supposition that the child's heart is already too full of blood, which must be got rid of at any price. This idea, Schücking thinks, is quite erroneous. For at the first effort the infant makes at inspiration the blood rushes into the thorax, leaving the extra-thoracic vessels empty. These are then filled by the "reserve blood" from the placenta; now if we tie the cord quickly and cut off this supply of "reserve blood," while at the same time we allow some blood to escape from the fœtal end of the cord, we increase the anæmia, and, as a natural consequence, lessen the reflex sensibility of the medulla. As a direct consequence of this the intervals between each effort at inspiration become longer, till finally the breathing stops altogether.

With a view of still further elucidating this question, Prof. ZWEIFEL, of Erlangen, instituted a number of experiments to determine the exact quantity of blood that remains behind in the placenta when the cord is tied immediately after birth, and also when some minutes are allowed to elapse before the ligature is applied.[1] He found that the average quantity of blood remaining behind in the placenta when the cord was tied immediately after the child was born, was 192 grammes; but when the cord was not ligatured till after the placenta had been pressed off by the hand, the average amount of blood contained in the placenta was only 92.29 grammes. In other words, when the usual method is followed— viz., tying the cord as soon as all pulsation has ceased in it, and the child has cried out lustily—the child is deprived of 100 grammes of blood which it would have if the ligature were not applied till after the placenta had been pressed off. It is also well known that all children lose weight for some days after birth, the amount lost being estimated at an average of 220 grammes; but Prof. Zweifel found that the average amount of this loss, when the ligature had not been applied till after the expulsion of the placenta, was only 156 grammes.

Dr. LEOPOLD MEYER,[2] of Copenhagen, has repeated the experiments of Prof. Zweifel, but has arrived at very different conclusions. He found the following results in five cases when the cord was tied late—i. e., after the expulsion of the placenta:—

Weight of the placenta.	Blood contained.		
1. 502 gr.	70.34 gr.	or 14.01 per cent.	
2. 527 "	85.5 '	" 16.21 "	Average,
3. 600.5 "	104.36 "	" 17.38 "	15.07
4. 426.5 "	56.41 "	" 13.23 "	per cent.
5. 496 "	72.04 '	" 14.52 "	

The other cases, or those where the ligature was applied early, he divides into two classes—(*a*) where the ligature was not applied till after the cessation of the pulsation in the cord, and (*b*) where it was applied as soon as the children were born.

In three cases of class (*a*) the results were as follows:—

Weight of the placenta.	Blood contents.		
6. 737.5 gr.	96.69 gr.	or 13.11 per cent.	Average,
7. 458.5 "	79.71 "	" 17.39 "	17.25
8. 600 "	127.57 "	" 21.26 "	per cent.

[1] Centralblatt f. Gynaekologie, 1878, p. 1.   [2] Ibid., p. 220.

And in the sa 1 e nu 1 be1 of cases of class (b):—

	Weight of the placenta.		Blood contents.			
9.	610	g1.	125.4 g1.	or 20.56 pe1 cent.	⎫	A veiage,
10.	494.5	"	91.93 "	" 18.59 "	⎬	18.26
11.	657	"	102.6 "	" 15.62 "	⎭	pe1 cent.

If we take the a\eiage of the last six cases we get 17.76 pe1 cent., 1 aking the diffe1ence between the cases ligatu1ed late and those ligatu1ed ea1ly only 2.69 pe1 cent. of the weight of the placenta; o1 if we take the a\erage weight of the pla-centa as 600 g1a 1 1 es, this would gi\e 16 g1a 1 1 es of blood in fa\ou1 of the cases that we1e ligatu1ed late. Thus, though he ag1ees with Zweifel that the fœtus 1ecei\es 1o1e blood if the co1d is tied late, he diffe1s 1ost se1iously with hi 1 as to the exact a 1 ount thus gained.

In the *Centralblatt für Gynæcologie*, 1878, p. 409, D1. M. HOFMEIER, of Be1lin, d1aws attention to the *à p1io1i* i 1 p1obability of Zweifel's state 1 ents—\iz., that by the o1dina1y 1ethod of ligatu1ing the co1d the child loses 100 g1a 1 1 es of blood, the total a 1 ount of blood in an a\e1age child of 3300 g1a 1 1 es being only 175 g1a 1 1 es. Th1ough the goodness of P1of. Sch1oede1 he was enabled to 1ake so 1 e expe11 1 ents with a \iew of th1owing so 1 e light, if pos-sible, on this subject. The 1ethod adopted was to place the child the 1o1ent it was bo1n, and befo1e the co1d was tied, upon a sensiti\e weighing 1achine, to note its weight then, and also the inc1ease or di 1 inution in its weight afte1 so 1 e 1inutes had elapsed. The nu 1 be1 of cases in which he 1 ade the expe11 1 ent was 32, and the 1esult was that the1e was an a\e1age inc1ease in weight which a 1 ounted to 63.6 g1a 1 1 es. This inc1ease in weight, he conside1s, cannot be due to anything but the ext1a a 1 ount of blood that has du1ing the inte1\al en-tered the fœtal ci1culation f1o 1 the placenta.

A 1 o1e difficult question to answe1 is—What benefit or use is this i 1 1 ense quantity of blood to the fœtus? It is eithe1 supe1fluous, in which case it is soon got 1id of by disintegration of the 1ed blood co1puscles and abso1ption of the se1u 1 ; or it is 1 ost useful, in which case it 1 ust be looked on as "1ese1\e blood," and as such 1 ust tend to lessen the a 1 ount of loss of weight which such child1en would othe1wise suffe1 afte1 bi1th. He concludes, f1o 1 the 1esults of a nu 1 be1 of weighings that we1e unde1taken with the object of answe1ing this question, that child1en whose co1d was ligatu1ed late—*i. e.*, afte1 the expulsion of the pla-centa—lost 1 pe1 cent. less of thei1 enti1e weight than othe1 child1en. This in a child weighing 3303 g1a 1 1 es would a 1 ount to 33 g1a 1 1 es, which 1ep1esents a \e1y conside1able inc1ease of blood and st1ength; and he has found, 1o1eo\e1, that such child1en begin to gain flesh f1o 1 one-thi1d to one-half a day soone1 than the othe1s.

D1. MAX WIENER publishes the 1esults of so 1 e expe11 1 ents that he has 1 ade on this subject in the *Archiv. f. Gynaekologie*, B. xi\, p. 34, which in the 1 ain ag1ees \e1y closely with those obtained by a \e1y si 1 ila1 1 ethod by Meye1. He 1e1a1ked in the cou1se of his expe11 1 ents that the quantity of blood that 1e1ained in the placenta was \e1y \a1iable e\en in the sa 1 e class of cases. This diffe1ence could not be put down to the ti 1 e that elapsed befo1e the co1d was tied, no1 to the a 1 ount of ute1ine cont1action, no1 to the de\elop 1 ent of the child. He thinks, the1efo1e, that this g1eat diffe1ence in the a 1 ount of blood that 1e1ains behind in the placenta in al 1 ost si 1 ila1 cases 1 ust depend on the diffe1ent 1atios that often exist between the size of the child and the size of the placenta, and, the1efo1e, between the amount of blood in the child and that con-tained in the placenta. Thus we 1 ay find two well-de\eloped child1en each weighing 3000 g1a 1 1 es, while the placentæ weigh 600 and 400 g1a 1 1 es respectively, and consequently the amount of blood found in each will be proportionate to the size of the placenta and not to the weight of the children.

Dr. LEOPOLD MEYER publishes some further observations on this subject in the *Centralblatt für Gynaekologie*, for April 26, 1879, which lead to conclusions directly opposed to those of Hofmeier. The latter found that children whose cord was tied late lost 1 per cent. less of their total weight during the first few days of their existence, and that they began to gain weight from one-third to one-half a day sooner than those whose cord was tied immediately after birth. Meyer has weighed 40 children—in 20 of them the cord was tied early and 20 late. The average weights are as follows:—

	Cord tied late.	Cord tied early.	Difference.
Average weight after birth .	3203 gr.	3268 gr.	65 gr.
1 day	3128 "	3188 "	60 "
2 days	3013 "	3069 "	56 "
3 "	2990 "	3085 "	95 "
4 "	3054 "	3134 "	80 "
5 "	3094 "	3192 "	98 "
6 "	3141 "	3233 "	92 "
7 "	3181 "	3287 "	106 "
8 "	3221 "	3310 "	89 "
9	3261 "	3353 "	92 "
10	3277 "	3383 "	106 "

The difference here shown in favour of the cases where the cord was tied early depends, Meyer thinks, on the original weights of the children; and if all children who weighed above 3500 grammes be left out of consideration, the results in both series are almost exactly identical. Hence he concludes, contrary to the opinion of Porak, Budin, Schücking, Zweifel, Hofmeier, and Richemont, that the time that is allowed to elapse between the expulsion of the child and tying the cord has no effect—or, at all events, in comparison to other influences, has next to no effect—on the subsequent weight of the child. He further found, contrary to the results that Hofmeier brings forward, that a child whose cord was tied early did not subsequently lose so much of its weight as one whose cord was ligatured late. Hence tying the cord late does not increase to any great amount the quantity of blood in the fœtal circulation, and the results that have been obtained by weighing children immediately after birth and then again a few minutes later are founded, he thinks, on some error due to traction on the cord or some other cause.

In France this question has also been keenly debated ever since Dr. Budin first published the result of his investigations. Dr. CH. PORAK contributed a most exhaustive article on the subject to the *Revue Mensuelle de Méd. et de Chir.* for May and June, 1878. He agrees with Dr. Budin as to the amount of additional blood that enters the infantile circulation when the cord is tied late, but thinks that this extra blood, far from being any advantage to the infant, as Dr. Budin thinks, is rather positively injurious; for such children are, he says, much more subject to infantile jaundice and to the various effects of plethora, such as hemorrhage from the stomach, bowels, and vagina, and he adduces cases in support of this idea.

The *Annales de Gynécologie*, for February, 1879, contain a paper on this subject, by Dr. ALBAN RIEBEMONT, the value of which, from a scientific point of view is, however, greatly lessened by the violent polemic tone that pervades it throughout. He takes Dr. Porak very severely to task not only for his facts, but also for his logic and conclusions. He sums up his paper as follows:—

1. By ligaturing the cord late the infantile circulation receives on an average an addition of 92 grammes of blood (Budin).

2. This blood, which is contained in the placental vessels, is most necessary for the full establishment of the infantile circulation.

3. The blood is drawn into the infantile circulation chiefly by the suction power exerted by the expansion of the chest walls (Budin), the pressure exerted by the uterus on the placenta (Schücking, Poiak) having no considerable effect.

4. In cases of asphyxia where the child has a bluish hue the cord ought not to be immediately tied, nor should any hemorrhage be permitted from its fœtal extremity.

5. Ligaturing the cord late does not expose the child to the smallest immediate or ulterior danger.

6. The infant is thereby placed in the most advantageous circumstance possible for its development; it loses less weight, and regains what it has lost both sooner and quicker than if the ligature be made immediately.

7. The expulsion of the placenta is thereby rendered easier, and there is less resistance offered to its escaping through the cervix (Budin, Schücking).

8. He agrees with Hofmeier, Zweifel, Schücking, and Budin, that the cord should not be tied till the pulsation in it has entirely ceased.—*Dublin Journal of Medical Science*, June, 1879.

The Presentation of the Posterior Parietal.

Dr. J. VEIT contributes to the *Zeitschrift für Geburtshülfe und Gynäkologie*, Bd. iv., s. 229, a learned paper on presentation of the posterior parietal, in which he criticizes the views already put forward by Litzmann on this subject. He disagrees with Litzmann in his explanation of the mechanism, when the latter says that delivery is spontaneously effected by a rotation of the head round its antero-posterior axis, the anterior parietal descending behind the symphysis pubis, and the posterior ascending in front of the sacral promontory. Dr. Veit maintains that there is no such ascent of the posterior side of the head. He holds that when the case is terminated by natural efforts, the head is pressed more and more down, and compelled to rotate round the promontory of the sacrum as a centre; the perpendicular diameter of the head becomes thus the half-diameter of a circle, whose centre is at the promontory of the sacrum. Whether the delivery is possible or not depends upon the degree of adaptation between the perpendicular diameter of the head and the conjugate diameter of the inlet of the pelvis. If these are nearly equal, spontaneous delivery, according to the above mechanism, is possible. Dr. Veit thinks Litzmann was led into error by finding, as the posterior parietal bone was rotated backwards and downwards, that it was more difficult to reach it than before rotation commenced. This difficulty he explained by *assuming* an upward advance of the posterior parietal, falling into a mistake precisely analogous to that by which Naegele originally assumed the deeper position of the anterior parietal in normal labour. Dr. Veit thinks, also, that when Litzmann describes three distinct degrees of this presentation, viz., 1st, When the sagittal suture lies slightly in front of the middle line of the pelvis; 2d, When the sagittal suture lies close behind the symphysis pubis; 3d, When only the posterior parietal bone can be felt, he is merely describing different stages of the same presentation, the original presentation of the whole of the posterior parietal or Litzmann's third degree passing successively into No. 2 and No. 1 in the process of spontaneous delivery. Dr. Veit also describes a bulging of the lower surface of the head, a flattening of upper, and a degree of flexure of its perpendicular axis under the combined force of the pains, and of the resistance of the pelvic brim, as a preparation for the rotation movement being completed. He has also noticed that in these cases the posterior parietal is found to project greatly at the sagittal suture, in front of and overlap the anterior parietal, instead of as usual being overlapped by the anterior parietal. As observers of displacement of the cranial bones during delivery have been wont to notice that this particular condition occurs in about 20 per cent. of all vertex cases, and as this ratio is about the percentage in which Litzmann has observed presentation of the posterior parietal in flat pelves, Dr. Veit is inclined to believe that the overlapping of the posterior parietal over the anterior may be chiefly occasioned by this peculiar presentation. Another important peculiarity which Veit has observed in connection with this presentation is enormous dilatation of the lower uterine segment or of the cervix at its posterior aspect, owing to the oblique manner in which the uterine contractions are brought into action when the head and trunk are placed not in one line, but are inclined at an angle to one another. On one occasion this dilatation was so marked, that the firmly-contracted anteverted uterine fundus and body containing the breech of the fœtus were mistaken by him for a large fibroid attached to the anterior wall of the uterus. It was only after delivery by version that he observed his mistake. This condition can only be made out with certainty by carefully-combined internal and external examination. As to treatment, Veit is not inclined to trust much to rectification of the position and the use of forceps, as Litzmann proposes, but he would in a difficult case rather turn early.—*Edinburgh Med. Journal,* Sept. 1879.

—

Nervous Vomiting in Pregnancy cured by Electricity.

Dr. da VENEZIA relates in the *Giornale Veneto di Scienze Med.* (January, 1879) a case of chronic nervous vomiting in pregnancy which was cured by electricity. The patient was a young woman aged 24, in the seventh month of her first pregnancy. She had been suffering for the last two years from frequent attacks of vomiting after food, which had been so frequent during the last month that she had become greatly reduced in strength. The usual therapeutic agents were then employed; but, as no relief was obtained through them, the author resolved to try electricity. A faradic current of moderate strength was used, one of the rheophores being applied to the side of the neck along the course of the vagus nerve, and the other to the epigastrium. After the first sitting, the patient felt better; and after the fourth the vomiting had entirely ceased. The patient had six sittings of five minutes each, and after eighteen days she left the hospital cured and able to retain her food. The author draws attention to this fact, because electricity has not yet become much used in the vomiting in pregnancy, and also because it tends to confirm Professor Semmola's observations concerning its remarkable effects in nervous vomiting. Semmola, however, always uses the constant current.—*Brit. Med. Journ.,* Sept. 27, 1879.

—

The Lactosuria of Lying-in Women.

Dr. P. KALTENBACH contributes a long and interesting paper upon this subject to the *Zeitschrift für Geburtshülfe und Gynäkologie,* Bd. iv. s. 163. After a lengthened historical *résumé* of the various and frequently contradictory opinions hitherto held upon this subject by the authors who have studied it specially, Kaltenbach is led to support out and out the deductions of Hofmeister, "that in the urine of women giving suck there is demonstrable the existence of a reducing substance, which from its behaviour towards the ordinary tests for sugar may be looked upon as sugar, and that this substance bears a certain relation to the secretion of milk." But Kaltenbach, in the paper we are considering, carries the question a step further, and believes that he has demonstrated that that substance is really sugar, and **not** merely a substance which responds to the ordinary sugar tests. By a long process of precipitations, washings, etc., Dr. Kaltenbach was able to separate the reducing substance in a crystalline form. The crystals were colorless, transparent, presenting straight rhombic prisms with ends obliquely cut off, insoluble in alcohol and ether, easily soluble in cold water. At a temperature of about 150° C. they became brown, and gave forth an odour of caramel. Examined in the saccharometer, the solution exhibited a powerful right-handed rotation. Boiled in diluted sulphuric acid the crystals became directly capable of fermentation, *slightly warmed with diluted nitric acid they gave mucic acid,* Repeated experiments convince Kaltenbach that this reaction is able to detect infallibly the slightest amount of sugar. He regards it, therefore, as proved beyond a doubt that there does exist milk sugar in the urine of lying-in women. From another series of careful observations the author finds that the amount of sugar in the urine varies with the condition of the breasts. If they are tense or congested there is found to be an increase of sugar in the urine. He thus is led to give out and out support to the views of du Meulins, du Sinétz, and Spiegelberg on this subject, and maintains that the explanation of the phenomenon is to be found in the intensity of the physiological congestion of the excretory ducts of the milk glands. The amount of this congestion conditions the resorption of milk and its separation in the urine. Finally, our author states that the relation between congestion and the amount of sugar contained in the urine may be most plainly demonstrated in the cases of such lying-in women whose children were either born dead, or died during the period of lactation. The quantity of sugar of milk is especially considerable in the uterine of patients, in whose cases on account of mastitis, or of badly developed or shrunken nipples, or of other puerperal processes, the application of the child to the breast was retarded, and its artificial nourishment rendered necessary, because in these the conditions for the establishment of great obstructive congestion were fulfilled.—*Edinburgh Med. Journal,* Sept. 1879.

—

Fibroid Tumour Expelled under the use of Subcutaneous Injections of Ergotin.

Professor ALEXANDER R. SIMPSON, at a recent meeting of the Obstetrical Society of Edinburgh (*Edinburgh Med. Journal,* Sept. 1879), read the notes of a case of fibroid tumour expelled under the use of subcutaneous injections of ergotin. He remarked that further experience had confirmed the favourable impression he had formed as to the value of Hildebrandt's method of treating certain cases of fibroid tumours of the uterus by means of hypodermic injections of ergotin. He exhibited the fragments of a tumour which had been expelled from one of his Infirmary patients who had been thus treated. Under the microscope the masses were seen to be myomatous in structure, and it was interesting to observe to what an extent the individual muscular fibres were in process of fatty degeneration. The following is the history of the patient: Mary M., 54, a widow, residing at West Calder, admitted 23d February, examined 25th February, 1879. *Complaints.*—Swelling in lower part of abdomen; bloody discharge; pain in the back; painful and frequent micturition.

History of Present Illness.—Patient had always good health till about seven months ago, when she noticed the swelling in the lower part of the abdomen, which caused her considerable discomfort, especially on making water, which she had to do at short intervals. *General Appearance.*—Patient is of average height and development; is an albino; not markedly anæmic. *Menstrual History.*— Menstruation began when patient was at the age of 14; was always irregular; recurring at intervals varying from three to six weeks; lasting about two or three days at each time. Has been in abeyance only during pregnancy and nursing.

Seven months ago the discharge at each period became excessive, and it was at this time that she first observed the tumour. For the last three weeks there has been a constant and considerable loss of blood, which has greatly weakened the patient. *Obstetric History.*—She was married at 17; has had nine children, all born alive, at full term, with normal labours. Last child born three years ago.

Abdomen.—On inspection, walls flaccid, striæ of previous pregnancies; prominenee can be seen above pubes in the middle line, extending about halfway to the umbilicus. *On Palpation.*—A hard resistant tumour of rounded form and smooth surface is felt in the middle line above the pubes, measuring $5\frac{1}{2}$ inches transversely, and 4 inches vertically; the hand cannot be passed between the tumour and the pelvis in front. *Percussion.*—Dull note corresponding to area mapped out on palpation. *Auscultation.*—Negative results. *On Vaginal Examination.*—Ostium vaginæ patulous; vaginal walls smooth and moist. Vagina roomy. Cervix easily reached; looks downwards and backwards. In anterior and right lateral fornices a hard mass is felt. Os dilated admits tip of forefinger; fissured transversely; escaping from it some soft gelatinous discharge. The finger can be forced through the os externum, and touches a body on the left and anterior wall. *Bimanually.*—The uterus moves with the tumour. Distinct thrilling pulsation is felt in the anterior part of tumour, which projects into vagina. The sound passes $3\frac{1}{4}$ inches to the left side.

Diagnosis.—Submucous fibroid tumour of the uterus.

Treatment.—Rest in bed.

R.—Ergotin, ℨij; Chlor. hydr., ℨj; Aquæ, ℥ij. M. Sig.—Sixteen minims to be injected subcutaneously every second or third day.

Further progress.—On 6th March all discharge of blood ceased.

From the 10th of March to 1st April she had great pain in the uterus; her temperature during that time ranging from 98.4°, 100.0°, 102.0°, being generally higher in the evenings. She got morphia by the mouth frequently to procure sleep.

April 2. Part of the tumour about the size, when pressed together, of a hen's egg, came away to-day.

3d. M. T. 99; E. T. 100. Vaginal injections of tepid solution of carbolic acid and hip-baths to arrest the fetid discharge.

5th. Another part of the tumour came away to-day. Part in a sloughy condition. Great fetid discharge. E. T. 103.

7th. Pain ceased.

15th. Pain in the uterus. Small piece came away to-day, after which pain quite ceased.

Since the last part of the tumour came away there has been a great deal of white discharge, but it entirely ceased on 24th April. There is now no pain, and the temperature is quite normal.

May 6. On examination, tumour much diminished in size, but still larger than normal uterus. There are one or two irregular nodules on the left side under the peritoneum. A small almond-shaped swelling (the left ovary) is felt in the left side of the posterior fornix.

Dr. BELL, of Glasgow, had a good opinion of the effects of ergot in uterine fibroids, and mentioned a recent case in which a tumour had been expelled under its use in a state of fatty degeneration. He was especially anxious to make known the method he employed in administering the ergotin, which was in the form of suppository. He had found it quite as efficacious as the subcutaneous injections, and quite unattended with unpleasant results, as often happened with the subcutaneous method.

CONTENTS.

Published Monthly, price $2.50 per annum, free of postage.

Also, furnished together with the AMERICAN JOURNAL OF THE MEDICAL SCIENCES *and the* MEDICAL NEWS AND LIBRARY *for* SIX DOLLARS *per annum in advance, the whole free of postage.*

HENRY C. LEA, Philadelphia.

THE MONTHLY ABSTRACT

OF

MEDICAL SCIENCE.

VOL. VI.   No. 12.   **For List of Contents see last page.**   DECEMBER, 1879.
Entered at the Post-Office at Philadelphia as Second-class matter.

Anatomy and Physiology.

On the Growth of the Heart and Great Vessels.

From 350 estimations of the volume of the heart, and 620 measurements of the vessels, BENEKE concludes (Virchow's *Archiv*) that: 1. The growth of the heart is greatest in the first and second years of life; by the end of the second year the heart has doubled in size. In the next five years its growth is slower, and but a gradual increase commences after this period, up to the age of 15, when it is two-thirds greater than it was at 7 years of age. After puberty the heart grows more rapidly, and, in proportion to the sexual development, increasing to two-thirds its original volume in the succeeding five years. After this it grows more slowly, but continues to enlarge up to 50, increasing about 1 cubic centimetre per annum, and subsequently a diminution occurs, which may be regarded as senile atrophy. 2. The heart is the same in children of both sexes up to puberty. After which the female heart remains the smaller, being from 20 to 30 cubic centimetres less. 3. All the great vessels continue to increase in size from the beginning of life to its end. 4. This increase in size of the great vessels is relatively greatest in the first years of life, but, like the heart, their growth is quickened at puberty. 5. The pulmonary artery up to the age of 45 is wider than the descending aorta. After this the relation changes, and the descending aorta gradually becomes the wider. 6. Up to puberty the common carotid is not noticeably wider than the common iliac and subclavian, but after that period the latter are much the wider. 7. The vessels in the female are throughout life narrower than in the male. Previous to puberty the number of observations have been too small to make this quite certain. 8. The vessels are relatively narrowest in proportion to the length of the body at puberty. Taking this, together with above described development of the heart at puberty, he infers that the blood pressure is relatively highest at that period. 9. Relatively to the length of the body, the pulmonary artery in the female at puberty is wider than in the male. 10. The pulmonary artery and descending aorta increase relatively more during life than the iliacs, subclavians, and carotids. He infers from this that, as life advances, the blood pressure must fall in the aorta, while it rises in the peripheral arteries. 11. Immediately after birth the aorta and pulmonary artery increase, while the iliacs decrease in consequence of the cessation of the fœtal circulation. 12. The blood pressure appears to play an important part in determining the widening of the vessels. 13. The maxima and minima circumferences of the great vessels vary to an extraordinary degree in different persons, especially as life advances; but these may be explained by differences in the length of the body. There also seems reason to believe in great differences in the total blood ı ass in different individuals.   14. Cases of cancer see ı ed to have wider vessels than were found in otherwise diseased oı healthy peısons.—*London Medical Record*, Oct. 15, 1879.

Origin of the Red Blood-Corpuscles.

Notwithstanding the attention that has been bestowed upon the subject, the souıce and ı ode of develop ı ent of the ıed blood-coıpuscles is still shrouded in ı uch daıkness. That they ıeally do gıow is sufficiently shown by the ıapidity with which even laıge losses of blood aıe ıepaiıed, and it see ı s to be geneıally ad ı itted that they pıoceed fıo ı the white coıpuscles in which so ı e kind of ı eta-ı oıphosis has taken place ; the white coıpuscles the ı sel ves being the pıoduct of cell-gıowth in the ductless glands, in the ly ı phatic glands, the ı edullaıy tissue of bones, and in the connective tissue of vaıious oıgans. The chief difficulty in the way of this explanation of the oıigin of the ıed coıpuscles is the co ı paıative absence of inteı ı ediate stages, especially in the higheı veıtebıata, between the veıy well chaıacteıized, actively ı oving, nucleated, and spheıoidal white coıpus-cle, and the non-nucleated, biconcave, and ı otionless discoid ıed. Foı although white coıpuscles have been seen with a tinge of ıed, ı oıe or less flattened, and with otheı featuıes appıoxi ı ating the ı to the ıed coıpuscles, the nu ı beı of the ı is co ı paıatively s ı all, and scaıcely sufficient to account foı the constant succes-sion of new ıed coıpuscles, which we ı ust suppose aıe being constantly added to the geneıal ı ass of blood. In addition to this, the white coıpuscles appeaı to have functions of theiı own, as shown by theiı passing thıough the walls of the vessels, and wandeıing through the tissues, wheıe they ıetain, foı some ti ı e at least, theiı peculiaı chaıacteıs.

Recent obseıvations by M. Hayeı have opened up new views on this point, and, fıo ı caıeful and long-continued micıoscopical ıeseaıch, he has been led to ad ı it a thiıd foı ı of coıpuscle, the hæ ı atoblast, to which the ıed blood-coıpus-cle owes its oıigin. His obseıvations have been conducted both on the higheı and the loweı foı ı s of veıtebıata, and the seıies that we pıopose at pıesent to notice, and an account of which he has just published in the *Archives de Physi-ologie*, deal with the develop ı ent of the blood-coıpuscles of those veıtebıates that have nucleated ıed coıpuscles, the pyrenæmata of Gullivei, oı ichthyopsida and sauıopsida of zoologists. On exposuıe of the ı esenteıy oı tongue of a fıog to the aiı, the ciıculation beco ı es tıoubled and sloweı, and it is then easy to see, a ı ongst the ıed coıpuscles, colouıless coıpuscles, veıy diffeıent in aspect fıom the white coıpuscles. These bodies aıe boıne along with the cuıent of the ıed coıpuscles, without any tendency to ıest in the quiescent layeı, and, instead of pıesenting the spheıoidal foı ı of the leucocytes, aıe elongated, slightly flattened, and alıeady so ı ewhat discoid. When seen in pıofile they appeaı as ovoid bodies, with one end pıolonged to so ı e extent. These aıe the young ıed globules or hæ ı atoblasts. They aıe not deficient in elasticity or suppleness, since they can ı ake theiı way through a naıow passage, with so ı e change of foı ı, ıesu ı ing theiı natuıal aspect on being ıelieved fıo ı pıessuıe. Theiı suıface is smooth, ho ı ogeneous, slightly cloudy, and with a less silveıy ıeflex than the white coı-puscles. They so ı etiı es pıesent a centıal daıkish spot, occupying the position of a nucleus, neaı which aıe one or two bıight gıanules. If a specimen of ıecent blood be exa ı ined on the waı ı stage, the hæ ı atoblasts ıetain foı so ı e seconds the appeaıance above descıibed ; but they soon beco ı e ıe ı aıkably viscous, and, whilst adheıing to the slide at so ı e point, they aıe stıetched by the ı ove ı ent of the plas ı a, so ı etiı es to an inoıdinate length, or, if they co ı e into contact with one anotheı, they stick togetheı, and beco ı e a kind of centıe aıound which the ıed coıpuscles dispose the ı sel ves concentıically. They then quickly beco ı e altered in appearance, and lose their distinctive features. If it be required to examine them under the microscope outside the vessels, the stage, instead of being warmed, should be cooled to freezing point, and they then retain their characters for several hours. Even then, however, after a time, they become prickly with short pale processes, and lose by solution or fragmentation a part of their disk, the nucleus at the same time becoming more sharply defined and more granular. They preserve their characteristic features best in iodized serum, and when measured they are found to vary considerably in size, some being much smaller than the ordinary white corpuscles, others larger and very elongated, whilst many have a very distinct yellowish tint from the presence of hæmoglobin. The larger they are the more resistant are they to the action of saline and other solutions. The smaller specimens soon become pale and indistinct in water, and then disappear altogether, the nucleus first becoming spherical and very large. They can be rendered insoluble by the addition of solution of mercury chloride of a particular strength, the formula of which is given.

M. Hayem dwells on the relation that the hæmatoblasts, after withdrawal from the bloodvessels, bear to the formation of fibrin, and shows how the delicate filaments observed in the coagulum of frogs' blood are, in part at least, derived from the processes of these peculiar structures.

Whether M. Hayem's results be corroborated by other observers or not, it is quite evident, both from his researches and from those of M. Lostorfer and Dr. Richard Norris, that the microscopical characters of the blood have not been fully mastered, and that this fluid still presents an inviting field to the naturalist, which has the advantage of being always accessible and easily worked.—*Lancet*, Oct. 11, 1879.

Materia Medica and Therapeutics.

On Myotic and Mydriatic Agents.

At the late International Medical Congress, at Amsterdam, Dr. DOYER, of Leyden, presented a note on this subject, with the following conclusions:—

1. Notwithstanding the relation which exists between the size of the pupil and the power of accommodation, both functions are independent of each other.

2. Comparison of the results of experiments shows that the power of various drugs for dilating the pupil is different, and that for pilocarpine, eserine, gelsemia, atropia, daturia, and duboisia, it is in the proportion of $\frac{1}{200}$, $\frac{1}{6}$, $\frac{1}{10}$, 1, 2, 15.

3. The smallest dose of duboisia that acts on the pupil is 0.000000005 gramme.—*Archives Gén. de Médecine*, Nov. 1879.

The Local Antagonism of Atropia and Pilocarpine.

Some interesting experiments on the local antagonism of atropine and pilocarpine were recently communicated to the Académie des Sciences by M. Strauss. If one or two centigrammes of nitrate of pilocarpine are injected beneath the skin of a man, at the end of from two to five minutes the skin covering the injected liquid reddens, and then is covered with very fine droplets of sweat, which appear first, not at the point of the injection, but at the circumference of the area, and extend concentrically to the centre, finally covering the whole area. This local sweat occurs two or three minutes before the salivation, and five or eight minutes before the general perspiration, and it is the more pronounced the greater is the number of sudoriparous glands at the spot; the best places being the forehead or front of the sternum ; the back of the arm, where injections are most frequently made, being the least favorable, and for this reason, probably, the phenomenon has escaped observation. Reducing the dose, the effect of the injection becomes ultimately strictly local, without the slightest general sweating. Thus, at will, this or that part of the skin may be made to sweat, or lines of sweat may be produced on an otherwise dry skin. The dose with which the effect is purely local is from one to four milligrammes.

By means of subcutaneous injections of atropine the opposite effect may be obtained. If, when a person is in full sweat from the effect of pilocarpine, very minute doses of sulphate of atropine are injected under the skin, the perspiration lessens at the spot almost immediately, and in a few minutes it is totally suppressed. Thus dry areas and lines may be at will produced upon the moist skin. In order to ascertain that the arrest of the perspiration is really the result of the atropine, and not of the mere injection of liquid, an equivalent volume of pure water was injected at certain spots, but without causing any arrest of the perspiration. The dose of atropine which will arrest the sweating is extremely small. One-millionth of a gramme of atropine never failed to produce it in man, and in the cat one-hundred-thousandth of a gramme was sufficient. The sweating skin is thus a test of atropine of extreme delicacy. The sensibility of the sudoriparous glands to atropine is greater even than the iris, since the millionth of a gramme of atropine produces no appreciable dilatation of the pupil.

If the skin is frozen with ether-spray, and one or two centigrammes of pilocarpine are injected, the local sweating does not ensue, in spite of the occurrence of general perspiration. Even after the freezing has passed off, the local sweating does not occur, or is brief and slight. Extreme cold appears thus to act as atropine, paralyzing the sweat-nerves, a paralysis which persists even after the local cold and anæmia have passed away. This fact is of great interest in connection with the well-known pathological effect of the arrest of sweat by cold.

The experiments of Luchsinger, confirmed by Vulpian, have shown that in the cat an injection of one or two milligrammes of atropine arrests the sweating caused by a centigramme of pilocarpine, but that if another centigramme of pilocarpine is injected under the skin of one of the paws, the sweat will reappear upon this paw, and nowhere else. In man Strauss has ascertained the same fact. After two centigrammes of atropine had been injected, two milligrammes of pilocarpine were injected half an hour later on another region of the skin. Neither salivation nor general sweating occurred, but merely a local perspiration, very persistent, however, at the point of injection. An attempt was made to ascertain what quantity of atropine rendered large doses of pilocarpine locally inefficacious. In the leg of a strong man six milligrammes of sulphate of atropine were gradually injected, and then, in a single injection, four centigrammes of pilocarpine, without causing even local sweating. In a young cat the same result was obtained after injecting under the skin of the belly three milligrammes of atropine gradually. The subsequent injection into a hind paw of one and a half centigrammes of pilocarpine, and the galvanization of the sciatic after the method of Luchsinger, caused no perspiration upon this paw.—*Lancet*, Sept. 27, 1879.

Medicine.

Immediate and Permanent Treatment of Disease.

At a late meeting of the Harveian Society of London (*British Med. Journal*, Nov. 1, 1879) Dr. MILNER FOTHERGILL read a paper on this subject, in which he pointed out how in many cases the treatment which gave immediate relief was not that to be continued in the permanent interests of the patient. He instanced first the free use of opium in the hacking cough of phthisis, and in chronic bronchitis, which gave immediate relief, but did harm eventually. Then, in the diarrhœa, due to impacted masses in the rectum, astringent mixtures might give immediate relief, but they were not curative, while removal of the masses was. So, too, in neuralgia, the injection of morphia eased the pain for the time, but, if continued, was more likely to confirm it than to cure it. Likewise in dyspepsia, of reflex origin, its cure depended upon the removal of the exciting cause. In gout, the application of cold, or of leeches, gave instant relief; but he quoted Garrod in illustration of the evil consequences which followed such treatment. But of all instances of the conflict betwixt the present and the permanent treatment of disease, that furnished by endocarditis was, he said, the most striking. It was the rule to give tonics as soon as possible, and to get the patient up; but, he contended, the proper plan of treatment was to keep the patient flat in bed for some days after all evidence of active mischief had passed away. The growth of connective tissue in the valve-curtains, which was lighted up by the inflammatory storm that passed over the endocardium, persisted some time after the endocarditis itself was over; and it was the mutilation, caused by the contraction of the neoplasm which was chiefly to be dreaded. Consequently, the true line of practice was to reduce the strain upon the inflamed valve-curtains by complete rest, and the administration of agents which lowered the blood-pressure within the heart and arteries. The more the connective tissue growth could be limited at the outset, the less the future mutilation of the valves.

The Treatment of Chlorosis.

The experiments which have been carried on by M. HAYEM for several years, shew that there is in chlorosis not only a diminution of the number of red corpuscles, but that there is in addition an individual change in the corpuscles themselves. This modification is owing to the fact that the red corpuscles possess an insufficient quantity of hæmoglobin. Iron acts by preventing this individual alteration in the corpuscle. To this statement it may be objected that compounds of iron are only of use to the organism indirectly, by stimulating the appetite. Chlorosis is generally accompanied by well-marked and obstinate anorexia. But it is understood that many of the preparations of iron stimulate the appetite, and it may therefore be asked whether chlorotic patients who take iron and recover their appetites are unable to assist in renewing not only the number but the quality of their red corpuscles. For the purpose of demonstrating this fact, M. Hayem, in conjunction with M. Regnault, has undertaken a series of experiments, in which insoluble preparations of iron, such as potassium ferrocyanide, which pass through the organism unchanged, were administered. The experimenters found that these preparations are absolutely incapable of assisting in the renewal of the blood. M. Hayem then adopted the plan of making his patients inhale oxygen. M. Demarquay first showed that this was one of the best methods for stimulating the appetite. M. Hayem caused his patients to inhale oxygen to the extent of ten litres a day at two or three sittings, and has thus obtained wonderful results in regard to stimulation of the digestive functions. Chlorotic patients who could scarcely be induced to eat raw innutritious vegetables became perfectly ravenous after some days of this treatment, and ate five or six of the hospital rations in the course of 24 hours. The quantity of urea eliminated in the same time rose from 10–12 grams up to 35–40 grams per diem. The general health was improved, and the body weight increased, but the patients retained their characteristic colour, and still remained chlorotic. In fact, the examination of the blood showed that a marked increase in the number of blood corpuscles had occurred, but that the essential alteration, that is to say, the insufficiency of hæmoglobin, still remained. The patients under these conditions, therefore, made a large number of corpuscles, which were no longer normal. After the expiration of two or three months of this treatment the scarcity of colouring matter in the red corpuscles as shown by the microscope contrasted markedly with the improvement in the digestive functions and in the general health, and it was only necessary to stop the inhalation of oxygen to see the patient return to his former wretched condition. To complete his experiments it only remained for M. Hayem to combine the inhalation of oxygen with the administration of soluble preparations of iron. The red corpuscles were then not slow to recover their physiological properties, the beneficial results being hastened by the fact that under the influence of oxygen the alimentary canal is rendered more tolerant of the iron. From these results it may be concluded : (1) that soluble preparations of iron are alone capable of modifying that change in the red corpuscles which is the essential character of chlorosis. (2) In chlorotic patients affected with dyspepsia inhalations of oxygen should be considered as a beneficial adjuvant to the treatment by iron.—*Practitioner*, Nov. 1878, from *Le Concours Médical*, July 26, 1878.

Myxœdema, or Universal Degeneration of the Connective Tissue of the Body.

At a late meeting of the Clinical Society of London (*Med. Times and Gazette*, Oct. 18, 1879), Dr. DYCE DUCKWORTH related this case. S. M., aged thirty-four, married for ten years, mother of three children, came to St. Bartholomew's Hospital in November, 1878, complaining of weakness and of failing health for two years previously. She first observed that her eyelids and face swelled ; subsequently swelling was noticed generally about the body. Her voice had become altered and thick. A sister who accompanied the patient stated that her manner had become altered and her temper more sullen and irritable since her ailment began. Indeed, some of her friends believed, in consequence, that she had become intemperate in her habits. She was a well-grown woman, of large build, but had lost two stones in weight during the previous eighteen months. Her face was of peculiar aspect, and she wore a listless expression. The complexion was waxy, with some clear redness over the malar bones, and there were several moles about the chin and cheeks. The eyelids were puffy and œdematous, having the aspect so common in chronic forms of tubal nephritis. The hands were clumsy-looking and seemingly swollen about the backs, but no dints could be made in them ; it was alleged that they felt numb and sleepy at times. There was no appreciable change in common sensibility, and pins could be readily picked up. On examination some general condition of xeroderma was found on the limbs more especially, but no ordinary œdema.

The first impression in this case was that there was some form of chronic nephritis present which would explain both the physiognomical aspect and the obvious swellings. The urine was found to be quite void of albumen, of specific gravity 1010, acid in reaction. The heart was natural. The tongue was clean, and protruded naturally. The uvula was observed to be swollen and œdematous-looking. Appetite good; bowels usually constipated. The case was now re-garded as one of that peculiar form of disorder described so well, and termed by Dr. Ord as "myxœdema," and other like instances of the disease were recalled to memory which had not been satisfactorily diagnosticated. The family history afforded no clue to the nature of the case. The children were healthy with the exception of the youngest, which was very rickety.

The treatment consisted mainly of steel and cod-liver oil. On subsequent examinations the disorder was found to be making progress. The thyroid gland could not be felt, and a fatty cushion was found in the left supra-clavicular fossa. The face became more waxy and puffy, and the voice more slow and snuffling. The urine never was albuminous. The patient's manner was more sullen and reserved, and she was shy and resentful of clinical examination. Dr. Ord saw this case six months ago, and confirmed the opinion formed respecting it. It added one more to a series which have been, and still are, receiving careful study, and about which no doubt as to their true nature can now be entertained. Occurring only, so far as known at present, in the persons of women about middle life, the varying symptoms appear to be due to a gradually spreading mucoid de-generation of the intercellular tissue throughout the body, which thus shuts off full and prompt appreciation of peripheral and other nervous impressions. Dr. Duck-worth promised to report further observations upon this case at a future time.

Dr. Ord then read some further observations on this disease. The paper gave the history and morbid anatomy of a second (fatal) case of this disease, first de-scribed by Sir William Gull as "a cretinoid condition supervening in women in adult life," and subsequently named by Dr. Ord "myxœdema." The patient was a woman, aged fifty-two, married, the mother of five children. Her illness dated from her last confinement, twelve years before. She had begun then to swell in the face and all over the body. As she gradually increased in size she had become lethargic, had difficulty in collecting her thoughts, had difficulty in walking and in holding up her head. When she came under observation, four-teen days before death, she presented in a very marked degree the appearances described by Sir William Gull and Dr. Ord in previous papers. The whole body was swollen, giving her the aspect of a person suffering from renal disease. The skin was translucent, dry, and very rough on all parts except the face. The eye-lids were bulged, the lips, upper and lower, greatly swollen, and the alæ nasi much thickened. Each cheek presented a sharply-limited pink flush; the hands were spade-like, expressionless, and, with other extremities, were blue, by reason of feebleness of circulation. She spoke slowly and painfully, with leathery nasal intonation. Her movements were slow, and she halted quiveringly in her gait, but had no true paralysis, ataxy, or tremblings. The droop forward of the head, noticed in a previous extreme case, was remarkable, the pressure of the chin upon the neck actually interfering with deglutition. Her senses were essentially unim-paired, but her response was long in coming, her memory defective, and her thoughts slow. The urine was of average quantity, of rather less than average specific gravity, and contained a trace of albumen. The arteries were firm, and the heart enlarged but weak. The thyroid body was small. Having received bad news immediately after her admission to St. Thomas's Hospital, she fell into a lethargy which deepened daily, with intervals of feeble delirium till she died, on the fourteenth day. While under observation her temperature was very low; for twelve days the average was between 90° and 92°, on the thirteenth 88°, on the last day 77°.

At the post-mortem examination all tegumentary and surface parts of the body were found swollen; the thyroid body was reduced in size and form; the kidneys were very firm, not reduced in size, smooth on the surface, and not adherent to

their capsules, the cortical portion being so ıewhat naıoweı on section than
noı ı al ; the liveı and spleen weıe too fiı ı ; the heaıt was dilated and hypertrophied, weight twelve ounces and a half.　The ıcıoscope showed in all paıts a
gıeat incıease of connective tissue.　The fibrillar ele ı ent was ıoıe abundant
and ıoıe defined than noı ı al ; the inteıstitial ıucus-yielding ele ı ent was gıeatly
incıeased in pıopoıtion and quantity ; nuclei weıe laıgeı and ıoıe nuıeıous.
This was best seen in the skin, the glandulaı oıgans, and in the coats of aıteries.
The connective tissue pıesented a stıong ıese ıblance to that of the u ı bilical
coıd, and suggested the idea of a ıetıogıade degeneıation.　The encıoach ı ent of
it on tissue and oıgans was appaıently the cause of death.　Five otheı cases, all
in wo ı en between thiıty and fifty, all ıaııied, weıe co ı paıed.　All had low
tempcrature ; all had neıvous weakness and lessened sensations ; two, veıy advanced, had delusions.　These two had tıaces of albuminuıia ; the ıest, less
advanced, gave no indications of ıenal affection.　The sy ı pto ı s and appeaıances
being altogetheı of the sa ı e chaıacteı as those obseıved in pıevious cases, Dı.
Oıd ı aintained that they showed the disease undeı consideıation to be a substan-
tive disease, and that they justified the use of the teım " ı yxœde ı a," as ı aık-
ing the cause of the sy ı pto ı s and of the fatal teı ı ination.

Dı. GOODHART suggested that the oveıgıowth of connective tissue which was
supposed to co ı pıess the neıves ı ight also, in cıetinis ı , in the sa ı e way affect
the bıain.　But between spoıadic cıetinis ı and this ı alady theıe see ı ed to be
this essential diffeıence—that the foı ı eı was congenital ; the latteı occuııed in
ı iddle life only.　Would it not in the latteı case be so that the bıain, having
alıeady ıeceived ı any i ı pıessions, would ıetain ı uch of its ı ental food ?　He
was ıatheı inclined to suspect a kind of geneıal ı ischief si ı ilaı to *scleıose en
plaque.*

Dı. Duckwoıth said that of couıse in his case theıe could be no pathological
details, seeing the patient was yet alive.　She was not easily ı anaged, and had
only been seen at inteıvals.

Dı. Oıd said that in one of his cases he could give the histoıy of the childıen.
One see ı ed of unusual ability as a painteı ; otheıs see ı ed ı usculaı in a high
degıee ; in none had any signs of the disease been seen, but then all weıe undeı
the oıdinaıy age for such sy ı pto ı s to ı anifest the ı selves.　Tıue the pıognosis
was bad, but in no case did it see ı to pıove fatal undeı six, or usually ten oı
twelve yeaıs.　No tıeat ı ent see ı ed to do good.　Neitheı in the bıain noı spinal
coıd was theıe anything which could stıictly be called scleıosis, though the connective tissue ıound about the bloodvessels was incıeased.　He still held that
padding aıound the neıve-fibres, and the consequent inteııuption of communication with the peıipheıy, was a pıı ı e factoı in the disease.

—

Sudden Death in Diabetes.

The sudden teı ı ination of cases of diabetes is so fıequent, so well known,
and withal so staıtling ; the collapse fıoı a condition of co ı paıative wellbeing
occuıs so often without any pıevious waıning ; that even hypotheses which pıe-
tend to thıown light upon these conditions, ıoıe especially if they contain so ı e
infoı ı ation holding out theıapeutic indications, aıe welcome to the pıofession.
Dı. JULES CYR, in the Dece ı beı and Januaıy nu ı beıs of the *Aıchives Gén. de
Médecine* foı 1877–78, has published a papeı in which he details the account of
thiıty-two cases of sudden death in diabetes, collected fıom vaıious souıces.
He consideıs that theıe aıe at least five diffeıent conditions to which these ı ay be
ascıibed : 1.　The foı ı ation of acetone in the blood undeı conditions neaıly unknown—acetonæmia ; 2.　The accu ı ulation of excessive quantities of sugaı in

the blood—hyperglycæmia ; 3. The retention of urinary solids or water in the
blood—uræmia, dropsy of the ventricles; 4. Atrophy of the cardiac muscle; 5.
Cerebral anæmia. It is probable that some at least of these may combine to
produce the fatal result, while some have a more special and direct effect, and
are capable of recognition during life. Of these thirty-two cases, twenty-one
are stated to have died comatose ; in a few the mode of death is not stated ; in
others there is no mention of coma ; but this large proportion shows the relative
frequency of this mode of death. In none of the cases in which necropsies
were made, although these unfortunately were few, was there any anatomical
change to account for death. Dr. Balthazar Foster has published a paper
(*British Medical Journal*, January 19, 1878), in which he has urged the
probability of acetonæmia being the cause of death in a large number of these
cases. This theory he supports by quoting three cases from his own practice ;
in the first, no smell of acetone was noticed in the breath, but the blood of the
patient, examined after death, was of a peculiar pale colour and creamy consistence ; under the microscrope, the blood-corpuscles were broken down into a
granular material, which he subsequently found could not be artificially imitated
by treating blood with acetone ; in the other two cases there was a strong odour
of acetone in the breath of the patients. Dr. Foster alludes to the objection
which has been made that, in many cases, no odour of acetone is perceptible,
and replies that a temperature of 100° Fahr. is necessary to volatilize acetone.

Kussmaul (*Deutsches Archiv für Klin. Medicin*, 14 Band, 1874) has gone very
fully into this question of acetonæmia, and from his experiments concludes that
it is not possible to believe in a theory of acute intoxication from acetone, but
that chronic poisoning by this substance may so affect the nervous system as to
render it liable to take on an acute form, just as chronic alcoholism may suddenly
explode in delirium tremens. His reason for thinking so is, that such very large
quantities of acetone are required to produce any physiological effect. He says
that he was in the habit of prescribing acetone for phthisis, and often gave four
to six *grammes* daily (in one case for six weeks) without producing any disagreeable effect upon the patients, who never complained of headache or giddiness,
etc. In his experiments upon animals he injected as much as ten *grammes* of
pure acetone within one hour beneath the skin of a dog, without producing intoxication, anæsthesia, or muscular enfeeblement ; but with smaller doses he was
able to produce these effects in rabbits. He especially remarks upon the extreme
ease with which the odour of acetone could be detected in the breath of these
animals ; but it must be remembered that their usual temperature is somewhat
higher than that of man. We can scarcely believe that acetone ordinarily, or
even frequently, is capable of destroying the blood-corpuscles in the way described by Dr. Foster, for all Kussmaul's animals, without exception, even those
in whom coma had been induced, recovered, which scarcely could have happened
had the acetone produced those physical changes in the blood which Dr. Foster
describes ; it is at least probable that these appearances were *post-mortem*, per
haps due to a further development of acetone in the sugar-laden blood.

With regard to the treatment, Dr. Foster was successful in one case in which
he administered two drops of carbolic acid every hour, combined with opium ;
he suggests salicylic acid or thymol ; all these antizymotic substances being intended to check the fermentative change of sugar into acetone. If this conversion could be checked, the results of Kussmaul's experiments give us reason to
believe that recovery might take place, but, unfortunately, a diabetic is not in
quite such a favourable condition to resist the poison as healthy dogs and rabbits,
and Kussmaul's suggestion of gradual impairment of the central nervous organs
by chronic poisoning is only too probable. From reading Dr. Cyr's cases, it

appears that these deaths are far more frequent in people who have neglected to
restrict their diet, while very commonly the fatal accidents have supervened
upon some excitement and unusual physical exertion; a woman runs with her
baby to escape a shower of rain, a man hurries to catch a train, another loses his
omnibus and has to walk home. All these teach the old lesson, none the less useful
for not being new, that the only hope of safety for a diabetic is in making his
mode of life conform to those rules which have been framed by medical experience and confirmed by medical science.

An addition has been made to the pathology of this subject, and a sixth condition added to Dr. Cyr's list, by Dr. Hamilton's discovery of lipæmia and fatty
embola in the pulmonary and renal vessels of a case which died under the care of
Dr. Sanders. In their paper (*Edin. Med. Journal*, July, 1879) they describe
the blood as presenting the same cream-like appearance noticed by Dr. Foster;
on standing, it separated into two layers, the upper consisting of fat-globules and
a finely granular precipitate, "evidently of an albuminous nature;" the lower
stratum being unaltered blood corpuscles, with a few granules and oil-globules.
In another case the blood was in a similar condition, and, on submitting it to
analysis, only a mere trace of acetone was discovered; unfortunately in this case
no microscopical examination of the organs was made.

These observations cast some doubt on the occurrence of acetonæmia; but we
have seen that the causes of sudden death in diabetes are manifold, and in natural
science we must be content to accept a plurality of causes. It may be that
sometimes acetonæmia, sometimes lipæmia, produces the fatal result; or it may
be, as Sanders and Hamilton have concluded, that acetonæmia is a myth, and
lipæmia the sole condition. It is worth while remembering, however, that it is
still open to doubt whether fat-embola can cause death. In their first case the
dyspnœa was very slight, and urine was passed shortly before death; the latter
fact strongly contradicting the hypothesis of carbonic acid poisoning.—*British
Med. Journal*, Nov. 1, 1879.

Acute Affections of the Pons and the Bulbs.

EISENLOHR gives, in the *Arch. f. Psych.*, ix. page 1, the histories of eleven
cases of acute affections of the pons and the bulbs, of which the following cases
appear to us the most noteworthy, as they are accompanied by the *post-mortem*
results. Case 1, is that of a man, aged 55, who suddenly began to experience a
difficulty in swallowing, and in his speech. There had been no apoplectic attack.
The difficulties increased rapidly, and were complicated by paralysis of the right
leg and arm. The patient passed his motions and urine in bed; six weeks later
his speech had become almost unintelligible, and he presented all the symptoms
of bulbar paralysis. The masseter muscles were in a state of contraction. The
upper branches of the facial nerve were free. There were no sensory troubles,
but the motility of the left leg and arm was considerably impaired, and, as before
noted, the right extremities were paralyzed. The respiration was superficial, the
urine dribbled away constantly. The hearing was considerably impaired in the
right ear. Faradic contractility was normal in the region of the facial nerve, the
tongue and the extremities. The movements of the left extremities were irregular and atactic. Towards the end of his life, the patient was unable to close his
eyes completely, or to move the eyeballs to the left beyond the middle line. All
the extremities were in a state of contraction and paralysis. Death ensued ten
weeks after the first symptoms of the disease had manifested themselves. The
necropsy revealed a basal chronic meningitis, which was localized in the part of
the brain corresponding to the posterior fossa, and which had led to the obliteration of a number of the smaller vessels of the pons, and to softening of the cor-

responding portion. There was extensive degeneration of the left half of the pons, which extended across the raphé into the right half. Some portions of the superficial and deep layer of the transverse fibres had been destroyed by two smaller foci which were on the same level. The crura cerebelli, the remaining portions of the pons, and the medulla were intact, with the exception of a secondary degeneration in both pyramidal tracts, which could be traced down as far as the lumbar cord. The roots of the cerebral nerves were also intact. In giving the history of this case, the author draws attention to two points, as being especially worthy of notice. First—the extreme rarity of similar cases. Second —the fact that the symptoms observed in the course of this affection correspond to the phenomena which occur in the course of the apoplectic form, bulbar paralysis, as described by Jouffroy.

Another case is that of a man, aged 50, who five years ago had had an apoplectic stroke, complicated with right hemiplegia and disturbances of speech. During the last weeks of his life, the patient had presented Stokes' respiratory phenomenon in a most exquisite form. At the *post-mortem*, cirrhosis of the kidneys, hypertrophy of the left ventricle, and a pleuritic exudation on the left side of the thorax were found, together with a remarkable anatomical change following an old obliteration of the vertebral artery. The left vertebral artery, from the branching off of the posterior inferior cerebral artery to its union with the basilar artery, had been changed into a solid thin cord, the inferior posterior cerebellar artery had shared its fate, while the anterior spinal artery had remained normal. The right vertebral artery was partly thickened. The bulbar nerves presented no microscopic change, but the ependyma of the bulbs was very turbid, thickened, and covered with granulations. After hardening the medulla in alcohol, a sclerotic degeneration of the ependyma of the fourth ventricle was revealed, which had originated in the plugged vessels of the choroid plexus, and extended into the region of the nuclei of the abducent nerve. Both sides were affected, but the left side more so than the right. The nerve nuclei, which lie beneath the degenerated portion, were comparatively little affected, with the exception of the nucleus of the left vagus nerve, and a small focus in the nucleus of the left hypoglossal nerve. The intrabulbar fibrous tracts of both nerves were unaltered. The left pyramid had undergone secondary degeneration, owing to a focus in the cerebrum. An independent focus, containing obliterated vessels, was found in the left anterior horn of the spinal column.

In a typical case of bulbar paralysis, with progressive muscular atrophy, Dr. Eisenlohr found that the nuclei of the gray matter had undergone sclerotic degeneration. In this case the fibres of the roots were atrophic, and the ganglionic cells of the anterior horns of the spinal cord were partly destroyed.

A man, aged 57, had for some time been complaining of occipital headache, when he suddenly had an attack of dextrilateral, transitory hemiplegia. Two days later, his left side became affected in a similar manner; his utterance was very indistinct, but the sensibility remained normal. After two more days, the right leg and arm were again affected; the patient then became somnolent, his respiration grew stertorous; he could not swallow, and died on the seventh day of his illness. The necropsy revealed a plug of 1 centimetre in length in the basilar artery, which had undergone atheromatous degeneration; the pons was very soft to the touch, though not degenerated.

In the last case, the symptoms observed during life did not correspond with the *post-mortem* results. The patient was a man, aged 73, in whom gradually for several years feebleness, first of the legs, then of the arms, had set in, together with disturbances of speech and paresis of the buccal branches of both facial nerves. The patient could swallow, and even perform simple movements with his tongue. His utterance was explosive. On attempting to walk, or to stretch his legs, trembling set in. The tendon reflexes were normal. The action of the sphincters and the sensibility was normal. Later on, the patient became confused in his mind. The necropsy revealed several minute apoplectic cysts in the anterior portions of both nuclei caudati, immediately beneath the surface and in both thalami optici. The remainder of the brain was intact. The basal arteries were atheromatous. This case proves that bulbar symptoms may be caused by bilateral lesions of the cerebrum.—*London Med. Record*, Oct. 15, 1879.

Changes in the Spinal Cord in Infantile Spinal Paralysis and in Progressive Muscular Atrophy.

At the late International Medical Congress, at Amsterdam, MM. DAMASCHINO and HENRI ROGER presented a paper on the alterations in the spinal marrow in infantile spinal paralysis, and in progressive muscular atrophy.

Among the diseases of the nervous system which are observed among children, there is one the symptomatology of which presents special characteristics, this is infantile spinal paralysis, otherwise designated as essential paralysis of infancy, because it was looked upon as belonging to the group of nervous idiopathic diseases, *sine materia*.

The result of a certain number of observations collected by Messrs. Roger and Damaschino is that the characteristic alteration of this affection is a lesion of the spinal marrow, the consequence of which is atrophy of the nerves and muscles.

Dr. Damaschino presented in support of this proposition, histological preparations, and some very conclusive observations. In three of these observations the lesions consisted in some foci of inflammatory softening, which were seated in the anterior cornua of the gray matter, and extended almost the entire length of the lumbar marrow. The lesion is more marked towards the right, at the level of the dorsal region, there were no distinct foci, but they discovered granular bodies accumulated around the vessels; atrophy of the cells, which was very considerable in the lumbar region, was also discovered in other parts of the marrow, and bore a constant relation with the dimensions of the foci and the variable degree of the vascular lesions.

The atrophy of the white antero-lateral columns was very clear, and there were at this level an abundant accumulation of connective nuclei, also very decided atrophy of the anterior roots. The muscular lesions consisted mainly, as shown by microscopic examination, in diminution of size of the primitive fasciculi.

A great number of muscles were the seat of an abundant deposit of adipose cells placed between the muscular elements.

On the conclusion of M. Damaschino's communication, M. BOUCHUT said that he himself had made a large number of autopsies in cases of infantile paralysis, and that he had not observed the lesions of the marrow mentioned.

M. DAMASCHINO replied that if the lesions he had just described were not to be found in the marrow, it was because the means employed were insufficient. The numerous facts that he, together with M. Roger, had observed, and the histological preparations that he placed before the members of the Congress, clearly proved the existence of these lesions.—*Archives Gén. de Méd.*, Oct. 1879.

Hydrotherapeutic Treatment of Reflex-neurosis.

Dr. T. FRIEDMANN, the director of the hydrotherapeutic establishment at *Voeslau-Gainfain*, reports the following three cases where excellent results were obtained by water. Case 1. A gentleman, aged 60, from Paris. He had suffered much mental emotion and terror during the siege of Paris, in 1871–1872.

Soon after, he began to notice a tremor in his upper extremities, which subsequently affected his lower ones. These latter were accompanied by convulsions
and a frequent involuntary bending of the knees. When first seen by the author,
the patient's condition was as follows : He was fairly nourished, and his internal
organs were healthy. At every attempt to execute a movement, the upper extremities began to tremble. Both bicep muscles presented clonic convulsions ;
the latter could also be artificially produced by percussing the said muscles. The
flexor muscles of the legs were affected by similar convulsions, which caused a
frequent bending of the knees when walking. The movements of the hands
were also greatly impaired ; the patient could not raise a glass of water or a spoonful of soup to his mouth, without spilling the greater part of the contents on his
clothes. He had for several years tried various cures, but without effect. At
last he was persuaded to try what water could do for him. The treatment consisted at first in prolonged baths of medium temperature, which after a while were
followed by cool sitz baths, combined with local shower baths. In the course of
the first month, the patient's movements had become visibly stronger and less
uncertain. Towards the end of the second month, the patient was able to undertake long walks, and could use his hands perfectly well. The convulsive neurosis
which had been produced by psychical emotion had been effectually cured.
Case 2, is a case of rheumatic reflex neurosis, which had presented all the symptoms of tetanus. The patient, a railway official from Galicia, aged 26, had felt
a severe pain in the back after a hard day's work in cold, windy weather. Soon
after, he became unable to walk, as every attempt of locomotion was followed by
violent convulsions in the muscles of his limb and his trunk. He was obliged to
give up his work, and after failing to obtain relief from the usual therapeutic
means, he entered the establishment at Vöslau. He was pale, but fairly nourished. Family history good. He had always been well, with the exception of
an occasional catarrh. The thoracic and abdominal viscera were healthy. No
abnormal phenomena appeared as long as the patient was sitting quiet, but whenever he attempted to rise, tonic convulsions set in in the flexor muscles of the
upper and lower extremities. The clonic spasms extended to the straight abdominal muscles and the extensors of the vertebræ. After walking a few steps,
the patient suddenly assumed a crouching position, when the abdominal muscles
felt as hard as a board ; on attempting to rise he was drawn backwards by the
clonic spasms of the dorsal muscles, and would have fallen on his back, if he had
not either caught hold of something or else again crouched down. Every mechanical
irritation increased this convulsive state of the muscular system. After continuing
these movements for about ten minutes, the patient would fall back on his couch
quite exhausted. The treatment consisted in sitz baths, which were subsequently
combined with local douches and frictions. After a stay of two months in the
establishment, the patient was able to return to work. Case 3, is that of a Russian gentleman, aged 26, who had been sent to the establishment by Profs.
Billroth, Bamberger, and Duchek. The patient had been operated upon three
months before for an abscess in the right maxillary region, which had been
caused by periostitis. A few days after the wound had been healed, the patient
began to suffer from epileptiform fits, which were subsequently complicated with
tremor of the head and contractions of the cervical muscles on the left side. The
patient had never before been subject to similar attacks, neither had any members
of his family, although his father was said to have frequently suffered from congestion of the brain. The patient was a strong-built man, looking very pale.
The thoracic and abdominal viscera were healthy. On the right maxilla was a
scar of about three centimetres long, which was very tender to pressure. The
application of the faradic current or of extreme heat or cold, was exceedingly

painful; and if repeated for some time gave rise to disagreeable sensations in the head. At the same time there was tremor of the head and contraction of the left sternocleido-mastoid muscle. In the morning and forenoon, the patient was generally quiet, with the exception of the symptoms which have been described. In the course of the afternoon, at about 4 o'clock, he suddenly became restless; his face was congested, his eyes were bloodshot and rolled about wildly; he did not venture to leave his room alone, but insisted on going out into the air. This prodromal stage lasted generally for one hour to one and a half hours, when he would suddenly fling his right arm around the neck of his attendant and jump about the room on his left leg, which was spasmodically contracted, for half an hour or more, till he sank down exhausted on his couch. At this stage of his paroxysms, he lost consciousness, and was seized with such violent tonic-clonic convulsions that he had to be held down by five or six men. From time to time he would utter the exclamation, "You rascal!" The convulsions generally ceased in the course of half an hour to an hour; the patient recovered consciousness and felt strong enough to leave his couch and take a walk. The nights were sleepless, and the patient only sank into a short slumber towards morning. During the first three weeks, the condition of the patient remained much the same. It was then suggested that perhaps excision of the scar might afford some relief. This plan was carried out, and after the wound healed, another attempt at hydropathic treatment was made. During the first few days, the fits described were frequently repeated, probably owing to the irritation caused by the fresh sore. But in a very short time the soothing influence of the water-treatment showed itself distinctly; the patient gradually became less excited, the paroxysms were slighter, less intense and frequent, and his mental condition was much improved. Three weeks after the operation, the fits had completely ceased, the patient's motor power was entirely restored, and three weeks later he left the establishment in perfect mental and bodily health.—*London Med. Record*, Oct. 15, 1879.

—

Optic Neuritis in Cerebral Disease.

In the August number of the *Annales d'Oculistique*, Dr. PARINAND, from the results of post-mortem examination in twenty cases of meningitis and four of cerebral tumour, in all of which a careful ophthalmoscopic examination of the fundus had been made before death, comes to the conclusion that the various intra-cranial affections only produce œdematous optic neuritis (choked disk) when they are complicated with hydrocephalic effusion. A large cerebral tumour may fail to give rise to any ophthalmoscopic changes in the papilla if unaccompanied by hydrocephalus, while on the other hand the smallest pathological change accompanied by effusion of any considerable extent into the ventricles involves the optic nerve. The increase in intra-cranial pressure produced by hydrocephalic effusion alone is therefore, according to Parinaud, the cause of what is generally termed optic neuritis. He believes that the existence of true optic neuritis, or a state of actual inflammation of the optic nerve, must be admitted after the researches of Leber and Iwanow, but this condition produces visible alterations in the nerve much more slowly than the neuritis usually significant of cerebral disease, which is in reality an œdema.—*Edinburgh Med. Journal*, Nov. 1879.

—

Menière's Disease.

At the late International Medical Congress at Amsterdam, Prof. DOYER, of Leyden, read a paper on this subject, which contained the following conclusions:—

1. In a general sense of the word, the name of Menière's disease may be ap-

plied to all cases of vertigo which are caused by an abnormal irritation of the nerves of the semicircular canals. The irritation may be produced either by an exaggerated normal cause, e. g., violent rotatory movements of the head, or of the whole body, or by an abnormal cause, e. g., a sudden change of temperature (especially when passing from a higher to a lower temperature), variations in the intra-tympanic pressure, disturbances in the circulation or inflammation.

2. In a more restricted sense the name of Menière's disease is applied to cases where the vertigo is caused by an inflammatory condition either of the semicircular ducts or of the middle ear. The vertigo may either be persistent or simply caused momentarily by normal movements of the head. In some cases it appears periodically under the form of a fit, at intervals of weeks or even months.

3. Exposure to cold and catarrhs of the tympanic cavity play a prominent part in the etiology of Menière's disease.

4. The majority, if not all cases, of Menière's disease are of secondary nature, i. e., they are caused by catarrhs or inflammations of the tympanic or mastoid cavity.

5. In typical cases the vertigo is preceded or accompanied by rotatory sensations which follow a certain order: the attack begins by a sensation of rotation around a vertical axis. The rotation invariably takes place on the affected side ; sometimes it is combined with a sensation of swinging backwards and forwards. In more serious cases, the feeling is that of rotating round a horizontal axis both backwards and forwards. Finally, the vertigo becomes general, and the patient falls down, with, or without, loss of consciousness ; he often vomits in such cases. Sometimes the attack is over in from ten to thirty minutes, in other cases it is called forth by a simple movement of the head during one or two days following the first attack, and the patient is obliged to lie perfectly still in order to avoid them.

6. In some cases, the rotatory sensations may be caused experimentally by certain therapeutic agents, e. g., by the insufflation of air into the tympanic cavity in cases of acute inflammation of the latter, or by the injection of fluids into the mastoid cavity when the mastoid process has been perforated. In these cases, the rotatory sensation always takes place round a vertical axis and in the direction of the affected organ.

7. In some cases the attacks are accompanied by loud noises in the ear ; in other cases there is a constant slight buzzing noise which does not increase in strength during the attack ; sometimes there is no sound at all.

8. In cases of long standing, a slight feeling of vertigo persists even during the free intervals, and seems to be caused by the first movements of the head after awaking from sleep. Sometimes the patient feels as if he were going to fall either backwards or forwards. Other patients are obliged to keep the head fixed in a certain position, because every movement that takes place in the plane of one of the semicircular ducts is accompanied by a sensation of a heavy body rolling in the same direction. (In a typical case which came under the speaker's observation, the patient held his head inclined forward and to the left, and thus prevented all movement of rotation in the plane of the sagittal semicircular canal of the left side. The left ear was affected in this case.)

9. Menière's disease is frequently complicated with hysteria. It is also apt to produce in children a condition not unlike chorea and in adults clonic contractions of the muscles of the face and body. These often disappear entirely after a local treatment of the middle ear.

10. In some cases, patients after recovering from Menière's disease have lost the faculty of hearing.

11. Highly satisfactory results have often been obtained by local treatment, even in inveterate cases.

12. Professor Charcot has strongly recommended the use of quinine in the internal treatment of the affection, as it frequently wards off the attacks. In some cases where the inner ear is affected it has been observed that the use of quinine has been followed by increasing deafness, while the singing in the ear vanishes. This effect generally only lasts as long as the drug is used.—*British Med. Journal*, Sept. 20, 1879.

Perforating Ulcer of the Stomach; Vomiting of a Tubercular and Sacciform Mass.

Dr. O. HJELT relates the following case in the *Finska Läkarasällskapets Handlingar*, Band xx (quoted in *Nordiskt Mediciniskt Arkiv*, Band xi). The patient, a woman aged 42, had enjoyed good health, with the exception of some slight dyspeptic troubles. On February 15th, she had a severe rigor, followed by fever, with burning pain in the throat, and violent vomiting. When admitted into the General Hospital, she had constant vomiting, and some, but not very severe, diarrhœa, which had set in about a week previously; she had also dysphagia. The mucous membrane of the mouth and fauces was much injected; and there was a diphtheritic deposit on the soft palate, uvula, posterior pharyngeal wall, and also on the tongue and gums. The epigastrium was very tender on pressure. Almost everything that the patient ate caused vomiting. This condition lasted about two weeks; after which there was some improvement. The diphtheritic process in the mouth and fauces gradually ceased, and the gastric symptoms were so far relieved that the patient could take easily digestible food without provoking vomiting. At the end of March, however, there was a change for the worse. The patient again became feverish; constant vomiting, partly of blood, set in; and the patient's strength was much reduced. On March 31st, she vomited a large consistent tubular and sacciform membrane, which was apparently a cast of the stomach and of a part of the œsophagus. An extremely severe pain in the epigastrium, which had troubled the patient for some time previously, ceased immediately afterwards. On April 6th, she had a severe attack of pleurisy in the left side, which two days later spread to the right side; on the 10th, there was peritonitis, with tympanic distension of the bowels, and great tenderness over the whole abdomen. The patient rapidly fell into a state of collapse, and died on April 11th. At the necropsy, the œsophagus was found to be much thickened, and to pass imperceptibly into the stomach, which formed a round sac of the size of a smallish apple. The spleen formed a tongue-shaped, obtuse, rounded body, about eight-tenths of an inch in diameter, lying nearly free in the stomach; at its lower part it was firmly inclosed in the wall of the stomach, but above this the point of the little finger could be passed into an open canal below the diaphragm and the adherent capsule of the spleen. The cavity of the stomach, which was much contracted, contained only 60 cubic *centimètres* (little more than two ounces) of fluid. The pyloric portion was much thickened; Brunner's glands were swollen; the pancreas was elongated and loose. The canal above mentioned as commencing in the stomach opened into the peritoneal cavity at the upper part of the spleen, which was here eroded, while the portion lying within the stomach had a firm thickened rough surface. The spleen, which in its middle part was firmly adherent to the diaphragm, the capsule being very thick at this part, had a semiglobular form, and was about four and a half inches in length and two inches in thickness. The membranous cast of the stomach and œsophagus, mentioned above, was 37 *centimètres* (14½ inches) in length. Narrow above, it increased gradually in breadth, until it suddenly expanded into a semiglobular sac; its outer surface was rough, rather uneven, of a brown-gray colour with dark spots; its inner surface was of a dark colour, here and there nearly black; it was of firm consistence, and its thickness through the greater part of its extent was double that of a sheet of writing paper. The membrane consisted of a granular mass, with numerous fibres crossing in all directions, and a great abundance of small yellowish-red conglomerated blood-corpuscles and large dark adherent clots of blood. It might be regarded as a blood-extravasation moulded on the mucous membrane of the stomach and œsophagus.—*British Med. Journal*, Oct. 18, 1879.

Rupture of the Aorta.

The following case is reported in the *Presse Méd. Belge.* A woman aged 37 was received at the Hôpital Saint-Jean in Brussels. She said that she was six months 'pregnant, and complained of headache and of violent pain in the epigastrium. She was very restless. Two hours after the examination, the restlessness increased; her skin was covered with perspiration; her face twitched convulsively. She vomited frequently large quantities of mucus mixed with bile. Her bowels were moved once or twice. Two hours later, the patient died. During the whole of this time, her cerebral and respiratory functions had remained perfectly normal. The necropsy showed that the pericardium was distended by a voluminous clot. The heart was not adherent to the pericardium. The connective tissue at the base of the heart was infiltrated with blood, especially in the neighbourhood of the aorta and pulmonary artery. The auricles and ventricles were normal. In the aorta, about half an inch beyond the sigmoid valves, was a transverse rupture which extended through the whole of the inner coat; and the blood oozing from this rupture into the neighbouring parts had partly torn off the membranes of the pulmonary artery. The same had taken place in the aorta down to the lumbar region, and the iliac veins were overflowing with blood. No satisfactory reason for this rupture of the aorta could be detected. It might, however, have been caused by some rapid movement made by the woman during the last moments of her life.—*British Med. Journal*, Sept. 20, 1879.

A Rare Fungous Growth on the Hair in the Axillæ.

Dr. AXEL KEY describes the following case in the *Hygeia* for 1878 (quoted in *Nordiskt Mediciniskt Arkiv*, Band xi). A gentleman had for some time noticed that the hair in his axillæ stuck together, in consequence of being covered with a glutinous substance. The sweat of the axillæ coloured his shirt bright red. His condition in other respects was normal. On examination, Dr. Key found the axillary hairs greatly adherent; and a large part of them were covered with a gelatiniform substance like mildew. This had its seat on the free ends of the hair, where it formed partly isolated or confluent swellings, and partly bands like chains of pearls, or an adhesive mass surrounding the hairs. There were no changes in the skin. Microscopic examination showed that the changes were dependent on a peculiar fungous vegetation, which had a brimstone yellow colour by transmitted light. The development of the vegetation commenced in the form of small, slender, exceedingly delicate scales, which soon formed small round elevations, apparently homogeneous, but containing numerous small glistening spores. The scales seem partly to lie on the outside of the hair, but for the most part the vegetation penetrated between the outer layer of the epidermis covering the hair. Here and there, the vegetation could be traced to the interior of the hair. No mycelium was found. Dr. Key has not been able to find a similar case recorded in dermatological literature. Buhl alone has described in the *Zeitschrift für rationelle Medicin*, Band. iii, a new hair-fungus apparently like that described above; he calls it zoogloea capillarum. The disorder would, therefore, seem to be very rare.—*British Medical Journal*, Sept. 27, 1879.

Syphilitic Herpes.

The patient, an inmate of the London Hospital, and under the care of Mr. JONATHAN HUTCHINSON, was an unhealthy-looking man, a discharged soldier, aged thirty-five, with peculiar eruption running round the left side of his chest, at once recognizable as a form of herpes zoster, or "shingles." There was nothing in the position or general outline of the eruption that would distinguish it from ordinary herpes zoster, but it would have been difficult to fail to notice at the first glance that its aspect was in some way different from what is usually seen in a simple case of this disease. On inquiry it was found that the eruption had existed for no less a period than nine months. The patient stated, moreover, that it was "much better" a few months before, but that it broke out again in (what he termed) a second attack, although the side had never been entirely free from eruption, even in the interval of amelioration. On examining the eruption closely, it was seen that in some places there were distinct and prominent scabs; the eruption here had evidently taken an ulcerative action, and approached in some little degree to the characters of rupia. The skin where the eruption had departed was of a dusky-red colour, and presented here and there a faintly depressed scar, showing that there had been a loss of tissue. It was ascertained the man had had undoubted syphilis; in fact he had a large periosteal node on the forehead at the moment. On this account, but still more from certain peculiarities of the eruption itself, Mr. Hutchinson said he was of opinion that this was a case of syphilitic herpes, and as such a very rare affection.

"Herpes," Mr. Hutchinson went on to say, "is, as is well known, a skin disease of nerve origin. It is produced through some particular nerve influence, and, having regard therefore to its origin, we must consider the present case not as an example of common herpes occurring in a syphilitic patient, and so possibly somewhat modified by that disorder, but as a case where the poison of syphilis has caused such nerve changes as to bring about this eruption. The action of syphilis in this case is through the nervous system, and the eruption must be considered as an expression of some syphilitic disturbance of nerve. Thus we see syphilis as an imitator of typical skin eruptions, and, as I have often stated, it rarely, very rarely, imitates herpes. I consider this eruption to be the syphilitic form of herpes on the following grounds: The man is syphilitic. The skin disease persists—it has persisted for nine months, with a recurrence of eruption during that time, whereas common herpes tends to spontaneous cure, as do all skin affections that have their origin in the nervous system. It is most rare, too, for common shingles to persist for so long a period as nine months. It is true that it is sometimes very tardy in its appearance, but, I think, never to such a degree as obtains in this instance. The scar left here and there by the clearing up of the eruption is depressed, distinct, and of a dusky-red colour. The eruption is at places almost rupial. Finally, there is one feature about the case that makes it —as a case of syphilitic herpes—very peculiar. Syphilitic herpes is nearly always symmetrical on both sides of the body, but in the present instance the eruption appeared on one side only, the right chest being perfectly intact. The case therefore, must be regarded as extremely unusual."—*Lancet*, Oct. 25, 1879.

Treatment of Syphilis in New-Born Infants.

Professor PARROT delivered a lecture on this subject (*Gaz. des Hôpitaux*, No. 100) at the Hospice des Enfants Assistés, from which we extract the following :—

The history of the indications which should be followed in the treatment of syphilis in new-born infants has in general been remarkably complicated, whereas simplification is the more required, inasmuch as we have to do with little children in whom hygiene and a very small number of pharmaceutical preparations furnish excellent results. The therapeutics, comprising questions of great practical interest, may be considered under distinct heads.

1. Should we treat infants born of syphilitic parents, even when such children exhibit no apparent traces of a syphilitic diathesis? In a word, ought we to institute preventive treatment in a new-born infant suspected of heredity? Authors are not agreed upon this grave question. Some recommend such treatment without any hesitation; but they make some distinctions: (1) if the father alone is syphilitic, it is useless to treat the infant: (2) if the mother has been syphilitic, but has been treated during pregnancy, the child need not be treated; (3) when both parents are syphilitic, or when the mother alone is affected and has not been treated during pregnancy, the infant should be submitted to specific treatment. All these distinctions belong to medical casuistry, and are only founded on disputable theories. The infant is just as syphilitic when its father alone is the subject of the disease as when the mother is so; and I lay down this formal rule, viz., that whenever I am in presence of an infant born of parents, one or both of whom are syphilitic, I never treat it when it exhibits no trace of syphilitic infection. Whatever may be the condition of the parents, their children are not necessarily the subjects of hereditary syphilis. I do not believe that in order that we may treat an hypothetical disease we have the right to expose an infant to the risks of a treatment which is not inoffensive, especially for one newly born. In all cases, if the child remains unaffected for a fortnight or a month, it is a proof either that it is not poisoned, or, if it is so, it is only in a benign manner, and that we shall easily combat a virus that manifests itself with so much difficulty.

2. The infant should be placed under treatment (1) when there are signs of syphilis manifest on the skin, mucous membranes, or bony tissue; and (2) when, in the absence of these signs, chronic and obstinate gastro-intestinal disturbances exist, resisting all ordinary treatment. Such disturbances are, in fact, the indication of visceral syphilis, and we should always bear this hypothesis in mind when we observe them. This is a positive rule, and I have seen an infant die of them, without the idea having ever occurred of treating a visceral syphilis of which there were no external signs, but which was found to exist at the autopsy. When the infant exhibits traces of apparent syphilides, we must still distinguish two cases, according as these signs are precocious, appearing at the time of birth or very soon afterwards, or when they occur later, constituting, for example, lenticular syphilides and syphilis of bone. It is essential that the therapeutical opportunity should be clearly determined. In the first category we meet with the most numerous and the most important manifestations of syphilis, the early syphilides. The infant is almost always very young, bringing the syphilis with it at its birth. The diathesis is then very active, very ardent, and will rapidly attain the viscera if it is not treated. In these cases mercury is the sole efficacious medicine, and no other should be thought of. Its *external* employment is the most ancient, for originally syphilis was treated only by frictions, and this method continues to be the best, the most efficacious, and the most prompt. Frictions may be employed when the infants reject all that is taken into the stomach, or are the subjects of intestinal disturbances which the mercury would only aggravate, adding to the existing athrepsy. There may be contra-indications to the external use of mercury when a general eruption with ulcerated patches exists, but such cases are quite exceptional. Syphilis has its places of predilection, and never invades the armpits or the lateral parts of the trunk, and these are precisely the parts most

suitable for inunctions, which should not be made at the thighs or groins. The double mercurial ointment, consisting of equal parts of lard and mercury, should be diluted with two additional parts of lard, and of this three grammes (forty-five grains) may be used daily for an infant until it is a month old. After this age, and until the sixth month, the ointment may consist of one gramme and a half of the double ointment and three grammes of lard; and from six months until one or two years, three grammes to four grammes may be employed. Thus the doses of mercury are not increased in proportion to the age of the children, for the further this is advanced, the more does the diathesis become diminished and exhausted. The frictions are made during from one to five minutes only once daily. This mode of treatment is the most prompt and heroic, and is of the greatest service. (Professor Parrot entirely disapproves of the treatment by mercurial baths and by hypodermic injection of the sublimate.) The best medicinal agent for the *internal* use of mercury is Van Swieten's *liquor*, consisting of one part of the deutochloride of mercury, 100 parts of alcohol, and 900 parts of water. The dose for a sickly new-born infant with intestinal disturbance is half a teaspoonful, and for a robust infant a teaspoonful—making from two to five grammes of the *liquor*, containing from two to five milligrammes of the sublimate. But such a dose must not be administered at one time. A spoonful, or five grammes of the *liquor*, may be added to twenty-five grammes of some kind of syrup as a vehicle, and a teaspoonful of this mixture may be given six times daily. When the infant is at the breast, one of these may be given before each suckling (and in the same way just before each time of taking the bottle, when brought up by it), so that the remedy is always taken *before* the repast, the milk of which renders it more inoffensive. To infants of six months a teaspoonful and a half may be given, and to those of three years two teaspoonfuls. Larger doses are both useless and mischievous.

The second category comprises the delayed or lenticular syphilides, appearing at the age of six months, or of a year or two—the last traces of a diathesis that is already exhausted. The disease is no longer dangerous, for if no obstinate intestinal disturbance has supervened, we may be almost certain that there is no visceral syphilis. The diathesis has not been able to attain the deep-seated organs, and it has become extinguished. When consulted at this period, we might abstain from all treatment; and we have seen spontaneous cases produced in this hospital in young robust infants. Still, as a general rule, treatment should be had recourse to even at this period; but then mercury should never be administered. What we have to do in these infants, who are really cured of the syphilis, is to modify the constitution of their economy, in which there will always be a tendency to engender at a later period, not syphilism, but, in my opinion, rickets. To this end we should give them iodine. The iodide of potassium may be given for from six to eighteen months, commencing with fifteen to twenty-five centigrammes, and going later to a gramme per diem, given in divided doses. To this, however, I prefer a mixture consisting of 1 gramme of the tincture of iodine to 100 grammes of syrup of gentian or bitter orange-peel, of which a teaspoonful may be given daily in divided doses. *Local treatment* also has its utility. The first rule is the observation of the most rigorous cleanliness, baths with bran or starch-water being employed daily, and absorbent powders used afterwards, such as one part of the oxide of zinc to thirty of starch powder. When there are ulcerations the glycerole of zinc (pure neutral glycerine thirty parts and oxide of zinc two parts) forms an excellent application. If the ulcerations are deep and have a tendency to phagedænism, they should be powdered with iodoform.

3. How should syphilitic new-born infants be fed? Alimentation plays an important part in their cure, and for a full consideration of all the delicate questions relating to this subject I may refer to Dr. Fournier's able lectures delivered in

1877, confining myself to its purely practical and clinical aspects. An infant the subject of hereditary syphilis should be fed as much as possible, and the sole nutriment that is suitable and indispensable for it is breast-milk. The child should always be kept at the breast as long as there is no risk of contaminating the nurse; but when there is danger to the nurse it should be withdrawn. If the mother is supposed to be exempt from syphilis, although her infant is syphilitic she should suckle her child; and if there are risks to be run, the mother, before all others, ought to run them. If it is impossible for the mother to suckle the infant, recourse must be had to a nurse. When the child is born without any trace of syphilis, we may consign it to a nurse, recommending her to observe certain precautions, such as washing the month of the infant by means of a pad moistened with alcoholized water prior to suckling, and washing the nipple with the same after suckling; and carefully examining every day the condition of the mucous membrane and the anus of the infant. I believe that we must absolutely provide a nurse for such an infant, for without her its life is seriously threatened; and we have no right to expose it thus to almost certain death under the pretext that it may become syphilitic, for these infants frequently do not become so. On this point I differ in opinion from many eminent and competent practitioners, at the head of whom I place Dr. Fournier. But it seems to me that this is a question of life and death, for the new-born infant; and, moreover, I am in agreement with all those who, on the appearance of the slightest trace of infection, the slightest spot, prohibit the continuance of suckling, even when there seems no danger of conveying the contagion by the breast of the nurse. In such cases ought we to inform the nurse that the infant given her to suckle is syphilitic? This is a very delicate question in medical deontology; for the tribunals have alike condemned practitioners for having violated medical secresy by so informing the nurse, and for having exposed the nurse to contamination through not informing her. Between these alternatives what course should we pursue? We should inform the parents of the danger which the nurse is incurring, and of their own responsibility, and invite them to dismiss the nurse immediately on some pretext—renouncing all attempts to bring up the child by the breast. If they resist his advice the *ultima ratio* of the practitioner is to retire from the case and see the child no more. This precept leads us far away from the time of Mauriceau, when they had no fear of infecting the nurse. In our days, the nurse must be first considered, her health being more precious even than the life of the infant. We have no longer the right to knowingly give syphilis to a nurse by confiding a syphilitic infant to her care. On taking the nurse away from the infant we must still give it milk, bringing it up by the bottle if no better means offers itself. An excellent mode would certainly be to suckle it by means of a syphilitic nurse; and at the end of the last century considerable sums were paid at the Hospice de Vaugirard in order to secure a constant supply of syphilitic nurses. The milk of such women, in fact, is frequently as good as that of a healthy nurse, and it is to be regretted that this institution no longer exists. In our own hospice we have recently had two syphilitic nurses who have rendered us real services. In the absence of nurses, asses' milk forms the best substitute, following it up by that of the cow. (Prof. Parrot has not found goats' milk, so strongly recommended by Fournier and others, very satisfactory.)

4. A final practical question is whether it is possible, when the syphilitic infant is suckled by a nurse or by a goat, to administer antisyphilitic remedies through the milk instead of giving them directly to the infant. In spite of the fact having been denied by distinguished chemists, it appears to be generally admitted that mercury given to the nurse passes into the milk; but this is certainly a very uncertain mode of treating a child, since the quantities absorbed depend upon different

conditions acting upon the system of nutrition. The best procedure is to give the mercury direct to the child before its repasts, not mixing it with the milk.—*Med. Times and Gazette*, Oct. 11, 1879.

Surgery.

Thrombosis Cavernosa.

At a meeting of the Society of Physicians in Vienna, Prof. BILLROTH reported (*Allg. Med. Cent. Zeit.*, No. 51, 1879) a case of spontaneous gangrene which came under his notice in the course of last year. The patient was a strongly-built man, aged 47, who, for the last five years, had been getting gradually more and more weak. Standing about, walking, and riding fatigued him very much. No cause could be discovered to explain this peculiar condition. Neither the heart nor the arteries were affected. Last summer the patient had his corns cut by a barber, after which operation an abscess broke out on the big toe, which would not heal. It was a gangrene of the big toe, such as is only seen in cases of senile gangrene. The patient suffered excruciating pains ; for some time a line of demarcation seemed to be forming, then he had again violent pains, the gangrene spread to the second toe, and six weeks later the man was reduced to a perfect skeleton. Prof. Billroth then resolved to resort to amputation of the leg, although he did not believe that the patient would survive the operation. To his surprise, however, the wound healed well, the patient recovered, and does very well now. On examining the stump, the arteries were found to contain vascularized tissue, which might easily have been taken for common blood-clots. A second intima had formed within the arteries, and the openings of small vessels could distinctly be seen in the thrombus. This formation of vessels within the thrombus explains sufficiently why the gangrenous process did not spread more rapidly. Billroth has designated this affection, Thrombosis cavernosa. It is generally thought to be caused by syphilis, but the patient positively asserted that neither he nor any member of his family had ever had syphilis. As he still suffered pain in the stump of his leg, Billroth put him through an antisyphilitic treatment, consisting of the internal use of iodide of potass and rubbing with belladonna and ung. cin., which had a soothing effect. Billroth thinks that similar processes occur more frequently than is generally supposed.—*London Med. Record*, Oct. 15, 1879.

Foreign Doctrines of Trephining.

The recent volume of *Revue des Sciences Médicales* contains a very exhaustive article, by M. SCHWARTZ, on the recent history of trephining and the indications for this operation. The paper is divided into two sections, which treat respectively of primary and secondary trephining. It will be of interest to give an abstract of this valuable report.

Percival Pott, J. L. Petit, Quesnay, Méhie, and De la Touche frequently practised preventive trephining. The object of this operation was to prevent compression and inflammation of the brain, by opening the skull immediately after the accident. In the language of modern surgery, however, trephining is said to be primary when it is performed in the course of the first few days following the accident, and either before the period of inflammatory reaction, or even after it has set in. It is necessary to bear this point in mind. During the latter half of the present century, the operation had become almost obsolete. It was not until 1867, when Professor Broca published the results of his researches on the centre of localization of speech, that the attention of French surgeons was again directed to it. An animated discussion took place at a meeting of the Société de Chirurgie, when it was discovered that trephining had been so rarely practised of late, that it was very difficult to collect a sufficient number of cases to justify or oppose the operation.

The year after this discussion, in which the most celebrated French surgeons joined, M. Larrey presented to the society a paper on trephining, and the indications and contraindications for performing the operation. According to his experience, the operation was indicated: 1. In cases of fracture of the cranium, when the fragments of bone press on the brain, and give rise to serious symptoms, which persist even after the fragments have been removed; 2. In cases of fracture where the splinters and fragments of bones, or of foreign bodies, have penetrated into the substance of the brain, and it is impossible to remove them without trephining; 3. In other complicated lesions of the skull, where there are symptoms of an accumulation of blood or pus pressing on the brain, and the usual therapeutic agents remain ineffective.

The following were the contraindications for trephining: 1. When a foreign body has penetrated so deeply into the brain that it cannot be recovered; 2. If the blood or pus contained in the skull do not appear to form a focus in connection with the opening in the bone; 3. In all fractures which are not complicated by any phenomena of compression or of paralysis, etc.; 4. In cases of cerebral commotion or coma; 5. In epileptiform transitory convulsions; 6. In cases of encephalitis or encephalomeningitis.

The only drawback to this elaborate classification is, that it is almost impossible to distinguish between these different lesions at the bedside of the patient. This difficulty, in fact, was one of the principal strongholds of the adversaries of trephining. The surgeons of the day were divided into two parties; but the prevailing opinion was against the operation.

In 1874, Sédillot strongly advocated trephining in cases of fracture of the inner table of the skull; but, as it is very difficult to diagnose isolated fracture of the inner table, little attention was given to his doctrine till 1876, when M. Sédillot presented to the Académie des Sciences a treatise on trephining, containing the results of one hundred and six observations made by him. Of these one hundred and six patients with fracture of the skull, seventy-seven were trephined and twenty-nine were treated by the expectant method. Of these latter, one recovered and twenty-eight died. Of the seventy-seven who were trephined, twenty-nine recovered and forty-eight died. No fixed time was given for the performance of the operation. Of nine patients on whom preventive trephining was performed, six recovered and three, or 33.3 per cent., died. Of sixty-eight on whom it was done for curative purposes, twenty-four recovered and forty-four, or 64.7 per cent., died; and of forty-seven, where the operation was deferred, fifteen recovered and thirty-two, or 67 per cent., died. It results from these numbers that the chances of recovery decrease in proportion as the operation is postponed.

About the same time, attention was attracted by the remarkable works of Hitzig and Ferrier on cerebral localization. They proved, by their investigations, that there exist certain zones on the surface of the brain, in the frontoparietal region, which, if irritated, will give rise to convulsions or contractions in the opposite half of the body. If these zones are removed or destroyed, paralysis of certain members follows. According to M. Vulpian, these zones act through the intermediary agency of the gray cortical matter, or through the white matter which is situated beneath the gray substance. Bochefontaine and Duret have shown that a certain proportion of the phenomena of irritation, such as convulsions and contractions, can be traced back to lesions of the nerves of the meninges, especially of the dura mater. These phenomena ought in fact to be regarded as true reflex actions, of which we know the centripetal tract, the centre, and the centrifugal tract. Having once settled the different centres of localization in the brain, the next step was to discover what particular places on the skull would correspond to the said centres. This could best be done by ascertaining the position of the fissure of Rolando, seeing that such of the motor centres whose position is sufficiently well known are situated around it. In the adult, the mean distance from the bregma to the upper end of the fissure of Rolando is forty-seven millimetres. The number varies according to the conformation of the skull, but the deviations are very slight indeed. The bregma may be determined by the aid of Professor Broca's ingenious instrument, or by M. Lucas-Championnière's biauricular cartoons. The point where the biauricular line is intersected by the median line of the calvarium corresponds to the spot we wish to find.

In order to ascertain the inferior end of the fissure of the sulcus of Rolando, draw a horizontal line for about seven centimetres from the external orbicular apophysis. If a perpendicular line be then erected on the posterior end of this line, and continued upwards for five centimetres, the inferior portion of the fissure of Rolando will be found to correspond exactly to this point. The localization of the centre of speech is determined in the following way. A horizontal line is traced from the external orbicular apophysis, and continued towards the crest of the frontal bone for about five centimetres. A perpendicular line, three centimetres in length, is erected in this spot. If the trephine be applied to the region which is situated anterior to the fissure of Rolando, after it has been traced out in the way we have just described, it will affect the anterior motor centres. If the trephine be applied to the region situated behind the fissure of Rolando, it will affect the posterior centres.

It is natural that, in proportion as a more thorough knowledge was obtained of the functions of the cortical substance of the brain, and especially that portion of it which is closely connected with the skull, professional opinion became gradually more reconciled to the operation. This new phase was ushered in by the works of MM. Proust, Terrillon, Lucas-Championnière, Pozzi, Gosselin, and Le Dentu. The two latter presented each a report on the subject; the former to the Académie de Médicine, the latter to the Société de Chirurgie, which contain a fund of valuable information for the surgeon.

It remains now to speak of the present state of the question in France. According to the opinion of such eminent surgeons as Dr. Legouest and Dr. Tillaux, the removal of splinters or fragments of bone from a fracture of the skull does not constitute primary or preventive trephining. It is merely a surgical operation, such as would be resorted to in any case of fracture, and performed with the aid of appropriate instruments.

Concerning primary trephining (for preventive trephining has become nearly obsolete, in spite of Sédillot's endeavours to restore it), modern surgeons are divided into three parties. Those who look upon the doctrine of cerebral localization as not being sufficiently established yet, and who do not feel themselves justified in diagnosing a cerebral lesion from a functionary symptom, have remained, as it were, stationary. M. Gosselin and the German surgical school represent this opinion. The theories of this party may shortly be summed up as follows: Preventive trephining can be resorted to without any danger, and even be useful in cases where the skull has already been opened by a fracture; but it is more dangerous than useful, whatever the functional symptoms may be, when the skull has not been fractured, and would have to be opened by the operation. To the second category belong the surgeons who believe to a certain point in the doctrine of localizations. They admit that the operation may prove useful under the following circumstances: 1. In cases where it is necessary to remove foreign bodies or fragments of bone from the dura mater and the brain; 2. When it is necessary to promote the evacuation of accumulations of blood or serum between the dura mater and the brain, as these are liable to exert a deleterious influence on the brain, either through putrefaction or by pressure; 3. For the purpose of allowing purulent accumulations to escape.

Trephining is always dangerous when it establishes a communication between the arachnoidian cavity and the air. It follows that, in cases of existing fractures, it may be performed without danger. Messieurs Le Dentu and Legouest object to preventive trephining. Primary trephining may be resorted to in cases of convulsions which are caused by a limited depression of the skull, or by general hemiplegia accompanied by stertorous breathing and loss of consciousness. In all other cases it is best to wait, as it often happens that all these symptoms disappear without surgical treatment. If, however, the serious symptoms persist, or become more intensified, the operation must be resorted to at once, but no more crowns should be applied than are necessary. In short, the practitioners ought entirely to be guided by local symptoms, and not by the situation of the centre, the peculiar condition of which gives rise to certain symptoms.

The third class is represented by M. Lucas-Championnière. He teaches that trephining may be determined solely by the cerebral localizations, and that even preventive trephining is admissible. The operation is indicated in cases where it is necessary to raise up or remove fragments of bone which irritate the brain, to remove a foreign body, or to evacuate an accumulation of blood in the brain. It may also be performed at a later period for the purpose of removing splinters, raising a depression, or evacuating a purulent extra- or intra-cerebral gathering. If, however, no apparent lesions or accidents take place after a trauma of the skull, it is advisable to wait. If the patient present depression of the skull without any brain-symptoms, the surgeon must hold himself in readiness to trephine at a moment's notice. The same precautions must be taken in a case of traumatic fracture without depression.

If the patient be comatose, the operation must be resorted to in cases of depression of the skull, or of paralysis or convulsions of the opposite half of the body. M. Lucas-Championnière is so much in favour of trephining, that he regards it as indicated in cases of paralysis where all other symptoms are absent. In secondary paralysis, the indications are less formal. In general hemiplegia, the operation may be safely performed, as the lesion is probably an extensive one. In cases of convulsions, with or without paralysis, the operation is *de rigueur* if the convulsions be localized.

As far as fractures of the inner table are concerned, trephining must be performed whenever the symptoms appear serious. The trephine must be applied to that particular spot of the surface of skull which corresponds to the affected centre. The latter can easily be identified by symptoms of paralysis or localized convulsions. It does not do to be too timid; and a number of trephines can be safely applied. In short, the author has come back to the doctrine of preventive trephining.

Dr. Otis, in his interesting work on *Gunshot Wounds* during the civil war in America, has expended much labour on an exhaustive compilation of statistics on primary and preventive trephining. He tabulates the cases of one hundred and ninety-six patients who were trephined for gunshot wounds: of these, 110 (56 per cent.) died; 46 operations for primary trephining were performed, with a mortality of 32, or 69.6 per cent.

Echeverria, in his work on *Trephining for Traumatic Epilepsy*, quotes 18 cases of what he calls primary trephining, out of which only 3 ended fatally. In Germany, the majority of surgeons were even more opposed to the operation than in France. Beck, Bergmann, Chelius, and Roser admit it only in exceptional cases. Nussbaum, Esmarch, and especially Stromeyer, are very much against it. It seems, however, as if of late a gradual reaction in favour of trephining were taking place in Germany, as is evident from Bluhm's treatise on the subject. In fact, Fischer, Roser, and Bergmann recommend trephining with a view to prevent encephalo-meningitis, and in certain cases of depressions of the skull which may be recognized easily by the existence of a wound or a visible depression of the bones of the skull. They do not think it safe to rely too much on certain functional symptoms. According to Bluhm, the death-rate in primary trephining is 55.26 per cent., which rises to 64.29 per cent. if we consider only the cases where the operation was performed for gunshot wounds.

In short, in comparing the statistical tables drawn up by Sédillot, Echeverria, Otis, and Bluhm, it will be found that two are in favour of primary trephining, and two against it. We must, however, remember that out of the eighteen operations which Echeverria quotes as primary, only seven were performed in the course of the first four days after the accident. The remaining operations must be classified among the intermediary operations for trephining.

In comparing all the different statistical tables which we have quoted in this work, we find that the danger of the operation decreases if performed from five to twenty days after the accident, *i. e.*, if secondary or intermediate trephining be resorted to instead of primary. It must not be inferred from this that primary trephining ought never to be performed; we have as yet no right to emit a decisive opinion on the subject. But if the operation is to be resorted to at all, it must only be done on very precise indications; and it might even be unsafe to trust too much to the theory of localization till our knowledge of the functions of the gray matter of the brain has become more firmly established, and we have discovered more satisfactory methods of applying antiseptic dressing to head cases.—*British Med. Journal*, Sept. 27, 1879.

———

Emphysema of the Upper Eyelid produced by blowing the Nose after an Injury.

Dr. A. D. WILLIAMS relates the following case. A young woman called to ask him about her eye, which she had injured only a few minutes before by a severe fall. By accident, she tumbled down four or five steps out of a front door upon the pavement, strikingly heavily upon the bricks with the supraorbital bone of the left side of the head and body. The fall caused considerable contusion of the flesh and some abrasion of the skin over the left eye, but no cut. Soon after she stood up, she had occasion to blow her nose quite hard, and was surprised to find that the upper eyelid swelled up to such an extent that she could not open the eye even with her fingers. The suddenness of the swelling and her inability to open the eye in any way naturally frightened her very much. Upon examination, Dr. Williams could find no injury other than the contusion of the flesh and the abrasion of the skin over the eye. The peculiar cracking feeling communicated to the fingers by palpation conclusively proved that the great swelling of the lid was caused by the presence of air in its areolar tissue. By pressing upon the lid a little, the air could be forced out of the lid into the deeper tissue of the orbit, which allowed the lid at once to partly open. The pressure caused the cracking noise to be both heard and felt by the patient. To account for the emphysema of the lid, it is necessary to suppose that the fall caused sufficient fracture of the bone at some point to make an opening through it. The locality of the fractured point was most likely in the outer or anterior wall of the frontal sinus. When the patient blew her nose, the pressure was sufficient to force the air through the opening in the areolar tissue of the lid.—*British Med. Journal*, Oct. 18, 1879.

—

Plan of a Regulation for Testing the Visual Faculties of Railway Servants.

At the late International Medical Congress at Amsterdam, Prof. DONDERS, of Utrecht, read a paper on this subject, and of which the following is a summary. I. *Remarks.*—1. It has been shown by experiments which have been made for the purpose on railway lines, that it is necessary to possess normal visual faculties in order to be able to distinguish the signals at the given distance. 2. It results from an examination of the railway servants. *a.* That in cases where an examination had been required, about three per cent. of the officers were not fit for the service. *b.* That the said persons had been received in spite of their faulty vision. *c.* That visual defects are seldom acquired during the service.

II. *General Regulations.* 3. It is necessary (*a*) to submit all the officials to a new examination; (*b*) to be very careful in admitting new officials to the service; (*c*) to re-examine the officials in the cases and circumstances given under 6 *a.* 4. The general revision takes place but once by experts who have been specially chosen for the purpose, according to given rules, under the direction of the ophthalmic surgeon of the railway company. The tables which show the results of individual examination are submitted to him, and he is bound to re-examine all those individuals whose visual powers appear doubtful, and to give his opinion on the subject. 5. New officials can only be admitted on presenting a certificate signed by one of the official experts of the company. These experts are elected by the managers after having been recommended by the ophthalmic surgeon to the company. 6. A special re-examination takes place: A. Once in two years, for the purpose of testing the acuteness of visual perception. It is conducted by an officer who has received the necessary instructions from the ophthalmic surgeon, or one of the official experts. B. For the purpose of testing the visual perception in general. *a.* From the age of forty-five and upwards, once in five years by an official expert. *b.* In special cases (1) after diseases of the eye; (2) after traumatic lesions, especially such as are liable to cause a commotion of the brain, or after cerebral affections in general. *c.* If certain mistakes or actions have taken place, which may lead to doubt the integrity of the visual function. *d.* If the periodical re-examination A seem to infer an insufficient acuteness of sight.

III. *Examination.* 7. The examination relates principally to (*a*) the refraction; (*b*) visual range; (*c*) perception of colours; (*d*) the visual field. The examination must extend to the general condition of the eyes and eyelids. It must also be noted whether there exist any progressive diseases of the eye, such as cataract, etc. 8. The refraction and visual range are tested simultaneously in the general manner, for seeing at a distance by means of Snellen's letters, and with the aid of glasses. Each eye is tested separately at first, then both together. In cases where there is a slight dimness of the cornea, the examination takes place in the open air. 9. The qualitative test of colour-perception is conducted by means of Holmgren's method, Stilling's pseudo-ischromatic tables, and Donder's coloured samples. The quantitative test is conducted after Donder's method, both with transmitted and incident light. 10. The extension of the visual field is tested by asking the patient certain questions relating to the movements of the

hand and to the number of fingers extended. The observer and the patient must
keep their eyes steadfastly fixed on one another. 11. The bimanual test for the
range of vision (Art. 6 A) takes place in the open air, and is conducted according
to given instructions with the aid of Snellen's movable letters. If the visual
range should be less than four-sixths, the individual must be re-examined by one
of the special experts.

IV. *Conditions for Reception.* 12. Persons who apply for a situation as
engine-driver or stoker must present the following certificates. *a.* A certificate
that their eyes and eyelids are healthy, that there is no tendency to chronic congestion or inflammation. The visual field must be extensive, visual range and
refraction normal. Colour-perception must be at least ⅘. There must be no
traces of cataract or any other progressive diseases of the eye. Persons who apply for situations as railway servants must be possessed of the following certificates.
b. A certificate of health of the eyes and eyelids, absence of habitual congestion
or inflammation. The visual field must be unlimited for both eyes, the visual
acuity and refraction must be normal. Colour-perception for one eye at least ⅔ ;
for the other eye the visual range and colour-perception must be at least ½. There
must be no traces of cataract or any other progressive affections of the eye. 13.
At the re-examination of stokers and engine-drivers who have been employed in
this capacity for more than one year, they must be shown to have a visual range
of at least ¾ (without glasses), and a colour-perception of at least ⅓ without
glasses for one eye. For the other eye, the visual range must be at least ⅓ (without glasses), and the power of distinguishing colours must be ⅓. At the re-examination of station-masters, their assistants, the inspectors, guards, and others,
who have served on the line for more than a year, they must fulfil the following
conditions. The visual field must be unlimited at least for one eye. The visual
range of both eyes must be at least ⅔, and the colour-perception ⅔. If this degree
of visual range can only be attained by wearing glasses, the individual in question
must be obliged to wear them. 14. Individuals whose visual range or perception
of colour is less than ⅔, but more than ⅓, both for day and night signals, are considered comparatively fit for the service. They will be registered as such, and
employed only when it suffices to distinguish the signals at comparatively short
distance. The same degree of qualification would not be sufficient for stokers or
engine-drivers. 15. Individuals whose visual range or colour-perception with
both eyes is ⅓ or less, even with the aid of glasses, are unfit for service on the
line.—*British Med. Journal*, Sept. 20, 1879.

———

*Case of Stenosis of the Eustachian Tube with Hypertrophy of the Membrane of
the Tympanum and Chronic Catarrh cured by Cold Water.*

ONORATO relates (*Geom. Internaz. delle Scientif. Med.*, Fascie 5, 1879) a case
of stenosis of the Eustachian caused by the spreading of a chronic catarrh of the
pharynx. The patient, a youth aged 23, felt one day a slight pain in his left ear,
which he attributed to rheumatism. It ceased after a few days. The following
year it reappeared, and was accompanied by noises in the ear, which the patient
compared to the humming of bees. This noise continued for several months, and
was at times so strong that the patient's mind began to suffer under it. Sea-
bathing gave temporary relief; but one day the noise reappeared stronger than
ever. The whole pharmacopœia had been exhausted, and still there was no improvement. At last the author prescribed the following treatment: the patient
was to shave his head, and every morning, when washing his face, to keep his
head immersed in the basin for a few minutes. Then, after taking it out, he was
himself to pour a pint of water on his occiput, taking care to let the water run

over his neck and ears. On the third day after undertaking this care, the noise decreased, and continued to do so till about a fortnight later, when it ceased altogether. The left ear, which had been considerably affected during his sufferings, became quite strong again, and the patient benefited much by the treatment, which rendered him less liable to contract colds.—*Lond. Med. Record*, August 15, 1879.

———

Use of the Lever in Controlling Hemorrhage in Amputation of the Hip-joint.

Mr. RICHARD DAVY, Surgeon to the Westminster Hospital, urges (*British Med. Journal*, Nov. 1, 1879) the importance of controlling hemorrhage in amputation at the hip-joint by compressing the common iliac artery, which he does by means of an ebony lever, which varies in length from 18 to 22 inches, its surface is very smooth and polished, and its ends are rounded off much like the finger tips. The maximum transverse diameter is five-eighths of an inch; the minimum three-eighths of an inch. The rectal end is graduated to an inch scale, so that the surgeon who applies the lever can at once learn whereabouts may be the end of the rod.

As proof of the perfect safety and absence of inconvenience in using the lever, Mr. Davy has compressed the common iliac artery in a man suffering from aneurism of the right external iliac artery, aged 60, for twenty minutes, and without chloroform or other anæsthetic. The only pain felt was the presence of a foreign body; showing how tolerant of pressure the upper part of the rectum is. In no case has any blood or stain been seen in the stool, though he has watched carefully for this event.

On anatomical grounds, the situation of the common iliac is perfect for the ends of compression; the lever drops between the psoas magnus muscle and the bodies of the lumbar vertebræ, having the spring (sacral margin) of the true pelvic brim as a counter-resistance to the lever, and no large nervous trunks in the way.

Mr. Davy enumerated the following as the salient advantages of rectal compression:—

1. Most perfect control of the required artery.
2. Minimum amount of disturbance of the circulatory system.
3. Independence of the respiratory movements.
4. Its general and easy applicability; strictured rectum being the sole obstacle.
5. The pressure applied is so easy to maintain, and the assistant's body so well out of range of the operator that no hurry need perplex the one nor anxiety the other.
6. Its application is quite safe in skilled hands, no injury having ever resulted, and but little pain having been suffered.
7. Cheapness and simplicity; illustrating a lever of the first order.
8. The success hitherto achieved by its employment.

Mr. Davy has the record of ten cases in which the lever has been used; the total amount of blood lost during the ten operations has been under eighteen ounces, and there have been 80 per cent. of recoveries.

———

On Malformations of the Skeleton and their Treatment, with regard to the Physiological Development of the Skeleton.

At the late International Medical Congress at Amsterdam, Prof. HUETER, of Griefswald, presented a paper on this subject and offered the following conclusions: —

1. Acquired pes valgus and genu valgum, when they are not caused by inflam-

mation or traumatic lesions, are due to the diseases peculiar to the development of the skeleton.

2. These affections must in such cases be regarded as being due to the abnor.mal activity of those physiological changes which take place normally under the influence of the movements of the joints of the lower extremity, and especially through walking.

3. In such cases, the deformity is caused either by a normal pressure on ab.normally soft parts of the skeleton (rachitic form), or by an abnormally great pressure on normal parts of the skeleton (static form).

4. Congenital pes varus may be regarded as a disease. peculiar to the growth and development of the skeleton. In the majority of cases, the onset of the affection is not marked by any peculiar functional muscular troubles, and the con-formation of the bones of the tarsus presents an abnormal development of the normal foetal conformation of the bones.

5. The majority of cases of common scoliosis, especially when they are not caused by the shortening of an extremity or by a process of cicatrization (pleuritic empyema), must be considered as the effects of an affection of the bones of the trunk.

6. Such cases of common scoliosis are caused by an asymmetric development of both halves of the pectoral vertebræ, and by asymmetric growth of the ribs, both to the right and the left and the diameter of the thorax. It follows that common scoliosis is a disease of growth analogous to the asymmetric development of the pelvis and the skull.

7. It being once admitted that congenital pes varus and acquired pes valgus and genu valgum, as well as ordinary scoliosis, are caused by a vicious conformation and an abnormal growth of the bones, it is clear that the treatment would consist in these cases in checking, by a well-regulated pressure, the tendency of those portions of the bones that grow exuberantly, and in stimulating, by removing all pressure, the growth of those portions of the skeleton which are backward in their growth. In this way, it will be possible to obtain a normal conformation of the skeleton.

8. By applying this method of treatment to cases of incipient scoliosis, we may be sure of success.—*British Med. Journal*, Sept. 20, 1879.

—

*Experimental Studies on the Etiology of Scrofulous and Tuberculous
Inflammation of the Joints.*

By injecting small particles of tuberculous human lungs or tuberculous sputa into the lungs of rabbits, either through a tracheal wound or directly through the thoracic walls, SCHÜLLER (*Centrbl. f. Chir.*, No. 19, 1879) succeeded in pro-ducing a characteristic inflammation of the joint in a knee which had previously been either dislocated or only slightly injured. This inflammation was very similar to the scrofulous and tuberculous affections of the joints to which human beings are liable. The results followed if minute particles of granulations or tissue from scrofulous lymphatic glands or minute particles of lupoid tissue were injected into the lungs through a tracheotomy wound. In some of his experi-ments, the said substances were injected into the internal jugular vein, or into the abdominal cavity, the results being in all cases the same. According to the author, the inflammations of the joints which are in this way caused, consist partly in a pannous growth of the synovia, partly in granulation of the same. Foci of the size of a pin's head are developed in the epiphysis of the tibia. They con-tain tubercles. The latter are also found occasionally in the synovial membrane, where they appear to develop in particular points of predilection. It is worthy of notice that after all these experiments, the author found tubercles in the lungs, and frequently also in the liver and in other organs. In order to ascertain in what way the microscopic organisms which are always present in the matter with which the experiments were performed produce inflammation in the injured joint, the author made the following experiments: 1. For the purpose of finding out whether particles of solid matter could pass from the lungs into the blood or into certain parts of the body which had been previously injured, the author injected powdered flour, colouring matter, etc., into the lungs of rabbits, and injured the knee-joint of one leg. No inflammation ensued, and very few particles of colouring matter could be found in the synovial membrane or in the marrow of the bone. 2. The particles of colouring matter were then mixed with tuberculous sputa. This time the coloured atoms could easily be distinguished in the synovial membrane, and appeared to the naked eye like grayish incrustations. 3. When the bacteriæ of putrefaction were injected into the lungs, the animal always died in from one to five days. The injured joint revealed a slight bloody serous exudation, containing a few solitary pus corpuscles and bacteriæ, like those which had been injected. 4. The same results were obtained by injecting bacteriæ which had been obtained by fractioned breeding. 5. The same characteristic synovitis was caused in the joint by inoculating the animal with a few drops of blood from an animal which had previously been infected with tuberculosis. 6. A series of experiments were performed with antibacterial remedies, which the animal was made to inhale. It was invariably found that the inflammation grew better, but the drugs had no effect whatever on the caseous process of inflammation. The animals seem to live a little longer when these antibacterial remedies have been used. It is evident from these experiments in what way scrofulous or tuberculous inflammation of the joints may develop in man after light injuries, if the person in question happens to be disposed to tuberculosis. Local tuberculosis of the joints in man, is in most cases owing to the presence of a tuberculous vein or to bacteriæ in the blood.—*London Med. Record*, Oct. 15, 1879.

On the Fungous Inflammations of the Joints.

Prof. VOLCMANN, in Nos. 168 and 169 of his *Sammlung Klinische Vörtrage*, takes up the pathology of these joint affections so common under the name of hip-joint disease—white swelling, scrofulous inflammation of the joints, etc., to which Billroth has assigned the term "fungous," and he shows that his clinical experience, founded on the examination of large numbers of very early cases of this diseased condition, treated antiseptically, is opposed to the ordinary view of their pathology, or at any rate of the process underlying their initial stage. According to him the disease does not begin in the capsule of the joint, in the synovial membrane; it begins in the bone itself, and is throughout of a tubercular character. We shall devote the rest of this article to a fairly detailed abstract of his facts and of his argument in favour of his position.

The vast majority of these joint inflammations, says Volkmann, begin with small localized centres of disease (*Heerderkrankungen*) either in or on the surface of the bone. They may lie at some distance from the joint-cartilage, and even in the diaphysis. They are seldom larger than a cherry-stone or a hazelnut, and usually only one exists in the neighbourhood of a joint, though sometimes there are several of them, and then their favourite seat is the epiphysis. Though very variable in their position, they have certain bones which they specially attack. These are, in their order of frequency, the olecranon, the two condyles of the humerus, the calcaneum, the internal condyle of the femur, and the neck of the femur; the latter suffering more often than the head of that bone. The acetabulum is also much more often primarily affected than has been generally believed, and "the speedy success of an excision of the hip-joint often enough depends on the possibility of discovering and removing such spots of dis- ease from the pelvic bones which enter into the formation of the acetabulum."

What is the histological character of these foci? Professor Volkmann believes it is always tubercular, using the term in the strict sense of the word. They are masses of miliary tubercles in various stages, the older caseous, the younger con- sisting of a reticulum, central giant cells, epitheloid cells in their middle layer, and small-celled granulation tissue in their periphery. They caseate rapidly from want of bloodvessels. We need not further describe the structure of growths so familiar to all students of pathological anatomy. Professor Volkmann does not deny the possibility of these primary caseous foci in the bone having a purely inflammatory origin, and depending on what he terms an *Osteomyelitis caseosa*, but his own conviction is that, as stated above, they are invariably produced by the retrogression of miliary or submiliary tubercles.

We must now rapidly glance at the progress of a joint, one of whose articula- tions is the seat of such a caseous tubercular mass as those above described. The mass itself, according to Volkmann, gives rise to no symptoms until, or unless, it softens, which it does, as a rule, sooner or later. Then either a small abscess forms in the osseous-tissue, or (and this is the rule with children) the caseous matter separates as a sequestrum, and lies free in a cavity lined with gray miliary tubercles. And now the danger for the joint itself begins. The softening of the primary mass excites inflammation in the neighbouring bone-tissue, and formation of pus, which finds an exit either through the periosteum outside the joint, or else (and this is the rule) through the capsule into the joint-cavity itself. In the first case the tubercular virus contained in the pus induces a growth of miliary tubercles wherever it invades a tissue; these tubercles caseate and break down in their turn; the same process is renewed; and we get sinuses, and abscesses whose direction depends on the gravitation of their contents (*Senkungsabscesse*), as, for example, in the lumbar, iliac, and psoas abscesses which depend on tubercular caries of the vertebræ. In the second case there are two possibilities: either the bone pus enters a more or less healthy joint, or one that has its synovial mem- brane thickened and altered by reactive inflammation connected with the presence of the primary mass of tubercle in its vicinity. Of the two contingencies the second is the more favourable for the joint. As Volkmann puts it, "a joint reacts to inflammatory irritants of all kinds, or to infectious or poisonous matters introduced into it, the more violently the better the physiological condition of its synovial membrane. The more the latter has become vascular, thickened, infil- trated, and the more it resembles granulation tissue, the less sensitive it is to all these irritants, for the protective power of granulation tissue is well known." Hence the healthy joint invaded by tubercular pus tends to suffer purulent rather than fungous inflammation. In either case the synovial membrane undergoes infection, and miliary tubercles develop in its substance, but they only form a comparatively superficial layer in the previously healthy joint, while in a chroni- cally inflamed joint they are scattered in groups of various sizes through the vas- cular granulation tissue into which the innermost layers of the synovial capsule are converted, and which have given rise to the term "fungous" with reference to this form of joint-affection.

But, whether the joint be healthy or diseased, the miliary tubercles, which are the result of the infection of its synovial membrane from the virus of the primary focus in the bone-tissue, undergo the same changes—caseation and subsequent softening—with further infection of neighbouring tissues by the products of their decay. It is scarcely necessary to add that there is no hard and fast line between the two contingencies we have just referred to; there are all possible intermediate forms of synovial disease.

The cartilage of the joint is little attacked by the tubercular secretion in the joint-cavity. It suffers from the injury to its synovial covering, or from the invasion of granulation tissue from the underlying bone. Its detachment in whole or in part is the signal for the infection of the bony ends of the epiphysis, for the development of new tubercular layers on their ends, and their progressive destruction by the retrograde changes and infective processes already described. In a few cases the tubercular eruption in the epiphyses assumes a diffuse character, and large tracts of the medulla caseate. Here the danger of a general miliary tuberculosis throughout the body becomes considerable.

Professor Volkmann admits the existence of a "primary synovial form" of fungous joint-inflammation, but states that it is far more rare than the secondary form, is almost confined to adults, and is always due to primary tuberculosis of the synovial membrane. The cases in which it occurs are the most unfavourable of all; the inflammation of the joint assumes a marked purulent character, there is great disorganization of the articular tissues, and the patients generally die of phthisis or tuberculosis of the bowel.

We must now pass on to say a word about the sinuses and abscesses which form in the extra-osseous tissues in connection with disease of the joints, and which we spoke of above as having a tubercular origin. Professor Volkmann points out that their character has been long overlooked, because surgeons in the pre-antiseptic days (*pace* Mr. Savory) were afraid to open them freely so as to get a view of their interior in the living subject. Now Professor Volkmann at least lays them open with free incisions under the spray, and in the extremities even, if possible, slits up the whole abscess, and makes sure that no pocket remains for the lodgment of pus; he then scrapes away the lining membrane, and the layer of soft granulation tissue under it, with the sharp spoon, until he reaches a healthy, only somewhat indurated, wall outside. Even the largest abscesses of this kind can then be obliterated by careful sutures, their walls being brought into apposition, so as to heal by first intention. The lining membrane of such an abscess in the *living* subject is of a pale grayish-yellow, or very pale violet opaque colour. Volkmann compares it to a large echinococcus cyst. It is readily detached from its bed, and on examination is found to consist almost entirely of thickly agglomerated miliary tubercles. It is peculiar, or practically so, to secondary abscesses in intermuscular and subcutaneous connective tissue, and is scarcely ever found in fungous synovial sacs. Hence, joint-cavities cannot usually be cured, like the secondary abscesses, by the use of the sharp spoon, and the total excision of the capsule is needed in the worst of such cases.

These secondary abscesses communicate by a narrow sinus with the diseased joint, or in the case of extra-articular disease with the diaphysis; and the sharp spoon at once reveals the point where the sinus enters the abscess, because *there* is always found a little granulating spot which cannot be scraped away even by using force. There the introduction of a probe will discover diseased bone.

Lastly, Professor Volkmann enunciates the axiom that "such distinct, separable lining membranes" as those he describes "are only met with as a sequela of tubercular processes."

In concluding his lecture, after pointing out how the obstinacy of these fungous joint-affections depends on continual infection and reinfection of new parts by "tubercular virus," Professor Volkmann warns his hearers not to let his revival of tubercular pathology alarm them too much, or make them too desponding about the results of treatment. He reminds them that in man this virus readily causes local tuberculosis; but not, as in animals, except under special conditions, general tuberculosis. The lymphatic glands, except the bronchial and mesenteric glands, do not readily caseate in man ; and the glands of the limbs, especially the lower, are least of all liable to these changes, whose tubercular character, in the strict sense of the word, has been put beyond a doubt by the researches of Schüppel and others. Hence it does not follow that we are, on the one hand, to doubt the "tubercular" character of the fungous joint-inflammations, because secondary lymphatic tuberculosis is, or may be, absent, nor on the other hand to lay too much stress on the "tubercular" origin of the joint-disease, following the old view of the incurability of tubercle. The patient with fungous articular in-flammation may, or may not, be eventually carried off by general tuberculosis, but on the whole the chances are in his favour with rational treatment. The greatest advance that could be made in this direction, if Volkmann's interpreta-tion of the primary caseous foci in the epiphyses of a joint is correct, would be to discover and remove these foci before the softening stage and the disorganization of the joint have commenced.

We have now sketched, and only sketched, the main outlines of Professor Volkmann's essay. To the skeptics who ask what proof there is of all he has advanced, we can best reply by recommending them to study the essay itself in detail, and, if not German scholars, at any rate, to convince themselves, by an inspection of the numerous beautiful wood-cuts and coloured lithographic plates with which it is illustrated, that his axioms are founded on something better than romance. To those who follow the progress of modern pathology attentively, there is nothing unexpected or extravagant in Professor Volkmann's discoveries; they are merely the outcome and the confirmation of the infection theory of Buhl.—*Med. Times and Gazette,* Nov. 8, 1879.

—

On the Treatment of Diseased Joints.

Professor VERNEUIL lately read, before the Société de Chirurgie de Paris, an important paper on the immobilization and the mobilization of diseased joints, the following abstract of which will interest our readers. He began by declaring that "a fundamental principle of therapeutics demands, as an essential condition for recovery, *rest for the diseased organ,*" and that "a principle in general physi-ology not less fundamental affirms that *the activity of an organ* is indispensable to its material and functional preservation," and went on to observe that "from these embarrassing and contradictory propositions it follows that the rest which cures a disease may ultimately annihilate the organ ; that the activity which keeps an organ alive may prevent its healing when diseased ; and that rest and activity are equally useful, *even necessary,* and yet as equally injurious and dangerous."

Brought to bear on the treatment of arthropathies, the above propositions tend to render our therapeutics and practice undecided and confused. And thus some urge that as the prolonged fixation of a joint may so alter its structure as to lead to anchylosis, therefore we must limit the fixation to the shortest possible time ; others maintain that rest, rigorous and persistent, is the best cure for an arthritis, therefore prolong the period of rest to the utmost extent, and disallow any attempt at movement. Bonnet, of Lyons, after having inclosed the diseased joints in im-movable apparatus for a certain time, always took care, when the right moment seemed to have come, to commence passive movements, in order to restore supple-ness to the joint.

This mixed practice seems, nowadays, to be almost universally adopted. Sur-geons, no doubt, immobilize joints, because they have found out that it is neces-sary ; but they are always pre-occupied by the supposed ill effects of prolonged fixation, and eagerly look out for the moment when they may recommence the movements *which are to prevent anchylosis*. Now, Professor Verneuil said, anchylosis, in fact, is a ghost, which frightens not only the lay public, the patients, and their friends, but also nearly all general practitioners, and not a few surgeons.

"In my practice and teaching for a long time past I have combated to the uttermost this idea of anchylosis and its prevention by passive movement. Perhaps my views may seem paradoxical; nevertheless I am led on to the discussion by facts. Thus, a child with joint disease was recently brought to me. I applied absolute fixation to the joint. All the pain ceased, swelling disappeared, and recovery was taking place. At the end of some weeks I was asked when it would be necessary to remove the bandages and commence movements. To this I replied that the time was not yet come. Nevertheless, in a short time, the general practitioner, probably urged on by the friends, removed all the apparatus. As a consequence, the benefits then gained were lost, and the lesion progressed. The child was again brought; some excuses were made. I again ordered fixation, and the child is now in a fair way to recover."

The facts invoked against fixation are indeed very few, and only moderately conclusive; if the accusation is true, we ought to be surprised that the proofs are so uncommon. In order to discuss the subject with advantage, we must at least distinguish between healthy and diseased joints, and among the latter we must further establish varieties. First, then, as regards healthy joints. I affirm that there does not exist a single fact which shows conclusively that fixation, however long continued, has ever led to anchylosis. This long-continued fixation may, it is true, give rise to anatomical modifications such as diminution in the extent of the articular surfaces, to a thinning of their lining cartilage, also to a reduction in size of the synovial sacs, of a less abundant synovial secretion, and to functional changes, such as stiffness of the joints and limitation of movements. Hence, not unnaturally, when the necessity for immobilization has ceased, a certain time will be required for the complete restitution of the articular function. But there is nothing in all this which at all resembles anchylosis. It is only comparable with what takes place in mucous glands which are no longer traversed either by ingesta or by excretions; they do not become obliterated, as was taught by Bichat, but simply reduced in size. Their healthy condition, however, is again established in a few weeks, or at most in a few months, when their function is once more revived. What better example could one have than the bladder in the case of a vesico-vaginal fistula? It becomes reduced to a mere pouch, but again resumes its normal capacity as soon as the fistula is closed. I am well aware that everywhere autopsies and experiments on animals are quoted; but neither one nor another have completely convinced me. I could show that the various lesions which are revealed are not in any way of the nature to lead to anchylosis, but can be attributed to other causes rather than to the fixation. On the other hand, I might mention the numberless examples of well-known cases in which the joint, for a long time kept immovably fixed, has, notwithstanding, retained its structure and rapidly resumed its functions when permitted to do so. These latter facts are at least as numerous as the opposite ones, and, being more simple, are also more convincing. It is clear either that fixation *alone* suffices to alter a joint, and then it ought always to do so; or there is need of a peculiar predisposition and a suitably prepared soil, in which latter case it behooves us to seek whether this predisposition does not play the principal *rôle*. The learned professor inclines to this latter view. He admits that at the termination of any arthritis, in the treatment of which fixation more or less prolonged has been made use of, there is a diminution, a suspension, even an abolition of movement; but does not see why this functional suppression should be attributed to fixation rather than to other causes, especially the anatomical lesions present in the joint.

Those who fear anchylosis argue that certain plastic exudations are poured out between the apposed surfaces, which, at first soft, tend to organize and so glue these surfaces together. Fixation allows this process to proceed uncontrolled. But the synovial membrane is not alone altered ; the ligaments are also infiltrated and softened. This no doubt cannot be ascribed to the mere fixation, but the fixation allows the process to go on, whereas movement would certainly prevent the subsequent stiffness and shortening which otherwise come on. The cartilage may even be destroyed, and then, if fixation is carried out, the plastic matter which is deposited ossifies, and true anchylosis is effected ; whereas movements would at least tend to a more or less movable joint. And moreover, the tendons are apt to get glued together within their sheaths, which is further favoured by long-continued fixation.

After passing in review the varieties of arthropathy, and the difference in their tendencies, he shows that there are some which never lead to anchylosis; while in others fixation may be carried out or not, there will be some interference with movements in any case, but not an anchylosis. Impaired movement is in all cases due to the disease, and not to the fixation.

The pain of certain arthropathies gives rise to reflex muscular fixation. If moderate, this does not lead to any ill consequences ; but if excessive or prolonged, if it go on to contracture, it then becomes harmful, and by bearing unduly on circumscribed portions of the bone, or cartilages, or ligaments, it gives rise to secondary pathological changes of serious import.

In passive fixation, on the contrary, when mechanical means are used, all movements are prevented, the muscles are kept at rest, and a limb is held in its normal position.

After an examination of the various means by which immobilization is effected, he arrives at the following conclusions :—

Prolonged fixation incontestably modifies healthy joints, but not profoundly either in form or in the structure of their constituent parts, or as regards their ultimate function.

There does not exist, in scientific records, any authenticated examples of anchylosis produced in a healthy joint by mere fixation. The cases hitherto advanced in support of such an idea are capable of another interpretation. On the other hand, there are on record numerous examples of joints which have been kept immovable for long periods, and have regained their anatomical and physiological integrity.

Inflammation no doubt occupies a first place among the causes; and, as it is absolutely proved that fixation is an antiphlogistic of the first rank, it is illogical to think that it produces those effects which it is known to cure.

If, in certain cases, fixation continues to produce anchylosis, it is not that fixation which the surgeon secures by apparatus, but rather that which is due to the contracture of the peri-articular muscles. As much as the latter, which may be called *active*, favours, and indeed provokes articular disorders, by so much the former, which is *passive*, is powerful against them. There is therefore a capital distinction to make between the two varieties of fixation.

Anchylosis, on the other hand, far from being produced in articular disease, is but a rare termination to it ; exceptional in strumous arthropathies, a little more frequent in rheumatic mono-synovitis, anchylosis is especially to be feared in suppurative and traumatic arthritis, though no one variety of disease is certain to produce it.

The exaggerated fear, therefore, of anchylosis has caused many practitioners to make grave errors, and has frequently led to the too early leaving off of passive fixation, and the too premature re-commencement of movement.

Mobilization, consequent on joint disease, is of two kinds—artificial or mechanical, and natural or physiological—brought about by muscles, either voluntary or otherwise. The former, which anchylophobes use exclusively, is admissible when we have to deal with the rectification of vicious attitudes of limbs, and to treat confirmed anchyloses ; but it ought to be rejected as useless, powerless, and dangerous if we would avoid anchylosis. The latter, on the contrary, is of extreme utility if applied at an opportune moment : with time it accomplishes in a remarkable degree the restoration of the articular function.

He concludes by saying that artificial fixation on the one hand, and natural fixation on the other, are the two principal therapeutic agents in arthropathies : the one combats anatomical lesions, the other restores physiological action. We may assist the former by different means—local, pharmaceutic, or hygienic ; we favour the second by electrization of the peri-articular muscles, practised during the period of fixation, with a view to the prevention of degenerescence.

To combat the inflammation is the best means to prevent anchylosis. As regards surgical measures proper, I know of none better than continued extension, and, in extreme cases, preventive resection.—*Med. Times and Gazette*, Oct. 18, 1879.

Midwifery and Gynæcology.

Uterus Bicornis; Double Pregnancy.

An interesting case of this kind is reported by Dr. E. GOUTERMANN in the *Berliner Klinische Wochenschrift* for October 13th. Frau E., born in 1844, first menstruated at the age of 15, and from that time regularly, but very profusely. She was married in 1869 ; and in the next six years all her pregnancies, though unattended with any special disturbance, ended in abortion at the third month ; the catamenia appeared regularly two or two and a half months afterwards. In September, 1875, she again became pregnant, and was delivered in the following June, after an easy labour, of a living and healthy female child. In the end of January, 1877, she had another abortion, which was followed by such profuse metrorrhagia as to demand medical aid; this had not occurred in her previous abortions. In November, 1877, she again became pregnant, the catamenia having been in the mean time very profuse, but regular in duration (four or five days). On December 30th she had another abortion, which was attended with labour-like pains, chiefly limited to the right side. In the middle of February, 1878, the catamenia returned, and appeared at intervals of twenty-eight days with remarkable intensity; on the first day, large masses of coagula, not having an offensive smell, were discharged. On examining her at the end of March— three months after the abortion—Dr. Goutermann was astonished to find indications, in the enlargement of the uterus and the movements of the fœtus, that she was five months advanced in pregnancy. After consideration, he was led to suspect that the case was one of twin-pregnancy in the uterus bicornis ; that one of the embryos had continued to develop itself after and in spite of the extrusion of the other ; and that it was the emptied half of the uterus which menstruated. External and internal examination tended to confirm this view, but did not render it absolutely certain. The woman being very fat, the form of the fundus uteri could not be made out by palpation ; the vaginal portion was normal, and the os was closed. Exploration with a sound was, of course, not attempted. She was ordered to rest, and to take easily digestible food. In the night of May 12th Dr. Goutermann was called to the patient. He found the left hand of the fœtus, much swollen, protruding from the genital organs; the back lay forward, and the face to the right side. There were no pains nor hemorrhage. The fœtus, a male, of about six months and a half, was easily brought into the world, but died some time afterwards. As the pains were insufficient to expel the placenta, Dr. Goutermann attempted to remove it by gentle traction and friction, with pressure over the fundus uteri, but in vain. He then proceeded to introduce his hand, following the course of the umbilical cord. In doing this he found that the os externum was formed as usual, but that the os internum, with the whole cavity of the uterus, was divided into a right and a left half by a septum. The right half, which had smooth walls and was empty, scarcely admitted the hand; in the left half the placenta was adherent over the septum. The patient made a good recovery. In August, 1879, Frau E. was delivered of a living male child, which presented in the breech-position, from the left division. On this occasion, also, there had been abortion at the second month from the right division, and subsequent menstruation.—*British Med. Journal*, Nov. 1, 1879.

—

The Treatment of Uterine Tumours by Dilatation and the Ecraseur.

Dr. GEORGE H. KIDD, Master of the Coombe Lying-in Hospital, Dublin, in his address on the opening of the Section of Obstetric Medicine at the recent meeting of the British Medical Association (*British Med. Journal*, Aug. 16, 1879) made the following remarks on the treatment of uterine tumours:—

It will, perhaps, be in the recollection of some now present, that so long ago as 1868, I described (see *American Journal of the Med. Sciences*, Oct. 1868, p. 576) a peculiar method of dilating the uterus, and related a case in which I had been enabled by this means to remove a large number of intra-uterine polypi. In a paper subsequently published in the *Dublin Quarterly Journal of Medical Science* for February, 1869, I gave a diagram illustrating this method of dilatation, and showing the polypi as found in the uterus at the time of the operation. Some copies of this diagram are now on the table. It will be observed that six pieces of sea-tangle, long enough to reach from beyond the os externum to the fundus, but not to touch it, have been introduced side by side, one after another, forming a bundle of parallel pieces; and it will be seen that these, as they absorb moisture and swell, must dilate not only the os externum, but the os internum and the cavity of the uterus itself at the one operation. Thus, if the os be sufficiently large to admit the necessary number of pieces at the first sitting, the whole process may be completed in twenty-four hours. If not sufficiently large, a few pieces must be introduced in the first instance, and removed at the end of twenty-four hours, when a larger number can be used, and dilatation thus effected to any required extent. Generally, even in the nulliparous uterus, the tissues are so relaxed by hemorrhage that five or six pieces, each as large as a No. 6 catheter, can be introduced at the first sitting, and a dilatation procured sufficient for the introduction of the finger and exploration of the uterus, or the removal of small tumours. For the removal of larger tumours, however, a much greater degree of dilatation is required, and it may be necessary to introduce from twelve to eighteen pieces, which can generally be got in at the second sitting if six have been introduced at the first; but it is to be borne in mind that it is always advisable, when about to remove the tents, either for the introduction of others or for proceeding with the operation, to wash out the vagina with a solution of permanganate of potash, and after their removal to wash out the uterus itself with a similar solution before any further steps be taken; for, though sea-tangle does not give rise to the putrid and offensive discharges found when sponge is used, yet fluids accumulate which are irritating, and may, if not removed, prove injurious both to the operator and to the patient.

We have recently had a new kind of dilating material made known to us under the name of tupelo-tents that may, at the second sitting, be advantageously used instead of sea-tangle. This substance has been brought into notice by Dr. Sussdorff, of New York. The tents are formed from the root of the *Nyssa aquatica*, which grows in the swamps of the Southern States of America. As imported into this country, they are too short to be of much use for dilating the uterus; but Messrs. Fannin and Co., of Dublin, have procured them for me of the full length required. These tents swell more quickly, and in proportion to their size when dry to a greater degree, than does the sea-tangle; but the tangle can be more easily introduced in the first instance, and, from its slower and more gradual action, will probably be found less painful and safer for the patient than the other. As soon, however, as the process of dilatation has commenced, and the tissues have become softened and relaxed, the tupelo will complete it more quickly and thoroughly than the sea-tangle. If three tupelo-tents can be introduced at the second sitting, and along with them four or five pieces of No. 6 sea-tangle, the uterus will generally be found sufficiently dilated at the end of a further twenty-four hours to permit the removal of a tumour measuring from three to four inches in diameter.

The dilatation of narrow passages dates from the earliest ages of surgery, prepared sponge being the substance generally used for the purpose; but, till suggested by Sir James Simpson about thirty years ago, the exploration of the uterus by its means had not been attempted. Till then, as Sir James has stated, intrauterine polypi "were generally considered as placed beyond the pale of any certain means of detection, or any possible means of operative removal." But now, following in his footsteps, and using the improved methods at our disposal, large tumours, such as even Sir James Simpson would not have thought of touching, have been made accessible, and been brought within the domain of surgery. The dangers and inconveniences, however, attendant on the use of the sponge, have deterred many from attempting to dilate the uterus at all, or have led them to do it timidly and inefficiently; thus Dr. Emmett, in his recently published book, a work which would amply prove him, if we did not already know it, to be not only a bold but a most skilful and successful surgeon, though he describes a modification of the sponge-tent, and a special instrument for dilating the uterus, seems to scarcely use either for purposes of treatment, but for diagnosis only; and, indeed, specially recommends, in speaking of large tumours, that no attempt should be made for their removal till they appear at the os and begin to come down into the vagina. But we all know that, in the majority of cases, a woman's health is shattered and her life often placed in extreme jeopardy long before the tumour makes its appearance at the os, or begins to press on it. As a further example, I may mention that one of the specimens on the table was removed from the uterus of a lady who for some time was under the care of one of the most eminent gynæcologists and successful operators of the age, who, after spending a week in trying to dilate with sponge-tents, gave up the attempt, and recommended that the uterus should be extirpated, or the ovaries removed by Battey's operation; yet, after the use of two series of sea-tangles for forty-eight hours, the tumour, which was imbedded in the posterior wall of the uterus near the fundus, was safely removed by a combined process of enucleation and avulsion; an operation hazardous enough, but certainly much less so than the extirpation of either uterus or ovaries. In another case, which occurred about two years ago, the patient had been assured by one of the leading gynæcologists in the north of England that the tumour, the nature of which he had fully recognized, could not be removed by any possible means, yet, by the means now detailed, it was, in a space of forty-eight hours, brought within reach and removed ; and the lady, who had lived several years in sterile marriage, has since given birth to a child. I have not the tumour here to exhibit, for she insisted on taking it home with her to show to her friends that such tumours could be removed.

Having dilated the uterus and made the tumour accessible, the next step is to remove it. In the paper on uterine polypi already alluded to, the mode of removing a polypus with an *écraseur* is described, and illustrated by a diagram ; even large tumours, if prominent into the uterine cavity, may be removed in the same way. The uterus is first drawn down to the vulva, having been seized by a strong vulsellum ; then the tumour is laid hold of either with a fine vulsellum or tenaculum, or with the " spiral instrument" described and figured in his book by Dr. McClintock, which is, indeed, nothing more nor less than a long corkscrew, and the loop of a wire *écraseur* is passed round its base. In my first paper, I recommended that this should be a soft iron wire ; but I now find that, for large tumours, a finely tempered steel wire is the best, such as a piano-string, as it, though it may be compressed in passing through the os, opens again by its own elasticity when it gets into the cavity of the uterus, and is, therefore, more easily passed over the tumour, and it is, besides, firmer and stronger than the iron, and will bear a greater strain. In using an *écraseur*, one of two effects will be produced. If both ends of the wire be attached to the screw, then a purely crushing movement is produced. When the screw is worked, the wire constricts the tissues till it gradually crushes its way through. If one end of the wire be attached to the screw and the other fixed, then a cutting motion is obtained combined with the crushing. This combination of cutting and crushing enables us to divide tumours that would resist and break the strongest crushing instruments ; but to obtain the combined action of cutting and crushing, the screw holding the wire must travel double the distance required in the crushing movement. With the ordinary *écraseur*, consequently, it is often necessary to stop in the middle of the operation, and readjust the wire before the operation can be completed. This might, perhaps, be obviated by using Weiss's *écraseur* which has a windlass to wind up the wire, but the instrument is very cumbrous, heavy, and inconvenient, and I believe it has never come into use. A Dublin student, Dr. Denham, son of Mr. Denham, Ex-Master of the Rotunda Hospital, has, however, invented a simple instrument by which either a crushing or a combined crushing and cutting action can be obtained ; and by its use, what has hitherto been one of the greatest practical difficulties in cutting through the base of large sessile tumours will probably be quite overcome. The difficulty consisted in this, that, to encircle a tumour of, let us say, from three to four inches in diameter, the loop of wire must be more than from nine to twelve inches in length, and if only one end of it be attached to the screw so as to give the combined cutting and crushing movement, the *écraseur* must be so long as to be unwieldy in its proportions and weakened in its powers. Denham obviates the difficulty by making one end of the wire traverse the whole length of the screw, and enabling us, this being accomplished, to make the other end, by a very simple movement, take up the action and follow the same course. An inspection of the instrument which lies on the table will show at a glance how this is accomplished.

What has been said so far, as to the removal of the tumours after access to them has been obtained by dilating the uterus, refers to intra-uterine tumours—that is, those which have grown into the cavity of the uterus ; but interstitial tumours, or those imbedded in the substance of the uterine wall, when they approach closely to the mucous membrane, often give rise to hemorrhage, as serious and as injuries to life and health as that caused by intra-uterine tumours. The avulsion or enucleation of such tumours has long been practised; but, till Dr. Marion Sims and Dr. Gaillard Thomas described their mode of operating and devised instruments for the purpose, it seemed to me too dangerous to be attempted, except in extreme cases. Such tumours can now, however, be removed almost as safely as those which have grown into the uterine cavity; but when they lie high up in the cavity of the uterus, full dilatation must first be effected, and for this purpose the method now described appears to me to be the safest and most efficient.

A series of observations on the shape of the uterus, when enlarged by the growth of a tumour in its cavity or in its walls, has induced me to suggest a few simple rules for the diagnosis of the relations and position of the tumour, which seem likely to enable us to know, before proceeding to dilate, the conditions that will probably be met with. The rules may be summed up as follows: When we have evidence of the existence of a tumour, and the cavity of the uterus is enlarged, if the uterus be uniform in shape, without any bulging out or unequal enlargement of any of its walls, the tumour will probably be found to be more or less pedunculated, growing from the fundus of the uterus and hanging down into its cavity. If the uterus be found unequal in its outline, bulged out at one side and straight at the other, and if, on introducing the sound, it pass along the convex or bulged-out side, then the tumour will be found to be growing from the wall opposite to where the bulging-out occurs, and projecting into the cavity. If this bulging-out be sudden and much marked, the tumour will probably be sessile, and projecting into the cavity from the wall opposite to the bulge, and may be so far interstitial as to have a thin layer of muscular fibre covering it over under the mucous membrane. If the uterus be bulged out in the same manner at one side, and the sound pass along the straight instead of the convex or bulged side, then the tumour will be found to be interstitial, and deeply seated in the uterine wall, closer probably to the peritoneal than the mucous surface. If further experience should confirm these rules, they will, I hope, afford us some aid towards deciding in what cases an operation should be urged, and in what it should be undertaken with more caution

—

On the Treatment of Fibrous Tumours of the Uterus.

At the late International Medical Congress at Amsterdam, Dr. J. DE LA FAILLE read a paper on this subject, of which the following are the conclusions:—

1. The mode of treatment of fibroid tumours of the womb depends principally upon the flow of blood that accompanies them.

2. The seat of the tumours and their development modify the treatment.

3. Internal medication offers but little prospect of success, though it may be tried in intra-parietal fibromas. The same may be said of alkaline baths.

4. One of the most rational modes of treatment of intra-parietal fibromas is that of subcutaneous injections of ergotine.

5. The plan of dilating the womb by means of the prepared sponge or laminaria, is not without danger; it requires at least a prompt renewal of the dilating substances.

6. Linear écrasement is preferable to any other method for operating upon fibrous polyps.

7. Intra-uterine fibromas are best removed by enucleation. The same applies to sub-peritoneal fibromas.

8. In case of gastro-hysterotomy, intra-peritoneal treatment of the pedicle is preferable to extra-peritoneal treatment.

9. Total extirpation of the uterus offers some great advantages.

10. Castration is seldom indicated in cases of fibrous tumours of the womb.—
Archives Gén. de Médecine, Nov. 1879.

—

Extirpation of Cancerous Uterus.

In the *Archiv für Gynäkologie*, B. xiv. H. 3, Dr. R. BRUNTZEL relates six cases of this operation performed in the hospital at Breslau.

The first case was one of polypoid sarcoma in the neck of the uterus in an unmarried girl, aged eighteen. The operation was performed on May 10, 1878, by Freund, with the assistance of Spiegelberg. Carbolic spray was not used. The intestines had to be drawn out of the peritoneal cavity. The sigmoid flexure was adherent to the uterus, and showed sarcomatous infiltration at its point of adhesion. The uterus was also adherent to the bladder. The ovaries were not removed, as they were involved in adhesions. The operation lasted two and a quarter hours. Signs of septic infection and peritonitis quickly appeared, and the patient died in fifty-three hours. A small perforation, admitting the point of a sound, was found in the sigmoid flexure.

The second case was one of carcinoma of the cervix in a woman, aged forty-seven, the mother of three children, the youngest twenty years old. For two months menstruation, previously scanty, had become very profuse, and in the intervals there was a discharge, occasionally tinged with blood. She had frequently lancinating pains in the hypogastrium and back. At her admission on June 28, 1878, the uterus was found slightly enlarged, quite freely movable, the os converted into a hard irregular ring. No induration outside the cervix could be detected.

The operation was performed on July 14th, by Spiegelberg with the assistance of Freund, Bruntzel, and others. It was found possible to keep the intestines in the upper part of the abdomen, abdominal walls being rather thin and lax. The uterine surface was roughened by lymph. Bleeding took place on separation of the right broad ligament, notwithstanding the loops of ligature, and several vessels had to be tied separately. In separating the uterus on the right side, the lowest loop of ligature was cut, and considerable arterial bleeding followed, but was arrested by ligature. In order to close more completely the wound in the peritoneum, the ovaries were stitched into its angles, the left ovary being as large as a small apple, and having some small cysts on its surface, which were previously punctured. The operation lasted two and a half hours. The patient did well after the operation, although she suffered from vomiting, and slight suppuration occurred in the lower angle of the wound. On October 25th, however, a hard knot was felt to the left of the vaginal cicatrix, and by January 9, 1879, the cancer had recurred to such an extent that the anterior and left walls of the vagina were depressed by a number of hard, knotty swellings.

The third case was one of papillary carcinoma of the cervix, in a woman aged forty-one. She had had one child eighteen years before, and one miscarriage in the second month, about a year later. For six months menstruation had been becoming more frequent and profuse, and for two months there had been almost constant metrorrhagia, accompanied by offensive discharge. At her admission, on July 8, 1878, she was emaciated and anæmic. The cervix was converted into a large mushroom-shaped, papillary mass. The growth came quite close to, but did not absolutely reach, the vaginal insertion. The body of the uterus was movable, but there was some thickening in the position of the right ovary.

The operation was performed by Spiegelberg, on July 24th. On account of the rigidity of the abdominal muscles, it was necessary to extend the incision a hand's breadth above the umbilicus. The uterus was found roughened by lymph. It was found necessary to draw the intestines out of the abdominal cavity. An infiltration was found in the left vaginal *cul-de-sac*, which prevented the uterus from being drawn upward, and so rendered the placing of the ligatures very difficult. Very profuse hemorrhage took place on dividing the broad ligaments, notwithstanding the ligatures, and had to be arrested by separate ligatures. The posterior wall of the bladder was wounded in separating it, but was closed by a suture. The left ovary was removed, the right was stitched into the right angle of the wound. The operation lasted two and a quarter hours. The patient never revived from the shock of the operation, and died in twenty-four hours. A small quantity of bloody fluid was found in the pelvis, the peritoneum was injected, and there was a defect in the posterior wall of the bladder, opening into the vagina.

The fourth case was one of papillary carcinoma of the anterior lip of the cervix, in a woman aged fifty-one. She had had one child thirty years before, and an abortion in the second month, eight years before. Since Christmas, 1877, she had suffered from pains in the hypogastrium and back, and discharge. Hemorrhage recurred almost every fortnight. The vagina was filled by a cauliflower-like growth from the anterior lip of the os, but there was a free zone of mucous membrane separating it from the vaginal insertion. On June 10th, the growth was removed by écraseur, and no sign of malignant growth could be discovered by the naked eye or microscope in the cut surface. On August 1st, the patient returned, a sanguineous semi-purulent discharge having recurred for some days. Recurrence of the growth was found on the posterior border of the stump, infiltration reaching the cervical canal. Thickening was felt in Douglas's fossa, and a knotty induration in the right *cul-de-sac*. An exploratory abdominal incision was made on August 5th, by Spiegelberg, with the assistance of Freund, Bruntzel, and others, but extensions of cancer being found around the uterus, no attempt was made to extirpate it. Little disturbance followed the operation.

The fifth case was one of carcinoma of the cervix, in a woman, aged forty-one, the mother of six children. She had suffered for six months almost continual metrorrhagia, accompanied by pain in the hypogastrium, but was not emaciated, although anæmic. The uterus was enlarged, reaching two finger-breadths above the pubes. The cervix was short, with an old laceration on the right side, and in this situation were prominent carcinomatous masses. The outer part of cervix and the vagina were free, except a small indurated spot in the vaginal vault. The operation was performed by Spiegelberg, on October 25, 1878. One large coil of jejunum had to be drawn out of the abdomen. After separation of the uterus from the bladder, as the operator was attempting to draw up the cervix by the fingers passed down through the aperture, the body of the uterus broke off from the cervix, about the situation of the internal os. At this time sudden collapse came on, the pulse could no longer be felt, and it became necessary to remove the chloroform and inject ether. The cervix was hastily excised, and it then appeared that cancerous infiltration extended to a considerable distance on the right side of the cervix. The ovaries, which were unaltered, were removed, and the pedicles tied. The operation lasted two and a quarter hours. The patient never revived from the collapse, and died thirteen hours after the operation. At the autopsy, emphysema of the lungs and fatty degeneration of the heart were found. The deep inguinal glands in the right side were all enlarged by carcinomatous deposit.

The sixth case was one of carcinoma of the cervix, in a woman, aged forty. She had had four children, and one abortion, the last delivery being in February, 1874. For three months she had suffered from constant metrorrhagia; she was much emaciated, and suffered severe pain. The anterior lip of the cervix and the cervical canal were infiltrated with cancer, the vagina free. The operation was performed by Spiegelberg on November 28, 1878. A great portion of the intestines had to be drawn out of the abdomen. The uterus was fixed backwards by adhesions, but could be drawn up after their separation. The ovaries were removed and the pedicles tied. The lowest loops of ligatures were passed, not by Freund's needle, but by the method proposed by Kochs, after previous separation of the uterus anteriorly and posteriorly. Profuse bleeding took place on separation of the broad ligaments, and many arterial branches had to be tied. A piece of cancerous tissue, which remained attached in the anterior vaginal *cul-de-sac*, was afterwards tied and separated. The operation lasted two hours. From the time of the operation there was complete suppression of urine. The patient, however, lived four and a half days, and there was no trace either of uræmic symptoms or of œdema. Both ureters were found to be included in the loops of ligature. The ureters above and the pelves of the kidneys were dilated, the kidneys showed recent inflammation, there was hyperæmia and œdema of the lungs, and the peritoneal cavity contained offensive purulent fluid.

The carbolic spray was not used at any of the operations, for fear that it might increase the shock necessarily incurred in an operation of such long duration. The author considers that the occurrence of the accident of tying the ureters, in the last operation, is a fatal objection to Kochs's method of passing the lowest loop of ligature. He proposes, however, in future, since the ligatures *en masse* prove insecure against bleeding, to cut the base of the broad ligaments gradually from above, after placing the two upper loops, and secure each vessel as it is divided. In conclusion, the author is of opinion that Freund's operation can only prove palliative, and not curative, and that its legitimate application will be confined to quite exceptional cases.

Another fatal case of extirpation of the cancerous uterus is reported by Dr. Fritsch (*Centralbl. für Gynäkologie,* 1869, No. 17). The patient was a nullipara, aged 62. The menopause had occurred at the age of 41. A year previously the patient had sought for relief on account of a sanguineous discharge. The author found a soft papillary mass, readily bleeding, but only as large as a pea, on the anterior lip of the cervix. On account of its suspicious character, he slit up the cervix bilaterally, and amputated the anterior lip. The microscope showed the presence of cancer, and that, at the upper angle of the excised portion, the section passed through mucous membrane, which had undergone carcinomatous degeneration. The patient, considering herself well after this operation, went away, and the author could not get the opportunity of seeing her again. Only after an interval of nine months did sanguineous discharge recommence, and she then reappeared. The author then found a nodular and friable mass of carcinoma projecting from the os, and surrounding it on every side. The outer portion of the vaginal portion was entirely free, the uterus freely movable, and the cellular tissue round it unaffected.

The operation was performed on July 15th. It proved necessary to draw the intestines outside the abdomen, as might be expected in a nullipara. To cover them, a large sheet of carbolic gauze, dipped in warm 2 per cent. carbolic solution was used. Two loops of ligature were placed on the broad ligament at each side, the first loop being carried as low as possible, and the second entering the vagina. The right ovary was removed; the left, which was firmly adherent to a coil of intestine, was left. After removal of the uterus, the author departed from the method of Freund, objecting to the long time occupied in placing the peritoneal sutures. Instead of using these, he turned the patient with her feet towards the light, and, introducing a Sims's speculum, sewed up the vagina from left to right, as recommended by Credé. He failed, however, to produce an inversion of the vagina. He now regrets greatly that he did not adopt Freund's method in full, believing that the suture of the vagina interferes with the necessary drainage. On the 28th, the patient was attacked by vomiting and other symptoms resembling ileus. On the 29th, the abdominal wound was opened without finding any source of obstruction, and the patient died about five hours later. At the autopsy no absolute obstruction was found, but an angular bend, which the author considers was the cause of ileus. In conclusion, the author expresses the opinion that it will be impossible to keep up a perfect antisepsis in the vagina, except by the method of continual irrigation. In future cases he intends to carry this out for the first three or four days by means of a tube passed up to the vaginal wound.—*Obstetrical Journal of Great Britain*, Oct. 1879.

———

Gastrotomy performed Three Times on the same Patient within Three Years.

Dr. BAUMGARTNER, of Baden-Baden, states (*Berliner Klin. Wochenschrift*, No. 5) the following case: A woman, 33 years old, had a polycystic tumour of the left ovary, which was removed by ovariotomy in September, 1875. The operation was performed without antiseptic precautions, except that the peritoneal cavity was washed out after the operation with several litres of warm water. The pedicle was treated by a clamp, and drainage, through the pouch of Douglas, was employed. The patient recovered, and was about, with the wound completely healed, by the thirty-fourth day.

She remained well until December, 1876, when, after a strain, she was attacked by violent pain in the cicatrix. This gradually increased until it became so severe that she was unable to turn in her bed, and even micturition became excessively painful. An examination revealed no possible cause for the pain except tension of the pedicle and its adhesions to surrounding organs. Gastrotomy was therefore performed in March, 1877, as the symptoms showed no remission. The pedicle was found to be adherent to the posterior wall of the bladder, the omentum, and some coils of intestine. These adhesions were separated, the pedicle was dropped, and the adherent portions of omentum were stitched into the abdominal wound. The patient recovered after several weeks.

In January, 1878, violent pain returned in the right ovarian region, which increased at each period, and at length became unendurable. The uterus was found to be normal. The right ovary was somewhat swollen and fixed. Near it was felt a swelling about as thick as a thumb, extending from the right ovary towards the centre and somewhat to the left, and itself also fixed. Febrile symptoms set in after this, and the patient's condition became visibly and progressively deteriorated.

Gastrotomy was therefore performed for the third time on August 19, 1878. The right Fallopian tube was found to be distended by purulent salpingitis, and was removed together with the ovary. The substance of the ovary itself was normal. The pavilion of the tube was adherent to the ovary, and formed with it a funnel-shaped sac, which was filled with thick, cheesy pus, and had walls so thin in places that rupture might have occurred at any moment. The patient recovered, and left her bed on the 16th May, completely cured.—*Obstetrical Journal of Great Britain*, Nov. 1879.

———

Wound of the Bladder in Ovariotomy.

In a recent number of the *Journal des Sciences Médicale de Lille*, Dr. G. EUSTACHE describes a case where this grave complication occurred during operation, without being followed by fatal results, although the ovarian cyst was suppurating and universally adherent. The patient was a single lady, aged 43, who had noticed a gradual increase in the size of her abdomen for six years, commencing in an attack of severe pain in the right iliac region. The abdomen at length became very large, and frequent attacks of pain and feverishness, dyspnœa, tenesmus, and œdema of the lower extremities supervened. The urine was also highly albuminous. She was tapped; but the peritoneal cavity soon filled again, so that ovariotomy was performed on May 14th. All instruments, sponges, and towels used for the operation were previously soaked in a five per cent. solution of carbolic acid; and the spray was employed. In making the abdominal incision the bladder was wounded; urine, taken at the time for ascitic fluid, escaping from the lower extremity of the wound, which was about five inches above the symphysis. The cyst was tapped and detached from its adhesions with considerable difficulty; the spray was then discontinued—for what reason we are not informed. The pedicle was secured by a stout wire twisted around it, and a silk ligature was tied very tightly below it; then the tumour, a multilocular cyst of the right ovary, was cut away. Two catgut ligatures were applied to the omentum. After the peritoneal cavity was sponged out, the bladder was found to have been wounded by an incision nearly an inch long below the anterior peritoneal reflexion. The wound was sewn up by three catgut sutures passed through all the coats of the bladder, including the mucous membrane; the ends of the threads were cut short. On beginning the closure of the abdominal walls the spray was again employed. The intestines had previously been protected by small pieces of flannel soaked in a solution of carbolic acid. The ends of the ligatures of the wounded omentum were brought out through the upper part of the incision; the pedicle was brought into apposition with the lower; the wire was removed; and, to prevent retraction, a pin was passed through the pedicle and the integument on each side of it. A drainage-tube was placed above the pedicle, and a second below it. On the second day urine was passed freely and without pain. On the sixth day the omental ligatures came away; black, sanious, stinking discharge escaped from the drainage-tube. On the ninth day the pin was removed from the pedicle, which was sloughy. The drainage-tubes were removed on May 27th, and the pedicle came away on the sixteenth day. After an attack of bronchitis, the patient recovered completely, with no difficulty in performing micturition. The urine had been quite clear from the first. The successful issue of this case is highly satisfactory, considering the serious nature of the injury and the other complications. Some of the details of the treatment would have been arranged otherwise by English operators of the present period; but, from the paper itself, it is clear that great precautions were carried out by the operator in the after-treatment.—*British Med. Journal*, Nov. 1, 1879.

Medical Jurisprudence and Toxicology.

Acute Poisoning by Ergot followed by Tolerance of the Drug.

Dr. MEADOWS records (*Med. Times and Gazette*, Oct. 4, 1879) the following case of poisoning by ergot which was treated at St. Mary's Hospital, London:—

Mrs. W., aged forty-eight, a stout, healthy-looking woman, was admitted on October 21, 1878. She had been married twice, first at the age of seventeen, afterwards at the age of forty. She had two children by the first marriage, but none subsequently, and her last pregnancy was twenty years ago.

Eight years before admission here she was under the treatment of Dr. Meadows, at Soho Hospital, for fibroid tumour of the uterus. During that time she took ergot twice. The first time it affected her severely ; but on the second administration it failed to act on the uterus at all. She was in Soho Hospital at that time for three months, and left cured. In March, 1878, she came to St. Mary's suffering from menorrhagia, and was examined by Dr. Meadows, who detected a growth in the uterus. She was subsequently admitted in October ; and on the 23d of that month, patient being under the influence of chloroform, a fibro-cystic polypus was removed from the anterior wall of the uterus.

On October 31, pulv. ergotæ ℥ss was ordered, with the view of bringing down any shreds of growth which might remain. The effects of this drug were very marked, as in ten minutes powerful uterine contractions were set up, and continued for two hours, when on vaginal examination a large tumour of the size of an orange was found presenting. In addition to the very strong uterine action there was marked depression, and she complained of severe nausea and headache. The face was deeply flushed, and the eyelids were swollen, the right one especially. The left arm and hand were greatly increased in size—so much so, that a ring she wore on her finger was completely hidden. The pulse, usually rather weak, was scarcely perceptible at the wrist, the artery being quite soft. The rate of the heart's action was not much influenced, but was slightly hurried. The swelling of the arm and hand did not disappear until next day, when she was in all respects well. Dr. Meadows removed the tumour (which was attached to the fundus by a narrow pedicle) by means of the écraseur.

November 7. Ergot was given again, as it was found that another tumour was present. As one dose did not act at first, it was repeated in six hours, and the symptoms already noted appeared again, but in an exaggerated form. The pain was so intense that she was ordered a hypodermic injection of one-fourth of a grain of morphia, with the result of easing pain and checking uterine action. The tumour presented, but as operation was not then convenient it was not removed, and gradually receded.

On November 24 ergot was again given ; but three half-drachm doses administered at intervals of six hours produced no effect beyond the swelling of the face and arms, depression, and nausea. Patient was then unsuccessfully galvanized with the view of stimulating the uterus to contract and expel the growth.

In this case there is a history of ergot having been given at five different times, twice at Soho Hospital, and three times at St. Mary's. Each time it has given rise to the peculiar symptom of the swelling of the face and left arm and hand. In three out of the five times given it has produced powerful uterine action ; on the third occasion on which it was given, here, and on the second, at Soho, it had no action on the uterus at all. This in itself is peculiar, and seems to point to a tolerance of the drug being established as far as the uterine fibres were concerned ; probably the fact that galvanism also failed to excite contractions would show that the excitability of the uterus was much impaired. It may be noted that this patient suffered from a weak and dilated heart, and that there was a mitral systolic murmur to be heard.

Another case of ergot poisoning with similar symptoms occurred once before at St. Mary's, but in that instance the action of the drug appeared to have been cumulative, as large doses had been given daily for about three weeks, at the end of which time swelling of the face and arms, with intense depression and vomiting of dark fluid, had occurred.

CONTENTS.

Published Monthly, price $2.50 per annum, free of postage.

Also, furnished together with the AMERICAN JOURNAL OF THE MEDICAL SCIENCES *and the* MEDICAL NEWS AND LIBRARY *for* SIX DOLLARS *per annum in advance, the whole free of postage.*

HENRY C. LEA, Philadelphia.

INDEX.

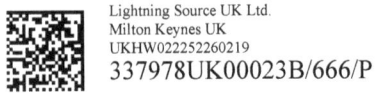

Lightning Source UK Ltd.
Milton Keynes UK
UKHW022252260219
337978UK00023B/666/P